Myles
Textbook for Midwives

For Churchill Livingstone:

Senior Commissioning Editor: Mary Seager
Project Development Manager: Mairi McCubbin
Project Manager: Pat Miller
Designer: Judith Wright
Illustrations Manager: Bruce Hogarth
Page Layout: Jim Hope / Alan Palfreyman (PTU Elsevier)

Myles
Textbook for Midwives

FOURTEENTH EDITION

Edited by

Diane M. Fraser

BEd MPhil PhD RGN RM MTD
Professor of Midwifery and Head of Academic Division of Midwifery,
School of Human Development,
University of Nottingham, Nottingham, UK

Margaret A. Cooper

BA RGN RM MTD
Director of Pre-Registration Midwifery Programmes,
Academic Division of Midwifery – Lincolnshire, School of Human Development,
University of Nottingham, Lincoln, UK

Foreword by

Gillian Fletcher

MCSP
President, National Childbirth Trust, London, UK

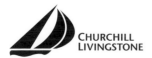

CHURCHILL
LIVINGSTONE

EDINBURGH LONDON NEW YORK OXFORD PHILADELPHIA ST LOUIS SYDNEY TORONTO 2003

First edition 1953   Eighth edition 1975
Second editon 1956   Ninth edition 1981
Third edition 1958   Tenth edition 1985
Fourth edition 1961   Eleventh edition 1989
Fifth edition 1964   Twelfth edition 1993
Sixth edition 1968   Thirteenth edition 1999
Seventh edition 1971   Fourteenth edition 2003

ISBN-13: 978–0–443–07234–5
ISBN-10: 0–443–07234–5
   Reprinted 2004 (twice), 2006, 2007

International edition ISBN-13: 978–0–443–07235–2
International edition ISBN-10: 0–443–07235–2
   Reprinted 2004 (twice), 2005, 2006, 2007

British Library Cataloguing in Publication Data
A catalogue record for this book is available from the British Library

Library of Congress Cataloging in Publication Data
A catalog record for this book is available from the Library of Congress

Note
Medical knowledge is constantly changing. Standard safety precautions must be followed, but as new
research and clinical experience broaden our knowledge, changes in treatment and drug therapy may
become necessary or appropriate. Readers are advised to check the most current product information
provided by the manufacturer of each drug to be administered to verify the recommended dose, the
method and duration of administration, and contraindications. It is the responsibility of the
practitioner, relying on experience and knowledge of the patient, to determine dosages and the best
treatment for each individual patient. Neither the Publisher nor the author assumes any liability for
any injury and/or damage to persons or property arising from this publication.

The Publisher

Contents

Contributors

Robina Aslam MSc PGCEA RGN RM ADM
Midwife Teacher, Academic Division of Midwifery –
Lincolnshire, School of Human Development,
University of Nottingham, Lincoln, UK

52 *Risk Management*

Jean Evelyn Bain BN RN
Clinical Nurse Specialist, Neonatal Unit, Ninewells
Hospital, Dundee, UK

42 *Recognising the Ill Baby*

Diane Barrowclough BA(Hons) MMedSci RN RM ADM
Course Leader, School of Nursing and Midwifery,
University of Sheffield, Sheffield, UK

12 *Preparing for Pregnancy*

V. Ruth Bennett BA MEd RN RM MTD
Formerly Lecturer, European Institute of Health
and Medical Sciences, University of Surrey, UK

 7 *The Female Pelvis and the Reproductive Organs*
 8 *The Female Urinary Tract*
 9 *Hormonal Cycles: Fertilisation and
    Early Development*
10 *The Placenta*
11 *The Fetus*
55 *Vital Statistics*

Kuldip Kaur Bharj BSc MSc RN RM MTD DipN(Lond)
IHSM RSA
Senior Lecturer in Midwifery, School of Healthcare
Studies, University of Leeds, Leeds, UK

 2 *The Social Context of Childbirth and Motherhood*

Karen Blakey MSc RGN RN RM ADM MTD CertEd
Midwife Teacher, University of Manchester,
Manchester, UK

14 *Parent Education: a New Dimension*

Eileen Brayshaw MSc Grad Dip Physiol MCSP SRP FETC
Clinical Associate and Clinical Physiotherapy
Specialist in Women's Health, Huddersfield
University, Huddersfield, UK

15 *Special Exercises for Pregnancy, Labour and the
    Puerperium*

Linda K. Brown BA MEd RN RSCN RM MTD
Formerly Course Director for Midwifery Courses
by Distance Learning, South Bank University,
London, UK

 7 *The Female Pelvis and the Reproductive Organs*
 8 *The Female Urinary Tract*
 9 *Hormonal Cycles: Fertilisation and Early Development*
10 *The Placenta*
11 *The Fetus*
55 *Vital Statistics*

Sue Brydon MSc RM RGN
Midwife, Supervisor of Midwives, Maternity Unit,
Queen's Medical Centre, University Hospital,
Nottingham, UK

52 *Risk Management*

Terri Coates MSc DipEd RN RM ADM
Freelance lecturer and writer; practising Midwife;
Formerly Midwifery Course Director, Distance
Learning Centre, South Bank University, London, UK

30 *Malpositions of the Occiput and Malpresentations*
32 *Midwifery and Obstetric Emergencies: 'Shoulder Dystocia'*

Margaret A. Cooper BA RGN RM MTD
Director of Pre-Registration Midwifery Programmes,
Academic Division of Midwifery – Lincolnshire,
School of Human Development, University of
Nottingham, Lincoln, UK

 1 *The Midwife*
 2 *The Social Context of Childbirth and Motherhood*

Helen Crafter MSc PGCEA FPCert RGN RM ADM
Senior Lecturer in Midwifery, Thames Valley
University, London, UK

Margaret A. Crichton BA MSc DipN(Lond) RN RM MTD
Midwife Teacher, School of Nursing, Midwifery and
Health Visiting, University of Manchester,
Manchester, UK

Susan Dapaah MA BSc(Hons) RN RM ADM CertEd
Senior Lecturer, School of Health, Staffordshire
University, Stafford, UK

Victor E. Dapaah MD FRCOG
Consultant Obstetrician & Gynaecologist,
Staffordshire General Hospital,
Stafford, UK

Margie Davies RGN RM
Midwifery Liaison Officer, Multiple Births
Foundation, Queen Charlotte's & Chelsea Hospital,
London, UK

Soo Downe RM BA(Hons) MSc PhD
Principal Lecturer (Research), Department of
Midwifery Studies, University of Central Lancashire,
Preston, UK

Jean Duerden MBA RN RM RSCN
Local Supervising Authority Responsible Midwifery
Officer, Yorkshire and North Lincolnshire
Consortium of Local Supervising Authorities,
Leeds, UK

Carole England BSc(Hons) RGN RM ENB405 CertEd(FE)
Nurse/Midwife Teacher, Academic Division of
Midwifery – Derby, School of Human Development,
University of Nottingham, Derby, UK

Philomena Farrell RN RM
Clinical Midwife Manager, Regional Neonatal
Intensive Care Unit, Royal Maternity Hospital, Belfast,
Northern Ireland

Diane M. Fraser BEd MPhil PhD RN RM MTD
Professor of Midwifery and Head of Academic
Division of Midwifery, School of Human
Development, University of Nottingham,
Nottingham, UK

Alison Gibbs RGN AdvDip Neonatal Care ENB A19 405 931
C&G 7307
Advanced Neonatal Practitioner, Neonatal Intensive
Care Unit, Queen's Medical Centre, Nottingham, UK

Claire Greig BN MSc PhD RGN SCM ADM MTD Neonatal
Certificate
Lecturer, Faculty of Health and Life Sciences, Napier
University, Edinburgh, UK

Adela Hamilton BSc(Hons) MA CertMgt CertTch SRN SCM
Lecturer in Practice, City University, London, UK

Sally Inch RN RM
Breast Feeding Advisor, Breastfeeding Clinic,
Women's Centre, Oxford Radcliffe Hospital NHS
Trust, Oxford, UK

Beverley Kirk BA(Hons) PGCE
English Teacher/ Pastoral Head, Ashfield School,
Kirby-in-Ashfield, Nottinghamshire, UK

Jennifer Lennox BSc(Hons) RN(M) RN RM ADM CertEd ENBR71
Senior Lecturer; Family Planning Practitioner, School of Health, Community and Family Studies, Northumbria University, Newcastle Upon Tyne, UK

36 Family Planning

Carmel Lloyd MA PGCEA RN RM ADM
Lecturer, Midwifery and Womens Health, Florence Nightingale School of Nursing and Midwifery, King's College London, London, UK

19 Common Medical Disorders Associated with Pregnancy
20 Hypertensive Disorders of Pregnancy

Rosemary Mander MSc PhD RGN SCM MTD
Reader, School of Nursing Studies, University of Edinburgh, Edinburgh, UK

5 Evidence-Based Practice
37 Bereavement and Loss in Maternity Care

Sally Marchant RN RM PhD DipEd
Editor, MIDIRS, Midwifery Digest, Bristol, UK

33 Physiology and Care in the Puerperium
34 Physical Problems and Complications in the Puerperium

Carol McCormick RN RM ADM BScHons (PGDL)
Consultant Midwife, Labour Ward, Nottingham City Hospital NHS Trust, Nottingham, UK

24 The First Stage of Labour: Physiology and Early Care
25 The First Stage of Labour: Management

Chris McCourt BA PhD
Centre for Midwifery Practice, Wolfston School of Health Science, Thames Valley University, London, UK

50 Community, Public Health and Social Services

Sue McDonald BAppSc PhD RN RM CHN FACM
Professor of Midwifery and Women's Health, Graduate Clinical School of Midwifery and Women's Health, Kathleen Syme Education Centre, La Trobe University, Melbourne, Australia

28 Physiology and Management of the Third Stage of Labour

Mary McGowan
Registrar of Births, Deaths and Marriages, Hatfield Register Office, Hatfield, UK

55 Vital Statistics

Irene Murray BSc(Hons) RN RM MTD
Teaching Fellow (Midwifery), Department of Nursing and Midwifery, Highland Campus, University of Stirling, Inverness, UK

13 Change and Adaptation in Pregnancy

Margaret R. Oates MB ChB DPM FRCPsych
Senior Lecturer in Psychiatry, University of Nottingham, Queen's Medical Centre, Nottingham, UK

35 The Psychology and Psychopathology of Pregnancy and Childbirth

Dora Opoku BSc(Hons) MA RM RGN MTD
Head of Department, Midwifery Department, City University, London, UK

6 The History and Regulation of Midwifery

Lesley Page BA MSc RM RN RNT RMT
Head of Midwifery and Maternity Services, The Royal Free, Hampstead NHS Trust, London, UK; Visiting Professor, Thames Valley University, London, UK

3 Woman-Centred, Midwife-Friendly Care: Principles, Patterns and Culture of Practice

Patricia Percival RN RM BAppSc(NAdmin) BAppSc MAppSc PhD RN RM CHN FRCNA
Registered Nurse, Registered Midwife, Ascot, Perth, Australia

46 Jaundice and Infection

Maureen D. Raynor MA PGCEA RMN RN RM ADM
Midwife Teacher, Academic Division of Midwifery – Nottingham, School of Human Development, University of Nottingham, Nottingham, UK

35 The Psychology and Psychopathology of Pregnancy and Childbirth

Nancy M. Riddick-Thomas MA RM RGN ADM CertEd
Midwifery Team Leader, School of Care Sciences,
University of Glamorgan, Pontypridd, UK

4 *Ethics in Midwifery*

Jane M. Rutherford DM MRCOG
Consultant in Fetomaternal Medicine, Obstetrics
and Gynaecology, Queen's Medical Centre,
Nottingham, UK

48 *Pharmacology and Childbirth*

Della Sherratt BEd(Hons) MA RN RM MTD NDNCert FETCert
Midwife, Making Pregnancy Safer, Reproductive
Health Research, World Health Organization,
Geneva, Switzerland

54 *International Midwifery*

Christine Shiers MSc PGCEA RGN RM ADM
Senior Lecturer, Institute of Nursing and Midwifery,
University of Brighton, Conquest Hospital,
St Leonard's-on-Sea, UK

17 *Abnormalities of Early Pregnancy*
29 *Prolonged Pregnancy and Disorders of Uterine
    Action*
32 *Midwifery and Obstetric Emergencies*

Norma Sittlington BSc(Hons) MSc RN RSCN RM ANNP
Advanced Practitioner, Neonatal Unit, Liverpool
Women's Hospital, Liverpool, UK; Formerly
Advanced Neonatal Nurse Practitioner, Regional
Neonatal Intensive Care Unit, Royal Maternity
Hospital, Belfast, Northern Ireland

38 *The Baby at Birth*
39 *The Normal Baby*

Amanda Sullivan BA(Hons) PhD P/GDip RM RGN
Consultant Midwife, Antenatal Clinic, Maternity Unit,
Nottingham City Hospital NHS Trust, Nottingham, UK

23 *Specialised Fetal Investigations*

Denise Tiran MSc PGCEA RGN RM ADM
Principal Lecturer – Complementary
Medicine/Midwifery, School of Health and Social
Care, University of Greenwich, London, UK

49 *Complementary and Alternative Medicine in
    Maternity Care*

Tom Turner MB FRCP FRCPCH
Consultant Paediatrician, Queen Mother's Hospital,
Yorkhill, Glasgow, UK

45 *Congenital Abnormalities*

Anne Viccars BSc(Hons) MA PGDipEd RM RGN
Senior Lecturer in Midwifery, Institute of Health and
Social Care, Bournemouth University, Bournemouth,
UK

16 *Antenatal Care*

Stephen P. Wardle MB ChB MRCPCH MD
Consultant Neonatologist, Queen's Medical Centre,
University Hospital Nottingham, Nottingham, UK

47 *Metabolic Problems, Endocrine Disorders and Drug
    Withdrawal*

Yvonne S. Watson MSc MTD RN RM ENB901
Senior Lecturer, Family Planning Practitioner, School
of Health, Community and Family Studies,
Northumbria University, Newcastle Upon Tyne, UK

36 *Family Planning*

Foreword

The birth of a baby is a momentous occasion: tiny details of the experiences surrounding the whole event are etched in the memory forever. Midwives carry a huge responsibility in helping women through the hard work and pain that is labour, yet what a privilege it is to help women and their partners capture the excitement of bringing a new human being into the world.

Murray Enkin defined the relationship between the art and the science involved in care during pregnancy and childbirth in this way:

'Art: those essential but unmeasurable components of care that count even though they cannot be counted: the empathy and judgement that permits care to be personalized for each woman and her family.

Science: the extent to which care is based on evidence that it is effective; that it achieves the desirable effect.'

This is the challenge that faces every midwife in practice today: how to utilise the science when appropriate and in ways that do not undermine the complex physiological and sociological aspects of childbirth. How does the midwife enable women to feel special and confident in their ability to give birth in an environment where there is increasing emphasis on safety and risk management? This is especially difficult for midwives supporting women for whom the pregnancy or labour are not straightforward, and in settings where they have never met the couple before.

How does one empower women and their partners to have an experience of that 'birthday' that they will want to revisit time and again? In recent years much of the research on women's birth experience has highlighted that it is not so much what the midwife knows and her clinical skills but who she is as a person and how she relates to the couple that makes a difference to their experience and memories of the birth (Audit Commission 1997; Green, Coupland & Kitzinger 1998; Singh & Newburn 2000).

The editors of this new edition of *Myles Textbook for Midwives* have done an excellent job of weaving both the art and the science of midwifery throughout. The result is a textbook that draws the reader in. The editors have managed to maintain the individual approach of each author, while weaving all the chapters into a cohesive whole, full of essential information, as well as brimming with up-to-date research.

The anatomical and physiological information is very easy to access. There are so many clear diagrams and pictures, making the information much more accessible.

Having been an NCT antenatal teacher and tutored student NCT teachers for over 20 years, it is especially interesting to see how the issue of pain relief and comfort in labour are addressed. Many of the women attending antenatal classes today seem much more frightened of the pain of labour and less confident in their ability to cope with it than women in the past, perhaps because of the images fed through the media. Midwives and antenatal teachers need to address those fears and instill confidence. This chapter contains much food for thought, drawing together up-to-date research on the physiology of pain as well as the facts about a wide range of pain-relief options.

There is much current debate in the midwifery world about the continued rise in medicalisation of birth and the erosion of 'normality' centring around what we mean by 'normal labour'. Recent research has shown that this definition can be differently interpreted, resulting in a high proportion of women whose labours were listed as normal having all kinds of interventions. The RCM has set up a Virtual Institute on Normal Birth to take this debate forward within the UK and internationally. This dilemma, relating to fundamental principles of midwifery and patterns of care, is explored on numerous occasions within the book. There is also a wealth of detailed information about the specific needs of those women with existing medical conditions and the very special role of the midwife in caring for these women.

The chapter entitled 'The Social Context of Childbirth and Motherhood' deals with many of the challenges facing midwives in trying to provide services that are sensitive and appropriate to all women, their babies and families, whatever their culture, race or religion. This book should provide much of what will be needed by those starting out on a midwifery career.

In meeting the challenge for change, midwives should embrace the renewed enthusiasm within the NHS for real partnership with those who use the health services. At all levels and in all areas of health, service users are working alongside health professionals to improve services and monitor those improvements.

The current proposed changes to Patient and Public Involvement and the setting up of Patient Advice and Liaison Services (PALS) and patients' forums, will mean that existing multidisciplinary specialist forums such as Maternity Service Liaison Committees (MSLCs) will be reviewing their remit and ways of working. With the National Service Framework for Children, which includes a section on the maternity services, on the horizon, there will be more need than ever for a specialist maternity multidisciplinary forum that enables both those who use and provide maternity services to work closely together towards providing the kind of services that women and midwives deserve. Exciting and challenging times lie ahead.

Gillian Fletcher

REFERENCE

Audit Commission 1997 First class delivery: improving maternity services in England and Wales, Audit Commission for Local Authorities and National Health Service for England and Wales: London.

Enkin MW 1989 Effective care of the low risk woman in pregnancy and childbirth. In: van Hall E, Everaerd W (eds) The Free Woman: Womans' Health in the 1990s. 9th International Congress of Psychosomatic Obstetrics and Gynaecology Conference Proceedings. Parthenon, Carnforth: pp. 48–61

Green J, Coupland V, Kitzinger J 1998 Great expectations: a prospective study of women's expectations and experiences of childbirth. Books for Midwives Press, Hale.

Singh D, Newburn M 2000 Women's experiences of postnatal care. National Childbirth Trust, London.

Preface

The celebration of 100 years of midwifery legislation seemed a very appropriate point in history for chapter authors to make revisions to *Myles Textbook for Midwives*. With the increase in e-learning it might be questioned whether there is still a place for substantial textbooks such as this; however, the response from students and midwives was overwhelmingly in favour of continuing to bring together in book form the subjects that contribute to the art and science of midwifery.

Evaluations received from students, their mentors and teachers have all contributed to this Fourteenth edition. Given the high profile of evidence-based practice in the new NHS, it has been important to keep a balance between adequate and extensive referencing so that understanding of essential content is not lost in a plethora of reference sources. Readers need therefore to be aware that source materials referenced can only be examples of the extensive literature available. Annotated bibliographies have been provided to give some indication of the value of material available elsewhere.

We remain particularly grateful to the many midwives who have continued to contribute to revised editions of this valuable textbook. A number of new authors are included in the Fourteenth edition and whilst the majority of expertise comes from midwives, the multi-professional and user contributions reflect the imperative for us to learn and work together in the maternity services.

Childbearing women, their babies and families remain the focus of this book. The order of material has, for the most part, remained unchanged to continue to reflect that emphasis. However, a compromise has been made in the ordering of the section on anatomy and physiology. Reviewers of the Thirteenth edition found it unhelpful to study physiological changes without having an overview of normal anatomy first. This therefore forms the second section of the book, being preceded by chapters on midwifery and the context in which the midwife practises. Given the rapid changes in society and health care at the turn of the millennium, this context will no doubt evolve rapidly too.

Midwives have opportunities to work in a variety of maternity service organisations, in women's homes and overseas. Whatever the context and the culture of these settings it is the intention of this text to convey the importance of woman-centred midwife-friendly care. For the majority of women childbirth will be a normal although life-changing experience. When women do experience complications the quality of individualised care becomes even more important. The midwife has a key role to play in assisting women make choices and feel in control even when presented with difficult options and dilemmas. This edition has therefore retained the integrated nature of sections of the Thirteenth edition to continue to reduce the false impression that women fall into a 'normal' or 'abnormal' category for the whole of the childbearing continuum. The chapters on postnatal care have been expanded in an attempt to address perceived differences in the standard of care women say they receive during the first few weeks of motherhood. The book also includes a new chapter on pharmacology to provide midwives with an overview of the safety requirements when prescribing and administering drugs in pregnancy and postnatally. A major revision to the chapter on professional regulation was needed when legislation required the five statutory bodies for nursing, midwifery and health visiting to be replaced by a Nursing and Midwifery Council (NMC) in April 2002. During 2002 the NMC began to replace a number of UKCC publications and readers need to be aware that other UKCC publications quoted by chapter authors might well have been replaced during the lifetime of this Fourteenth edition.

A particularly valuable aspect of Myles textbook has been the very clear and easy to understand illustrations. Where these have evaluated positively they have been retained but new ones have been added to enhance clarity and illustrate less common conditions more effectively. A new addition is a colour section to the book that we believe will be welcomed by new readers and those who possess earlier editions.

Grounding the material in research and authoritative opinion continues to be essential where good evidence exists. In contrast the reader is at times presented with dilemmas and uncertainties of practice as we do not always know the right answers. A challenge must be for midwives to share with women the best knowledge to date to help them in their decision making. This book cannot provide all that knowledge, but we hope it will provide a comprehensive framework for maternity practice and act as a catalyst for life-long learning.

We hope that in the next century of midwifery regulation, students and midwives will continue to enjoy and value Myles textbook. The contents of this Fourteenth edition should play an important part in enhancing midwifery care for childbearing women and their families.

Nottingham 2003   Diane M. Fraser
                                                   Maggie Cooper

Note: Wherever the female gender is used, the male is also implied, where appropriate, and vice versa.

Acknowledgements

The volume editors wish to record their thanks to Ruth Bennett and Linda Brown who significantly revised the 13th edition and made the task of editing this 14th edition considerably easier. They also wish to thank those authors who originated some of the chapters in earlier editions and whose work has provided the foundation for the current volume. These include:

Jo Alexander
Jean Ball
Thelma Bamfield
Anne Bent
Greta Beresford
Ruth Bevis
Tricia Murphy-Black
Patricia Cassidy
Sarah Das
Chloe Fisher
Liz Floyd
Jocelyn Franey
Annie Halliday
Edith Hillan
Deborah Hughes
Lea Jamieson
Rosemary Jenkins
Margaret Lang
Victoria Lewis
Alison Livingston
Anne Matthew
Sinead McNally
Maureen Michie
Jean Proud
Sarah Rankin
Sarah Roch
Carolyn Roth
Jennifer Sleep
Helen Stapleton
Valerie Thomson
Anne Thompson
Valerie Tickner
Elizabeth Torley
Josephine Williams
Jane Winship

They also wish to thank those critical readers whose constructive comments and suggestions facilitated the task of editing. Encouragement and support of relatives, friends and colleagues has been much appreciated. Finally, the hard work and co-operation of the chapter authors must be very warmly acknowledged and a particular thanks must go to Dawn Glen for her invaluable administrative support.

Section 1
Midwifery

SECTION CONTENTS

1

The Midwife

Diane M. Fraser   Margaret A. Cooper

The midwife is recognised worldwide as being the person who is alongside and supporting women giving birth. However, the midwife also has a key role in promoting the health and well-being of childbearing women and their families before conception, antenatally and postnatally, including family planning.

In the UK the midwife's skills are increasingly valued and midwives are being urged to expand their role even further in the field of public health. Their responsibilities are to diagnose and monitor pregnancies, labours and postpartum progress, to work with childbearing women and other health care professionals to achieve the best possible outcomes for each individual family. This demands a wide range of skills, knowledge and personal attributes.

This chapter aims to:

- define the midwife in terms of expectations of her capabilities, from both the perspectives of childbearing women, the UK statutory body; World Health Organization (WHO) and the European Union (EU)

- discuss the continuing education and professional development of practising midwives

- identify the chapters of the book that cover the different aspects of midwifery practice.

Midwives, women and their partners

Midwife means 'with woman', or, in France, 'wise woman'. Throughout the ages women have depended upon a skilled person, usually another woman, to be with them during childbirth. In the past men were excluded from the birthing room, being allowed in only once the baby was born. Now pregnant women are encouraged to choose a birth partner, male or female, to support them in labour. Midwives had therefore to develop their skills of 'being with woman' to include and involve the woman's chosen birth partner(s). At times this requires the midwife to stand back, observe, listen and intervene only when invited to do so or when it is in the best interests of the woman, fetus or baby. At other times the midwife will need to ensure that the woman's partner is appropriately informed about childbirth and parenting so that they can make sound decisions together. On occasions the midwife might need to act as the woman's advocate when the partner's/friend's/relative's actions are unlikely to enhance, or could harm, the health and safety of mother and child (see Lewis & Drife (2001) for details of the 12% of all women included in the maternal deaths in 1997–1999 self-reporting that they had been subjected to domestic violence). In the past midwives have been criticised for neglecting the needs of fathers, ignoring them or pressurising them to become more involved than they would choose if allowed to make their own decision (Bartels 1999).

To understand and empathise with each woman's individual needs and encourage her to have confidence in her own body and capabilities for parenting, the midwife needs a high level of knowledge and decision-making abilities. It is this thorough grounding in knowledge, experience and personal insight that enables her to refrain from taking control away from the mother while being at hand to step in when assistance is needed.

Alliances between childbearing women and midwives were pivotal in stemming the tide of technologically dominated, actively managed labours of the 1970s and 1980s (O'Driscoll & Meagher 1980). In 1992 the government's Select Committee report (known as the Winterton report) on the maternity services was published (House of Commons Health Committee 1992). Evidence from women cited the importance of their having more choice, control and continuity of care when using the maternity services. Government responses in each of the four countries in the UK, of which Changing Childbirth (DoH (Department of Health) 1993) is perhaps the best known, set standards for health care providers to make their maternity services 'woman centred'. Chapter 3 discusses some of the ways in which midwives and maternity services have responded.

Midwives and normal childbirth

Midwives are recognised as the experts and lead caregivers in normal childbirth, but this is not as simple as it sounds. Alongside the move to provide women with more choice, control and continuity has been the debate about what is 'normal' and how much choice should be available to women in a resource-limited National Health Service (NHS) and increasingly litigious society (see Ch. 52 Risk management). In 2001 (Downe et al 2001) the Association for Improvement in the Maternity Services (AIMS) and the Trent Research Midwives Group conducted an exploratory survey to establish whether women recorded as having had a 'normal birth' had received any interventions. Given that 62.3% of the 956 births classified as 'normal' actually received what AIMS would define as an 'obstetric delivery' (Beech 1997), discussions sprung up around the country to try to define 'normal' birth. A difficulty of definition arises over whether any interventions can be classed as being 'normal' and from whose perspective. For example an ultrasound scan in early pregnancy has become routine but can change an anticipated pleasurable event to a stressful pregnancy (see Chs 23 and 37). At the other extreme, views are polarised as to whether women whose pregnancy is uncomplicated should be able to demand a caesarean rather than a vaginal birth (Kaufman & Liu 2001).

Midwives will find themselves working as independent practitioners with their 'normal' caseload for much of the time yet, perhaps on the same day participating in a multiprofessional team when complications develop. There are strong arguments for providing women whose care becomes more complicated with as good, if not even better, continuity of midwifery care if it can really be claimed that midwives are 'with woman' (Gould 2002). At times this will give midwives dilemmas in prioritisation and on occasions their own views will not always coincide with those of their clients or other health care professionals. Chapter 4 may help in the resolution of ethical dilemmas whilst the book as a whole will assist midwives in diagnosing and providing care both when childbirth is straightforward and when it is less so. No book nor current best evidence can provide all the answers and midwives need to learn to cope with uncertainty, be knowledgeable about what is known and not known and have the confidence to engage effectively in multiprofessional discussions about best practice, audit and research. Although intellectual and clinical skills and competencies are essential for safe midwifery practice, the midwife's interpersonal skills are likely to be what makes a difference to women's experiences and memories of childbirth.

Definition and capabilities of the midwife

Midwives need to be aware of the legislation and guidelines defining their role, describing their scope of practice and specifying standards of competence. Some of the most significant are highlighted in this chapter.

In 1972 a definition of the midwife was developed by the International Confederation of Midwives (ICM). A year later it was adopted by the International Federation of Gynaecology and Obstetrics (FIGO) followed by the WHO. In 1990 at the Kobe Council meeting, the ICM amended the definition, which was later ratified by FIGO in 1991 and by WHO in 1992 (Box 1.1).

At the European level, member states of the EU, (known at the time as the European Community (EC)), prepared a list of activities that midwives should be entitled to take up within its territory (EC Midwives Directive 1980). Although midwives must learn about all of these activities, in the UK it is recognised that it is highly unlikely that midwives would be expected to be proficient in them all – for example the manual removal of the placenta would be carried out by a doctor unless no doctor is available and the mother's life is at risk (Box 1.2).

Fitness for practice, award and purpose

It might be expected that if midwives are fit to practise they will also be fit to work in any setting and be eligible to receive the appropriate award from the university where they were educated. This is, however, a simplistic assumption.

> **Box 1.1** International definition of the midwife (ICM 1992)
>
> A midwife is a person who, having been regularly admitted to a midwifery educational programme, duly recognised in the country in which it is located, has successfully completed the prescribed course of studies In midwifery and has acquired the requisite qualifications to be registered and/or legally licensed to practise midwifery.
>
> She must be able to give the necessary supervision, care and advice to women during pregnancy, labour and the postpartum period, to conduct deliveries on her own responsibility and to care for the newborn and the infant. This care includes preventative measures, the detection of abnormal conditions in mother and child, the procurement of medical assistance and the execution of emergency measures in the absence of medical help. She has an important task in health counselling and education, not only for the women, but also within the family and the community. The work should involve antenatal education and preparation for parenthood and extends to certain areas of gynaecology, family planning and child care. She may practise in hospitals, clinics, health units, domiciliary conditions or in any other service.

Fitness for practice

Midwives' rule 33 of the United Kingdom Central Council for Nursing, Midwifery and Health Visiting (UKCC 1998) specifies the outcomes to be achieved before a student is eligible to register as a midwife on part 10 of the Nursing and Midwifery Council (NMC) register. This rule has remained the same for a considerable period of time. In an evaluation study of preregistration programmes of midwifery education it was found, however, that rule 33 did not adequately capture the essence of a competent midwife (Fraser et al 1998). In an attempt to demonstrate the need for a more holistic definition of a competent midwife at the point of registration, a three-dimensional model was developed (Fig. 1.1). This model, with its overlapping dimensions, should not be seen as static but rather as a way of illustrating that the midwife needs to integrate

Box 1.2 Activities of a midwife: the European Directive (UKCC 1998, p. 26)

Member states shall ensure that midwives are at least entitled to take up and pursue the following activities:

- to provide sound family planning information and advice
- to diagnose pregnancies and monitor normal pregnancies; to carry out examinations necessary for the monitoring of the development of normal pregnancies
- to prescribe or advise on the examinations necessary for the earliest possible diagnosis of pregnancies at risk
- to provide a programme of parenthood preparation and a complete preparation for childbirth including advice on hygiene and nutrition
- to care for and assist the mother during labour and to monitor the condition of the fetus in utero by the appropriate clinical and technical means
- to conduct spontaneous deliveries including where required an episiotomy and in urgent cases a breech delivery
- to recognise the warning signs of abnormality in the mother or infant which necessitate referral to a doctor and to assist the latter where appropriate; to take the necessary emergency measures in the doctor's absence, in particular the manual removal of the placenta, possibly followed by manual examination of the uterus
- to examine and care for the newborn infant; to take all initiatives which are necessary in case of need and to carry out where necessary immediate resuscitation
- to care for and monitor the progress of the mother in the post-natal period and to give all necessary advice to the mother on infant care to enable her to ensure the optimum progress of the new-born infant
- to carry out the treatment prescribed by a doctor
- to maintain all necessary records.

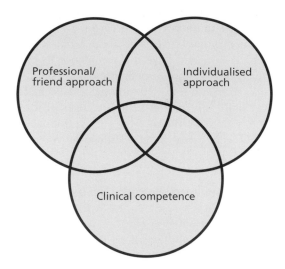

Fig. 1.1 An holistic, integrated model of a competent midwife. (From Fraser et al 1998 p. 32, reproduced by permission of the English National Board for Nursing, Midwifery and Health Visiting (ENB).)

a variety of different abilities and recognise that there will be different emphases according to context and over time. From this an assessment matrix was developed as a guide to universities in providing students with realistic learning and assessment opportunities (ibid pp 93–98). This was seen to be particularly relevant as the dimension of most importance to childbearing women, 'professional/friend', was the least effectively assessed from evidence obtained during the evaluation study (Berg et al 1996, Fraser 1999, Waldenstrom et al 1995).

In 1999 the former professional body's Commission for Education produced a report discussing fitness for nursing, midwifery and health visiting practice (UKCC 1999). Following on from this report the UKCC decided to interpret rule 33 in the form of competency statements (UKCC 2000). These 29 competencies will now have to apply to all programmes in the future, whether or not rule 33 is amended.

Fitness for award

While the UKCC were developing professional competencies, the DoH commissioned the Quality Assurance Agency for Higher Education (QAAHE) to prepare subject benchmark statements for all 11 university health care programmes (not including dentistry and medicine). During this work an overarching health professions framework emerged under the following three main headings:

- expectations of the health profession in providing patient/client services
- the application of practice in securing, maintaining or improving health and well-being
- the knowledge, understanding and skills that underpin the education and training of health care professionals.

This framework illustrates the academic and practitioner features that are held in common. These are developed more fully in each subject's benchmark statement and standards to describe the profession specific expectations and requirements. Thirty-four midwifery standards have been specified to set out the different expectations of midwives entering their first post immediately on completion of a diploma or honours degree preregistration programme of midwifery (QAAHE 2001).

Fitness for purpose

Although NHS Trusts can now refer to national competency and benchmark standards to clarify their expectations of new midwives, there are still likely to be local variations. This might include variations in opportunities, for example to suture perineums (Ch. 27), 'top-up' epidurals (Ch. 26) or assist women birth in water. What is more important than small variations in learning opportunities and the development of specific psychomotor skills is a midwife's personal insight including the recognition of her capabilities and when it is necessary to learn new skills.

When taking up employment it is essential for midwives to discuss their development needs and ensure that they are not expected to undertake activities for which they have not been prepared or are inappropriate for their level of expertise. Each midwife is allocated, or chooses a person to be her supervisor of midwives. This person is invaluable in assisting with a midwife's personal development plan and providing support in difficult contexts (Ch. 51).

Autonomous midwifery practice

Once qualified as a midwife there are a variety of employment opportunities. However, whichever type of midwifery organisation provides employment, the midwife, even at the point of registration, has responsibility for and autonomy within her sphere of practice. Professional autonomy for midwives does not, however, mean that midwives should create professional boundaries and exert powers to protect their territory. Instead autonomy means having freedom to act on behalf of childbearing women, working in partnership with them and having the knowledge and capability to provide continuity of carer for women with straightforward pregnancies as well as working in partnership with other members of the health care team when this is in the best interests of the woman, fetus or newborn.

The UKCC describes seven guiding principles which establish their philosophy and values in relation to expected outcomes of midwifery programmes. The relevance of these principles is outlined below.

Provision of women-centred care

Every woman expects to be treated as though she is special and important. Although at times maternity units and community workloads can be busy, individual women want midwives to be there for them, not for someone else. It is essential that midwives have an understanding of social, cultural and context differences (see Ch. 2) so that they can respond to the needs of women and their families in a variety of care settings and prioritise and manage work appropriately. Of particular importance is working with families to draw up a plan of care and support and then evaluate and modify that care as circumstances warrant. To do this midwives need knowledge of available resources and expertise so that members of the multidisciplinary team and other organisations can be drawn upon as required to meet the holistic needs of individual women.

Ethical and legal obligations

The practice of a midwife is controlled by law. In the UK legislation was first enacted in 1902. Since then there have been a number of Midwives Acts until 1979 when three professional groups were brought together under the Nurses, Midwives and Health Visitors Act (amended more recently by the Nursing and Midwifery Order in 2001, which abolished the UKCC and four National Boards) (see Ch. 6). Midwives also need to be familiar with other Acts of Parliament and Statutory Instruments that impact on their practice.

Dimond has written extensively on the interpretation and application of law in midwifery in journals and in her own book (Dimond 1994).

The Code of professional conduct (NMC 2002) sets requirements for the behaviour of midwives and nurses in relation to such things as confidentiality, respect and personal responsibility for ethical choices (see Ch. 4). Midwives may find themselves expected to care for women who have decided to terminate their pregnancy. Whilst midwives may exercise a conscientious objection in relation to participating in the termination, they cannot refuse to provide care for the woman because they disagree with her decision to terminate. Counselling services are normally provided for women and staff facing these sort of ethical dilemmas and stressful situations.

Respect for individuals and communities

Society is composed of people from many cultural, ethnic and religious backgrounds. Midwifery care must be provided in a non-discriminatory way and without prejudice. Where midwives find they do not have the skills or expertise to provide effective care for individuals or groups then they need to seek assistance. In areas where there are a number of residents who do not speak the local language, link workers or an interpreting service can be more appropriate than asking another family member, especially a child, to communicate between the woman and the midwife (see Chs 2 and 54).

Quality and excellence

Individual midwives should strive for continual improvement and excellence in midwifery practice. To protect the health and well-being of mothers and babies, supervision of midwives is enshrined in statute. Clinical governance has more recently been established to assure the quality of all the health services provided by an individual NHS Trust and has many principles that mirror statutory supervision of midwives (Ch. 51). Auditing of standards and discussion of difficult maternity care scenarios are ways in which all professional groups can work together to improve the quality of the service. Involvement of mothers in evaluating care and suggestions for areas that need improvement have become even more important in contributing to quality and excellence in the maternity services.

The changing nature and context of midwifery practice

The pace of change is likely to increase throughout the new millennium and midwives need to be prepared to adapt accordingly. This is likely to include embracing new technologies, provided they enhance the quality of care, working in new ways as patterns of care change and listening to mothers to understand what matters to them (see Chs 3 and 23). What will be essential is for midwives to discriminate between change that is likely to benefit the woman and her family and change that is for administrative or other non-care-related convenience. Midwives need to be flexible and also become change agents when necessary. This might necessitate learning new skills or further developing existing ones and having the initiative to identify when change is needed.

Evidence-based practice and learning

The use of the term 'evidence-based' rather than 'research-based' practice has been growing (Proctor & Renfrew 2000, Renfrew 1997). This is intended to draw practitioners' attention to the need for sound evidence for effective care and not assume that all research is of value but that it must be critically analysed. It is also intended to foster the use of systematic reviews such as Effective care in pregnancy and childbirth (Chalmers et al 1989) and the regularly updated guides and more recently the electronic Cochrane Library to which most universities and NHS Trusts subscribe. Assistance with accessing the literature can normally be obtained from librarians as well as from journals and books (e.g. Stanton & Fraser 2000).

Chapter 5 will provide more information on evidence and research and midwives need to be aware that there are now many good qualitative studies that add to the body of midwifery knowledge and understanding. The midwife has a responsibility to make use of all available resources to inform her practice, including experiential knowledge. It is recognised that some areas of practice are difficult to research or are underresearched and evidence is unavailable. The midwife will never be absolved from the duty to weigh up the clinical evidence elicited by her personal observations and to take account of her experiences and client's wishes.

Lifelong learning

Development of different learning styles can aid effective lifelong learning. Laurillard (1994) and Miller et al (1994) believe that it is important to encourage students to vary their learning style according to context or goal. Whereas some might learn best by adopting a surface or memory style of learning, this alone will be inadequate unless students can also develop a deep level of processing information. The 'fire drills' that are suggested to help midwives respond rapidly and effectively to emergency situations (Ch. 32) lend themselves to surface styles of learning, but when situations are complex and require much investigation and reflection then problem-solving skills become essential. With so much information available it can be difficult for midwives to know where to go to keep up to date. Databases are invaluable for searching for topics of relevance but it can be difficult just from a title or abstract to assess the value of a piece of information. Critiquing skills are of utmost importance in ensuring time is used productively when accessing new information (Crombie 1996).

As well as learning from the literature, midwives also need to grasp opportunities to learn from each other by observing and discussing different ways of practising and, where necessary, seeking out an education or training event. Working and learning together are seen by the Government as key to delivering patient centred care in the NHS (DoH 2001). Although evidence of learning is required, in the form of a professional profile, for 3-yearly renewal of professional registration, this is likely to be insufficient to meet the requirements for competent midwifery practice in a constantly changing health service.

Continuing professional development (CPD)

Since the middle of the twentieth century midwives in the UK have been required to attend statutory refresher courses every 5 years. Although these ensured a minimum amount of professional development, they were not always adequate in meeting professional development needs. Furthermore it was argued that nurses, as well as midwives, need to 'be refreshed' to maintain professional competence. From April 2001 all midwives and nurses have had to meet PREP (postregistration education and practice) requirements to renew their professional registration (UKCC 1997). Evidence to fulfil these requirements has to be presented in the form of a personal professional profile which demonstrates that practitioners have been developing their knowledge and expertise during the previous 3 years. Formally the expectation is that practitioners will have completed at least 5 days (or 35 hours) of study during this time. Those practitioners who are registered on more than one part of the professional register need to fulfil the PREP requirements for each part if they wish to remain on the 'live' register in each of these parts.

Midwives who are also neonatal nurses have been particularly challenged by these requirements. Some have decided to keep just their nursing qualification 'live', others have decided to keep their midwifery and not their nursing qualification 'live', whilst others have found it is possible to keep both 'live'. Decisions in these areas need to be made alongside longer term career aspirations.

Professional profiles

There are many commercially produced guides to assist in preparing a professional profile as well as folders that can be purchased to record evidence of CPD. However, a ring binder and set of dividers can equally well fulfil a practitioner's needs and lends itself to being individually stylised. Alternatively the profile can be maintained electronically but a hard copy will be needed if requested for audit purposes by the Nursing and Midwifery Council.

Midwives are required to record evidence of study and learning relevant to their sphere of practice. The UKCC defined five categories that they believed would cover all possible fields of professional practice:

- care enhancement e.g. developments in practice, standard setting, empowering women
- reducing risk e.g. health promotion and screening, identification of health problems, protection of individuals
- client/patient and colleague support e.g. counselling, leadership, supervision
- practice development e.g. personal research and study, change agent, visiting other practice areas
- education development e.g. mentorship and lecturer/practice educator programmes.

As well as being a mandatory requirement for maintaining professional registration, a personal profile can be useful when applying for a job, providing evidence when claiming non-standard entry or advanced standing for a course of study as well as aiding personal development through reflection.

APL and APEL

Accreditation of prior learning (APL) and accreditation of prior experiential learning (APEL) are often possible for a number of postregistration courses. These involve matching what you have done before with the course you are now interested in studying. If there is evidence of equivalence, then exemption from certain modules and units might be permitted. Credit will then be awarded provided there is evidence that prior study or learning is authentic, relevant, had appropriate depth and breadth and was relatively recent. APL/APEL schemes vary between universities and just because one university will allow perhaps a third of the course to be exempt through APL/APEL there is no guarantee that another will allow the same sort of percentage exemption. Normally there will be advisors to guide prospective students through the process.

It is obviously essential that resources are not wasted and hence the NHS is keen to ensure that midwives supported by the Workforce Development Confederations (the NHS bodies responsible for workforce planning and commissioning education programmes and events with education providers) receive value for money and are not required to engage in repetitive learning.

Career pathways

There are a number of different possibilities for midwives to consider when planning their longer term careers. Whichever route is intended, all will require evidence of high motivation and lifelong learning. The ENB undertook some useful projects during the 1990s that included the identification of the following nine hallmarks of a lifelong nurse/midwife learner (ENB 1994):

- responsible and accountable for their work
- self-reliant in their way of working
- adaptable to changing health care needs
- flexible to changing demands
- challenging and creative
- innovative
- resourceful
- able to work as change agents
- able to share and promote good practice and knowledge.

This can be a helpful framework when identifying training and education needs for development alongside acquiring new skills to meet service needs. Midwives now have an exciting array of career opportunities, which include: caseload practice; a career as expert/leader in specific areas of midwifery practice such as consultant midwife, birth centre lead midwife, hospital labour ward coordinator and ventouse practitioner; a career in management, whether in midwifery or more general management in the NHS; a career as midwife researcher on midwifery and collaborative projects; a career in education as a midwife lecturer in universities or practice educator in the NHS; a career in standard setting and audit; a career as the midwife expert in multiprofessional teams such as teenage pregnancy, drug addiction, domestic violence, fetomaternal medicine and also opportunities to work in developing countries (see Ch. 54). In addition a midwife learns a multitude of valuable transferable skills.

As you pursue your midwifery career it is essential to reflect in and on your practice (some useful guidance can be found in Church & Raynor 2000). By so doing you will not only understand more about your own learning capabilities, but most importantly will see how you can make a difference to the childbirth experiences of women and their families. Reflection is not, however, sufficient; it needs to be followed by appropriate action and understanding that different actions may be required in different contexts. The next two chapters provide a discussion of some of the varying contexts in which a midwife practices.

REFERENCES

Bartels R 1999 Experience of childbirth from the father's perspective. British Journal of Midwifery 7:681–683

Beech B A L 1997 Normal birth – does it exist? Association for the Improvement in the Maternity Services Journal 9:4–8

Berg M, Lundgren I, Hermansson E et al 1996 Women's experience of the encounter with the midwife during childbirth. Midwifery 12:11–15

Chalmers I, Enkin M, Keirse M J N C (eds) 1989 Effective care in pregnancy and childbirth. Oxford University Press, Oxford

Church P, Raynor M D 2000 Reflection and articulating intuition. In: Fraser D (ed) Professional studies for midwifery practice. Churchill Livingstone, Edinburgh, p 23–43

Crombie I K 1996 The pocket guide to critical appraisal. BMJ Publishing, London

Dimond B 1994 Legal aspects of midwifery. Books for Midwives Press, Hale, Cheshire

DoH (Department of Health) 1993 Changing childbirth: report of the Expert Maternity Group. HMSO, London

DoH (Department of Health) 2001 Working together – learning together. A framework for lifelong learning for the NHS. DOH, London

Downe S, McCormick C, Beech B L 2001 Labour interventions associated with normal birth. British Journal of Midwifery 9:602–606

EC Midwives Directive 1980 EC Council Directive 80/155/EEC Article 4. Official Journal of the European Communities L33/28

ENB (English National Board for Nursing Midwifery and Health Visiting) 1994 Creating lifelong learners. Partnerships for care. ENB, London

Fraser D M 1999 Women's perceptions of midwifery care: a longitudinal study to inform curriculum development. Birth, Issues in Perinatal Care 26:99–107

Fraser D, Murphy R, Worth-Butler M 1998 Preparing effective midwives: an outcome evaluation of the effectiveness of pre-registration programmes of education. ENB, London

Gould D 2002 One-to-one midwifery – making it happen. British Journal of Midwifery 10:17

House of Commons Health Committee 1992 Second report, Maternity services, vol 1. HMSO, London

ICM (International Confederation of Midwives) 1992 Definition of the midwife. ICM, London

Kaufman T, Liu D 2001 Should caesareans be performed only on the basis of medical need? Nursing Times 97:17

Laurillard D 1994 Rethinking university teaching. Routledge, London

Lewis G, Drife J (eds) 2001 Why mothers die 1997–1999. The fifth report of the Confidential Enquiries into Maternal Deaths in the United Kingdom. RCOG Press, London

Miller C, Tomlinson A, Jones M 1994 Learning styles and facilitating reflection. ENB, London

NMC (Nursing and Midwifery Council) 2002 Code of professional conduct. NMC, London

O'Driscoll K, Meagher D 1980 Active management of labour. W B Saunders, London

Proctor S, Renfrew M (eds) 2000 Research and practice in midwifery. A guide to evidence-based practice. Baillière Tindall, Edinburgh

QAAHE (Quality Assurance Agency for Higher Education) 2001 Subject benchmark statements: health care programme – midwifery. QAAHE, Gloucester

Renfrew M J 1997 The development of evidence based practice. British Journal of Midwifery 5:100–104

Stanton W, Fraser D 2000 Accessing the literature. In: Fraser D (ed) Professional studies for midwifery practice. Churchill Livingstone, Edinburgh, p 2–3

UKCC (United Kingdom Central Council for Nursing, Midwifery and Health Visiting) 1997 PREP and you. UKCC, London

UKCC (United Kingdom Central Council for Nursing, Midwifery and Health Visiting) 1998 Midwives rules and code of practice. UKCC, London

UKCC (United Kingdom Central Council for Nursing, Midwifery and Health Visiting) 1999 Fitness for practice: the UKCC Commission for Nursing and Midwifery Education (Peach report). UKCC, London

UKCC (United Kingdom Central Council for Nursing, Midwifery and Health Visiting) 2000 Requirements for pre-registration midwifery programmes. UKCC, London

Waldenstrom U, Borg I M, Olsson B 1995 The childbirth experience: a study of 295 new mothers. Birth 23:144–153

2 The Social Context of Childbirth and Motherhood

Kuldip Kaur Bharj   Margaret A. Cooper

CHAPTER CONTENTS

In this chapter the context within which maternity services are organised and delivered will be highlighted. The midwife has a key role in the provision of appropriate and sensitive care to all women, their babies and families. To do so effectively, midwives need to understand how factors such as culture, race, religion, social exclusion may impinge upon the quality of services provided so that they might work towards providing greater equality for all childbearing women and their families.

The chapter aims to:

* discuss the social context of childbirth in contemporary Britain

* explore basic terminologies used when caring for people from diverse backgrounds and debate their implication for midwifery practice

* discuss the factors that need consideration in the delivery of appropriate and sensitive maternity services

* discuss the strategies that the midwife may utilise to provide and deliver maternity care to women from vulnerable groups.

Introduction

Contemporary British maternity services are based on the premise that all women want a service that offers safety, that is flexible and responsive to their individual linguistic, religious and cultural needs, that communicates effectively and provides the information that allows informed choices for evidence-based care. The previous government, having acknowledged the need to respond to the individual needs of all consumers, proposed many radical changes through the

NHS reforms. Proposals in policy documents (e.g. the NHS and Community Care Act 1990, the 'Changing Childbirth' report (DoH 1993), The Patient's Charter (DoH 1991, 1995), and Maternity Services (DoH 1994) required many radical changes in the way health services are planned, purchased and provided. In particular they emphasised the need for NHS provider units to be more responsive to the needs of the local population, more sensitive to the needs of all users, and to offer greater choice, higher standards and better quality of health care provision. The central themes of consumerism, individualism and holism, which underpin these policies, have been further strengthened by Department of Health initiatives to modernise the NHS (DoH 1997, 2000a). The present government's quest for the provision of high quality care that is individualised and holistic depends on the recognition of individuals as having unique needs and organisations that place the needs of their local populations in the centre when planning and delivering services.

Britain's maternity services and woman-centred care

Although generally there is overall satisfaction with the NHS, public concerns with regards to the wide variation in the quality of service provision and delivery continue to persist (DoH 2000a). Women, in the main, express satisfaction with the maternity services; however, some, particularly those from diverse backgrounds such as young single women, those with disabilities, women from lower socioeconomic classes, women from the black and minority ethnic communities amongst many other groups, continue to have poor experiences (Audit Commission 1997, DoH 1992, 1993). Whereas women from middle classes are somewhat reluctant to have intervention imposed on to them and may seek a less clinical environment for intrapartum care, women from disadvantaged backgrounds complain that they are more likely to receive less favourable treatment because services fail to take account of their linguistic, religious and cultural needs (Cartwright 1979; Larbie 1985, Pearson 1985, Phoenix 1990). Many of the reasons given by women for the dissatisfaction with maternity services includes fragmented care, long waiting times, insensitive care, lack of emotional support, inadequate explanations, lack of information, medical control, inflexibility of hospital routines, and dehumanising aspects of hospitalisation and reproductive technologies (Kitzinger J 1990, Kitzinger S 1978, Oakley 1979, Reid & Garcia 1989). Women from disadvantaged backgrounds, however, claim that they experience additional difficulties owing to stereotypes and discrimination (Phoenix 1990).

Changes in society and dissatisfaction with the way the maternity services were organised and delivered led to campaigns for better access to effective and appropriate obstetric and midwifery care, tailored to meet consumer needs. Women are not a homogeneous group and midwives should emphasise the provision of flexible services that meet individual needs of the women. Britain is made up of groups of people from a wide range of diverse backgrounds and many of these groups experience disadvantage. Maternity services therefore need to be relevant and responsive to the individual needs of the women and their families, listening to their views and respecting their ethnic, cultural, social and family backgrounds. Women need to be cared for by midwives who exhibit a respectful and caring attitude to women and provide a holistic approach to care that recognises cultural and social diversity and the different skills required to meet the needs of women using the maternity services (UKCC 2001).

A woman-centred philosophy promotes greater control for childbearing women with a move towards a model of increased partnership (DoH 2001a). However, providing woman-centred care is a complex issue, particularly in a multiethnic society where individuals and families have diverse health needs. The health needs of groups that experience disadvantage have been given a priority by the government in a number of policy documents such as the Independent Inquiry into Inequalities in Health report (DoH 1998), Saving Lives: Our Healthier Nation (DoH 1999) and The NHS plan (DoH 2000a).

Understanding terminologies

Organisations and midwives need to understand some of the common terminologies in use, for example 'race', 'culture', 'ethnicity', and 'social exclusion', as well as their implication for professional practice so that they are better placed to deliver culturally congruent care in the maternity services.

Concept of 'race'

The term 'race' is underpinned by the premise that people are differentiated by specific genetic and physical characteristics (e.g. caucasian, negroid, etc.) and are connected by common descent and origin. However, the term has been a subject of controversy for some time amongst anthropologists, biologists and social scientists. With the developments in the scientific world, the notion that there was a biological difference in the 'races' has been rejected on the grounds that there is little genetic difference between different 'races' and, more so, that genetic differences within 'races' are greater than the differences between 'races' (Rose & Rose 1986). 'Race', though, is a term in wide use in the social and political context and is associated with concepts such as discrimination and racism. Some of the related terminologies are:

Prejudice. This refers to holding an unfavourable opinion or feeling, formed without knowledge, thought or reason. It is often based on personal beliefs and stereotypes operating at an unconscious level – for example, assuming that all Asian women cannot speak English or read their own mother tongue.

Discrimination. This is a process whereby one person is treated less favourably than another and occurs when the prejudice is brought into action, often to the disadvantage of particular groups or individuals. Discrimination can operate in two forms. Direct discrimination operates at an individual level and indirect discrimination is usually at an institutional level.

Direct discrimination arises where an individual is treated less favourably, on the grounds of gender, 'race', disability, sexual orientation, religion, culture or age, than another person would be treated in the same or similar circumstances. An example from the Commission for Racial Equality is (CRE 1994, p. 22):

> A receptionist at a community health clinic tells a black woman that there are no appointments available for at least 2 weeks. She then proceeds to offer a white woman an appointment for the next day.

Indirect discrimination occurs when a requirement or condition that applies to everyone has the effect of excluding a significantly greater proportion of people from a particular group than others. An example adapted from the CRE (1994) is:

> An antenatal clinic offers classes on breathing and relaxation techniques for expectant mothers. These classes are also open to their partners. Women from some ethnic groups who experience difficulty in discussing childbirth issues in male company often drop out or do not attend. They miss out on these facilities, as there are no classes for women only.

Racism. This is a doctrine or ideology or a dogma that is underpinned by the assumptions that some groups are superior to the others and is interpreted as the systematic oppression of individuals or groups based on their skin colour or ethnic origin (Fernando 1991). Racism is associated with power, that is individuals, or institutions' ability to make things happen or prevent them from happening. In other words, racism is the ability to enact prejudice and discrimination, either at an individual or institutional level, by those who are in power either by an act of deliberation or unintentionally.

Individual racism operates through the behaviour of people at a personal level, leading to discrimination. An example of individual racism is where a health care practitioner does not provide translating or interpreting services because she believes that whilst in England everyone should speak English. This in fact will lead to a poorer quality of service.

Institutional racism, on the other hand, is 'the collective failure of an organisation to provide an appropriate and professional service to people because of their colour, culture or ethnic origin. It can be seen or detected in processes, attitudes and behaviour which amount to discrimination through unwitting prejudice, ignorance, thoughtlessness and racist stereotyping, which disadvantages ethnic minority people' (Macpherson 1999, p. 28). This suggests that institutional racism is essentially a situation when racial prejudice becomes part and parcel of institutions and is set in the structures of the society, so that long-standing practices can cause organisations to discriminate unintentionally.

Notwithstanding legislation that prohibited racial discrimination, evidence continues to demonstrate that discrimination continues to exist at disturbing levels in employment and service provision and service delivery. The Stephen Lawrence Inquiry (Macpherson 1999) accelerated the revisions to the Race Relations Act 1976, which were long overdue and led to its amendments, which came into force in April 2000. The Race

Relations (Amendment) Act 2000 strengthened its application to public authorities. This legislation requires all organisations to produce race equality schemes encompassing a raft of policies and procedures, which would go a long way to assist midwives and organisations in promoting equal opportunities in employment and service provision and delivery. Bharj & Khan (1995) argue that such policies, aiming to promote sensitive and appropriate care, must be comprehensive and take into account consumer needs to ensure equitable provision and delivery of services. The statutory obligations placed by the Race Relations (Amendment) Act upon organisations will mean some radical changes to the way organisations and midwives respond to the people for whom they provide and deliver maternity services.

Concept of 'culture'

When planning and delivering individualised care, account should be taken of clients' cultural prescriptions, which should contribute to the delivery of responsive care. When referring to multicultural societies, the basic understanding of the culture is often assumed to mean the way of life of a society or a group of people and is used to express social life, food, clothing, music and behaviours. However since the classical definition of culture as 'a complex whole, which includes knowledge, beliefs, art, morals, customs and other capabilities and habits acquired by *man* as a member of society' (Taylor 1871), the term culture within anthropological discourses has been subject to many revolutions and there is no consensus about how the term should be used (Barley 1995). Culture is hence a difficult term to define.

Linton (1945), for instance, describes culture as a 'way of life of its (society's) members; the collections of ideas and habits which they learn, share and transmit from generation to generation'. Lewis (1976) further develops the concept through giving recognition to its dynamic and socially inherited nature, emphasising that 'subject to the vagaries of innovation and change' culture is conveyed 'in a recognisable form from generation to generation'. Leininger (1978), arguing from a nursing perspective, suggests that 'culture is the learned and transmitted knowledge about a particular culture with its values, beliefs, rules of behaviour, and life-style practices that guides a designated group in

their thinking and actions in patterned ways'. This definition highlights the fact that culture is a multifaceted concept and cannot be limited to any one aspect. Some authors, like Helman (1994), take a broader perspective making reference to possible genetic links as well as mystical elements in the sense that some aspects are both explicit and implicit, and arguing that culture is 'a set of guidelines … which an individual inherits as a member of a particular society and which tells *him* how to view the world and learn how to behave in it in relation to other people. It also provides *him* with a way of transmitting these guidelines to the next generation – by the use of symbols, language, art and ritual.'

Although this plethora of definitions provides a variety of insights into the concept, there are a number of commonalities – namely that culture is learned, it is shared and it is passed on from generation to generation. Culture is learned; members of the society inherit or learn a set of guidelines through which they attain concepts of role expectancies, values and attitudes of society. It is therefore not genetically inherited (i.e. it is not a manifestation of particular genetic constitution) but is socially constructed through the process of socialisation. This is a process through which human beings learn to behave within the society where individuals learn the values and attitudes that are acceptable to the environment in which they exist. As a result members of a cultural group share similar beliefs and systems. This is a lifelong process usually initiated by the family, but then influenced by other institutions such as education, religion and the media as well as being shaped by historical, geographical, economic, social and political factors. Culture therefore evolves over time and is not a static entity.

Behaviour of individuals is shaped by the values and attitudes they hold as well as the physical and geographical surroundings in which they interact. Practitioners therefore should remain mindful that individuals perceive and respond to stimuli from economic, social and political factors in different ways and they will be affected differently according to age, gender, social class, occupation and many other such factors. Their interactions are complex, as well as the way they influence cultural changes. Culture changes as a result of forces both from 'within' and from 'outside'. Therefore to explain a culture of a particular group or explain the cultural health beliefs of a group is problematic.

When closely examining people from any one cultural group, a wide variation within them can be noted, which might be a result of personal experiences dictating a different attitude or a perception to particular aspects of a shared culture. Culture is very much a dynamic state; culture influences individuals, and individuals in turn contribute to culture, enriching or modifying it. Culture therefore is not a group phenomenon and to treat it as homogeneous can be quite dangerous as it can lead to generalisations. When considering people from one cultural group some aspects can be true for some and not for others. Another commonality of culture is that it is transmitted and it therefore constitutes a heritage or social tradition.

In a multicultural, multiethnic society valuing diversity is an important aspect. An understanding of some of the cultural differences between social groups is essential in ensuring that professional practice is closely matched to meet the needs of individual clients and should go a long way in the delivery of culturally congruent care. Practitioners of health and social care must understand the role culture plays in determining health, health behaviours and illness so that services are planned and delivered to meet the health needs of the population they serve. However, some writers caution the role of culture in explaining patterns of health and health-related behaviour, arguing that emphasis on culture diverts attention away from the role of broad structural process in discrimination and the role that racism plays in health status (Ahmad 1993, 1996, Stubbs 1993). In practice, then, emphasis on culture could lead to attributing inequalities entirely to cultural differences, diverting attention from the real causes of discrimination and racism often faced by women from diverse backgrounds.

Concept of 'ethnicity'

The term 'ethnicity' has largely replaced the term 'race', encompassing all of the ways in which people from one group seek to differentiate themselves from other groups. 'Ethnicity is an indicator of the process by which people create and maintain a sense of group identity and solidarity which they use to distinguish themselves from others' (Smaje 1995, p. 16). People of a particular group have a common sense of belonging to a group, and have shared beliefs and values and a sense of relationship. In general, people use these terms to identify the 'other' but it must be remembered that all people have a culture and ethnicity.

The 'objective' view about ethnicity is that it is dominant in traditional literature and that 'markers' exist which demonstrate the nature of ethnicity. These markers include cultural traditions such as language, religion, history, geographical origins such as region, land, nation, as well as biological characteristics. In opposition to this traditional view, more recent literature emphasises the 'subjective' view of ethnicity, which includes three key concepts: 'ethnic consciousness' is where people belonging to an ethnic group are conscious of some of the factors in social interaction; 'ethnic awareness' is something that is heightened by ethnic mobilisation and finally 'ethnic identity' is personal experience of the way someone views various aspects of their ethnicity. This view emphasises the flexible nature of the concept.

The objective and subjective views suggest that people have a sense of identity with a particular group and it is more than shared characteristics; it is about creating an identity through practice. The 'outsiders' of the group, which the group members themselves do not necessarily associate with, impose some markers based on physical characteristics. For example the term 'Asian', which is often used to refer to people of South Asian origin, does not differentiate between Pakistani and Indian communities. It is such categorisation that leads to fixed differences and gives a sense of the 'outsider', 'not one of us', leading to stereotypes and discrimination.

When people value their own culture more highly than that of the other ethnic group, perceiving their cultural ways to be the best, they devalue and belittle other ethnic groups, by perceiving others culture as bizarre and strange; this is referred to as *ethnocentrism*. Ethnocentric behaviour, in particular when other individuals' cultural requirements may be ignored or dismissed as unimportant, would do very little to meet the tenets of woman-centred care and hinders the delivery of sensitive care.

Ethnicity therefore is a way people identify themselves as part of a group through self-identification of characteristics as well as categorisation by others. Ethnicity, like culture, is learned; it is not fixed and rigid. It is shaped by the social and political relationships between other ethnic groups and is a result of a socialisation process and not of genetic inheritance.

Ethnic groups are not homogeneous; such groups comprise people with wide variation in culture, lifestyle, language and religion. Concepts of 'ethnicity' have come under criticism for failing to acknowledge this aspect and for seeing ethnicity as a key determinant of human behaviour, and also for ignoring the fact that other dimensions of inequality (such as class, age, gender, etc.) cut across ethnicity.

Concept of 'social exclusion'

'Social exclusion' is a term introduced by the government to describe groups of people or communities who are likely to experience social marginalisation as a result of a number of interrelated problems such as unemployment, poor or limited skills, low income, poor housing, high crime environment, poor or ill health and family breakdown. All these factors add to social isolation and are key determinants of inequalities of health, contributing to health and ill health of the communities.

The present government has established a 'Social Exclusion Unit' to address the issue of social exclusion with the aim of improving the health of the nation as well as reducing inequalities of health.

Socially excluded: disadvantaged groups

Despite a number of quality initiatives, the issues of equality in service provision and service delivery continue to persist; evidence continues to illustrate that there is variation in the quality of experience amongst some sectors of the community, as well as in the outcomes of maternity services in terms of infant and maternal mortality (Audit Commission 1997, Lewis & Drife 2001). In a broad sense, the government has affirmed its commitment to addressing the issue of equal opportunities in service provision and delivery for some time, responding through a number of health policies (DoH 1995, 2000b, NAHA 1988) and more recently, by giving the health of some community groups as a designated priority area (DoH 1998, 1999, 2000a, 2001a). Organisations and individuals are charged to develop and deliver maternity services in such a way that they give an important consideration to the needs of people from 'disadvantaged' groups as well as to reducing inequality and inequity.

Defining disadvantage

Hart et al (2001, p. 31), in their attempt to define the term 'disadvantage' to mean 'individuals whose identities may be constructed in relation to such concepts as impairment, discrimination, prejudice, poverty, social exclusion, inequality, membership of minority group, of low educational achievement', argue that use of the term is controversial and means different things in different contexts, depending upon the historical, social and political situation. They go on to suggest that, whereas every woman during pregnancy is at risk of being disadvantaged, there are in the main five categories in which disadvantage may be located. The first two categories, related to the 'person', are mental or physical impairment, or particular characteristics no longer attributed to mental or physical impairment that have historically led to individuals experiencing prejudice and discrimination (e.g. ethnicity, gender, etc.). A further two categories are concerned with the manner in which either other individuals or organisations interact with those in the first two categories (i.e. women who experience prejudice and those who experience discrimination). The final category they claim may be a consequence of any of the above, and refers to women who live in material poverty. In light of these, women who are most likely to experience most disadvantage include those who are:

- young
- with disability (physical, sensory or learning)
- living in relative poverty
- from black and minority ethnic backgrounds (The use of terminology to describe different groups in the community is an extremely sensitive issue and there is no single acceptable term that embraces all members of the minority ethnic groups. The term black and minority ethnic communities has been used here to include all individuals who experience discrimination and disadvantage associated with 'race' and ethnicity.)
- users of drugs
- from travelling communities
- lesbians.

Women who fall into any one of these categories may be viewed as disadvantaged not because they have, for example, a disability or are from travelling communities, but because they are more likely to be socially excluded. They are more likely to experience discrimination or be unemployed and it is the detrimental impact of these circumstances on health that is of concern. There is strong evidence that the disadvantaged groups have poorer health and poorer access to health care, with clear links between inequality in social life and inequality in health, demonstrating that inequality exists in both mortality and morbidity not just in the United Kingdom but also in Europe (Townsend & Davidson 1982, Whitehead 1987, 1992). People from these groups have not enjoyed the health gains from wider social and environmental improvements, and are less likely to adopt healthier lifestyles or obtain fair access to services at the same level as the most affluent sectors of the community. Many people from the black and minority ethnic communities have been equally vulnerable (DoH 2001b).

Women from the above groups not only experience dissatisfaction with maternity services but as a consequence of the 'disadvantage' are at an increased risk of ill health and premature death. Evidence from the Confidential Enquiry into Maternal Deaths 1997–1999 (Lewis & Drife 2001) demonstrates that maternal mortality rates among the socially excluded are 20 times higher than in the population as a whole. Women from the lower socio-economic groups, those who are very young and some specific groups of women from the black and minority ethnic communities are more likely to die than their 'white' counterparts. One of the main underlying factors that may have contributed to premature deaths of these women is their inability to access maternity services. Many women from black and minority ethnic communities spoke little English and in a large number of cases there were inadequate interpreting services, which meant that health care professionals did not have appropriate and relevant information on which to base care.

A number of models of care have been introduced, particularly in nursing, to deliver culturally congruent care. However, in midwifery the philosophy of 'woman-centred care' is much used to meet individual needs of the women who experience disadvantage. To facilitate care that is responsive to the needs of the women, health professionals need to understand women's social, cultural and historical backgrounds so that care is tailor-made to meet their needs (see Ch. 3).

Women from socially excluded groups: implications for practice

Young mothers

Britain has the highest rate of teenage pregnancy and teenage parenthood in Europe. Ninety thousand teenagers in England become pregnant every year; of these nearly 8000 are under the age of 16 years. Approximately three-fifths of teenage conceptions will result in livebirths (Social Exclusion Unit 1999). Many young mothers do achieve a successful outcome to their pregnancy and parenting; it should, however, also be recognised that mortality and morbidity amongst babies born to these mothers is increased and that the mothers show a higher risk of developing complications such as hypertensive disorders and intrapartum complications (Lewis & Drife 2001). Young teenage mothers tend to present late for antenatal care and are disproportionately likely to have some risk factors associated with poor antenatal health (e.g. poverty and smoking).

For many young mothers, pregnancy and parenthood means an early conclusion to their education with consequent reduced career opportunities and increased likelihood that they will find themselves socially excluded and living in poverty. The Government's Social Exclusion Unit report on teenage pregnancy, published in June 1999, set two major targets: to halve the pregnancy rate in under 18-year-old teenagers by the year 2010 and to achieve a reduction in the risk of long term exclusion for teenage parents and their children. Midwives have a role to play in the achievement of both these targets through their public health role and the provision of appropriate, accessible services (see Ch. 50).

With appropriate support, young mothers can make an effective transition to parenthood. They can be assisted to develop good parenting and life skills and be helped out of this potential downward spiral. MacKeith & Phillipson (1997), writing about young mothers, argue that being judgmental achieves nothing positive but it reduces self-esteem, engenders resentment and destroys the relationship between the midwife and her client.

Women with disabilities

Women with disability are increasingly becoming users of the maternity services as they seek to live full and autonomous lives. The midwife needs to allow sufficient time to assess how the disability may impact on the woman's experience of childbirth and parenting and to work with her in identifying any resources that may alleviate perceived difficulties. Assumptions should not be made on visual observation alone. Where possible the woman should have a named midwife with whom she can build a trusting relationship and have continuity of carer. An introduction to other professionals who may be involved in the care should be considered early in pregnancy. Comprehensive record keeping will reduce the likelihood of repetitive questioning.

The woman will probably be well informed about her disability but may need the midwife to provide advice on the impact that the physiological changes of pregnancy and labour may have on her, for example the increased weight and change to her centre of gravity. Some women and their partners may raise concerns regarding a genetic condition that could be passed on to their baby and need referral to specialist services such as a genetic counsellor. Midwives and other health care professionals should recognise the need to approach antenatal screening in a sensitive manner. Midwives need to be aware of local information pertaining to professional and voluntary organisations and networks and adopt a multidisciplinary approach to planning and provision of services.

A birth plan will help the woman to identify her specific needs alongside the issues that most pregnant women are concerned with, such as choice of pain relief and views on interventions. Midwives should empower women with a disability to make informed choices about all aspects of their antenatal, intrapartum and postnatal care (RCM 2000a). If the woman is to give birth in hospital it may be helpful for her to visit the unit, meet some of the staff and assess the environment and resources in relation to her special needs. A single room should be offered to her to facilitate the woman's control over her immediate environment and, where appropriate, to adapt it to accommodate any equipment that she may wish to bring with her. The woman who is blind or partially sighted may prefer to give birth at home where she is familiar with the environment. If she has a guide dog then consideration needs to be given to its presence in the hospital environment (see Plate 1).

Women with learning difficulties may need a friend or carer to help with the birth plan but the midwife should not overlook who is the client; she must involve her as much as possible and recognise that she may have feelings and anxieties that she is less able to articulate.

The Changing Childbirth report (DoH 1993, p. 53) states 'It is important that services reflect the needs of women who have disabilities and ensure that action is taken to overcome the obstacles that confront them. While physical obstructions are of course a frustrating problem, there are other equally daunting barriers resulting from the prejudice and ignorance of able-bodied professionals.'

Women living in relative poverty

It is well documented that women living in poverty are more likely to suffer health inequalities and have a higher rate of maternal and perinatal mortality (Lewis & Drife 2001, Townsend & Davidson 1982, Whitehead 1987).

Tackling inequality is high on the public health agenda and the midwife has an important role in targeting women in need. The Sure Start scheme has contributed to the development of social support and health promotion opportunities for some women. Other initiatives such as 'Pregnant in Cowgate' have been successful in improving contact with women, building trust, reducing preterm labour, increasing smoking cessation and improving nutrition (Davies 1997).

Salmon & Powell (1998) recognise that midwives should be sensitive to the financial difficulties that some women face and should not give inappropriate advice that may reinforce an already vulnerable situation. They also recognise that concepts such as continuity and choice, advocated in reports such as Changing Childbirth (DoH 1993), may be viewed as secondary for women struggling with the daily reality of managing poverty.

Women from the black and minority ethnic communities

According to the 1991 census there are an estimated 3 million people of black and minority ethnic origin residing in England and Wales, accounting for up to 6% of the total population. Since 1999, however, Britain has undergone further changes in the population profile and these statistics underestimate the contemporary profile. For example, the political instability within Eastern Europe and Asia has contributed significantly to the increase in migration of political and religious refugees into Britain. However, Britain's black and minority ethnic population is unevenly distributed; variations exist within regions and within districts, with representation in some areas being up to 60% of the population. Of the total population nearly 50% are of South Asian ethnic origin, people of Indian origin being the largest group. The second largest group comprises people of African–Caribbean origin. Chinese is the smallest ethnic group. Consequently, there is a wide variation in culture, lifestyle, language and religion; they differ not only from the majority of the population but also from each other.

Such changes in the demographic profile as well as the diversity in cultural requirements have created major challenges for maternity services, and is a most likely cause for the services' inability to respond to the individual needs of the women from diverse backgrounds (Darr & Bharj 1999). Through recognition of this inadequacy, an attempt to redress this discrepancy has been made by recent health policy, placing the responsibility for responding to ethnic diversity explicitly on organisations and health care professionals (DoH 1997, 2000a). In addition to this, the emphasis is on ensuring that all health care practitioners are prepared in a manner to enable them to provide high quality antidiscriminatory care that is accessible, appropriate and responsive to the varied health needs of the diverse population (Gerrish et al 1996).

People from black and minority ethnic communities are included in the 'disadvantaged' or in the 'socially excluded' category for two main reasons. First, they are visible minorities as a result of their skin colour and ethnic origin; they are more likely to experience racial harassment, discrimination and social inequalities. Secondly they are predominantly residents of deprived inner cities and more likely to have poor housing, be at risk of high employment, and have low paid occupations, poor working conditions, poor social security rights, and low income, all of which lead to poverty. As a result of these factors they are more likely to be categorised into lower socioeconomic status. Additional factors such as lifestyle, environmental factors and genetic determinants are often cited as indicators of poor maternity and health outcomes; however, key determinants are poverty, poor housing and poor education (Nazroo 1997, Proctor & Smith 1992).

Although some women from the black and minority ethnic communities express satisfaction with the maternity services, literature as well as testimonies from many has indicated that inaccessibility of maternity services, inappropriate service provision, insensitive service delivery and overall discrimination within the NHS remain major issues that underpin their experiences of maternity services. The following two key elements can assist in the provision of equitable maternity services:

- ensuring that women from the black and ethnic minority communities understand the maternity service, what it offers and when and how they can use it
- ensuring that all health services, including maternity and preventive services, are appropriate to the health care needs of the local population, including the black and ethnic minority population, and that they are delivered in a manner that is culturally sensitive.

Women from travelling families

It would be wrong to categorise travelling families as a homogeneous group; this umbrella term merely serves to describe the nomadic nature of their lifestyle but fails to recognise their origins or the social context of their lives. Travellers may belong to a distinct social group such as the Romanies, their origins may lie in this country or elsewhere such as Ireland or Eastern Europe, or they may be part of the social grouping loosely termed 'New Age' travellers or part of the Showman's Guild travelling community. As with all social groups, their cultural background will influence their beliefs about and experience of health and childbearing.

A common factor, which may apply to all, is the likelihood of prejudice and marginalisation. Midwives need to examine their own beliefs and values and develop their knowledge to address the needs of travelling families with respect and provide a service which is non-judgmental. An informed approach to lifestyle interpretation may stop the midwife identifying the woman as an antenatal defaulter with the negative connotations that accompany that label.

Moving on may be through choice related to lifestyle, but equally it may be the result of eviction from unofficial sites.

Some health authorities have designated services for travelling families that contribute to uptake and continuity of care. These carers understand the culture and are aware of specific health needs; they can also access appropriate resources, for example a general practitioner (GP) who is receptive to travellers' needs. A trusting relationship is important to people who are frequently subjected to discrimination. Handheld records contribute to continuity of care and communication between care providers, but the maternity service also needs to address communication challenges for individuals who do not have a postal address or who have low levels of literacy.

Women who are lesbian

Evidence suggests that an increasing number of women are seeking motherhood within a lesbian relationship; the exact numbers are unclear as it is the woman's choice as to whether she makes her sexual orientation known. The midwife can, however, create an environment in which she feels safe to do so. Communication and careful framing of questions can reduce the risk of causing offence and assist the midwife in the provision of woman-centred care.

Wilton & Kaufmann (2001) identify the booking interview as the first time, as a user of the maternity service, that the woman must consider how she will respond to questions such as 'when did you last have sex?' or 'what is the father's name?' Issues such as parenting, sex and contraception may have different meanings for the midwife and the woman and therefore careful use of non-heterosexist language by the midwife will help to promote a climate for open communication (Hastie 2000). Hastie argues that the 'realities of lesbian experiences are hidden from the mainstream heterosexist society and so stereotypes are rife among health practitioners' (p. 65); she goes on to say that oppression and invisibility damage health. The RCM (2000b) position paper 22 on maternity care for lesbian mothers states that midwives should take a lead in challenging discriminatory language and behaviour, both positively and constructively. Wilton & Kaufmann (2001) suggest that this can be achieved by developing awareness and understanding, signalling acceptance and improving service delivery.

A framework for analysis

There is a dearth of evidence around women's experiences of maternity services. Five themes emerge from analysis of this literature as well as that of midwives' experience in caring for women from disadvantaged backgrounds:

- knowledge and understanding
- communication and language
- relationship
- discrimination
- insensitive and inappropriate services.

Each of these themes will be considered in turn.

Knowledge and understanding

Knowledge and understanding have been identified as issues that need to be addressed by both midwives and women themselves if organisations are to achieve delivery of responsive maternity care to all women. Midwives need some knowledge and understanding of cultures and lifestyles of the women for whom they care. It is only then that they can feel confident in working with these women to plan the services and care that the women require and deserve. Several texts provide health care professionals with such background relating to black and minority ethnic communities, for example Schott & Henley (1996). However, although such background information reading is helpful, it is suggested that midwives should adopt a critical approach to reading such material and applying it to individual women in order to avoid generalisations, which may lead to stereotypical responses. It is evident that prior knowledge of information is helpful; however, midwives should develop sensitive approaches through which they can ascertain this information from the women, which will assist with delivery of responsive care as well as assist the development of relationships between the women and the midwives.

Midwives need to understand the worldview of the women with disabilities in order to shape the maternity services to meet individual needs of these women. They need to value key principles of rights, independence, choice and inclusion. Many women with disability may have been educationally disadvantaged, as they may have had to miss compulsory education in school years because of receiving medical treatment for their disability. The disability may have led to social isolation, which in turn could have restricted the woman's awareness of services available. Midwives also need to have knowledge of the potential effect that disability may have on the individual woman as a recipient of maternity care.

Clearly midwives need to have knowledge and understanding of all women they care for. They need to understand and interpret, with the woman's help, her lifestyle so that service delivery meets individual requirements.

Similarly, women from disadvantaged backgrounds, in particular, for a number of reasons lack knowledge and understanding of the maternity services. Evidence from a number of small scale studies has identified that women from disadvantaged backgrounds are offered little or no information regarding options of care during pregnancy and labour; lack of effective communication and language is cited as a major hindering factor (Coombs & Schonveld 1992, DoH 1993, Katbamna 2000, LFHSA 1992, PCHC 1992, Ullah 1994). Because of inadequate information such women are not aware of the range of maternity services and choices available to them. For example, a video plus leaflet on hospital delivery in Bengali will tell only half the story with respect to birth options if the leaflet on home birth is available only in English (CRE 1994). Women who do not have full and appropriate information cannot easily access health services; the consequence is poor uptake of maternity and other preventative services.

Communication and language

Communication difficulty, due either to linguistic limitations or to other forms of disability, is cited as a major challenge by both midwives and childbearing women. There is well-documented evidence indicating that communication and language act as a barrier in effectively accessing and utilising maternity services. As a consequence the quality of services is poor, resulting in adverse maternity outcomes (DoH 1993, Lewis & Drife 2001, Woollett & Dosanjh-Matwala 1990a,b). Other carer groups have found maternity services inaccessible, for example, fathers who are the sole carers for their babies have identified that the majority of information on pregnancy and childbirth is aimed at women and does not cater for them.

Midwives claim that communication and language difficulties hinder the delivery of effective maternity services and have expressed dissatisfaction with the care they provide when they cannot effectively communicate with women whose first language is not English, or women with hearing or visual impairment. They state that inability to understand the women as well as explain themselves leaves them frustrated (Audit Commission 1995). Often midwives unintentionally exhibit these frustrations in their behaviour and attitude; these are negatively perceived by the women, which affects their experience of maternity services. Conversely, there are circumstances when women whose level of competence in English is generally low have been characterised as unresponsive, rude and unintelligent by staff (Bowler 1993a, b). Consequently women in such environments feel that the reception and handling they receive is less than adequate and are left feeling humiliated. Arguably women who have poor experiences of maternity services as a result of the above attitudes are less likely to access maternity and preventative services readily.

Women's testimonies also recognise that communication and language act as a barrier to accessing and utilising services effectively. Their experiences of hospitalisation or health services have been greatly exacerbated by inadequate information. They are not always given adequate information about the full range of maternity services; information is not available in appropriate formats to reach women who have visual or hearing impairment or who cannot speak English fluently or understand it well. Equally these women experience difficulties in finding out about the availability of the services as well as their rights to these. Many women from lower socioeconomic groups feel less confident than others in actively participating in the decisions about the care they receive and indeed are less able to make 'informed choices'; to this end they are unable to give informed consent. These factors essentially leave the women feeling frustrated and isolated, marring their experience of maternity services as well as their relationships with midwives.

Often women are encouraged to bring their own interpreters (e.g. adults, family members, neighbours and children). Relying on such measures leads to 'making do' and 'making the best of the situation'. Although such interpreter or translator contributions can be useful in overcoming communication difficulties, they can be major barriers during the consultation process, especially when discussing sensitive and personal issues. Voluntary interpreters or relatives and friends are often untrained in the art of interpreting, have little or no knowledge of the NHS and are often confused themselves by medical terminology; therefore organisations and midwives need to look towards professional qualified interpreters or liaison workers.

Communication is a bedrock of accessible and woman-centred services, for two reasons. First, women can access and use services only if they are aware of their existence. Midwives can overcome this issue by communicating appropriately and giving timely information to women to enable them to access maternity services. Secondly, many women from disadvantaged backgrounds, for social and political reasons, are not confident and are unable to express their needs and preferences to the midwives and so fail to utilise services effectively (Beech 1991). Consequently, exercising choice and control over the care they receive becomes a challenge and women-centred care will remain a myth for them (Hunt & Symonds 1995, Neile 1997, Stapleton 1997). Midwives can play an important role here in facilitating environments to enable women to participate in the decisions about the care they want, need and receive.

Indeed, in circumstances where women cannot effectively communicate with the midwives and other health care professionals, they are unable to fully participate in the decisions about the care they receive. These women feel that professionals and hospitals 'take over' and make decisions about them without first discussing all the options, or informing them of their rights. It is therefore vital that women are provided with relevant and appropriate information, so that they can actively participate in the decisions about the care they receive. Box 2.1 provides suggestions for developing a communication and information strategy.

Relationship

A positive relationship between women and midwives is the cornerstone of appropriate and sensitive service delivery. Health care professionals acknowledge that they have difficulty in developing 'good relationships' with some users and carers, in particular with those

---

Box 2.1 Communication and information strategy

- Provide information in appropriate community languages and formats to all consumers regarding choices and the services available.
- Explore different mediums of communication, for example audiotapes, videotapes, appropriate and sensitive pictorial information, Braille and large print.
- During the translation process, ensure that translators are experienced in the appropriate field, and are familiar with medical terminology used.
- Take into consideration sensitivity of cultural/religious beliefs when presenting information.
- Ensure that publicity/information materials project positive images of people from the black and minority ethnic communities, women with disabilities and other groups who are at risk of being socially excluded.
- Explore various channels for the dissemination of information to members of socially excluded groups, for example, local ethnic press, radio, television and local community road shows.

---

who are unable to speak English fluently (Murphy & Clark 1993). When providing care to people from these groups, staff provide the necessary care but do not really get to know them. Often when there is no feedback from these users the staff get frustrated and angry. Consumers' testimonies acknowledge this poor relationship and the negative effect it has on their experience of childbirth (Woollett & Dosanjh-Matwala 1990a, b). Good relationships between women and midwives promotes trust and confidence, thus providing a conducive environment where the midwife can ascertain the needs and preferences of the women as well as providing appropriate information so that the woman can make informed choices. Midwives need to develop their ability to develop relationships with all women including those at risk of exclusion. To this end, Kirkham (2000) offers useful guidance to midwives.

Discrimination

There is well-documented evidence illustrating the detrimental effect of discrimination and racism on people's health (Virdee 1997), which can operate at different levels. Several studies confirm that midwives commonly use stereotypes of women in determining their needs and preferences and utilise these to make judgements about the kind of care women deserve, as well as what a particular woman is likely to want in labour and delivery (Bowler 1993a, b; Green et al 1998, Pope et al 2001). Midwives' behaviour is informed by these stereotypes and prejudices. For example, women with disabilities are cared for in a paternalistic manner, which hinders their empowerment; women from travelling families are viewed by society as a threat, dishonest scroungers and dirty; women from South Asian backgrounds are seen as thick, smelly, attention seeking, making too much noise during labour and having low pain threshold (Bowler 1993a, b). Many of these stereotypes are not substantiated, given that there are many similarities between many women from the dominant groups. However, when professional practices are based on these stereotypes there can be harrowing consequences. For example, in Bowler's study (1993a, b), based on the assumption that Asian women have low pain threshold it was found that midwives often withheld pain relief from Asian women, whom they considered were not in real need nor deserving of such care.

Many writers, having examined how discrimination is institutionalised in maternity services, argue that it is part and parcel of an organisation's policies, practices and procedures (Phoenix 1990, Torkington 1991). Phoenix in her analysis examines the role of stereotypes in the area of reproduction, where attempts to reduce fertility rate for women from the black and minority ethnic communities can be seen as a form of institutional discrimination. Some of the assumptions held about women from the black and minority ethnic communities are they: 'have too many children', 'breed like rabbits', 'drain resources' and 'swamp British culture'. These stereotypes held by the health care professionals feed into reproductive ideologies in determining service provision. Often, when delivering services based on these assumptions, staff have made racist and derogatory comments; these have been a cause of dissatisfaction to the women and has prevented them seeking care.

Institutional discrimination may also result from policies and procedures that unintentionally exclude some groups of women. Many organisations and health care professionals claim that they treat everyone the same; care delivery is based upon normal policies and routine practices and 'race' makes no difference. This 'colour blind' approach is arguably based upon the premise that equal provision is made for all women and the women are expected to integrate and make use of the pre-existing services. This approach in itself can lead to discriminatory practices, where universal provisions fail to meet specific health requirements of women from disadvantaged groups.

Women from socially excluded groups are often seen to have 'special needs', making extra demands on the service. Emphasis on cultural differences that account for ill health, for example tuberculosis, rickets, hepatitis, has contributed towards pathologising culture. Hence government initiatives such as the 'stop the rickets' and the 'Asian mother and baby' campaigns have been criticised by many from the black and minority ethnic communities who claim their communities are singled out, with the blame on their cultural dietary habits or lifestyles, or even their inability to care for their children (Rocherson 1988, Torkington 1984). These approaches focus on cultural idiosyncrasies with particular emphasis on linguistic or cultural differences and quite effectively obscure power differentials between minority ethnic groups and the majority.

Some forms of discrimination are difficult to identify, particularly when they are institutionalised. Discriminatory attitudes and hostility, however, will affect negatively the standard of care and support provided to women from socially excluded groups. They are therefore less likely to make full and confident use of maternity provision in future. Arguably women from some groups, for example those from the black and minority ethnic communities and those with disabilities, are 'more visible'; they are more likely to be negatively stereotyped and therefore their care adversely affected. Negative experiences may be significant factors in reducing women's confidence and prevent them from exercising choice and control over the care they receive.

Insensitive and inappropriate maternity services

There is abundant literature that continues to indicate that the quality of maternity services offered to women from socially excluded groups is often insensitive and inappropriate in meeting individual maternity needs of these women (Bowes & Domokos 1996, Coombs & Schonveld 1992, DoH 1993, LFHSA 1992, PCHC 1992, Ullah 1994).

There does not appear to be sufficient staff (bilingual speakers, signers, etc.) to overcome communication difficulties experienced by women who are unable to communicate in English or who have disabilities such as hearing or visual impairment. In their attempt to communicate with these women, midwives in many cases make use of relatives or friends as interpreters during sensitive consultations. In addition, women have reported many incidences of insensitive services, such as women being denied the option to see a female doctor, insensitivity during postnatal examination, or an intrauterine contraceptive device being fitted in the presence of a group of male medical students, which they found extremely distressing but often did not complain about as they were unaware of their rights.

Often many maternity and preventative services are inappropriate and preclude women from socially excluded groups from effectively utilising these services. Many maternity services are still provided based on an ethnocentric model, which is based on the principle of providing services to meet the needs of a mainly white homogeneous society. Such services are unlikely to meet the diverse needs of the women from disadvantaged backgrounds. Women from the black and minority ethnic communities constantly argue that current services do not take into account their lifestyles, cultural and religious prescriptions in terms of diet where advice is often based on traditional British food. Health education and education for parenthood is often not culturally sensitive where women and their partners are positively encouraged to attend jointly; maternal and neonatal health screening is also not always appropriate (Coombs & Schonveld 1992, Katbamna 2000, LFHSA 1992).

Users and carers of maternity services, regardless of their race, colour, class, creed, national origin, disability, gender or sexual preference, should have equal access to services. As far back as 1988, the National Association of Health Authorities claimed that 'equal access' does not mean 'treating everyone exactly the same' or providing the 'same services'; 'equal access' means rather that services need to be provided and delivered in a manner that is flexible, adequate, appropriate and sensitive to diverse needs. Users and carers should be able to use maternity services with ease and have confidence that they will be treated with respect.

Maternity services: putting equity in quality

There are moral, ethical and legal frameworks governing organisations and individuals, placing professional and statutory obligations to provide relevant and responsive maternity services for all users and carers. Organisations and individuals are charged to develop and deliver maternity services in such a way that they give an important consideration to the needs of people from 'disadvantaged' groups as well as to reducing inequality and inequity.

Midwives play a key role in bringing about change. They have responsibility to facilitate an environment to provide all women and their carers with appropriate information and encourage more active participation in the decision-making process, including ensuring 'informed consent' prior to any medical intervention.

Role of the midwife

Midwives are in a unique position to exploit the opportunities created by the NHS reforms and government proposals to deliver equitable services, and to create culturally sensitive organisations and practice. Midwives have a moral, ethical and professional responsibility to provide culturally sensitive care to all women as well as to develop equitable service provision and delivery. The Code of professional conduct (NMC 2002, p. 3) requires a midwife to 'respect the patient or client as an individual' and holds the practitioner 'personally accountable for ensuring that you promote and protect the interests and dignity of patients, irrespective of gender, age, race, ability, sexuality, economic status, lifestyle, culture and religious or political beliefs'.

Midwives need to be knowledgeable and understand their own values, attitudes, norms and expectations that affect their professional practice, as well as their consumers' diverse cultures and religions, to enable them to respond equitably. Midwives also need to be aware of issues of prejudice, discrimination and racism and how these manifest themselves in the provision and delivery of health care and may act as a barrier to seeking health care.

Midwives should take account of the difficulties encountered by women who are less familiar with the health services and less confident, and ensure that they are able to create a conducive environment that will enable the women to explain their views and wishes regarding their maternity care. For many, the use of interpreters will be fundamental in the communication process. To this end, midwives should be adequately prepared to utilise interpreters effectively, taking into account the need for privacy and dignity. Midwives should also effectively utilise interpersonal skills and be sensitive to the communication process between themselves and the women who experience communication difficulties so as to create an opportunity for effective and efficient exchange of information. This would serve to provide women with clear, balanced and evidence-based information that they can understand, enabling them to make appropriate informed choices and exercise control over the care they receive.

Midwives play a key role in bringing about change. As advocates of women, they should ensure that the needs and wishes of consumers, in particular women who may not be able to effectively communicate, are taken into consideration during the planning and delivery of services. As change agents, they will need to utilise skills of adaptability, flexibility and political awareness in the development and implementation of innovatory practices to ensure that they are available equitably to all women. Midwives should actively participate in raising awareness of the available services amongst all women.

Conclusion

This chapter has focused on a raft of issues that need to be taken into account by midwives and organisations when providing and delivering maternity and preventative services to all users and carers, in particular those who are most at risk of being excluded. The NHS reforms and government proposals for Britain's maternity services have created exciting opportunities for practitioners to respond to major changes in developing and implementing equitable services, as indeed many are demonstrating. However, midwives cannot achieve this huge agenda on their own. Organisations have to create a culturally sensitive environment, and the issues identified in this chapter need to be addressed strategically. The needs of users and carers from disadvantaged backgrounds must be brought into the mainstream and integrated into the planning and commissioning processes through effective consultation with members of all sectors of the communities. The voices of the members who are most at risk of exclusion should be listened to at every point of the planning and commissioning cycle. It is only then that we can provide relevant and appropriate services to meet the needs of all users and carers. Midwives are in a unique position to take this opportunity for implementing change, so that we as a profession can provide a high quality service that is sensitive, accessible, appropriate and responsive to all users and carers of maternity services. This will go a long way to improve in general the health status of the nation as a whole.

REFERENCES

Ahmad W I U (ed) 1993 'Race' and health in contemporary Britain. Open University Press, Buckingham

Ahmad W I U 1996 The trouble with culture. in: Kelleher D, Hillier S (eds) Researching cultural differences in health. Routledge, London, p 190–219

Audit Commission 1995 What seems to be the matter: communication between hospitals and patients. Audit Commission for Local Authorities and National Health Service for England and Wales, London

Audit Commission 1997 First class delivery: improving maternity services in England and Wales. Audit Commission for Local Authorities and National Health Service for England and Wales, London

Barley S R 1995 'Culture'. In: Nickolson N (ed) Encyclopaedic dictionary of organisational behaviours. Blackwell, New York

Beech B 1991 Who's holding your baby? Bedford Square Press, London

Bharj K, Khan D 1995 Pregnancy, loss and culture: responding to the need. British Journal of Midwifery 3(11):600–602

Bowes A M, Domokos T M 1996 Pakistani women and maternity care: raising muted voices. Sociology of Health and Illness 18:45–65

Bowler I 1993a 'They're not the same as us': midwives' stereotypes of south Asian descent maternity patients. Sociology of Health and Illness 15(2):157–178

Bowler I 1993b Stereotype of women of Asian descent in midwifery, some evidence. Midwifery 9:7–16

Cabinet Office 1999 Teenage pregnancy: report by the Social Exclusion Unit. HMSO, London

Cartwright A 1979 The dignity of labour? Tavistock, London

Coombs G, Schonveld A 1992 Life will never be the same again. Health Education Authority, London

CRE (Commission for Racial Equality) 1994 Race relations code of practice in primary health care services. CRE, London, p 22

Darr A, Bharj K 1999 Addressing cultural diversities in health care – the challenge facing community nursing. In: Atkin K, Lunt N et al (eds) 1999 Evaluating community nursing, Baillière Tindall, London, Ch 2, p 23–43

Davies J 1997 Them and us: poverty, deprivation and maternity care. In: Kargar I, Hunt S C (eds) Challenges in maternity care.

DoH (Department of Health) 1992 Health Committee second report, session 1991–92: maternity services. Winterton report. HMSO, London

DoH (Department of Health) 1993 Changing childbirth: report of the Expert Maternity Group. HMSO, London

DoH (Department of Health) 1994 The patients' charter and maternity services. HMSO, London

DoH (Department of Health) 1991, 1995 The patients' charter. HMSO, London

DoH (Department of Health) 1997 The new NHS: modern, dependable, DoH, London

DoH (Department of Health) 1998 Independent inquiry into inequalities in health report (chairman: Sir Acheson). HMSO, London

DoH (Department of Health) 1999 Saving lives: our healthier nation. White Paper. HMSO, London

DoH (Department of Health) 2000a The NHS plan. A plan for investment, a plan for reform. Stationery Office, London

DoH (Department of Health) 2000b The vital connections: an equalities framework for the NHS. DoH, London

DoH (Department of Health) 2001a Shifting the balance of power within the NHS: securing delivery. DoH, London

DoH (Department of Health) 2001b The annual report of the Chief Medical Officer of the Department of Health. DoH, London

Fernando S 1991 Mental health, race and culture. Macmillan/MIND, London, p 24

Gerrish K, Husband C, MacKenzie J 1996 Nursing for a multi-ethnic society. Open University Press, Buckingham

Green J, Curtis P, Price H, Renfrew M J 1998 Continuity to care: the organisation of midwifery services in the UK: a structured review of the evidence. Hochland & Hochland, Hale, Cheshire

Hart A, Lockey R, Henwood F, Pankhurst F, Hall V, Sommerville V 2001 Researching professional education. Addressing inequalities in health: new directions in midwifery education and practice. Research report series number 20. ENB, London, p 31

Hastie N 2000 Cultural conceptions. In: Fraser D (ed) Professional studies for midwifery practice. Churchill Livingstone, Edinburgh, p 63–75

Helman C G 1994 Culture, health and illness, 3rd edn. Butterworth-Heinemann, Oxford

Hunt S, Symonds A 1995 The social meaning of midwifery. MacMillan, Basingstone, Hampshire

Katbamna S 2000 'Race' and childbirth. Open University Press, Buckingham

Kirkham M (ed) 2000 The midwife–mother relationship. MacMillan, Basingstone, Hampshire

Kitzinger J 1990 Strategies of the early childbirth movement: a case study of the National Childbirth Trust. In: Garcia J, Kilpatrick R et al (eds) The politics of maternity care. Oxford University Press, New York, ch 5, p 92–115

Kitzinger S 1978 Women as mothers. Fontana, London

Larbie J 1985 Black women and the maternity services. Health Education Council and the National Extension College for Training in Health and Race, London

Leininger M M 1978 'Trans-cultural nursing: concepts, theories and practice. John Wiley, New York

Lewis G, Drife J (eds) 2001 Why mothers die 1997–1999. The fifth report of confidential enquiries into maternal deaths in the United Kingdom. RCOG, London

Lewis I M 1976 Social anthropology. Penguin, Harmondsworth

LFHSA (Leeds Family Health Services Authority) 1992 Research into the uptake of maternity services as provided by primary health care teams to women from black and ethnic minorities. LFHSA, Leeds

Linton R 1945 cited in Haralambos M, Holborn M 1995 Sociology themes and perspectives. Collins, London, p 3

MacKeith P, Phillipson R 1997 Young mothers. In: Kargar I, Hunt S C (eds) Challenges in maternity care. Macmillan, Basingstoke, Hants

Macpherson W 1999 The Stephen Lawrence inquiry: report of an inquiry. Home Office, London

Murphy K, Clark J M 1993 Nurses, experience of caring for ethnic minority clients. Journal of Advanced Nursing 18:442–450

NAHA (National Association of Health Authorities) 1988 Action not words – a strategy to improve health services for black and minority ethnic groups. NAHA, Brimingham

National Health Service and Community Care Act 1990. HMSO, London

Nazroo J 1997 The health of Britain's ethnic minorities: findings from a national survey. Policies Studies Institute, London

Neile E 1997 Control for black and ethnic minority women: a meaningless pursuit. In: Kirkham M J, Perkins E R (eds) 1997 Reflections on midwifery. Baillière Tindall; London, ch 6, p 114–134

NMC (Nursing and Midwifery Council) 2002 Code of professional conduct. NMC, London, p 3

Oakley A 1979 Becoming a mother. Martin Robertson, Oxford

Pearson M 1985 Racial equality and good practice in maternity care. Health Education Council and the National Extension College for Training in Health and Race, London

PCHC (Parkside Community Health Council) 1992 Women speak out. PCHC, London

Phoenix A 1990 Black women and the maternity services. In: Garcia J, Kilpatrick R et al (eds) The politics of maternity care. Oxford University Press, New York, ch 15, p 274–299

Pope R, Graham L et al 2001 Woman-centred care. International Journal of Nursing Studies 38:227–238

Proctor S R, Smith I J 1992 A reconsideration of the factors affecting birth outcome in Pakistani Muslim families in Britain. Midwifery 8:76–81

Race Relations (Amendment) Act 2000 Stationery Office, London

Race Relations Act 1976, HMSO, London

RCM (Royal College of Midwives) 2000a Position paper 4a: woman-centred care, reprinted in RCM Midwives Journal 2001 4(2), p 46–47

RCM (Royal College of Midwives) 2000b Maternity care for lesbian mothers. Position paper no. 22. RCM, London

Reid M, Garcia J 1989 Women's views of care during pregnancy and childbirth. In: Chalmers I, Enkin M, Keirse M J N C (eds) Effective care in pregnancy and childbirth. Clarendon Press, Oxford, p 131–142

Rocheron Y 1988 The Asian mother and baby campaign: the construction of ethnic minorities 'health needs'. Critical Social Policy 22:4–23

Rose S, Rose H 1986 Less than human nature. Race and Class 27(3):47–66

Salmon D, Powell J 1998 Caring for women in poverty: a critical review. British Journal of Midwifery 6(2):108–111

Schott J, Henley A 1996 Culture, religion and childbearing in a multiracial society: a handbook for health care professionals. Butterworth-Heinemann, London

Smaje C 1995 Health, race and ethnicity: making sense of the evidence. King's Fund Institute, London, p 16

Social Exclusion Unit 1999 Teenage pregnancy. Stationery Office, London

Stapleton H 1997 Choice in the face of uncertainty. In: Kirkham M J, Perkins E R (eds) Reflections on midwifery. Baillière Tindall, London, ch 3, p 47–69

Stubbs P 1993 'Ethnically sensitive' or 'anti-racist'? Models for health research and service delivery. In: Ahmad W I U (ed) 1993 'Race' and health in contemporary Britain. Open University Press, Buckingham, ch 3, p 34–47

Taylor E B 1871 cited in Helman C G 1994 Culture, health and illness, 3rd edn. Butterwork-Heinemann, Oxford, p 2

Torkington P 1984 Blaming black women – rickets and racism. In: O'Sullivan S (ed) 1987 Women's health, a spare rib reader. Pandora, London, ch 2, p 82–85

Torkington P 1991 Black health – a political issue. Catholic Association for Racial Justice and Liverpool Institute of Higher Education, London and Liverpool

Townsend P, Davidson N 1982 Inequalities in health: the Black report. Penguin, Harmondsworth

UKCC (United Kingdom Central Council for Nursing, Midwifery and Health Visiting) 2001 Strenghening and supporting the midwifery contribution to maternity care for women and their families. Registrar's letter 23/2001 31 August 2001. UKCC, London

Ullah S 1994 The health needs of Bangladeshi women for maternity care. Family Health Services Authority, Bradford

Virdee S 1997 Racial harassment. In: Modood T, Berthoud R, Lakey J et al (eds) 1997 Ethnic minorities in Britain: diversity and disadvantage, Fourth National Survey of Ethnic Minorities. Policies Studies Institute, London, ch 8, p 259–289

Whitehead M 1987 The health divide: inequalities in health in the 1980s. Health Education Council, London

Whitehead M 1992 The health divide (revised edn). Penguin, Harmondsworth

Wilton T, Kaufmann T 2001 Lesbian mothers' experiences of maternity care in the UK. Midwifery 17:203–211

Woollett A, Dosanjh-Matwala N 1990a Pregnancy and antenatal care: the attitudes and experiences of Asian women. Child Care, Health and Development 16(1):63–78

Woollett A, Dosanjh-Matwala N 1990b Postnatal care: the attitudes & experiences of Asian women in east London. Midwifery 6:178–184

FURTHER READING

Karger I, Hunt S 1997 Challenges in midwifery care. Macmillan, Basingstoke, Hants

Midwives frequently encounter challenging situations in practice; this text provides a useful resource to help them meet the special needs of women such as the traveller or the woman with a hearing impairment.

Kirkham M (ed) 2000 The midwife–mother relationship. Macmillan, Basingstone, Hants

This book examines the midwife–mother relationship that underpins maternity care. It includes examples of practice in different social contexts and addresses some of the challenges that a midwife may face, such as difficulties of communication.

Schott J, Henley A 1996 Culture, religion and childbearing in a multiracial society. Butterworth Heinemann, Oxford

This book provides a valuable resource for midwives and other health professionals involved in the care of women and their families from diverse racial and religious backgrounds. It invites readers to examine their own cultural beliefs and become sensitive to others who may hold different beliefs.

3

Woman-Centred, Midwife-Friendly Care: Principles, Patterns and Culture of Practice

Lesley Page

Midwives hold an important key to positive care around the time of childbirth that will contribute to a good start for the baby and parents during this critical period of human life. Where care is appropriately organised, and midwives hold interpersonal, clinical skills and knowledge, care is more likely to be positive. If care is fragmented, oriented to technology rather than human relationship, where midwives do not have professional autonomy and the culture of care is institutionalised, even if they hold the best skills, attitudes and knowledge, midwives will not be able to do their best for families and communities in their care. The way that care is organised, including the pattern and culture of practice, is probably one of the most important factors in creating effective, sensitive and individual care.

This chapter aims to examine:

- the background to recent changes to the patterns and culture of practice

- the principles of woman-centred practice

- key characteristics of different patterns of practice

- how different patterns of practice may support these principles

- two examples of successful developments and advice on how to practise within different patterns

- how to manage situations in which neither midwives nor women have a range of choices about how and where to give birth, or the pattern of practice.

Background

The roots of midwifery lie in the care of childbearing women by other women from their own community or family. Even after the professionalisation of midwifery with the registration of midwives, the majority were community based. The majority of births were home births, with the balance of home versus hospital births being altered over the last half century. This brought about a division between hospital and community midwifery; where midwives were hospital based they were organised on a model of acute care nursing. Thus care became highly fragmented. In addition, as maternity care became more and more technical and medical in its nature, it became more difficult for midwives to practise autonomously. Thus, the potential for an ongoing relationship between the woman and her midwife was eroded, and the ability for midwives to use all their skills and knowledge and to manage care was diminished.

Since the early 1980s much work has been undertaken to redevelop continuity in the relationship between women and their midwives, and to enable midwives to practise more autonomously. This work has happened in many parts of the world. It has consisted of changes in midwifery regulation, and in policy at governmental and local level, of developments of innovative practice and of research and evaluation. In some countries, for example The Netherlands, New Zealand and Canada, midwives are not employees of a health service but work in publicly or insurance-funded independent practices. Ideally, although practising independently, these midwives have access to local health services with mechanisms for consultation, referral and transfer when problems occur. In two of the Provinces of Canada, for example, midwives have admitting privileges to local hospitals where they are part of medical departments (Page 2000a).

The new midwifery

What has arisen from these developments in policy and practice is a reformation of midwifery that takes in some of the historical values and functions of midwifery while adapting it to the needs of the modern world and more complex health services. What has been called the 'new midwifery' has emerged over recent years.

The internationally accepted definition of a midwife is a basis for understanding the scope of practice of midwifery (UKCC 1998). However, it is only a starting point. This definition provides no ideas on how midwifery is similar to medical maternity practice, and how it differs. There are two aspects of effective midwifery that make it unique. First, midwives are the specialists in normal labour and birth, and hold the potential to support normal healthy outcomes. Secondly, midwives have the potential to work through a personal relationship with women (the original meaning of midwife) through the whole of pregnancy, birth and the early weeks of life, including labour; this relationship has been described in a number of ways that include one of friendship, of partnership, and of skilled companion. Such a relationship is the basis for achieving the aims of midwifery.

The aims of midwifery

The aims of midwifery are far wider than physical health of mother and baby. They include the following:

- to help the mother and her family make the transition to parenthood in the best way possible; that is, to emerge from childbirth physically and emotionally intact, with the relationships within the family, particularly the attachment between the mother and baby and parents, as strong as possible, and to have the confidence, knowledge and commitment to care for her child until adulthood
- to support and protect physiological processes and healthy outcomes
- to provide comfort and alleviate the distressing symptoms of pregnancy, labour and birth and the postpartum period.

Principles of patterns of practice for the new midwifery

The principles of patterns of practice that support development of the new midwifery are as follows:

- woman-centred care, including choice, control and continuity for women
- the potential for the development of a personal continuous relationship between the woman and her midwife

- community-based care
- midwifery autonomy and a clear expression of the distinct nature of midwifery practice, including the support of normal or physiological birth
- appropriate support for midwives
- a positive organisational culture
- an interface with other professionals, midwives, doctors, nurses and health visitors, and hospitals and mechanisms for consultation, referral and transfer
- cost effectiveness.

I will discuss each of these principles in detail before moving on to the patterns of practice that will support them.

Woman-centred care, choice control and continuity

The term 'woman-centred care' is often used to describe the philosophy of care promoted from the report Changing Childbirth (DoH 1993) and other reports from all parts of the UK (House of Commons 1992, SOHHD 1993). This term means that women and their families should be at the heart of everything midwives do in practice. They should be given choice in the place of birth, caregiver and care, and be given control over their own care and experience. Two keys to achieving these principles are the provision of continuity of carer – a professional who they could get to know and trust over time who would provide and manage most care – and the restoration of autonomous midwifery. These ideas may sound perfectly sensible. However, in reality the majority of women give birth in large institutions. In such institutions there is always a tendency to start to develop routines, practices and attitudes that move away from the central purpose of the organisation. In the case of maternity services this means that they may not be in the best interests of women and their families. Sometimes such institutions unconsciously attend to the needs of staff before families. Often they are arranged in such a way that it is very difficult for staff to provide the best care. Any group of people is likely to develop a life of its own. In many health services there is a rigid hierarchy or an informal power structure that may give some groups like midwives little professional autonomy. This is not simply a matter of a hierarchy in which midwives have less power than

other professionals because, although it is the case that midwives are often lower in the health service hierarchy than doctors, much of the oppression of midwifery comes from within midwifery itself.

The work of Kirkham & Stapleton (2001) has been invaluable in helping to understand the prevailing culture of midwifery in the NHS. They described how, in less than a century, English midwives became 'regulated, professionalized and medically controlled. The values reflected in the organization of midwives were those of an organizational vision culturally coded as masculine. The domestic, caring female values became increasingly invisible, although remained essential, in the support of individual childbearing women. Adjusting to profound changes, midwives manifest the classic responses of an oppressed group, internalizing the powerful values of medicine and exercising "horizontal violence" towards colleagues seen as deviant' (p. 157). It is easy to see then, that the support of women in having choice and control of their own care, pregnancy and birth by midwives may be limited in a profession that sees itself as powerless, and this will control other members of the profession who are seeking change and to empower childbearing women.

To talk about giving women choice uses a consumer concept that may not do justice to the complex process that occurs when a midwife develops a relationship with a woman so that they may share information, discuss it properly and reach a decision. Choice is not, as Leap reminds us, a matter of providing women with a menu and letting them get on with making the choice (Leap 2000). I have heard midwives say to women 'it is up to you – it is your choice' without understanding their role in providing information and aiding discussion and consideration of decisions that are especially complex in today's world, and difficult even for trained educated professionals to understand when evidence needs to be taken into account.

In addition, genuine choices are often limited by what is available and acceptable to local services and communities. To give women genuine choice requires a change to health services so that choices are actually available. It also requires that all professionals, including medical staff, are encouraged to look their beloved beliefs, practices and rituals in the eye and question them to see if they are genuinely likely to be beneficial to individual women and families. This is not an easy thing for any of us to do.

Giving women choice and control requires that information from a number of sources be taken into account. This information should be taken not only from good evidence, but also from the personal values and preferences of the woman, her clinical history and examination, and the context of care. This process requires a balance of many skills and much knowledge and is not easy. It helps tremendously if the midwife has a continuous and ongoing relationship with a woman, and if she is confident that she has the professional autonomy to make decisions together with the woman.

A personal relationship between the woman and her midwife

'Midwives can do a better job if their work is structured in such a way as to enable them to become acquainted with and take responsibility for their patients' (Freely 1995). Freeley described the care she received from a team of midwives as 'care with a face and a memory and an ever open ear. It made me feel like an active participant'. In comparison, the care she experienced in the conventional system was from a 'faceless institution'. It is through the development of relationships between caregivers and childbearing women and their families that we make the change from faceless institution to humanistic supportive care.

The relationship between women and their midwives is seen by women as important in itself, and not only as an instrumental means of leading to other outcomes (Wilkins 2000). However, the development of a relationship is also the basis of the ability to give women choice and control, and helps in the support of physiological birth and in the comforting role of the midwife. Importantly, this relationship is the medium for the support the midwife may give the family in their journey to their new roles and responsibility, the transition to parenthood. As the skilled companion (Campbell 1984) the midwife acts as a guide and supporter, helping the woman through rough and difficult terrain, enjoying the pleasures and excitement of the journey, while allowing the woman and her partner to make their own journey and learn the lessons and gather a sense of their own strength from the journey and its completion.

If midwives know and understand the women they are caring for, and where trust has grown between them, they will find it easier to respond to individual needs, to comfort and to encourage women through some of the difficulties, not only of pregnancy and after the birth but also through labour and birth. Women describe the importance of knowing their midwife, particularly during labour and birth, and of the confidence and trust this brings (McCourt et al 2000).

Women who have received 'continuity' of care do not use the term continuity. These women talk about the value of knowing their caregivers and why this is important to them. Women tend to link supportive care with knowing their midwife (McCourt et al 2000).

In the study by McCourt et al (2000), women who had received one-to-one care described the importance of the availability of the midwife both directly and over time; they described the trust that develops and the way that knowing the midwife is reassuring as follows:

> I knew exactly what was going to happen, when and how, that was one bit of it. Another thing is you knew the person there, and she was there only herself, no one else (p. 282).

There is a sense of intimacy, of feeling that the midwife was accessible, on the same level as the woman:

> Well I could talk to her about anything and say to her everything, that's how much confidence I had in her.

Women also described the way midwives become a part of the experience:

> well they do know me, they recognize me, but my midwife, she was part of it, part of the birth, the baby (p. 282).

Women talked about the midwife as a friend, as being like family. They described midwives they had come to know as 'my midwife' in contrast to 'the midwife' or 'they'. There was a sense of closeness to the midwife, of a special relationship.

It is this 'with woman' aspect of midwifery that many midwives have tried to reintroduce to midwifery practice over recent years: the relationship that allows a spirit of 'being with' rather than 'doing to'. Midwives have explained the great lengths they go to in order to develop the relationship that puts women at the heart of care, and seeks and supports their active involvement in their pregnancy and birth (Pairman 2000).

Midwives who describe the relationship, like women, describe it in terms of friendship, partnership, professional friendship and professional servant (Kirkham 2000). It is a relationship in which midwife and woman contribute equally, and is one of sharing, involving trust, shared control and respect, and shared meaning through understanding (Pairman 2000). It acts as a foundation for shared decision making, and facilitates communication. Although called a friendship, it is not exactly a friendship because the midwife enters as an expert, and the relationship is usually terminated at the end of care. It can be seen as a friendship with a purpose.

The relationship is used intentionally to shift power towards the woman, what Cronk (2000) has described as the professional servant, but midwives cannot empower women unless they themselves are empowered (Kirkham 2000). The trust is not only by the woman from the midwife but requires that the midwife believes in or trusts the woman (Leap, 2000). It is recognised that the most powerful help for a woman may come from doing as little as possible, as Leap (2000, p. 2) puts it, 'the less we do the more we give'. Although there are times, particularly in labour, when a midwife may need to take charge or take control, this works better when there is a previously formed relationship (Anderson 2000).

Importance of continuity and what it means. It is difficult to form the kind of relationship described unless the pattern of practice allows the provision of what has become known as 'continuity of carer'. The term 'continuity of carer' is a description of the structure that is set up to enable the relationship between the woman and her midwife to develop over time. This structure should organise care so that individual women may receive most of their care from a named midwife. This named midwife provides and manages most of the midwifery care for a woman, and is likely to be available for critical events in the woman's pregnancy including labour and birth. This is not the same as solo practice. In the most effective organisations the midwife has a partner or small number of partners who will stand in for the named midwife when she is unavailable, and who will also have formed a relationship with the woman. Essentially in this system of care midwives follow women through the service, rather than having women progress through a number of teams of people – an assembly line or conveyer belt of sorts.

The development of patterns of practice that allow true continuity of caregiver may require radical change. It will also require a system of on call for a large number of midwives. It is the need for these radical changes that has led to the development of tremendous controversy and debate around the need for continuity of carer, particularly amongst midwives. It has been claimed that what women really want is continuity of care – a shared philosophy. This denies the importance of the relationship in itself to women, and the use of self that a midwife may give in supporting and comforting and encouraging women. It also denies the difficulty of large numbers of people making complex decisions in the same way as others, given their own personal values and knowledge. In addition, the lack of a real knowledge of the medical history and personal values and preferences of the individual woman makes it very difficult to make personally sensitive and appropriate decisions.

It has also been argued that women have other priorities, such as the health of their baby and good information, as though such desires could be ranked in a hierarchy (Page 1995). Some have interpreted evidence in such a way that they argue women do not really want continuity of carer. In reality, evidence to refute or support the idea that it is important for women to have continuity of caregiver, or that particular outcomes are the direct outcomes of continuity of carer, is not easy to develop or interpret from the dominant paradigm of research: the randomised controlled trial. In addition, finding out about what women want from care around birth is difficult. Women tend to expect what is on offer (DeVries et al 2001). Even so, when surveys of women who have experienced 'continuity of carer' are undertaken, the majority indicate that it is important to them, and even in surveys of women who have not experienced 'continuity of carer' the majority indicate that it would be helpful to them. Moreover, qualitative research is beginning to explain why it is so important to so many women (McCourt et al 2000).

The development of a high level of continuity of carer may be the most difficult change to achieve, but is probably the most fundamental or important change to bring about. It is helped tremendously if community and hospital services can be integrated, and if most of a woman's care is moved away from centralised institutions and given in the community.

Community-based care

Moving away from centralised institutions. In most of the Western world, maternity services have been centralised into acute care hospitals. This is despite the fact that pregnancy is a normal part of the life of the majority of women, and that childbearing is in general a healthy life event. Instead it would be more appropriate for care to be given in the primary care sector of the health service, rather than by specialists in an acute care setting.

The problems of centralised birth. There are two problems with the centralisation of birth into acute care. First, there is a tendency, referred to earlier, in all large organisations of people to move towards institutionalisation. Kirkham wrote, 'with the centralization of birth into hierarchically organized and increasingly large hospitals, midwifery increasingly adopted the responses and values of those institutions. All these responses served to protect the status quo which reinforced the values of obstetrics not midwifery.' Kirkham drew on the work of Raphael Leff who 'sees the fragmented care given in maternity hospitals as part of a social defence system … constructed to help individual professionals avoid experiencing anxiety, guilt, doubt and uncertainty. Both caring and gratitude are diminished in a system where people are treated in a depersonalized way and any activities which threaten the status quo are intensely resisted' (Kirkham 2000, p. 157).

If the midwife can become a part of the woman's community, getting to know the woman and her family more personally, learning to understand their lives and the nature of the life around them, she will be able to be more responsive to them as individuals, and may be released from the depersonalisation of the institution. This is also important in allowing midwives to respond to the needs and characteristics of different neighbourhoods and communities, and to understand the racial and ethnic mix and level of poverty or affluence of 'her' patch (see Ch. 2). Such knowledge helps in deciding whether the development of different community services, for example a shopfront practice or premises within a housing estate, are appropriate (Davies 2000). It takes health care to the community rather than expecting women to visit for health care. Increasing accessibility and attractiveness are important parts of good health care. Community-based care can be provided either in the home (for example antenatal visits at home, or a genuine choice of home birth) or in community centres, midwives' or doctors' surgeries or offices situated in the community. Small hospitals, and out-of-hospital birth centres, will provide care that is both near the woman's own home and less acute care for at least a small group of women.

Secondly, when the care of childbearing women takes place in an acute care setting, in the main by specialists or consultants, there will be a tendency to use more medical and surgical interventions. Care provided by skilled, confident and experienced primary practitioners (midwives and family doctors or GPs) is more likely to support physiological processes and less likely to lead to unnecessary intervention. It is for these reasons that policy documents such as Changing Childbirth (DoH 1993) proposed a shift to community-based care as fundamental to effective provision of maternity care.

Home birth will lead to a more profound change from hospital birth than any other change in the organisation of care. The best evidence on the outcomes of home birth and the experience of home birth for women without complications or real risk factors shows persistently that there is a lower rate of interventions, and that women who ask for a home birth generally enjoy the experience (Page 2000b). Birth at home means that the woman can relax in her own environment, and that she is in a different power relationship with professionals, who are invited into her home. Although there are exceptions (Edwards 2000), in general the relationship is of a higher quality. Home birth brings with it its own pattern of practice, and on the whole it is easier to provide the woman with midwives she can get to know and trust.

Midwifery autonomy – expressing the unique nature of midwifery in practice

To practice the new midwifery the midwife needs professional autonomy. This does not mean, however, that the midwife should practise in isolation. She needs to work in an interface with other members of the health care team, while knowing that the contribution she makes is unique and cannot be made by any other member of the team. The midwife has specialist approaches and skills that no other member of the health care team has, even though some of her role will overlap with that of doctors, both GPs and obstetricians (Page 2001).

Professional autonomy requires that:

- the midwife is responsible for all care unless she makes a referral to another health professional
- any guidelines and policies should have been developed and approved by midwifery after a proper process of consultation.

The worldview of midwifery is to have confidence in normal or physiological processes, rather than feeling that these could fail at any moment. This worldview requires a different knowledge base, research interest, and skill set in midwives. During pregnancy and birth there should be sufficient focus on the woman's experience, and help and support for distressing aspects of pregnancy and birth, as well as sharing the enjoyment and joy. Presence, comfort and appropriate touch, reassurance and encouragement are central aspects of midwife-led care. Particularly during labour and birth, midwifery autonomy allows the midwife to take into account the woman as an individual in making decisions about care, and to provide more flexible care. I have never been able to see how midwife-led care or autonomous midwifery can be effective without some basis of continuity. However, there is considerable debate about this matter and midwife-led care rather than continuity has been the aim of a number of innovations.

Support and satisfaction for midwives

One of the most effective ways of helping midwives to move away from institutionalised and hierarchical structures is to break the working groups into smaller groups or practices, and to enable them to manage themselves and their own resources, while ensuring that they have some mechanisms for support and development. This may happen in some health services (such as Canada and New Zealand) by having midwives own their own practices, while receiving public funding for care provided and access to local maternity services for consultation, referral and transfer. The best form of practice may be a small group of midwives in which each midwife is the named or primary midwife for individual women. Some midwives enjoy solo practice, especially if there are colleagues they can call on to cover on call occasionally. However, for the majority of midwives perpetual on call may be too much.

The development of a 'woman-centred' organisation is sometimes seen as being at odds with developing a supportive organisation for midwives. Yet this need not be the case. It can be seen from the work of Stevens & McCourt (2001) and Sandall (1997) that what provides satisfaction to women can be a mutual source of satisfaction to midwives, in particular the development of a meaningful relationship with women. In the one-to-one service the midwives' positive views and their comments on strengths focused on:

- enabling the development of relationships with women and families and with other professionals
- greater autonomy of practice
- considerable professional and personal development
- flexibility, variety and mutual support (Stevens & McCourt 2001, p. 12).

Sandall (1997) describes the characteristics of occupational autonomy, developing meaningful relationships with women, and social support as important factors in work satisfaction for midwives.

The development of continuity-of-carer schemes and close relationships with women gives midwives a sense of primary loyalty to women and can release a midwife from feeling that her main allegiance is to the profession or her employer (Brodie 1997, Page 1995). This may be one of the most empowering aspects of working with women. Yet the recognition of the prevailing culture of midwifery shows how difficulties may arise in changing patterns of practice and in creating greater midwifery autonomy. Kirkham & Stapleton (2001) undertook a study related to supervision in midwifery. They found what they described as a caring, self-sacrificing client-centred culture with an overwhelming helplessness and lack of support. There is evidence of horizontal violence, and where change is sought it is often done quietly and secretly, 'doing good by stealth' (p. 150). Only on rare occasions did midwives and supervisors seek change in more open ways. Amongst the NHS midwives studied there was little evidence of reflection, analysis or planning to meet their support needs. So, any changes need to be developed together with the development of support for midwives.

The needs that midwives have of supervisors or managers have been identified as the need for listening and being there, vulnerability and the need for protection, advocacy and facilitation, facilitation towards empowerment, and the danger of dependency. Kirkham (2000) identifies what she describes as two conflicting discourses of support and trust. There is a need for trust but there are many ways in which midwives felt unable to trust supervisors, managers and colleagues. In many ways these needs parallel almost completely the needs of childbearing women. As women need strong midwives to enable their growth and development through the process of birth, so midwives need structures and appropriate leadership that allow them to support each other and to be challenged to grow and develop. Kirkham (2000) proposes ways of starting to change this culture; she includes the development of continuity of carer, and the approach of listening to midwives while helping them to ask themselves the questions from which they can develop a support strategy. Simple interventions such as praising, thanking and recognition of achievement are important. More complex approaches include the development of equality of esteem, and specific skills to develop power sharing and to encourage reflection.

A positive organisational culture

Woman-centred care *need* not be at conflict with the needs of midwives or indeed other staff; neither *should* it be at conflict. Retention of midwives and work satisfaction are crucial to an effective and 'positive' organisational culture. A positive culture is, in other words, a place that 'feels good' and supports good work.

Organisational culture here means the atmosphere, aims, values and expectations, and relations between people (professionals and those being cared for) within the structure that is the context for practice. Culture is reflected in the priorities we choose, the way we spend our time, our language and behaviour. In the maternity services the culture should:

- be woman centred – that is, staff behaviour, policies, guidelines, and buildings are focused on the individual needs of women
- be supportive of staff, with attention to midwives
- support continuous learning and professional and personal development – that is, priority is given to learning and provision of resources, including time; there is evidence of discussion, questioning, reflection, challenge and review; practice is seen as an opportunity to learn; there is comfort in senior

staff learning from junior staff and vice versa; care is evidence based
- accept that physiological pregnancy and birth are the normal base of practice and should be supported (this last characteristic is explained in depth in the report from the Caesarean Section Working Group of the Ontario Women's Health Council (2000))
- demonstrate relationships between staff that are respectful with an understanding of the strength of the role of each professional group and the distinct contribution to be made by each.

Connection with the health services and mechanisms for consultation and referral

Some of the patterns of care we will review include independent or private practice. Possibly these patterns hold the greatest potential for professional autonomy. However, it is crucial that autonomy is not confused with separation or isolation of practice. In today's world, women are entitled to more complex and medical care if it is needed. Perhaps one of the highest level skills of any midwife is to be able to differentiate between situations in which she can support physiological birth and those when consultation or referral is needed.

Autonomous midwifery needs a strong interface with colleagues and the health service or hospital. I have seen at first hand the results of a hospital service that treats midwives antagonistically, does not recognise them as professionals and where this antagonism results in delays in care for mother and baby. The worst situations are when a mother or baby has to be transferred to hospital because of acute problems at a home birth, and antagonism to home birth or the midwife are allowed to result in emotional responses that affect care. This may easily result in death or severe disability, or a very negative experience for the woman and her family.

A connective supportive interface will be helped by multiprofessional guidelines and policies for practice, discussion and active negotiation with colleagues, and help in understanding roles, particularly around a time of change. It is recognised in the discussions about relative safety of home and hospital birth that the safety net of the system is crucial (Olsen 1997). Sometimes guidelines are seen as a hazard to midwifery autonomy, but guidelines such as the 'Kloosterman list' in The Netherlands may serve to protect the autonomy of midwives and the right to home birth (Sandall et al 2001).

Balancing the needs to redevelop a distinct identity and a sense of purpose that goes beyond being doctor's assistant, yet still working together cooperatively with medical colleagues, may not be easy. It is for this reason that the profession needs strong leaders who can articulate the unique nature of midwifery practice, maintain effective relationships and negotiate a safe environment for midwives who will challenge current boundaries of practice.

Cost effectiveness

There is no such thing as a health service with unlimited resources, nor will it ever be possible, or even right, to develop innovations that take a disproportionate share of the health service budget. Innovations should be cost effective – this means that resources should be used appropriately and provide value for money; they should add something to the quality of care. In most health care systems there are choices made between priorities. In today's world it may be that technology or the use of technology will be funded before something like an increase in the number of midwives. This choice reflects the values of the dominant culture. A tool for assessing the number of midwives required is important (Ball & Washbrook 1996).

One problem is that it is often assumed that the current way of organising things is the most cost effective, and anything that improves the quality of care of necessity costs more. However, the current system of standard care as it is provided in countries like the UK is actually very wasteful; it is not cost effective. First, although midwives may not be paid enough for what they do, the numbers are so great that salaries take up the largest part of the midwifery budget. When the role of midwives is restricted, as it is by present culture and structures, this is a huge waste of money and resources. Secondly, the traditional organisation of midwives on shifts is an inflexible system that does not follow the ebb and flow of midwifery workload. Innovations such as one-to-one midwifery have reduced length of stay, have the potential to reduce beds, have reduced the intervention rate and have also increased the number of births per midwife post (Piercey 1996, Piercey et al 2001). Yet still, even after a thorough evaluation, it is often viewed as being too expensive.

Patterns of practice

It is important to recognise that the patterns of practice and culture of our midwifery services, whether traditional or innovative, are always a product of the wider social environment and nature of the health service. Thus, for example the nature of midwifery in The Netherlands has arisen because of a number of broad social factors like the nature of the family, the place of women in the family, attitudes to health care, and geography. In addition, the structure and culture of the health service, and laws, have established a strong base for the maintenance of midwifery as a profession (Sandall et al 2001). Likewise, the development of midwifery in the UK, its strengths and problems, must be viewed in the light of the nature of the NHS. However, as in all other parts of life, a process of globalisation has meant that many of the industrialised countries share similar trends. For example most of these, with the exception of The Netherlands, have centralised maternity services. Many have a very high operative and assisted birth rate.

Four key characteristics of patterns of practice

The pattern of practice is defined here as the structure or organisation of care around four key characteristics. These characteristics are:

- employee or independent practitioner
- community, integrated or centralised care
- continuity or fragmented care
- midwifery autonomy or medicalised approaches.

First I will define and describe these key characteristics, and then I will give two examples of different patterns of practice that integrate these characteristics.

Publicly or insurance-funded independent practice

In some parts of the world (e.g. The Netherlands, New Zealand) midwives practise as independent practitioners, having their services funded for each course of care either by the health service or health insurance. There is a big difference between publicly funded or privately funded independent midwifery practice because a publicly funded practice, if widely enough available, will give access to the majority of women rather than the small numbers who are able or willing to pay for their midwifery care. In general, publicly funded independent midwives may find it easier than privately funded midwives to form an interface with the maternity services for back-up, consultation, referral and transfer.

Midwives who are an employee of an organisation will inevitably find some limitations on practice, as the midwife must follow the policies and guidelines of the institution or employer. However, with enlightened and strong midwifery leadership this may not be too much of a problem, and there is usually greater security for the midwife in such a position. In services that are not progressive, or where there is not strong and enlightened midwifery leadership, the situation can be very frustrating and will severely limit the ability of any midwife to give of her best.

Community-based or integrated care or centralised care

At one end of the continuum the woman may have all of her care at home, including the birth and care after birth. Some women will have all of their care in pregnancy and most of the care after birth in the community – either at home or in the midwife's or doctor's surgery or office. Some services will integrate community and hospital so that the emphasis is on having a midwife follow women through the system of care from start to finish. At the other extreme, women receive all their care in an acute care centralised hospital setting. The place of care and birth will have a profound effect on the nature of care, outcomes of care and the ability of the midwife to use her abilities to the full.

Continuity of caregiver or fragmented care

The highest level of continuity of caregiver is to have one practitioner who provides all the care, including care during labour and birth. A few women receive this from midwives in solo practice. However, this is impractical for many midwives as it places permanent on-call demands on them. Close to this is a system whereby the woman has most of her care from one named midwife who is responsible for all care and provides most hands-on care. This midwife is supported by another midwife, or small number of midwives, who will get to know the women in their partner's caseload and provide cover when the named

midwife is unavailable. Practices such as one-to-one midwifery, the Birth Under Midwife project and Shrewsbury maternity service provided a very high level of continuity of caregiver with this approach. This is often called a *personal caseload*.

Some patterns, usually called team midwifery, will offer continuity from a team of midwives. This is often known as a *team caseload* rather than a personal caseload (Page et al 2000). In general, the level of continuity achieved is not so high. Some teams, if they are too large, or extend only to hospital or community care, may even break down continuity.

For a time in the UK there was an emphasis on providing *shared care*. This was aimed at making the services of a specialist or consultant obstetrician available to all women. Some use the term 'shared care' differently. Canadian midwives may use the term to describe sharing care with a partner or colleague, another midwife. In the UK the principle of shared care led to complete fragmentation, and moved much care into the hospital. There are still a number of women who have not met the consultant who is a name on the notes, and who see a different person at nearly every visit.

The shift from a standard midwifery system, where midwives work shifts and are allocated to hospital or community, ward or department rather than to individual women, to continuity of carer is a radical one. It requires radical changes not only in the service but also to the lives of midwives who will be expected to do on call. The pattern of on call should be considered carefully. Experience and logic teach that, if the midwife provides a high level of continuity, she may be on call more often but called out less when she is on call than if she shares call with a large team. In addition, she is more likely to know the women she is called out for and most midwives report that this is easier than when the woman is a stranger. Although some midwives may not want an on-call commitment, it may offer greater flexibility than a shift system for midwives who wish to work in this way.

Midwifery autonomy versus medicalised midwifery

The upper end of midwifery autonomy will be found in independent midwifery, and in home births and out-of-hospital birth centres. It is important to repeat that this term implies professional control over how practice is organised, values of practice and the use of interventions. It does not imply practising in isolation or antagonism with others in the health service. Midwifery, as discussed at length earlier in the chapter, has a distinct and unique approach to childbirth care. Midwifery autonomy allows this to be expressed in practice. However, in many parts of the world midwifery follows the obstetric model and approach. Care has become technocratic – that is, focused on technology rather than human care.

Examples in practice

Having discussed the key characteristics of different patterns of practice I will now describe two examples of successful patterns of practice that integrate many of the key principles discussed earlier.

One-to-one midwifery

How it works. This is a very simple form of practice in which one named midwife is responsible for the care of individual women. This named midwife works with a midwife partner who gets to know the women in her caseload and provides on-call cover when the named midwife is unavailable. This pattern of practice integrates a high level of continuity with midwifery-led care. Care is organised in group practices of six to eight midwives to provide support, allocation of the caseload and peer review of practice. The pilot was set up to provide for the requirements of the Changing Childbirth report (DoH 1993), specifically to provide a service that is sensitive to the needs of individual women and their families, and to give women choice, continuity and control.

Midwives meet the woman at the beginning of pregnancy and provide care throughout. Because it is geographically based the midwives are situated in a local community and provide much care in the woman's own home. All women in the local neighbourhood are cared for by the service, including low and high risk women. Where the woman has a low risk pregnancy the midwife is the lead professional and responsible for all care. Where the woman has complications or is high risk the midwife works with the medical team but is still responsible for all midwifery care. Women choose whether to give birth in the home or in the hospital.

Outcomes of One-to-One Midwifery. One-to-one midwifery was first implemented in November 1993.

Two cohort studies have been undertaken to assess one-to-one midwifery and to compare it with standard care (Page et al 1999, 2001). The first was undertaken soon after implementation, and the second when the service was well established. So far as we know it is the only study of an innovation once it had been running for some time. The study focused on:

- women's responses to their care
- clinical interventions and outcomes for both mothers and babies
- standards of care
- continuity of care
- use of economic resources.

There was a lower rate of clinical interventions associated with one-to-one care, and the differences between the groups were increased in the second cohort. The high level of continuity through all the processes of pregnancy and birth, and after birth, was maintained in the second cohort (Page et al 1999, 2001). Standards of care were also maintained, despite the newness of the service in the first cohort (McCourt & Page 1996).

Women receiving one-to-one care were far more satisfied with their care, and had a closer relationship with those midwives caring for them. In general the responses to pregnancy and birth were more positive. Many women in both groups felt it was important to have continuity of carer through the whole process including labour and birth; the majority of women who had received one-to-one care felt that it was very important (76%) or quite important (10%) (Beake et al 2001).

Especially if the savings from the reduced interventions are taken into account, one-to-one promises to be a very cost-effective pattern of care. Midwives who chose to practise in this way were highly satisfied with this approach to practice (Beake et al 2001, McCourt & Page 1996, Page et al 2001).

Edgware birth centre

The Edgware Birth Centre (EBC) is a stand-alone birth centre situated 5 miles from the nearest acute maternity unit. It was funded directly by the Department of Health to evaluate this model of stand-alone midwife-managed care. I have chosen this as an example of a successful development in part because it demonstrates the power that can be achieved by having a protected environment in which midwives are free to use and develop their skills. The birth centre takes self-selected low risk women, in contrast to one-to-one, which provides midwifery care to both low and high risk women for a complete geographical area. The emphasis is on creating a home-from-home environment that aims to develop holistic individualised care and construct a shared ethos based on a social model of care, to be truly responsive to the needs of child-bearing women and their families (Walker 2001, p. 8).

Women who use EBC give birth in a homely room, attended by a midwife and midwife assistant, who wear casual clothes (no uniform). Many, around 50%, use a birth pool. There is an emphasis on encouraging physiological birth, and the use of technology is avoided. Midwives in this situation need to be able to anticipate and manage problems while having confidence in 'normal' birth. The skills required are specified in the job description that was developed as a part of the risk management profile of the centre. There is an emphasis on skill sharing and professional development. Clinical guidelines are a part of clinical governance and are tested in day-to-day practice as part of a reflective critical incident analysis. These have been termed 'living guidelines' (Walker 2001, p. 11).

What are the outcomes? An independent external evaluation was carried out. Outcomes were compared with 'low risk' women who had their babies at main obstetric units. Analysis was by intention to treat. Women who booked to have their baby at the birth centre were significantly less likely to have induced labours, instrumental deliveries, epidurals and planned caesarean sections. Of those women booked to use the centre, 19% were transferred antenatally and a further 12% were transferred in labour, 85% of women breastfed, labours were an average 15% shorter, and used much less pharmaceutical analgesia. The cost analysis indicated that care was approximately 30% cheaper than for those delivering at local consultant-led units.

Evidence from qualitative data suggested that women were satisfied with their care even if they had to be transferred (98% of women said they would recommend it to their friends). What women valued from this model was the informal individualised approach, which extends to all parts of the care cycle. Evaluation of responses of midwives indicates an appreciation of the need to use all skills, and decision making. Although challenging and needing individual responsibility and decision-making skills, midwives did not find the work stressful; rather it boosted confidence and the realisation that there was 'a lot more to give' (Walker 2001).

The overall organisation and choice for midwives

It may not be feasible for all midwives to provide on-call services. In any maternity service the midwives should be able to choose their pattern of practice – that is, whether they carry a caseload or do shifts. Thus the overall organisation will require ward- or hospital-based midwives as well as midwives following women through the system of care (i.e. carrying a caseload). With the majority of women being cared for by caseload midwives, staffing in the hospital can be reduced to core or minimal staffing levels.

Evaluations of clinical outcomes associated with different patterns of care

Many innovations in the pattern of practice have been introduced in different parts of the world over the last 20 years. Some of these have been evaluated (Table 3.1). Evaluation of a complex change, such as a change in the pattern of practice of midwives, may be undertaken in a number of ways. Unlike trials of new drugs, or simple changes in treatment, which are appropriately evaluated by randomised controlled trials, a change in the organisation of care requires an appropriate evaluation for a change that is highly complex. The evaluation will need to take into account the responses of participants, including staff, any change in the use of economic resources and an assessment of safety and other clinical outcomes. It is particularly important in such evaluations that the innovation in the organisation of care (or the intervention) is thoroughly understood and described. Evaluation of a new organisation of care may entail different forms of research that may include different methods and methodology, for example social science and anthropological methodology. The collection, analysis and interpretation of quantitative and qualitative data are required. Such evaluations are complex and costly.

Table 3.1 Intervention rates associated with some different patterns of practice (where differences are shown these are all significant; studies differ in outcomes assessed)

Aim and type of study	[1] Home-like birth environment	[2] Continuous support	[3] Continuity of care	[4] One-to-one v. standard care	[5] One-to-one v. standard care	[6] Evaluation of caseload	[7] Partnership v. conventional care	[8] Randomised controlled trial
Differences in rates of analgesia/epidural	Lower	Lower	Lower	Lower	Lower	Lower	Lower	Lower
Differences in rates of augmented labour	Lower	Lower		Lower		Lower		Lower
Differences in rates of normal birth					Higher		Higher	
Differences in rates of operative delivery	Lower	Lower			Lower			
Differences in rates of caesarean section	Lower	Lower			Lower			
Differences in rates of intact perineum				Higher	Higher		Higher	
Differences in rates of reproductive tract trauma/episiotomy	Lower episiotomy rate/higher vaginal perineal tear rate	Lower in individual trials	Lower rates of episiotomy/ higher rates of tears	Lower	Lower			Lower
5 minute Apgar of less than 7		Lower						
Resuscitation of newborn			Lower					

[1] Cochrane review to assess the effects of care in a home-like birth environment on labour and birth involving outcomes (Hodnett ed 2002b)
[2] Cochrane review to assess the effects of continuous support during labour; 14 trials involving more than 5000 women (Hodnett 2002a)
[3] Cochrane review to assess continuity of care during pregnancy and childbirth and the puerperium with usual care by multiple caregivers (Hodnett 2002c)
[4] First cohort study to assess differences between one-to-one care (with a high level of continuity) and standard care (Page et al 1999)
[5] Second cohort study to assess differences between one-to-one midwifery and standard care (Page et al 2001)
[6] Evaluation of caseload midwifery (a high level of continuity) in comparison with traditional shared care (North Staffs Changing Childbirth Research Team 2000)
[7] A comparison of partnership caseload midwifery care with conventional team midwifery care (Benjamin et al 2001)
[8] Randomised controlled trial of midwifery care in a tertiary level obstetric service (Biro et al 2000)

One of the difficulties of such studies is that they evaluate a package of change, and it may be difficult to disentangle the important elements of the innovation. For example, even where a high level of continuity has been achieved and interventions are lower, we cannot say with certainty that this is because of the continuity. Actually, this may not be important; what is important is that a number of studies have shown that women see the relationship with a caregiver or small number of caregivers as important.

Understandably although regrettably some innovations have not been evaluated at all, and others have had more limited evaluations. In the evaluation of one-to-one midwifery referred to earlier (McCourt & Page 1996), all those aspects described have been evaluated at two separate times: first when the innovation was introduced, and then when the innovation had become a more standard part of the service. Any further discussion of methodology that is appropriate for the evaluation of new patterns of practice is outside of the scope of this chapter. The reader is advised to scrutinise Cochrane reviews for a synthesis (meta-analysis) of the outcomes of all current studies. It is apparent from evidence in these reviews that constant support in labour is effective (Hodnett 2002a) and this evidence has been accepted into policy at local and national level in a number of countries. Home-like settings are associated with lower rates of intrapartum analgesia/anaesthesia, augmented labour, operative delivery and greater satisfaction with care. Hodnett (2002b) warns that it may be the increased support rather than the surroundings that is important. The Cochrane review of continuity of care indicates an association with a lower rate of uptake of drugs for pain relief during labour, with newborns less likely to need resuscitation, and mothers less likely to have an episiotomy but more likely to have a vaginal or perineal tear (Hodnett 2002c).

Four more recent evaluations of innovations where there is a high degree of continuity of carer on a caseload basis, or from a team of midwives providing continuity from start to finish (not included in the Cochrane review) indicate that there is an association with lower levels of medical interventions, such as epidural (Benjamin et al 2001, Biro et al 2000, North Staffs Changing Childbirth Group 2000, Page et al 1996, 2001) and augmentation rates (Benjamin et al 2001, Biro et al 2000, North Staffs Changing Childbirth Group 2000), an increase in normal births (Benjamin et al 2001, Page et al 2001), an intact perineum (Benjamin et al 2001, Page et al 1996, 2001) and lower rates of episiotomy (Benjamin et al 2001, Biro et al 2000, Hodnett 2002a, b, c, Page et al 1996, 2001). In the second evaluation of one-to-one midwifery practice there was also a significant difference in the caesarean section rate, with a lower rate of assisted births (forceps and ventouse) and caesarean section associated with one-to-one midwifery practice (Beake et al 2001, Page et al 2001). All these studies showed that the new pattern was associated with a higher level of satisfaction amongst women.

In a team midwifery scheme where continuity of carer was not increased (and may even have decreased), although satisfaction was improved there were no apparent differences in clinical outcomes (Waldenstrom et al 2000). Many women favour the provision of continuity of carer through the whole process of care, including labour and birth. Where women have experienced continuity of carer they recognise it as an advantage and would want the same kind of care again (McCourt et al 2000). Qualitative research shows us why women appreciate continuity of carer. It is found to give women confidence in their midwives, and is seen as more sensitive and personal care. Continuity of carer transforms the experience of birth for women and for midwives. Those midwives who choose to practise in this way are intensely satisfied with the form of practice (Stevens & McCourt 2001). It has also been demonstrated that even radically different patterns of practice may be introduced into a traditional setting without any compromise in standards of care (McCourt & Page 1996).

Evaluations of midwifery-led care indicate that some are associated with a lower intervention rate and some are not. However, it seems that women who have received midwife-led care are more satisfied than those women who are receiving standard care, shared care or medical care (Waldenstrom et al 2000).

Freestanding birth centre care may also be associated with a lower rate of medical interventions, and intense satisfaction with care in both women and practising midwives (see the Edgware Birth Centre).

What evaluations (Callwood & Thomas 2001, North Staffs Changing Childbirth Group 2000) do show is that there is a marked difference between different services in intervention rates, including caesarean births, that is not accounted for by differences between the populations. This may be explained by the study of four different types of hospitals in Ontario, Canada with low caesarean section rates. The common characteristics of these four units included a strong belief in supporting normal birth and a commitment to providing one-to-one constant care in labour (known to affect intervention rates and psychological outcomes positively), as well as a number of other characteristics such as strong leadership and encouragement of learning and development (Caesarean Section Working Group of the Ontario Women's Health Council 2000). Again, it seems that both pattern of practice and culture of care may be an important part of effective care.

How to work in different patterns of practice

Working in one-to-one and continuity of caregiver schemes

Particularly for midwives who have worked only in standard care, or for students on their first experience of caseload practice, there are a number of things to be considered. First, in this pattern of practice you will be called on to provide skilled and knowledgeable care through all the periods of pregnancy and birth. Many midwives will feel the need to refresh skills in a particular area. You should talk to an experienced midwife, and look at your job description or requirements of practice carefully, thinking through areas in which you need development. A good orientation and support for the first weeks, plus an orientation manual, are very important for midwives starting out in this pattern of practice (Stevens & McCourt 2001). Having confidence and competence in these clinical skills will reduce the stress of starting out. But remember that one of the advantages of this form of practice is that you will learn very quickly.

You also need to think about time management. There are a number of patterns of on call and it is important to find one that suits you and your partners. You will need to work flexibly, but ensure that you keep enough time for personal life, family friends and rest and relaxation. Good administrative support is invaluable. Some times will be very busy, and some very quiet; it is important to use the quiet time for rest

and relaxation. Accessories that will allow organisation and enhance security include a filofax, a mobile phone, a security alarm and a good map. You will be required to travel for some of your time. It is important to have a good tour of your patch, and learn about one-way streets and parking, about safe and less safe areas and about weather patterns if in more remote or northerly areas. You need to think about how you might safeguard your personal security on the streets and in homes.

Relationships with women

Your skills will be integrated through your relationship with individual women and their families, making them central to the decision-making process and using evidence to inform decisions. This takes considerable experience and good interpersonal skills. You will wish to find out about the groups of people in your area; are there different racial or ethnic groups, and are there pockets of poverty? Although your care will be very important to the women and families in your practice you will need to recognise that you cannot sort out a long or complex background of difficulties, nor will you be able to ameliorate all social situations. Although you should seek to form a supportive relationship that may feel like friendship, it is important to ensure that there are boundaries around your life so you may meet your own needs for a healthy balanced life. Having your own network of support at home and at work is important.

Relationships with other staff

One of the rewards of working in a small practice is the possible camaraderie with your colleagues. These practices can be supportive, stimulating and fun. However, when there are severe tensions between members of the group it can be very difficult. Even if you have chosen your partners you may find difficulties in working together. It is important to talk through and agree values and practices as far as is possible, and to hold regular meetings (Stevens & McCourt 2001). Establishing a process of peer review that is both challenging but supportive is important. You will work with a number of other professionals in the health service. As in all relationships, a level of trust is crucial to effective working relationships. You may wish to take some assertiveness training because trust is often established not only because you are competent but also because you appear confident.

Constraints and how to handle them

When there are no choices

Many maternity services will not offer midwives a choice of patterns of practice and many midwives will not be free to move to find a maternity service of their choice. Some midwifery services will make good care very difficult to achieve; even if you can achieve good care it may take a lot out of you. When practising in less than ideal situations it is important to do the best you can, while recognising that there are some factors out of your control and accepting that your contribution is limited. It is important, though, not to give up completely. Work out your most important principles and how to put them into practice. For example, giving women choice and control when you meet them for the first time in active labour is not easy. But still you can make sure you spend even a little 'contracted' time in establishing a relationship, and in finding out about the woman's central values and preferences, even if this has to be done between contractions. Watching body language is more important than ever in this situation.

The politics

Everyone is a potential leader, not just those in management positions. Sometimes suggesting and helping to make a small change can make a big difference. Perhaps you could suggest, for example, moving the furniture in the birth room around so that it is easier for the woman to move. Or you might get furniture, such as rocking chairs and birth balls, in place. Often there is a manager or managers who will feel empowered knowing that midwives at the grass roots are seeking change. Do not be frightened to make suggestions. Enthusiasm amongst students and staff is infectious and adds more than can be imagined to the work situation. If you find problems be ready to describe them to the appropriate people, but be ready to propose a solution and if possible to contribute to it.

Doing the best you can

Few midwives practice in the perfect environment. Frustrations may arise in any pattern of practice. When they do it is important to be clear on what is the most important value to you, and that you know that you are doing no harm to those in your care. If circumstances lead you to believe that any situation is unsafe, it is a professional responsibility to seek help and to report the situation.

Conclusion

Midwives have the potential to make a big difference to the start of life for the family. This difference may be good or harmful. The pattern and culture of practice will affect the ability of midwives to give of their best. Careful consideration and development of the most effective, efficient and humane pattern of practice may be the most important part of health care.

REFERENCES

Anderson T 2000 Feeling safe enough to let go: the relationship between a woman and her midwife during the second stage of labour. In: Kirkham M (ed) The midwife–mother relationship. Macmillan, London, p 92–118

Ball J, Washbrook M 1996 Birthrate plus. A framework for workforce planning and decision making for midwifery services. Books for Midwives Press, Cheshire

Beake S, McCourt C, Page L 2001 Evaluation of one-to-one midwifery second cohort study. Hammersmith Hospitals NHS Trust/Thames Valley University, London

Benjamin Y, Walsh D, Toub N 2001 A comparison of partnership caseload midwifery care with conventional team midwifery care: labour and birth outcomes. Midwifery 17:234–240

Biro M, Waldenstrom U, Pannifex J H 2000 Team midwifery care in a tertiary level obstetric service: a randomized controlled trial. Birth 27:168–173

Brodie P 1997 Being with women: the experiences of Australian team midwives (thesis). University of Technology, Sydney

Caesarean Section Working Group of the Ontario Women's Health Council 2000 Attaining and maintaining best practices in the use of caesarean sections: an analysis of four Ontario hospitals. Ontario Women's Health Council, Ontario, p 5–81

Callwood A, Thomas J 2001 The national sentinal caesarean section audit. RCOG/Clinical Effectiveness Support Unit, London

Campbell A 1984 Moderated love: a theology of professional care. SPCK, London

Cronk M 2000 The midwife: a professional servant. In: Kirkham M (ed) The midwife–mother relationship. MacMillan, London, p 19–27

Davies J 2000 Being with women who are economically without. In: Kirkham M (ed) The midwife–mother relationship. MacMillan, London, p 120–141

DeVries R, Salvelson H B, Wiegers T A, Williams A S 2001 What (and why) do women want? The desires of women and the design of maternity care. In: Devries R B C, Teijlingen E R V, Wrede S (ed) Birth by design: pregnancy, maternity care, and midwifery in North America and Europe. Routledge, New York, p 243–266

DoH (Department of Health) 1993 Changing childbirth. The report of the Expert Maternity Group, vol 1 (the Cumberlege report). DOH, London

Edwards N 2000 Women planning homebirths: their own views on their relationships with midwives. In: Kirkham M (ed) The midwife–mother relationship. MacMillan, London, p 55–84

Farquhar M, Camilleri-Ferrante C, Todd C 2000 Continuity of care in maternity services: women's views of one team midwifery scheme. Midwifery 16:35–47

Freely M 1995 Team midwifery – a personal experience. In: Page L (ed) Effective group practice in midwifery: working with women. Blackwell Science, Oxford, p 3–11

Hodnett E 2002a Caregiver support for women during childbirth (Cochrane Review). In: The Cochrane Library. Issue 1. 2002. Update Software, Oxford

Hodnett E 2002b Home-like versus conventional institutional settings for birth (Cochrane Review). In: The Cochrane Library. Issue 1. 2002. Update Software, Oxford

Hodnett E 2002c Continuity of caregivers for care during pregnancy and childbirth (Cochrane Review). In: The Cochrane Library. Issue 1. 2002. Update Software, Oxford

House of Commons (Winterton report) 1992 Maternity services: the second report from the Health Committee session 1991–92. HMSO, London

Kirkham M 2000 The midwife–mother relationship. MacMillan, London

Kirkham M, Stapleton H 2001 Midwives support needs as childbirth changes. MIDIRS Midwifery Digest 11:157–163

Leap N 2000 The less we do, the more we give. In: Kirkham M (ed) The midwife–mother relationship. Macmillan, London, pp 1–17

McCourt C, Page L 1996 Report on the evaluation of one-to-one midwifery. Centre for Midwifery Practice, Thames Valley University, London

McCourt C, Hirst J, Page L A 2000 Dimensions and attributes of caring: women's perceptions. Churchill Livingstone, Edinburgh, p 269–287

North Staffordshire Changing Childbirth Research Team 2000 A randomised study of midwifery caseload and traditional 'shared care'. Midwifery 16:295–302

Olsen O 1997 Meta-analysis of the safety of home birth. Birth 24:4–13

Page L 1995 Effective group practice: working with women. Blackwell Science, Oxford

Page L 2000a Midwifery in Canada. International Midwifery 13:6–7

Page L 2000b Putting science and sensitivity into practice. In: Page L A (ed) The new midwifery: science and sensitivity in practice. Churchill Livingstone, Edinburgh, p 7–42

Page L 2001 The midwife's role in pregnancy and labour. In: Chamberlain G S P (ed) Turnbull's obstetrics. Churchill Livingstone, Edinburgh, p 473–486

Page L A, McCourt C, Beake S, Hewison J, Vail A 1999 Clinical interventions and outcomes of one-to-one midwifery practice. Journal of Public Health Medicine 21(3):243–248

Page L, Cooke P, Percival P 2000 Providing one-to-one practice and enjoying it. In: Page L A (ed) The new midwifery: science and sensitivity in practice. Churchill Livingstone, Edinburgh, p 123–140

Page L, Beake S, Vail A, McCourt C, Hewison J 2001 Clinical outcomes of one-to-one midwifery practice. British Journal of Midwifery 9:700–706

Pairman S 2000 Women-centred midwifery: partnerships or professional friendships. In: Kirkham M (ed) The midwife–mother relationship. Macmillan, London, p 207–225

Piercey J 1996 Report on the evaluation of one-to-one midwifery practice. Thames Valley University, London

Piercey J, Page L A, McCourt C 2001 Evaluation of one-to-one midwifery second cohort study/midwives responses. Hammersmith Hospitals NHS Trust/Thames Valley University, London, p 31–43

Sandall J 1997 Miwives' burnout and continuity of care. British Journal of Midwifery 5:106–111

Sandall J, Bourgeault I L, Meijer W J, Schueking B A 2001 Deciding who cares winners and losers in the late twentieth century. In: Devries R B C, Teijlingen E R V, Wrede S (ed) Birth by design: pregnancy, maternity care, and midwifery in North America and Europe. Routledge, New York, p 117–138

SOHHD (Scottish Office Home and Health Department) 1993 Provision of Maternity Services in Scotland. A policy review. HMSO, Edinburgh

Stevens T, McCourt C 2001 Midwives' responses. In: Beaks S, McCourt C, Page L (eds) Evaluation of one-to-one midwifery second cohort study. Hammersmith Hospitals NHS Trust/Thames Valley University, London, p 8–15

UKCC (United Kingdom Central Council) 1998 Midwives rules and code of conduct. UKCC, London, p 25

Waldenstrom U, Brown S, McLachlin H, Forster D, Brennecke S 2000 Does team midwife care increase satisfaction with antenatal, intrapartum and postpartum care? A randomized controlled trial. Birth 27:156–167

Walker J 2001 Edgware Birth Centre: what is the significance of this model of care? MIDIRS Midwifery Digest 11:8–12

Wilkins R 2000 Poor relations: the paucity of the professional paradigm. In: Kirkham M (ed) The midwife–mother relationship. Macmillan, London, p 28–52

4

Ethics in Midwifery

Nancy M. Riddick-Thomas

Modern midwifery involves many different practices and conflicts. The days of clinical practice being clear-cut, right or wrong are long gone. Increasingly uncertainties are growing, causing midwives to make decisions in the absence of robust evidence. There is a need to explore what it is about current practice that causes dilemmas. Changes in society over the last two decades have meant changes in health care provision. The publication of the patient's charter (DoH 1991) and more recently Your Guide to the NHS (DoH 2001) has raised public awareness to the choices available as well as raising people's expectations regarding involvement in care decisions.

This chapter aims to:

- raise awareness of ethical theories and their use in supporting clinical practice

- explore aspects of clinical practice that health professionals face on a daily basis

- clarify areas of potential conflict

- offer a degree of direction for further discussion or study.

Introduction

Beliefs and values are very personal. They are dependent on many things, not least an individual's background, society and personal views developed over time. Time for reflection to explore these issues is important. It is also essential for health professionals to be open and honest about practice dilemmas.

Another potential area of conflict is that of law. Law and ethics are often seen as complementary to one another, yet at times they are also seen to be placed on opposite sides of a coin. Any exploration of ethics should also be able to guide the reader to the areas of overlap or conflict. The study of ethics will provide the framework for exploration and aid resolution of dilemmas. However, it will not provide a quick fix, or an easy answer.

The area of ethics is complex, difficult and could be seen as off-putting by some. This need not be so. It should be used as a daily tool to support decision making and to enable rather than disable practice. If used like this it should be liberating and empowering. Being ethically aware is a step towards being an autonomous practitioner. It means taking responsibility, empowering others and facilitating professional growth and development.

When attempting to explore a new area, one of the initial problems is often the terminology used. Consider for a moment your first experiences within a clinical setting. The language used may have been familiar but the terminology was so new you may have felt lost. Ethics is the same; some of the terminology used is different and the words need greater explanation and understanding. Other parts of the terminology appear on the surface to be easier and more common place (Box 4.1). Even so, when asked to clarify or explain your understanding of these words, it is often not so easy.

What is found is there is more than one interpretation for a word. Different people may understand different things from the same words. So ethics is often about clarifying what people understand, think and feel in a given situation, often from what they say as much as what they do. Jones (2000, p. 8) has outlined ethics as 'the basic principles and concepts that guide human beings in thought and action'. The same could be said of philosophy, in that moral philosophy is often the foundation of modern ethical decision making and ethics itself is the application of philosophical principles to everyday situations. To understand this better there is a need to explore the theories surrounding ethics and their supportive philosophical frameworks.

Framework and theories

When first exploring the ethics of a situation it is helpful to have a framework with which to work. There are many ethical frameworks that could be adopted to use in clinical situations. Edwards (1996) advocates a four-level system based on the work of Melia (1989, pp. 6–7). Edwards believes that there are four levels of moral thinking that can help formulate arguments and discussions and ultimately assist in solving moral dilemmas (Box 4.2).

Such a framework can be used to help midwives work through situations that arise in daily practice. Take the case of Mary (Box 4.3). Using Edward's four

---

Box 4.2 Edward's levels of ethics

Level one	Judgements
Level two	Rules
Level three	Principles
Level four	Ethical theories

(After Edwards 1996).

Box 4.1 Terminology

• Informed consent	Information regarding options for care/treatment
• Rights	Justified claim to a demand
• Duty	A requirement to act in a certain manner
• Justice	Being treated fairly
• Best interests	Deciding on best course for an individual

Box 4.3 Case Scenario: Mary

Mary is 23 years old and is pregnant with her second child. She has requested that she have minimal interventions during the pregnancy and a natural birth, no intervention, no drugs and a quiet environment. Her previous pregnancy was complicated by raised blood pressure, which culminated in Mary having a caesarean section. Mary is adamant that nothing will go wrong this time. Her midwife is anxious to ensure safety of mother and fetus/child, while also building Mary's trust.

levels, the midwife supporting Mary during her pregnancy can work through what she should do. On talking to Mary and discovering her wishes for pregnancy and birth it is clear that she holds strong views about pregnancy and childbirth. It would be easy for the midwife to make an immediate *judgement* about both Mary and her reasons for wanting a low technology pregnancy and birth. During the course of the meeting between Mary and her midwife it would be important for the ground rules to be set and the midwife would have to outline the legal and moral *rules* that govern her practice. One such moral rule that would be vital is that of *truth telling*. In order for Mary and her midwife to build a trusting relationship that would be of benefit throughout the pregnancy it is important that honesty is established and both parties are truthful with each other. What the midwife has to acknowledge and promote in this relationship is the *principle* of *autonomy*. Principles are rather general, but autonomy is based on the understanding of respect for choices made by people.

The midwife needs to establish that what is being asked for is Mary's choice; it is important that this is an informed and rational request, one based on sound judgements and beliefs. This having been established, the midwife then has a duty to uphold that choice if she is to respect Mary's autonomy and earn her trust. (The issues of choice and informed consent will be explored more fully later in this text.) Providing this relationship continues to be founded on the above judgements, rules and principles then the midwife would be seen to be demonstrating the *ethical theory*. The midwife may be taking a position that she sees as her duty to care for Mary, acting in the best interests of both her and her unborn child. In moral philosophy this would be called a deontological stance, as outlined by Beauchamp & Childress (2001), and Thompson et al (2000).

It can be seen that in working with Mary a midwife would call on all four of Edward's levels. It would be useful to examine these levels in more detail.

Level one: judgements

Judgements are frequently made readily, based on information gained. Judgements may have no real foundation except the belief of the individual who made it. In this case scenario the midwife could have made a judgement about Mary before any real information had been gained. That judgement may have been based on past experiences of requests like Mary's that may not have been as well founded or as well thought through. We all make judgements every day; it can be helpful to reflect on past judgements and consider whether, in retrospect, they were well founded or based on personal bias or prejudice.

Throughout our daily lives we make judgements about each other, whether it is on the bus, in the supermarket or during a shift on a busy ward. What is important to remember is that it is an instant judgement that has been made, possibly biased, and it may not necessarily have been well thought through and based on all available evidence. How judgements are made is interesting. What informs a judgement is often linked to personal values and beliefs, society, as well as experiences of similar past events. All these and more shape the decision-making processes and to be aware of them is the first step to understanding yourself and your own moral values.

Level two: rules

Rules govern our daily lives. When looking at ethics, rules are what guide our practice and control our actions. Rules come in many forms and from many sources. Beauchamp & Childress (2001) outline different types of rules. These include *substantive rules* covering such things as privacy, truth telling or confidentiality, *authority rules* determined by those in power and enforced on a country or section of society, and *procedural rules* defining a set course of action or line to be followed. In the case scenario in Box 4.3 the midwife may have considered the rule of truth telling to be an important part of building Mary's trust.

Level three: principles

Principles are based on four main aspects that underpin general morality. Beauchamp & Childress (2001) have explained these in considerable detail. The first of these is *respect for autonomy*. This term has been used extensively over the last few years. The focus of health care has been around the professional's duty to respect individuals' autonomy and whenever possible to promote or enable them to exercise their autonomy. This is what the midwife will need to do if she is to help Mary have the type of pregnancy and birth the latter has requested. The second principle is *non-maleficence*, interpreted as avoiding harm. It could be said that most health care professionals would be trying to do this. Brown et al (1992) advised us that this principle is a strong one and as such should not be taken lightly. The midwife in the case scenario needs to establish that no harm is likely to occur from Mary's request and that it is an informed one based on facts and sound information. She could have harmed Mary by either not respecting her wishes and insisting she have interventions or not checking that Mary's information was sound.

The third principle is that of *beneficence* – doing good or balancing the benefits against the harms in a given situation (Beauchamp & Childress 2001). This entails positive action on one person's part to benefit another person. The midwife has not only to acknowledge Mary's right to non-intervention, but also to ensure autonomy is preserved by actively promoting Mary's interests, supporting her chosen type of care. This can be difficult for health professionals when they may believe a course of action is not in a client's best interests. A large part of the midwife's role in such situations will be to ensure appropriate, timely and up to date information and advice is available.

The fourth principle, *justice*, means to be treated fairly. In many instances this is all people want. It is important that health care professionals are seen to be acting fairly and treating all clients as equals. Within the case scenario, fair play would mean Mary being listened to, being supported in her choice of care and being treated as an equal in any decision-making process. It can be seen that the practice and thought processes outlined by the case scenario can encompass all four of the principles of level three. This may not always be the case.

Level four: ethical theories

Theories are taken to mean the two main ethical theories of utilitarianism and deontology. Many texts outline these two theories as they are the most widely used and form the foundation of much ethical decision making (Beauchamp & Childress 2001, Jones 2000, Thompson et al 2000).

Utilitarian theory. Utilitarian theory has been widely adapted over the years. It is based on the idea of balancing the consequences of following certain actions or rules. This can be thought of as a very large pair of scales, with the benefits of an action on one side and the harm or consequences of taking the

action on the other. There is a need to tip the scales in favour of the benefits over the possible harms that could occur. This theory stems from the work of Jeremy Bentham and later John Stuart Mill in the nineteenth century (Raphael 1989). They believed that pleasure was more desirable than pain and that anything that increased pleasure for the majority of people must be a morally right action. Practically this theory is attractive in that it can aid decision making for the masses; an action is good if it provides benefits for the many. Scarce resources within the NHS have meant that very difficult decisions have to be made. Determination of where the greatest good lies and how to do the least harm in any given situation have become important. Such decision making may be made easier by applying ethical theories (Tschudin 1994).

Many aspects of midwifery care have been organised on utilitarian principles. Antenatal clinics allow many women to be seen by skilled professionals under one roof. Many screening tests are offered to all irrespective of need or individual assessment, and team midwifery often means what fits with the midwives rather than with individual women (Flint 1993, p. 59). There may be times when such practices are appropriate; for example for some safety issues everyone should follow set procedures to ensure standards of care are maintained. When you are next called on to make a decision ask yourself how the balance of benefits and harms would weigh on scales.

Deontology. Deontology is the second of these theories. Jones (2000) tells us this term is from the Greek word 'deon' meaning duty. As health professionals you would all say you have a duty towards your clients/patients. But there is a need to explore where else your duty lies. This list could be quite long (Box 4.4).

The list could be longer if you added personal duties (i.e. family, friends, etc.). Recognising that you have a duty of care is one thing, balancing the competing demands of those duties is quite another. Conflicting duties can cause dilemmas in deciding the best course of action. It is often difficult to prioritise such duties, but some prioritisation needs to occur to enable decision making to be meaningful. The midwife looking after Mary has a duty to both Mary and her baby, she has a duty to her profession via the NMC and she has a duty to her employer.

> **Box 4.4** Duty of care to...
>
> - Self
> - Colleagues
> - Clients/patients
> - Relatives
> - Fetus/baby
> - Employer
> - Profession (NMC)

There are no easy answers here. This work is based on that of Immanuel Kant (Hollis 1985) and there have been a number of interpretations of his writings over time (Edwards 1996). Kant emphasised that to do one's duty is the most important thing, irrespective of any consequences that carrying out this duty may produce.

This is where there is seen a difference between utilitarianism and deontology. In following a utilitarian theory it would be essential to consider the consequences and choose the best course of action – that is, the one that produces the best outcome for the most people. Following a deontological approach on the other hand would require the person to carry out something that is a duty irrespective of any consequences. This would be very hard in practice for most people as it suggests certainties of actions, and an attitude of irrelevance towards consequences of actions. Life is often more complicated, however, and as such many other factors need to be considered.

Another aspect of Kant's work was the emphasis on *respect for persons*. To this end he believed that people are individual and should be treated with respect, not merely as a means to an end. Beauchamp & Childress (2001) believe that if an action necessitates treating someone in this way then it is the action that is wrong. Respect for persons is important within maternity care, as was seen in the case situation in Box 4.3. In order for the midwife to build a relationship of trust she had to show respect for Mary's wishes, reinforcing the fact that Mary was respected as an individual.

Having outlined the levels of decision making (Edwards 1996), it is important that we now explore some other influences on the midwife's role. There are aspects that are either part of or develop from the basic moral frameworks outlined above. These are aspects of ethics that are seen daily in professional life, but they could still cause problems, dilemmas or conflicts in one form or another.

Consent/information giving

Informed consent is a relatively recent term; indeed, Beauchamp & Childress (2001, p. 77) suggest that it was not until the mid 1970s that the term was explored in any real detail. It has been claimed that within ethics informed consent means 'giving patients and clients as much information as they need' (Jones 2000, p. 104). This is traditionally what ethical consent is held to be. This principle is very different, however, to the legal standpoint in that 'consent' within legal frameworks is taken to be based on the reasonable person standard, or the 'Bolam' test (Dimond 1994, p. 49). Consent within ethics means that the client has listened, understood and agreed to the procedure or treatment being proposed. For many reasons this may not be realistic. Johnstone (1989, p. 181) outlines six reasons why consent may not be realistic in everyday clinical practice. These are:

- lack of time
- clients will forget
- most clients do not want to know
- most clients would not understand
- it could be harmful if clients refused treatment based on information given
- considering all these, gaining informed consent is impracticable.

These reasons seem plausible; there will always be situations where a client has said 'what do you think?' or you find the client has asked two or three of your colleagues for the same information after you have spent 10 minutes explaining things. One aspect not on Johnstone's list that is also important is that of the professional's knowledge base. To be able to provide information and then gain a valid consent the professional attempting to gain that consent has to be at least as knowledgeable as the client from whom consent is being sought. With increasing use of the World Wide Web this is becoming an almost impossible task. Health professionals have a duty to keep up to date and be able to inform their clients to the best of their ability (NMC 2002, point 6, UKCC 1998).

Consider once again the case scenario in Box 4.3. There will be many times during Mary's pregnancy when consent may be required. To ensure that the consent given is valid the midwife will have to hold wide-ranging discussions on such things as antenatal screening tests, ultrasound scanning, birth choices and birth interventions such as pain relief, positions for birth and active management of the third stage of labour. The midwife must also be sure that Mary understands the options and alternatives open to her. Mary has asked for minimal interventions, so without being judgmental or coercive the midwife will have to explore Mary's views and recommend what she believes is 'best practice'. Respecting a person's right to exercise choice and decision making can be difficult. What if Mary was requesting something that did not meet the standard of best practice? How would the midwife be expected to react then? The Midwives rules and code of practice (UKCC 1998) can be used in such a situation to inform and enable the midwife to act in the woman's best interests. The midwife would have backup support systems from both her supervisor of midwives (see Ch. 51) and her immediate line manager.

Enabling informed consent to occur and empowering women to decide what is best for them are fundamental parts of 'respect for autonomy' (Brown et al 1992). When attempting to support the midwife in such situations there is an apparent need to fall back on the legal definition of a 'reasonable person'. However, Brown et al (1992) have explored this issue and advise caution in following a reasonable person standard. They argue that if all reasonable people would choose one procedure but Mary chooses another then Mary could be seen as being unreasonable because she is the only one to choose the first type of procedure. It may be easier and possibly more desirable for some in today's litigation-conscious health service to abide by a legal definition of competence that Maclean (2001, p. 46) outlines as an ability to 'comprehend, retain and use information and weigh it in the balance'. (See also NMC 2002, section 3.)

For a health professional it can be very difficult to respect a person's autonomy when current evidence tells you their request is not best practice. At times the courts have been called on to decide; for example in the case of Re S (Savage 1998) both mother and fetus's lives were at risk, yet the mother refused treatment that could have saved the fetus and lessened the risk of morbidity or mortality for herself. These cases are rare, but they can damage the client–professional relationship.

There is potential, in the case scenario in Box 4.3, for Mary's wishes to conflict with the midwife's professional judgement. The fact that Mary had previously suffered raised blood pressure could suggest that she is at risk of developing complications in this pregnancy. The midwife may choose to play down these potential risks, however, preferring to build a relationship of trust and respect for Mary's autonomy. Once trust is present then mutual respect for each person's views will grow, and with that can develop a sharing of viewpoints and exchange of information around the risks and benefits of any chosen course of action.

Caring

The public sees those who work in the health services as belonging to the caring profession. It is usually accepted that health professionals care for their clients and as such would always have their best interests in mind. But caring can mean different things to different people. There is a need to be clear on what those involved in providing care understand by the term *caring*.

It is suggested that doctors and nurses/midwives may have different ideas on what constitutes caring (Brown et al 1992). Doctors have traditionally followed the medical model of care. This means that principles of beneficence and paternalism are more likely to be followed by doctors in preference to the principle of autonomy, which is more frequently associated with nurses' and midwives' style of care (Brown et al 1992).

It might be argued that paternalism, or making decisions on behalf of others, *is* caring for clients because health professionals' education and training enables them to 'know best' (Brown et al 1992, p. 57). This does not, however, give health professionals the right to override someone's views and wishes. In the case of Mary, caring for her means making decisions in partnership with her, not exerting pressure to coerce her into agreeing to have interventions in labour that she really does not want, because both midwives and doctors believe them to be in her or the baby's best interests.

When advocating one course of action over another the midwife has to be clear why one particular option is best for any individual and be prepared to step back if it is not the chosen type of care. Stepping back does not mean opting out or abdicating responsibility, as midwives still have an ethical and legal duty to care for their clients (UKCC 1998). It is, rather, having the ability to recognise when a client has made an informed and rational decision. It also has to be remembered that the midwife, if put into the position of not agreeing with a course of action chosen by a client, has the support and guidance of the supervisor of midwives (Kirkham & Stapleton 2000, UKCC 1998).

Autonomy is an individual's right to make choices on their own behalf. Being able to exercise autonomy is seen as having the ability to understand, reason, evaluate options and make decisions for yourself (Brown et al 1992). For health professionals to enable or promote a client's autonomy there is a need to support, inform and accept that person's views and value systems, irrespective of whether they differ from their own. This is where decision making becomes difficult. It is very difficult to stand by and watch someone make what you feel is a wrong decision, and even more difficult to support someone through a course of action when you feel it is fundamentally wrong.

As mentioned earlier there have been situations where the legal system has been brought in to decide the best course of action (Dimond 1994). Supporting an individual's decision is respecting their autonomy; it is also the start to a trusting relationship – a partnership where both sides should feel free to voice their views and beliefs knowing they will be listened to and supported. Within such relationships a client will know that when a professional speaks against a course of action it is for sound and justified reasons and not something that was done lightly.

Empowerment and advocacy

It has already been seen that an important part of the midwife's role is supporting women and enabling them to exercise their autonomy. This is seen as empowerment. This term is difficult to find in many ethical textbooks and a dictionary definition is, 'to give power' and 'authorise' (Sykes 1976, p. 339). Power is often a perception of another's influence over someone or something. It has also been said that knowledge is

power (Collins 1988, p. 223). As health professionals, midwives are perceived as being knowledgeable in the subject of midwifery and related health issues. It is understandable then that many of their clients would see them as powerful people, having influence over them and their pregnancies.

Whether power is real or perceived is irrelevant; the fact that someone *feels* less powerful than someone else means that any relationship that develops is unequal. Those with less power (real or perceived) will always react differently and there is the very real risk of coercion and latterly paternalism creeping into a relationship. Clients may be heard to say 'what would you do?' or 'you decide; I don't know what to do'. Handled properly these are opportunities to inform, educate and empower clients to act autonomously. Handled poorly there could be a potential area of conflict where the professional overrides autonomy and paternalism creeps into the provision of care.

Being able to empower others to act and decide for themselves is what midwifery should be about. A large part of a midwife's role is education and support (UKCC 1998). This role is going to become far more important in the coming years as more emphasis is placed on public health and health promotion (DoH 1992a, 1997, Welsh Office 1998).

When faced with clients who, despite all information, support and encouragement, are still reluctant to act or speak up for themselves, many midwives are finding they need to take on an advocacy role on their behalf. Advocacy is seen as speaking out on another's behalf (Gates 1994). There is, again, a fine dividing line between advocacy and paternalism. Put simplistically, paternalism is acting on another's behalf whereas advocacy is speaking out on another's behalf.

Johnstone (1989) has examined the notion of advocacy and suggests it to be useful in situations where clients have been unable to make their own choices. When taking on the role of advocate there is a need to be clear on a number of points. Acting as an advocate can be difficult and involves putting personal views or values aside. Advocacy means speaking out for someone's rights. Within the scenario in Box 4.3 Mary's requests were for minimal interventions in her pregnancy; if this is seen as a right then in such cases there is usually a corresponding duty on someone to provide care in accordance with that right. In Mary's case this would be both the midwife and hospital obstetric team.

However, speaking out on someone's behalf does not mean speaking up for what you think is best. Gates (1994) believes it means speaking up for what that person wants to happen. For this to occur the person speaking out has to know what is wanted and not just speak for what they think is in someone's best interests. It can be difficult to determine what is in someone's best interests. You must know either that person well enough to know what they would want or be sure that what the person wants to happen is a rational decision made following full and clear discussion of all alternatives.

Choices

Having explored informed consent and caring, we find that much of what has been said concerns the area of choices (see Ch. 3). Choices and decisions are made every day, most often without us thinking about them. Thompson et al (2000) suggest that life events often influence how we make decisions and also how we react to them. This is often true in our professional lives also, with past experience playing a large part in our decision-making processes.

How decisions are made has been the focus of many books and studies. There are equally as many models to assist in this process. Thompson et al (2000, pp. 272–273) outline the 'problem-solving approach' as well as the 'nursing process model', Walsh (2001, p. 498) uses a model adapted from Thompson & Thompson (1985) called the 'bioethical decision-making model'. These are just a few from many. Whatever model is used, the important things are to:

- Be clear what the problem or decision is. This may take some time to sort out. There is a need to discuss the issues with a wide range of people.
- Collect all relevant information. This may mean talking to many people to gain an insight into the facts of a situation.
- Weigh up the benefits or harms of a situation. Here it may help to call on the principles of beneficence and non-maleficence: trying to do good while avoiding harm.

Only when such things have been done can a decision be made on the best course of action in any situation. Tschudin (1994) suggests that you may even ask yourself if you are the right person to be making such decisions. You can only decide that when you have all the facts.

Having considered as many aspects as possible, discussing your views with others involved with the situation may also help. This not only provides an alternative viewpoint, it also aids your reflective processes (John 1996) and ensures that you consider views that may be opposite to your own.

Collaborative relationships

Within any decision-making process there is a need to work with others, to collaborate in attempting to come to the right decision. There have been many calls for health professionals to work together (Audit Commission 1997); such calls are now also being extended to public health and social care (Welsh Office 1998).

For any partnership to work there is a need to build a trusting relationship. Mutual trust and respect for each other's views and practices is important. For some there is a need to break through the power barrier. According to Brown et al (1992) working practices have historically been built on power and coercion.

Trust and truthfulness are fundamental aspects of the work of any health professional. Within ethics these are seen as virtues to be commended in a person (Beauchamp & Childress 2001). When someone is trusted it is believed that the person will act in a proper manner and make decisions for the right reasons. In the case scenario in Box 4.3, it was vital that the midwife built up trust between Mary and herself for their relationship to work. Being truthful was an important part of the trusting relationship. Other virtues, such as honesty and reliability, sometimes go alongside these. Mary has to be able to trust her midwife and believe that everything that happens is open for discussion and negotiation. It takes time and a willingness to work together to build such relationships, but care should be taken as such relationships can also be broken down in seconds. Professional relationships are just as important as those we develop with clients. To be able to work together there is a need to understand the other profession's values and codes. Thompson et al (2000) have outlined a number of codes and declarations that are seen as influencing practice. Of particular interest would be the International code of medical ethics (Thompson et al 2000, p. 340), and the

International code of ethics for midwives (Charity & Ord 2000, p. 92, Thompson et al 2000, p. 345).

The International code of medical ethics outlines the duties of physicians in general, to the sick and to each other, while the International code of ethics for midwives talks about midwives' relationships, midwifery practice, responsibilities of midwives and the advancement of knowledge and practice. It can be seen that both concern the scope and practice of its practitioner, while the midwifery code also called for advancement of knowledge. Both the medical and midwifery professions would benefit from examining, sharing and in part adopting each other's codes and values. If more sharing were to take place, a new collaborative model of supportive health care may emerge – one that places the client at the centre and provides the type of care that respects rights, promotes autonomy and protects the vulnerable. In the mean time, ways of working together, promoting mutual respect and understanding need to be developed.

Law and ethics

The position of law, ethics and reproductive health has been widely explored (Callahan 1995; Dimond 1994; Mason & McCall Smith 2000). There are times when these seem to work together to support each other and when calling on one may clarify the position of the other. There are also times when there appears a great divide between the two and no middle ground can be found. In relation to informed consent, within law this is taken to mean the reasonable person standard, or Bolam test (Dimond 1994). This means a person should be given as much information as any reasonable person could be expected to understand. In ethics, informed consent means 'full information before treatment' (Johnstone 1989); this is taken to mean that a person should be given as much information as they may require to make a decision. Johnstone (1989) goes on to highlight that there are some practical reasons why gaining informed consent from clients could prove difficult, lack of time being one important factor in the information-giving process.

To examine these issues more closely there is a need to look towards modern society. Many of the modern laws are developed from and stand firmly in the foundations of society (Mason & McCall Smith 2000). The values and practices of society often inform the development of laws, although Mason & McCall Smith (2000) suggest that the laws take such a considerable time to change, and that the health care professions often are left unsure of their legal position.

A real dilemma for maternity service staff is that of consent for caesarean sections. A pregnant woman cannot legally be forced to have a caesarean section for a risk to the fetus because she is normally deemed as competent and the fetus has no rights in law until it is born. In trying to save the life of a fetus, therefore, health professionals are constrained by the law that protects its mother (Dimond 1994). This may sound clear cut, but it is an uncomfortable position for those responsible for the care of a woman who refused the intervention. While accepting the law, one's personal code of ethics may be saying it is wrong to sit back and let a fetus die.

It may be seen that in being supported by the law you may also be constrained by it. Fear of litigation appears to be a guiding principle of modern practice. Risk management and clinical governance are high on most health service agendas. The underlying reason for the development of these within clinical practice has been improvement in practices and the establishment of common standards. It is important that midwives also become involved in these initiatives if collaboration and cooperation between disciplines are to be promoted.

Research

Any examination of ethics would not be complete without also looking into the ethical implications of research in the maternity services. Robson (1997, p. 470) has outlined the British Psychological Society's research involving human participants, while Cormack (2000) contains a chapter by Hazel McHaffie that uses two case scenarios to emphasise the issues to be considered. Whichever approach is taken there are some common aspects that most authors emphasise. These can be summarised as the 'five Cs' (Box 4.5).

Caring. Any research that is undertaken should be performed in a caring manner. Those who are subjects of research should be able to expect the highest standards of care and their care would not be adversely affected if they chose not to participate.

Consent. This has to be gained prior to any research being undertaken. Those involved in research should

---

Box 4.5 'Five Cs' of ethical research

1. Caring
2. Consent
3. Confidentiality
4. Codes
5. Committees

Box 4.6 Ten questions to ask

1. What is the scientific background of the research?
2. What are the qualifications of the person/s leading the project?
3. Are there any circumstances that could cause bias for a researcher?
4. Is there any foreseeable effect on health?
5. If any hazards or discomforts exist, are there plans to accommodate them?
6. How is consent gained? Is it clear and in writing?
7. How are confidentiality and anonymity assured for all subjects?
8. Is there an information sheet for subjects to read?
9. Have subjects been given the opportunity of opting out?
10. Are there contact details if staff or subjects require more information or are concerned regarding any aspect of the research?

(Adapted from DoH 1992b.)

---

know what the research is about, what it entails and the risks, benefits and alternatives. Robson (1997) recommends that the subjects must also be clear that they should be able to retain the ability to opt out of the research should they change their minds.

Confidentiality. All research should maintain confidentiality of its subjects. Taking part in research should not put any individual under the spotlight, or highlighting the person in any way. If there were any need to disclose information Cormack (2000) advises that permission would have to be sought in advance of any disclosure occurring.

Codes. These are guidelines for practice. They make recommendations about how practice should be governed in certain situations. There are ethical codes related to research on human subjects. The Department of Health issues advice on these (DoH 1992b, p. 20); in particular they highlighted the code of practice on the use of fetuses and fetal material in research and treatment, and the World Medical Association Declaration of Helsinki (Thompson et al 2000, p. 340).

Committees. There are statutory committees set up to monitor and control research involving human subjects within health care. These are called the Local Research Ethics Committees (LREC), as outlined in the above DoH report (DoH 1992b). Since the publication of this all health authorities have a duty to establish such a committee to review, monitor and control the research carried out within their areas. Any health research carried out must be submitted to this committee within the area it is to be carried out. If the research covered more than three health authority areas a 'Multi-centred Research Ethics Committee' (MREC) should be consulted (for details see the website www.corec.org.uk).

The fundamental principle when considering whether research is ethical is that of protection of the vulnerable; this may be the staff, clients or the researchers themselves (Cormack 2000). Although advancement of knowledge is important, it should not be made at the cost of compromising any one group of society. It is not only those involved in carrying out research who should be aware of the research protocols but also those involved in it and those who may simply be working within the same clinical area. To this end, it can be helpful to ask the very simple questions given in Box 4.6.

Current ethical issues

When studying ethics you become aware of so many aspects of life that have ethical implications that can and do make working within the maternity services challenging. The media, in their many forms, play an important role in today's society and often force us to become ethically aware of issues we may not have particularly thought about, or may not have become 'public' until they became headline news.

At times like this it is to professionals that clients turn for answers to their many questions. This has been seen on a number of occasions in the last few years. Diane Blood (Mason 1998) became headline news when she wanted artificial insemination by her dead husband's sperm. The Siamese twins from Malta sparked a national debate over whether they should be separated (Bennett 2000). The investigation into the Bristol heart babies (Maisey 2000) also led to the organ retention national inquiry. This last case in particular saw midwives manning telephone help-lines to offer counselling to bereaved parents, in some cases many years after the events.

Such events can be very distressing for any health professional involved. Having a structured framework to work through the issues can help. But having open and meaningful discussions with colleagues is vital if a deeper understanding of the situation is to be gained. Such things as rights of individuals, protection of the vulnerable, duty of care and where the best interests lie should be explored openly and safely away from the client's bedside (Dimond 1993). That is not to say that clients should not be involved, but the moment of crisis may not be the best time to explore sensitive issues, and sometimes a client representative may be better placed to speak out in a time of distress.

Conclusion

The area of ethics is growing and the need for health professionals to become more aware of the issues involved is escalating. This chapter has raised the possibility of using a framework (Edwards 1996) to organise your thoughts and decision-making processes.

A starting point must be the clarification of personal values, beliefs and moral principles. Without this it will be difficult to move forward and assist others with their problems and dilemmas. Many things, family, friends, society and professional life (Jones 2000) will have shaped your individual values and beliefs. By examining and reflecting on these you will be able to acknowledge any biases you may hold and start to work through them. Reflection skills have become important in modern professional life (UKCC 2001) as a means of critically reviewing events and learning from them.

Moving forward may not be easy, but it is important if care is to improve and standards are to be maintained. Many reports in recent years have recommended that the midwifery profession include its client group in decision making. Pregnant women should have an increased number of choices, they should have more control over events and midwives should be providing them with continuity of care (DoH 1993). But in providing women with these things midwives are also having to confront the fact that women need more information. The quality of information giving is dependent, in part, on midwives' knowledge base. Midwives must also ensure that once women have the options for care the choices they make are informed and are based on sound research-based evidence (Price 2001, RCM 2000).

Another aspect of moving forward is that of collaborative care. There have been many calls for health professionals to work more closely together (Audit Commission 1997; UKCC 1998). To work together means to resolve a number of differences between professions. Doctors and midwives might have different starting points, but this should not mean that a middle ground cannot be found. Sharing codes of practice and developing a joint code may be the first step towards closer relationships.

Studying ethics will raise many questions, some of which will not lend themselves to satisfactory answers. Although that is frustrating, sharing of dilemmas and gaining a different viewpoint on it may help. Multidisciplinary case conferences, seminars and study sessions could be one way forward. Medical, midwifery, health visiting and social work professionals are just some of those whose viewpoints could be included to broaden the discussion and add to the overall quality of care provided.

Midwives may find their PREP profile (UKCC 2001) provides a tool to reflect upon many private dilemmas and conflicts. Within the profile there is an opportunity to address a number of ethical questions. Such questions could be: 'who has rights in a situation?', 'was there a duty of care?', 'what was in the client's best interests?', and 'how can one balance the good of one action against any possible harm it could cause?'. These may help you explore the issues and organise your thoughts in preparation for the next time that you are faced with a similar issue.

REFERENCES

Audit Commission 1997 First class delivery: improving maternity services in England and Wales. Audit Commission, London

Beauchamp T L, Childress J F 2001 Principles of biomedical ethics, 5th edn. Oxford University Press, Oxford

Bennett J 2000 Siamese twins: both lives must be equally respected. British Journal of Nursing 9(17):1122

Brown J M, Kitson A L, McKnight T J 1992 Challenges in caring. Chapman & Hall, London

Callahan J C 1995 Reproduction ethics and the law: feminist perspectives. Indiana University Press, Bloomington

CESDI (Confidential Enquiry into Stillbirths and Deaths in Infancy) 1999 Confidential Enquiry into Stillbirths and Deaths in Infancy annual report. University Hospital of Wales, Cardiff

Charity J, Ord B 2000 Ethical dilemmas in midwifery practice. In: Fraser D (ed) Professional studies for midwifery practice. Churchill Livingstone, Edinburgh, p 92

Collins 1988 Dictionary of quotations. Collins, London, p 223

Cormack D 2000 The research process in nursing, 4th edn. Blackwell Science, Oxford

Dimond B 1993 Patients' rights, responsibilities and the nurse. Quay Publishing, Lancaster

Dimond B 1994 The legal aspects of midwifery. Books for Midwives, Hale, Cheshire

DoH (Department of Health) 1991 The patient's charter. HMSO, London

DoH (Department of Health) 1992a Health of the nation. HMSO, London

DoH (Department of Health) 1992b Local Research Ethics Committees. HMSO, London, p 2

DoH (Department of Health) 1993 Changing childbirth: report of the Expert Maternity Group. HMSO, London

DoH (Department of Health) 1997 The new NHS: modern dependable. HMSO, London

DoH (Department of Health) 2001 Your guide to the NHS. HMSO, London

Edwards S D 1996 Nursing ethics a principle based approach. Macmillan, Basingstoke, Hants

Flint C 1993 Midwifery teams and caseloads. Butterworth Heinemann, Oxford, p 59

Gates B 1994 Advocacy: a nurses guide. Scutari Press, London

Hollis M 1985 Invitation to philosophy. Blackwell Sciences, Oxford

John C 1996 The benefits of a reflective model of nursing. Nursing Times 92(27):39–41

Johnstone M-J 1989 Bio ethics a nursing perspective. Baillière Tindall, London

Jones S 2000 Ethics in midwifery, 2nd edn. Mosby, New York

Kirkham M, Stapleton H 2000 Midwives support needs as childbirth changes. Journal of Advanced Nursing 32(2):465–472

Maclean A 2001 Briefcase on medical law. Cavendish, London, p 46

Maisey M 2000 I do have faith in nurses' professional judgement. Nursing Standard 14 (32):29

Mason J K 1998 Medico-legal aspects of reproduction and parenthood, 2nd edn. Ash Gate, Dartmouth

Mason J K, McCall Smith R A 2000 Law and medical ethics. Butterworth, London

Melia K 1989 Everyday nursing ethics. Macmillan, London, p 6–7

NMC (Nursing and Midwifery Council) 2002 Code of professional conduct. NMC, London

Price S 2001 Using the MIDIRS informed choice leaflets in clinical practice. MIDIRS Midwifery Digest 11(2):261–263

Raphael D D 1989 Moral philosophy. Oxford University Press, Oxford

RCM (Royal College of Midiowes) 2000. Vision 2000. RCM, London

Robson C 1997 Real world research. Blackwell Science, Oxford

Savage W 1998 The right to choose. Nursing Standard May 2–26:12(35)14

Sykes J B 1976 The concise Oxford dictionary. Oxford University Press, Oxford, p 339

Thompson I E, Melia K M, Boyd K M 2000 Nursing ethics, 4th edn. Churchill Livingstone, London

Thompson J E, Thompson H O 1985 Bioethical decision making for nurses. Appleton Century-Crofts, Norwalk

Tschudin V 1994 Deciding ethically: a practical approach to nursing challenges. Baillière Tindall, London

Walsh L V 2001 Midwifery community-based care during the childbearing year. Harcourt, London, p 498

Welsh Office 1998 Better health better Wales. Welsh Office, Cardiff

UKCC (United Kingdom Central Council for Nursing, Midwifery and Health Visiting) 1998 Midwives rules and code of practice. UKCC, London

UKCC (United Kingdom Central Council for Nursing, Midwifery and Health Visiting) 2001 The PREP handbook. UKCC, London

FURTHER READING

Frith L 1996 Ethics and midwifery: issues in contemporary practice. Butterworth Heinemann, Oxford

An interesting book focussing on a variety of aspects related to midwifery practice. Clearly discusses midwifery issues and relates to the ethical theories that underpin them. This is an easy book to read and would be useful as a supportive text for midwifery students

Beauchamp T L, Childress J F 2001 Principles of biomedical ethics, 5th edn. Oxford University Press, Oxford

An ethical theories book that most readers will find useful to dip into. Not a book for bedtime reading, rather a text that is essential to support any enquiry into ethics. It is nicely linked to health care and uses case studies to apply the theories to clinical practice

Jones S 2000 Ethics in midwifery, 2nd edn. Mosby, London

A good basic introduction to ethics in the midwifery setting. Easy to read and compact enough to carry around. Divided into two sections this book firstly outlines the main theory standpoints and uses a case study approach in the second section to lead the reader through the process of ethical enquiry and decision making.

Thompson I E, Melia K M, Boyd K M 2000 Nursing ethics, 4th edn. Churchill Livingstone, London

A comprehensive text written from a nursing perspective but has many good aspects that the student midwife will find useful. Easy to read and navigate, it is a good reference text, which is well referenced.

5

Evidence-Based Practice

Rosemary Mander

When she provides care during childbearing, the midwife is able to do so only by virtue of her expert knowledge. It is this knowledge that distinguishes her from the multitude of people who offer their opinions to the childbearing woman and her family. The midwife's unique knowledge that, in turn, determines her practice, may be based on or developed from a number of sources. Traditionally, the midwife has drawn on her own personal experience of childbearing. In more recent times, the midwife's occupational experience has assumed greater significance. Precedent has been quoted as having been an important influence (Thomson A 2000) and this may have been enforced by those in authority, such as senior midwives or even medical personnel. Another factor in influencing midwifery practice has been ritual (Rodgers 2000). It is only relatively recently that research, and more recently still evidence, has been required as the basis of midwifery practice.

This chapter aims to:

- examine the meaning of the term 'research'

- introduce the concepts underpinning research

- consider the research basis of midwifery

- encourage critical reading of research

- indicate the steps necessary prior to the utilisation of research in practice.

Research

Although research may carry a range of implications, a dictionary definition is useful: 'systematic investigation towards increasing the sum of knowledge'
(Macdonald 1981, p. 1148)

Clearly, research is about asking questions, but not in a casual or haphazard way. Systematic or organised questioning is crucial to research. Thus planning, in the form of what may be known as the 'research process', underpins research activity. The purpose of this activity is also encompassed in the above definition, in that research aims to improve knowledge by increasing it. In caring situations, such knowledge is intended to be utilised in order to ensure more effective care.

Evidence

Relatively recently the term 'evidence' has been introduced to refer to a particular form of research. This is what has been referred to by Chalmers as 'strong research' (1993, p. 3). The introduction of the need for 'evidence' was initiated by the observations made by Cochrane (1972). He identified the lack of scientific rigour in medical clinical decision making, and went on to single out obstetricians for merciless criticism because of their want of such rigour. A group of obstetricians, with other colleagues practising in the maternity area, responded to this scathing condemnation by attempting to correct the situation. In order to develop an evidence base for practitioners who lacked the time or the opportunities to search and evaluate the literature, this group set about reviewing the research systematically. This resulted, first, in the publication of two highly significant edited volumes (Chalmers et al 1989) and, later, the ongoing development of the Cochrane database.

Unsurprisingly, evidence is meant to provide the basis for evidence-based practice, which has been defined in the following terms:

> the conscientious, explicit and judicious use of current best evidence in making decisions about the care of individual patients
>
> (Sackett et al 1996, p. 71)

Audit

Another term used all too frequently in the maternity area, 'audit', is widely misunderstood. Unlike research in the maternity area, audit differs in that it has not been subjected to the scrutiny of a research ethics committee (Maresh 1999). Occasionally, one may be forgiven for wondering whether this is the only

difference. The more acceptable criteria, however, for the audit are as follows (Brandom 1996, Campbell 1997, p. 6, Rees 1997, p. 8):

- it is well localised functionally or geographically, or both
- it is a continuing activity
- it has measurable objectives to ensure relevant comparisons
- it is intended that an action will ensue, such as a change in service provision.

The crucial role of the clinical environment becomes apparent when one considers the three aspects of an audit as traditionally undertaken – that is, with a focus on structure or process or outcome. This role and the focus on outcomes is well illustrated by an audit of water birth (Garland & Jones 2000).

Although it is the process that is most frequently addressed by an audit, it is, conversely, this aspect that is least likely to be satisfactorily audited (Walsh 1999, p. 430). The problem, according to Walsh, is that the audit loop is unlikely to be completely closed. By this is meant that guidelines are set and data are collected, but strategies to correct any shortfall may not be implemented and there is no evaluation of any change in practice when it is implemented. Thus, the audit process is effectively stalled, and the audit cycle is unable to proceed to develop into the continuing audit spiral which leads to improvement in health care (Maresh 1999, p. 137).

Although numerical approaches are often assumed to be fundamental to audit, Maresh maintains that this is not necessarily the case (Maresh 1999, p. 140). He argues that hard-edged statistical approaches are not always necessary for audit. His example of this 'softer' approach appears in his example, in which he suggests that obtaining women's views about their care is an 'alternative method of auditing maternal morbidity' (Maresh 1999, p. 140). Such data may be obtained through qualitative research methods, rather than quantitatively, in order to learn of women's perspective on their experience of pregnancy.

Some of the problems inherent in audit manifested themselves in a study of a change in maternity care based on the recommendations of the Changing childbirth report (Beake et al 1998, DoH 1993). One example is that the demarcation between audit, which addresses ongoing practice, and research, which features a new intervention, appears to have become blurred in the context of this study. Thus, my opening criticism of audit may still be justified, rather than being only a historical problem as Walsh states (1999, p. 430). Another of the problems that Beake and colleagues encountered in the course of their audit related to data collection. They relied on women's medical case notes to provide the data that they planned to utilise for audit purposes. These auditors found that the instruments that they were using as data collection tools had, in practice, been developed for quite a different purpose – that is, as records of care. Thus, these researchers were able to draw only limited conclusions about the effects of the woman-centred intervention that they introduced.

Rationale for research-based and evidence-based practice

Research-based practice in nursing and midwifery has long been regarded as a means of ensuring that quality care is provided. Additionally, some consider that the status of these professions may be enhanced by this level of intellectual activity. The introduction of evidence-based practice, however, was initiated by medical personnel. It followed on from Cochrane's withering criticism of his obstetric colleagues' abysmal record of research utilisation, as mentioned above (1972).

Evidence-based practice has been advocated and supported by a multiplicity of UK policy documents. These recommendations have largely been on the grounds that it may facilitate the solution of long term resource allocation problems in the UK health service, by increasing both effectiveness and efficiency. Effectiveness has been defined as 'how successfully an aim is achieved', whereas efficiency is 'how well one does something' (Paton 1995, p. 31). Evidence-based practice forms the mainstay of 'clinical governance', which is being implemented in the UK in a government initiative to improve the quality of health care (Hundley et al 2000, Viccars 1998).

Randomised controlled trial

The strength of the research or quality of the evidence utilised to build evidence-based practice is clearly crucial. For this reason, the research design that is usually regarded as the most powerful, the randomised controlled trial (RCT), is the one most frequently recommended in this context.

The RCT overcomes the biases inherent when past experience, single case studies or case series without comparison groups are used as the basis of care (Enkin et al 1995). The reasons for the power of the RCT are found in its objectivity or freedom from bias, which are likely to affect the results when other research designs are utilised. The bias that often materialises, possibly inadvertently, is associated with the sampling or selection of subjects for the experimental treatment or intervention and the control group, who receive either no treatment, a placebo intervention or the standard care. As the name of this design indicates, the allocation of eligible people to either the intervention or the control group is by randomisation. In this way all have an equal chance of being recruited to either group and systematic differences between the groups are avoided.

An example of randomisation is in the groundbreaking RCT on episiotomy (Sleep 1984) in which randomisation was by the opening of an opaque, sealed envelope when the woman was in the second stage of labour, in order to determine the perineal management.

These precautions mean that the findings are relevant or generalisable to a far wider target population than just the sample involved. Enkin and colleagues maintain that the logic underpinning the RCT, if implemented conscientiously, makes this research design 'the gold standard for comparing alternative forms of care' (1995, p. 70). Bias may be further reduced by ensuring that, as far as possible, the woman and baby, those caring for them and those collecting data are 'blind' or unaware of the treatment group to which allocation has been made.

The principles of conducting a RCT which justify confidence in the results have been listed by Sleep (1991) (Box 5.1).

After data have been collected to measure the outcomes in both or all of the treatment groups, these data are subjected to demanding statistical tests. Thus, an assessment is made of the possibility that any differences in outcomes are due to chance, rather than the experimental intervention. The application of these tests must be rigorous. When the research report is published a full account of the procedures is included, as well as details of whether there was ever

> **Box 5.1** Principles of conducting a randomised controlled trial
>
> - The number of subjects should be adequate to ensure that differences are not due to chance.
> - Randomisation of the subjects happens before the intervention and there is no withdrawal.
> - The allocation must not be predictable.
> - Compliance with the intervention should be complete.
> - When the data are analysed, each subject is retained in the allocated group, regardless of the actual treatment.
>
> (After Sleep 1991, p. 201)

any deviation from this protocol. Because the researcher follows the research protocol conscientiously, the findings may be checked by other researchers by replicating the study, either partially or else in its entirety.

Despite the power of the RCT, it is none the less necessary for the practitioner to scrutinise the research report to ensure that the context and intervention are relevant to the present situation. This scrutiny is vital in maternity care, where systems of care differ greatly and where cultural values are fundamental to the attitudes of women and, perhaps, to staff. Such scrutiny is likely to take account of not only the research findings and the local situation, but also the midwife's intimate knowledge of the woman and the midwife's personal and professional experience, as well as her intuition.

The RCT is the research method that underpins evidence-based practice. Other forms of evidence may be utilised in practice, but these other forms are often considered to be of lesser value. In this way, hierarchies of evidence may be drawn up (Jennings & Loan 2001). The RCT is an important example of the quantitative approaches to research.

Research methods

Quantitative research

The research that has been mentioned up to this point in this chapter has focused on areas of care amenable to scientific measurement, or quantification. For this reason the methods used are known as quantitative methods (Hicks 1996). In the next section there will be some discussion of another approach, which is known as qualitative research. If the researcher's area of interest involves phenomena that may be counted, numbered or otherwise measured then a quantitative approach is likely to be the more appropriate.

When I undertook a study examining student midwives' employment decisions and practice, I decided that quantitative methods were suitable (Mander 1994). These methods permitted counting the number of students and midwives who planned to practise as midwives and the number who had other plans. It was also possible to count the number and to measure the length of time that the midwives practised as such. In this research on employment decisions, as in all quantitative research, it was essential for the researcher to maintain objectivity as far as possible. In this way the researcher tries to remain impartial and to reduce the possibility of bias by avoiding becoming personally involved with the data or the respondents. The researcher must also attempt to limit the scope for personal or subjective interpretation of the data, as was described in the account of RCTs above. In my research on student midwives I undertook scrupulous pretesting of the research instrument (a postal questionnaire) to ensure its reliability and validity (see below). A pilot test may be used to test the complete research protocol, rather than a pretest of a particular aspect.

Quantitative research usually employs quite a structured format, thus giving rise to one of its strengths, being easily replicated. This structure invariably begins with a literature search, on the basis of which the researcher formulates a hypothesis and possibly some research questions. The researcher then seeks to test the hypothesis and to answer the research questions by using the research approach or design that is most appropriate. Following on from the design are various methods of sampling, data collection and statistical data analysis; the researcher needs to consider a wide range of possibilities before deciding which of these will best answer the research questions (Hicks 1996, Rees 1997).

Reliability and validity

The issues of reliability and validity are crucially important when considering the methods and the instruments to be used.

- *Reliability* refers to the constancy or accuracy of a measurement or observation. At a simple level this might refer to ensuring that a sphygmomanometer had been accurately calibrated.
- *Validity* is the extent to which the research is measuring what it is supposed to be measuring, or whether it is inadvertently measuring another closely related phenomenon.

Quantitative research has been criticised on the grounds that it may be reductionist. This is because, in order to make sense of the respondents' behaviour or responses, the researcher must simplify or reduce the events to their most basic component parts. The appropriateness of such a reductionist approach in research into a topic as humanely complex as child-bearing is a problem that the researcher must consider carefully when choosing the research method. It is possible that a quantitative research approach may neglect some important aspect of the phenomenon under study. This may be because the researcher is unaware of its existence or possibly because it is too complex, or otherwise challenging, to cope with.

Qualitative research

Qualitative approaches to research may sometimes be more appropriate to help the midwife researcher to find answers to complex and challenging questions (Morse 1992, Morse & Field 1996). Although some critics may regard the qualitative research approach as 'soft', it may be more suitable for examining the human situations that are fundamental to childbearing. A crucial feature of all forms of qualitative research is their ability to understand the person's experience, which is known by the German term 'verstehen' (Leininger 1985). To achieve this understanding, the researcher must observe the actions and listen to or read the thoughts of the person. In this way the perspective of the person experiencing the phenomenon becomes apparent. This approach has been described as 'emic', and is clearly different from the 'etic' or quantitative approach mentioned above. The qualitative researcher makes no attempt to achieve objectivity; in fact the reverse applies as the researcher seeks to interact personally with the informant and the data. In this way, the researcher seeks a complete understanding of the phenomenon, event or experience; this is in marked contrast to the reduction-ist tendency in quantitative research.

There are a number of different forms of qualitative research, such as grounded theory, phenomenology and ethnography, which differ in their theoretical basis, the involvement of the researcher and the degree of structure. The qualitative method that is chosen will depend on the extent of existing knowledge about the topic, as determined by the preliminary search of the literature, and the researcher's expertise.

The analysis of qualitative data tends not to use statistical tests, although computer programs are increasingly frequently used (Dey 1993). As with other stages, the data analysis involves the researcher's profound involvement. This personal input may be challenging, as the topics may be quite emotional – as I found during my study of the midwife's care of the mother who relinquishes her baby for adoption (Mander 1995).

The exploratory nature of qualitative research makes it ideally suited to areas where knowledge is scanty or underdeveloped (Leininger 1985). For this reason, this type of research may sometimes be regarded as a basic building brick of midwifery theory. A further strength of qualitative research is that it is able to provide fresh perspectives on phenomena that the 'experts' regard as well understood. Clearly this is important when the midwife needs a comprehensive understanding of the woman's experience of some aspect of childbearing or care.

Triangulation

Qualitative and quantitative are the two main approaches to research, which have much to offer midwifery. These two approaches do not need to be regarded as discrete entities, however, as both qualitative and quantitative aspects may be combined in a single research project. This combination is one form of 'triangulation', which may, for example, incorporate a multiplicity of methods, theoretical approaches or sources of data (Denzin 1978). Whereas the quantitative approach tends towards the 'scientific' aspects of care, qualitative research tends towards the more human. The exploratory nature of qualitative research means that it has the capacity to 'open up' new areas of knowledge, which is facilitated by its lack of external structure. In the same way, qualitative approaches are likely to provide in-depth detail, rather than the large-scale statistically significant evidence that is provided by quantitative studies.

Although some researchers regard the gap between these two research approaches as unbridgeable (Carr 1994, Clarke 1995), there are more constructive ways of viewing the situation. Rather than a right or wrong research method, the reader or consumer of research should be thinking in terms of the appropriateness of the research approach for the question that is being asked. It may be that a postal questionnaire and tests of significance are not entirely suitable for studying intimately human matters.

The research process

A systematic approach of research is what differentiates it from any other form of questioning or enquiry. This systematic approach may be termed 'the research process'. In his book on research for midwives, Rees (1997, p. 21) outlines the stages of the research process, beginning with the development of the research question. For Rees this process ends with the 'communication of the findings'. This may be in the form of a written report, a journal article or a verbal presentation to colleagues or at a conference. It may be, however, that the process does not end with the dissemination of the research findings. Following on from the 'publication' of the findings in whatever form, it may be suggested that each practitioner has a responsibility to be aware of the research and to take an interest in the utilisation of the material. This stage may, in turn, be followed by the evaluation of the implementation of the research and the resulting change in practice.

Research ethics

The woman and baby for whom the clinical midwife provides care, seek her help for precisely that reason – that is, to obtain care. Because of this rather obvious statement, it is necessary to question whether researchers should be permitted to recruit this woman and baby as research subjects in the course of that care. This question, and others that emerge in using and undertaking research, raise certain ethical issues that the midwife should consider (Beauchamp & Childress 1994). These and other ethical issues were addressed in Chapter 4. One ethical principle that is fundamentally crucial to research and deserves some attention in this chapter, though, is the principle of autonomy.

Autonomy, meaning 'self-rule', is one of the most basic and inalienable of human rights. It means that the woman has the right to decide what does or does not happen to her and to her body. A woman seeking midwifery care has no obligation to participate in any research associated with that care, but should be able to choose freely whether to do so. Both the researcher and the midwife do have an obligation to ensure that the woman is aware that she is under no compulsion whatever to participate in any research and that, if she does agree to become involved, she is able to withdraw at any point.

It may be that pressure on the woman to be involved in research is subtle, and information about involvement should be provided in writing for her to keep. To enable the woman to make this decision she needs to be informed about the details and implications of the study before agreeing to participate. Researchers are usually required to obtain the woman's consent in writing, but the consent form *per se* is of little significance compared with the information which allows that consent, if given, to be fully informed. The researcher should also allow the woman sufficient time to consider, and perhaps discuss, whether to be involved; a period of at least 24 hours is recommended. This removes the possibility of recruiting women who are especially vulnerable, such as those who are in labour or those who have recently given birth to a baby who is unwell.

A crucial extension of autonomy is the researcher's responsibility to ensure that the anonymity and confidentiality of each informant or respondent are maintained. This means that not only is the person not named but also that she and any data she provides are normally in no way identifiable. The concept of confidentiality tends to be more elusive, especially when a small number of informants may be involved in a study focusing on an easily recognised activity, such as having given birth or the birth of a baby with a disability.

Research critique

The term 'critique' is often used to indicate the need to examine carefully or criticise research, such as when it is published in the form of a report. Unlike the usual meaning of the word 'criticism', the critique is not necessarily imbued with negative overtones. Critique does, however, comprise a fair and balanced judgement, seeking the strengths as well as any limitations inherent in the research. Using the framework of critique and having already mentioned its strengths, I here consider whether evidence-based practice has any limitations.

The evidence base has been criticised appropriately for its incompleteness. Evidence exists only on those aspects of care that have been subjected to research scrutiny. It has been estimated that only about 12% of the care provided by midwives is able to be informed by sound evidence. Thus it may be argued that the evidence base is inadequate to permit the midwife to provide comprehensive care.

The incomplete nature of the evidence base is an aspect of evidence-based practice (EBP) that is being addressed by ongoing research. Such ongoing research, though, is also producing new evidence that may conflict with or contradict that which was previously used (Kim 2000). This possibility places a great responsibility on the practitioner, who must ensure that she utilises the current best evidence. To do this she should understand how to make this assessment (see below).

Some practitioners consider that EBP may be less than appropriate in a setting that involves a uniquely human activity such as midwifery. Some consider that EBP may remove the human aspect from care. This danger has been referred to as 'routinisation' or even as 'cookbook care' (Kim 2000). This argument about reducing the humanity of providing care has been extended to include the effects of EBP on the practitioner's occupational group. In this way, the likelihood of achieving or maintaining professional status among EBP practitioners has been said to be reduced (Bonell 1999).

Some therefore consider that EBP may serve to reduce either the significance of care or the role of the carer. However, it may be that this latter point is the opposite of the truth. This is because, in order to use EBP effectively, the practitioner is required to employ certain skills in addition to the knowledge, personal experience, occupational experience, empathy and intuition which the midwife is accustomed to using. These additional skills required of the midwife practising EBP include the need to understand the evidence on which her practice is based. She must understand the strengths and weaknesses of the research and must be able to select the evidence that is to be utilised as against that not to be utilised.

Research utilisation by the practitioner

Having established the crucial significance of research to midwifery in general, and to midwifery practice in particular, it may be helpful to consider the reality of the midwife's utilisation of research. This phase is one of the final stages of the research process but, perhaps for that reason, it may be neglected by practitioners. The utilisation of research has attracted considerable attention, especially for nursing (Rodgers 2000). When this problem was first examined among nurses, Hunt (1981) found that their difficulties related largely to their education. She identified the nurses' lack of knowledge about research findings. Even when this difficulty did not apply, the nurse encountered difficulty in, first, understanding and, second, believing the research. Any chance of utilising the research was further hampered by the nurse's ignorance about how it might be applied. An even more sinister phenomenon was also highlighted by the study; this involved organisational difficulties preventing the nurse from being allowed to utilise research findings.

The problems identified by Hunt among nurses were endorsed more recently by a study of midwives' attitudes to research utilisation (Meah et al 1996). This study involved 32 midwives taking part in group interviews to elicit the themes that mattered to them. Educational deficits again manifested themselves. The midwives were unable to evaluate research, found difficulty in interpreting statistical material and could not understand research methods. The sinister organisational impediment found by Hunt was again identified, as Meah and colleagues found that midwives lacked autonomy in implementing research findings and that they had no role models from whom they could learn research-based practice. Clearly, as these researchers correctly observed, many of these faults are at least partly the responsibility of the researchers.

A perplexing phenomenon that also limits the midwife's use of midwifery research was found by Hicks (1992). Using a cross-over technique 18 midwives were asked to evaluate two research reports. Half were told that the reports were by a midwife and an obstetrician respectively, and the other half were told that they were by an obstetrician and a midwife respectively. The midwives consistently judged the report that they thought to be by the midwife as poorer than the other. Thus, Hicks concludes that midwives have an inappropriately low opinion of other midwives' research; it is likely that this low esteem is another factor serving to inhibit utilisation of research.

Another study that further illuminates the problem of midwives' research utilisation was undertaken by Harris (1992). Using research into perineal pain control as her example, she asked 76 staff what research they knew about and what research they utilised. She identified profound ignorance relating to the plentiful and authoritative research on this fundamentally important topic. In contrast, Harris revealed the staff's better knowledge and enthusiastic implementation of other research that is of questionable authority and relevance; the research in question recommended the withdrawal of air-rings from frail, infirm elderly patients, but the staff were applying it to new mothers.

An important intervention study that attempted to resolve these problems was undertaken by Hundley and colleagues (2000). These researchers employed a quasiexperimental research design to assess the changes in research awareness and practice among a sample of midwives and nurses. The intervention, which was applied to the experiment group but not the control group, involved a programme of education on certain policy and practice topics for 'ward sisters'. The researchers found that staff attitudes to research, their knowledge of research and their involvement in research significantly improved in the group to whom the educational intervention had been applied. Quite appropriately, however, these researchers remind us that a change in practice is not easily achieved. The change that they engendered and measured involved a considerable change in the culture of the clinical settings in which the research was undertaken, as has been identified by other researchers (Rogers et al 2000).

The consumer of research

It may have become apparent by this point in this chapter that there is little value in undertaking research – that is, beginning the research process – unless that process is completed. The most important aspect of the completion of the process is the utilisation of research. Although the researcher clearly plays a crucial role in the dissemination of research findings, the actual decision about the utilisation of research must be made by the research consumer.

It is necessary to consider, at this point, who the research consumer is (Tallon et al 2000). In an otherwise admirable book, Buggins & Nolan (2000) define the consumer simply as the consumer of health care. The consumers of health care research, however, comprise a far wider group.

The ultimate consumer of research is the person who receives or, preferably, participates in care. In midwifery this is the childbearing woman and her family. It is likely, though, that for the woman to experience research-based or evidence-based care, the staff involved should practice EBP. For this reason, the midwife also becomes a consumer of research. To extend further the range of consumers of research, we should also include the midwifery student. This is because her midwifery education provides the foundation for her subsequent midwifery practice.

The midwifery student

The midwifery student learns about research in a number of ways. First, research is integrated into her formal education by those who teach (Thomson P 2000). In this way, she learns the techniques that are outlined below to evaluate or make a critique of the relevant studies. The student also learns about the current research evidence, and the areas of practice that have yet to be subjected to research scrutiny. Secondly, in her experience of clinical practice, the student is able to observe the utilisation of research by her mentor, who acts as a role model in this respect. Thirdly, the student may actually become involved in research. This is likely to be by attending journal clubs that are organised by active researchers and by meeting researchers at research seminars and conferences. Additionally the involvement may be associated with participating in ongoing research in the clinical settings where the student experiences her placements. Finally, the student may find that she is presented with opportunities for undertaking research. This is an immense responsibility, which may not be available to all midwifery students. The rationale is that, for the research to be valuable or at least not harmful in any way, the student requires close supervision from an experienced researcher with a considerable amount of time (Mander 1988).

> **Box 5.2** Actions following reading a research report
>
> • Implementation
> • Rejection as inappropriate
> • Replication to test appropriateness

The midwife

The midwife is likely to encounter research reports in a wide range of midwifery, nursing and other journals as well as at meetings and conferences. Following the midwife's critical reading of a research report in a journal or another publication, she has a number of choices open to her (Box 5.2):

• The midwife may be convinced that the research findings are likely to resolve a problem that has been identified in her own clinical setting. On the basis of this she may seek to implement it in her own clinical area and subsequently evaluate the change in care.
• The midwife may decide to reject the study on the grounds that:
  — it does not relate to her working situation
  — the work is too seriously flawed to be of any value
  — the research was undertaken in a country with a different system of maternity care and is not easily transferable.
• Although the research has some limitations or was undertaken in a different country, some of the problems identified may relate to those in the midwife's clinical area. For these reasons, a researcher will be approached to assist the midwifery staff in further investigating this work by replicating this study locally and with a suitably sized sample.

The woman

The childbearing woman, who is the ultimate consumer of research, may be involved in a number of ways. Increasingly women are becoming involved in the earlier stages of research. This is through the need for this specialised input into planning and implementing the study. Women have for a long time acted as the subjects of research. The information and advice that the midwife gives to the woman during her childbearing experience should, as far as possible, be research based. This information may be provided verbally, in the form of evidence-based leaflets (MIDIRS 1996/7), or both. With the increasing availability of research evidence through the internet, the woman is often able to find her own information.

Critical reading

The consumer's reading of a research report should involve critical reading; this term means that the report should be judged well, in the sense of fairly, rather than harshly or excessively negatively. Similarly, reading research requires an objective examination, in order to identify its strengths and any limitations. It may be argued that even the best research has some weak points, but the reverse may also be true in that even a weak study is likely to provide some points from which the consumer is able to learn.

As has been mentioned already, asking questions is fundamental to research. This obviously applies to the researcher, but it also applies to the research consumer such as the midwife in clinical practice. Many of the midwife's questions will relate to her practice, especially to those routines that may have become established as 'unit policy' and over the use of which she may feel that she has little control. It may be that some of her questions will be answered by the research literature, but whether this is so depends on her critical reading. Thus the consumer should adopt a questioning approach to care in childbearing, an example of which is her reading of research. The following points should be included in this reading.

The complete research

The consumer should consider the material in its entirety, rather than taking a piecemeal approach. This complete picture will illuminate points that might otherwise be missed; for example, a small sample might be inappropriate to permit conclusions to be drawn, but if an in-depth qualitative study is being undertaken a small sample would be reasonable. Similarly, in a quantitative study, the tables and statistical tests may appear daunting to some readers, but they are a crucial part of the findings and need to be read in conjunction with the text.

A further advantage of reading the complete report lies in the likelihood of the reader observing any points that may have been neglected or even omitted. In this way the reader would be in a position to question why this information has been neglected or omitted. This may be because of an error or oversight, but may alternatively be because the researcher wishes to minimise or disguise some less than satisfactory aspect of the study. An example would be when the response rate to an invitation to participate is not stated. The reader would be justified in being cautious about the quality of this work and may even suspect that this information was omitted because the rate was unacceptably low. The response rate is a good reflection of the suitability of the instrument and may indicate the importance of the research to the sample.

Specific points

While examining the complete report the midwife should question whether the various parts of it form a unified whole, whether they are discrete entities or whether there are gaps in the presentation. A problem that may emerge is that one part does not lead into the next; for example, the research questions may bear little relation to the literature review from which they should have arisen. This would lead the reader to wonder how these questions originated. Another example would be when the conclusions are not clearly derived from the findings. In this case the reader might question the possibility of the researcher having decided on the conclusions in advance of doing the research.

Author's details

The author's name, designation and qualifications may be helpful initially in evaluating the research. This may be because of knowledge of and respect for this researcher's previous work or because an examination of this particular problem is sought from, for example, a midwifery or organisational point of view. The place where the researcher is based or employed may assist in deciding its relevance if, for example, the report was written in a country where maternity care differs from the reader/consumer's.

Introduction

The introduction should explain the significance of the research topic and allow the reader to decide whether the report is likely to be helpful.

Literature review

The literature review leads the reader through the development of knowledge about the chosen topic up to the present time to indicate why this current research project was necessary. If recent research is not mentioned, the reader has to question whether the project was undertaken some time previously and is out of date. Additionally, if earlier important research is not mentioned, the question 'why' must be asked; the omission may have been due to ignorance or perhaps there was another agenda. The literature review should show how the research is based on a relevant theoretical framework; such a framework, which is based on a high level of knowledge, often helps the researcher to frame questions and to design the study (Cormack & Benton 2000, p. 80). However, in some research approaches, such as grounded theory, it is usual to undertake the literature review alongside rather than prior to the data collection.

Hypothesis/research questions

The hypothesis or research questions, or both, should emerge inevitably out of the literature review. These statements or questions should be phrased precisely to exclude all possibility of any ambiguity.

Research approach/design

The research approach or design should include a discussion of the possibilities that were considered and the reasons why one approach was chosen in preference to another. The researcher should show understanding of the issues relating to the differing approaches and of having read the important literature on research design. The reader must at this point question whether this approach is likely to be able to answer the research questions that are being asked.

Research method

The research method describes, with some discussion of the literature and the alternatives that were not selected, the complete research as it was planned. This usually begins with the subjects and the sample. In a quantitative study it would be necessary to give details of the calculations to produce the number of subjects for findings to be statistically significant The reader could then question whether the subjects in the sample would be able to provide the information to answer the research questions. An example of when this is not done is if certain groups such as children or people with learning difficulties are not allowed to speak for themselves, but the researcher instead focuses the project on their parents or carers.

Details of how the sample was identified and recruited are also necessary. A random sample may lend strength to a research project, but a sample of convenience needs to be identified as such.

Data collection

The data collection should be detailed in terms of how the research instrument was chosen and how it was designed, tested and applied. This applies particularly to questionnaires, but may also be relevant to interview schedules or observation checklists. The reader must consider whether these aspects are appropriate to answer the research questions, bearing in mind the strengths and limitations of the various instruments. Some critical discussion by the researcher of the reliability and validity of the research method would be expected in this section.

Data analysis

The data analysis planned should be explained. This includes a discussion of the relevance of the statistical tests used and an explanation of these.

Ethical implications

Ethical implications of the research should be considered, with some discussion of how any dilemma was resolved. The obtaining of ethical approval is usually reported.

Research findings

The findings should begin with any aspect of the research deviating from that described in the method section. Then response rates and other relevant data should be provided. In this section the reader should be aware of any omission, which might indicate that some aspects of the study were not completed.

This section may include some discussion of the findings or the discussion may be in a separate section. This discussion relates the findings to the research questions. The researcher would be expected to identify in this section whether there were any aspects of the research questions that were not answered and the reasons for this. This discussion hence may include the researcher's *own* criticism of the research undertaken (Benton & Cormack 2000).

Conclusions

The conclusions should relate closely to the findings and should be well substantiated. This section may include recommendations which, again, must be well supported by the research.

Conclusion

The requirement for the midwife's practice to be 'evidence based' is constantly impressed on her. The meaning of 'evidence' and 'evidence-based' care is less frequently considered. It is important to examine carefully the meaning of evidence and the forms in which evidence may be employed in midwifery practice. The methods used to obtain this evidence also deserve attention. The difference between evaluative research and audit is important in that audit is compared with predetermined standards. It is hoped that this material will be utilised by students and midwives in their midwifery practice as well as by childbearing women. In this way it may encourage some to embark on their own research projects.

REFERENCES

Beake S, McCourt C, Page L, Vail A 1998 The use of clinical audit in evaluating maternity services reform: a clinical reflection. Journal of Evaluation in Clinical Practice 4(1):75–83

Beauchamp T L, Childress T F 1994 Principles of biomedical ethics, 4th edn. Oxford University Press, Oxford

Benton D C, Cormack D F S 2000 Reviewing and evaluating the literature. In: Cormack D F S (ed) The research process in nursing, 4th edn. Blackwell Science, Oxford, ch 9, p 103–113

Bonell C 1999 Evidence-based nursing: a stereotyped view of quantitative and experimental research could work against professional autonomy and authority. Journal of Advanced Nursing 30(1):18–23

Brandom E 1996 Audit and research – basic principles. Midwives 109 (1304):255

Buggins E, Nolan M 2000 Involving consumers in research. In: Proctor S, Renfrew M (eds) Linking research and practice in midwifery: a guide to evidence-based practice. Baillière Tindall, New York, ch 5, p 89–102

Campbell R 1997 Evaluating maternity care. In: Campbell R, Garcia J (eds) The organization of maternity care. Hochland & Hochland, Hale, Cheshire, ch 1, p 1–13

Carr L T 1994 Strengths and weaknesses of quantitative and qualitative research: what method for nursing? Journal of Advanced Nursing 20(4):716–721

Chalmers I 1993 Effective care in midwifery: research the professions and the public. Midwives Chronicle 106(1260):3–12

Chalmers I, Enkin M, Keirse M J N C 1989 Effective care in pregnancy and childbirth. Oxford University Press, Oxford, vols 1, 2

Clarke L 1995 Nursing research: science visions and telling stories. Journal of Advanced Nursing 21(3):584–593

Cochrane A L 1972 Effectiveness and efficiency. Nuffield Provincial Hospitals Trust, London

Cormack D F S, Benton D C 2000 Asking the research questions. In: Cormack D F S (ed) The research process in nursing, 4th edn. Blackwell Science, Oxford, ch 7, p 77–88

Denzin N K 1978 The research act: a theoretical introduction to sociological methods, 2nd edn. McGraw-Hill, New York

Dey I 1993 Qualitative data analysis: a user-friendly guide for social scientists. Routledge, London

DoH (Department of Health) 1993 Changing childbirth: report of the Expert Maternity Group. DoH, London

Enkin M, Keirse M J N C, Chalmers I 1995 A guide to effective care in pregnancy and childbirth, 2nd edn. Oxford University Press, Oxford

Garland D, Jones N 2000 Waterbirth: supporting practice with clinical audit. MIDIRS Midwifery Digest 10(3):333–336

Harris M 1992 The impact of research findings on current practice in relieving postpartum perineal pain in a large district general hospital. Midwifery 8(3):125–131

Hicks C 1992 Research in midwifery: are midwives their own worst enemies? Midwifery 8(1):12–18

Hicks C 1996 Undertaking midwifery research. Churchill Livingstone, Edinburgh

Hundley V, Milne J, Leighton-Beck L, Graham W, Fitzmaurice A 2000 Raising research awareness among midwives and nurses: does it work? Journal of Advanced Nursing 31:78–88

Hunt J M 1981 Indicators for nursing practice: the use of research findings. Journal of Advanced Nursing 6(4):189–194

Jennings B M, Loan L A 2001 Misconceptions among nurses about evidence-based practice. Journal of Nursing Scholarship 33(2):121–127

Kim M 2000 Evidence-based nursing: connecting knowledge to practice. Chart 97(9):1,4–6

Leininger M M 1985 Nature rationale and importance of qualitative research methods in nursing. In: Leininger M M (ed) Qualitative research methods in nursing. Grune & Stratton, Orlando, p 1–26

Macdonald A M 1981 Chambers' twentieth century dictionary. Chambers, Edinburgh, p 1148

Mander R 1988 Encouraging students to be research minded. Nurse Education Today 8(1):30–35

Mander R 1994 Midwifery training and the years after qualification. In: Robinson S, Thomson A (eds) Midwives, research and childbirth. Routledge, London, vol 3, ch 9, p 233–259

Mander R 1995 The care of the mother grieving a baby relinquished for adoption. Avebury, Aldershot

Maresh M 1999 Auditing care. In: Marsh G, Renfrew M (eds) Community-based maternity care. Oxford general practice series. Oxford University Press, Oxford, ch 9, p137–152

Meah S, Luker K A, Cullum N A 1996 An exploration of midwives' attitudes to research and perceived barriers to research utilisation. Midwifery 12(2):73–84

MIDIRS 1996/7 Informed choice for women (leaflets 1–10). MIDIRS and the NHS Centre for Reviews and Dissemination, Bristol and York

Morse J M (ed) 1992 Qualitative nursing research: a contemporary dialogue. Sage, London

Morse J M, Field P A 1996 Nursing research: the application of qualitative approaches, 2nd edn. Chapman & Hall, London

Paton C 1995 Competition and planning in the NHS. Chapman & Hall, London, p 31

Rees C 1997 An introduction to research for midwives. Books for Midwives, Hale, Cheshire, p 8

Rodgers S E 2000 The extent of nursing research utilization in general medical and surgical wards. Journal of Advanced Nursing 32(1):182–193

Rogers S, Humphrey C, Nazareth I, Lister S, Tomlin Z, Haines A 2000 Designing trials of interventions to change professional practice in primary care: lessons from an exploratory study of two change strategies. British Medical Journal 320(7249):1580–1583

Sackett D, Rosenburg W, Gray J A, Haynes B, Richardson W S 1996 Evidence based medicine: what it is and what it isn't. British Medical Journal 312(7023):71–72

Sleep J 1984 The West Berkshire episiotomy trial. In: Thomson A M, Robinson S (eds) Research and the midwife conference proceedings for 1983. Department of Nursing, Manchester University, Manchester, p 81–95

Sleep J 1991 Perineal care: a series of five randomised controlled trials. In: Robinson S, Thomson A M (eds) Midwives research and childbirth. Chapman & Hall, London, vol 2, p 199–251

Tallon D, Chard J, Dieppe P 2000 Relation between agendas of the research community and the research consumer. The Lancet 355(9220):2037–2040

Thomson A 2000 Is there evidence for the medicalisation of maternity care? MIDIRS Midwifery Digest 10(4):416–420

Thomson P 2000 Implementing evidence-based health care: the nurse teachers' role in supporting the dissemination and implementation of the SIGN clinical guidelines. Nurse Education Today 20(3):207–217

Viccars A 1998 Clinical governance: just another buzzword of the '90s? MIDIRS 8(4):409–412

Walsh D 1999 Demystifying clinical audit. MIDIRS Midwifery Digest 9(4):430–431

FURTHER READING

General research texts
Abbott P, Sapsford R 1998 Research methods for nurses and the caring professions. Open University Press, Buckingham

This book draws on a range of relevant and recognisable examples.

Cormack D F S (ed) 2000 The research process in nursing, 4th edn. Blackwell Science, Oxford

This authoritative edited book discusses important issues in considerable depth.

Rees C 1997 An introduction to research for midwives. Books for Midwives, Hale, Cheshire

This book is highly accessible and utilises examples of situations and studies that are familiar to the midwife.

Quantitative research
Hicks C 1996 Undertaking midwifery research. Churchill Livingstone, Edinburgh

Relatively challenging topics are addressed in a reader-friendly style.

Feminist research
Oakley A 1993 Essays on women, medicine and health. Edinburgh University Press, Edinburgh

The issues relevant to research for and by women are analysed comprehensively.

Implementation of research
Proctor S, Renfrew M 2001 Linking research and practice *in* midwifery: a guide to evidence-based practice. Baillière Tindall, Edinburgh

The challenges and benefits of evidence-based midwifery practice are addressed by these well-recognised midwife researchers.

Qualitative research
Rice P L, Ezzy D 1999 Qualitative research methods: a health focus. Oxford University Press, Oxford

These methods are highly appropriate in midwifery and are becoming increasingly important. Their place is fully demonstrated.

Evidence-based practice
Walsh D 2000–1 Evidence-based care series. British Journal of Midwifery May 2000–Feb 2001

A range of issues as well as examples are covered in an accessible style in this series of journal articles.

USEFUL WEB ADDRESSES

Bandolier – a bulletin that summarises RCTs in an easy to access and easy to read format: http://www.jr2.ox.ac.uk/bandolier/

Cochrane database – often considered the last word in locating evidence: http://hiru.mcmaster.ca/COCHRANE/DEFAULT.HTM

DARE (Database of Abstracts of Reviews of Effectiveness) – NHS Centre for reviews and dissemination, York University: http://www.york.ac.uk/inst/crd/

NHSEED – NHS Economic Evaluation Database comprises cost–benefit and cost effectiveness analyses: http://nhscrd.york.ac.uk/nhsdhp.htm

MIRIAD – the Midwifery Research Database includes current research relevant to midwives, although it no longer accepts new studies: http://www.leeds.ac.uk/miru/miriad/miriad.htm

National Electronic Library for Health – an excellent resource with many links and NICE guidelines. It also has a primary care specific site: http://www.nelh.nhs.uk/midwife/default.asp

6

The History and Regulation of Midwifery

Dora Opoku

CHAPTER CONTENTS

The main purpose of midwifery regulation is to articulate the laws concerning what is expected from midwifery professionals, their practice and the legal safeguards in place to protect the public. The regulatory body of nursing and midwifery, the Nursing and Midwifery Council (NMC) makes secondary rules and sets standards for dealing with registrants facing charges of misconduct.

In setting out the new legal framework for midwifery regulation, this chapter makes linkages between regulation of midwives, nurses and other key health care professionals. It looks at the new direction in which midwifery regulation is being taken by the government.

The chapter aims to:

- cover current regulation governing practice, including the Nursing and Midwifery Order 2001

- trace the historical context

- set into a sociopolitical context the emerging issues in health and social care

- describe the structure of the NMC

- identify some key objectives and differences between the NMC and its predecessor

- discuss the driving principles to keep the NMC streamlined, simple and cost effective

- discuss in broad terms relevant articles in the Nursing and Midwifery Order 2001

- highlight aspects of regulation concerning midwifery and other NMC registrants still under development.

New legislation relating to midwifery

On 1 April 2002, the Nursing and Midwifery Council came into existence as the new statutory regulatory body responsible for overseeing the self-regulation of nurses, midwives and health visitors in the United Kingdom. This continues the combined regulation arrangement for midwives and nurses, a trend which first started with the Nurses, Midwives and Health Visitors Act 1979 and became effective in 1983. As then, the status of midwifery as a separate and distinct profession is safeguarded, a theme which will be developed further in this chapter. The legal basis for the creation of the NMC is Article 3(1) of the Nursing and Midwifery Order 2001 (referred to as the Order), which stated that 'there shall be a body corporate known as the Nursing and Midwifery Council…'.

The main purpose of the Order is to provide a stronger framework for public protection and to implement important reforms to the system of professional regulation by making regulation simple, streamlined and more effective in dealing with the many complex issues affecting the modern day health services, users of the service and the key professions of nursing and midwifery so vital to it.

The most visible expression of the new streamlined approach is the combination of the five statutory bodies into a single regulatory body, the NMC. Thus at the end of March 2002, the UKCC (United Kingdom Central Council), the national boards for England, Scotland, Wales and Northern Ireland, ceased to exist having completed the handing over of their various functions to the NMC. This brought an end to the UKCC era and heralded in the NMC, which had hitherto worked alongside the UKCC for 11 months in 'shadow' preparing for assumption of regulatory functions. Although the impending changes to statutory regulation were extensively trailed in the professional journals, the full impact of the change on the 640 000 nurses, midwives and health visitors whose registration at the time was inherited by the NMC will fully emerge only during the first 3 years of the passage of the Order.

Previous survey findings of the UKCC indicate that midwives as a professional group have tended to develop a strong commitment to new regulations (Asbridge 2002). Within the first year of the Nursing and Midwifery Order, every practising midwife fulfilled a statutory function by notifying her intention to practise to the local supervising authority (LSA) in the usual way – a practice that has continued since the first Midwives Act (1902).

The development of regulation in the UK – historical context

Early years

In Britain, following 12 years of almost non-stop controversy among the medical profession, who opposed the registration of midwives, the first Midwives Act was finally passed in 1902. As with all the previous failed Midwives Bills, the passage of the 1902 Bill was promoted by individual Members of Parliament through Private Members' Bills and supported in the House of Lords by others who supported midwife registration. At no time did the government take the initiative to enable the progress of a Midwives Bill through both Houses, even though the movement campaigning for registration of midwives at the time had gained much public support.

In some European countries legislation governing the control of midwives had been adopted as early as 1801, having been initiated by their governments, as was the case in Austria, Norway and Sweden. The struggles for legislation to control the practice of midwives in the UK prior to the first Midwives Act and since have been well documented in recent years, particularly by Cowell & Wainwright (1981), Donnison (1988), Heagerty (1996) and Towler & Bramall (1986). However, it is interesting to note that from 1889 eight Bills were introduced but did not succeed. The reasons for this included:

- opposition from the medical profession as doctors thought that midwives would encroach upon their practice
- opposition from the nursing profession, which wanted nurses included in the legislation (the Nurses Registration Act was passed 17 years later in 1919)
- lack of interest by members of parliament
- lack of parliamentary time.

The midwifery statutory bodies

The Midwives Act 1902 established the Central Midwives Board (CMB) with jurisdiction over midwives in England and Wales. This was followed by the Midwives (Scotland) Act 1915 and the Midwives Act (Ireland) 1918, which established similar bodies in Scotland and Ireland. After the partition of Ireland in 1922 the Republic of Ireland continued with the Central Midwives Board for Ireland until legislation established An Board Altranais in 1951, which became responsible for the statutory control of both nurses and midwives. In Northern Ireland the Joint Nurses and Midwives Council (Northern Ireland) Act 1922 made provision for a Joint Council to take over responsibility for nurses and midwives and the Nurses and Midwives (Northern Ireland) Act 1970 established the Northern Ireland Council for Nurses and Midwives (NICNM).

It can therefore be seen that prior to 1983 four separate bodies were responsible for the regulation of midwifery in the UK and Republic of Ireland. As there was a generally similar pattern in those regulatory systems and there was reciprocity among them, this section will mainly describe the situation in England and Wales.

The main provisions of the Midwives Act 1902 were as follows:

1. Prohibition of unqualified practice – unqualified women were prohibited from using any title implying that they were midwives certified under the Act and from attending women in childbirth other than under the direction of a qualified medical practitioner. This was to ensure that a doctor was present when there was an unqualified person in attendance.

2. *The CMB* – this was established with the statutory functions of:

- keeping a register of properly certified midwives
- framing rules to regulate, supervise and restrict within due limits the practice of midwives
- arranging for the training of midwives and the conduct of examinations
- setting up professional conduct proceedings with power to remove from the register any midwife found guilty of misconduct and also to restore the name of anyone so removed if judged appropriate.

3. *Rules regulating the practice of midwives* – the Midwives Act 1902 conferred powers on the CMB to make rules regulating practice to keep the public safe. The rules used to be much more detailed, partly because of the then poor educational standards of midwives. As the standard of education and practice of midwives improved, the rules were modified accordingly. In 1947 a Midwife's code of practice was introduced to reduce the detail in the rules (CMB 1948); however, the code remained fairly prescriptive even in its last CMB edition in February 1983. The CMB for Scotland and the NICNM, although reducing detail in the midwives' practice rules, did not produce a code of practice. The rules have at all times identified the sphere of practice of the midwife as being related to midwifery care of a woman in whom there are no complications.

4. *Local supervising authorities and the supervision of midwives* – these were also empowered by the Midwives Act 1902. In accordance with the Act, LSAs were appointed to supervise the practice of midwives and ensure that midwives obeyed the midwives' rules. Local government bodies, approved by the CMB, were nominated as LSAs until the reorganisation of the National Health Service in 1974. At that time the regional health authorities in England, area health authorities in Wales, area health boards in Scotland and social services boards in Northern Ireland became the LSAs. The LSAs were given powers to appoint inspectors of midwives. In 1936 the title 'inspector' was changed to supervisor of midwives and a circular from the Ministry of Health in 1937 stated that the supervisor of midwives should be the counsellor and friend of midwives. Practising midwives have been required to give notice of intention to practise to the LSA since the inception of the CMB.

There are some remarkable issues to be noted here and especially for those who would advocate a return to the days of the CMB. 'This powerful body was not, as was the case with other professional statutory bodies, to be largely constituted of members of the occupation to be regulated, but to be in the hands of medical practitioners' (RCM 1991, p. 6). What is more, the CMB was not required to include even one midwife. At no time did the midwifery statutory bodies have a majority of midwives but they were dominated by doctors who also held the chairmanships until the last decade prior to dissolution in 1983.

In the intervening years, the legislation was amended and changed to address the improved education of midwives and differences in health care needs. There is a general acknowledgement among midwives that the midwives involved with the development of this legislation represented the profession well and made some advancement towards the establishment of safe parameters of care in the midwifery services in the UK.

At the handover of functions of the three existing UK midwifery statutory bodies (England and Wales, Northern Ireland, Scotland) in July 1983, the UKCC took over the three sets of existing rules, and for England and Wales also the code of practice.

The UKCC years

On 1 July 1983 the statutory control of the practice, education and supervision of midwives became the responsibility of the UKCC and four National Boards for Nursing, Midwifery and Health Visiting (Boards), one in each of the four countries of the UK. These five bodies are referred to as statutory bodies as they were established with the Nurses, Midwives and Health Visitors Act 1979, which was later amended by the Nurses, Midwives and Health Visitors Act 1992 and consolidated in the Nurses, Midwives and Health Visitors Act 1997.

The UKCC was, until 31 March 2002, the regulatory body for nursing, midwifery and health visiting. Its mission was to establish and improve standards of nursing, midwifery and health visiting in order to serve and protect the public. Its key tasks were to:

- maintain a register of qualified nurses, midwives and health visitors
- set standards of nursing, midwifery and health-visiting education, practice and conduct
- provide advice for nurses, midwives and health visitors on professional standards
- consider allegations of misconduct or unfitness to practice due to ill health.

The UKCC promoted safe practice by nurses, midwives and health visitors through the development and promotion of professional standards. In its policy work, health and social trends were identified and strategies developed for anticipating change in the fields of education and practice, health and social policy. Further public protection was provided through the professional conduct work. Much of the UKCC's effort was put into the development of safe practice. However, when a complaint was made, professional conduct officers investigated it thoroughly and fairly.

In this way the UKCC regulated the professions, assisting practitioners to develop and understand their personal and professional accountability (UKCC 1997).

The primary legislation in the context of the statutory control of the midwife under the UKCC were the two Nurses, Midwives and Health Visitors Acts 1979 and 1992. These two Acts were consolidated in the Nurses, Midwives and Health Visitors Act 1997. Two underlying principles of the Act were the protection of the public and the government *of* the three professions *by* the three professions *for* the three professions.

It was argued at the time the Nurses, Midwives and Health Visiting Bill was being debated that, in order to achieve the latter principle, a majority of the Council and National Board members were to be nurses, midwives and health visitors. As it will be seen later, this view had gone out of favour when the 2001 Order was drafted. The majority of members on the Council of the UKCC were elected by the three professions from the four countries of the UK.

In 1992 the UKCC became the elected body, whereas formerly elections had been to the National Boards, which then nominated members to the Council. Responsibility for investigation of alleged professional misconduct was transferred from the National Boards to the Council. The National Boards became smaller, executive bodies concerned with the approval and monitoring of education and training and retained responsibility for the supervision of midwives in accordance with UKCC Midwives rules (UKCC 1993).

During the passage of the 1979 Act, midwives determinedly sought for and succeeded in establishing a special clause to be inserted into the Act enshrining in legislation the requirement for a statutory midwifery committee that must be consulted on all midwifery matters. This clause went some way to addressing their concerns about retaining control of the practice of midwives and, even though some midwives remained unhappy with the loss of a separate Midwives Act, this clause strengthened the Act for midwives. The other strength of the Act was that the supervision of midwives continued to be a statutory requirement for midwives specified in the primary and in the secondary legislation and it was the UKCC Midwifery Committee that had the responsibility for formulating the rules to control the practice of midwives, which includes the supervision of midwives.

Context of the change from UKCC to the NMC

The Nursing and Midwifery Order 2001 and subsequent establishment of the NMC as the new regulator of nurses and midwives in the UK from April 2002 has to be seen within the wider sociopolitical context in order to appreciate fully the far-reaching nature of the new professional regulatory framework.

Problems with the existing arrangements

The delivery of health care has been through a period of tremendous change during the last decade and continues to do so. Professional regulation needed to adapt and change to keep abreast with the new public expectation. The change process in the context of the new Order started some 6 years earlier under a Conservative Government, when Baroness Cumberledge, a Minister of Health, commissioned the J. M. Consulting Group to review regulations of health professionals, of which the UKCC was one, for the Department of Health. The reasons for the review are perhaps best summed up by the person who initiated it. Contributing to the debate that preceded the passage of the Order in the House of Lords in December 2001, Baroness Cumberledge recalled her own experiences as a lay member of the UKCC prior to becoming a Minister in 1992. Her own perception and that of others was that, in spite of the very best intentions and hard work of its leaders to protect the public, the UKCC was burdened with processes and procedures that made it cumbersome, rigid, slow, bureaucratic and very demanding on members' time (Hansard 2001). Perhaps the most critical leverage for reform was a need to make explicit the laws intended to protect the public. For midwives, this may come as an important oversight or omission since almost 80 years earlier the Midwives Act of 1902 was explicitly grounded in a desire to protect poor mothers from incompetent and dangerous midwives (Donnison 1988). In spite of public protection being implied rather than explicitly stated in law, the UKCC took public protection as its most important reason for existence and devised standards and procedures to effect this.

The report of the J. M. Consulting Group, which came out in 1996 (JM Consulting 1996), affirmed the primary purpose of regulation of the professions as being that of protecting the public. Among a number of recommendations for achieving greater public protection, it called for regulations to be simplified and a return to the basics of ensuring safe practice and minimum standards, rather than aiming continually to improve practice. It suggested a single regulatory body that, in time, should aim for a majority of lay members.

Other groups were also unhappy about the regulation of health care professionals. For many years, similar criticisms had been levelled at the UK system of self-regulation arrangements of the health professions. Writers such as Robinson (1988) and the influential National Consumer Council (NCC 1999) have long criticised the UK approach, mainly the General Medical Council (GMC) but other health professions as well, where each profession is allowed to regulate itself and have a separate regulatory body. They argued that such fragmentation failed to protect the public from unsafe and incompetent practitioners, protecting instead the interests of the profession they represented. J. M. Consulting's report echoed similar conclusions about the system under the UKCC and the other health regulatory bodies it reviewed. It recommended that statutory regulatory changes were necessary in order to put patients at the heart of the regulatory process. Baroness Emerton, a nurse and chairman of the UKCC until 1993, commented thus about the UKCC during the House of Lords debate in 2001: 'There is no doubt that large bodies are not effective and efficient at working speedily and it has been apparent that professional conduct work has been slowed down by procedure' (Hansard 2001). Furthermore, the UKCC's powers to deal with registrants whose fitness to practise was impaired was made difficult by an unhelpful and opaque definition of misconduct, as 'conduct unworthy of a nurse, midwife or health visitor' (SI 1993). With these sentiments, the outlook for continuation of the 1997 Act looked bleak. Predictably, J. M. Consulting recommended a simplified system of regulation for nurses and midwives – a recommendation that was accepted by the government of the day.

Changing times

Many of the recommendations made by J. M. Consultants were accepted by the Labour Government in 1998. Leading up to their election in 1997, Labour gave a strong manifesto pledge, later included in the Queen's speech, to reform and improve the NHS.

During its long period in opposition during the whole of the 1980s and until it was returned to power, Labour had often criticised the Conservative Government for what it perceived as inadequate funding of the NHS and questioned their credentials as supporters of a publicly funded health service.

The Health Act 1999

Contrary to what many in the profession expected, and indeed urged for in order to bring about major changes, the Labour administration chose to enact the Health Act 1999 as the overarching primary act to cover a number of health-related matters. The Health Act 1999 included an agreement that changes to professional regulations would be effected by the affirmative order procedures.

The Health Act 1999 is thus the major umbrella legislation with powers for bringing into effect a number of strategies intended to modernise the health service, including how best to achieve the type of professional regulation recommended by J. M. Consulting. The Health Act 1999 gave additional powers to the Secretary of State for Health to introduce change under these procedures without further primary legislation and, perhaps most significantly, without the agreement of the professional bodies in question.

Context of change to nursing and midwifery regulation

In considering the wider context of the time leading up to the drafting and consultation of the Nursing and Midwifery Order (2001) and it finally getting on to the statute books, brief mention needs to be made of some of the significant drivers that interacted with health professional self-regulation. It is argued here that the significance of some of these drivers cannot be underestimated.

Devolution

Although its impact on midwifery regulation specifically is yet to be gauged at the early stages of the implementation of the Nursing and Midwifery Order, no discussion of the context of the change can be complete without some reference to devolution in the United Kingdom. Heralded as a major part of its programme for constitutional reform, the incoming

Labour Government in 1997 set into motion a number of processes that culminated in the Scotland Act 1998, the Government of Wales Act 1998 and the Belfast (Good Friday) Agreement (The Agreement 1998). In the referenda in 1997 and 1998 that preceded the passage of these Acts of Parliament, the electorates of Scotland, Wales and Northern Ireland decided in favour of devolution and voted in their Members of Parliament and National Assemblies.

Certain existing powers were formally transferred from the Westminster Parliament in Whitehall to the devolved administrations. These include responsibility for the administration of the National Health Service in the different countries.

The four health departments became accountable to their NHS Executives for overseeing services provided locally by health boards and NHS Trusts to patients and their communities. How devolution will impact on these provisions and services including midwifery and public health will emerge in different ways in the four countries as they meet their local health, public health and social care needs. Up until April 2002 the National Boards were responsible for several aspects of regulation including the approval of educational institutions providing preregistration education and ensuring that such courses met the UKCC requirements as to their kind, content and standard. As discussed earlier in the chapter, the four National Boards ceased to exist when the new Order came into effect.

However, as existed previously under the UKCC, the health departments will continue to work closely in partnership with the NMC to safeguard the health and well-being of their communities. Although devolution created a system of greater accountability to the local electorate, the principles that underpin the Nursing and Midwifery Order apply across the UK and are therefore not devolved to national governments. The Order sets out the higher level rules and regulations that need to apply throughout the UK. It was important that, if fragmentation was to be avoided, a common standard needed to apply. In this respect, the Westminster Parliament in England acted as the lead for bringing the Nursing and Midwifery Order 2001 to the statute books. With the exception of quality assurance arrangements for education, which has been contracted to the four Departments of Health, the NMC retains all other powers of regulation of nursing and midwifery.

Rising public concerns about professional self-regulation

Another important context where the Order can be seen to be interacting with the prevailing evidence concerns public disquiet about professionals regulating themselves. Self-regulating professional bodies are funded by the professionals themselves, so in the case of nurses and midwives their periodic registration payment is the sole funding of the functions of the regulator, as was the case with the UKCC and will continue under the NMC. They elect professional members to their council and are largely autonomous and enjoy little external interference. Self-regulation and professional freedom are based on the assumption that professionals can be trusted to work without supervision and, where necessary, to take action against colleagues (Hogg 2000). In its publication on professional self-regulation and clinical governance, the UKCC (2000a) set out the requirements for professional self-regulations as being underpinned by three principles:

* promoting good practice
* preventing poor practice
* intervening in unacceptable practice.

The UKCC (2000) acknowledged self-regulation as a privilege rather than a right of the professions; it works by the creation of a contract between the public and the professions, which are allowed to regulate their own members in order to protect the public from harm that could be caused by poor or unsafe professional practice.

In the late 1990s, however, public trust in health professions' abilities, and indeed their willingness, to sanction their colleagues and remove them from positions where they can cause further damage to the public was found to have failed abysmally. Although many of the headline-grabbing cases involved doctors, and therefore the GMC, the UKCC came in for some criticism as well. The length of time it took to deal with cases of professional misconduct was one area of major cause for concern. Perhaps the most notorious case of a health professional causing immense damage to his patients involved Harold Shipman, a GP who killed many elderly patients. Having first come to the attention of the GMC in 1976 for conviction of falsifying morphine prescriptions, he was let off with a warning and went back to practice. In 1998, while a criminal investigation was under way for the high number of deaths among his patients, on the advice of

their lawyer the GMC Council was unable to suspend Shipman from the medical register. It will be wrong to judge all doctors and indeed health care professionals on the basis of what Shipman did. Shipman has become a landmark case and its effect on professional self-regulation will reverberate well into the future.

Bristol Royal Infirmary (BRI) Inquiry

July 2001 saw the publication of the BRI Inquiry, also known as the Kennedy report because it was chaired by Professor Ian Kennedy, which also very much influenced the government's thinking and approach to professional regulation. The inquiry panel conducted a public inquiry into the management of the care of children receiving complex cardiac surgery in that hospital between 1984 and 1995. The report revealed a catalogue of cases where health care professionals working in Bristol at that time failed to protect children who entered the cardiac unit for surgery.

Due to what the report called the 'club culture', there existed an imbalance of power, with too much control in the hands of a few individual health care professionals and managers. The inquiry found that no standards existed for evaluating performance, and a lack of teamwork and confusion throughout not just BRI but the NHS as a whole as to who was responsible for monitoring the quality of care. The combination of all these factors is strongly implicated as having contributed to the deaths of 30–35 more children in Bristol than might have been expected in a comparable unit elsewhere.

The influence of the Kennedy report went far beyond the local Trust. A sizable number of its 198 recommendations concern the regulation of healthcare professionals. Although the report was published after the initial draft and consultation on the Nursing and Midwifery Order in 2000, there was much evidence in the Order of merging of ideas on professional self-regulation between what the Kennedy report recommended later and the direction of the draft Order. For example, there was also much evidence of the government's drive to link the different health regulatory bodies within a quality assurance framework.

Kennedy stated that: 'regulation of healthcare professionals is not just about disciplinary matters. It should be understood as encapsulating all of the systems which combine to assure the competence of healthcare professionals: education, registration, training, CPD and revalidation as well as disciplinary matters.'

The full BRI Inquiry report can be found on the DoH website, details of which are included in the references. It gives an account of a failure of regulatory systems to protect the public and an organisational culture that also failed because of, among other factors, poor leadership and a lack of standards-monitoring mechanism at both local and national levels.

It was against this background that the Nursing and Midwifery Order was drafted. The Order encompassed the main recommendations made by J. M. Consulting but, as indicated, there is also evidence of how the government attempted to respond to concerns about professional self-regulation. Accountability of the professions to patients and the public in general, especially around fitness to practice, was highlighted by both the Shipman case and the Bristol Inquiry to be tilted too much in favour of the professions.

The Order also addresses some of the arrangements of parity across the professions. The GMC, General District Council (GDC) have also, rather late in the day, incorporated rule amendments to bring the rules in line with those existing in the UKCC, and had rewritten into the new Order the ability to suspend practitioners pending investigations. Unfortunately, the introduction of the suspension powers was too late to protect Shipman's patients. This change came about with a recent regulatory amendment.

Nursing and Midwifery Order 2001

The final stages to enable the handover of statutory control of nursing, midwifery and health visiting from the UKCC to the NMC came about following the passage of the Nursing and Midwifery Order 2001 through the House of Lords on 13 December 2001. The Order came before Parliament under Section 62 (9) of the Health Act 1999, which, as previously stated, gave powers to the Secretary of State for Health to introduce this among other Orders.

Why a Nursing and Midwifery Order and not an Act?

It may be helpful before going further to clarify the difference between primary and secondary legislation, into which all legislation is divided. *Primary legislation is enshrined in Acts of Parliament*, which have been debated in the House of Commons and the House of Lords before receiving the Royal Assent. Such legislation is expected to last at least one or two decades before being revised. With the pressure that exists on parliamentary time, Acts of Parliament are frequently designed as 'enabling legislation' in that they provide a framework from which statutory rules may be derived, otherwise known as *secondary or subordinate legislation*. *All secondary legislation is published in statutory instruments (SIs)*. *Statutory rules* (secondary legislation) do not generally require parliamentary time as they are, when agreed, endorsed by the Secretary of State in the past but will now be transferred to the Privy Council and laid before the House of Commons for formal and generally, automatic approval. Statutory rules can therefore be implemented or amended much more quickly.

The Nursing and Midwifery Order 2001 is neither of the above. It came under what is known as the *affirmative Order procedure*. It is an ancient and by all accounts an infrequently used law-making process with its roots going as far back as to Henry VIII. Because of this association, it is sometimes known as the Henry VIII rule. It differs from primary legislation in the sense that, unlike primary legislation, it is not debated in either the House of Commons or the House of Lords before receiving the Royal Assent. This procedure is more amenable for rule amendments without the need for a major discussion and passage through the Parliamentary process. Statutory rules can emanate from an Order and this is an important difference between an Order and secondary rules.

Although the affirmative Order procedure shares many similarities with secondary legislation, which as has been noted are published in SIs, there is an important difference between the two. It is this: The Nursing and Midwifery Order 2001 has written within it secondary law-making powers, which will be made by SI. For example, the new Midwives rules will come about via SI, as will the new rules and procedures governing fitness to practise (formerly known as professional conduct rules and procedures). There are a fair number of other rules all to be made by SIs, such as the rules necessary to establish the new professional register and those to be brought in for election to the next Council that is to take over in 2005. Affirmative Orders have in common with secondary rules the facility to adapt, amend and implement rule changes more quickly than an Act of Parliament. Their appeal for the government in a time of rapidly changing health and social scene may well lie in their amenability to be changed quickly and bypass lengthy Parliamentary procedures.

The progress of the Order in all other ways was akin to the way statutory rules are made. The draft order was 'laid' before each House of Parliament for a period of 1 month. Though points for clarification and objections could be raised, there could be no amendments once it was 'laid' and had to be accepted in its entirety or the whole Order was in danger of falling.

In fact, this nearly happened with the Nursing and Midwifery Order during its passage in the House of Lords. Having been the subject of extensive consultation going back some time, it came rather unexpectedly when Lord Clement-Jones tabled a motion that threatened the passage of the whole Order. After declaring a family interest in the Order, Lord Clement-Jones indicated that he was representing the views of a small group of health visitors who dissented from the position of the Community Practitioners and Health Visitors Association (CPHVA).

It would not have escaped the attention of midwives, and indeed other UK registrants, that neither the title of the Order nor the regulatory body included the words 'health visiting'. At a crucial stage, Lord Clement-Jones moved a motion for an amendment to the Order on the grounds that:

- the NMC does not contain health visiting in the title
- health visiting is not recognised as a distinct profession outside nursing.

He went on to develop his argument that 'Health visiting is not recognised as a different profession outside nursing, as there are no provisions under the Order for a compulsory register of specialists in community and public health including health visitors' (Hansard 2001, column 1498). Lord Clement-Jones' interjection was rather unexpected as the final draft Order had initially seemed to have the support of the key professional organisations – the Royal College of Midwives (RCM), Royal College of Nursing (RCN), Unison and the CPHVA.

Had the Order not been passed in December 2001, the professions would, in all likelihood, still be under the auspices of the UKCC, a body which had started preparing to wind up. It would also have seriously derailed the government's election pledge to modernise regulation as set out in the NHS plan (England)

in July 2000 (DoH 2000) and with it the three tests this set out for the regulatory bodies: to make them smaller, with much greater patient and public representation, and with faster and more transparent procedures with clearer accountability to the public and health service.

Speaking against the amendment, Baroness Howells of St Davids succinctly summarised the situation as follows: 'All these organisations would have liked more for themselves, but they have all recognised that a fully consultative process has taken place and the best formula has been found to accommodate all parties' (Hansard 2001, vol 11213, column 1506). In her opinion, an acceptable solution to a very complex situation had been found after a long drawn-out process. She went on to say that the long process of consultation had led to an acceptable solution to a complex situation. Following assurances from the government Health Minister, Lord Hunt, that the status of health visitors would not be diminished under the Order, Lord Clement-Jones withdrew his motion and the Order was passed on 13 December 2001.

Many registrants may be used to the more familiar Acts of Parliament providing the legal basis of their professional regulation and the temptation will be to continue referring to an Act of Parliament in the context of the new rule change. It is worth noting that the correct terminology is to refer to it as the Nursing and Midwifery Order 2001. The Order is as binding as previous Acts of Parliament regulating the midwifery and nursing professions.

Not for the first time leading to the passage of rules affecting midwifery, midwifery representations, mainly the RCM and Association of Radical Midwives (ARM), came together with maternity groups in a determined way to ensure that midwifery as a profession is strongly represented in the Order. They made strong representation at each stage of the consultation process and, although their collective influence in shaping the final Order cannot be quantified, on balance midwives should feel satisfied that mothers and babies will continue to be protected by the provisions in the Order.

The Nursing and Midwifery Council

There are certain functions necessary for regulation of nurses and midwives and these were automatically continued by the NMC when they took over the regulatory functions in April 2002. Like the UKCC before, it is required to:

- maintain a professional register
- give advice to practitioners and others
- set standards for conduct and practice
- deal with allegations of misconduct.

These key functions of the regulator remain unchanged and will continue through the transitional phase. However, some important changes can be seen when the UKCC is compared with the NMC in both the responsibilities and style of working set out in the Order.

A number of these changes have come about as a result of the new Council assuming some of the roles and responsibilities previously carried out by the National Boards for nursing, midwifery and health visiting. Where, for example, the National Boards monitored the UKCC standards for quality assurance arrangements for programmes leading to registration and recordable qualifications, this function has now been assumed by the NMC. As noted earlier, the NMC has the powers to delegate and has indeed delegated aspects of quality assurance monitoring locally to the four countries.

Specifically for midwifery, one of the key changes resulting from the Order concerns advice and guidance for LSAs. The provision of guidance and standards for LSA formerly came under the remit of the National Boards; however, from 1 April 2002, the NMC assumed this function. It is interesting to note that there are no provisions under the Order for the delegation of this function, a function which is widely seen as an effective mechanism for public protection. In time, the NMC will provide guidance on how this aspect of its new responsibility will be carried out uniformly across the whole of the UK. There were some methodological differences regarding advice and monitoring of LSA functions under the National Boards, but these will disappear.

The core business therefore remains largely unchanged in substance. The next section turns to changes introduced in the Order.

Additional objectives for the NMC

As noted earlier, the main purpose of the new Order, which came out of the Health Act 1999, was to bring changes and reform to statutory regulatory bodies in order to address a number of concerns and modernise it. Some of these concerns were highlighted by J. M. Consulting, while others came from other events such as the conduct of misbehaving professionals and ways in which their regulating bodies dealt with them.

It is perhaps not surprising to find that the greatest proposals for change in the Order were in areas where problems had occurred or perceived to have existed under the old regulatory arrangement.

As the regulatory body set up to regulate nursing and midwifery, the NMC's ruling Council has also been given the responsibility of overseeing the implementation of additional objectives set out in the Order. Some of these are expanded here for clarity. Setting up of the Council sought to achieve the following:

- explicit requirement for public protection
- a streamlined Council with a streamlined committee structure to improve its efficiency and reduce bureaucracy
- power for Council to design procedures to make and maintain efficiency
- a greater representation of public and patient interest and involvement
- increase in lay participation balanced with professional representation
- faster and more transparent procedures
- a wider definition of unfitness to practise of a nurse or midwife for reasons of misconduct
- more powers to deal with these in a fair and effective manner
- greater transparency and accountability to the public
- consistency across professional boundaries
- greater cooperation and partnership with different professions, the NHS and private sectors.

Implementing the new self-regulation framework

As will be noted from these new responsibilities imposed by the Order on the NMC, a number of the structures and committees that operated under the UKCC will either disappear altogether or be replaced. The Order identifies the setting up of four statutory committees, which will be discussed in greater detail later. Apart from the four statutory committees, the NMC has the power to structure itself as it sees fit to enable it to carry out its functions effectively and efficiently.

Members of the Council are accountable to the public and professions for effecting these changes and reform.

Membership of the Council

The first Council is referred to in the Order as the Transitional Council. The Transitional Council members were appointed by the Privy Council some months before the demise of the UKCC, which it 'shadowed' to orientate new members of the Council so as to ensure that the regulation of nurses and midwives continued smoothly and uninterrupted.

During its term in office, the Council has many important changes and reforms to implement. Among the most pressing will be consulting and agreeing on rules for operating an election scheme in fulfilment of Article 3 of the Order. Election of registrant members is scheduled to take place in time for the next Council to take over in 2005. The term of future Councils shall be 4 years.

The Members. The Council is made up of 12 registrant members and 11 lay members. Both registrant and lay members of the first Council were appointed by the Privy Council, which will continue to appoint the lay members in future Councils.

The 12 registrant members are made up of four from each of the parts of the register for nurses, midwives and community and public health workers. Each of the four UK countries are equally represented.

The Order stipulates that, in the rules regarding elections, only a registrant may seek election, however, and they may be elected to only one part of the register. A new category of membership to Council is introduced: that of alternate member. For each registrant member appointed as either in the first Council or in future Councils, there is an alternate member. Therefore, midwifery will be represented on the Council by eight midwives in total: four members and four alternate members.

Comparison between UKCC and NMC membership structure. The numbers in each category are shown in Table 6.1. On balance, midwifery comes out positively in a number of significant aspects, including increased representation on the ruling Council where midwifery is represented by eight out of the 24 registrant members.

Table 6.1 Comparison between UKCC and NMC membership structure

	UKCC	NMC
Members	60	35
Lay people	4	11
Nurses	28	8
Midwives	8	8
Health visitors	4	8

The Council members will normally elect a President from among themselves, but for the first Council an appointment was made; although the President is a nurse, the Order does not prevent non-registrants from the position of President of Council.

The position of the alternate member may not be a concept familiar to most practitioners and a brief explanation of their function is given here. An alternate member has the same function as a registrant member and may attend Council meetings, but can vote only if his or her corresponding practitioner member is unable to do so.

A number of conclusions fall out of analysis of the composition of membership of the NMC when compared with that of the UKCC. Whereas the latter had 40 elected registrant members and 20 appointees by the Secretary of State for Health, it is immediately obvious that the NMC represents a significantly reduced Council with much greater prominence given to lay participation. The difference between members with voting powers is only one in favour of the registrants. Reference to the points made earlier about the drivers and objectives of the new Order should give some pointers to what is being attempted here. The composition of the membership of the Council could be said to provide the foundations for a greater lay participation and representation in the regulation of nurses and midwives.

Lay members are carefully selected to eliminate anybody who is a nurse or midwife or has at any time been on any part of the professional register kept by the UKCC. They must also not belong to a profession or have qualifications that in the opinion of the Privy Council will favour the nursing and midwifery professions in their performance on Council. This is a significant departure from previous memberships of Nursing, Midwifery and Health Visiting regulatory councils where written into the Acts were stipulation for a number of representatives from the medical colleges. The first group of lay members come from education, consumer groups and nonmedical health employers.

Executive support

For most practitioners, contact with the statutory body is normally with the base from where the Council conducts most of its business, in other words the Headquarters of the NMC. This is where the team supporting the function of the Council is housed. It is headed by the Registrar who, as the Chief Executive, is responsible for overseeing the day-to-day running of the systems and structures that ensure that the apparatus of regulation works and is Secretary to Council meetings.

Past Registrars and Chief Executives under the UKCC have all been registrants but, like the position of the President of Council, there is again no stipulation under Article 4 of the Order for the appointee to be a registered nurse or midwife and in fact the first person to be appointed Registrar of the NMC is neither.

This discussion of the membership of the new Council highlights another demonstration of how the Order interacts with evidence to bring into the statute a new and contemporary set of ideas around statutory framework of self-regulation of nurses and midwives.

Framework for coordinating health regulators

It has already been noted in the preceding discussion on the BRI Inquiry (BRI Inquiry 2001, DoH 2002a) and Shipman that the system of separate self-regulation of the different health care professions which exists in the UK has been found wanting on a number of counts in providing effective and efficient public protection. Differences between one professional regulator and another, gaps between services, poor and uncoordinated systems for communications between different groups delivering health and social care have been cited as examples of disruption to effective and safe patient care. The Kennedy report (BRI Inquiry 2001) was one such major enquiry to highlight the many flaws that it saw as having contributed to, among other things, practices that put professional interest above those of the patient; lack of transparency and accountability, lack of integration and transparency were other problems highlighted.

In short, in future regulators are required to ensure that they inform the public about what they do, how they plan to do it, give the public a say and, finally, must be subject to scrutiny and questions about what they have done.

The government's NHS plan (England) published in 2000 already included a proposal for an overarching body to oversee all the health regulators. Following the publication of the Kennedy report in 2001, which called for the setting up of such a body as a matter of urgency, the Secretary of State for Health (England) accepted to act on this recommendation. Following consultation, the government announced in March 2002 that it had reached agreement to progress the statutory requirements to bring about a new independent council which will coordinate the work of the regulators of doctors, nurses, midwives and other health care regulators and improve the consistency and accountability to Parliament of the regulators' work.

In order to assume the legal powers necessary to undertake the functions entrusted in it, an Act of Parliament was necessary for the creation of such a body. Because the Kennedy report and other developments requiring rule change came about subsequent to the Health Act of 1999 they, unlike the Nursing and Midwifery Order, were not included in the raft of changes to professional regulations that could be effected by the affirmative Order procedure. To facilitate its passage through Parliament, this was included in the NHS Reform and Healthcare Professions Act (2002), which will lead to the creation of the Council for the Regulation of Healthcare Professionals (section 25) early in 2003. This Council will have nine members from the professions it will oversee and ten members representing public interest and the NHS.

The UKCC stated in 2000 (UKCC 2000a) that professional self-regulation is a privilege rather than a right of the professions. This still remains the case and, in order for nursing and midwifery to continue to enjoy a professional self-regulatory system that meets the public and government agendas for today and the future, many changes to the laws governing regulation have been necessary. Some are included in the Nursing and Midwifery Order 2001; other ideas are already part of the health service and regulatory bodies agendas. Since the Labour Government came into power in 1997, the concept of clinical governance has been introduced and developed as a framework through which practitioners are accountable for improving the quality of their clinical care and ensuring high standards of practice. As a process, it involves all members of the health care team and incorporates quality assurance aspects such as evidence-based practice, research and complaints and clinical incident reporting. Employers have also got a major public protection role and are brought into the loop of cooperating with regulatory bodies. Professional self-regulation is a central component of the whole clinical governance initiative, which lies with employers in the main. The proposed new Council for the Regulation of Healthcare Professionals is intended to give the necessary authority, backed by the law, for a body to add the missing piece of the jigsaw to modern regulation of health care professions.

Other developments in self-regulation

The introduction of an additional layer of regulatory arrangement was a cause for concern for the professions broadly, on two counts: first the possible erosion of their independence as self-regulating bodies independent from government and, secondly, that they were in danger of being weighed down with too much regulation and bureaucracy. Following representation of these concerns during the consultation, amendments were made to the Bill that sought to satisfy the professional bodies on these counts by stressing that in future their independence from government will be maintained. It is envisaged that though the proposed new Council will oversee the individual regulators; it will not get involved in the direct regulation of health care professionals. Assurances were also given that the Council's main purpose is to ensure consistency in the work of health care regulators and encourage the adoption of best practice by all. Not surprisingly perhaps, the most contentious aspect of the powers for the proposed Council concerned powers to require a regulator to change its rules in the interest of the public. Following consultation, it has been agreed that, before the Council could use its reserve right to direct a regulator to change its rules, the direction will need to be approved by both Houses of Parliament, this time by affirmative order procedures.

The nine professional regulators affected were given further assurances that Whitehall Ministers will not select any of the members of this new Council although it remains to be seen how the eventual membership will be arrived at. (The regulators affected are the GMC, General Dental Council, General Optical Council, Royal Pharmaceutical Society, NMC, General Osteopathic Council, General Chiropractic Council, Pharmaceutical Society of Northern Ireland, and Health Professions Council.) It will have become obvious from this discussion that nursing and midwifery regulation is entering a new phase in its existence; no longer can one health professional regulator function in isolation with regard to how its rules and regulations affect its registrants, patients and clients. Each health regulator now needs also to have regard for how any changes they propose fit in with the whole unified system of health care professions. Evidence of health care regulators already working together in quite important ways is provided by the latest edition of the Code of professional conduct (NMC 2002). This key document, which provides the reference for determining allegations of professional misconduct by a nurse or midwife, is built around value statements agreed by all the United Kingdom health care regulatory bodies. The code gives a clear and unambiguous statement on the expectations of registered nurses and midwives and will eventually be translated by the other regulatory bodies into their various standards and guidance documents.

The values speak directly to the practitioner who as an accountable person responsible for his or her own practice is expected to comply with these shared values along with all registrants with a United Kingdom health care regulatory body. These values (NMC 2002) require registrants to:

- respect patients or clients as individuals
- obtain consent before giving any treatment or care
- protect confidential information
- cooperate with others in the team
- maintain professional knowledge and competence
- be trustworthy
- act to identify and minimise risk to patients and clients.

The exercise of working towards a common consensus on their values highlighted some of the divergence between the various professions. Another value regarding the need for each registrant to carry a personal indemnity as a prerequisite to being an accountable practitioner has not been agreed by the nursing and midwifery professions as of the time the NMC issued its Code of professional conduct in April 2002. The Council has received legal advice pointing out that, in advising, treating and caring for patients, registered practitioners must be indemnified against claims for professional negligence and its inclusion in the NMC's Code of professional conduct is recommended. This has potential implications for independent midwifery in particular owing to the difficulty they have experienced in the past decade or so in obtaining indemnity at reasonable prices. So here we see an early problem with assimilation of ideas and values surrounding health care regulation. Such issues will no doubt be of great importance to the proposed overarching regulating Council.

Speaking of the agreement between government and the regulators on the proposed new Council, Mr Hutton, a Health Minister, said (DOH 2002b/0114): 'The new Council will be a guardian of the Public interest, totally independent from Government and answerable to Parliament. … we expect the new Council will be able to achieve its goals by persuasion and agreement with regulators on any necessary reform.' Nurses, midwives, the other professions and indeed the public will be unfamiliar with what seems like a multilayered arrangement of professional self-regulation. The full extent of its impact and powers will emerge as the Council starts its work. Regulation is changing rapidly and all midwives will be part of this change. It is incumbent therefore on each midwife to keep abreast of these changes.

Hogg (2000) captures the essence of this far-reaching concept of regulation when she argued in the Consumer's Association consultation document that statutory professional self-regulation is a contract between the government and the professions. She developed her argument further by saying that professionals accept some restrictions in exchange for the right to control who enters and leaves the profession.

Bridging the regulatory/quality assurance gap

Current government thinking, supported by recommendations from other sources, proposes the need for unifying mechanisms intended to give greater public protection and accountability in the NHS.

The Kennedy report said (BRI Inquiry 2001):

A Council for the Regulation of Healthcare Professionals should be created to bring together those bodies which regulate healthcare professionals … in effect, this is the body currently referred to in the NHS Plan as the council of Healthcare Regulators … [It] must ensure that there is an integrated and co-ordinated approach to setting standards, monitoring performance, and inspection and validation. Issues of overlap and of gaps between the various bodies must be addressed and resolved.

…The Department of Health should establish and fund Councils and set their strategic framework, and thereafter periodically review them.

Following publication of the report, Professor Kennedy has stressed that professional regulation and quality-assuring delivery are separate functions. They are both necessary although they are different in the way they operate; they are linked in delivering a safer quality practice for the public.

Rules in the Nursing and Midwifery Order relating to midwifery

Earlier in the chapter, a claim is made that the status of midwifery as a separate and distinct profession is protected in the Order. Evidence of this can be found in Article 3 where it is stated that 'there shall be four statutory committees', these are the:

- Investigating Committee
- Conduct and Competence Committee
- Health Committee
- Midwifery Committee.

The identification of a statutory Midwifery Committee in the Order is a strong position for midwifery and, as will come to light later, the committee is invested with a lot of clout.

Being a statutory committee means that a Midwifery Committee has to be in existence as long as the Order remains unchanged, unlike other committees that the Council may establish as it considers appropriate to discharge its functions and, as such, may or may not choose to delegate some of its functions to such committees. Under the Order, the Midwifery Committee must be consulted by Council on any matter regarding midwifery practice and LSA advice and guidance, and it has greater authority than was the case under the UKCC.

The most important parts of the Order specifically concerning midwifery are set out under Article 41 of the Order.

Article 41 – the Midwifery Committee

Under (1) and (2) of this article, the role of the Midwifery Committee is defined. The Midwifery Committee shall advise the Council, at the Council's request or otherwise, on any matter affecting midwifery.

Council is also charged with consulting the Midwifery Committee on the exercise of its functions as far as it affects midwifery, 'including any proposals to make rules'. It therefore has responsibility for drafting new standards and rules under statutory rules procedure on behalf of Council and once the due process of consultation has taken place will be approved of by the Privy Council. In legal terms, 'shall' is a powerful word and the use of 'shall' in this context prohibits the Council from taking any decisions about midwifery without first consulting and seeking advice from the Midwifery Committee. The Midwifery Committee is made up of the eight midwifery members of Council, lay members and nominated individuals.

Article 42 – rules as to midwifery practice

Provisions under this article allows Council to make rules specifically to regulate midwifery practice beyond those rules that affect all registrants. As discussed earlier, the Order empowers the NMC to draw up secondary legislation in the form of rules. Midwives rules are passed under this procedure and the rules referred to in this article will be made by SI. It has been the practice in the past for the midwives rules to be supplemented by a code of practice; although these requirements do not have a legal status, they have provided information and standards intended to assist safe practice. Its continuation as a document in future is yet to be decided.

It states in Article 42(1) that Council regulate the practice of midwifery with rules that may address:

- the circumstances that may lead to a midwife being suspended from practice

- a requirement for midwives to give notice of their intention to practise to the local supervision authority in which they intend to practise
- a requirement for midwives to attend courses.

Finally, in Article 42(2), LSAs are required in turn to inform Council of any midwives notifying them of their intention to practise.

There is no specific requirement under the Order for midwifery education to come under the remit of the Midwifery Committee. During the consultation phase of the draft Orders, this non-inclusion of midwifery education in the Midwifery Committee's remit caused a great deal of concern to organisations representing midwifery, such as the RCM. They argued that one of the basics of autonomy of any profession includes having control of educating and training of its members. Although the final Order did not reflect this wish, the first Council indicated that the Midwifery Committee will have included in its remit matters relating to midwifery education.

Article 43 – local supervision of midwives

Article 43(1). Under this subsection of Article 43 is to be found details of how the LSA is to exercise general supervision over all midwives practising within its area according to the Council's rules; this means every practising midwife, whether employed or self-employed. Under this article, LSAs are required to report to the Council any situation where it is of the opinion that the fitness to practise of a midwife in its area is impaired. In such situations, as happened previously, LSAs will continue to have the power under NMC midwives rules when they are formulated to suspend a midwife from practice. In the interim period, the UKCC Midwives rules and code of practice (UKCC 1998) continue to apply.

Article 43(2). This requires the Council to prescribe the qualifications of individuals whom the LSA can appoint as supervisors of midwives. These qualifications will be spelt out in the midwives rules, which the Midwifery Committee will have responsibility for drafting. The process to bring about the new NMC midwives rules and code of practice will be a major task undertaken by the Midwifery Committee on behalf of Council in its first term of office.

Article 43(3). This is a new provision that locates all matters relating to advice and guidance on supervision with the NMC. Council is required to establish the standards and provide guidance for the LSAs to exercise their functions. Previously, the advice and guidance was given by the National Boards in fulfilment of UKCC standards.

Article 45 – attendance by unqualified persons at childbirth

This is an important section and restricts those who may attend a woman in childbirth. This restriction was retained in spite of representation by the Association for the Improvement in Maternity Services (AIMS) for a fine for this offence to be dropped altogether. They maintained that, given the debate about midwifery attendance at home births, a woman may at least have the attendance of a partner, or as a last resort a relative, in cases where a woman wanting to give birth at home has no qualified midwife available to attend her – their argument being that having someone unqualified is better than having no one in attendance at all. During the House of Lords debate (Hansard 2001, column 1515), Lord Hunt stated that the point of the offence is to protect the function of midwifery in the interest of public safety, an offence that has been in force since the first Midwives Act of 1902.

Article 45(1) and (2). This states that only a registered midwife or a registered medical practitioner, or a student midwife or a medical student as part of a statutorily recognised course, may attend a woman in childbirth. There is an exemption for anyone acting in cases of sudden or urgent necessity; otherwise anyone attending or assuming responsibility for care outside of these categories is committing an offence.

Article 45(3). This lays down a fine not exceeding level 5 on the standard scale to a person who contravenes this article.

Taking on board advice from J.M. Consulting, which thought that the level of the fine should reflect the seriousness of the offence, the fine has in fact been raised within the Order, from level 4 in the previous legislation under the UKCC to a level 5.

The register

Article 5 – establishment and maintenance of register

Article 5(1). This requires the Council to establish and maintain a register of qualified nurses and midwives. This important function is a continuation of what previous regulators have done. In the case of the NMC, it inherited the register kept by the UKCC unchanged. In future, however, many changes can be anticipated before the eventual shape and parts of the register are agreed. The size of the programme of work around the new register cannot be underestimated and it will start with a draft consultation document from the NMC. The Council has promised to take cognisance of the many sensitivities and country-specific historic issues (Asbridge 2002). It has also indicated that, given the enormity of the task surrounding the setting up of a new register, Council may phase in the changes over time rather that in one go.

All registrants will have the opportunity to participate in the consultation process and contribute to shaping the future of their professional register.

Over the past two decades, all registered midwives have become familiar with Part 10 of the UKCC Register as the part where their registration is held. At this point, the only certainty is that the final register will be streamlined to a degree and therefore there is a high probability that the familiar 'Part 10' will be replaced with another title.

Article 5(2). This requires the Council to establish the standards of proficiency necessary for admission to the different parts of the register. In determining these standards the Order requires that the overriding consideration should as previously be standards most likely to achieve safe and effective care for patients and clients.

The Order stipulates additional qualities an individual seeking admission to any part of the register must satisfy.

The requirement for evidence of good character as a pre-requisite for admission to the professional register is retained. As previously, there is no attempt to define what constitutes a good character compatible with safe and effective practice as a nurse or midwife. A new quality requirement is introduced additionally, which, on the face of it, could prove problematic in its implementation. The Council is required to prescribe the requirements to be met by an applicant to demonstrate that they are in good health to make them capable of safe and effective practice.

As with all the standards Council will establish, a full consultation will take place before publishing the final requirement.

Article 5(4). This authorises the Council to prescribe details such as address and others that may be shown on the register with regards to each registrant. Throughout the consultation period leading to passage of the Nursing and Midwifery Order, the inclusion of this requirement perhaps more than any provoked much negative response from students and practitioners about the possibility of such details being made available to anyone.

Article 8(1–4) – access to register

Some safeguards are given here regarding the Article 5(4) in that, although the Council is bound by law to make the register available for inspection by members of the public, it is up to the Council to maintain and publish the register in such a manner it considers appropriate.

Article 9 – registration

Midwives who qualify in the UK on successful completion of a Council's approved education programme may apply for registration on payment of the prescribed fee and should satisfy the Council's requirement of good health and good character.

Midwives whose registration were in accordance with EU Midwifery Directive are eligible without a requirement to obtain further education, training or experience.

During the life of the transitional Council, it has set itself the objective of reviewing the processes and standards for overseas registration and will in due course publish these. Until that time, the rules made under the UKCC remain in force. Progress on these and other aspects of the NMC's progress can be found on their website at www.nmc-uk.org.

Article 15 – education and training

This is a key function of the NMC and its obligations are defined in Article 15(1–10). As has been noted, the demise of the four national boards meant a number of important functions around approval of education, training and monitoring of these programmes, which collectively are referred to as quality assurance arrangements for NHS-funded education for nurses, midwives and health visitors, now come under the remit of the NMC.

Article 15 of the Order sets out the broad principles of quality-assuring pre-registration midwifery and nursing education and training and gives permission to Council to delegate these functions within their standards. The NMC has contracted with the individual national bodies to deliver the NMC's educational quality assurance.

Article 16 – visitors

In delivering the educational quality assurance, the Council may appoint appropriately qualified and suitable persons known as 'visitors' to undertake the actual visits to institutions in England to review compliance with the Council's quality assurance processes. Scotland, Wales and Northern Ireland quality assurance processes will differ methodologically but will be governed by the same principles of partnership between the NMC, NHS and higher education to deliver a collaborative quality assurance.

A number of important issues regarding pre- and post-registration continuing professional development were handed down from the UKCC to the NMC. Among the most pressing matters include developing the agenda for Fitness for practice, which came out of the UKCC's Commission for Nursing and Midwifery Education under Sir Leonard Peach (UKCC 1999). The Commission was charged with undertaking a review to prepare a way forward for pre-registration nursing and midwifery education that enables fitness for practice based on health care need.

The majority of the report's 33 recommendations addressed pre-registration nursing education and were able to be implemented during the term of the UKCC.

However, there were important recommendations that went across both professions. On midwifery education specifically, the following was recommended (recommendation 12): 'Consideration should be given as to whether pre-registration midwifery education should move to a competency-based approach'.

The UKCC finalised the competencies for preregistration midwifery, which are now incorporated into most curricula. Total conversion by all higher education institutions to the competency-based framework was completed in September 2002 in all four countries (UKCC 2002b).

Article 19 – postregistration training

The Council is required to make rules regarding the standards registrants need to meet with respect to their continuing professional development. The rules will articulate the implications of failure to comply with the requirements for their registration status of an individual failing to meet their standards. The postregistration framework is cited as one of the major issues passed from the UKCC to the new Council and will in due course become widely publicised.

Articles 21–38 – fitness to practise

Council's functions in respect of fitness to practise, ethics and other matters. The Order sets out the legal obligations required of the NMC in fulfilling its duties regarding professional conduct. The requirements set out in the Order could involve many potential changes to professional conduct compared with what operated under the UKCC and will continue for the first 3 years of the new Council's term of office.

Although the Order contains many potential rule changes to those that operated under the UKCC, a number of these are permissive; in other words, the Council is free to set aside those that, in its opinion, would not enhance the achievement of its objective of protecting the public in a speedy and effective manner. For example, under Article 21(1) the Council is required to establish standards of conduct, performance and ethics expected of registrants and students and give them guidance on these matters as it sees fit. Although a code of conduct as a guidance for registrants is a well-established concept in nursing and

midwifery regulation, and is the basis for determining allegations of professional misconduct, performance and ethics expected of registrants and prospective registrants are new additions.

The competence expected of potential registrant nurses and midwives up to the point of registration has been defined as a result of the Fitness for practice recommendation (UKCC 1999). It will be quite another task here to define what constitutes lack of or diminished competence of a practitioner and it is suggested that this activity will be a major undertaking before the Council is eventually able to publish its standards on competence and how to deal with practitioners found to be incompetent.

The Order gives greater professional conduct powers to the NMC, which, if they choose to adopt all of them, has the potential of producing even longer delays than the UKCC found itself struggling with in dealing with allegations against practitioners. Increased bureaucracy and higher registration fees to meet the cost of a very complex process can also be expected. Should this happen, it will be counter to the stated objective of the Order to streamline professional regulations and deal with allegations of poor conduct, poor performance and ethics in a swift manner in order to remove incompetent practitioners from doing further harm. All interested parties will have an opportunity to contribute to discussions around any code of behaviour before it is introduced if the NMC chooses to adopt and implement this section of the Order. Cases of poor performance will be considered by the Conduct and Competence Committee, one of the new statutory committees to be set up under the NMC.

Some of the greater professional conduct powers the Order bestows on the NMC are summarised here. The Council is required to establish new professional conduct rules within the next 3 years, which are designed to enhance public protection by giving the Council greater flexibility in the powers it can use to protect the public. It has the powers to deal with lack of competence as well as registrants who commit misconduct, or are unsafe to practise on health grounds. Unlike the previous arrangement where professional misconduct investigations could not be instigated until a complaint was received, the NMC can launch their own investigations without needing to wait for a complaint to be submitted. They can also force the disclosure of evidence and impose conditions on individuals' practice if it is necessary to protect the public. Reading the Order, the sections dealing with fitness to practise can be read as conveying the potential for very harsh rules for the professions. It will be of great interest to all registrants to follow these and other developments over the next 3 years.

Conclusion

This chapter has given an outline of the regulation governing the profession of midwifery and to a degree nursing and other professions who provide health care in the UK. It has grounded much of the discussions within the context of modernising the systems of health care, which seeks to avoid fragmentation and gaps that in the recent past have been found to have been inefficient in protecting the public.

REFERENCES

Asbridge J 2002 The NMC: new, modern and effective. Royal College of Midwives Journal 5(4):139

BRI (Bristol Royal Infirmary) Inquiry 2001 Learning from Bristol: the report of the public inquiry into children's heart surgery at the Bristol Royal Infirmary, 1984–1995 (chairman Ian Kennedy). Command paper CM5207, July 2001. Bristol Royal Inquiry. Stationery Office, London

CMB (Central Midwives Board) 1948 CMB rules framed under the Midwives Acts 1902–1936: Notice concerning midwives code of practice, Section 96–103. CMB, London

Cowell B, Wainwright D 1981 Behind the blue door: the history of the Royal College of Midwives. Baillière Tindall, London

DoH (Department of Health) 2000 The NHS plan. HMSO, London

DoH (Department of Health) 2002a Learning from Bristol: the response to the report of the public inquiry into children's heart surgery at the Bristol Royal Infirmary, 1984–1995. DOH, London

DoH (Department of Health) 2002b Better protection for the patient. Government meets Kennedy report recommendation for independent regulatory Council. Press Release reference 2002/0114. DoH, London

Donnison J 1988 Midwives and medical men, a history of the struggle for the control of childbirth, 2nd edn. Historical Publications, p. 162

EU (European Union) Midwives Directive 80/155EEC Article 4 amended by the European Union Directive 89/594/EEC. EU, Brussels

Government of Wales Act 1998 HMSO, London

Hansard (Lords) 2001 Vol 011213, 13 December. HMSO, London

Heagerty B V 1996 Reassuring the guilty: the Midwives Act and control of English midwives in the early 20th century. In: Kirkham M (ed) Supervision of midwives. Books for Midwives Press, Hale, Cheshire

Health Act 1999 HMSO, London

Hogg C 2000 Professional self-regulation: a patient-centred approach. A consultation document. Consumers' Association, London

J M Consulting 1996 The regulation of health professionals conducted for the UK Health Department. J M Consulting, Bristol

Joint Nurses and Midwives Council (Northern Ireland) Act 1922, HMSO, London

Midwives Act 1902 HMSO, London

Midwives Act (Ireland) 1918 HMSO, London

Midwives (Scotland) Act 1915 HMSO, London

MoH (Ministry of Health) 1937 Supervision of midwives. Circular 1620. MOH, London

NCC (National Consumer Council) 1999 Self-regulation of professionals in health care. NCC, London

NHS Reform and Healthcare Professions Act 2002 Stationary Office, London

NMC (Nursing and Midwifery Council) 2002 Code of professional conduct. NMC, London

Nurses and Midwives (Northern Ireland) Act 1970 HMSO, London

Nurses, Midwives and Health Visitors Act 1979, 1992, 1997 HMSO, London

Nurses Registration Act 1919 HMSO, London

Nursing and Midwifery Order 2001 HMSO, London

RCM (Royal College of Midwives) 1991 Report of the Royal College of Midwives' commission on legislation relating to midwives. RCM, London

Robinson J 1988 A patient voice at the GMC. A lay member's view at the GMC. Health Rights, London

Scotland Act 1998 HMSO, London

SI (Statutory Instrument) 1993 No 893 The Nurses Midwives and Health Visitors (Professional Conduct) Rules 1993. Approval Order. HMSO, London

The Agreement (1998) The agreement reached in the multi-party negotiation on Northern Ireland, 10 April 1998/Command paper No 3883. HMSO, Belfast. Online. Available: www.nio.gov.uk

Towler J, Bramwall J 1986 Midwives in history and society. Croom Helm, England

UKCC (United Kingdom Central Council for Nursing, Midwifery and Health Visiting) 1983 Midwives code of practice. UKCC, London

UKCC (United Kingdom Central Council for Nursing Midwifery and Health Visiting) 1992 Code of professional conduct. UKCC, London

UKCC (United Kingdom Central Council for Nursing, Midwifery and Health Visiting) 1993 Midwives rules. UKCC, London

UKCC (United Kingdom Central Council for Nursing, Midwifery and Health Visiting) 1997 This is the UKCC. UKCC, London

UKCC (United Kingdom Central Council for Nursing, Midwifery and Health Visiting) 1998 Midwives rules and code of practice. UKCC, London

UKCC (United Kingdom Central Council for Nursing, Midwifery and Health Visiting) 1999 Fitness for practice. UKCC Commission for Nursing and Midwifery Education. UKCC, London

UKCC (United Kingdom Central Council for Nursing, Midwifery and Health Visiting) 2000a Professional self-regulation and clinical governance. UKCC, London

UKCC (United Kingdom Central Council for Nursing, Midwifery and Health Visiting) 2000b Requirements for midwifery registration programmes. Registrar's letter 35/2000. UKCC, London

USEFUL ADDRESSES

Bristol Royal Infirmary Inquiry (BRI Inquiry) www.bristol-inquiry.org.uk/index

British Studies Web Pages (Quick Guide to UK Devolution) http://elt.britcoun.org.pl/g guide.htm

Departments of Health
www.doh.gov.uk/modernisingergulation
http://ccta.gov.uk/doh/intpress.nsf
www.doh.gov.uk/healthad

Department of Health response to the BRI Inquiry www.doh.gov/bristolinquiryresponse/

Health Professions of Wales www.wnb.org.uk

National Health Service Education for Scotland www.hebs.scot.nhs.uk or www.sosig.ac.uk

Northern Ireland Practice and Education Council for Nursing and Midwifery (NIPEC) www.ni-assembly.gov.uk

Nursing and Midwifery Council www.nmc-uk.org

Quality Assurance Agency www.qaa.ac.uk

The NHS plan (July 2000) www.nhs.uk/nationalplan

2

Section 2
Human Anatomy and Reproduction

SECTION CONTENTS

7

The Female Pelvis and the Reproductive Organs

V. Ruth Bennett   Linda K. Brown

A woman is first and foremost a person and, when she bears a child, a mother. Many societies define her through her fertility and her body is adapted for this by its shape and function. The midwife needs to be familiar with the anatomical features of the woman and to understand the processes of reproduction but must never forget the social significance of childbearing or that a woman's body is unique, personal and private. The physiology of the various organs is described in appropriate chapters throughout the book.

Female pelvis

Functions

The primary function of the pelvic girdle is to allow movement of the body, especially walking and running. It permits the person to sit and kneel. The woman's pelvis is adapted for childbearing, and because of its increased width and rounded brim women are less speedy than men.

The pelvis transmits the weight of the trunk to the legs, acting as a bridge between the femurs. This makes it necessary for the sacroiliac joint to be immensely strong and virtually immobile. The pelvis also takes the weight of the sitting body on to the ischial tuberosities.

The pelvis affords protection to the pelvic organs and, to a lesser extent, to the abdominal contents. The sacrum transmits the cauda equina and distributes the nerves to the various parts of the pelvis.

The normal female pelvis

The female pelvis (Fig. 7.1), because of its characteristics, gives rise to no difficulties in childbirth, providing the fetus is of normal size. A knowledge of pelvic anatomy is needed for the conduct of labour as one of the ways to estimate the progress made is by assessing

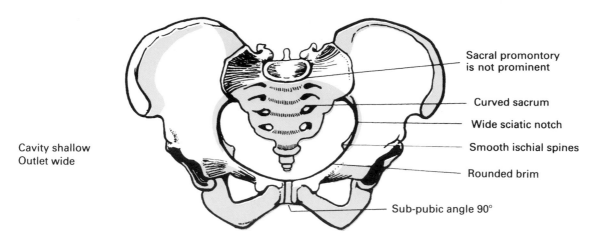

Cavity shallow
Outlet wide

Sacral promontory
is not prominent

Curved sacrum

Wide sciatic notch

Smooth ischial spines

Rounded brim

Sub-pubic angle 90°

Fig. 7.1 Normal female pelvis.

the relationship of the fetus to certain pelvic landmarks. A midwife must be competent to recognise a normal pelvis in order to be able to detect deviations from normal and refer them to the doctor.

Pelvic bones

There are four pelvic bones:

- two innominate ('nameless') or hip bones
- one sacrum
- one coccyx.

Innominate bones

Each innominate bone (Fig. 7.2) is composed of three parts:

The ilium. The ilium is the large flared-out part. When the hand is placed on the hip it rests on the iliac crest, which is the upper border. At the front of the iliac crest can be felt a bony prominence known as the anterior superior iliac spine.

A short distance below it is the anterior inferior iliac spine. There are two similar points at the other end of the iliac crest, namely the posterior superior and the posterior inferior iliac spines. The concave anterior surface of the ilium is the iliac fossa.

The ischium. The ischium is the thick lower part. It has a large prominence known as the ischial tuberosity, on which the body rests when sitting. Behind and a little above the tuberosity is an inward projection, the ischial spine. In labour the station of the fetal head is estimated in relation to the ischial spines.

The pubic bone. This bone forms the anterior part. It has a body and two oar-like projections, the superior ramus and the inferior ramus. The two pubic bones meet at the symphysis pubis and the two inferior rami form the pubic arch, merging into a similar ramus on the ischium. The space enclosed by the body of the pubic bone, the rami and the ischium is called the obturator foramen.

The innominate bone contains a deep cup to receive the head of the femur. This is termed the acetabulum. All three parts of the bone contribute to the acetabulum in the following proportions: two-fifths ilium, two-fifths ischium and one-fifth pubic bone.

On the lower border of the innominate bone are found two curves. One extends from the posterior inferior iliac spine up to the ischial spine and is called the greater sciatic notch. It is wide and rounded. The other lies between the ischial spine and the ischial tuberosity and is the lesser sciatic notch.

The sacrum

The sacrum is a wedge-shaped bone consisting of five fused vertebrae. The upper border of the first sacral vertebra juts forward and is known as the sacral promontory. The anterior surface of the sacrum is concave and is referred to as the hollow of the sacrum. Laterally the sacrum extends into a wing or ala. Four pairs of holes or foramina pierce the sacrum and, through these, nerves from the cauda equina emerge to supply the pelvic organs. The posterior surface is roughened to receive attachments of muscles.

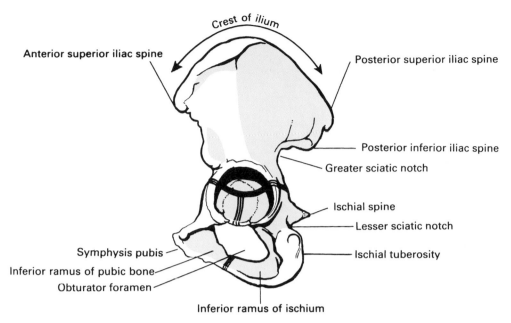

Fig. 7.2 Innominate bone showing important landmarks.

The coccyx

The coccyx is a vestigial tail. It consists of four fused vertebrae, forming a small triangular bone.

Pelvic joints

There are four pelvic joints:

- one symphysis pubis
- two sacroiliac joints
- one sacrococcygeal joint.

The symphysis pubis. The symphysis pubis is formed at the junction of the two pubic bones, which are united by a pad of cartilage.

The sacroiliac joints. These are the strongest joints in the body. They join the sacrum to the ilium and thus connect the spine to the pelvis.

The sacrococcygeal joint. This joint is formed where the base of the coccyx articulates with the tip of the sacrum.

In the non-pregnant state there is very little movement in these joints, but during pregnancy endocrine activity causes the ligaments to soften, which allows the joints to give. This may provide more room for the fetal head as it passes through the pelvis. The symphysis pubis may separate slightly in later pregnancy. If it widens appreciably, the degree of movement permitted may give rise to pain on walking. The sacroiliac joints allow a limited backward and forward movement of the tip and promontory of the sacrum, sometimes known as 'nodding' of the sacrum. The sacrococcygeal joint permits the coccyx to be deflected backwards during the birth of the head.

Pelvic ligaments

Each of the pelvic joints is held together by ligaments:

- interpubic ligaments at the symphysis pubis
- sacroiliac ligaments
- sacrococcygeal ligaments.

There are two other ligaments important in midwifery:

- the sacrotuberous ligament
- the sacrospinous ligament.

The sacrotuberous ligament runs from the sacrum to the ischial tuberosity and the sacrospinous ligament from the sacrum to the ischial spine (Fig. 7.3). These two ligaments cross the sciatic notch and form the posterior wall of the pelvic outlet.

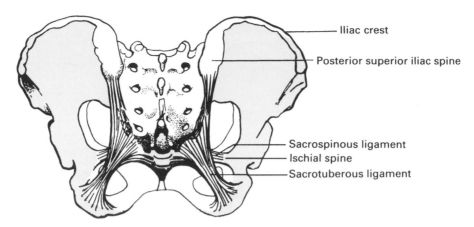

Fig. 7.3 Posterior view of the pelvis to show ligaments.

The true pelvis

The true pelvis is the bony canal through which the fetus must pass during birth. It has a brim, a cavity and an outlet.

The pelvic brim

The brim (Fig. 7.4) is round except where the sacral promontory projects into it. The promontory and wings of the sacrum form its posterior border, the iliac bones its lateral borders and the pubic bones its anterior border. The midwife needs to be familiar with the fixed points on the pelvic brim that are known as its landmarks. Commencing posteriorly these are (see Fig. 7.4 for numbers):

- sacral promontory (1)
- sacral ala or wing (2)

- sacroiliac joint (3)
- iliopectineal line, which is the edge formed at the inward aspect of the ilium (4)
- iliopectineal eminence, which is a roughened area formed where the superior ramus of the pubic bone meets the ilium (5)
- superior ramus of the pubic bone (6)
- upper inner border of the body of the pubic bone (7)
- upper inner border of the symphysis pubis (8).

Diameters of the brim

Three diameters are measured (Figs 7.5 and 7.8):

The anteroposterior diameter. This diameter is a line from the sacral promontory to the upper border of the symphysis pubis. When the line is taken to the uppermost point of the symphysis pubis it is called the

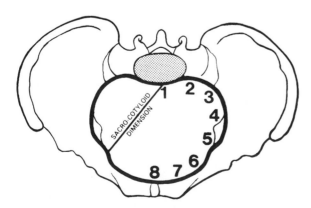

Fig. 7.4 Brim or inlet of female pelvis.

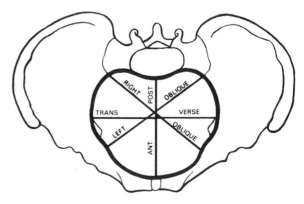

Fig. 7.5 View of pelvic inlet showing diameters.

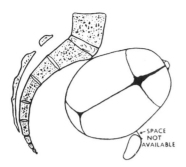

Fig. 7.6 Fetal head negotiating the narrow obstetrical conjugate.

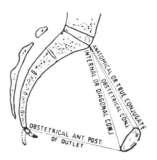

Fig. 7.7 Median section of the pelvis showing anteroposterior diameters.

anatomical conjugate and measures 12 cm; when it is taken to the posterior border of the upper surface, which is about 1.25 cm lower, it is called the *obstetrical conjugate* and measures 11 cm. The reason for this is that the obstetrical conjugate represents the available space for passage of the fetus (Fig. 7.6). The term *true conjugate* may be used to refer to either of these measurements and the midwife should take care to establish which is meant.

The *diagonal conjugate* is also measured anteroposteriorly from the lower border of the symphysis to the sacral promontory. It may be estimated on vaginal examination as part of a pelvic assessment and should measure 12–13 cm (Fig. 7.7).

The oblique diameter. This diameter is a line from one sacroiliac joint to the iliopectineal eminence on the opposite side of the pelvis and measures 12 cm. There are two oblique diameters. Each takes its name from the sacroiliac joint from which it arises, so the left oblique diameter arises from the left sacroiliac joint and the right oblique from the right sacroiliac joint.

The transverse diameter. This diameter is a line between the points furthest apart on the iliopectineal lines and measures 13 cm.

Certain structures pass through the pelvic brim, which may affect the space available for the fetus: for instance, the descending colon enters the pelvis near the left sacroiliac joint.

Another dimension is described, the *sacrocotyloid* (see Fig. 7.4). It passes from the sacral promontory to the iliopectineal eminence on each side and measures 9–9.5 cm. Its importance is concerned with posterior positions of the occiput when the parietal eminences of the fetal head may become caught (see Ch. 30).

The pelvic cavity

The cavity extends from the brim above to the outlet below. The anterior wall is formed by the pubic bones and symphysis pubis and its depth is 4 cm. The posterior wall is formed by the curve of the sacrum, which is 12 cm in length. Because there is such a difference in these measurements the cavity forms a curved canal. Its lateral walls are the sides of the pelvis, which are mainly covered by the obturator internus muscle.

The cavity is circular in shape and although it is not possible to measure its diameters exactly, they are all considered to be 12 cm (Fig. 7.8).

The pelvic outlet

Two outlets are described: the anatomical and the obstetrical. The *anatomical outlet* is formed by the lower borders of each of the bones together with the sacrotuberous ligament. The *obstetrical outlet* is of greater practical significance because it includes the narrow pelvic strait through which the fetus must pass. The narrow pelvic strait lies between the sacrococcygeal joint, the two ischial spines and the lower border of the symphysis pubis. The obstetrical outlet is the space between the narrow pelvic strait and the anatomical outlet. This outlet is diamond-shaped. Its three diameters are as follows (Fig. 7.8):

The anteroposterior diameter. This is a line from the lower border of the symphysis pubis to the sacrococcygeal joint. It measures 13 cm. As the coccyx may be deflected backwards during labour, this diameter indicates the space available during delivery.

The oblique diameter. This is said to be between the obturator foramen and the sacrospinous ligament, although there are no fixed points. The measurement is taken as being 12 cm.

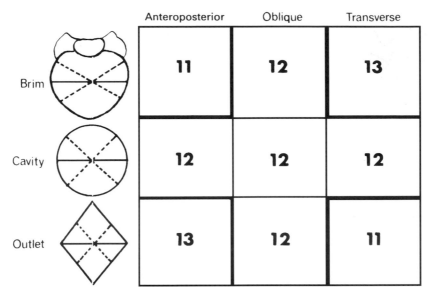

	Anteroposterior	Oblique	Transverse
Brim	11	12	13
Cavity	12	12	12
Outlet	13	12	11

Fig. 7.8 Measurements of the pelvic canal in centimetres.

The transverse diameter. This is a line between the two ischial spines and measures 10–11 cm. It is the narrowest diameter in the pelvis. The plane of least pelvic dimensions is said to be at the level of the ischial spines.

The false pelvis

This is the part of the pelvis situated above the pelvic brim. It is formed by the upper flared-out portions of the iliac bones and protects the abdominal organs, but is of no significance in obstetrics.

Pelvic inclination

When a woman is standing in the upright position, her pelvis is on an incline. The anterior superior iliac spines are immediately above the symphysis pubis in the same vertical plane. The brim is tilted and if the line joining the sacral promontory and the top of the symphysis pubis were to be extended, it would form an angle of 60° with the horizontal floor. Similarly, if a line joining the centre of the sacrum and the centre of the symphysis pubis were to be extended, the resultant angle with the floor would be 30°. The angle of inclination of the outlet is 15° (Fig. 7.9). When the woman is in the recumbent position the same angles are made with the vertical, which should be kept in mind when carrying out an abdominal examination.

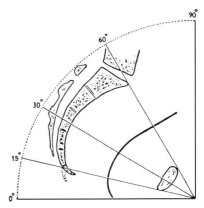

Fig. 7.9 Median section of the pelvis showing the inclination of the planes and the axis of the pelvic canal.

Pelvic planes

These are imaginary flat surfaces at the brim, cavity and outlet of the pelvic canal at the levels of the lines described above (Fig. 7.10).

Axis of the pelvic canal

A line drawn exactly half-way between the anterior wall and the posterior wall of the pelvic canal would trace a curve known as the *curve of Carus*. The midwife needs to become familiar with this concept in order to make accurate observations on vaginal examination and to facilitate the birth of the baby.

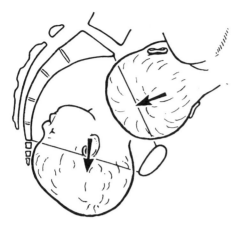

Fig. 7.10 Fetal head entering plane of pelvic brim and leaving plane of pelvic outlet.

The four types of pelvis (Table 7.1)

Classically, pelves have been described as falling into four categories according to the shape of the brim (Fig. 7.11). It is unlikely that a woman's pelvis is classified in life unless she encounters difficulties in childbirth. Of much more importance is the individual woman's pelvic capacity and whether it is adequate for the passage of the child she is carrying (Williams et al 1995). It is a common saying that the fetal head is the best pelvimeter. If one of the important measurements is reduced by 1 cm or more from the normal, the pelvis is said to be contracted and may give rise to difficulty in labour (see Chs 29 and 32) or necessitate caesarean section.

The gynaecoid pelvis

This is the ideal pelvis for childbearing. Its main features are the rounded brim, the generous forepelvis (the part in front of the transverse diameter), straight side walls, a shallow cavity with a broad, well-curved sacrum, blunt ischial spines, a rounded sciatic notch and a sub-pubic angle of 90°. It is found in women of average build and height with a shoe size of 4 or larger.

The justo minor pelvis. This pelvis is like a gynaecoid pelvis in miniature. All diameters are reduced but are in proportion. It is normally found in women of small stature, less than 1.5 m in height, with small hands and feet, but is occasionally found in women of normal stature.

The outcome of labour in this situation depends on the fetus. If the fetal size is consistent with the size of the maternal pelvis, normal labour and birth will take place. Often these women have small babies and the outcome is favourable. However, if the fetus is large, a degree of cephalopelvic disproportion will result. The same is true when a malpresentation or malposition of the fetus exists.

The android pelvis

This is so called because it resembles the male pelvis. Its brim is heart shaped with a narrow forepelvis, and has a transverse diameter that is towards the back. The side walls converge, making it a funnel shape with a deep cavity and a straight sacrum. The ischial spines are prominent and the sciatic notch is narrow. The sub-pubic angle is less than 90°. It is found in short and heavily built women who have a tendency to be hirsute. This type of pelvis predisposes to an occipito-posterior position of the fetal head and is the least suited to childbearing.

The heart-shaped brim favours a posterior position of the occiput as a result of insufficient space for the biparietal diameter in the narrow forepelvis, combined

Table 7.1 Features of the four types of pelvis				
Features	**Gynaecoid**	**Android**	**Anthropoid**	**Platypelloid**
Brim	Rounded	Heart-shaped	Long oval	Kidney-shaped
Forepelvis	Generous	Narrow	Narrowed	Wide
Side walls	Straight	Convergent	Divergent	Divergent
Ischial spines	Blunt	Prominent	Blunt	Blunt
Sciatic notch	Rounded	Narrow	Wide	Wide
Sub-pubic angle	90°	<90°	>90°	>90°
Incidence	50%	20%	25%	5%

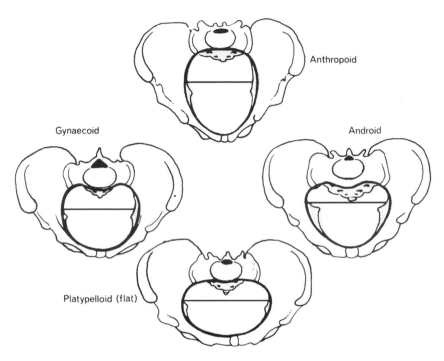

Fig. 7.11 Characteristic inlet of the four types of pelvis.

with the fact that the greater space lies in the hind-pelvis. Funnelling in the cavity may hinder progress in labour. At the pelvic outlet, the prominent ischial spines sometimes prevent complete internal rotation of the head and the anteroposterior diameter becomes caught on them, causing a deep transverse arrest. The narrowed sub-pubic angle cannot easily accommodate the biparietal diameter and this displaces the head backwards (Fig. 7.12). (Posterior positions of the occiput are described in Ch. 30.)

The anthropoid pelvis

This has a long, oval brim in which the anteroposterior diameter is longer than the transverse. The side walls diverge and the sacrum is long and deeply concave. The ischial spines are not prominent and the sciatic notch is very wide, as is the sub-pubic angle. Women with this type of pelvis tend to be tall, with narrow shoulders. Labour does not usually present any difficulties, but a direct occipitoanterior or direct occipitoposterior position is often a feature and the position adopted for engagement may persist to delivery.

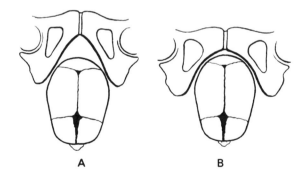

Fig. 7.12 (A) Outlet of android pelvis. The head does not fit into the acute pubic arch and is forced backwards on to the perineum. (B) Outlet of the gynaecoid pelvis. The head fits snugly into the pubic arch.

The platypelloid pelvis

This flat pelvis (Fig. 7.11) has a kidney-shaped brim in which the anteroposterior diameter is reduced and the transverse increased. The side walls diverge, the sacrum is flat and the cavity shallow. The ischial spines are blunt, and the sciatic notch and the sub-pubic angle are both wide. The head must engage with the sagittal

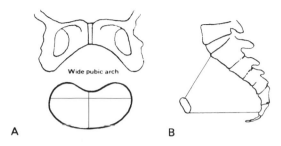

Fig. 7.13 Rachitic flat pelvis. (A) Note wide pubic arch and kidney-shaped brim. (B) The lateral view shows the diminished anteroposterior diameter of the brim and the increased anteroposterior diameter of the outlet.

suture in the transverse diameter, but usually descends through the cavity without difficulty. Engagement may necessitate lateral tilting of the head, known as *asynclitism*, in order to allow the biparietal diameter to pass the narrowest anteroposterior diameter of the brim (Box 7.1).

Other pelvic variations

High assimilation pelvis. This occurs when the 5th lumbar vertebra is fused to the sacrum and the angle of inclination of the pelvic brim is increased. Engagement of the head is difficult but, once achieved, labour progresses normally.

Deformed pelvis. Deformation of the pelvis may result from a developmental anomaly, dietary deficiency, injury or disease (Box 7.2).

Pelvic floor

The pelvic floor is formed by the soft tissues that fill the outlet of the pelvis. The most important of these is the strong diaphragm of muscle slung like a hammock from the walls of the pelvis. Through it pass the urethra, the vagina and the anal canal.

Functions

The pelvic floor supports the weight of the abdominal and pelvic organs. Its muscles are responsible for the voluntary control of micturition and defecation and play an important part in sexual intercourse. During childbirth it influences the passive movements of the fetus through the birth canal and relaxes to allow the exit of the fetus from the pelvis.

Box 7.1 Negotiating the pelvic brim in asynclitism

Anterior asynclitism
The anterior parietal bone moves down behind the symphysis pubis until the parietal eminence enters the brim. The movement is then reversed and the head tilts in the opposite direction until the posterior parietal bone negotiates the sacral promontory and the head is engaged.

Posterior asynclitism
The movements of anterior asynclitism are reversed. The posterior parietal bone negotiates the sacral promontory prior to the anterior parietal bone moving down behind the symphysis pubis.

Once the pelvic brim has been negotiated, descent progresses normally accompanied by flexion and internal rotation.

Muscle layers

The superficial layer. This layer is composed of five muscles (Fig. 7.14):

- The *external anal sphincter* encircles the anus and is attached behind by a few fibres to the coccyx.
- The *transverse perineal muscles* pass from the ischial tuberosities to the centre of the perineum.
- The *bulbocavernosus muscles* pass from the perineum forwards around the vagina to the corpora cavernosa of the clitoris just under the pubic arch.
- The *ischiocavernosus muscles* pass from the ischial tuberosities along the pubic arch to the corpora cavernosa.
- The *membranous sphincter of the urethra* is composed of muscle fibres passing above and below the urethra and attached to the pubic bones. It is not a true sphincter since it is not circular, but it acts to close the urethra.

The deep layer (Fig. 7.15). This layer is composed of three pairs of muscles, which together are known as the *levator ani muscles*. They are so called because they lift or elevate the anus. Each levator ani muscle (left and right) consists of the following:

- The *pubococcygeus muscle* passes from the pubis to the coccyx, with a few fibres crossing over in the perineal body to form its deepest part.

Box 7.2 Deformed pelves

Developmental anomalies

Naegele's and Robert's pelves. Both these rarities are due to failure in development. In the Naegele's pelvis one sacral ala is missing and the sacrum is fused to the ilium, causing a grossly asymmetric brim. The Robert pelvis is similar but bilateral. In both instances the abnormal brim prevents engagement of the fetal head.

Dietary deficiency

Deficiency of vitamins and minerals necessary for the formation of healthy bones is less frequently seen today than in the past but might still complicate pregnancy and labour to some extent. The midwife must be alert for them especially in immigrant or poor populations.

Rachitic pelvis. Rickets in early childhood can lead to gross deformity of the pelvic brim. The weight of the upper body presses downwards on to the softened pelvic bones. The sacral promontory is pushed downwards and forwards and the ilium and ischium are drawn outwards. This results in a flat pelvic brim similar to that of the platypelloid pelvis (see Fig. 7.13). The sacrum tends to be straight with the coccyx bending acutely forward. Because the tuberosities are wide apart, the pubic arch is wide. With the improvements in child care seen throughout the world, this type of pelvis should be infrequently seen. The clinical signs of rickets, bow legs and spinal deformity can occasionally be seen.

If severe contraction is present caesarean section is required to deliver the baby. The fetal head will attempt to enter the pelvis by asynclitism.

Osteomalacic pelvis. The disease osteomalacia is rarely encountered in the UK. It is due to an acquired deficiency of calcium and occurs in adults. All bones of the skeleton soften as a result of gross calcium deficiency. The pelvic canal is squashed together until the brim becomes a Y-shaped slit. Labour is impossible and caesarean section would be performed. In early pregnancy incarceration of the gravid uterus may occur because of the gross deformity.

Injury and disease

Trauma. A pelvis that has been fractured will develop callus formation or may fail to unite correctly. This may lead to reduced measurements and therefore to some degree of contraction. Conditions sustained in childhood such as fractures of the pelvis or lower limbs, congenital dislocation of the hip and poliomyelitis may lead to unequal weightbearing, which will also cause deformity. The child puts her weight on the stronger leg and that side of the pelvis is pressed inwards, leading to flattening of the pelvic brim. With the expert orthopaedic care today, this should be less frequently seen.

Spinal deformity. If kyphosis (forward angulation) or scoliosis (lateral curvature) is evident, or is suggested by a limp or deformity, the midwife must refer the woman to a doctor. Pelvic contraction is likely in these cases and the outcome of pregnancy is dependent on the degree of deformity.

- The *iliococcygeus muscle* passes from the fascia covering the obturator internus muscle (the white line of pelvic fascia) to the coccyx.
- The *ischiococcygeus muscle* passes from the ischial spine to the coccyx, in front of the sacrospinous ligament.

Between the muscle layers, and also above and below them, there are layers of pelvic fascia. This is loose areolar tissue that is used like packing material in the spaces. The tissue that fills the triangular space between the bulbocavernosus, the ischiocavernosus and the transverse perineal muscles is known as the *triangular ligament.*

The perineal body

This is a pyramid of muscle and fibrous tissue situated between the vagina and the rectum. It is made up of fibres from the muscles described above. The apex, which is the deepest part, is formed from the fibres of the pubococcygeus muscle, which cross over at this point; the base is formed from the transverse perineal muscles, which meet in the perineum, together with the bulbocavernosus in front and the external anal

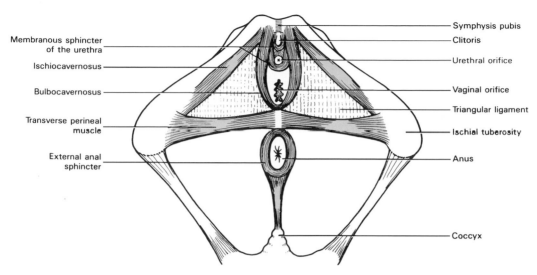

Fig. 7.14 Superficial muscle layer of the pelvic floor.

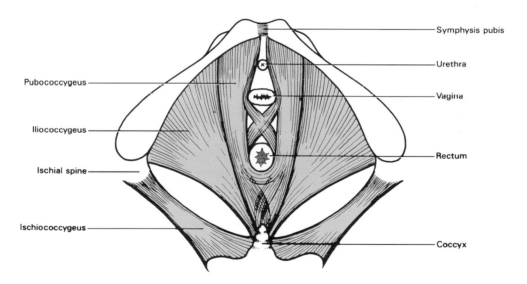

Fig. 7.15 Deep muscle layer of the pelvic floor.

sphincter behind. The perineal body measures 4 cm in each direction. (See also Chs 27 and 15 for the perineum in labour and for pelvic floor exercises.)

The vulva

The term 'vulva' applies to the external female genital organs (Fig. 7.16). It consists of the following structures:

The mons veneris ('mount of Venus') or mons pubis. This is a pad of fat lying over the symphysis pubis. It is covered with pubic hair from the time of puberty.

The labia majora ('greater lips'). These are two folds of fat and areolar tissue, covered with skin and pubic hair on the outer surface. They arise in the mons veneris and merge into the perineum behind.

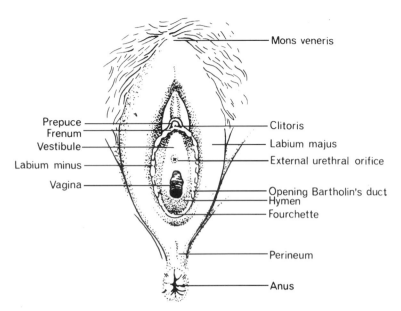

Fig. 7.16 Female external genital organs, or vulva.

The labia minora ('lesser lips'). These are two thin folds of skin lying between the labia majora. Anteriorly they divide to enclose the clitoris; posteriorly they fuse, forming the fourchette.

The clitoris. This is a small rudimentary organ corresponding to the male penis. It is extremely sensitive and highly vascular and plays a part in the orgasm of sexual intercourse.

The vestibule. This is the area enclosed by the labia minora in which are situated the openings of the urethra and the vagina.

The urethral orifice. This orifice lies 2.5 cm posterior to the clitoris. On either side lie the openings of Skene's ducts, two small blind-ended tubules 0.5 cm long running within the urethral wall.

The vaginal orifice. This is also known as the introitus of the vagina and occupies the posterior two-thirds of the vestibule. The orifice is partially closed by the *hymen*, a thin membrane that tears during sexual intercourse or during the birth of the first child. The remaining tags of hymen are known as the 'carunculae myrtiformes' because they are thought to resemble myrtle berries.

Bartholin's glands. There are two small glands that open on either side of the vaginal orifice and lie in the posterior part of the labia majora. They secrete mucus, which lubricates the vaginal opening.

The vulval blood supply

This comes from the internal and the external pudendal arteries. The blood drains through corresponding veins.

Lymphatic drainage

This is mainly via the inguinal glands.

Nerve supply

This is derived from branches of the pudendal nerve. The vaginal nerves supply the erectile tissue of the vestibular bulbs and clitoris and their parasympathetic fibres have a vasodilator effect.

The vagina

Functions

The vagina is a passage that allows the escape of the menstrual flow, receives the penis and the ejected sperm during sexual intercourse and provides an exit for the fetus during delivery.

Position

It is a canal running from the vestibule to the cervix, passing upwards and backwards into the pelvis along a line approximately parallel to the plane of the pelvic brim.

Relations (Figs 7.17 and 7.18)

A knowledge of the relations of the vagina to other organs is essential for the accurate examination of the pregnant woman and her safe delivery.

Anterior. In front of the vagina lie the bladder and the urethra, which are closely connected to the anterior vaginal wall.

Posterior. Behind the vagina lie the pouch of Douglas, the rectum and the perineal body, each occupying approximately one-third of the posterior vaginal wall.

Lateral. On either side of the upper two-thirds are the pelvic fascia and the ureters, which pass beside the cervix; on either side of the lower third are the muscles of the pelvic floor.

Superior. Above the vagina lies the uterus.

Inferior. Below the vagina lie the external genitalia.

Structure

The posterior wall is 10 cm long whereas the anterior wall is only 7.5 cm in length because the cervix projects at a right angle into its upper part.

The upper end of the vagina is known as the *vault*. Where the cervix projects into it, the vault forms a circular recess that is described as four arches or fornices. The posterior fornix is the largest of these because the vagina is attached to the uterus at a higher level behind than in front. The anterior fornix lies in front of the cervix and the lateral fornices lie on either side. The vaginal walls are pink in appearance and thrown into small folds known as *rugae*. These allow the vaginal walls to stretch during intercourse and childbirth.

Layers

The lining is made of squamous epithelium. Beneath the epithelium lies a layer of vascular connective tissue.

The muscle layer is divided into a weak inner coat of circular fibres and a stronger outer coat of longitudinal fibres.

Pelvic fascia surrounds the vagina, forming a layer of connective tissue.

Contents

There are no glands in the vagina. It is, however, moistened by mucus from the cervix and a transudate that seeps out from the blood vessels of the vaginal wall.

In spite of the alkaline mucus, the vaginal fluid is strongly acid (pH 4.5) owing to the presence of lactic acid formed by the action of Döderlein's bacilli on glycogen found in the squamous epithelium of the lining. These lactobacilli are normal inhabitants of the vagina. The acid deters the growth of pathogenic bacteria.

Blood supply

This comes from branches of the internal iliac artery and includes the vaginal artery and a descending branch of the uterine artery. The blood drains through corresponding veins.

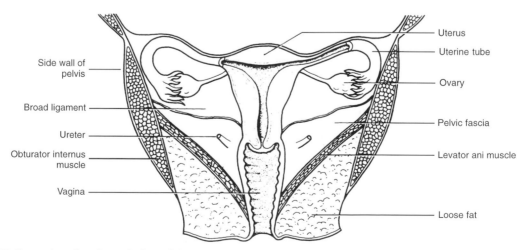

Fig. 7.17 Coronal section through the pelvis.

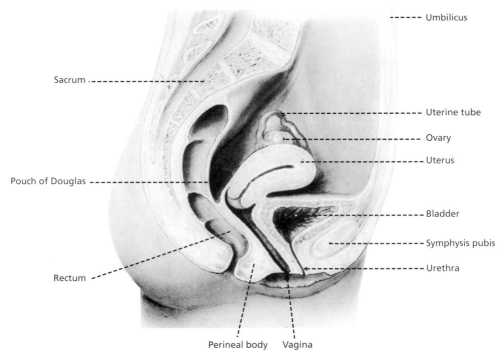

Fig. 7.18 Sagittal section of the pelvis.

Lymphatic drainage

This is via the inguinal, the internal iliac and the sacral glands.

Nerve supply

This is derived from the pelvic plexus. The vaginal nerves follow the vaginal arteries to supply the vaginal walls and also the erectile tissue of the vulva.

The uterus

Functions

The uterus exists to shelter the fetus during pregnancy. It prepares for this possibility each month and following pregnancy it expels the uterine contents.

Position

The uterus is situated in the cavity of the true pelvis, behind the bladder and in front of the rectum. It leans forward, which is known as *anteversion*; it bends forwards on itself, which is known as *anteflexion*. When the woman is standing this results in an almost horizontal position with the fundus resting on the bladder.

Relations (Figs 7.17 and 7.18)

Anterior. In front of the uterus lie the uterovesical pouch and the bladder.

Posterior. Behind the uterus are the rectouterine pouch of Douglas and the rectum.

Lateral. On either side of the uterus are the broad ligaments, the uterine tubes and the ovaries.

Superior. Above the uterus lie the intestines.

Inferior. Below the uterus is the vagina.

Supports

The uterus is supported by the pelvic floor and maintained in position by several ligaments, of which those at the level of the cervix (Fig. 7.19) are the most important.

The transverse cervical ligaments. These fan out from the sides of the cervix to the side walls of the pelvis. They are sometimes known as the 'cardinal ligaments' or 'Mackenrodt's ligaments'.

The uterosacral ligaments. These pass backwards from the cervix to the sacrum.

The pubocervical ligaments. These pass forwards from the cervix, under the bladder, to the pubic bones.

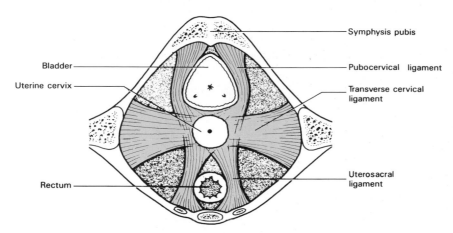

Fig. 7.19 Supports of the uterus, at the level of the cervix.

The broad ligaments. These are formed from the folds of peritoneum, which are draped over the uterine tubes. They hang down like a curtain and spread from the sides of the uterus to the side walls of the pelvis.

The round ligaments. These have little value as a support but tend to maintain the anteverted position of the uterus. They arise from the cornua of the uterus in front of and below the insertion of each uterine tube and pass between the folds of the broad ligament, through the inguinal canal, to be inserted into each labium majus.

The ovarian ligaments. These also begin at the cornua of the uterus but behind the uterine tubes and pass down between the folds of the broad ligament to the ovaries.

It is helpful to note that the round ligament, the uterine tube and the ovarian ligament are very similar in appearance and arise from the same area of the uterus. This makes careful identification important when tubal surgery is undertaken.

Structure

The non-pregnant uterus is a hollow, muscular, pear-shaped organ situated in the true pelvis. It is 7.5 cm long, 5 cm wide and 2.5 cm in depth, each wall being 1.25 cm thick (Fig. 7.20). The cervix forms the lower third of the uterus and measures 2.5 cm in each direction.

The uterus consists of the following parts:

The body or corpus. This makes up the upper two-thirds of the uterus and is the greater part.

The fundus. This is the domed upper wall between the insertions of the uterine tubes.

The cornua. These are the upper outer angles of the uterus where the uterine tubes join.

The cavity. This is a potential space between the anterior and posterior walls. It is triangular in shape, the base of the triangle being uppermost.

The isthmus. This is a narrow area between the cavity and the cervix, which is 7 mm long. It enlarges during pregnancy to form the lower uterine segment.

The cervix or neck. This protrudes into the vagina. The upper half, being above the vagina, is known as the supravaginal portion while the lower half is the infravaginal portion.

The internal os (mouth). This is the narrow opening between the isthmus and the cervix.

The external os. This is a small round opening at the lower end of the cervix. After childbirth it becomes a transverse slit.

The *cervical canal* lies between these two ora and is a continuation of the uterine cavity. This canal is shaped like a spindle, narrow at each end and wider in the middle.

Layers

The uterus has three layers, of which the middle muscle layer is by far the thickest.

The endometrium. This layer forms a lining of ciliated epithelium (mucous membrane) on a base of connective tissue or stroma.

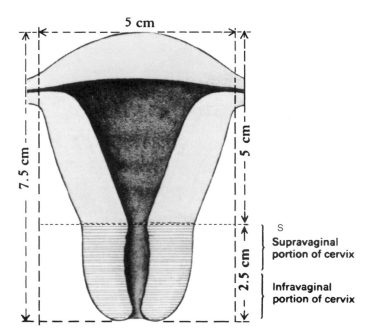

Fig. 7.20 Measurements of the uterus.

In the uterine cavity this endometrium is constantly changing in thickness throughout the menstrual cycle (see Ch. 9). The basal layer does not alter, but provides the foundation from which the upper layers regenerate. The epithelial cells are cubical in shape and dip down to form glands that secrete an alkaline mucus.

The cervical endometrium does not respond to the hormonal stimuli of the menstrual cycle to the same extent. Here the epithelial cells are tall and columnar in shape and the mucus-secreting glands are branching racemose glands. The cervical endometrium is thinner than that of the body and is folded into a pattern known as the 'arbor vitae' (tree of life). This is thought to assist the passage of the sperm. (The portion of the cervix that protrudes into the vagina (see Fig. 7.20) is covered with squamous epithelium similar to that lining the vagina. The point where the epithelium changes, at the external os, is termed the squamo-columnar junction.)

The myometrium, or muscle coat. This layer is thick in the upper part of the uterus and is more sparse in the isthmus and cervix. Its fibres run in all directions and interlace to surround the blood vessels and lymphatics that pass to and from the endometrium. The outer layer is formed of longitudinal fibres that are continuous with those of the uterine tube, the uterine ligaments and the vagina.

In the cervix the muscle fibres are embedded in collagen fibres, which enable it to stretch in labour.

The perimetrium. This is a double serous membrane, an extension of the peritoneum, which is draped over the uterus, covering all but a narrow strip on either side and the anterior wall of the supravaginal cervix from where it is reflected up over the bladder.

Blood supply (Fig. 7.21)

The uterine artery arrives at the level of the cervix and is a branch of the internal iliac artery. It sends a small branch to the upper vagina, and then runs upwards in a twisted fashion to meet the ovarian artery and form an anastomosis with it near the cornu. The ovarian artery is a branch of the abdominal aorta, leaving near the renal artery. It supplies the ovary and uterine tube before joining the uterine artery. The blood drains through corresponding veins.

Lymphatic drainage

Lymph is drained from the uterine body to the internal iliac glands and also from the cervical area to many

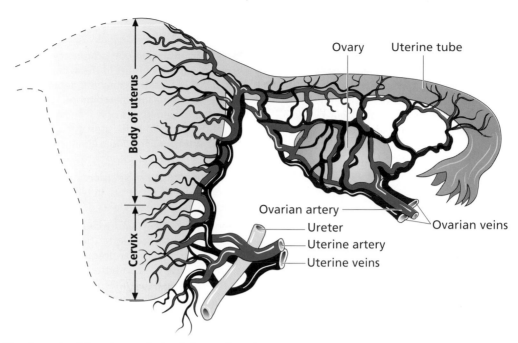

Fig. 7.21 Blood supply of the uterus, uterine tubes and ovaries.

other pelvic lymph glands. This provides an effective defence against uterine infection.

Nerve supply

This is mainly from the autonomic nervous system, sympathetic and parasympathetic, via the inferior hypogastric or pelvic plexus.

Uterine malformations

For pregnancy and labour to be achieved with minimal difficulty, a woman must have normal reproductive anatomy. When structural abnormality of the pelvic organs exists, problems arise that can place an extra burden on mother and fetus. The possible effects of such abnormalities are explained in Box 7.3.

The uterine tubes

Functions

The uterine tube propels the ovum towards the uterus, receives the spermatozoa as they travel upwards and provides a site for fertilisation. It supplies the fertilised ovum with nutrition during its continued journey to the uterus.

Position

The uterine tubes extend laterally from the cornua of the uterus towards the side walls of the pelvis. They arch over the ovaries, the fringed ends hovering near the ovaries in order to receive the ovum.

Relations

Anterior, posterior and superior. In front of, behind and above the uterine tubes are the peritoneal cavity and the intestines.

Lateral. On either side of the uterine tubes are the side walls of the pelvis.

Inferior. The broad ligaments and ovaries lie below the uterine tubes.

Medial. The uterus lies between the two uterine tubes.

Supports

The uterine tubes are held in place by their attachment to the uterus. The peritoneum folds over them, draping down below as the broad ligaments and extending at the sides to form the infundibulopelvic ligaments.

Box 7.3 Uterine malformations

Embryological development of the uterus

The female genital tract is formed in early embryonic life when a pair of ducts develop. These paramesonephric or Müllerian ducts come together in the midline and fuse into a Y-shaped canal. The open upper ends of this structure lead into the peritoneal cavity and the unfused portions become the uterine tubes. The fused lower portion forms the uterovaginal area, which further develops into the uterus and vagina.

Types of uterine malformation

Various types of structural abnormality can result from failure of fusion of the Müllerian ducts. Three of these abnormalities can be seen in Figure 7.22. A double uterus with an associated double vagina will develop where there has been complete failure of fusion. Partial fusion results in various degrees of duplication. A single vagina with a double uterus is the result of fusion at the lower end of the ducts only. A bicornuate uterus (one with two horns) is the result of incomplete fusion at the upper portion of the uterovaginal area. In rare cases, one Müllerian duct regresses and the end result is a uterus with one horn – termed a unicornuate uterus.

Effect of abnormality on pregnancy

When pregnancy occurs in the woman with an abnormal uterus, the outcome depends on the ability of the uterus to accommodate the growing fetus. A problem exists only if the tissue is insufficient to allow the uterus to enlarge for a full-term fetus lying longitudinally.

If there is insufficient hypertrophy, the possible difficulties are abortion, premature labour and abnormal lie of the fetus. In labour, poor uterine function may be experienced.

Minor defects of structure cause little problem and might pass unnoticed with the woman having a normal outcome to her pregnancy. Occasionally problems arise when a fetus is accommodated in one horn of a double uterus and the empty horn has filled the pelvic cavity. In this situation, the empty horn has grown owing to the hormonal influences of the pregnancy, and its size and position will cause obstruction during labour. Caesarean section would be the method of delivery.

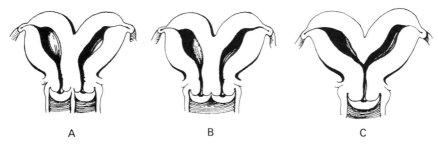

| A | B | C |

Fig. 7.22 Uterine malformations: (A) Double uterus with duplication of body of uterus, cervix and vagina. (B) Duplication of uterus and cervix with single vagina. (C) Duplication of uterus with single cervix and vagina.

Structure

Each tube is 10 cm long. The lumen of the tube provides an open pathway from the outside to the peritoneal cavity. The uterine tube has four portions (Fig. 7.23):

The interstitial portion. This is 1.25 cm long and lies within the wall of the uterus. Its lumen is 1 mm wide.

The isthmus. This is another narrow part that extends for 2.5 cm from the uterus.

The ampulla. This is the wider portion where fertilisation usually occurs. It is 5 cm long.

The infundibulum. This is the funnel-shaped fringed end that is composed of many processes known as *fimbriae*. One fimbria is elongated to form the ovarian fimbria, which is attached to the ovary.

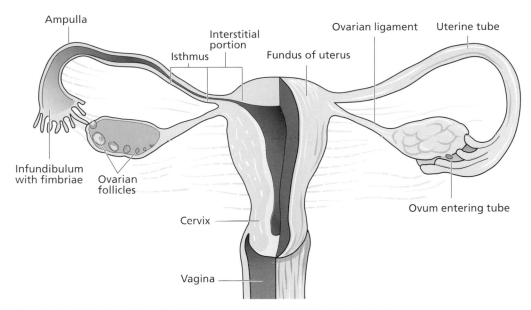

Fig. 7.23 The uterine tubes in section. Note the ovum entering the fimbriated end of one.

Layers (Fig. 7.24)

The lining. This is a mucous membrane of *ciliated cubical epithelium* that is thrown into complicated folds known as plicae. These folds slow the ovum down on its way to the uterus. In this lining are goblet cells that produce a secretion containing glycogen to nourish the ovum.

Beneath the lining is a layer of *vascular connective tissue*.

The muscle coat. This consists of two layers, an inner circular layer and an outer longitudinal layer, both of smooth muscle. The peristaltic movement of the uterine tube is due to the action of these muscles.

The tube is covered with *peritoneum* but the infundibulum passes through it to open into the peritoneal cavity.

Blood supply

This is via the uterine and ovarian arteries, returning by the corresponding veins.

Lymphatic drainage

This is to the lumbar glands.

Nerve supply

This is from the ovarian plexus.

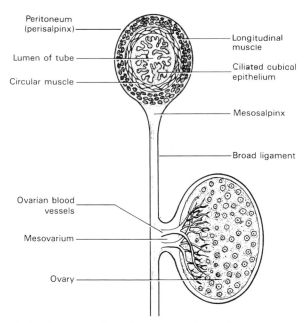

Fig. 7.24 Cross-section of a uterine tube and ovary.

The ovaries

Functions

The ovaries produce ova and the hormones oestrogen and progesterone.

Position

The ovaries are attached to the back of the broad ligaments within the peritoneal cavity.

Relations

Anterior. In front of the ovaries are the broad ligaments.

Posterior. Behind the ovaries are the intestines.

Lateral. On either side of the ovaries are the infundibulopelvic ligaments and the side walls of the pelvis.

Superior. Above the ovaries lie the uterine tubes.

Medial. In between the ovaries lie the uterus and the ovarian ligaments.

Supports

The ovary is attached to the broad ligament but is supported from above by the ovarian ligament medially and the infundibulopelvic ligament laterally.

Structure

The ovary is composed of a medulla and cortex, covered with germinal epithelium.

The medulla. This is the supporting framework, which is made of fibrous tissue; the ovarian blood vessels, lymphatics and nerves travel through it. The hilum where these vessels enter lies just where the ovary is attached to the broad ligament and this area is called the *mesovarium* (Fig. 7.24).

The cortex. This is the functioning part of the ovary. It contains the ovarian follicles in different stages of development, surrounded by stroma. The outer layer is formed of fibrous tissue known as the tunica albuginea. Over this lies the germinal epithelium, which is a modification of the peritoneum.

The cycle of the ovary is described in Chapter 9.

Blood supply

The blood supply is from the ovarian arteries and drains by the ovarian veins. The right ovarian vein joins the inferior vena cava, but the left returns its blood to the left renal vein.

Lymphatic drainage

This is to the lumbar glands.

Nerve supply

This is from the ovarian plexus.

The breasts

The breasts are also linked with the female reproductive system and are described in Chapter 40.

Male reproductive system

(Fig. 7.25)

The scrotum

Function

The scrotum forms a pouch in which the testes are suspended outside the body. It lies below the symphysis pubis and between the upper parts of the thighs behind the penis.

Structure

It is formed of pigmented skin and has two compartments, one for each testis.

The testes

Function

The testes are the male gonads and produce spermatozoa and the hormone testosterone. Testosterone is responsible for the development of secondary sex characteristics. Together with follicle-stimulating hormone (FSH), it also promotes production of sperm.

Position

The testes are situated in the scrotum. In order to achieve their proper function they must be kept below body temperature, and this is why they are situated outside the body.

Structure

Each testis is 4.5 cm long, 2.5 cm wide and 3 cm thick.

Layers

There are three layers to the testis:

Tunica vasculosa. This is an inner layer of connective tissue containing a fine network of capillaries.

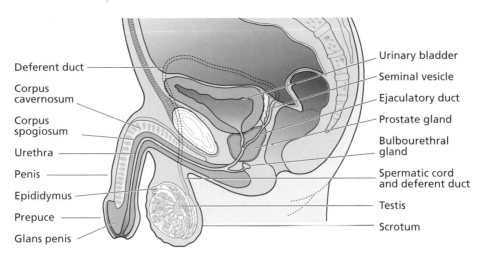

Fig. 7.25 Male reproductive system.

Tunica albuginea. This is a fibrous covering, ingrowths of which divide the testis into 200–300 lobules.

Tunica vaginalis. This is the outer layer, which is made of peritoneum brought down with the descending testis when it migrated from the lumbar region in fetal life.

The duct system is highly intricate:

The seminiferous ('seed-carrying') tubules. These are where spermatogenesis, or production of sperm, takes place. There are up to three of them in each lobule. Between the tubules are interstitial cells that secrete testosterone. The tubules join to form a system of channels that lead to the epididymis.

The epididymis. This is a comma-shaped, coiled tube that lies on the superior surface and travels down the posterior aspect to the lower pole of the testis, where it leads into the *deferent duct* or vas deferens.

The spermatic cord

Function

The spermatic cord transmits the deferent duct up into the body, along with other structures. The function of the deferent duct is to carry the sperm to the ejaculatory duct.

Position

The cord passes upwards through the inguinal canal, where the different structures diverge. The deferent duct then continues upwards over the symphysis pubis and arches backwards beside the bladder. Behind the bladder it merges with the duct from the seminal vesicle and passes through the prostate gland as the ejaculatory duct to join the urethra.

Structure

The spermatic cord consists of the deferent duct, the testicular blood vessels, lymph vessels and nerves.

Blood supply

The testicular artery, a branch of the abdominal aorta, supplies the testis, scrotum and attachments. The testicular veins drain in the same manner as the ovarian veins (see The ovaries, above).

Lymphatic drainage

This is to the lymph nodes round the aorta.

Nerve supply

This is from the 10th and 11th thoracic nerves.

The seminal vesicles

Function

The function of the seminal vesicles is production of a viscous secretion to keep the sperm alive and motile.

Position

The seminal vesicles are two pouches situated posterior to the bladder.

Structure

The seminal vesicles are 5 cm long and pyramid shaped. They are composed of columnar epithelium, muscle tissue and fibrous tissue.

The ejaculatory ducts

These small muscular ducts carry the spermatozoa and the seminal fluid to the urethra.

The prostate gland

Function

The prostate gland produces a thin lubricating fluid that enters the urethra through ducts.

Position

It surrounds the urethra at the base of the bladder, lying between the rectum and the symphysis pubis.

Structure

It is 4 cm transversely, 3 cm in its vertical diameter and 2 cm deep. It is composed of columnar epithelium, a muscle layer and an outer fibrous layer.

The bulbourethral glands

These are two very small glands, which produce yet another lubricating fluid that passes into the urethra just below the prostate gland.

The penis

Functions

It carries the urethra, which is a passage for both urine and semen. During sexual excitement it stiffens (an erection) in order to be able to penetrate the vagina and deposit the semen near the woman's cervix.

Position

The root lies in the perineum, from where it passes forward below the symphysis pubis. The lower two-thirds is outside the body in front of the scrotum.

Structure

There are three columns of erectile tissue:

The **corpora cavernosa.** Two lateral columns form the corpora cavernosa; there is one on either side in front of the urethra.

The **corpus spongiosum.** This is a posterior column that contains the urethra. The tip is expanded to form the glans penis.

The lower two-thirds of the penis is covered in skin. At the end, the skin is folded back on itself above the glans penis to form the prepuce or foreskin, which is a movable double fold. The penis is extremely vascular and during an erection the blood spaces fill and become distended.

The male hormones

The control of the male gonads is similar to that in the female, but it is not cyclical. The hypothalamus produces gonadotrophin-releasing factors. These stimulate the anterior pituitary gland to produce FSH and luteinising hormone (LH). FSH acts on the seminiferous tubules to bring about the production of sperm, whereas LH acts on the interstitial cells that produce testosterone.

Testosterone. This hormone is responsible for the secondary sex characteristics – namely deepening of the voice, growth of the genitalia and growth of hair on the chest, pubis, axilla and face.

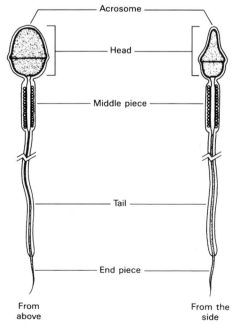

Fig. 7.26 Spermatozoon.

Formation of the spermatozoa

Production of sperm begins at puberty and continues throughout adult life. Spermatogenesis takes place in the seminiferous tubules under the influence of FSH and testosterone. The process of maturation is a lengthy one and takes some weeks. The mature sperm are stored in the epididymis and the deferent duct until ejaculation. If this does not happen, they degenerate and are reabsorbed. At each ejaculation, 2–4 ml of semen are deposited in the vagina. The seminal fluid contains about 100 million sperm per ml, of which 20–25% are likely to be abnormal. The remainder move at a speed of 2–3 mm per minute. The individual spermatozoon has a head, a body and a long, mobile tail that lashes to propel the sperm along (Fig. 7.26). The tip of the head is covered by an acrosome; this contains enzymes to dissolve the covering of the ovum in order to penetrate it.

REFERENCE

Williams P L, Bannister L H, Berry M M et al 1995 Gray's anatomy, 38th edn. Churchill Livingstone, New York

FURTHER READING

Brayshaw E, Wright P 1994 Teaching physical skills for the childbearing year. Books for Midwives Press, Hale, Cheshire

This book, which aims to teach exercises suitable for pregnancy and the puerperium, begins with information on the musculature of the lower body including the abdomen. The second chapter gives details of the changes to the musculoskeletal system during and following pregnancy. Chapter 7 is also worth referring to for postnatal problems.

Beischer N A, Mackay E V, Colditz P B 1997 Obstetrics and the newborn. W B Saunders, London

This book offers photographic as well as line illustrations and some comparative anatomy, for example of the sheep's pelvis as compared with that of the human female.

Burnett C W F 1992 The anatomy and physiology of obstetrics, 7th edn (rev. Anderson M). Faber & Faber, London

This classic text addresses all the physical anatomy relevant to the midwife and is a useful reference.

Coad J with Dunstall M 2001 Anatomy and physiology for midwives. Mosby, Edinburgh

Information in this comprehensive text is similar to that presented in the above chapter. Students may value additional diagrams, text boxes and a fuller account of gametogenesis.

Hinchliff S, Montague S, Watson R (eds) 1996 Physiology for nursing practice, 2nd edn. Baillière Tindall, London.

A good general anatomy text that may be helpful as reference, though the section on reproductive anatomy and physiology is inevitably shorter than that needed for midwives.

Johnson M, Everitt B 2000 Essential reproduction, 5th edn. Blackwell Science, Oxford

In all respects this text is an unsurpassed source of up-to-date explanation of the physiology of reproduction.

Rutishauser S 1994 Physiology and anatomy: a basis for nursing and health care. Churchill Livingstone, Edinburgh.

This is a very clear text that gives a full account of reproduction including aspects of fertility, sexuality and psychological factors. The diagrams are tinted, which may help the student to understand some aspects more clearly.

Stables D 1999 Physiology in childbearing with anatomy and basic sciences. Baillière Tindall, Edinburgh

This is a comprehensive text aimed at midwives. It offers a little more detail than the chapter above and in addition supplies background information such as the structure of the cell and the nature of bone and muscles, which may be helpful to students pre-registration.

Verralls S 1993 Anatomy and physiology of obstetrics, 3rd edn. Churchill Livingstone, Edinburgh

This text for student midwives is popular because of the very simple line drawings that show structures in diagrammatic fashion. It also addresses application of the knowledge in specific areas.

Williams P L, Bannister L H, Berry M M et al 1995 Gray's anatomy, 38th edn. Churchill Livingstone, New York

A large volume with detailed information about the anatomy of every part of the human body that will provide the reader with much more insight into the structure and function of the reproductive organs.

8 The Female Urinary Tract

V. Ruth Bennett   Linda K. Brown

The urinary system is chiefly thought of in connection with its elimination function and the production of urine. It also has important functions in connection with the control of water and electrolyte balance and of blood pressure.

In the female the urinary tract has an importance associated with its proximity to the reproductive organs. When the woman is not pregnant, her uterus lies just behind and partly over the bladder. When she is pregnant the enlarging uterus affects all the parts of the urinary tract at various times and the hormones of pregnancy have an even greater influence than the mechanical effects. The normal, healthy woman may perceive these changes as a minor nuisance created by frequency of micturition and her kidneys continue to function well. A few may experience complications and those who already have diseased kidneys may undergo deterioration in their condition: some women suffer impairment of the function of part of the urinary tract as a direct result of pregnancy. The midwife may have an important part to play in minimising any ill-effect.

The urinary tract begins at the two kidneys, which are linked up to the blood supply by the large renal arteries and veins. It continues as a passage for urine in the two ureters, the bladder and the urethra.

The kidneys

The kidneys are two bean-shaped glands that have both endocrine and exocrine secretions. Their function is to extract soluble wastes from the blood and to excrete such water and minerals as are surplus to the body's requirements. They also prevent substances that are needed by the body from being lost. They have a part to play in red cell production and in maintaining blood pressure.

Position and supports

The kidneys are positioned at the back of the abdominal cavity, high up under the diaphragm. The right kidney is displaced a little downwards by the liver, so the two kidneys are not quite level. They are maintained in position by a generous packing of perinephric fat and by the closeness of neighbouring organs, particularly parts of the gastrointestinal tract in front and the musculature of the posterior abdominal wall behind (Fig. 8.1).

Appearance

The gland is recognisable by its dark red appearance and typical shape, so that other similarly shaped objects may be called 'kidney-shaped'. It is about 10 cm long, 6.5 cm wide and 3 cm thick. It weighs around 120 g. It is covered with a tough, fibrous capsule.

The inner border of the organ is indented at the hilum; here the large vessels enter and leave and the ureter is attached by its funnel-shaped upper end to channel the urine away.

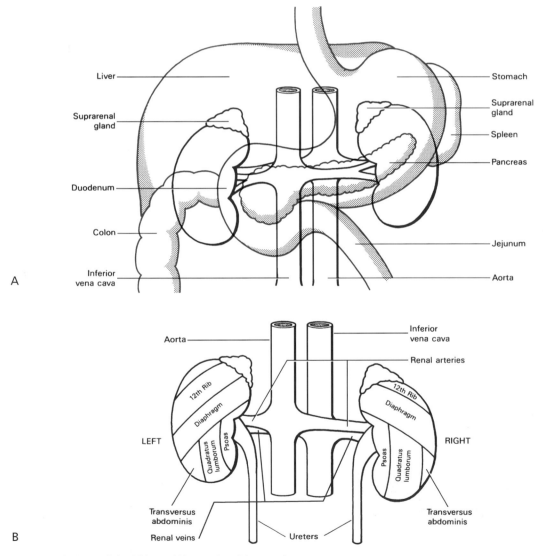

Fig. 8.1 Relations of the kidney: (A) anterior; (B) posterior.

Inner structure

The glandular tissue is formed of *cortex* on the outside and *medulla* within. The cortex is dark with a rich blood supply, whereas the medulla is paler. A collecting area for urine merges with the upper ureter and is called the *pelvis*. It is divided into branches or calyces and each calyx cups over a projection from the medulla known as a *pyramid*. There are some 12 pyramids in all and they contain bundles of tubules leading from the cortex. The tubules create a lined appearance and these are the *medullary rays*. The base of each pyramid is curved and the cortex arches over it (Fig. 8.2) and projects downwards between the pyramids forming columns of tissue (*columns of Bertini*).

The nephrons

When the tissue of the kidney is examined under the microscope, it is found to be formed of about 1 million nephrons, which are its functional units.

The manufacture of urine depends on a constant and generous supply of blood. Each nephron starts at a knot of capillaries called a *glomerulus* (Fig. 8.3). It is fed by a branch of the renal artery, the *afferent arteriole*, and the blood is collected up again into the *efferent arteriole*. Afferent means 'carrying towards' and efferent 'carrying away'. This is the only place in the body where an artery collects blood from capillaries. The blood vessel continues alongside the nephron.

Surrounding the glomerulus is a cup known as the *glomerular capsule*, into which fluid and solutes are exuded from the blood. The glomerulus and capsule together are the *glomerular body* (Fig. 8.3). The pressure within the glomerulus is raised because the afferent arteriole is of a wider bore than the efferent arteriole and this factor forces the filtrate out of the capillaries and into the capsule. At this stage there is no selection; any substance with a small molecular size will filter out.

The cup of the capsule is attached to a tubule as a wine glass to its stem. The tubule initially winds and twists, then forms a straight loop which dips into the medulla, rising up into the cortex again to wind and turn before joining a *straight collecting tubule*, which receives urine from several nephrons. The first twisting portion of the nephron is the *proximal convoluted tubule*, the loop is termed the *loop of Henle* and the

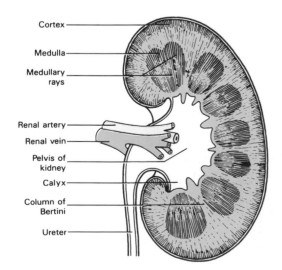

Fig. 8.2 Longitudinal section of the kidney.

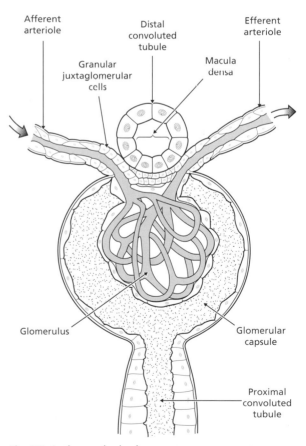

Fig. 8.3 A glomerular body.

second twisting portion is the *distal convoluted tubule*. The whole nephron is about 3 cm in length (Fig. 8.4). The straight collecting tubule runs from the cortex to a medullary pyramid; it forms a medullary ray and receives urine from over 4000 nephrons along its length.

Juxtaglomerular apparatus. The distal convoluted tubule returns to pass alongside granular cells of the afferent arteriole and this part of the tubule is called the *macula densa* (see Fig. 8.3). The two are known as the *juxtaglomerular apparatus*. The granular cells secrete renin (see Endocrine activity), whereas the macula densa cells monitor the sodium chloride concentration of fluid passing through.

Blood supply

The renal arteries are early branches of the descending abdominal aorta and divert about a quarter of the cardiac output into the kidneys. The artery enters at the renal hilum between the ureter behind and the renal vein in front. It sends numerous branches into the cortex and forms a glomerulus for each nephron. Blood is collected up and returned via the renal vein (see Fig. 8.1).

Lymphatic drainage

A rich supply of lymph vessels lies under the cortex and around the urine-bearing tubules. It drains into large lymphatic ducts that emerge from the hilum and lead to the aortic lymph glands.

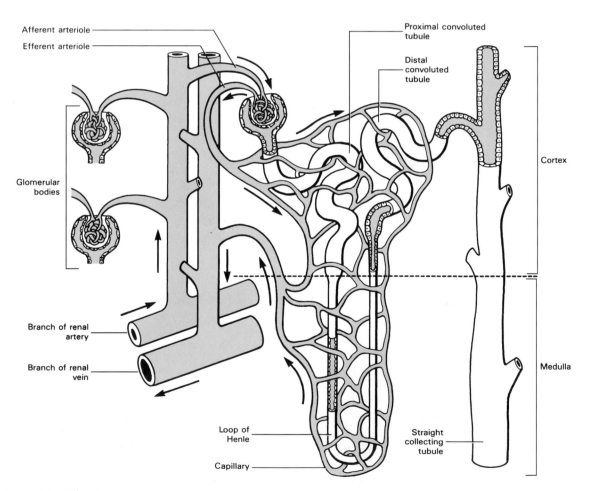

Fig. 8.4 A nephron.

Nerve supply

Nerves enter by the renal hilum and provide a sympathetic and parasympathetic nerve supply.

The making of urine

This takes place in three stages:

- filtration
- reabsorption
- secretion.

Filtration. This is the simple process of water and the substances dissolved in it being passed from the glomerulus into the glomerular capsule as a result of the raised intracapillary pressure. Blood components such as corpuscles and platelets as well as plasma proteins, which have a large molecule, are kept in the blood vessel; water, salts and glucose escape through the filter as the *filtrate* (Fig. 8.5). A vast amount of fluid passes out in this way, about 2 ml per second or 120 ml per minute. Ninety-nine per cent of this must be recovered, or the body would be totally drained of fluid within hours. Filtration is increased in pregnancy as it helps to eliminate the additional wastes created by maternal and fetal metabolism.

Reabsorption. The body selects from the filtrate the substances which it needs: water, salts and glucose.

Normally all the glucose is reabsorbed; only if there is already more than sufficient in the blood, for example after eating sweet or sugary foods, will any be excreted in the urine. The level of blood glucose at which this happens is the *renal threshold* for glucose. In the non-pregnant woman, the threshold is 10 mmol/l and in the pregnant woman 8.3 mmol/l. It is more likely, therefore, that glucose will appear in the urine during pregnancy.

The water is almost all reabsorbed. If the body has lost fluid by other means, such as sweating, or if fluid intake has been low, then more water is conserved, less urine is passed and the urine appears more concentrated. In the opposite circumstances, when the individual has drunk a lot of water and is sweating little, the urine is more copious and dilute. Note that drinking alcohol does not have this effect. The posterior pituitary gland controls the reabsorption of water by producing antidiuretic hormone (ADH). The more ADH produced, the more water is reabsorbed. Newborn babies are poorly able to concentrate and

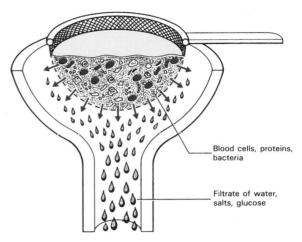

Fig. 8.5 Filtration: larger molecules stay in the sieve (glomerulus) and smaller molecules filter out (into the glomerular capsule).

Labels in figure:
Blood cells, proteins, bacteria
Filtrate of water, salts, glucose

dilute their urine, and preterm infants even less so. For this reason they are unable to tolerate wide variations in their fluid intake. Pregnant women pass a greater amount of urine than when non-pregnant.

Minerals are selected according to the body's needs. The reabsorption of sodium is controlled by aldosterone, which is produced in the cortex of the adrenal gland. The interaction of aldosterone and ADH maintains water and sodium balance. The pH of the blood must be controlled and if it is tending towards acidity then acids will be excreted. This is commonly the case. However, if the opposite pertains, alkaline urine will be produced. Often this is the result of an intake of an alkaline substance.

Secretion. Certain substances, such as creatinine and toxins, are added directly to the urine in the ascending arm of the loop of Henle.

Endocrine activity

The kidney secretes two hormones. One, renin, is produced in the afferent arteriole and is secreted when the blood supply to the kidneys is reduced and in response to lowered sodium levels. It acts on angiotensinogen, which is present in the blood, to form angiotensin, which raises blood pressure and encourages sodium reabsorption. The second hormone, erythropoietin, stimulates the production of red blood cells.

Summary of functions

The kidney functions may be summarised as follows:

- elimination of wastes, particularly the breakdown products of protein, such as urea, urates, uric acid, creatinine, ammonia and sulphates
- elimination of toxins
- regulation of the water content of the blood and indirectly of the tissues
- regulation of the pH of the blood
- regulation of the osmotic pressure of the blood
- secretion of the hormones renin and erythropoietin.

The urine

Urine is a yellow colour ranging from pale straw colour when very dilute to dark brown if very concentrated. In the newborn baby it is almost clear. It has a recognisable smell, which in health is not unpleasant when freshly passed. It should never be cloudy.

An adult passes between 1 and 2 litres of urine daily, depending on fluid intake. Less is produced during the night than in the day. Pregnant women secrete large amounts of urine because of the increased glomerular filtration rate and they often have to rise at night to empty the bladder (see Ch. 13). In the first day or two postpartum a major diuresis occurs and urine output is copious.

The specific gravity of urine is 1.010–1.030. It is composed of 96% water, 2% urea and 2% other solutes. Urea and uric acid clearance are increased in pregnancy. Urine is usually acid and contains no glucose or ketones, nor should it carry blood cells or bacteria. Women are susceptible to urinary tract infection but this is usually an ascending infection acquired via the urethra. A low count, less than 100 000 per ml, of bacteria in the urine (bacteriuria) is treated as insignificant.

The ureters

The tubes that convey the urine from the kidneys to the bladder are the ureters. They assist the passage of the urine by the muscular peristaltic action of their walls. The upper end is funnel shaped and merges into the pelvis of the kidney where the urine is received from the renal tubules.

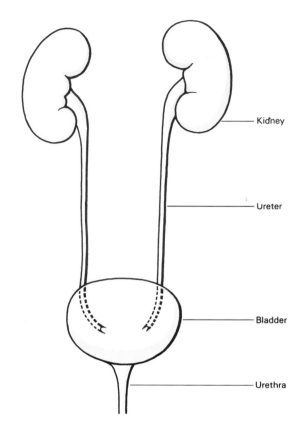

Fig. 8.6 The renal tract.

Each tube is about 25–30 cm long and runs from the renal hilum to the posterior wall of the bladder (Fig. 8.6). In the abdomen they pass down the posterior wall, remaining outside the peritoneal cavity. On reaching the pelvic brim, they descend along the side walls of the pelvis to the level of the ischial spines and then turn forwards to pass beside the uterine cervix and enter the bladder from behind. They pass through the bladder wall at an angle (Fig. 8.7) so that when the bladder contracts to expel urine the ureters are closed off and reflux is prevented.

Structure

The ureters have three main layers:

The lining. This is formed of transitional epithelium arranged in longitudinal folds. This type of epithelium consists of several layers of pear-shaped cells and makes an elastic and waterproof inner coat.

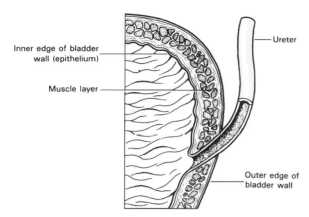

Inner edge of bladder wall (epithelium)

Muscle layer

Ureter

Outer edge of bladder wall

Fig. 8.7 Diagram to show the entry of the ureter into the posterior wall of the bladder.

The muscular layer. This is arranged as an inner longitudinal layer, a middle circular layer and an outer longitudinal layer. Waves of peristalsis pass along the ureter towards the bladder.

The outer coat. This is of fibrous connective tissue, which is protective. It is continuous with the fibrous capsule of the kidney.

Blood, lymph and nerve supply

The upper part of the ureter is supplied similarly to the kidney. In its pelvic portion it derives blood from the common iliac and internal iliac arteries and from the uterine and vesical arteries, according to its proximity to the different organs. Venous return is along corresponding veins.

Lymph drains into the internal, external and common iliac lymph nodes.

The nerve supply is sympathetic and parasympathetic.

The ureter in pregnancy

The hormones of pregnancy, particularly progesterone, relax the walls of the ureters and allow dilatation and kinking. In some women this is quite marked and it tends to result in a slowing down or stasis of urinary flow, making infection a greater possibility (Fig. 8.8; see also Ch. 13).

The bladder

The bladder is the urinary reservoir, storing the urine until it is convenient for it to be voided. It is described

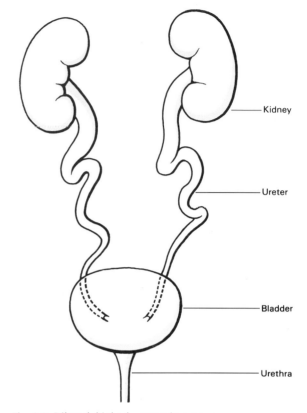

Kidney

Ureter

Bladder

Urethra

Fig. 8.8 Dilated, kinked ureters in pregnancy.

as being pyramidal; its base is triangular. When it is full, however, it becomes more globular in shape as its walls are distended. Although it is a pelvic organ it may rise into the abdomen when full, and during labour it is certainly abdominal. It is one of the organs that most greatly concern midwives because of its closeness to the uterus.

Position

In the non-pregnant female, the bladder lies immediately behind the symphysis pubis and in front of the uterus and vagina (Fig. 8.9). In addition, the anteverted, anteflexed uterus lies partially over the bladder superiorly. The intestines and peritoneal cavity also lie above. The ureters enter the bladder from behind; the urethra leaves it from below. Underneath the bladder is the muscular diaphragm of the pelvic floor, which forms its main support and on which its function partly depends.

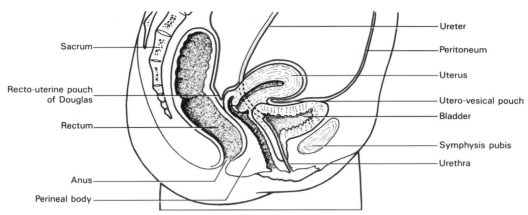

Fig. 8.9 Sagittal section of the pelvis showing the relations of the bladder.

Structure

The base of the bladder is termed the *trigone*. It is situated at the back of the bladder, resting against the vagina. Its three angles are the exit of the urethra below and the two slit-like openings of the ureters above. The apex of the trigone is thus at its lowest point, which is also termed the neck (Fig. 8.10).

The anterior part of the bladder lies close to the pubic symphysis and is termed the apex of the bladder. From it the urachus runs up the anterior abdominal wall to the umbilicus. In fetal life this is the remains of the yolk sac but in the adult is simply a fibrous band.

The empty bladder is of similar size to the uterus but when full of urine it becomes, of course, much larger. Its capacity is around 600 ml but it is capable of holding more, particularly under the influence of pregnancy hormones. The midwife will commonly observe a woman who has recently given birth voiding upwards of 1 litre on a single occasion.

Layers

The lining. The lining of the bladder, like that of the ureter, is formed of transitional epithelium, which helps to allow the distension of the bladder without losing its water-holding effect.

The lining, except over the trigone, is thrown into wrinkles or *rugae*, which flatten out as the bladder expands and fills.

The mucous membrane lining lies on a submucous layer of areolar tissue that carries blood and lymph vessels and nerves.

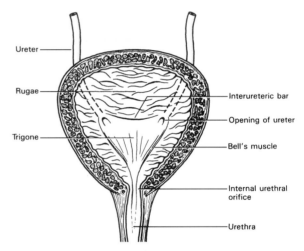

Fig. 8.10 Section through the bladder.

The epithelium over the trigone is smooth and firmly attached to the underlying muscle.

The musculature. The musculature of the bladder consists chiefly of the large detrusor muscle whose function is to expel urine. (To detrude is to thrust down to a lower place.) This muscle has an inner longitudinal, a middle circular and an outer longitudinal layer. Around the neck of the bladder, the circular muscle is thickened to form the *internal urethral sphincter*. The general elasticity of the numerous muscle fibres around the bladder neck tend to keep the urethra closed (Williams et al 1995).

In the trigone the muscles are somewhat differently arranged. A band of muscle between the ureteric apertures forms the *interureteric bar*. The urethral dilator muscle lies in the ventral part of the bladder neck and the walls of the urethra and is thought to be of significance in overcoming urethral resistance to micturition (Williams et al 1995).

The outer layer. This layer of the bladder is formed of visceral pelvic fascia, except on its superior surface, which is covered with peritoneum (see Fig. 8.9).

Blood, lymph and nerve supplies

The vesical arteries, superior and inferior, are the main suppliers of blood. A few small branches from the uterine and vaginal arteries also bring blood to the bladder. Corresponding veins return used blood.

Lymph drains into the internal iliac glands and into the obturator glands.

The nerve supply is parasympathetic and sympathetic and comes via the important Lee–Frankenhäuser pelvic plexus in the pouch of Douglas. The stimulation of sympathetic nerves causes the internal urethral sphincter to contract and the detrusor muscle to relax, whereas the parasympathetic nerve fibres cause the bladder to empty and the sphincter to relax.

The urethra

The final passage in the urinary tract is the urethra, which is 4 cm long in the female and consists of a narrow tube buried in the outer layers of the anterior vaginal wall. It runs from the neck of the bladder and opens into the vestibule of the vulva as the urethral meatus. During labour the urethra becomes elongated as the bladder is drawn up into the abdomen and may become several centimetres longer.

Structure

The lining. The urethra forms the junction between the urinary tract and the external genitalia. The epithelium of its lining reflects this. The upper half is lined with transitional epithelium whereas the lower half is lined with squamous epithelium. The lumen is normally closed unless urine is passing down it or a catheter is in situ. When closed, it has small longitudinal folds. Small blind ducts called urethral crypts open into the urethra, of which the two largest are Skene's ducts, which open just beside the urethral meatus. Their main significance is in the possibility of infection with an organism such as the gonococcus.

The submucous coat. The epithelium of the urethra lies on a bed of vascular connective tissue.

The musculature. The muscle layers are arranged as an inner longitudinal layer, continuous with the inner muscle fibres of the bladder, and an external circular layer. The inner muscle fibres help to open the internal urethral sphincter during micturition.

The outer layer of the urethra is continuous with the outer layer of the vagina and is formed of connective tissue.

The external sphincter. At the lower end of the urethra, voluntary, striated muscle fibres form the so-called membranous sphincter of the urethra. This is not a true sphincter but it gives some voluntary control to the woman when she desires to resist the urge to urinate. The powerful levator ani muscles, which pass on either side of the uterus, also assist in controlling continence of urine.

Blood, lymph and nerve supplies

The blood is circulated by the inferior vesical and pudendal arteries and veins. Lymph drains to the internal iliac glands.

The internal urethral sphincter is supplied by sympathetic and parasympathetic nerves but the membranous sphincter is supplied by the pudendal nerve and is under voluntary control.

Micturition

The urge to pass urine is felt when the bladder contains about 200–300 ml of urine, but also when psychological stimuli operate such as waking after sleep, arriving or leaving home, and from external stimuli such as the sound and feel of water and the feel of the toilet seat. Helpless laughter or paroxysmal coughing may also trigger a desire to empty the bladder.

In newborn babies there is no resistance to the spontaneous prompting of the bladder that it wishes to be emptied. The sphincters relax, the detrusor muscle contracts and urine is passed. After about 2 years a child learns to resist the urge to void and by adulthood it is taken for granted. Many women, particularly the pregnant and parous, experience difficulty in maintaining continence under the stress of coughing, laughing, sneezing and other factors that raise intra-abdominal pressure. Regular muscular exercise such as walking, swimming, running and pelvic floor exercises help to raise the tone of the voluntary muscles.

In summary, the bladder fills and then contracts as a reflex response. The internal sphincter opens by the action of Bell's muscles (see Fig. 8.10). If the urge is not resisted, the external sphincter relaxes and the bladder empties. The act of emptying may be speeded by raising intra-abdominal pressure either to initiate the process or throughout voiding. The act of micturition can be temporarily postponed but the full bladder becomes progressively more uncomfortable.

REFERENCE

Williams P L, Bannister L H, Berry M H et al 1995 Gray's anatomy, 38th edn. Churchill Livingstone, New York

FURTHER READING

Beischer N A, Mackay E V 1997 Obstetrics and the newborn, 3rd edn. W B Saunders, London

Chapter 38 in this book offers an account of changes in pregnancy with radiological/ultrasound illustrations, as well as addressing urinary tract problems associated with childbearing.

Coad J with Dunstall M 2001 Anatomy and physiology for midwives. Mosby, Edinburgh

Chapter 2 of this book gives a very accessible account of the urinary system and a number of examples of clinical applications. A stylised diagram of urine production may help the individual who learns best from visual representation.

McLaren S M 1996 Renal function. In: Hinchliff S, Montague S, Watson R (eds) Physiology for nursing practice, 2nd edn. Baillière Tindall, London

This excellent chapter amply describes the functioning of the human kidney with full explanations of chemistry and of hormonal control. There is discussion of many urinary problems. Illustrations are simple and enhanced with colour.

Rutishauser S 1994 Physiology and anatomy: a basis for nursing and health care. Churchill Livingstone, Edinburgh

A good text with clear explanations and illustrations that amplify this subject.

Stables D 1999 Physiology in childbearing with anatomy and basic sciences. Baillière Tindall, Edinburgh

This text offers a fuller account of the urinary system, including changes in pregnancy and a short account of the postnatal period.

9 Hormonal Cycles: Fertilisation and Early Development

V. Ruth Bennett   Linda K. Brown

CHAPTER CONTENTS

The biological cycles of a woman follow a monthly pattern and have a profound influence on her life and behaviour. When a woman is sexually active and no fertility control is used, recurring pregnancies will intervene and may obliterate the pattern for most of her fertile life. These cycles are first described without this interruption.

The hypothalamus is the ultimate source of control and it governs the anterior pituitary gland by hormonal pathways. The anterior pituitary gland in turn governs the ovary by hormones. Finally the ovary produces hormones that control changes in the uterus. All these changes occur simultaneously and in harmony. A woman's moods may change along with the cycle and emotional influences can alter the cycle because of the close relationship between the hypothalamus and the cerebral cortex.

The ovarian cycle

The ovarian cortex contains 200 000 primordial follicles at birth. Some of these become cystic and are then known as Graafian follicles. From puberty onwards, certain follicles enlarge and one matures each month to liberate an ovum.

Graafian follicle (Fig. 9.1). The ovum is situated at one end of the Graafian follicle and is encircled by the narrow *perivitelline space*. Surrounding this lies a clump of cells called the *discus proligerus*, the cells of which radiate outwards to form the *corona radiata*. The innermost cells of the corona are very clear and are referred to as the *zona pellucida*. The whole follicle is lined with granulosa cells and contains follicular fluid. The outer coat of the follicle is the *external limiting membrane* and around this lies an area of compressed ovarian stroma known as the *theca*.

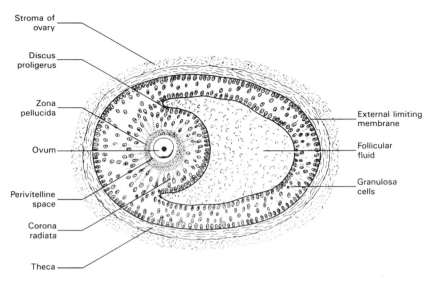

Fig. 9.1 A ripe Graafian follicle.

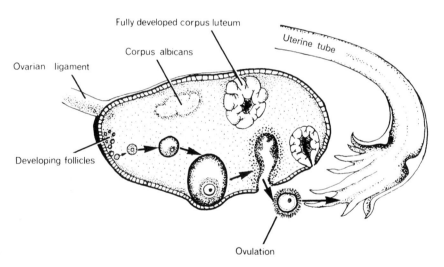

Fig. 9.2 The life cycle of a Graafian follicle.

Under the influence of follicle stimulating hormone (FSH) and, later, luteinising hormone (LH) the Graafian follicle matures and moves to the surface of the ovary. At the same time it swells and becomes tense, finally rupturing to release the ovum into the fimbriated end of the uterine tube, which is cupped underneath the ovary in readiness (Fig. 9.2). This is *ovulation*. Some women feel pain at this time; this may be related to a small loss of blood into the peritoneal cavity and is termed 'mittelschmerz'.

The empty follicle is known as the *corpus luteum* (yellow body).

Corpus luteum. After ovulation the follicle collapses, the granulosa cells enlarge and proliferate over the next 14 days and the whole structure becomes irregular in outline and yellow in colour. Unless pregnancy occurs, the corpus luteum will then atrophy and become the *corpus albicans* (white body) (Fig. 9.2). The ovary contains a number of these white bodies in varying stages of degeneration.

Ovarian hormones

Oestrogen. This comprises a number of compounds including oestriol, oestradiol and oestrone. They are produced under the influence of FSH by the granulosa cells and the theca in increasing amounts until the degeneration of the corpus luteum when the level falls.

The effects of oestrogen are widespread. It is responsible for the secondary sex characteristics such as the female shape, the growth of the breasts and the uterus and the female distribution of hair. It influences the production of cervical mucus and the structure of the vaginal epithelium. This in turn encourages the growth of Döderlein's bacilli, which are responsible for the acidity of the vaginal fluid. During the cycle, oestrogen causes the proliferation of the uterine endometrium. It inhibits FSH and encourages fluid retention.

Progesterone. This, with related compounds, is produced by the corpus luteum under the influence of LH. They act only on tissues that have previously been affected by oestrogen.

The effects of progesterone are mainly evident during the second half of the cycle. It causes secretory changes in the lining of the uterus, when the endometrium develops tortuous glands and an enriched blood supply in readiness for the possible arrival of a fertilised ovum. It causes the body temperature to rise by $0.5\,°C$ after ovulation and gives rise to tingling and a sense of fullness in the breasts prior to menstruation.

The changes caused by progesterone in pregnancy are listed in Chapter 13.

Relaxin. This is a hormone that has been measured in human blood and is at its maximum level between weeks 38 and 42 of pregnancy. It originates in the corpus luteum and is thought to relax the pelvic girdle, to soften the cervix and to suppress uterine contractions. Although it reduces oxytocin release it does not affect the increasing number of oxytocin receptors in the myometrium. The presence of these receptors is a more important factor in labour than the actual level of oxytocin (Steer 1990).

Pituitary control

Under the influence of the hypothalamus, which produces gonadotrophin-releasing hormone (GnRH), the anterior pituitary gland (adenohypophysis) secretes two gonadotrophins: FSH and LH. GnRH is released in a series of pulses about an hour apart and the gonadotrophins likewise are secreted in a pulsatile manner (Johnson & Everitt 2000). This appears to be crucial to the normal pattern of the menstrual cycle. The gonadotrophic activity of the hypothalamus and the pituitary is influenced by positive and negative feedback mechanisms from ovarian hormones.

FSH. This hormone causes several Graafian follicles to develop and enlarge, one of them more than all the others. FSH stimulates the granulosa cells and theca to secrete oestrogen. The level of FSH rises during the first half of the cycle and when the oestrogen level reaches a certain point its production is stopped.

LH. This is first produced a few days after the anterior pituitary starts producing FSH. Rising oestrogen causes a surge in both FSH and LH levels, the ripened follicle ruptures and ovulation occurs. Levels of both gonadotrophins then fall rapidly. Progesterone inhibits any new rise in LH in spite of high oestrogen levels, but if no pregnancy occurs the corpus luteum degenerates after 14 days. The negative feedback effect of progesterone ceases and FSH and LH levels rise again to begin a new cycle (Johnson & Everitt 2000).

Prolactin. This is also produced in the anterior pituitary gland, but it does not play a part in the control of the ovary. If produced in excessive amounts, however, it will inhibit ovulation, a phenomenon that occurs naturally during breastfeeding (see Ch. 40).

The uterine cycle or menstrual cycle (Fig. 9.3)

Although each woman has an individual cycle that varies in length, the average cycle is taken to be 28 days long and recurs regularly from puberty to the menopause except when pregnancy intervenes. The first day of the cycle is the day on which menstruation begins. There are three main phases and they affect the tissue structure of the endometrium, controlled by the ovarian hormones.

The menstrual phase. This phase, characterised by vaginal bleeding, lasts for 3–5 days. Physiologically this is the terminal phase of the menstrual cycle when the endometrium is shed down to the basal layer along with blood from the capillaries and with the unfertilised ovum.

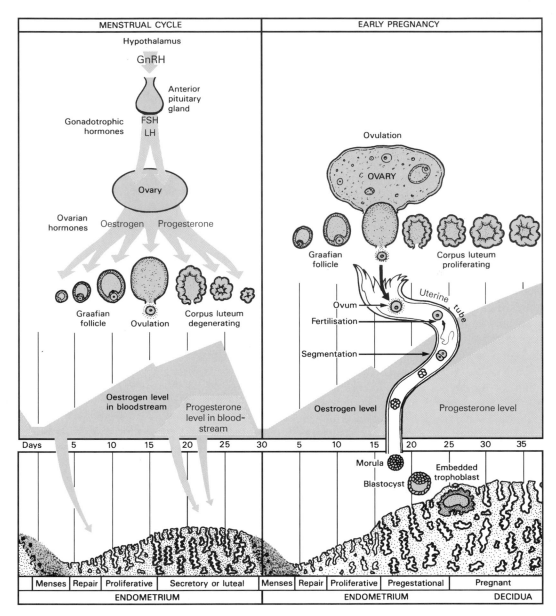

Fig. 9.3 Menstrual cycle (left half): diagrammatic representation of the action of the gonadotrophic hormones on the ovary and of the ovarian hormones on the endometrium. Early pregnancy (right half): diagrammatic representation showing ovulation, fertilisation, decidual reaction and embedding of the fertilised ovum.

The proliferative phase. This follows menstruation and lasts until ovulation. Sometimes the first few days while the endometrium is re-forming are described as the *regenerative phase*. This phase is under the control of oestrogen and consists of the regrowth and thickening of the endometrium. At the completion of this phase the endometrium consists of three layers:

A *basal layer* lies immediately above the myometrium, about 1 mm in thickness. This layer never alters during the menstrual cycle. It contains all the necessary rudimentary structures for building up new endometrium.

A *functional layer* which contains tubular glands and is 2.5 mm thick. It changes constantly according to the hormonal influences of the ovary.

A *layer of cuboidal ciliated epithelium* covers the functional layer. It dips down to line the tubular glands.

The secretory phase. This phase follows ovulation and is under the influence of progesterone and oestrogen from the corpus luteum. The functional layer thickens to 3.5 mm and becomes spongy in appearance because the glands are more tortuous.

Puberty

This is the period in life during which the reproductive organs undergo a surge in development and reach maturity. The first signs are breast development and the appearance of pubic hair. The body grows considerably and takes on the female shape. Puberty culminates in the onset of menstruation, the first period being called the *menarche*. The first few cycles are not usually accompanied by ovulation so that conception is unlikely before a girl has been menstruating for a year or two.

Menopause

The end of a woman's reproductive life is marked by the gradual cessation of menstruation, the cycles first becoming irregular and then ceasing altogether at the *menopause*. This time of life is known as the *climacteric*. It is often accompanied by physical symptoms like hot flushes and emotional changes such as mood swings. There is an increased tendency to obesity and in the following years signs of ageing will appear. These changes are due to a fall in the production of oestrogen because the ovary is no longer able to respond to pituitary gonadotrophins. The sexual drive may not be diminished but some women find it difficult to accept that they are no longer fertile. The menopause usually occurs around the age of 50 years but it should not be assumed that the climacteric is complete until 2 years have elapsed since the last period. In the intervening months the woman should continue to use contraception if appropriate.

Fertilisation

Following ovulation, the ovum, which is about 0.15 mm in diameter, passes into the uterine tube and is moved along towards the uterus. The ovum, having no power of locomotion, is wafted along by the cilia and by the peristaltic muscular contraction of the tube. At this time the cervix, under the influence of oestrogen, secretes a flow of alkaline mucus that attracts the spermatozoa. At intercourse about 300 million sperm are deposited in the posterior fornix of the vagina. Those that reach the loose cervical mucus survive to propel themselves towards the uterine tubes while the remainder are destroyed by the acid medium of the vagina. More will die on the journey through the uterus and only thousands reach the uterine tube where they meet the ovum, usually in the ampulla. It is only during this journey that the sperm finally become mature and capable of releasing the enzyme hyaluronidase, which allows penetration of the zona pellucida and the cell membrane surrounding the ovum (Fig. 9.4). Many sperm are needed for this to take place but only one will enter the ovum. After this, the membrane is sealed to prevent entry of any further sperm and the nuclei of the two cells fuse. The sperm and the ovum each contribute half the complement of chromosomes to make a total of 46 (Box 9.1). The sperm and ovum are known as the male and female *gametes*, and the fertilised ovum as the *zygote*.

Neither sperm nor ovum can survive for longer than 2 or 3 days and fertilisation is most likely to occur when intercourse takes place not more than 48 hours before or 24 hours after ovulation. It therefore follows that conception will take place about 14 days before the next period is due.

Development of the fertilised ovum (Fig. 9.5)

When the ovum has been fertilised, it continues its passage through the uterine tube and reaches the uterus 3 or 4 days later. During this time segmentation or cell division takes place and the fertilised ovum divides into 2 cells, then into 4, then 8, 16 and so on until a cluster of cells is formed known as the *morula* (mulberry). These divisions occur quite slowly, about

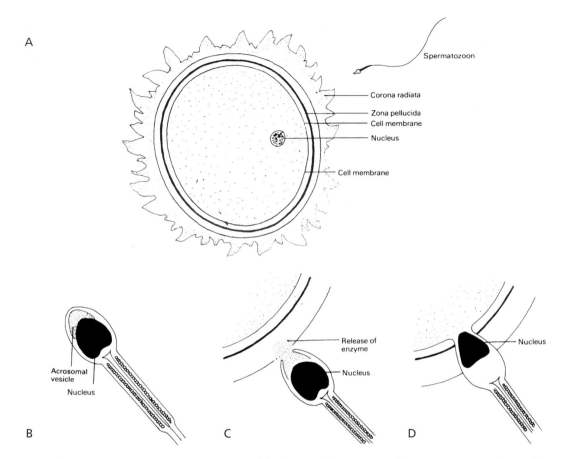

Fig. 9.4 Fertilisation. Diagrammatic representation of the fusion of the ovum and the spermatozoon. (Note that B, C and D are more greatly magnified than A.)

once every 12 hours. Next, a fluid-filled cavity, or *blastocele*, appears in the morula, which now becomes known as the *blastocyst*. Around the outside of the blastocyst there is a single layer of cells known as the *trophoblast*; the remaining cells are clumped together at one end forming the *inner cell mass*. The trophoblast will form the placenta and chorion, while the inner cell mass will become the fetus, amnion and umbilical cord. On its journey, the ovum is nourished by glycogen from the goblet cells of the uterine tubes and later the secretory glands of the uterus.

When the blastocyst first tumbles into the uterus, it lies free for 2 or 3 more days. The trophoblast, especially the part which lies over the inner cell mass, then becomes quite sticky and adheres to the endometrium. It begins to secrete substances that digest the endometrial cells, allowing the blastocyst to become embedded in the endometrium. *Embedding*, sometimes known as *nidation* (nesting), is normally complete by the 11th day after ovulation and the endometrium closes over it completely, the only evidence of the presence of the blastocyst being a small bulge on the surface.

The decidua

This is the name given to the endometrium during pregnancy. From the time of conception the increased secretion of oestrogens causes the endometrium to grow to four times its non-pregnant thickness. The corpus luteum also produces large amounts of progesterone, which stimulate the secretory activity of the endometrial glands and increase the size of the blood vessels. This accounts for the soft, vascular, spongy bed in which the fertilised ovum implants. Three layers are found:

> **Box 9.1** Chromosomes
>
> Each human cell has a complement of 46 chromosomes arranged in 23 pairs, of which two are sex chromosomes. The remainder are known as autosomes. During the process of maturation, both gametes (ovum and spermatozoon) shed half their chromosomes, one of each pair, during a reduction division called meiosis. Genetic material is exchanged between the chromosomes before they split up. In the male, meiosis starts at puberty and both halves redivide to form four spermatozoa in all. In the female, meiosis commences during fetal life but the first division is not completed until many years later at ovulation. The division is unequal; the larger part will go on to form the ovum while the remainder forms the first polar body. At fertilisation the second division takes place and results in one large cell, which is the mature ovum, and a much smaller one, the second polar body. At the same time, division of the first polar body creates a third polar body.
>
> When the gametes combine at fertilisation to form the zygote, the full complement of chromosomes is restored. Subsequent division occurs by mitosis where the chromosomes divide to give each new cell a full set.
>
> **Sex determination**
> Females carry two similar sex chromosomes, XX; males carry two dissimilar sex chromosomes, XY. Each spermatozoon will carry either an X or a Y chromosome, whereas the ovum always carries an X chromosome. If the ovum is fertilised by an X-carrying spermatozoon a female is conceived, if by a Y-carrying one, a male.

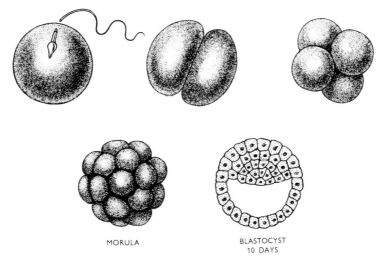

MORULA

BLASTOCYST
10 DAYS

Fig. 9.5 Diagrammatic representation of the development of the fertilised ovum.

The basal layer. This layer lies immediately above the myometrium. It remains unchanged in itself but regenerates the new endometrium during the puerperium.

The functional layer. This layer consists of tortuous glands, which are rich in secretions. The stroma cells are enlarged in what is known as the decidual reaction. This affords a defence against excessive invasion by the syncytiotrophoblast and limits its advance to this spongy layer. The advantage of this is that it provides a secure anchorage for the placenta and allows it access to nutrition and oxygen but as soon as the baby is born, separation can occur (see Ch. 28).

The compact layer. This layer forms the surface of the decidua and is composed of closely packed stroma cells and the necks of the glands.

The blastocyst embeds within the spongy layer and the different areas of decidua are identified according

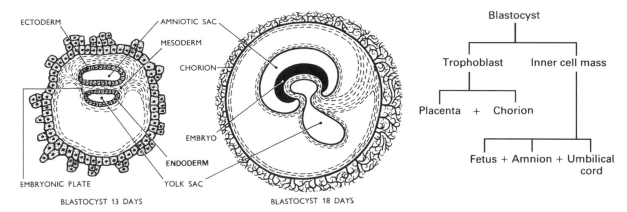

Fig. 9.6 The development of the blastocyst.

to their relationship to it. The decidua underneath the blastocyst is termed the *basal decidua*, that which covers it is the *capsular decidua*, and the remainder is called the *parietal* (or the *true*) *decidua*. Eventually, as the embryo grows and fills the uterine cavity, the capsular decidua meets and fuses with the parietal decidua.

The trophoblast

Small projections begin to appear all over the surface of the blastocyst (Figs 9.6 and 9.7), becoming most prolific at the area of contact. These trophoblastic cells differentiate into layers: the outer syncytiotrophoblast (syncytium), the inner cytotrophoblast and below this a layer of mesoderm or primitive mesenchyme.

The syncytiotrophoblast. This layer is composed of nucleated protoplasm, which is capable of breaking down tissue as in the process of embedding. It erodes the walls of the blood vessels of the decidua, making the nutrients in the maternal blood accessible to the developing organism.

The cytotrophoblast. The cytotrophoblast is a well-defined single layer of cells which produces a hormone known as human chorionic gonadotrophin (HCG). This hormone is responsible for informing the corpus luteum that a pregnancy has begun. The corpus luteum continues to produce oestrogen and progesterone. Progesterone maintains the integrity of the decidua so that shedding does not take place. In other words, menstruation is suppressed. The high level of oestrogen suppresses the production of FSH.

The mesoderm. This layer consists of loose connective tissue. There is similar tissue in the inner cell mass

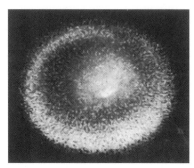

Fig. 9.7 Ovum in early pregnancy covered with chorionic villi (see Ch. 10).

and the two are continuous at the point where they join in the body stalk.

Further development of the trophoblast is discussed in Chapter 10.

The inner cell mass

While the trophoblast is developing into the placenta, which will nourish the fetus, the inner cell mass is forming the fetus itself. The cells differentiate into three layers, each of which will form particular parts of the fetus:

The ectoderm. This layer mainly forms the skin and nervous system.

The mesoderm. This layer forms bones and muscles and also the heart and blood vessels, including those in the placenta. Certain internal organs also originate in the mesoderm.

The endoderm. This layer forms mucous membranes and glands. The three layers together are known

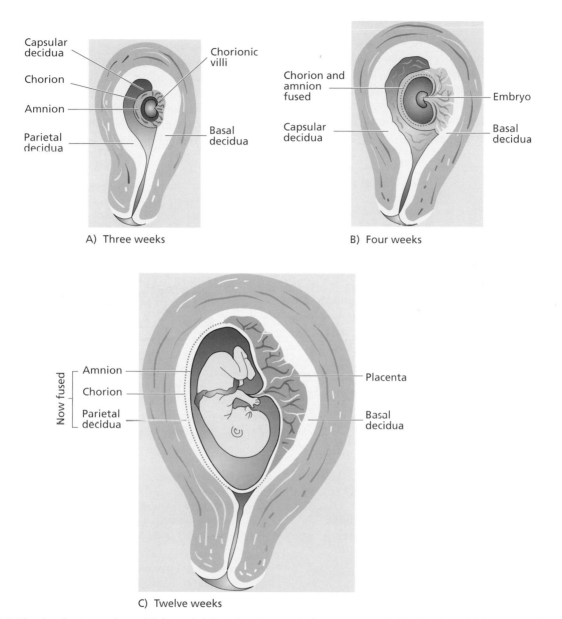

Fig. 9.8 The developing embryo: (A) (3 weeks) Showing the amniotic sac, surrounded by chorion which is covered with capsular decidua. (B) (4 weeks) The amnion is in contact with the chorion. The placenta is seen embedded in the basal decidua. (C) (12 weeks) The capsular decidua has thinned out and atrophied. The chorion is attached to the parietal decidua.

as the *embryonic plate*. Two cavities appear in the inner cell mass – one on either side of the embryonic plate.

The amniotic cavity. This cavity lies on the side of the ectoderm. It is filled with fluid, and gradually enlarges and folds around the embryo to enclose it. The *amnion* forms from its lining. It swells out into the chorionic cavity (formerly the blastocele) and eventually obliterates it when the amniotic and chorionic membranes come into contact. Details of the amniotic fluid are found in Chapter 10.

The yolk sac. The yolk sac lies on the side of the endoderm and provides nourishment for the embryo until the trophoblast is sufficiently developed to take over. Part of it contributes to the formation of the primitive gut; the remainder resembles a balloon floating in front of the embryo until it atrophies and becomes trapped under the amnion on the surface of the placenta. After birth, all that remains of the yolk sac is a vestigial structure in the base of the umbilical cord, known as the *vitelline duct*.

The embryo (Fig. 9.8)

This name is applied to the developing offspring after implantation and until 8 weeks after conception. During the embryonic period all the organs and systems of the body are laid down in rudimentary form so that at its completion they have simply to grow and mature for a further 7 months. The conceptus is known as a *fetus* during this time (see Ch. 11).

REFERENCES

Johnson M H, Everitt B J 2000 Essential reproduction, 5th edn. Blackwell Science, Oxford

Steer P J 1990 Endocrinology of parturition. In: Franks S (ed) Clinical endocrinology and metabolism. Baillière Tindall, London, vol 4, no 2 (June)

FURTHER READING

Coad J with Dunstall M 2001 Anatomy and physiology for midwives. Mosby, Edinburgh

A very full and clear explanation of endocrine activity is given in Chapter 3. Chapter 4 addresses the reproductive cycles in similar detail with clear diagrams to assist the reader. A number of clinical issues of relevance to midwives are highlighted. Related chapters include that on sexual differentiation and behaviour and that on genetics. Fertilisation is addressed in Chapter 6 with a detailed account including artificial reproduction methods.

Herbert R A 1996 Reproduction. In: Hinchliff S, Montague S, Watson R (eds) Physiology for nursing practice, 2nd edn. Baillière Tindall, London

This augments the material covered in this chapter and provides additional information on some aspects of menstruation and cell division in particular that will add to the understanding of these events.

Johnson M H, Everitt B J 2000 Essential reproduction, 5th edn. Blackwell Science, Oxford

This authoritative volume provides the interested reader with a much greater depth of information than is possible in the present book and is recommended for those who wish to study the hormonal patterns of reproduction in detail.

Rutishauser S 1994 Physiology and anatomy: a basis for nursing and health care. Churchill Livingstone, Edinburgh

This is a good basic textbook of anatomy and physiology. The chapter on sex and reproduction contains some useful, clear diagrams as well as one or two further details that may be of interest to the student midwife.

Stables D 1999 Physiology in childbearing with anatomy and basic sciences. Baillière Tindall, Edinburgh

The reproductive cycles are described and a detailed account of cell division is offered with a number of clear diagrams.

10 The Placenta

V. Ruth Bennett   Linda K. Brown

The placenta is a remarkable organ. Originating from the trophoblastic layer of the fertilised ovum, it links closely with the mother's circulation to carry out functions that the fetus is unable to perform for itself during intrauterine life. The survival of the fetus depends upon the placenta's integrity and efficiency.

Development

Initially the ovum appears to be covered with a fine, downy hair, which consists of the projections from the trophoblastic layer (see Ch. 9). These proliferate and branch from about 3 weeks after fertilisation, forming the *chorionic villi*. The villi become most profuse in the area where the blood supply is richest – that is, in the basal decidua. This part of the trophoblast is known as the *chorion frondosum* and it will eventually develop into the placenta. The villi under the capsular decidua, being less well nourished, gradually degenerate and form the *chorion laeve* (bald chorion), which is the origin of the chorionic membrane.

The villi erode the walls of maternal blood vessels as they penetrate the decidua, opening them up to form a lake of maternal blood in which they float. The opened blood vessels are known as sinuses, and the areas surrounding the villi as blood spaces. The maternal blood circulates slowly, enabling the villi to absorb food and oxygen and excrete waste. These are known as the nutritive villi. A few villi are more deeply attached to the decidua and are called anchoring villi.

Each chorionic villus is a branching structure arising from one stem (Fig. 10.1). Its centre consists of mesoderm and fetal blood vessels, and branches of the umbilical artery and vein. These are covered by a single layer of cytotrophoblast cells and the external layer of the villus is the syncytiotrophoblast. This means that four layers of tissue separate the maternal blood from

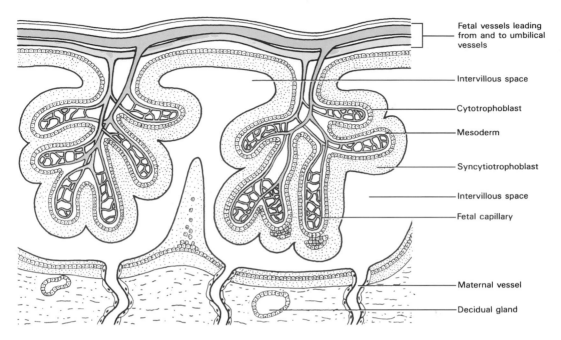

Fetal vessels leading from and to umbilical vessels

Intervillous space

Cytotrophoblast

Mesoderm

Syncytiotrophoblast

Intervillous space

Fetal capillary

Maternal vessel

Decidual gland

Fig. 10.1 Diagram to show chorionic villi.

the fetal blood and make it impossible for the two circulations to mix unless any villi are damaged.

The placenta is completely formed and functioning from 10 weeks after fertilisation. In its early stages it is a relatively loose structure, but becomes more compact as it matures. Between 12 and 20 weeks' gestation the placenta weighs more than the fetus because the fetal organs are insufficiently developed to cope with the metabolic processes of nutrition. Later in pregnancy some of the fetal organs, such as the liver, begin to function, so the cytotrophoblast and the syncytiotrophoblast gradually degenerate and this allows easier exchange of oxygen and carbon dioxide.

Circulation through the placenta

Fetal blood, low in oxygen, is pumped by the fetal heart towards the placenta along the umbilical arteries and transported along their branches to the capillaries of the chorionic villi. Having yielded up carbon dioxide and absorbed oxygen, the blood is returned to the fetus via the umbilical vein.

The maternal blood is delivered to the placental bed in the decidua by spiral arteries and flows into the blood spaces surrounding the villi. It is thought that the direction of flow is similar to a fountain; the blood

passes upwards and bathes the villus as it circulates around it and drains back into a branch of the uterine vein (Fig. 10.2).

The mature placenta

Functions

Respiration. During intrauterine life no pulmonary exchange of gases can take place so the fetus must obtain oxygen and excrete carbon dioxide through the placenta. Oxygen from the mother's haemoglobin passes into the fetal blood by simple diffusion and similarly the fetus gives off carbon dioxide into the maternal blood.

Nutrition. The fetus needs the same nutrients as anyone else and most of these are actively transferred across the placenta. Amino acids are required for body building, large quantities of glucose for energy and growth, calcium and phosphorus for bones and teeth, and iron and other minerals for blood formation. Food for the fetus derives from the mother's diet and has already been broken down into simpler forms by the time it reaches the placental site. The placenta is able to select those substances required by the fetus, even depleting the mother's own supply in some

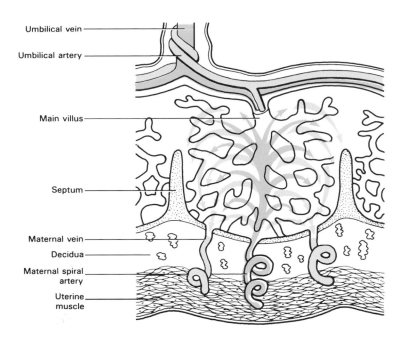

Fig. 10.2 Blood flow around chorionic villi.

instances. It can also break down complex nutrients into compounds that can be used by the fetus. Protein is transferred across the placenta as amino acids, carbohydrate as glucose, and fats as fatty acids. Water, vitamins and minerals also pass to the fetus. Fats and fat-soluble vitamins (A, D and E) cross the placenta only with difficulty and mainly in the later stages of pregnancy. Some substances, including amino acids, are found at higher levels in the fetal blood than in the maternal blood.

Storage. The placenta metabolises glucose, stores it in the form of glycogen and reconverts it to glucose as required. The placenta can also store iron and the fat-soluble vitamins.

Excretion. The main substance excreted from the fetus is carbon dioxide. Bilirubin will also be excreted as red blood cells are replaced relatively frequently. There is very little tissue breakdown apart from this and the amounts of urea and uric acid excreted are very small.

Protection. The placenta provides a limited barrier to infection. With the exception of the treponema of syphilis and the tubercle bacillus, few bacteria can penetrate. Viruses, however, can cross freely and may cause congenital abnormalities, as in the case of the rubella virus (see Ch. 46). It may be assumed that drugs will cross to the fetus although there are exceptions, for example heparin. Some drugs are known to cause damage, though many will be harmless and others are positively beneficial, such as antibiotics administered to a pregnant woman with syphilis (see Ch. 48).

Towards the end of pregnancy small antibodies, immunoglobulins G (IgG), will be transferred to the fetus and these will confer immunity on the baby for the first 3 months after birth. It is important to realise that only those antibodies that the mother herself possesses can be passed on.

Endocrine.

Human chorionic gonadotrophin (HCG). This is produced by the cytotrophoblastic layer of the chorionic villi. Initially it is present in very large quantities, peak levels being achieved between the 7th and 10th weeks, but these gradually reduce as the pregnancy advances. HCG forms the basis of the many pregnancy tests available, as it is excreted in the mother's urine. Its function is to stimulate the growth and activity of the corpus luteum.

Oestrogens. As the activity of the corpus luteum declines, the placenta takes over the production of oestrogens, which are secreted in large amounts throughout pregnancy. The fetus provides the placenta with the vital precursors for the production of oestrogens. The amount of oestrogen produced (measured as urinary or serum oestriol) is an index of fetoplacental well-being.

Progesterone. This is made in the syncytial layer of the placenta in increasing quantities until immediately before the onset of labour when its level falls. It may be measured in the urine as pregnanediol.

Human placental lactogen (HPL). HPL has a role in glucose metabolism in pregnancy. It appears to have a connection with the activity of human growth hormone, although it does not itself promote growth. As the level of HCG falls, so the level of HPL rises and continues to do so throughout pregnancy. Monitoring the level of HPL with the intention of assessing placental function has been disappointing in predicting fetal outcome.

Appearance of the placenta at term

The placenta is a round, flat mass about 20 cm in diameter and 2.5 cm thick at its centre. It weighs approximately one-sixth of the baby's weight at term, although this proportion may be affected by the time at which the cord is clamped owing to the varying amounts of fetal blood retained in the vessels.

The maternal surface (Fig. 10.3A). Maternal blood gives this surface a dark red colour and part of the basal decidua will have been separated with it. The surface is arranged in about 20 lobes, which are separated by sulci (furrows), into which the decidua dips down to form septa (walls). The lobes are made up of lobules, each of which contains a single villus with its branches. Sometimes deposits of lime salts may be present on the surface, making it slightly gritty. This has no clinical significance.

The fetal surface (Fig. 10.3B). The amnion covering the fetal surface of the placenta gives it a white, shiny appearance. Branches of the umbilical vein and arteries are visible, spreading out from the insertion of the umbilical cord, which is normally in the centre. The amnion can be peeled off the surface, leaving the *chorionic plate* from which the placenta has developed and which is continuous with the chorion.

The fetal sac

The fetal sac consists of a double membrane. The outer membrane is the chorion, which lies under the capsular decidua and becomes closely adherent to the uterine wall. The inner membrane is the amnion, which contains the amniotic fluid. As long as it remains intact, the fetal sac protects the fetus against ascending bacterial infection.

Chorion. This is a thick, opaque, friable membrane derived from the trophoblast. It is continuous with the chorionic plate, which forms the base of the placenta.

Amnion. This is a smooth, tough, translucent membrane derived from the inner cell mass. It is thought to have a role in the formation of the amniotic fluid (also termed liquor amnii).

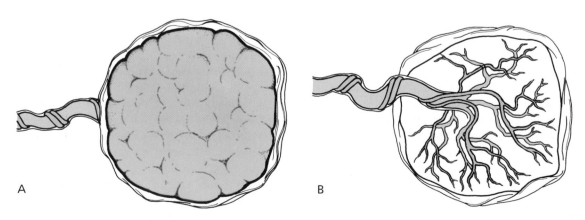

A   B

Fig. 10.3 The placenta at term. (A) Maternal surface. (B) Fetal surface.

Amniotic fluid

Functions

The fluid distends the amniotic sac and allows for the growth and free movement of the fetus. It equalises pressure and protects the fetus from jarring and injury. The fluid maintains a constant temperature for the fetus and provides small amounts of nutrients. In labour, as long as the membranes remain intact, the amniotic fluid protects the placenta and umbilical cord from the pressure of uterine contractions. It also aids effacement of the cervix and dilatation of the uterine os, particularly where the presenting part is poorly applied.

Origin

The source of amniotic fluid is thought to be both fetal and maternal. It is secreted by the amnion, especially the part covering the placenta and umbilical cord. Some fluid is exuded from maternal vessels in the decidua and some from fetal vessels in the placenta. Fetal urine also contributes to the volume from the 10th week of gestation onwards. The water in amniotic fluid is exchanged as often as every 3 hours.

Volume

The total amount of amniotic fluid increases throughout pregnancy until 38 weeks' gestation, when there is about 1 litre. It then diminishes slightly until term, when approximately 800 ml remains. However, there are very wide variations in the amount. If the total amount exceeds 1500 ml, the condition is known as *polyhydramnios* (often abbreviated to hydramnios), and if less than 300 ml, the term *oligohydramnios* is applied. Such abnormalities are often associated with congenital malformations of the fetus. The normal fetus swallows amniotic fluid, but if anything interferes with swallowing then an excessive amount of fluid will accumulate. Similarly, if the fetus is unable to pass urine then the amount of fluid will be reduced (see Ch. 45).

Constituents

Amniotic fluid is a clear, pale straw-coloured fluid consisting of 99% water. The remaining 1% is dissolved solid matter including food substances and waste products. In addition, the fetus sheds skin cells,

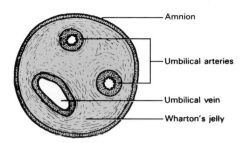

Fig. 10.4 Cross-section through the umbilical cord.

vernix caseosa and lanugo into the fluid. Abnormal constituents of the liquor, such as meconium in the case of fetal distress, may give valuable diagnostic information about the condition of the fetus. Aspiration of amniotic fluid for examination is termed amniocentesis (see Ch. 23).

The umbilical cord

The umbilical cord or *funis* extends from the fetus to the placenta and transmits the umbilical blood vessels: two arteries and one vein (Fig. 10.4). These are enclosed and protected by *Wharton's jelly*, a gelatinous substance formed from mesoderm. The whole cord is covered in a layer of amnion continuous with that covering the placenta.

The length of the average cord is about 50 cm. This is sufficient to allow for birth of the baby without applying any traction to the placenta. A cord is considered to be short when it measures less than 40 cm. There is no specific agreed length for describing a cord as too long, but the disadvantages of a very long cord are that it may become wrapped round the neck or body of the fetus or become knotted; either event could result in occlusion of the blood vessels, especially during labour. True knots should always be noted on examination of the cord, but they must be distinguished from false knots, which are lumps of Wharton's jelly on the side of the cord and are not significant.

Anatomical variations of the placenta and the cord

Succenturiate lobe of placenta (Fig. 10.5). This is the most significant of the variations in conformation

Blood vessels running
through the chorion
from the placenta
to the accessory
lobe

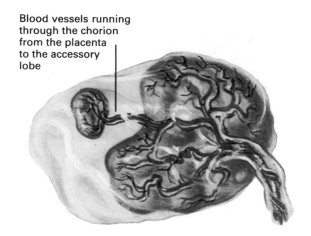

Fig. 10.5 Succenturiate lobe of placenta.

of the placenta. A small extra lobe is present, separate from the main placenta, and joined to it by blood vessels that run through the membranes to reach it. The danger is that this small lobe may be retained in utero after the placenta is born, and if it is not removed it may lead to infection and haemorrhage. The midwife must examine every placenta for evidence of a retained succenturiate lobe – a hole in the membranes with vessels running to it.

Circumvallate placenta (Fig. 10.6). In this situation an opaque ring is seen on the fetal surface of the placenta. It is formed by a doubling back of the chorion and amnion and may result in the membranes leaving the placenta nearer the centre instead of at the edge as usual.

Battledore insertion of the cord (Fig. 10.7). The cord in this case is attached at the very edge of the placenta in the manner of a table tennis bat. It is unimportant unless the attachment is fragile.

Velamentous insertion of the cord (Fig. 10.8). The cord is inserted into the membranes some distance from the edge of the placenta. The umbilical vessels run through the membranes from the cord to the placenta. If the placenta is normally situated, no harm will result to the fetus, but the cord is likely to become detached upon applying traction during active management of the third stage of labour.

If the placenta is low lying, the vessels may pass across the uterine os. The term applied to the vessels lying in this position is *vasa praevia*. In this case there is great danger to the fetus when the membranes rupture and even more so during artificial rupture, as the vessels may be torn, leading to rapid exsanguination of the fetus. If the onset of haemorrhage coincides with rupture of the membranes, fetal haemorrhage should be assumed and the birth expedited. It is possible to distinguish fetal blood from maternal blood by Singer's alkali-denaturation test, although, in practice, time is so short that it may not be possible to save the life of the baby. If the baby survives, haemoglobin levels should be estimated after birth.

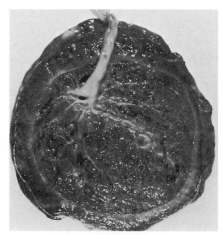

Fig. 10.6 Circumvallate placenta.

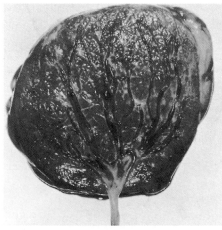

Fig. 10.7 Battledore insertion of the cord.

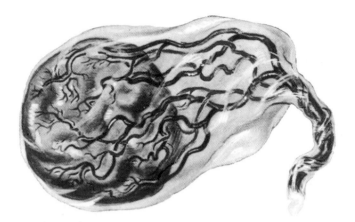

Fig. 10.8 Velamentous insertion of the cord.

Bipartite placenta (Fig. 10.9). Two complete and separate parts are present, each with a cord leaving it. The bipartite cord joins a short distance from the two parts of the placenta. This is different from the two placentas in a twin pregnancy, where there are also two umbilical cords, but these do not join at any point. Where there is a succenturiate lobe, the vessels are attached to the placenta directly and never join the cord.

A **tripartite placenta** is similar but with three distinct parts.

Except for the dangers noted above these varieties of conformation have no clinical significance.

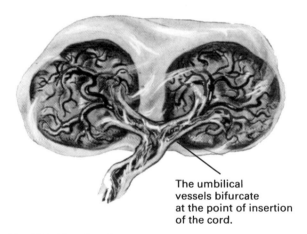

The umbilical vessels bifurcate at the point of insertion of the cord.

Fig. 10.9 Bipartite placenta.

FURTHER READING

Coad J with Dunstall M 2001 Anatomy and physiology for midwives. Mosby, Edinburgh

This reliable text presents a detailed account of the placenta.

Fox H 1991 A contemporary view of the human placenta. Midwifery 7(1 March):31–39

While this article is now several years old, it continues to provide an informative summary of knowledge about the placenta.

Johnson M H, Everitt B J 2000 Essential reproduction, 5th edn. Blackwell Science, Oxford

This volume provides much more detail, particularly about the development of the placenta and will help the reader to a fuller understanding of its function and the interdependence of maternal and fetal systems.

Llewellyn-Jones D 1999 Fundamentals of obstetrics and gynaecology, 6th edn. Mosby, London

This book has a useful section on the placenta and explains the processes of nutrition clearly. It also contains a chapter on placental abnormalities and diseases, which the reader may find useful.

Stables D 1999 Physiology in childbearing with anatomy and basic sciences. Baillière Tindall, Edinburgh

The placental hormones are explained in more detail and a diagram (11.4) gives a visual representation of different forms of placental transfer.

Williams P L, Bannister L H, Berry M H et al 1995 Gray's anatomy, 38th edn. Churchill Livingstone, New York

This authoritative and comprehensive volume provides the reader with detailed descriptions of the placenta and its functioning for the interested student.

11

The Fetus

V. Ruth Bennett   Linda K. Brown

The midwife needs to have an understanding of fetal development in order to estimate the approximate age of a baby born before term. It is also helpful to know the outline of organogenesis in order to appreciate the ways in which developmental abnormalities arise.

Time scale of development

The time scale of the pregnancy is important. When making reference to the age at which various prenatal events happen, it is important to distinguish between menstrual age (the time since the first day of the last menstrual period) and conceptional age (the interval since fertilisation). Embryologists use the latter whereas those involved with the pregnant woman tend to use the former. Figure 11.1 illustrates the comparative lengths of the different periods involved. The interval from the beginning of the last menstrual period (LMP) until conception is not strictly part of the pregnancy, although the as yet unfertilised ovum is already being prepared for release. For clinical purposes it is convenient to regard the pregnancy as beginning at the LMP because this is usually the only definitive date available. However, the midwife should be aware that an individual woman may know the exact date of conception and will rightly consider this as the beginning of her pregnancy.

For the first 3 weeks following conception the term *fertilised ovum* or *zygote* is used. From 3–8 weeks after conception it is known as the *embryo* and following this it is the *fetus* until birth, when it becomes a baby. Although when speaking to mothers the fetus in utero is usually referred to as a baby, the midwife should use the correct terminology during professional discussions and in her records.

Development within the uterus is summarised in Box 11.1.

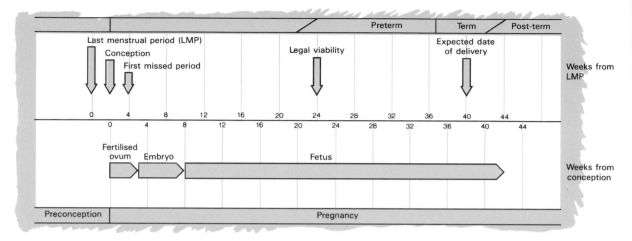

Fig. 11.1 Menstrual age, conceptional age and prenatal events.

Box 11.1 Summary of development (Fig. 11.2)

0–4 weeks after conception
Rapid growth
Formation of the embryonic plate (see Ch. 9)
Primitive central nervous system forms
Heart develops and begins to beat
Limb buds form

4–8 weeks
Very rapid cell division
Head and facial features develop
All major organs laid down in primitive form
External genitalia present but sex not distinguishable
Early movements
Visible on ultrasound from 6 weeks

8–12 weeks
Eyelids fuse
Kidneys begin to function and the fetus passes urine from 10 weeks
Fetal circulation functioning properly
Sucking and swallowing begin
Sex apparent
Moves freely (not felt by mother)
Some primitive reflexes present

12–16 weeks
Rapid skeletal development – visible on X-ray
Meconium present in gut
Lanugo appears
Nasal septum and palate fuse

16–20 weeks
'Quickening' – mother feels fetal movements

Fetal heart heard on auscultation
Vernix caseosa appears
Fingernails can be seen
Skin cells begin to be renewed

20–24 weeks
Most organs become capable of functioning
Periods of sleep and activity
Responds to sound
Skin red and wrinkled

24–28 weeks
Survival may be expected if born
Eyelids reopen
Respiratory movements

28–32 weeks
Begins to store fat and iron
Testes descend into scrotum
Lanugo disappears from face
Skin becomes paler and less wrinkled

32–36 weeks
Increased fat makes the body more rounded
Lanugo disappears from body
Head hair lengthens
Nails reach tips of fingers
Ear cartilage soft
Plantar creases visible

36–40 weeks after conception (38–42 weeks after LMP)
Term is reached and birth is due
Contours rounded
Skull firm

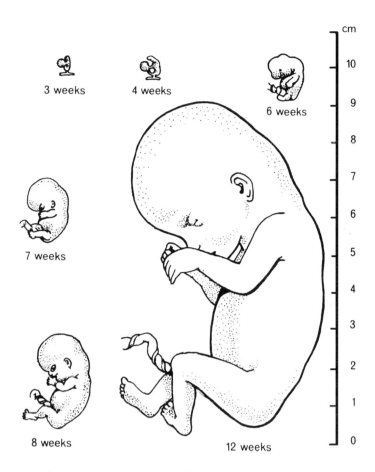

3 weeks

4 weeks

6 weeks

7 weeks

8 weeks

12 weeks

cm
10
9
8
7
6
5
4
3
2
1
0

Fig. 11.2 Sizes of embryos and fetus between 3 and 12 weeks' gestation.

Fetal organs

Some aspects of the development of fetal organs and their physiology are of special relevance to the midwife because of their effect on the newborn baby. A brief outline is given of the most important.

Blood

The origin of fetal blood is from the inner cell mass, along with all the other organs of its body. The fetus will inherit the genes that determine its blood group from both its parents; its ABO group and Rhesus factor may therefore be the same or different from those of its mother.

The fetal haemoglobin (Hb) is of a different type from adult haemoglobin and is termed HbF. It has a much greater affinity for oxygen and is found in greater concentration (18–20 g/dl at term). The reason for this is that oxygen must be obtained from the mother's blood in the placental site where the oxygen tension is lower than in the atmosphere. Towards the end of pregnancy the fetus begins to make adult-type haemoglobin (HbA).

In utero the red blood cells have a shorter life span, this being about 90 days by the time the baby is born.

The renal tract

The kidneys begin to function and the fetus passes urine from 10 weeks' gestation. The urine is very dilute and does not constitute a route for excretion, since the mother eliminates waste products, which cross the placenta. It is worth noting that the superior vesical arteries arise from the first few centimetres of the hypogastric arteries, which lead to the umbilical arteries, so that if a single umbilical artery is found then abnormalities of the renal tract are suspected.

The adrenal glands

The fetal adrenal glands produce the precursors for placental formation of oestriols. They are also thought to play a part in the initiation of labour, although the exact mechanism is not fully understood (see Ch. 24; also Johnson & Everitt 2000).

The liver

The fetal liver is comparatively large in size, taking up much of the abdominal cavity, especially in the early months. From the 3rd to the 6th month of intrauterine life, the liver is responsible for the formation of red blood cells, after which they are mainly produced in the red bone marrow and the spleen.

Towards the end of pregnancy, iron stores are laid down in the liver.

The alimentary tract

The digestive tract is mainly non-functional before birth. It forms from the yolk sac as a straight tube, later growing out into the base of the umbilical cord and subsequently rotating back into the abdomen. Sucking and swallowing of amniotic fluid containing shed skin cells and other debris begins about 12 weeks after conception. Most digestive juices are present before birth and they act on the swallowed substances and discarded intestinal cells to form meconium. This is normally retained in the gut until after birth when it is passed as the first stool of the newborn.

The lungs

The lungs originate from a bud growing out of the pharynx, which subdivides again and again to form the branching structure of the bronchial tree. The process continues after birth until about 8 years of age when the full number of bronchioles and alveoli will have developed. It is mainly the immaturity of the lungs that reduces the chance of survival of infants born before 24 weeks' gestation, owing to the limited alveolar surface area, the immaturity of the capillary system in the lungs and the lack of adequate surfactant. Surfactant is a lipoprotein that reduces the surface tension in the alveoli and assists gaseous exchange. It is first produced from about 20 weeks' gestation and the amount increases until the lungs are mature at about 30–34 weeks. At term the lungs contain about 100 ml of lung fluid. About one-third of this is expelled during birth and the rest is absorbed and carried away by the lymphatics and blood vessels as air takes its place.

There is some movement of the thorax from the 3rd month of fetal life and more definite diaphragmatic movements from the 6th month. Fetal breathing occurs in episodes of up to half an hour during rapid eye movement (REM) sleep (Johnson & Everitt 2000).

The central nervous system

This is derived from the ectoderm. It folds inwards by a complicated process to form the neural tube, which is then covered over by skin. This process is occasionally incomplete, leading to open neural tube defects.

The fetus is able to perceive strong light and to hear external sounds. Periods of wakefulness and sleep occur, both deep (slow wave) and REM sleep.

The skin

From 18 weeks after conception the fetus is covered with a white, creamy substance called *vernix caseosa*. This protects the skin from the fluid and from any friction against itself. At 20 weeks the fetus will be covered with a fine downy hair called *lanugo* and at the same time the head hair and eyebrows begin to form. Lanugo is shed again from 36 weeks and a full-term infant has little left.

Fingernails develop from about 10 weeks but the toenails do not form until about 18 weeks. By term the nails usually extend beyond the fingertips, but length of the nails is an unreliable guide to maturity.

The fetal circulation (Fig. 11.3)

The key to understanding the fetal circulation is the fact that oxygen is derived from the placenta. In addition, the placenta is the source of nutrition and the site of elimination of waste. At birth there is a dramatic alteration in this situation and an almost instantaneous change must occur. Therefore all the postnatal structures must be in place and ready to

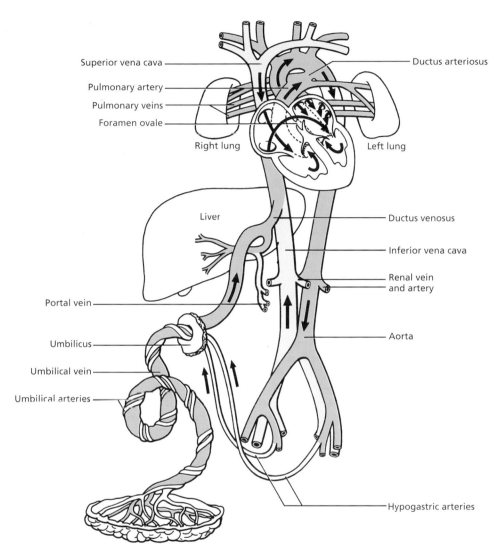

Superior vena cava
Pulmonary artery
Pulmonary veins
Foramen ovale
Right lung
Liver
Portal vein
Umbilicus
Umbilical vein
Umbilical arteries

Ductus arteriosus
Left lung
Ductus venosus
Inferior vena cava
Renal vein and artery
Aorta
Hypogastric arteries

Fig. 11.3 A diagram of the fetal circulation. The arrows show the course taken by the blood. The temporary structures are labelled in colour.

take over. There are several temporary structures in addition to the placenta itself and the umbilical cord and these enable the fetal circulation to take place while allowing for the changes at birth.

The umbilical vein. This vein leads from the umbilical cord to the underside of the liver and carries blood rich in oxygen and nutrients. It has a branch that joins the portal vein and supplies the liver.

The ductus venosus (from a vein to a vein). This connects the umbilical vein to the inferior vena cava.

At this point the blood mixes with deoxygenated blood returning from the lower parts of the body. Thus the blood throughout the body is at best partially oxygenated.

The foramen ovale (oval opening). This is a temporary opening between the atria that allows the majority of blood entering from the inferior vena cava to pass across into the left atrium. The reason for this diversion is that the blood does not need to pass through the lungs to collect oxygen.

The ductus arteriosus (from an artery to an artery). This leads from the bifurcation of the pulmonary artery to the descending aorta, entering it just beyond the point where the subclavian and carotid arteries leave.

The hypogastric arteries. These branch off from the internal iliac arteries and become the umbilical arteries when they enter the umbilical cord. They return blood to the placenta.

The blood takes about half a minute to circulate and takes the following course. From the placenta, blood passes along the umbilical vein through the abdominal wall to the under surface of the liver. This is the only vessel in the fetus that carries unmixed blood. The ductus venosus carries blood to the inferior vena cava where it mixes with blood from the lower body. From here the blood passes into the right atrium and most of it is directed across through the foramen ovale into the left atrium. Following its normal route it enters the left ventricle and passes into the aorta. The heart and brain each receives a supply of relatively well-oxygenated blood since the coronary and carotid arteries are early branches from the aorta. The arms also benefit via the subclavian arteries, which is why they are more developed than the legs at birth.

Blood collected from the upper parts of the body returns to the right atrium in the superior vena cava. This blood is depleted of oxygen and nutrients. This stream of blood crosses the stream entering from the inferior vena cava and passes into the right ventricle. The two streams remain separate because of the shape of the atrium but there is a mixing of 25% of the blood, allowing a little oxygen and food to be taken to the lungs through the pulmonary artery. This is necessary for their development. However, only a small amount of the blood entering the pulmonary artery is required by the lungs. The remainder passes through the ductus arteriosus to the aorta. Blood continues along the aorta and, although low in oxygen, has sufficient to supply the remaining body organs and legs. The internal iliac arteries lead into the hypogastric arteries, which return blood to the placenta via the umbilical arteries. The remaining blood supplies the lower limbs and returns to the inferior vena cava.

Adaptation to extrauterine life

At birth the baby takes a breath and blood is drawn to the lungs through the pulmonary arteries. It is then collected and returned to the left atrium via the pulmonary veins, resulting in a sudden inflow of blood. The placental circulation ceases soon after birth and so less blood returns to the right side of the heart. In this way the pressure in the left side of the heart is greater while that in the right side of the heart becomes less. This results in the closure of a flap over the foramen ovale, which separates the two sides of the heart and stops the blood flowing from right to left.

With the establishment of pulmonary respiration the oxygen concentration in the bloodstream rises. This causes the ductus arteriosus to constrict and close. For as long as the ductus remains open after birth, blood flows from the high pressure aorta towards the lungs, in the reverse direction to that in fetal life.

The cessation of the placental circulation results in the collapse of the umbilical vein, the ductus venosus and the hypogastric arteries.

These immediate changes are functional and those related to the heart are reversible in certain circumstances. Later they become permanent and anatomical. The umbilical vein becomes the *ligamentum teres*, the ductus venosus the *ligamentum venosum* and the ductus arteriosus the *ligamentum arteriosum*. The foramen ovale becomes the *fossa ovalis* and the hypogastric arteries are known as the *obliterated hypogastric arteries* except for the first few centimetres, which remain open as the superior vesical arteries.

Respiratory and circulatory changes are not the only ones involved. After birth the baby has to obtain nutrition through the establishment of breastfeeding or a breastfeeding substitute and to eliminate waste via the kidneys and gastrointestinal system. In addition, of course, other complex changes take place including the development of communication and the relationship between parents and child (see Ch. 38). Chapters 38 and 39 discuss further the physiology of the baby at term.

The fetal skull (Fig. 11.4)

The fetal skull contains the delicate brain, which may be subjected to great pressure as the head passes through the birth canal. It is large in relation to the fetal body (Fig. 11.5) and in comparison with the mother's pelvis; therefore some adaptation between skull and pelvis must take place during labour. The head is the most difficult part to be born whether it comes first or last.

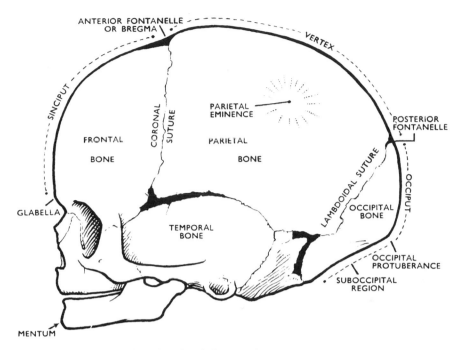

Fig. 11.4 Fetal skull showing regions and landmarks of obstetrical importance.

An understanding of the landmarks and measurements of the fetal skull enables the midwife to recognise normal presentations and positions and to facilitate birth with the least possible trauma to mother and baby. Where malpresentation or disproportion exists she will be able to identify it and take appropriate action.

Ossification. The bones of the fetal head originate in two different ways. The face is laid down in cartilage and is almost completely ossified at birth, the bones being fused together and firm. The bones of the vault are laid down in membrane and are much flatter and more pliable. They ossify from the centre outwards and this process is incomplete at birth leaving small gaps, which form the sutures and fontanelles. The ossification centre on each bone appears as a boss or protuberance.

Bones of the vault (Fig. 11.6)

There are five main bones in the vault of the fetal skull.

The occipital bone. This lies at the back of the head and forms the region of the occiput. Part of it contributes to the base of the skull as it contains the foramen magnum, which protects the spinal cord as it leaves the skull. At the centre is the *occipital protuberance*.

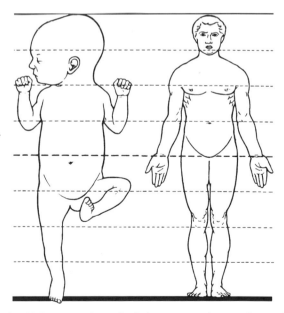

Fig. 11.5 Comparison of a baby's proportions to those of an adult. The baby's head is wider than the shoulders and one-quarter of the total length.

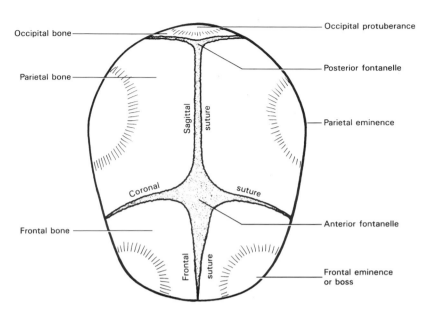

Fig. 11.6 View of fetal head from above (head partly flexed), showing bones, sutures and fontanelles.

The two parietal bones. These lie on either side of the skull. The ossification centre of each is called the *parietal eminence*.

The two frontal bones. These form the forehead or *sinciput*. At the centre of each is a frontal boss or frontal eminence. The frontal bones fuse into a single bone by 8 years of age.

In addition to these five the upper part of the *temporal bone* is also flat and forms a small part of the vault.

Sutures and fontanelles

Sutures are cranial joints and are formed where two bones adjoin. Where two or more sutures meet, a fontanelle is formed. There are several sutures and fontanelles in the fetal skull (see Fig. 11.6); those of most obstetrical significance are described below.

The lambdoidal suture. This suture separates the occipital bone from the two parietal bones.

The sagittal suture. This lies between the two parietal bones.

The coronal suture. This separates the frontal bones from the parietal bones, passing from one temple to the other.

The frontal suture. This runs between the two halves of the frontal bone. Whereas the frontal suture becomes obliterated in time, the other sutures eventually become fixed joints. Ossification of the skull is not complete until early adulthood.

The posterior fontanelle or lambda (shaped like the Greek letter lambda – λ). This is situated at the junction of the lambdoidal and sagittal sutures. It is small, triangular in shape and can be recognised vaginally because a suture leaves from each of the three angles. It normally closes by 6 weeks of age.

The anterior fontanelle or bregma. This is found at the junction of the sagittal, coronal and frontal sutures. It is broad, kite shaped and recognisable vaginally because a suture leaves from each of the four corners. It measures 3–4 cm long and 1.5–2 cm wide and normally closes by the time the child is 18 months old. Pulsations of cerebral vessels can be felt through it.

The sutures and fontanelles, because they consist of membranous spaces, allow for a degree of overlapping of the skull bones during labour and delivery.

Regions and landmarks of the fetal skull

The skull is divided into the vault, the base and the face (Fig. 11.7). The *vault* is the large, dome-shaped part above an imaginary line drawn between the orbital ridges and the nape of the neck. In the vault the bones are relatively thin and pliable at birth, which

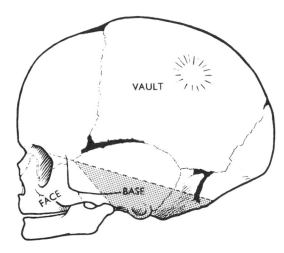

Fig. 11.7 Regions of the skull showing the large, compressible vault and the non-compressible face and base.

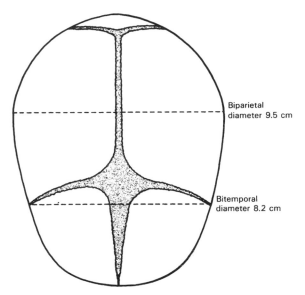

Fig. 11.8 Diagram showing the transverse diameters of the fetal skull.

allows the skull to alter slightly in shape during birth. The *base* is comprised of bones that are firmly united to protect the vital centres in the medulla. The *face* is composed of 14 small bones, which are also firmly united and non-compressible. The regions of the skull are described as follows:

The occiput. This region lies between the foramen magnum and the posterior fontanelle. The part below the occipital protuberance is known as the *suboccipital region*. The protuberance itself can be seen and felt as a prominent point on the posterior aspect of the skull.

The vertex. This is bounded by the posterior fontanelle, the two parietal eminences and the anterior fontanelle. Of the 96% of the babies born head first, 95% present by the vertex.

The sinciput or brow. This extends from the anterior fontanelle and the coronal suture to the orbital ridges.

The face. The face is small in the newborn baby. It extends from the orbital ridges and the root of the nose to the junction of the chin and the neck. The point between the eyebrows is known as the *glabella*. The chin is termed the *mentum* and is an important landmark.

Diameters of the fetal skull

The measurements of the skull are important because the midwife needs a practical understanding of the relationship between the fetal head and the mother's pelvis. It will become clear that some diameters are more favourable than others for easy passage through the pelvic canal and this will depend on the attitude of the head.

There are two transverse diameters (Fig. 11.8):

Biparietal diameter. This is 9.5 cm – the diameter between the two parietal eminences.

Bitemporal diameter. This is 8.2 cm – the diameter between the furthest points of the coronal suture at the temples.

The remaining diameters described are anteroposterior or longitudinal (Fig. 11.9):

Suboccipitobregmatic. This is 9.5 cm – the diameter from below the occipital protuberance to the centre of the anterior fontanelle or bregma.

Suboccipitofrontal. This is 10 cm – the diameter from below the occipital protuberance to the centre of the frontal suture.

Occipitofrontal. This is 11.5 cm – the diameter from the occipital protuberance to the glabella.

Mentovertical. This is 13.5 cm – the diameter from the point of the chin to the highest point on the vertex, slightly nearer to the posterior than to the anterior fontanelle.

Submentovertical. This is 11.5 cm – the diameter from the point where the chin joins the neck to the highest point on the vertex.

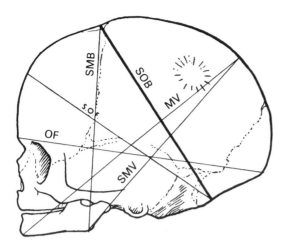

Fig. 11.9 Diagram showing the anteroposterior diameters of the fetal skull.

Diameter			Length
SOB	=	suboccipitobregmatic	9.5 cm
SOF	=	suboccipitofrontal	10.0 cm
OF	=	occipitofrontal	11.5 cm
MV	=	mentovertical	13.5 cm
SMV	=	submentovertical	11.5 cm
SMB	=	submentobregmatic	9.5 cm

Submentobregmatic. This is 9.5 cm – the diameter from the point where the chin joins the neck to the centre of the bregma.

Attitude of the fetal head

This term is used to describe the degree of flexion or extension of the head on the neck. The attitude of the head determines which diameters will present in labour and therefore influences the outcome.

Presenting diameters

The diameters of the head, which are called the presenting diameters, are those that are at right angles to the curve of Carus. There are always two: an anteroposterior or longitudinal diameter and a transverse diameter. The diameters presenting in the individual cephalic or head presentations are as follows:

Vertex presentation. When the head is well flexed, the suboccipitobregmatic diameter and the biparietal diameter present (Fig. 11.10). As these two diameters are the same length, 9.5 cm, the presenting area is circular, which is the most favourable shape for dilating the cervix. The diameter that distends the vaginal orifice is the suboccipitofrontal diameter, 10 cm.

When the head is not flexed but erect, the presenting diameters are the occipitofrontal, 11.5 cm, and the biparietal, 9.5 cm. This situation often arises when the occiput is in a posterior position. If it remains so, the diameter distending the vaginal orifice will be the occipitofrontal, 11.5 cm.

Brow presentation. When the head is partially extended, the mentovertical diameter, 13.5 cm, and the bitemporal diameter, 8.2 cm, present. If this presentation persists, vaginal delivery is extremely unlikely.

Face presentation. When the head is completely extended, the presenting diameters are the submentobregmatic, 9.5 cm, and the bitemporal, 8.2 cm. The submentovertical diameter, 11.5 cm, will distend the vaginal orifice.

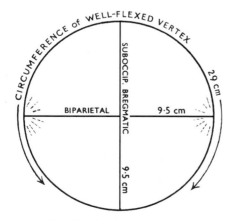

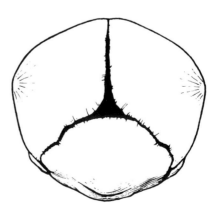

Fig. 11.10 Diagram showing the dimensions presenting when the fetal head is well flexed in a vertex presentation.

Box 11.2 Diameters of the fetal trunk

Bisacromial diameter 12 cm
This is the distance between the acromion processes on the two shoulder blades and is the dimension that needs to pass through the pelvis for the shoulders to be born. The articulation of the clavicles on the sternum allows forward movement of the shoulders, which may reduce the diameter slightly.

Bitrochanteric diameter 10 cm
This is measured between the greater trochanters of the femurs and is the presenting diameter in breech presentation.

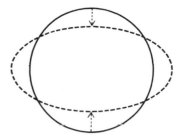

Fig. 11.11 Demonstration of the principle of moulding. The diameter compressed is diminished; the diameter at right angles to it is elongated.

Diameters of the fetal trunk are given in Box 11.2.

Moulding

This is the term applied to the change in shape of the fetal head that takes place during its passage through the birth canal. Alteration in shape is possible because the bones of the vault allow a slight degree of bending and the skull bones are able to override at the sutures. This overriding allows a considerable reduction in the size of the presenting diameters while the diameter at right angles to them is able to lengthen owing to the give of the skull bones (Fig. 11.11).

In a normal vertex presentation with the fetal head in a fully flexed attitude the suboccipitobregmatic and the biparietal diameters will be reduced and the mentovertical will be lengthened. The shortening may be by as much as 1.25 cm (Figs 11.12–11.17 illustrate moulding in various presentations).

Moulding is a protective mechanism and prevents the fetal brain from being compressed as long as it is not excessive, too rapid or in an unfavourable direction. The skull of the preterm infant, being softer and having wider sutures, may mould excessively; the skull of the post-term infant does not mould well and its greater hardness tends to make labour more difficult.

The intracranial membranes and sinuses (Figs 11.18 and 11.19)

The skull contains delicate structures, some of which may be damaged if the head is subjected to abnormal moulding during delivery. Among the most important are the folds of dura mater and the venous sinuses associated with them. These membranes are continuous with the dura mater that lines the cranium.

The falx cerebri. This is a sickle-shaped fold of membrane that dips down between the two cerebral hemispheres and runs beneath the frontal and sagittal sutures, from the root of the nose to the internal occipital protuberance.

The tentorium cerebelli. This is a horizontal fold of dura mater that lies in the posterior part of the skull at right angles to the falx cerebri. It is shaped like a horseshoe and situated between the cerebrum and the cerebellum, over which it forms a sort of tent. The membranes contain large veins or sinuses that drain blood from the brain.

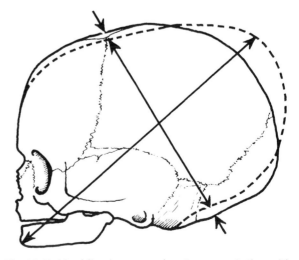

Fig. 11.12 Moulding in a normal vertex presentation with the head well flexed. The suboccipitobregmatic diameter is reduced and the mentovertical elongated.

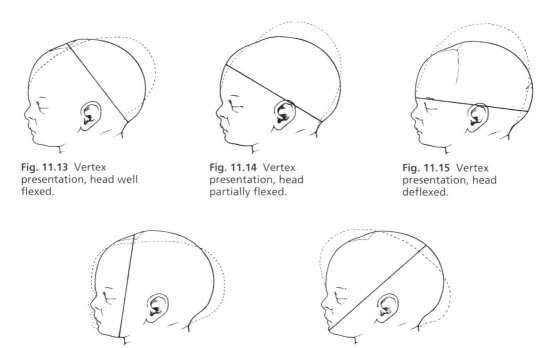

Fig. 11.13 Vertex presentation, head well flexed.

Fig. 11.14 Vertex presentation, head partially flexed.

Fig. 11.15 Vertex presentation, head deflexed.

Fig. 11.16 Face presentation.

Fig. 11.17 Brow presentation.

Figs 11.13–11.17 Series of diagrams showing moulding when the head presents. Moulding is shown by the dotted line.

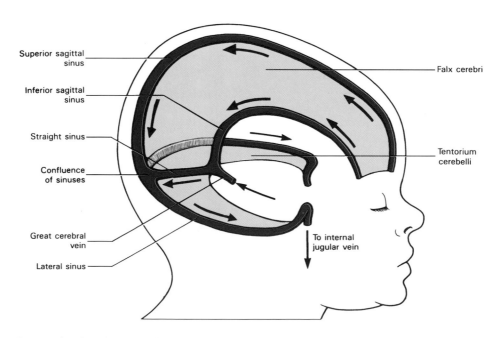

Fig. 11.18 Diagram showing intracranial membranes and venous sinuses. Arrows show direction of blood flow.

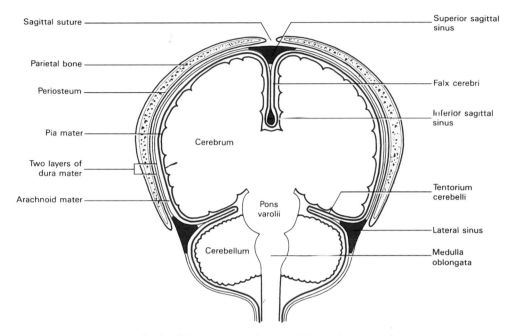

Fig. 11.19 Coronal section through the fetal head to show intracranial membranes and venous sinuses.

The superior sagittal sinus. This runs along the upper edge of the falx cerebri from front to back.

The inferior sagittal sinus. This runs along the lower edge of the falx cerebri in the same direction.

The great cerebral vein of Galen. This meets the inferior sagittal sinus at the inner end of the junction between the falx and the tentorium.

The straight sinus. This drains blood from both the great cerebral vein and the inferior sagittal sinus along the junction of the falx and the tentorium. The point where it reaches the skull and receives blood from the superior sagittal sinus is known as the *confluence of sinuses*.

The two lateral sinuses. These pass from the confluence of sinuses along the outer edge of the tentorium cerebelli and carry blood to the internal jugular veins.

The most vulnerable point of these structures is where the falx is attached to the tentorium. The tentorium is liable to tear and there is a danger of bleeding from the great cerebral vein.

REFERENCE

Johnson M H, Everitt B J 2000 Essential reproduction, 5th edn. Blackwell Science, Oxford

FURTHER READING

Coad J with Dunstall M 2001 Anatomy and physiology for midwives. Mosby, Edinburgh

A detailed discussion of embryonic and fetal development appears in Chapter 9. The fetal circulation and adaptation to neonatal life are addressed in Chapter 15 along with other adaptations at birth. Information is reliably presented and often clinical applications are given, which are helpful.

Johnson M H, Everitt B J 2000 Essential reproduction, 5th edn. Blackwell Science, Oxford

For the student who requires a detailed understanding of prenatal events and in particular the hormonal influences, this book is unsurpassed. It is important to be aware that it addresses reproduction in various species and discusses how much our knowledge of the physiology of sheep or goats can inform us of events in the human. Useful statements at the head of each small section give the principles that are relevant.

Moore K L, Persaud T V N 1998 The developing human, 6th edn. Saunders, London

Moore K L, Persaud T V N 1998 Before we are born, 5th edn. Saunders, London

These two books are very similar to one another and the reader will find a great deal of detail concerning the embryo and the developing fetus. There are numerous clear illustrations in colour as well as photomicrographs to show reproductive events.

Stables D 1999 Physiology in childbearing with anatomy and basic sciences. Baillière Tindall, Edinburgh

The equivalent information is scattered through the book in Chapters 13, 34 and 48 but the student may find some additional interesting details such as maternal influence on fetal size in Chapter 13.

Wolpert L 1991 The triumph of the embryo. Oxford University Press, Oxford

Originating in a series of Christmas lectures at the Royal Institution, this text explores the unifying principles that may account for the way embryos develop. Written for the non-specialist, it invites the reader to think broadly and aims to inspire as well as instruct.

3

Section 3
Pregnancy

SECTION CONTENTS

12 Preparing for Pregnancy

Diane Barrowclough

CHAPTER CONTENTS

Preparing for pregnancy is a positive step towards enhancing pregnancy outcome and provides prospective parents with options that may not be available once a pregnancy is confirmed. The midwife may need to support a couple as they embark on a programme that may include investigation, diagnosis and treatment in order to help them conceive, all of which may impact upon their physical, psychological and social well-being.

The chapter aims to:

- discuss the aims of preconception care

- review the health and environmental factors that have an effect on pregnancy outcome and describe methods of preconception screening

- give an overview of the management of the infertile couple and describe the assisted reproduction techniques available

- highlight the psychosocial, psychosexual and ethical issues associated with the management of infertility.

Preconception care

Unlike antenatal care the concept of preconception care has been around for less than 30 years; it has now been identified as a key area of health care. The aim of preconception care is 'to ensure that the woman and her partner are in an optimal state of physical and emotional health at the onset of pregnancy' (RCGP 1995, p. 3). It also provides prospective parents with a series of options that may not be available once a pregnancy is confirmed (Chamberlain 1995). Although pregnancy for some couples will be unplanned, the majority of couples who do plan a pregnancy could benefit from preconception care whether they just want to do the best for their baby or as an effort to

167

mitigate against conditions that can adversely affect the outcome of pregnancy.

Preconception advice is readily available particularly in the mass media and through the World Wide Web. However, the provision of preconception care is still not universal with the majority of services being provided by family planning clinics, well-woman clinics, general practitioners (GPs), practice nurses, midwives and health visitors, most of them opportunistic (Wallace & Hurwitz 1998). The preconception period refers to a time span of anything from 3 months to 1 year before conception (Bussell 2000) but ideally should include the time when both the ova and sperm mature, which is approximately 100 days before conception (Bradley & Bennett 1995).

The problem with preconception care is that the people who most need it rarely attend for such counselling. The people who do seek out such care are usually well-motivated educated couples. Even then, people find it hard to change their lifestyle and habits.

A preconception programme takes time to complete, therefore adequate time needs to be allowed for the initial consultation and the subsequent follow-ups where results, advice and treatment may be given. Box 12.1 outlines the information and investigations that may be included.

General health and fertility

Fertility and fatness

It has been well established that fertility and fatness are closely related with subfertility-related problems occurring in women below and above the desirable range of body weight. Where diet is restricted or accompanied by high levels of training such as in ballet dancers and athletes, or both, the menarche can be delayed, and secondary amenorrhoea and irregular cycles are common after the menarche (Frisch et al 1980). The average postpubertal woman has a body fat content of approximately 28%; a minimum of 22% is required for the maintenance of ovulation (Frisch & McArthur 1974). Conditions such as thyrotoxicosis, malabsorption syndromes, eating disorders such as anorexia nervosa and bulimia nervosa and psychological stress can result in secondary amenorrhoea (Thomas 2001). Weight gain as a result of increasing energy intake or reducing training regimes, or both, is usually sufficient to re-establish ovulation in

> **Box 12.1** Information and investigations in a preconception programme
>
> **History**
> - Family history
> - Medical history
> - Menstrual history
> - Obstetric history
> - Method of contraception
> - Medication
> - Occupation
> - Diet
> - Smoking
> - Alcohol
>
> **Observation-investigations**
> - Height and weight
> - Blood pressure
> - Urinalysis
> - Stool sample
> - Blood tests – haemoglobin
> - Folic acid and vitamin levels
> - Rubella immunity
> - VDRL (venereal diseases research laboratory)
> - Haemoglobinopathies
> - Lead and trace elements
> - Hair analysis (controversial)
> - Male – semen analysis
> - Female – cervical smear, high vaginal swab (HVS)

underweight women (Goldberg 2000). Fat distribution is also important as an increased waist–hip ratio, where fat distribution is predominantly around the abdomen as opposed to the hips and thighs, is associated with reduced chances of conception (Zaastra 1993). However, spontaneous ovulation and conception are possible when a programme of weight loss and exercise is adhered to (Clark et al 1998).

Body weight

Assessment of body type is done by the Quetelet or body mass index (BMI) and is calculated by dividing

Are you the correct weight for your height?

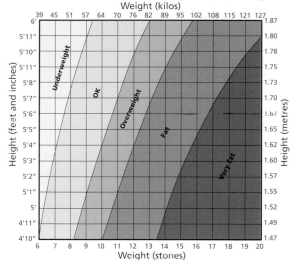

Fig. 12.1 'Are you the right weight for your height?' (Chart reproduced from the health guide by the Health Education Authority 2000. © Crown Copyright 2000.)

the weight in kilograms by the height in metres squared. It is a reflection of weight for height and therefore a high BMI identifies those people who are relatively overweight irrespective of their height.

Example. For someone who weighs 60 kg and is 1.65 m tall the BMI is calculated as follows:

$$\frac{(weight\ in\ kilograms)}{(height\ in\ metres\ squared)} = \frac{60}{(1.65 \times 1.65)} = 22.06$$

Alternatively a BMI chart as in Figure 12.1 can be used. The desirable or healthy range is between 20 and 24.9. The underweight, overweight and obese categories can lead to long term health hazards.

	BMI
Grade 0	< 20 (underweight)
Grade I	20–24.9 (healthy)
Grade II	25–29.9 (overweight)
Grade III	30–39.9 (obese)
Grade III	> 40 (severely obese)

A woman's nutritional status before pregnancy and during the first weeks before realising that she is pregnant may be more important than the diet she eats once her pregnancy is confirmed (Doyle 1992). By this time much of the cell organisation, differentiation and organogenesis will have taken place. Suboptimal conditions at this time can result in fetal damage and stunted growth. An optimum BMI for maximum fertility and for producing a healthy baby of normal birthweight appears to be around 23 (Wynn & Wynn 1983, 1990). Low maternal weight before conception is associated with an increased risk in low birthweight babies and symmetrical growth restriction (Bussell 2000) and for women with a BMI below 19.1 van der Spuy et al (1988) noted a fivefold increase in low birthweight.

Substantial evidence is accumulating that corroborates the relationship between the increased risk of pregnancy complications and adverse pregnancy outcomes in overweight and obese women. Even moderate overweight is a risk factor for gestational diabetes and hypertensive disorders of pregnancy, whereas overt obesity also includes a higher incidence of caesarean delivery, low Apgar scores, fetal macrosomia, neural tube defects (NTDs) and late fetal death (Baeten et al 2001, Cnattingius et al 1998, Galtier-Dereure et al 2000).

Obesity in the UK has doubled in the past decade and trebled in the last two decades. Today, 50% of British adults are overweight and by 2030 it is predicted that nearly half of the population will be obese, and up to 70% overweight (Haslam 2001). It is most likely that midwives will increasingly encounter women who are either overweight or obese prior to and during pregnancy. The aim of preconception care is to help such women achieve an appropriate BMI prior to conception to enhance pregnancy outcome. Overweight women should be encouraged to lose weight before conception; however, some caution is required as consuming an energy-deficient diet immediately prior to conception may result in nutritional deficiencies that could disadvantage the fetus. Dietary changes and weight loss should occur at least 3–4 months before attempting conception (Thomas 2001).

Principles of a healthy diet

It is well noted that fat consumption in the UK is above the current recommendations (DoH 1991), although according to the National Food Survey 1999 (MAFF 2000) the percentage of food energy derived from fat is falling. Fat is known to increase the palatability of food as well as being more energy dense and satisfying. Where food choices are abundant it is not easy to get people to change their eating habits and even though they may know what is good for them this does not induce them to alter their nutritional attitudes or behaviour (Bussell 2000).

When giving advice about a healthy diet a simple and easy guide is the 'balance of good health diagram from the Food Standards Agency (see Plate 2). The central tenet of this is to eat more starchy foods such as cereals and bread, at least five portions of fruit and vegetables daily and less fatty foods. Eating healthily is not always easy on a limited budget but foods such as baked beans, jacket potatoes, sardines and tuna are relatively cheap but nutritious foods (Ford et al 1994).

Folate, folic acid and neural tube defects

Folic acid is a water-soluble vitamin belonging to the B complex. The term 'folates' is used to describe the folic acid derivatives that are found naturally in food and the term 'folic acid' is used to refer to the synthetic form used in vitamin supplements and fortification of foods. The main sources of folate in the UK diet are dark green vegetables, potatoes, fruit and fruit juices, beans and yeast extract (Barrowclough & Ford 2000). Folates are vulnerable to heat and readily dissolve in water, therefore considerable losses can occur as a result of cooking or prolonged storage. Folic acid is more stable and better absorbed than folate and is added to many brands of bread and breakfast cereals in the UK. The Expert Advisory Group on Folic Acid and Neural Tube Defects (DoH 1992) recommended that, to reduce the risk of first occurrence of NTDs, all women should increase their daily folate and folic acid intake by an additional 400 μg prior to conception and during the first 12 weeks of pregnancy. This can be achieved by:

- eating more folate-rich foods
- eating more fortified foods such as bread and breakfast cereals
- taking a daily folic acid supplement of 400 μg.

Women with a history of a previous child with NTD should take a daily dose of 5 mg of folic acid to reduce the risk of recurrence (HEA 1996). The 400 μg folic acid supplements are reasonably priced and are readily available from pharmacies, health food stores and supermarkets but the 5 mg supplement is available on prescription only. However, as many as half of all pregnancies in some areas of the UK are unplanned, compliance with the recommendations is difficult (McGovern et al 1997). Fortification of flour used in food production with folic acid could prevent a significant proportion of NTD-affected births (DoH 2000a). The results of a consultation by the UK Health Departments and the Food Standards Agency on the universal fortification of flour in the UK are still awaited (DoH 2000b).

Vitamin A

Vitamin A is essential for embryogenesis, growth and epithelial differentiation, but a high intake of the retinol form of vitamin A is known to be teratogenic. In a study by Rothman et al (1995) a high dietary intake of vitamin A produced an increased frequency of birth defects that were concentrated among the babies born to women who had consumed high levels of vitamin A before the 7th week of pregnancy. The birth defects of these babies included: cleft lip, ventricular septal defect, multiple heart defects, hydrocephaly, craniosynostosis and transposition of the great vessels. High levels of retinol are found in the liver of farm animals so in 1990 the DoH recommended that women who are pregnant or planning a pregnancy should avoid eating liver and liver products such as pate or liver sausage as these contain large amounts of retinol.

Pre-existing medical conditions and drugs

Diabetes

Diabetes mellitus is the most prevalent chronic medical disease in the pregnant population. Infants of insulin-dependent diabetics have 10 times the general population risk of congenital malformation and five times the stillbirth rate (Casson et al 1997). Diabetic complications such as retinopathy and nephropathy may worsen during pregnancy, particularly if associated with hypertension. Women who have severe neuropathy or cardiovascular disease may even be advised against pregnancy (Cefalo & Moos 1995). In this respect, preconception counselling and family planning advice should be an important aspect of their diabetic management (American Dietetic Association 1998, Jantz et al 1995).

The aim of preconception care is to achieve normoglycaemia both pre- and periconception as many of the problems seen in the insulin-dependent diabetic mother are a direct result of hyperglycaemia (Cefalo & Moos 1995). However, Jantz et al (1995) found that only about one-third of diabetic women attend for preconception care.

The safety of currently available oral hypoglycaemic agents in pregnancy is not well established, therefore women with type II diabetes who are taking such treatments should be switched to insulin therapy both for the preconception period and for pregnancy (American Dietetic Association 1998).

Epilepsy

Epilepsy is the most common neurological problem seen during pregnancy (Cefalo & Moos 1995). The major anticonvulsant drugs used to treat epilepsy are known to have teratogenic effects and the newer antiepileptic drugs have not yet been sufficiently evaluated (Crawford 1997, Holmes et al 2001, Lloyd & Hunter 2001). Pregnancy is also known to alter the metabolism of antiepileptic drugs, with approximately one-third of women experiencing an increase in the number of seizures. However, this increase may be induced by deliberate non-compliance (Crawford 1997, Lloyd & Hunter 2001).

The aim of preconception care for the woman with epilepsy is to help her plan her pregnancies carefully and to keep her seizure free on the lowest possible dose of anticonvulsants. For some women this may mean withdrawal of therapy and for others a reduction from poly- to monotherapy (Crawford 1997). Some anticonvulsant drugs are folate antagonists. Therefore folic acid supplements are needed to protect against macrocytic anaemia and reduce the risk of NTDs (Lloyd & Hunter 2001). The daily dosage of folic acid requires individual counselling (DoH 1992) but is likely to be the higher dose of 5 mg (National Society for Epilepsy 2001).

There is concern that women with epilepsy are not getting the care and advice they need. Evidence suggests that information relating to contraception, teratogenicity of antiepileptic medication and folic acid supplementation is poor, and there is often poor seizure control and lack of preconception counselling (Fairgrieve et al 2000, Madden 1999).

Phenylketonuria (PKU)

Phenylketonuria is an inborn error of metabolism (see Ch. 47). Some women with PKU discontinue treatment during middle childhood. However, unless they resume careful dietary control around the time of conception, the toxic effect of phenylalanine (Phe) on the developing embryo/fetus results in a high rate of microcephaly, mental retardation and congenital heart defects (Hall 2000, Rouse et al 2000). Even through dietary control, it is not easy for some women to attain the recommended Phe levels of 120–360 μmol/L, but when dietary levels are achieved before conception or by 8–10 weeks of pregnancy the occurrence of congenital heart disease is significantly reduced (Platt et al 2000, Rouse 2000). Clearly, the woman with PKU needs specialist help and support throughout.

Oral contraception

Oral contraception should be stopped at least 3 months and preferably 6 months prior to planning a pregnancy to allow for the resumption of natural hormone regulation and ovulation. Also the oral contraceptive pill is associated with vitamin and mineral imbalances that may need correcting. Copper levels are raised whilst zinc levels are reduced and can result in a deficiency of the latter mineral. Vitamin metabolism is also affected, which may lead to deficiencies of folate, B complex and vitamin C and an increase in vitamin A, which can be teratogenic at high levels (Bradley & Bennett 1995). Other forms of contraception such as barrier methods will need to be advised during this time.

Drug abuse

The number of drug users is rising and the most frequently reported main drug of use is heroin followed by methadone, cannabis, cocaine and amphetamines, half of users being in their twenties (DoH 2000c). Disruption of the menstrual cycle is common among women using drugs like ecstasy, amphetamines, opiates and anabolic steroids, and heavy drug use during pregnancy is associated with miscarriage, preterm labour, low birthweight, stillbirth and abnormalities. Some women may be trying to come off tranquillisers that can take many weeks of withdrawal. Drug users are unlikely to present for preconception care as a high proportion of these women conceal their drug use (Illman 2001).

Environmental factors

Smoking

The evidence is substantial that pregnancy is adversely affected by smoking. In terms of fertility, in women smoking can induce early menopause and menstrual problems; in men it can cause abnormalities in sperm morphology and motility. During pregnancy, there is an increased risk of spontaneous abortion, preterm delivery, low birthweight and perinatal mortality because of antepartum haemorrhage and placental abruption (Sexton 1986). New evidence also shows that women who smoke during pregnancy pass harmful carcinogens on to their baby (DoH 1998).

Nutritional status tends to be compromised in smokers, characterised by higher intakes of energy, total fat, saturated fat, cholesterol and alcohol and lower intakes of most micronutrients and antioxidant vitamins (Dallongeville et al 1998).

More children and young people are starting to smoke; the prevalence of regular smoking of those aged 11 to 15 has increased in England from 8% in 1988 to 13% in 1996. Over this period the proportion of 15-year-old girls who smoke regularly has increased from just one in five to one in three (DoH 1998).

The addictive nature of smoking makes it very difficult for a woman to stop even when she knows it may harm her baby. The DoH (1998) has set a target to reduce the percentage of women who smoke during pregnancy to 15% by the year 2010; if successful this will mean that approximately 55 000 fewer women in England smoke during pregnancy.

The aim of preconception care is to help the woman stop smoking, and partner involvement is known to enhance success (Allen 2001). Raw et al (1999) advocate that all health professionals should ask about smoking at every opportunity where advice and assistance for smoking cessation can be given as well as arrangements for follow-up. This brief advice is designed to motivate attempts to stop smoking, although heavy smokers may need referral to specialist help. Midwives, general practitioners, obstetricians and other health professionals have regular, one-to-one contact with pregnant women and these contacts are ideal opportunities to offer support and practical advice on giving up smoking. The support needs to be continued throughout the antenatal period and even into the postnatal period as many women who do stop smoking in pregnancy go back to smoking within 1 month of the birth (DoH 1998). All advice should be consistent and well informed and staff may need specialist training.

Alcohol

Alcohol when drunk occasionally or in moderation is a very acceptable social activity, but when consumed in large quantities it can become problematic, reduce appetite and affect nutritional status (Goldberg 2000). High alcohol intakes in women have been associated with menstrual disorders and decreased fertility, even among women who had five or fewer drinks a week (Jensen et al 1998).

Alcohol is a teratogen and fetal alcohol syndrome (FAS) is used to describe the congenital malformations associated with excessive maternal alcohol intake during pregnancy. Although there is general agreement that women should not drink alcohol excessively during pregnancy, there is no consensus opinion as to what is a safe amount. A recent review by the Royal College of Obstetricians and Gynaecologists (RCOG 1999) found no conclusive evidence of adverse effects in either growth or IQ at levels of consumption below 15 units (120 g) per week. Even so, the recommendation is that women should remain cautious and limit alcohol consumption in pregnancy to no more than one standard unit of drink per day (Box 12.2).

Preconception advice can be given after taking a drinking history and women with a drink problem will need specialist referral for treatment and support. People with drinking problems are often very frightened at the thought of giving up alcohol and the effects it may have. Alcohol for some women may be

---

Box 12.2 Units of alcohol

1 unit of alcohol = $\frac{1}{2}$ pint of ordinary strength beer, lager or cider

$\frac{1}{4}$ pint of strong beer or lager

1 small glass wine

1 single measure of spirit

1 small glass sherry

just one part of a chronic lifestyle that includes low social status, poverty and poor nutrition; therefore she will need sensitive and supportive care (Plant 2000).

Exercise

Moderate exercise is known to be beneficial for health and the benefits of regular exercise for the healthy pregnant woman appear to outweigh the risks. According to Kardel & Kase (1998) exercise by physically fit women with uncomplicated pregnancies has no adverse effect on fetal growth. However, exercise intensity should be modified according to maternal symptoms and should not continue to fatigue or exhaustion. Also, exercise in the supine position should be avoided after the first trimester to avoid supine hypotension syndrome, and activities that require significant balance should be approached with caution (Bungum et al 2000).

Workplace hazards and noxious substances

Human are exposed to many environmental agents that may be hazardous to their reproductive capacity and much of this exposure may occur in the workplace even though employees are protected by the Control of Substances Hazardous to Health Regulations (COSHH 1999).

Exposure to solvents, ionising radiation and anaesthetic gases is known to be toxic and associated with central nervous system defects, microcephaly and an increased risk of miscarriage (Joffe 1986). Heavy metals are also known to be toxic (Table 12.1).

There has been concern about working with visual display units (VDUs) during pregnancy and there are reports of the risk of miscarriages or birth defects. However, to date the scientific studies that have been carried out and taken as a whole do not show any link (HSE 1998).

Genetic counselling

The decision to have a baby is not always straightforward for some couples. A family history of genetic disorders, a previous baby affected with a congenital abnormality and leaving childbearing until later years all increase the risk of giving birth to an abnormal child. For such couples, referral for genetic counselling will help them to decide what is best for them.

The risk of having a child with a genetic defect is something that only the couple can decide whether to take or not. It is essential therefore that the counsellor adopts a non-directive approach and that an undisturbed consultation allows adequate time for explanations, clarifying misconceptions and answering questions. When discussing genetic risks the terms

Table 12.1 Toxic effects of heavy metals

Metal	Source	Effect
Aluminium	Antacids Antiperspirants Food additives	Can compromise nutritional status
Cadmium	Cigarette smoking Processed foods Paint, batteries and fertilisers	Embryotoxic in animals
Copper	Contraceptive pill Copper kettles Swimming pools	Embryotoxic Teratogenic Premature birth in animals
Lead	Exhaust fumes from lead in petrol Lead piping	Miscarriage, stillbirth Malformations Retarded neurological development Low sperm count
Mercury	Pesticides Fungicides Dental fillings	Mental retardation Spasticity

'probabilities' and 'odds' are often used and this can be a source of confusion for some couples. Risk figures are often quoted as either odds or percentages. Harper (1998) states that many people do not have a clear idea about what constitutes a 'high' or 'low' risk and that it is very easy for odds to be reversed – for example where a 1 in 20 recurrence risk is interpreted as only a 1 in 20 chance of a normal child.

Mendelian inheritance

Genetic disorders can occur as a result of Mendelian inheritance and are either dominant or recessive. An *autosomal dominant* disorder occurs when the condition is present in the heterozygous state (i.e. only one gene of a pair of chromosomes need be affected); achondroplasia, neurofibromatosis and Huntington's disease are examples. The risks associated with this inheritance pattern are relatively straightforward – there is a 1 in 2, or 50%, risk in a couple where one of them is affected with the condition.

An *autosomal recessive* disorder occurs only in the homozygous state (i.e. both chromosomes of a pair must be affected), which means that any offspring of an affected individual are obligatory carriers given that the other partner is unaffected. Cystic fibrosis, inborn errors of metabolism and the haemoglobinopathies are common autosomal recessive disorders that the midwife is likely to encounter. Consanguinity is an important consideration in relation to autosomal recessive disorders as marriage between first cousins is legal in the UK (Harper 1998).

Genetic disorders can also be *x linked*. Such disorders are inherited through the female sex chromosome; this means that females are usually the carriers and any male offspring that they may have are affected with the disorder. Examples are muscular dystrophy, haemophilia and several types of colour blindness (Harper 1998).

Chromosome abnormalities

Chromosome aberrations include the trisomies, of which trisomy 21 (Down's syndrome) is the most common and trisomy 13 and 18 are more rare. Age factors are significant particularly in Down's syndrome, for which the risk is 1% for a woman around 40 years of age. Monosomies are usually lethal and non-viable autosomal trisomies are extremely common in spontaneous abortions. Sex chromosome abnormalities such as Turner's syndrome (XO) and Klinefelter's syndrome (XXY) have a rare recurrence rate in families.

Translocation is where extra chromosome material is translocated on to another chromosome and is regarded as balanced when the total amount of chromosome material is normal but only 45 chromosomes are present. Reciprocal translocations can also occur where there is exchange of chromosome material but no change in chromosome number, but the recurrence risk is low if neither parent is a balanced carrier for the translocation.

Non-mendelian disorders

The commoner congenital abnormalities such as NTDs and congenital heart disease do not follow the Mendelian inheritance pattern as there is no identified genetic locus and so they are referred to as *multifactorial*. These conditions arise as a result of a combination or interaction of environmental and genetic factors. The recurrence risk of such conditions depends upon the incidence of the disorder but is increased amongst close relatives (Harper 1998).

Prenatal diagnosis

Most prenatal diagnosis of a genetic condition occurs during pregnancy but ideally for a couple to truly benefit from the process such diagnosis should occur before a pregnancy is planned. This allows the couple time to consider the risk of genetic disorder, particularly when those risks are more accurately stated as is implicated in carrier status. The condition in terms of available treatments and consequences to the affected child can be discussed and the couple's perspective of the problem can be ascertained. Ultimately the goal of genetic counselling is to prevent or avoid a genetic disorder (Harper 1998). Preconception care involving a multidisciplinary team is the way to achieve this.

Infertility

The term 'infertility' is in most cases inappropriate, as it is only in extreme cases such as premature menopause or complete lack of sperm where there is no chance of conceiving at all. Most infertility is really some degree of subfertility and 1 in 7 couples needs specialist help to conceive, including some couples who have conceived before. The WHO (1992) defines subfertility as 'the inability of a couple to achieve conception or to bring a pregnancy to term after a year or more of regular, unprotected intercourse'. The prevalence of infertility has not changed greatly although more couples are now seeking help than previously (RCOG 2000).

Infertility is categorised as *primary* if there has been no prior conception and *secondary* if there has been a previous pregnancy irrespective of the outcome. Couples now have fewer than two children on average in most European countries and they tend to postpone these births until a later age when there is a natural reduction in fertility (European Society of Human Reproduction and Embryology (ESHRE) 2001). Under normal circumstances the chance of a couple conceiving within one menstrual cycle is 20–25% given that unprotected intercourse occurs at the optimum time, the female partner is ovulating regularly and the male partner is producing sperm of sufficient quality.

The factors responsible for infertility are many and varied, with an incidence in men up to 30% (Box 12.3) and in women up to 40% (Box 12.4). Approximately one-third of cases of infertility involve problems with both partners, and in one-third of couples the causes of infertility remain unexplained. The most common causes are ovulation failure and sperm disorders.

Initial management of the infertile couple

Much of the initial management of the infertile couple is via primary care, therefore the preliminary investigation of both partners and subsequent referral to specialist care will be through the general practitioner. Early referral should be instigated for couples where the female partner is over 35 years, and where there is amenorrhoea or significant pelvic infection (Hargreave & Mills 1998). The investigative process is aimed at achieving an accurate diagnosis and definition of any cause, an accurate estimation of the chance of conceiving without treatment and a full appraisal of treatment options.

It is important that both partners should be involved in the management of their infertility and that full explanations are given to the couple at each stage in the investigation and treatment. This should

---

Box 12.3 Causes of male infertility

Defective spermatogenesis

Endocrine disorders

- Dysfunction of:
  - —hypothalamus
  - —pituitary
  - —adrenals
  - —thyroid
- Systemic disease:
  - —diabetes mellitus
  - —coeliac disease
  - —renal failure

Testicular disorders

- Trauma
- Environmental (high temperature):
  - —congenital (hydrocele, undescended testes)
  - —occupational (furnaceman, long-distance lorry driver)
  - —acquired (varicocele, tight clothing)
- Cancer treatment

Defective transport

- Obstruction or absence of seminal ducts:
  - —infection
  - —congenital anomalies
  - —trauma
- Impaired secretions from prostate or seminal vesicles:
  - —infection
  - —metabolic disorders

Ineffective delivery

- Psychosexual problems (impotence)
- Drug-induced (ejaculatory dysfunction)
- Physical disability
- Physical anomalies:
  - —hypospadias
  - —epispadias
  - —retrograde ejaculation (into bladder)

Box 12.4 Causes of female infertility

Defective ovulation
Endocrine disorders
- Dysfunction of:
  —hypothalamus
  —pituitary
  —adrenals
  —thyroid
- Systemic disease:
  —diabetes mellitus
  —coeliac disease
  —renal failure

Physical disorders
- Obesity
- Anorexia nervosa or strict dieting
- Excessive exercise

Ovarian disorders
- Hormonal
- Ovarian cysts or tumours
- Polycystic ovary disease
- Ovarian endometriosis

Defective transport
Ovum
- Tubal obstruction:
  —infection (gonorrhoea, peritonitis, pelvic inflammatory disease)
  —previous tubal surgery
- Fimbrial adhesions:
  —previous surgery
  —endometriosis

Sperm
- Vagina:
  —psychosexual problems (vaginismus)
  —infection (causing dyspareunia)
  —congenital anomaly
- Cervix:
  —cervical trauma or surgery (cone biopsy)
  —infection
  —hormonal (hostile mucus)
  —antisperm antibodies in mucus

Defective implantation
- Hormonal imbalance
- Congenital anomalies
- Fibroids
- Infection

---

be backed up with written information that should include a list of addresses of relevant organisations. Rubella status should be confirmed and folic acid supplementation commenced for the female partner. A detailed drug history should be taken from both partners, including any history of drug abuse. Occupational factors should be noted. General advice regarding smoking and alcohol should be given to both partners and weight control advice, if appropriate, for the female partner (RCOG 1998). At this stage the couple should be advised to continue their normal sexual habit, as there is no evidence that attempts to time intercourse in the menstrual cycle improve conception rates (Hargreave & Mills 1998). The female partner should have measurement of serum progesterone levels in the midluteal phase and the male partner should initially have two semen analyses (Box 12.5) performed.

Further investigations

The more specialised investigations need to be undertaken in a dedicated, specialist infertility clinic where there is access to appropriately trained staff and a multiprofessional team. Both partners should be screened for *Chlamydia trachomatis* and the female partner investigated for tubal patency. The main factors that predict the chances of a successful pregnancy in infertile couples undergoing assisted conception are: the female partner's age, the length of time the couple have been trying to conceive, the previous ability to conceive and

> **Box 12.5** Semen analysis
>
> **Normal values** (WHO 1992):
> - semen volume > 2–5 ml
> - sperm concentration >20 million/ml
> - motility > 50% progressive motility
> - morphology > 30% normal forms
> - white blood cells < 1 million/ml

the quality of the sperm (Chambers 1999). The success rate for infertility treatment declines with increasing duration of infertility and increasing age (RCOG 2000).

Assisted reproduction techniques

A range of assisted reproduction techniques is available to treat the infertile couple and it is important that the appropriate treatment option is offered. The general practitioner, the local hospital or a licensed clinic may offer some treatments, but any centre that provides techniques that involves fertilisation outside the body has to be regulated by the Human Fertilisation and Embryology Authority (HFEA). The HFEA remains one of the few national statutory bodies of its kind in the world and was set up in 1991 to license and regulate clinics that provide:

- in vitro fertilisation (IVF) treatment
- donor insemination (DI) treatment
- gamete intrafallopian transfer (GIFT) where donated sperm or eggs are used in treatment
- storage of gametes or embryos.

Any clinic that carries out research involving human embryos is also subject to the HFEA licensing regulations. People seeking licensed treatments or wishing to donate or store gametes or embryos must be given the opportunity for counselling. This is to help them understand the implications of the proposed treatment for themselves and their families, for emotional support if needed and to help them cope with the consequences of infertility and treatment (HFEA 2001).

Ovulation induction

There are many reasons for ovulatory failure and although menstruation is strongly suggestive of ovulation it is not conclusive. Women with amenorrhoea or oliogomenorrhoea can be treated with ovulation-inducing agents provided that the male partner has an adequate sperm count. Clomifene is the most commonly prescribed drug but should be prescribed only when there are no other factors contributing to infertility and there is access to ovarian ultrasound monitoring. Clomifene works by inducing negative feedback that stimulates the release of GnRH, which in turn leads to an increase in FSH and ovarian follicular growth and can be effective in up to 80% of appropriately selected women. Treatment should be limited to six cycles with the lowest effective dose. The side-effects of clomifene include multiple pregnancy and ovarian hyperstimulation and a minority of women may experience symptoms such as hot flushes, abdominal distension, nausea, vomiting, breast tenderness, headache, hair loss and blurred vision (RCOG 2000).

Women with clomifene-resistant polycystic ovarian syndrome (PCOS) can be treated with human menopausal gonadotrophin (HMG) and FSH injections. Ultrasound scanning is undertaken throughout the treatment to monitor the number and size of developing follicles. If there were excess follicles or signs of ovarian hyperstimulation syndrome (OHSS), or both, the cycle would be cancelled (RCOG 2000).

Cabergoline, as opposed to bromocriptine, is rapidly becoming the treatment of choice for women suffering from anovulatory hyperprolactinaemia. This is because the latter is associated with the unpleasant side-effects of nausea, headache, vertigo and drowsiness whereas the former has significantly fewer side-effects (RCOG 2000).

Intrauterine insemination (IUI)

IUI is indicated where there are problems such as hostile cervical mucus, antisperm antibodies or male fertility problems such as a low sperm count, premature ejaculation, retrograde ejaculation, anatomical problems or impotence. It is also useful for cases of unexplained infertility. The tubal patency of the female partner must be assured. In order to increase the chances of success, ovulation is induced and the sperm prepared to maximise its fertilising ability before being inserted high into the uterus. If the sperm used for the procedure is freshly produced from the male partner then a licence is not required. If the sperm from the male partner has been previously frozen, then the clinic carrying out the procedure must be licensed by the HFEA for the storage of sperm.

Donor insemination (DI)

Donor insemination is a procedure in which sperm from an anonymous donor is used and may be indicated where the following factors are present in the male partner:

- azoospermia (absence of spermatozoa)
- oligospermia (reduced numbers of spermatozoa)
- vasectomy or failed reversal
- ejaculatory failure
- chemotherapy or radiotherapy
- a transmissible genetic disorder.

The issue of treating single women or lesbian couples with DI is controversial and fraught with ethical and religious dilemmas.

In vitro fertilisation/embryo transfer (IVF/ET)

'In vitro fertilisation' describes the technique where fertilisation occurs outside the body. IVF is indicated in cases where the female partner has fallopian tube occlusion, endometriosis or cervical mucus problems, or where male factors are the main problem. It may be appropriate for cases of unexplained infertility or when less invasive methods have been unsuccessful. It also provides an opportunity to detect specific sperm abnormalities and the fertilising ability of the sperm.

Ovulation induction follows a treatment protocol and includes down-regulation of the woman's own hormones followed by stimulation with FSH or HMG. Oestrogen levels are measured intermittently to indicate the level of response to the FSH and HMG and to observe for signs of OHSS, and frequent ultrasound scanning monitors the number and growth of the follicles. An injection of HCG is given 34–38 hours before egg collection. Retrieval is via ultrasound or laparoscopy under a mild sedative or general anaesthesia respectively. The oocytes are examined for maturity and if suitable are then placed with the prepared sperm from the male partner or donor and incubated. If successful fertilisation occurs and the embryos continue to develop normally, one or two embryos will usually be transferred into the woman's uterus, although up to three are permitted by the HFEA regulations. Any remaining embryos may be frozen for later use if the clinic is able to offer this facility.

Gamete intrafallopian transfer (GIFT)

This technique is indicated in cases where there is unexplained infertility and hostile cervical mucus, although tubal patency is necessary in the female partner and an adequate sperm count in the male. GIFT involves ovulation induction in the same manner as for IVF, but the eggs are then retrieved laparoscopically. The eggs are examined for maturity and a maximum of three are mixed with the prepared sperm and transferred into the fimbriated end of the uterine tube. Fertilisation then occurs in vivo (in the body). Unfortunately, the fertilising capacity of the gametes cannot be confirmed unless a successful outcome occurs or if IVF of the surplus oocytes is performed and the embryos frozen for future use. If donated eggs or sperm are used, or if embryos are stored, the clinic must be licensed by the HFEA.

Zygote intrafallopian transfer (ZIFT)

ZIFT is a variation of GIFT where fertilised eggs are placed in the uterine tubes at either the pronucleate or single cell (zygote) stage of embryo development.

Intracytoplasmic sperm injection (ICSI)

ICSI is a procedure that was developed in 1992 and is often a successful treatment of male infertility. It is used when IVF is not suitable and is performed with eggs obtained after ovulation stimulation as done in IVF. It involves injecting a single spermatozoon into an ovum. The sperms are prepared so that the most motile of these can be selected. It is a useful technique when there are very few normal sperms available or the fertilising ability of the sperm is dramatically reduced. However, there have been concerns over the use of this technique, particularly in relation to the potential for genetic abnormalities as well as the potential for chemical and mechanical damage or introducing foreign material into the oocyte during the injection process (Sutcliffe 2000). ESHRE (2001) has stated that ICSI is associated with a slightly increased risk of congenital malformations although this is not linked to problems with the technique itself but related to the prospective parents having the treatment.

Sperm and egg donation

Any person considering donation of either sperm or eggs must undergo an assessment and screening process before any gametes are provided, and be aged over 18 and under 45 and 35 years for men and women respectively. A medical and family history will be taken including details of any donations that have been made elsewhere. The HFEA has set a limit of 10 live birth events per donor. The donors are encouraged to write about themselves as well as provide non-identifying biographical information such as eye, hair and skin colour, hobbies and interests that is held on the register. The screening process aims to prevent the transmission of serious genetic disorders and includes screening for human immunodeficiency virus (HIV), cytomegalovirus (CMV) and hepatitis B antibodies. For sperm donation, semen analysis is carried out and if adequate the sperm is stored for a minimum of 180 days before use to allow for a second HIV test. The law states that the woman receiving the treatment and her husband or male partner being treated with her will be the legal parents although the donor will be the genetic parent. The donor does not have any legal relationship, legal rights or obligations to any child born. The donor will remain anonymous even when the child born as a result of the donation reaches adulthood and wishes to find out more information about his or her origins. People who consent to the donation or storage of gametes must be counselled so that they understand the implications and issues surrounding their proposed actions (HFEA 2001).

Surrogacy

The requirements in law for surrogacy arrangements are that the commissioning couple must both be over the age of 18, married to each other and the child genetically related to at least one of them. This means that either a fertile woman can be artificially inseminated with the sperm of the husband of the commissioning couple or the commissioning couple can undergo an IVF procedure and produce an embryo.

The surrogate mother then acts as a host as the embryo is placed in her uterus. The commissioning couple can then apply for a parental order within 6 months of the birth as long as the child is living with them. The surrogate mother must still register the birth, as consent to the parental order cannot be given until 6 weeks after the birth of the child and no money other than expenses must have been paid. When a court has granted the parental order the Registrar General will make an entry in a separate Parental Order Register reregistering the child. Adults who are the subject of parental orders are able to gain access to their original birth certificates after being offered counselling.

Psychosocial aspects of infertility

The psychological impact of infertility on a couple can be considerable. Commonly reported feelings are of guilt, anger, depression, anxiety, inadequacy, grief, loss of control, and low self-esteem (Daniluk 1997, Read 1999). Men and women react differently to the diagnosis of infertility. Women are reported to suffer greater psychosocial distress and higher levels of depression, whereas men report less distress and are able to adapt to childlessness better than their partners do. Only when male factors are diagnosed as the source of the fertility problem does the response become more negative with increased feelings of depression, social isolation and failure. The feelings of despair, anger and hopelessness can be profound particularly when the infertility is prolonged. Relationship difficulties may be encountered for various reasons. A fertile partner may feel angry, antagonistic or resentful toward an infertile partner or where conception has been delayed because of career aspirations or when one partner did not feel ready for parenthood. Ambivalence may be a problem when one partner already has a biological child or some men may not wish to consent to DI. The couple may have poor communication skills so that they are unable to express themselves and disclose their true feelings to each other. However, infertility can also have positive effects with couples feeling closer by improved communication, having increased sensitivity to partner's feelings and a sense of closeness (Leiblum 1997). Contact with other infertile couples and support groups can also prove helpful (McNaughton-Cassill et al 2000).

Fertility clinics should aim to address the psycho-social and emotional needs of their patients as well as their medical needs. The availability of appropriately trained counsellors is essential in the management of the infertile couple, as there are fundamental differences in their requirements from those of other disease-oriented consultations. The first is that the central focus is the couple's inability to fulfil their desire to have children. The second issue is that the interests of the child that may be conceived must be considered. Thirdly the treatment process often involves repeated therapies that if unsuccessful create further stress and disappointment, and finally the couple are obliged to share intimate details of their sexual behaviour (Boivin et al 2001).

One of the most difficult aspects of infertility treatment for a couple is deciding when to stop. The range of treatments available means that if one treatment fails then another one can be tried, which therefore can result in an endless cycle of treatment with disillusionment and despair at the end of it. Many couples are driven by the fact that the next treatment might be successful and making the decision to either remain childless or apply for adoption is something that they need help with.

Psychosexual aspects of infertility

The sexual demands that are placed on a couple are considerable particularly when the pressure to have intercourse is focused around the fertile days or at the culmination of an intense regimen of ovulation induction. The recreational aspect of sexual relations is often lost in the necessity for men to ejaculate at these key times, leading to the abandonment of sexual intimacy during the non-fertile times of the month. The same applies when the male partner has to produce a semen specimen as required for some of the assisted reproduction techniques.

Men can suffer from sexual difficulties such as erectile problems, sexual apathy and avoidance of sexual intercourse particularly if they are the source of the fertility problem (Leiblum 1997). Although infertility can be the source of sexual problems, the couple's infertility could conversely be associated with these. It is rare that sexual problems are the primary or single cause of reproductive failure but it is important that the sexual competency of both partners is assessed to ensure that the couple are engaging in full sexual intercourse, particularly in relation to frequency and timing (Read 1999).

Ethical issues associated with infertility

The reproductive technologies, although achieving the goal for many infertile couples, are fraught with ethical dilemmas for all concerned. Limited NHS resources result in decisions being made as to who can be treated and who cannot. Issues arise relating to the welfare of the child, the ages of the prospective parents, anonymity of donors, the child's rights to know about its genetic origins and surrogacy, to name but a few. Although these issues cannot be discussed in this chapter, everyone involved with infertility treatments must be aware of them (see Ch. 4).

The role of the midwife

It is unlikely that the midwife will be involved with couples whilst undergoing fertility treatment but when a successful conception is achieved the maternity services will then be involved. It is important that the midwife is aware of the types of treatments that are currently available and the stresses that the couple has endured during the process. It is likely that the couple will remain anxious throughout the pregnancy and in some cases will undergo fetal diagnostic screening.

REFERENCES

Allen H 2001 Helping pregnant smokers quit – a review for health professionals. Midirs Midwifery Digest 11(1):45–48
American Dietetic Association 1998 Clinical practice recommendations. Diabetes Care. Available: http://www.DiabetesCare/Supplement198/S56.htm 12 Sept 2001

Baeten J M, Bukusi E A, Lambe M 2001 Pregnancy complications and outcomes among nulliparous women. American Journal of Public Health 91(3):436–440
Barrowclough D, Ford F A 2000 Folic acid fortification: proposed UK recommendations. The Practising Midwife 3(6):32–33

Boivin J, Appleton T C, Baetons P et al 2001 Guidelines for counselling in infertility: outline version. Human Reproduction 16(6):1301–1304

Bradley S G, Bennett N 1995 Preparation for pregnancy. Glendaruel, Argyll, Scotland, p 23–32

Bungum T, Peaslee D L, Jackson A W, Perez M 2000 Exercise during pregnancy and type of delivery in nulliparae. Journal of Obstetric, Gynecologic, and Neonatal Nursing 29(3):258–264

Bussell G 2000. The dietary beliefs and attitudes of women who have had a low-birthweight baby: a retrospective preconception study. Journal of Human Nutrition and Dietetics 13(1):29–39

Casson I F, Clarke C A, Howard D V et al 1997 Outcomes of pregnancy in insulin dependent diabetic women: results of a five year population cohort study. British Medical Journal 215(7103):275–278

Cefalo R C, Moos M K 1995 Preconceptional health care a practical guide, 2nd edn. Mosby, London, p 98–164

Chamberlain G 1995 Turnbull's obstetrics. Churchill Livingstone, London, p 163–174

Chambers R 1999 Fertility problems a simple guide. Radcliffe Medical, Oxford, p. 39–61

Clark A M, Thornley B, Tomlinson L, Galletley C, Norman R J 1998 Weight loss in obese infertile women results in improvement in reproductive outcome for all forms of fertility treatment. Human Reproduction 13:1502–1505

Cnattingius S, Bergstom R, Lipworth L, Kramer M S 1998 Prepregnancy weight and the risk of adverse pregnancy outcome. New England Journal of Medicine 338(3):147–152

COSHH (Control of Substances Hazardous to Health Regulations) 1999 COSHH, London

Crawford P 1997 Epilepsy and pregnancy: good management reduces the risks. Professional Care of Mother and Child 7(1):17–18

Dallongeville J, Mare N, Fruchart J C, Amouyel P 1998 Cigarette smoking is associated with unhealthy patterns of nutrient intake: a meta-analysis. Journal of Nutrition 128:1450–1457

Daniluk J C 1997 Gender and Infertility. In: Leiblum S R (ed) Infertility: psychological issues and counselling strategies. John Wiley, New York, p 103–125

DHSS (Department of Health and Social Security) 1990 Vitamin A and pregnancy. PL/CMO (90) 11, PL/CNO (90). HMSO, London

DoH (Department of Health) 1991 Dietary reference values for food energy and nutrients for the United Kingdom. HMSO, London 8:85–89

DoH (Department of Health) 1992 Folic acid and the prevention of neural tube defects: report from an expert advisory group. DoH Publication Unit, Heywood

DoH (Department of Health) 1998 Smoking kills – a white paper on tabacco. Stationery Office, London

DoH (Department of Health) 2000a Folic acid and the prevention of disease: report of the Committee on Medical Aspects of Food and Nutrition Policy. Stationery Office, London

DoH (Department of Health) 2000b Consultation by the UK health departments and the Food Standards Agency on the report of the Committee on Medical Aspects of Food and Nutrition Policy on folic acid and the prevention of disease. Stationery Office, London

DoH (Department of Health) 2000c Statistical bulletin: statistics from the regional drug misuse databases for six months ending September. DoH, London

Doyle W 1992 Preconception care: Who needs it? Modern Midwife January/February:18–22

ESHRE (European Society of Human Reproduction and Embryology) 2001 Newsletter – congress highlights. ESHRE, Lausanne

Fairgrieve S D, Jackson M, Jonas P et al 2000 Population based prospective study of the care of women with epilepsy in pregnancy. British Medical Journal 321(16):674–675

Ford F A, Fraser R, Dimond H 1994 Healthy eating for you and your baby. Pan, London, p. 80–101

Frisch R E, McArthur J W 1974 Menstrual cycles: fatness as a determinant of minimum weight for height necessary for their maintenance or onset. Science 185:949–951

Frisch R E, Wyshak G, Vincent L 1980 Delayed menarche and amenorrhea in ballet dancers. New England Journal of Medicine 303(1):7–18

Galtier-Dereure F, Boegner C, Bringer J 2000 Obesity and pregnancy: complications and cost. American Journal of Clinical Nutrition 71(suppl):1242S–1248S

Goldberg G R 2000 Nutrition in pregnancy. Advisa Medica, London, 1(2):1–3

Hall J 2000 When is careless conception a form of child abuse? Lessons from maternal phenylketonuria. Journal of Pediatrics 136(1):12–13

Hargreave T, Mills J 1998 Investigating and managing infertility in general practice. British Medical Journal 316:1438–1441

Harper P S 1998 Practical genetic counselling, 5th edn. Butterworth Heinemann, Oxford, p 4–70

Haslam D W 2001 National obesity forum. In: Nutrition in practice. Advisa Medica, London, p 7

HEA (Health Education Authority) 1996 Folic acid and the prevention of neural tube defects guidance for health service purchasers and providers. HEA, London

HFEA (Human Fertilisation and Embryology Authority) 2001 Code of practice. HFEA, London

Holmes L B, Harvey E A, Coull B A et al 2001 The teratogenicity of anticonvulsant drugs. New England Journal of Medicine 344(15):1132–1138

HSE (Health Service Executive) 1998 Working with VDUs. HSE, Suffolk

Illman L 2001 Promoting a health lifestyle. In: Andrews G (ed) Women's sexual health, 2nd edn. Baillière Tindall, Edinburgh, p. 38–41

Jantz N K, William H, Becker M P et al 1995 Diabetes and pregnancy: factors associated with seeking preconception care. Diabetes Care 18(2):157–165

Jenson T K, Hjollund N H I, Henriksen T B et al 1998 Does moderate alcohol consumption affect fertility? Follow up study among couples planning first pregnancy. British Medical Journal 317(7157):505–510

Joffe M 1986 Women's work and pregnancy. In: Chamberlain G, Lumley J (eds) Prepregnancy care: a manual for practice. John Wiley, Chichester, p 245–261

Kardel K R, Kase T 1998 Training in pregnant women: effects on fetal development and birth. American Journal of Obstetrics and Gynecology 178(2):280–286

Leiblum S R 1997 Love, sex and infertility: the impact of infertility on couples. In: Leiblum S R (ed) Infertility: psychological issues and counselling strategies. John Wiley, Chichester, p 149–166

Lloyd C, Hunter E 2001 The care of pregnant women with epilepsy. Midirs Midwifery Digest 11(1):37–39

Madden V 1999 Women with epilepsy are not getting pregnancy advice. British Medical Journal 318(7195):1374

McGovern E, Moss H, Grewal G, Taylor A, Bjornsson S, Pell J 1997 Factors affecting the use of folic acid supplements in pregnant women in Glasgow. British Journal of General Practice 47:635–637

McNaughton-Cassill M E, Bostwick M, Vanscoy S E et al 2000 Development of brief stress management support groups for couples undergoing in vitro fertilisation. Fertility and Sterility 74(1):87–93

MAFF (Ministry of Agriculture Fisheries and Food) 2000 National Food Survey 1999. Stationery Office, London

National Society for Epilepsy 2001 http://epilepsynse.org.uk/pages/info/leaflets/women.cfg 9 Sept

Plant M 2000 Alcohol in pregnancy. Midirs Midwifery Digest 10(4):443–447

Platt L D, Koch R, Hanley W B et al 2000 The international study of pregnancy outcome in women with maternal phenylketonuria: report of a 12-year study. American Journal of Obstetrics and Gynaecology 182(2):326–333

Raw M, McNeill A, West R 1999 Smoking cessation: evidence based recommendations for the healthcare system. British Medical Journal 318:182–185

RCGP (Royal College of General Practitioners) 1995 The role of general practice in maternity care. Occasional paper 72: report of the RCGP Maternity Care Group. RCGP, London, p 3.

RCOG (Royal College of Obstetricians and Gynaecologists) 1998 The initial investigation and management of the infertile couple. Evidence based clinical guidelines. No. 2. RCOG, London

RCOG (Royal College of Obstetricians and Gynaecologists) 1999 Alcohol consumption in pregnancy. RCOG, London

RCOG (Royal College of Obstetricians and Gynaecologists) 2000 The management of infertility in tertiary care. Evidence based clinical guidelines. No. 6. RCOG, London

Read J 1999 Sexual problems associated with infertility, pregnancy and ageing. British Medical Journal 318(7183):587–589

Rothman K J, Moore L L, Singer M R, Nguyen U D T, Manning S, Milunsky A 1995 Teratogenicity of high vitamin A intake. New England Journal of Medicine 333(21):1369–1373

Rouse B, Matalon R, Koch R et al 2000 Maternal phenylketonuria syndrome: congenital heart defects, microcephaly, and developmental outcomes. Journal of Pediatrics 136(1):57–61

Sexton M 1986 Smoking. In: Chamberlain G, Lumley J (eds) Prepregnancy Care. John Wiley, Chichester, p 141–159

Sutcliffe A G 2000 Intracytoplasmic sperm injection and other aspects of new reproductive technologies. Archives of Disease in Childhood 83(2):98–100

Thomas B 2001 Pregnancy. Manual of dietetic practice, 3rd edn. Blackwell Science, Oxford, p 216–225

van der Spuy Z M, Steer P J, McCusker M, Steel S J, Jacobs H S 1988 Outcome of pregnancy in underweight women after spontaneous and induced ovulation. British Medical Journal 296:962–965

Wallace M, Hurwitz B 1998 Preconception care: who needs it, who wants it, and how should it be provided? British Journal of General Practice 48:963–966

WHO (World Health Organisation) 1992 Recent advances in medically assisted conception. Technical report series 820. WHO, Geneva

Wynn M, Wynn A 1983 The prevention of handicap of early pregnancy origin. Some evidence of good health before conception. Foundation for Education and Research in Childbearing, London

Wynn M, Wynn A 1990 The need for nutritional assessment in the treatment of the infertile couple. Journal of Nutritional Medicine 1:315–324

Zaastra B M 1993 Fat and female fecundity: prospective study of effect of body fat distribution on conception rates. British Medical Journal 306:484–487

FURTHER READING

Andrews G (ed) 2001 Women's sexual health, 2nd edn. Baillière Tindall, Edinburgh.

This is an excellent text that covers all aspects of women's health.

Tomlinson J (ed) 1999 ABC of sexual health. BMJ Publishing, London.

This is an informative text that covers male and female sexual health problems.

USEFUL ADDRESSES

Action on Smoking and Health (ASH)
102 Clifton Street
London EC2A 4HW
Tel: 020 7739 5902
Fax: 020 7613 0531

British Agencies for Adoption and Fostering (BAAF)
Sky-Line House
200 Union Street
London SE1 0LX
Tel: 020 7593 2000

British Epilepsy Association
New Anstey House
Gate Way Drive
Yeadon
Leeds LS19 7XY
Tel: 0113 210 8800
Fax: 0113 391 0300

British Infertility Counselling Association (BICA)
69 Division Street
Sheffield S1 4GE
Tel: 01342 843880

British Pregnancy Advisory Service (BPAS)
Austy Manor
Wootton Wawen
Solihull
West Midlands B95 6BX
Tel: 01564 793225
Fax: 01564 794935

Child
Charter House
43 St Leonards Road
Bexhill-on-Sea
East Sussex TN40 1JA
Tel: 01424 732361
Fax: 01424 731858

Diabetes UK
Central Office
10 Queen Anne Street
London W1G 9LH
Tel: 020 7323 1531
Fax: 020 7637 3644

FORESIGHT
The Association for the Promotion of Preconceptual Care
Mrs Peter Barnes
28 The Paddock
Godalming
Surrey GU7 1XD
Tel: 01483 427839
Hours 9.30 a.m.–6.00 p.m.

Human Fertilisation and Embryology Authority
Paxton House
30 Artillery Lane
London E1 7LS
Tel: 020 7377 5077

Issue (The National Fertility Association)
114 Lichfield Street
Walsall WS1 1SZ
Tel: 01922 722888
Fax: 01922 640070

Miscarriage Association
c/o Clayton Hospital
Northgate
Wakefield
W Yorks WF1 3JS
Tel: 01924 200799
Fax: 01924 298834

National Endometriosis Society
50 Westminster Palace Gardens
Artillery Row
London SW1P 1RL
Tel: 020 7222 2776
Fax: 020 7222 2786

QUIT,
Ground Floor, 211 Old Street
London EC1V 9NR
Quitline® 0800 00 22 00
NHS pregnancy smoking helpline 0800 169 9169

13 Change and Adaptation in Pregnancy

Irene Murray

CHAPTER CONTENTS

Physiological adaptation to pregnancy is dramatic and often underestimated. The timing and intensity of the changes vary between systems but all are designed to enable the woman to nurture the fetus and prepare her body for labour and lactation (Girling 2001). Recent advances in reproductive technology have led to changed perceptions of the effects of specific hormones and less certainty relating to the role of conventional endocrine glands. Genetic factors are now considered likely to underpin most of the physiological changes of pregnancy (Dunlop 1999). The focus on genetic influences will doubtless intensify in subsequent editions of this book.

The midwife's appreciation of the normal physiological changes of pregnancy will enable her to identify pregnancy-induced alterations, detect abnormalities, especially when affected by pre-existing illnesses, and provide appropriate midwifery care to all women (Burnett 2001).

This chapter aims to:

• provide an overview of the adaptation of each body system during pregnancy and the underlying hormonal changes

• identify physiological changes that mimic or mask disease, or cause discomfort or inconvenience to the woman

• review the diagnosis of pregnancy, distinguishing between possible, probable and positive signs of the condition.

The woman's psychological state is also affected by hormonal changes. These changes are discussed in Chapters 14 and 35.

Physiological changes in the reproductive system

The body of the uterus

After conception, the uterus develops to provide a nutritive and protective environment in which the fetus will develop and grow.

Decidua

After embedding of the blastocyst there is thickening and increased vascularity of the lining of the uterus, or *decidua* (see Ch. 9). Decidualisation, influenced by progesterone and oestradiol, is most marked in the fundus and upper body of the uterus (the usual sites of implantation) (Coad & Dunstall 2001).

The decidua is now believed to maintain functional quiescence of the uterus during pregnancy; spontaneous labour is thought to result from the activation of the decidua with resultant prostaglandin release following withdrawal of placental hormones. The decidua and trophoblast also produce relaxin, which appears to promote myometrial relaxation, and may have a role to play in cervical ripening and rupture of fetal membranes (Norwitz et al 2001).

Myometrium

In early pregnancy uterine growth is due to *hyperplasia* (increase in number due to division) and *hypertrophy* (increase in size) of myometrial cells under the influence of oestrogen. As gestation increases, hyperplasia is less important and hypertrophy accounts for most of the growth of the uterus. In the latter half of pregnancy the uterus expands mechanically owing to distension of muscle cells by the growing fetus and placenta (Cunningham et al 1997, p. 191):

	Prior to pregnancy	At term
• *Increase in weight of uterus*	50 to 60 g	1000 g
• *Increase in size of uterus*	7.5 × 5 × 2.5 cm	30 × 22.5 × 20 cm

The dimensions of the uterus vary considerably, however, depending on the age and parity of the woman (Cunningham et al 1997).

During the first few months of pregnancy the uterine walls become substantially thicker and less firm,

growing from 1 cm to 2.5 cm by 4 months. Then as gestation advances they gradually become thinner. By term the uterus has become a muscular sac with soft, readily indentable walls of 0.5–1 cm or less in thickness, making palpation of the fetus relatively easy (Cunningham et al 1997). Hyperplasia and hypertrophy of the myometrial cells leads to the three layers of myometrium becoming more clearly defined (Coad & Dunstall 2001) (Fig. 13.1).

Muscle layers. The outer longitudinal layer of muscle fibres is thin. It consists of a network of bundles of smooth muscles. These pass longitudinally from the front of the isthmus anteriorly over the fundus and into the vault of the vagina posteriorly, and extend into the round and transverse ligaments (Bennett & Cowan 2001).

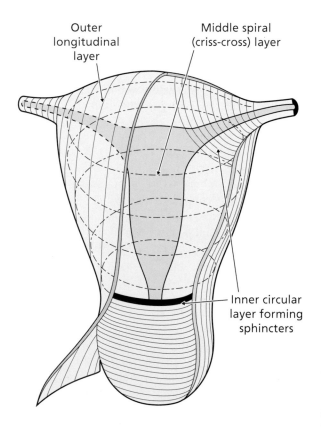

Fig. 13.1 Diagrammatic representation of differentiated muscle layers of uterus in pregnancy. (After Chamberlain et al 1991 p. 30, with permission of Gower Medical Publishing, London.)

The thicker middle layer comprises interlocked spiral myometrial fibres that are perforated in all directions by blood vessels. Each cell in this layer has a double curve so that the interlacing of any two gives the approximate form of a figure of eight. Due to this arrangement, contraction of these cells after delivery causes constriction of the blood vessels (see Ch. 28).

The inner circular layer is arranged concentrically around the longitudinal axis of the uterus and bundle formation is diffuse. It forms sphincters around the openings of the uterine tubes and around the internal cervical os (Cunningham et al 1997).

The myometrium is both contractile (can lengthen and shorten) and elastic (can enlarge and stretch) to accommodate the growing fetus and allow involution following the birth (Blackburn & Loper 1992). Thin sheets of connective tissue composed of collagen, elastic fibres, fibroblasts and mast cells separate the interconnecting bundles of 10–50 partially overlapping smooth muscle cells. The collagenous connective tissue supports the muscle fibres and provides a transmission network for the tension developed by contraction of the smooth muscle elements. Around the bundles of smooth muscle cells are blood and lymphatic vessels and nerve cells. The myometrial smooth muscle cells increase in pregnancy up to 15–20 times their non-pregnant length, or from 0.05 to 0.6 mm (Llewellyn-Jones 1999).

The contractile ability of the myometrium is dependent on the interaction between two contractile proteins, actin and myosin. The interaction of actin and myosin brings about contraction, whereas their separation brings about relaxation under the influence of intracellular free calcium. The coordination of synchronous contractions across the whole organ is due to the presence of gap junctions that connect myometrial cells and provide connections for electrical activity. Gap junctions are absent for most of the pregnancy but appear in significant numbers near term, manifesting themselves as *Braxton Hicks contractions*. Formation of gap junctions is promoted by oestrogens and prostaglandins. Progesterone, prostacyclin and relaxin, however, are all involved in inhibiting the formation of gap junctions by reducing cell excitability and cell connections and so limiting myometrial activity to small clumps of cells, thus maintaining uterine quiescence during pregnancy until the fetus is viable (Campbell & Lees 2000).

Uterine activity can be measured as early as 7 weeks' gestation, when Braxton Hicks contractions can occur every 20–30 minutes and may reach a pressure of up to 10 mmHg. These contractions facilitate uterine blood flow through the intervillous spaces of the placenta, promoting oxygen delivery to the fetus (Lowdermilk et al 1999). By the third trimester the contractions may become more rhythmic and noticeable, and may reach a pressure of 20–40 mmHg, occurring every 10–20 minutes, but usually cease with walking or exercise. Braxton Hicks contractions are usually painless but may cause some discomfort when their intensity exceeds 15 mmHg, accounting for the so-called *false labour* (Cunningham et al 1997).

Typically, in the last few weeks of pregnancy, *prelabour* occurs, in which further increases in myometrial contractions cause the muscle fibres of the fundus to be drawn up. The actively contracting upper uterine segment becomes thicker and shorter in length and exerts a slow, steady pull on the relatively fixed cervix causing the beginning of cervical stretching and ripening known as *effacement*, and thinning and stretching of the passive lower uterine segment. There is little rebound between contractions, however, hence there is no cervical dilatation at this time. These 'prelabour' contractions allow the pacemaker activity of the fundus to promote the coordinated, fundal-dominant contractions necessary for labour. The decreasing availability of progesterone to myometrial cells allows the effects of oestrogen to dominate (Campbell & Lees 2000) (see Ch. 24).

The perimetrium

The perimetrium is a thin layer of peritoneum that protects the uterus. It provides a relatively inelastic base upon which the myometrium develops tension to increase intrauterine pressure. It does not totally cover the uterus, being deflected over the bladder anteriorly to form the uterovesical pouch, and over the rectum posteriorly to form the pouch of Douglas (see Ch. 7). The double folds of perimetrium (broad ligaments), hanging from the uterine tubes and extending to the lateral walls of the pelvis, become longer and wider with increasing tension exerted on them as the uterus enlarges and rises out of the pelvis. The anterior and posterior folds open out so that they are no longer in apposition and can therefore accommodate the greatly enlarged uterine and ovarian arteries and veins

(Cunningham et al 1997). The round ligaments (contained within the hanging folds of perimetrium) provide some anterior support for the enlarging uterus and undergo considerable hypertrophy and stretching during pregnancy, which may cause discomfort or strain (Beischer et al 1997).

Blood supply

As a result of the increased cardiac output, the uterine blood flow progressively increases almost tenfold, from approximately 50 ml/min at 10 weeks' gestation and reaching a maximum of 450–700 ml/min at term. Eighty per cent perfuses the placenta and 20% perfuses the myometrium (Steinfeld & Wax 2001). The uterine arteries course along the lateral walls of the uterus giving off 9–14 branches, each of which penetrates the outer third of the myometrium. At this level the uterine arteries anastomose with the ovarian arteries. The resulting network of arteries then penetrates into the basal layer of the endometrium developing into spiral arteries to supply the decidua (Johnson & Everitt 2000). By about 16 weeks the spiral arteries are remodelled into uteroplacental arteries that decrease resistance to and promote the flow of maternal blood into the lacunae and intervillous spaces (Reiss 2001) (see Ch. 10). The coursing of blood through these enlarged and increasingly coiled arteries produces the uterine *souffle*, which may be heard with a sonicaid. As the uterus grows and stretches, however, the uterine spiral arteries become greatly increased in diameter and uncoiled to provide the necessary extra length and to accommodate the increased uteroplacental blood flow.

Changes in uterine shape and size

For the first few weeks the uterus maintains its original pear shape, but as pregnancy advances the corpus and fundus assume a more globular form in anticipation of fetal growth and also to accommodate increasing amounts of liquor and placental tissue. By 10 weeks the uterus is about the size of an orange (Lowdermilk et al 1999).

12th week of pregnancy

By 12 weeks the uterus is about the size of a grapefruit. It is no longer anteverted and anteflexed and has risen out of the pelvis and become upright. The fundus may be palpated abdominally above the symphysis pubis (Miller & Hanretty 1997). The uterus usually inclines and rotates to the right so that the left margin of the uterus faces anteriorly (*dextrorotation*), probably owing to the presence of the rectosigmoid colon on the left side of the pelvis (Cunningham et al 1997). The globular upper segment is sitting on an elongated stalk formed from the isthmus, which softens and which will treble in length from 7 to 25 mm between the 12th and 36th week (Lowdermilk et al 1999, Verralls 1993) (Fig. 13.2).

16th week of pregnancy

By 16 weeks the fetus has grown enough to put pressure on the isthmus, causing it to unfold so that the uterus becomes more spherical in shape (Coustan 1995) (Fig. 13.2). The isthmus and cervix develop into the lower uterine segment, which is thinner and contains less muscle and blood vessels than the corpus,

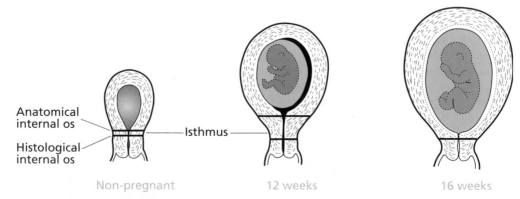

Fig. 13.2 Changes in the uterus from non-pregnant to 16 weeks' gestation. (After Miller & Hanretty 1997 p. 34, with permission of Churchill Livingstone, Edinburgh.)

and is the site of incision for the majority of caesarean sections (Campbell & Lees 2000).

20th week of pregnancy

At 20 weeks the fundus of the uterus can be palpated at the level of the umbilicus. From this stage of gestation until term the uterus becomes more cylindrical or ovoid in shape and has a thicker, more rounded, dome-shaped fundus (Llewellyn-Jones 1999). As the uterus continues to rise in the abdomen, the uterine tubes become progressively more vertical, which causes increasing tension on the broad and round ligaments (Cunningham et al 1997).

30th week of pregnancy

The lower uterine segment is still not complete but can be defined as the portion lying between the line of attachment of the uterovesical pouch of peritoneum superiorly and the internal os inferiorly (Llewellyn-Jones 1999). At 30 weeks the fundus may be palpated midway between the umbilicus and the xiphisternum (Beischer et al 1997).

Assessment of fetal size by abdominal palpation has been reported to be inaccurate as there is considerable variability in the site of the umbilicus. Consequently symphysis–fundal height measurements have become common practice (Neuberg 1995). However, a recent trial comparing the two methods found no differences in any of the outcomes measured, and concluded that there is insufficient evidence to evaluate the use of symphysis–fundal height measurement during antenatal care (Neilson 2002).

38th week of pregnancy

The uterus now reaches the level of the xiphisternum. The uterine tubes appear to be inserted slightly above the middle of the uterus (Cunningham et al 1997). As the upper segment muscle contractions increase in frequency and strength, the lower uterine segment develops more rapidly and is stretched radially, which, along with cervical effacement and softening of the tissues of the pelvic floor, permits the fetal presentation to begin its descent into the upper pelvis. This leads to a reduction in fundal height known as *lightening*, relieving pressure on the upper part of the abdomen but increasing pressure in the pelvis, which may lead to constipation, urinary frequency and sometimes increased vaginal discharge (Llewellyn-Jones 1999).

This also encourages further descent of the fetus into the pelvis. In the majority of multiparous women, however, engagement rarely occurs prior to labour (Campbell & Lees 2000).

The cervix

The cervix is composed of only about 10% muscular tissue, the remainder being collagenous tissue, with a marked difference in the ratio of smooth muscle to collagen between the different regions. Although the contractile strength is 40 times higher at the fundus than at the distal cervix, muscular activity of the cervix is sufficient to cause constriction during contractions in early labour. This may explain how the cervix does not dilate with Braxton Hicks contractions before the onset of labour (Steer & Johnson 1998).

During pregnancy the cervix remains firmly closed providing a seal against external contamination and holding in the contents of the uterus (Pollard 1994). It remains 2.5 cm long throughout pregnancy but becomes softer and swollen under the influence of oestradiol and progesterone. Its increased vascularity makes it look bluish in colour. Oestradiol stimulates growth of the columnar epithelium of the cervical canal. When this becomes visible at the external os it can give the appearance of an erosion, or an *ectropion*. This epithelium is less robust and is prone to contact bleeding. Under the influence of progesterone the mucous glands become distended and increase in complexity resulting in the secretion of a thick, viscous, mucoid discharge. It forms a cervical plug called the *operculum*, which provides protection from ascending infection (Campbell & Lees 2000, Cunningham et al 1997).

As uterine activity builds up during pregnancy the cervix gradually softens, or *ripens*, and the canal dilates. Some dilatation of the external os may be detectable clinically by 24 weeks, and in one-third of primigravidae the internal os will be open by the 32nd week (Steer & Johnson 1998). The enzyme collagenase and prostaglandins are both involved in cervical ripening; however, debate continues about whether the latter originates from local tissue or from amniotic fluid (Norwitz et al 2001).

Theoretically, *effacement* or *taking up of the cervix* normally occurs in the primigravida during the last 2 weeks of pregnancy but does not usually take place in the multigravida until labour begins. Clinically, however, there are many variations in the state of the cervix at the onset of labour (Llewellyn-Jones 1999, Steer & Johnson 1998). Effacement of the cervix is a mechanism whereby the connective tissue of the long firm cervix is progressively softened and shortened from the top downwards. The softened muscular fibres at the level of the internal cervical os are pulled upwards or 'taken up' into the lower uterine segment and around the fetal presenting part and the forewaters. The canal that was about 2.5 cm becomes a mere circular orifice with paper-thin edges. The mucus plug is expelled as effacement progresses (Calder 1999).

The vagina

During pregnancy the muscle layer hypertrophies and oestrogen causes the vaginal epithelium to become thicker and more vascular. Its violet colour is probably due to hyperaemia. The altered composition of the surrounding connective tissue increases the elasticity of the vagina making dilatation easier during the birth of the baby (Llewellyn-Jones 1999).

In pregnancy there is an increased rate of desquamation of the superficial vaginal mucosa cells. These epithelial cells release more glycogen, which is acted on by *Döderlein's bacilli*, a normal commensal of the vagina, producing lactic acid and hydrogen peroxide. This leads to the increased and more acidic (pH 4.5–5.0) white vaginal discharge known as *leucorrhoea*. While this provides an extra degree of protection against ascending infection by some organisms, others such as *Candida albicans* can more easily establish themselves, resulting in more frequent occurrence of vaginitis in pregnancy (Campbell & Lees 2000).

Changes in the cardiovascular system

Profound changes take place in the cardiovascular system that would normally be considered pathological but in pregnancy are physiological. Understanding of these changes is important in the care of women with normal pregnancies, as well as for the management of women with pre-existing cardiovascular disease whose health may be seriously compromised with the increased demands of pregnancy (Steinfeld & Wax 2001).

The heart

The heart enlarges by about 12% between early and late pregnancy. Distension of the heart chambers is due partly to increasing myometrial hypertrophy, but mostly to increased diastolic filling (particularly in the left ventricle) in parallel with the increasing blood volume. Echocardiographic studies of cardiac enlargement in pregnancy show that wall thickness increases very little (Steinfeld & Wax 2001). Cardiac enlargement does not appear to be associated with reduced myocardial efficiency as the proportion of blood ejected during systole (the ejection fraction) increases during early pregnancy. The improvement in myocardial contractility is thought to be due to lengthening of muscle fibres or to the reduction in afterload associated with the marked peripheral vasodilation that is characteristic of pregnancy. During late pregnancy the degree of vasodilation decreases and the ejection fraction also diminishes (Dunlop 1999).

The growing uterus elevates the diaphragm, the great vessels are unfolded and the heart is correspondingly displaced upwards, with the apex moved laterally to the left by about 15°. This can give an exaggerated impression of cardiac enlargement (de Sweit 1998a), and accounts for the left axial deviation seen on electrocardiograms (ECG) in pregnancy and for the apex beat appearing in the fourth rather than the fifth intercostal space (Steinfeld & Wax 2001). These ECG and radiographic changes are similar to those seen in ischaemic heart disease but are considered normal in pregnancy. The ECG also often reveals a Q wave and inverted T wave in lead III, which should not be misconstrued as suggesting pulmonary embolus (Girling 2001). Atrial or ventricular extrasystoles are frequent and there is increased susceptibility to supraventricular tachycardia (de Swiet 1998a).

By mid-pregnancy more than 90% of women develop an ejection systolic murmur, which lasts until the first week postpartum. If unaccompanied by any other abnormalities it reflects the increased stroke output (Burnett 2001). Twenty per cent develop a transient diastolic murmur and 10% develop continuous murmurs, heard over the base of the heart, owing to increased mammary blood flow (de Sweit 1998a).

Cardiac output

The increase in cardiac output ranges from 35 to 50% in pregnancy, from an average of 5 L/min before pregnancy to approximately 7 L/min by the 20th week; thereafter the changes are less dramatic (Fig. 13.3). The increased cardiac output allows blood flow to the kidneys, brain and coronary arteries to remain unchanged, while the distribution to other organs varies as pregnancy advances. The uterus, for example, receives 3% of the cardiac output in early pregnancy but 17% at term (400 ml/min extra). The breasts receive less than 1% of the cardiac output early in gestation and 2% at term (Burnett 2001, Steinfeld & Wax 2001).

The increased cardiac output is due to increases in both stroke volume and heart rate. The increase in heart rate begins in the 7th week and by the third trimester it has increased by 10–20%. Heart rates are typically 10–15 beats per minute faster than those of the non-pregnant woman, increasing from about 75 to 90 beats per minute. Women with normal hearts are often more aware of irregularities in heart rate in pregnancy. However, stroke volume (the amount of blood pumped by the heart with each beat) is not augmented until the plasma volume expands. The stroke volume increases by 10% during the first half of pregnancy, and reaches a peak at 20 weeks' gestation that is maintained until term (Girling 2001) (Fig. 13.4).

The cardiovascular system more than any other is extremely sensitive to change. Large variations in cardiac output, pulse rate, blood pressure and regional blood flow may follow trivial changes of posture, activity or anxiety. Inconsistencies in the literature about the timing of the changes of heart rate and stroke volume, and which factor is primarily responsible for the increased cardiac output at any given time in gestation, are therefore largely due to the difficulties of measurement techniques and the influence of posture on haemodynamics (Steinfeld & Wax 2001).

Up until the 1950s it was accepted that the cardiac output rose to a peak at 28–32 weeks, after which it declined towards non-pregnant values at term. Later it was concluded that cardiac output rose to a plateau well before the end of the first trimester and did not decline until after 32 weeks. The early studies that suggested a fall in cardiac output in the third trimester due to uterine compression of the inferior vena cava are now considered inaccurate because they are confounded by the use of the supine position and by vascular changes (Girling 2001). Studies into supine hypotensive syndrome have confirmed that the fall in

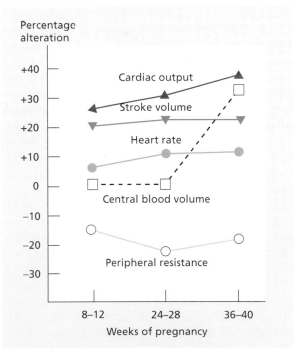

Fig. 13.4 Changes occurring in cardiac output, stroke volume, heart rate, central blood volume and peripheral vascular resistance during pregnancy, presented in percentages. (After Llewellyn-Jones 1999 p. 34, with permission of Mosby International Limited, London.)

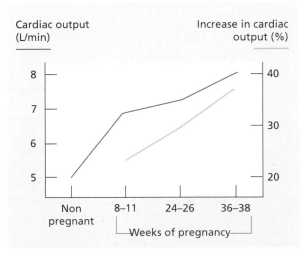

Fig. 13.3 Cardiac output in pregnancy. (From Llewellyn-Jones 1999 p. 34, with permission of Mosby International Limited, London.)

cardiac output in late pregnancy was spurious (de Sweit 1998a). This was demonstrated very thoroughly in a study by Robson et al (1989), which showed that the cardiac output had risen significantly 5 weeks after the missed period, and then had risen from a mean of 4.9 L/min prior to conception to a maximum of 7.2 L/min at 32 weeks, with no significant change thereafter until labour. Many other studies have subsequently examined this issue and current analysis suggests that cardiac output reaches its maximum level by about 24 weeks and is maintained at this level until term (Steinfeld & Wax 2001).

Blood

Blood pressure

As the cardiac output is raised but arterial blood pressure is reduced by 10%, it follows that resistance to flow must be decreased (de Sweit 1998a). The decrease in peripheral vascular resistance begins at 5 weeks' gestation, reaches a nadir in the second trimester (a 21% reduction) and then gradually rises as term is approached, but still remains slightly decreased at term to compensate for the increased cardiac output. It was formerly assumed that reduced peripheral vascular resistance was due to the addition of the low resistance uteroplacental circulation, which receives a large proportion of cardiac output. It now seems much more likely that it is caused by the mechanism controlling vascular activity (and therefore the vasodilation of early pregnancy). Agents that may be responsible for peripheral vasodilation include prostacyclin (a vasodilator) and thromboxane A_2 (a vasoconstrictor), endothelins (vasoconstrictors) and nitric oxide (a vasodilator). Continuing research in this area is extremely important in order to find explanations for pregnancy-induced hypertension and intrauterine growth restriction, both of which are associated with failure of vasodilation during pregnancy (Blackburn & Loper 1992, Dunlop 1999, Steinfeld & Wax 2001).

Early pregnancy is associated with a marked decrease in diastolic blood pressure but little change in systolic pressure. With reduced peripheral vascular resistance the systolic blood pressure falls an average of 5–10 mmHg below baseline levels and the diastolic pressure falls 10–15 mmHg by 24 weeks' gestation. Thereafter blood pressure gradually rises, returning to the prepregnant levels at term. Diastolic blood pressure

increases significantly during the second half of pregnancy to levels that are at least equivalent to those of women in the non-pregnant state (Burnett 2001, Steinfeld & Wax 2001) (Fig. 13.5).

Posture can have a major effect on blood pressure. The supine position can decrease cardiac output by as much as 25%. Compression of the inferior vena cava by the enlarging uterus during the late second and third trimesters results in reduced venous return, which in turn decreases stroke volume and cardiac output. If the paravertebral vessels and other vena caval collaterals are not well developed and perfused, the pregnant woman may suffer from *supine hypotensive syndrome*, which consists of hypotension, bradycardia, dizziness, light-headedness, nausea and even syncope if she remains in the supine position too long. This occurs in 10% of pregnant women. Loss of consciousness is due to reduced cerebral blood flow. By rolling the woman on to her left side the cardiac output can be instantly restored (Burnett 2001, Steinfeld & Wax 2001).

Blood flow

Blood flow in the lower limbs is slowed in late pregnancy (de Sweit 1998a). Poor venous return and increased venous pressure in the legs contribute to the increased distensibility and pressure in the veins of the legs, vulva, rectum and pelvis, leading to dependent oedema, varicose veins of legs and vulva, and haemorrhoids (Cunningham et al 1997).

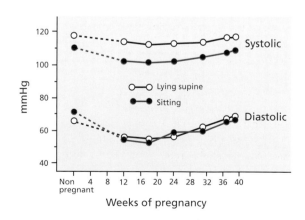

Fig. 13.5 Blood pressure changes as a result of pregnancy showing differences between sitting and lying positions. (From MacGillivray et al 1969 p. 395, with permission of Portland Press Ltd, London.)

The brain, kidneys and coronary arteries receive the same fraction (but a larger absolute amount) of cardiac output throughout pregnancy. Renal blood flow increases by as much as 70–80% (i.e. 400 ml per minute above non-pregnant levels) by the 16th week of pregnancy, which helps to enhance excretion. It remains at this high level until it declines at the end of pregnancy (de Sweit 1998a).

Blood flow is increased to the capillaries of the mucous membranes and skin, particularly in the hands and feet, reaching a maximum of 500 ml per minute by the 36th week. This helps to eliminate the excess heat produced by the increased metabolism of the maternal–fetal mass and cardiorespiratory work of pregnancy. The associated peripheral vasodilatation explains why pregnant women 'feel the heat', sweat profusely at times, have clammy hands and often suffer from nasal congestion (Cunningham et al 1997).

Blood flow to the breasts increases by about 2% throughout pregnancy. Evidence of this is seen in the dilated veins on the surface of the breasts as well as enlargement, heat and tingling from early pregnancy (de Sweit 1998a).

The uteroplacental circulation receives the greatest proportion of the cardiac output, with blood flow increasing from 1–2% in the first trimester to 17% by term. This translates into an increase in maternal blood flow to the placental bed of about 500 ml/min at term, although some studies have estimated uteroplacental blood flow to be as high as 700–900 ml/min (Burnett 2001, Steinfeld & Wax 2001). Such an increase can be accomplished only by the trophoblast converting the spiral arteries from narrow tortuous muscular vessels to wide-bored flaccid vessels, which reduces resistance to blood flow and permits increased perfusion. This begins after 12 weeks, when there is a sudden increase in blood flow to the intervillous space, and should be complete by 20 weeks. In maternal systole, blood flows through the spiral arteries into the choriodecidual space. The spiral nature of the arteries, together with their tendency to dilate terminally and a lack of responsiveness to vasoconstrictor transmitters, results in sluggish blood flow, which gives ample time for the exchange of metabolites at the placental interface (Johnson & Everitt 2000).

Techniques for accurate measurement of blood flow in the human uterus are fraught with problems because of its inaccessibility and the complexity of the blood supply. However, major advances have now been made using Doppler ultrasound. Reduced uteroplacental blood flow is found in women with pre-eclampsia or with fetuses with congenital abnormalities. Chronic reductions in placental perfusion result in smaller term babies (Johnson & Everrit 2000).

Blood volume

The two major components of blood – plasma and red cells – undergo dramatic adaptation. The total maternal blood volume increases 30–50% in singleton pregnancies, with a mean of 33%. In some women there may be only a modest increase in volume expansion, whereas in others it nearly doubles (Steinfeld & Wax 2001).

A higher circulating volume is required to:

- protect the mother (and fetus) against the harmful effects of impaired venous return in the supine and erect positions
- meet the demands of the enlarged uterus with a greatly hypertrophied vascular system and provide extra blood flow for placental perfusion at the choriodecidual interface
- supply the extra metabolic needs of the fetus
- provide extra perfusion of kidneys and other organs
- counterbalance the effects of increased arterial and venous capacity
- safeguard the mother against adverse effects of excessive blood loss at delivery.

The plasma volume, which corresponds with the increase in blood volume, increases by 50% over the course of the pregnancy (Burnett 2001). In a normal first pregnancy it may increase by about 1250 ml above non-pregnant levels and in subsequent pregnancies it may increase by about 1500 ml. The increase is related to the size of the fetus, being particularly large in multiple pregnancies. It starts in the first trimester, expands rapidly up until 32–34 weeks' gestation, then in the last few weeks of pregnancy it plateaus with very little change (Letsky 1998) (Fig. 13.6). The increase in plasma volume reduces the viscosity of the blood and improves capillary flow (Cunningham et al 1997) (Box 13.1).

Red cell mass, which represents the total volume of red cells in the circulation, increases during pregnancy in response to the extra oxygen requirements of maternal and placental tissue. Increased levels of erythropoietin and other hormones (prolactin, progesterone, human placental lactogen and oestrogen) are all involved in erythropoiesis. There is also an increase in F cells during pregnancy and reactivation of maternal haemoglobin F. The number of F cells reaches a peak at 18 to 22 weeks, usually returning to normal by 8 weeks postpartum (Steinfeld & Wax 2001).

There is still disagreement as to the exact increase in red cell mass and measurements have been influenced by iron medication. If it is accepted that the quantity of red cells in a healthy non-pregnant woman is about 1400 ml, then the rise in red cells for pregnant women not given iron medication is about 250 ml (18% increase) at term and for those given iron medication 400 ml (30% increase) at term. The effects of variables such as parity, age and other maternal characteristics on the red cell mass are not known (Burnett 2001).

The increase in red cell mass appears to be constant throughout pregnancy but it is most marked from about 20 weeks (Cunningham et al 1997). In spite of the increased production of red blood cells, the marked increase in plasma volume causes dilution of many circulating factors. As a result the red cell count, haematocrit and haemoglobin concentration all decrease (Letsky 1998) (Tables 13.1 and 13.2).

In healthy women with iron stores the mean haemoglobin concentration falls from 13.3 g/dl in the non-pregnant state to 11 g/dl in early pregnancy.

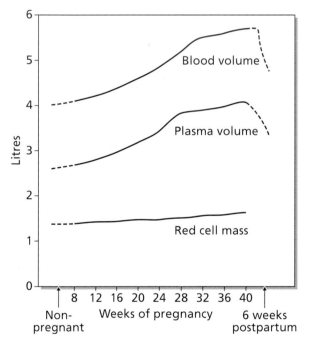

Fig. 13.6 Changes in blood volume, plasma volume and red cell mass during pregnancy. (From Llewellyn-Jones 1999 p. 33, with permission of Mosby International Limited, London.)

Box 13.1 Summary of changes caused by increased plasma volume in pregnancy

Haemodilution

- Physiological anaemia
- Decrease in concentration of plasma protein
- Decrease in concentration of immunoglobulins

Increased cardiac output

- Stroke volume increases
- Heart rate increases
- Heart enlarges

Table 13.1 Falling haemoglobin and haematocrit (PCV) in pregnancy despite rising blood volume and red cell mass

	Non-pregnant	Weeks of pregnancy 20	30	40
Plasma volume (ml)	2600	3150	3750	3850
Red cell mass (ml)	1400	1450	1550	1650
Total blood volume (ml)	4000	4600	5300	5500
Haematocrit (PCV) (%)	35.0	32.0	29.0	30.0
Haemoglobin (g/dl)	13.3	11.0	10.5	11.0

After Llewellyn-Jones 1999 p. 34, with permission of Mosby International Limited, London.

It is at its lowest at around 32 weeks' gestation when plasma volume expansion is maximal, and after this time rises by approximately 0.5 g/dl, returning to 11 g/dl around the 36th week of pregnancy. Anaemia in pregnancy has been defined as a haemoglobin of less than 11 g/dl in the first and third trimesters and less than 10.5 g/dl in the second trimester. The dated term *physiological anaemia* to describe this process is a misnomer and it has been suggested that such terminology should be abandoned (Campbell & Lees 2000).

In the past a lowered haemoglobin was mistaken for pathological anaemia and women were given prophylactic iron therapy. However, clinical experience has shown that many apparently healthy women are able to proceed through pregnancy with haemoglobins lower than 11 g/dl without complications (Letsky 1998). Pregnant women are known to be non compliant with iron therapy because of the unpleasant side-effects such as nausea and constipation. Most obstetricians nowadays do not consider iron therapy necessary unless serial estimations show that the haemoglobin has fallen below 10 g/dl or that there is a progressive reduction in mean cell volume (Campbell & Lees 2000) (see Ch. 19).

Apparent anaemia can be a sign of excellent physiological adjustment to pregnancy whereas a high haemoglobin level can be a sign of pathology (McFadyen 1995). A study by Steer et al (1995) showed that a mid-trimester fall in haemoglobin concentration to about 10 g/dl appears to be optimal, reflecting good volume expansion. Haemoglobin concentrations of 8.6–9.5 g/dl were associated with the highest mean birthweights, whereas levels above 14.5 g/dl were associated with an increase in preterm delivery and low birthweight babies.

Iron metabolism

The increased red cell mass and the needs of the developing fetus and placenta lead to increased iron requirements in pregnancy, with some increase in iron absorption. Iron demand increases from 2 to 4 mg daily. A healthy diet containing 10–14 mg of iron per day, 1–2 mg (5–10%) of which is absorbed, provides sufficient iron for the majority of pregnant women (Letsky 1998, p. 78).

The total iron requirements of pregnancy average about 1000 mg. About 500 mg are required to increase the red blood cell mass, and about 300 mg are transported to the fetus, mainly in the last 12 weeks of pregnancy. The remaining 200 mg are needed to compensate for insensible loss in skin, stool and urine. Practically all of the increased iron requirements occur in the last half of the pregnancy, averaging 6–7 mg per day. Since this amount is not available from body stores in most women, the red cell volume and haemoglobin level fall with the rising plasma volume. In spite of this, even if the mother has severe iron deficiency anaemia, the placenta is still able, mainly during the last 4 weeks of pregnancy, to provide the needed iron from maternal serum for the fetal production of haemoglobin. However, if the woman enters pregnancy with depleted iron stores, in spite of the moderate increase in iron absorption from the gut, the amount of iron absorbed from the diet plus that mobilised from stores may be insufficient to meet the demands imposed by pregnancy. The purpose of iron supplementation, therefore, is to maintain iron stores in order to prevent the development of true anaemia, rather than to raise the haemoglobin level. WHO recommendations since 1972 have been that supplements of 30–60 mg iron be given to women with iron stores, and 120–240 mg per day to women without stores (Letsky 1998).

There is evidence that absorption of dietary iron is enhanced in pregnancy from 10% in the first trimester to 66% by 36 weeks (Llewellyn-Jones 1999). The amount absorbed, however, depends very much on the rate of red cell production, the amount of iron stored, the iron content of the diet, and whether or not supplements are being taken. If stores are high then less iron will be absorbed (Letsky 1998).

It has been suggested that the estimation of serum ferritin concentrations to assess iron stores would be a more reliable screening test of iron deficiency anemia in the first trimester than haemoglobin levels, which lose their value as a result of haemodilution. Serum ferritin is stable, is not affected by recent ingestion of iron and appears to reflect the iron stores accurately. A serum ferritin of less than 50 g/L in early pregnancy would be an indication for daily iron supplements, whereas women with serum ferritin concentrations of 80 g/L are unlikely to need supplements (Letsky 1998). During the third trimester, however, serum ferritin levels in women without overt anaemia have been shown to vary widely, rendering the test unhelpful at this time (Campbell & Lees 2000).

Plasma protein

The total serum protein content falls within the first trimester and remains reduced throughout pregnancy. Albumin concentration falls quite abruptly in early pregnancy and then more slowly until late pregnancy (see Table 13.2). Albumin plays an important role, not only as a carrier protein for some hormones, drugs, free fatty acids and unconjugated bilirubin, but also because of its influence in decreasing colloid osmotic pressure. A fall in colloid osmotic pressure allows water to move from the plasma into the cells or out of vessels, and plays a part in the increased fragility of red blood cells, in oedema of the lower limbs and possibly also in the increased glomerular filtration rate. It is now accepted that peripheral oedema in the lower limbs in late pregnancy is a feature of normal, uncomplicated pregnancy and has therefore been removed from most definitions of pre-eclampsia (Girling 2001).

Clotting factors

Major changes in the coagulation system lead to the *hypercoagulable state* of normal pregnancy. The increased tendency to clot is caused by reduced plasma fibrinolytic activity and an increase in circulating fibrin degradation products in the plasma (Symonds & Symonds 1998).

From about the 3rd month of gestation there is a 50% increase in the synthesis of plasma fibrinogen concentration (factor I). This may be necessary for the body to deal with the frequent disruptions in the integrity of the vascular tree in the placental bed (Coustan 1995). It is also very important in the prevention of haemorrhage at the time of placental separation. The development of a fibrin mesh to cover the placental site to control the bleeding requires 5–10% of all the circulating fibrinogen. When this process is impaired, as for example in inadequate uterine action or incomplete placental separation, there is rapid depletion of fibrinogen reserves, which can lead to exsanguination and death (Campbell & Lees 2000).

Coagulation factors VII, VIII and X are also increased in pregnancy (Burnett 2001). Factors II (prothrombin) and V remain constant or show a slight fall. Both the prothrombin time (normal is 10–14 seconds) and the partial thromboplastin time (normal is 35–45 seconds) are shortened slightly as pregnancy advances. The clotting times of whole blood, however, are not significantly different in normal pregnancy. The platelet count declines slightly as pregnancy advances, which is explained partially by haemodilution. However, there is a substantial increase in platelet volume, which may be due to the hyperdestruction of platelets in pregnancy, and as young platelets are larger than old ones the balance is pushed towards an overall increase in size (Steinfeld & Wax 2001).

A decrease in some endogenous anticoagulants (antithrombin, protein S and activated protein C resistance) occur in pregnancy and are intended to reduce the risk of haemorrhage at the time of delivery; however, along with the physiological vasodilation of pregnancy, they contribute to a sixfold increase in the risk of thromboembolism in pregnancy (Girling 2001).

Table 13.2 Summary of common blood values and their changes

Normal range (non-pregnant)		Change in pregnancy	Timing
Protein (total)	65–85 g/L	↓10 g/L	By 20 weeks then stable
Albumin	35–48 g/L	↓10 g/L	Most by 20 weeks then gradual
Fibrinogen	2.5–4 g/L	↑ 2 g/L	Progressively from 3rd month
Platelets	150–400 × 10³/mm³	Slight decrease	No significant change until 3–5 days postpartum
Clotting time	6–10 min approx.	Little change	
White cell count	4–11 × 10⁹/L	9 × 10⁹/L	Peaks at 30 weeks then plateaus
Red cell count	4.5 × 10¹²/L	3.8 × 10¹²/L	Declines progressively to 30–34 weeks

White blood cells (leucocytes)

From 2 months the total white cell count rises in pregnancy and reaches a peak at 30 weeks, mainly because of the increase in numbers of neutrophil polymorphonuclear leucocytes (Letsky 1998). This enhances the blood's phagocytic and bactericidal properties. Numbers of eosinophils, basophils and monocytes remain relatively constant, and the lymphocyte count does not alter significantly. There is no change in the proportion of circulating T cells and B cells. The metabolic activity of granulocytes increases during pregnancy, possibly resulting from the stimulation of oestrogen (Steinfeld & Wax 2001).

Table 13.2 is a summary of changes in blood values in pregnancy.

Immunity

HCG and prolactin are known to suppress the immune response of pregnant women. Lymphocyte function is depressed. There is also decreased resistance to viral infections such as herpes, influenza, rubella, hepatitis, poliomyelitis and malaria. Serum levels of immunoglobulins IgA, IgG and IgM decrease steadily from the 10th week of pregnancy, reach their lowest level at 30 weeks and remain at this level until term (Letsky 1998).

Changes in the respiratory system

Pregnancy is associated with marked changes in respiratory physiology. Increased cardiac output leads to a substantial increase in pulmonary blood flow (Campbell & Lees 2000). The blood volume expansion and vasodilation of pregnancy result in hyperaemia and oedema of the upper respiratory mucosa, which predispose the pregnant woman to nasal congestion, epistaxis and even changes in voice. Nasal decongestant sprays should be used with caution because of their long term effect on the mucosa (Steinfeld & Wax 2001).

Knowledge of the changes in the mechanical aspects of ventilation in normal pregnancy is of particular importance for understanding the management of women with chronic respiratory diseases (Campbell & Lees 2000). Up to 70% of pregnant women with no underlying pre-existing respiratory disease experience some dyspnoea. Because the symptoms usually begin in the first or second trimester it is unlikely that the mechanical effects of the enlarging uterus are responsible. It may be that the conscious need to breathe, or shortness of breath, is influenced by the increased sensitivity of the respiratory centre to carbon dioxide owing to the effect of progesterone and oestrogen. Hyperventilation can be extremely uncomfortable and may lead to dyspnoea and dizziness. Although it is not usually associated with pathological processes, care must be taken not to dismiss it lightly and perhaps miss a warning sign of cardiac or pulmonary disease (Steinfeld & Wax 2001).

Alterations in the subdivision of lung volumes are largely due to alteration in thoracic anatomy during pregnancy. As the uterus enlarges, the diaphragm is elevated by as much as 4 cm, and the rib cage is displaced upwards. The shape of the chest changes as the anteroposterior and transverse diameters each increase by about 2 cm, resulting in a 5–7 cm expansion of the chest circumference. The lower ribs flare out and do not always fully recover their original position after pregnancy. Due to the elevation of the diaphragm the total lung capacity is reduced by 5% (Fig. 13.7). This

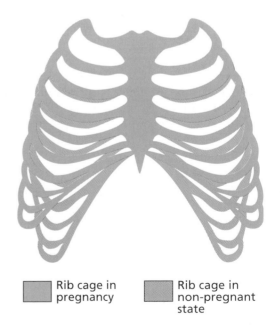

| | Rib cage in pregnancy | | Rib cage in non-pregnant state |

Fig. 13.7 Chest changes in pregnancy. The rib cage in pregnancy (pink) and non-pregnant state (grey) showing elevated diaphragm, increased chest circumference and lower ribs flaring out. (From de Swiet 1998b p. 115, with permission of Blackwell Science, Oxford.)

should improve air flow along the bronchial tree, and explains why women with respiratory problems in pregnancy do not deteriorate as much as women suffering from other chronic disorders (Campbell & Lees 2000, Steinfeld & Wax 2001).

Expansion of the rib cage causes the *tidal volume* to be increased by 30 to 40%. It rises early in pregnancy and continues to rise until term. Although the respiratory rate is little changed in pregnancy from the normal 14 or 15 breaths per minute, breathing is deeper even at rest, so that the *minute volume* rises by 40% in parallel with the tidal volume, from 7.5 L/min for a non-pregnant woman to 10.5 L/min in late pregnancy (de Sweit 1998b). The enhanced tidal volume contributes to an increase in *inspiratory capacity*. The *vital capacity* may remain the same or increase slightly from 100 to 200 ml (depending on body build), which represents the total functional capacity of the lungs (de Sweit 1998b). As a result the *expiratory reserve volume* and *residual volume* are decreased by 20%. The sum of these two volumes is known as the *functional residual capacity* and is decreased by 20% (Steinfeld % Wax 2001). The *minute ventilatory volume* that facilitates gas exchange is increased by 30–40%, from 7.5 to 10.5 L/min, and minute oxygen uptake increases appreciably as pregnancy advances (Cunningham et al 1997).

Both the alveolar oxygen partial pressure and the arterial oxygen partial pressure (P_aO_2) are increased from non-pregnant values of 98–100 mmHg to pregnant values of 101–104 mmHg. The rise in tidal volume and decrease in residual volume facilitates a 15–20% increase in oxygen consumption, which supports the additional metabolic requirements of mother and fetus. It is important to remember this maternal oxygen reserve when there is chronic lung disease or when general anaesthesia is required in pregnancy (Steinfeld & Wax 2001).

The 'hyperventilation of pregnancy' causes a 15–20% decrease in maternal arterial carbon dioxide partial pressure (P_aCO_2) from an average of 5 kPa (35 to 40 mmHg) in the non-pregnant woman to 4 kPa (30 mmHg) or lower in late pregnancy. Because fetal P_aCO_2 is 6 kPa, the carbon dioxide gradient from fetus to mother is increased, which facilitates the transfer of CO_2 from the fetus to the mother and causes carbon dioxide to be washed out of the lungs (Campbell & Lees 2000, Girling 2001).

The body has a considerable capacity for storing carbon dioxide in the blood, largely as bicarbonate. Renal excretion of bicarbonate is significantly increased and so the fall in P_aCO_2 is therefore matched by an equivalent fall in plasma bicarbonate concentration from the non-pregnant values of 24–30 mEq/L to the pregnant values of 18–21 mEq/L. Therefore, although maternal arterial pH changes very little, the resulting mild alkalaemia (arterial pH 7.40–7.45) further facilitates oxygen release to the fetus (Steinfeld & Wax 2001).

Changes in the urinary system

Striking anatomical changes are seen in the kidneys and ureters. The kidneys increase in weight and lengthen by 1 cm. Under the influence of progesterone the calyces and renal pelves dilate. The ureters also dilate and lengthen and are thrown into curves of varying sizes. The lumen in the distal third of the ureters may decrease in size because of hyperplasia, promoting compensatory dilatation in the upper two-thirds. The right ureter is usually more dilated than the left owing to the dextrorotation of the uterus, and as pregnancy advances the supine or upright posture may cause partial ureteric obstruction as the enlarged uterus compresses both ureters at the pelvic brim. All these factors can lead to urinary stasis and an increased risk of urinary tract infection in pregnancy (Steinfeld & Wax 2001) (Fig. 13.8) (see Ch. 19).

The ureters, however, should not be thought of as entirely toneless and floppy. Above the brim of the pelvis the upper ureters have increased tone with hypertrophy of the smooth muscle and hyperplasia of the connective tissue, and there is no decrease in ureteral peristalsis. Vesicoureteric reflux (VUR) occurs in at least 3% of pregnant women at or near term. The enlarging uterus displaces the ureters laterally so that as they pass through the muscle wall into the bladder they become shorter and perpendicular (instead of oblique) and therefore less efficient at the junction. It is yet to be established, however, whether VUR is a cause of ascending urinary tract infection (Baylis & Davison 1998).

After the 4th month of pregnancy the bladder trigone (base of bladder) is lifted and there is thickening of its intraureteric margin owing to the enlarging

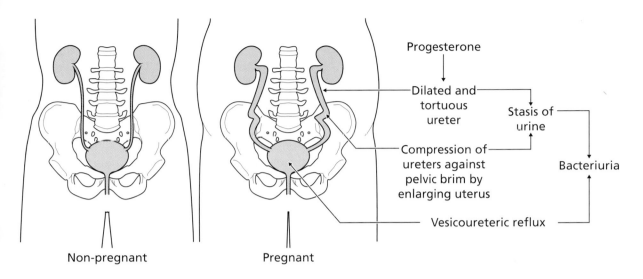

Fig. 13.8 Comparison of ureters in non-pregnant and pregnant women demonstrating factors predisposing to urinary tract infection in pregnancy.

uterus, hyperaemia of all the pelvic organs and hyperplasia of muscle and connective tissue. This process continues until term, resulting in a deepened and widened trigone. Bladder pressure increases and may result in reduced bladder capacity. To compensate for this, the urethra lengthens and intraurethral pressure increases. The muscles of the internal urethral sphincter relax, which, along with pressure from the pregnant uterus on the bladder, causes a significant number of women to experience some degree of stress incontinence. Antenatal teaching of pelvic floor exercises is important for helping to resolve this troublesome feature of pregnancy. Urgency of micturition and urge incontinence also increase in pregnancy, partly because of the effects of progesterone on the detrusor muscle. These all usually resolve spontaneously during the puerperium (Cardozo & Gleeson 1997).

It was formerly believed that frequency of micturition in early pregnancy was due to increased production of urine. The current view, however, is that in spite of the greatly increased workload of the kidneys the volume of urine excreted daily is not increased. Up to 80% of the filtrate received by the kidneys is reabsorbed in the proximal tubules independently of hormonal control. The urinary frequency and nocturia associated with pregnancy are probably a result of a combination of factors: the change in sleeping patterns,

pressure effects of the enlarging uterus on the bladder, and reduced bladder capacity due to increased pressure. Studies into the changes in bladder capacity, however, have produced contradictory results (Cardozo & Gleeson 1997, Cunningham et al 1997, Steinfeld & Wax 2001).

Numerous factors affect renal function in pregnancy, including increased plasma volume, increased glomerular filtration rate (GFR), increased renal plasma flow and alterations in hormones such as adrenocorticotrophic hormone (ACTH), ADH, aldosterone, cortisol, thyroid hormone and HCG (Steinfeld & Wax 2001).

The increase in blood flow is caused by vasodilation in the urinary tract (Campbell & Lees 2000). Early in pregnancy renal blood flow increases to levels 25–50% above non-pregnant values. There is disagreement, however, about whether this increase is sustained at the same level until term or whether some decrease occurs in the third trimester (Baylis & Davison 1998, Steinfeld & Wax 2001).

Although the increase in blood flow is mainly responsible for the 50% increase in GFR, the decrease in plasma oncotic pressure and enhanced permeability also increase glomerular filtration. The GFR returns to non-pregnant values close to term. As tubular reabsorption is unaltered the clearance of many solutes from the bloodstream is increased. Studies have shown a 45% increase in creatinine clearance by 9 weeks' gestation, a peak at about 32 weeks' gestation of about 50% above non-pregnant levels and a significant decrease towards non-pregnant levels prior to delivery. Plasma levels of urea and creatinine, which are conventionally used as markers for the severity of renal disease, decrease in proportion with the increase in GFR during normal pregnancy. Over the three trimesters, serum urea declines from non-pregnancy values of 4.3 mmol/L to 3.5, 3.3 and 3.1 mmol/L respectively, and mean serum creatinine levels decrease from 73 mmol/L before pregnancy to 65, 51 and 47 mmol/L respectively. As pregnancy advances a smaller proportion of uric acid is excreted by the kidneys, which is associated with the increasing serum uric acid concentration. There is a minimal increase in total protein excretion, with up to 500 mg in a 24 hour period being considered physiological – a factor that makes diagnosis of renal disease in pregnancy more difficult. Many women with proteinuria before pregnancy experience a progressive increase in the amount of protein spilled during pregnancy; however, the upper limit of normal is considered to be 300 mg over 24 hours. Amino acids and water-soluble vitamins are also found in much greater amounts in the urine of pregnant women (Baylis & Davison 1998, Girling 2001).

The increased GFR coupled with impaired tubular reabsorption capacity for filtered glucose results in excretion of glucose (*glycosuria*) at some time during pregnancy in 50% of women. It was previously believed that a reabsorptive mechanism in the proximal renal tubule became saturated so that the 'renal threshold' was exceeded. Glucose reabsorption is now known to occur secondarily to the absorption of sodium. It is, therefore, likely that other factors contributing to volume homeostasis and sodium retention are involved in the process. Whatever the true explanation, most obstetricians now accept that glycosuria is usually a physiological finding during pregnancy, reflecting neither renal impairment nor a malfunction of carbohydrate metabolism. However, because of its association with gestational diabetes and increased susceptibility to infection, glycosuria in pregnancy continues to require evaluation (Steinfeld & Wax 2001).

The urine is more alkaline owing to the presence of glucose and to the increased renal loss of bicarbonate caused by the alkalaemia of pregnancy (Baylis & Davison 1998). Stimulated by oestrogen secretion, there is increased renal production of the enzyme renin (which is also produced by the uterus and chorion). Renin rises early in pregnancy and continues to increase until term. It acts on angiotensinogen to form increased amounts of angiotensin I and II. Angiotensin II is a potent vasoconstrictor; however, healthy pregnant women do not respond with vasoconstriction and subsequent blood pressure elevation, as one would expect in the non-pregnant state, because in normal pregnancy there is selective loss of vascular sensitivity to angiotensin II (Steinfeld & Wax 2001) (Fig. 13.9). Increased production of angiotensin II also stimulates the release of increased levels of aldosterone. Aldosterone prevents the increased loss of sodium that could occur as a result of the increased GFR and the natriuretic effects of progesterone (Llewellyn-Jones 1999). Due to the increased GFR, the filtered load of sodium increases from non-pregnant levels of about 20 000 mmol/day to as much as 30 000 mmol/day. Tubular reabsorption increases in parallel with the GFR, with the retention of 3–5 mmol of sodium per day into the maternal and fetal stores. Despite elevated aldosterone levels, potassium excretion is decreased, possibly because of the effects of progesterone.

Water and sodium excretion are significantly reduced when the woman is in the upright position or changes from a recumbent to a supine position, owing to reduced venous return to the heart and therefore reduced renal perfusion. More recent studies suggest, however, that the impact of posture on glomerular filtration is variable and the decrease in renal plasma flow is not due simply to a positional effect (Baylis & Davison, 1998).

Posture does, however, affect the circadian rhythms of sodium excretion. At night while recumbent, fluid accumulated during the day as dependent oedema is mobilised and excreted via the kidneys. This reversal of the usual non-pregnant diurnal pattern of urinary flow causes nocturia and the urine is more dilute because of the excretion of extracellular fluid of relatively low osmolality (Cunningham et al 1997). It follows therefore that increased rest during the day in the

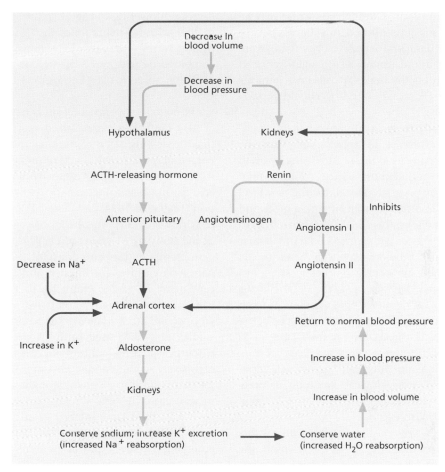

Fig. 13.9 The renin–angiotensin system. (From Hinchliff et al 1996 p. 226, with permission of Baillière Tindall, London.)

recumbent position will lead to excretion of maximum amounts of urine in the middle of the day (McFadyen 1995).

Changes in the gastrointestinal system

The gums become oedematous, soft and spongy during pregnancy, probably owing to the effect of oestrogen, which can lead to bleeding when mildly traumatised as with a toothbrush. Occasionally a focal, highly vascular swelling known as *epulis* (or gingivitis) develops; it is caused by growth of the gum capillaries. It usually regresses spontaneously after delivery. Most evidence indicates that pregnancy does not cause tooth decay. Profuse salivation, or ptyalism, is an occasional complaint in pregnancy; it is apparently caused by stimulation of the salivary glands due to ingestion of starch (Cunningham et al 1997).

Dietary changes in pregnancy, such as aversion to coffee, alcohol and fried foods, are very common in pregnancy, as are cravings for salted and spiced foods; these are perhaps due to a dulling of the sense of taste in pregnancy. Pica, the term given to the bizarre craving for and compulsive, secret chewing of food or ingestion of non-food substances (e.g. ice, coal, disinfectants) is also reasonably common, although some pica may be more to do with social tradition than with compulsive appetite. The mechanisms for these dietary changes are poorly understood and usually of no significance to the pregnancy unless the material consumed inhibits iron absorption (Edmonds, 1999; Steinfeld & Wax 2001).

Although in early pregnancy many women experience nausea, an increase in appetite may also be noticed, with the daily food intake increasing by up to 200 kcal. The hypothalamus, which controls total body fat, is reset by progesterone so that the new level of body fat store is achieved both by eating more and by expending less energy. This facilitates the woman to enter the third trimester with some 3.5 kg of fat store accumulated, which provides an energy bank for the last trimester when fat storage practically stops but energy is required for the growth of the fetus (Campbell-Brown & Hytten 1998). Many women notice an increase in thirst in pregnancy because of the resetting of osmotic thresholds for thirst and vasopressin. This contributes towards a fall in plasma osmolality, leading to increased water retention, which is a normal physiological alteration of pregnancy. HCG may influence osmoregulation in pregnancy (Baylis & Davison 1998).

As pregnancy progresses, the enlarging uterus displaces the stomach and intestines. As a result the appendix is displaced upwards and laterally so that appendicitis can be mistaken for pyelonephritis (Cunningham et al 1997, Edmonds 1999). At term the stomach attains a vertical position rather than its normal horizontal one. These mechanical forces lead to increased intragastric pressure and a change in the angle of the gastro-oesophageal junction, leading to greater oesophageal reflux (Ciliberto & Marx 1998). The upward displacement of the stomach when the uterus is unusually large (as in multiple pregnancy or polyhydramnios) makes many of the most annoying symptoms of pregnancy more difficult to treat (Steinfeld & Wax 2001).

Marked reduction of gastric and intestinal tone and motility plus relaxation of the lower oesophageal sphincter predispose to heartburn, constipation and haemorrhoids (Burnett 2001). Around 80% of women experience some degree of heartburn during pregnancy, usually in the third trimester. It is thought to be due to a small increase in intragastric pressure combined with decreased lower oesophageal sphincter tone, allowing gastric acid to reflux into the lower oesophagus. Although the true aetiology remains unclear, the combined influence of progesterone and oestrogen is probably responsible (Edmonds 1999, Steinfeld & Wax 2001).

Although an experimental study in rats by Shah et al (2001) implicates oestradiol, it is generally accepted that the slowing of gastrointestinal motility and gastric emptying is due to the effects of progesterone, producing an increased gastric volume with decreased gastric acidity, and beginning as early as 8–10 weeks' gestation (Levy et al 1994, Steinfeld & Wax 2001, Symonds & Symonds 1998). This belief has continued in spite of the study by Macfie et al (1991), which compared gastric emptying in non-pregnant women with pregnant women in each trimester, and found no significant delay in gastric emptying in any of the three trimesters of pregnancy compared with the control group. Ciliberto & Marx (1998) report on more recent studies that have shed further light on the subject; when peak plasma concentrations of drugs absorbed exclusively in the duodenum were measured in both pregnant and non-pregnant women at different times in gestation, it was shown that peak absorption occurred at the same interval in all women with the exception of those in labour. This suggests that gastric emptying is delayed only at the time of birth, and that the increased risk of aspiration due to endotracheal intubation associated with pregnancy results from an increase of oesophageal reflux and gastric acidity.

Following an extensive review of research studies published between 1966 and 1996 for the development of fasting guidelines, the American Society of Anesthesiologists supported the view that gastric emptying is normal in all three trimesters of pregnancy (Maltby 2000).

Although Girling (2001) suggests that the pH of gastric contents and the production of gastric acid remain unchanged in pregnancy, controversy continues over whether production of gastrin and gastric acidity increases, declines or remains the same. Since aspiration of gastric contents is an important cause of maternal morbidity and mortality in association with anaesthesia, the debate and the controversies will continue until irrefutable evidence is produced.

It is presumed that the relaxing effect of progesterone is responsible for slowing gut motility, resulting in longer transit time and for increased colonic water absorption, both of which contribute to the development of constipation, although studies to prove this are scant. Compression of the lower bowel by the uterus may also contribute to this problem, as may the administration of oral iron (Burnett 2001, Edmonds 1999).

The gall bladder becomes dilated during pregnancy and the rate of emptying is sluggish owing to the effects of progesterone. Bile may become thickened, with the increased risk of obstetric cholestasis (Campbell & Lees 2000). Incomplete emptying of the gall bladder may result in retention of cholesterol crystals – a prerequisite for gall stones, which are relatively common in asymptomatic pregnant women (Cunningham et al 1997).

Some studies suggest there is no change in liver size and blood flow, whereas others suggest an increase (de Sweit 1998a, Reynolds 1998). Although many changes occur in the liver in pregnancy that mimic liver disease, liver function tests should be interpreted with caution since there are considerable differences between laboratories with regard to 'normal ranges' (Ramsay et al 2000):

- serum albumin concentration falls quite abruptly in early pregnancy and then more slowly until late pregnancy (Cunningham et al 1997)
- serum alkaline phosphatase levels rise progressively during pregnancy and by late pregnancy are at approximately double non-pregnant values; the upper limit of normal for pregnancy is three times greater than the non-pregnant reference range (Girling 2001)
- serum cholesterol levels are doubled by the end of pregnancy (Ramsay et al 2000)
- many liver proteins are raised in response to oestrogen (Cunningham et al 1997)
- fibrinogen levels are increased from about the 3rd month of pregnancy by about 50% in the third trimester (Coustan 1995).

Changes in metabolism

In order to provide for increased basal metabolic rate and oxygen consumption, as well as the needs of the rapidly growing uterus, fetus and placenta, the pregnant woman undergoes many profound metabolic changes (Cunningham et al 1997). The increased dietary intake of approximately 200 kcal per day, in addition to the gastrointestinal changes of pregnancy, is accompanied by characteristic alterations in the metabolism of carbohydrate, protein and fat. Protein metabolism is enhanced to supply substrate for maternal and fetal growth. Fat metabolism increases, as evidenced by elevation of all lipid fractions in the blood. Carbohydrate metabolism, however, demonstrates the most dramatic changes (Ciliberto & Marx 1998).

The continuous supply of glucose required by the growing fetus is met first by the intake of glucose when the mother eats, and secondly by the enhanced secretion of insulin in response to glucose. During the first half of pregnancy the fasting plasma glucose concentrations are reduced in most women. As early as 15 weeks' gestation, maternal blood glucose levels after an overnight fast are considerably lower than in the non-pregnant state, but there is little change in plasma insulin levels. A standard oral glucose tolerance test at this time shows an enhanced response compared to the non-pregnant state with a normal pattern of insulin release, but reduced blood glucose values. In the second half of pregnancy, however, the pattern changes with further decreases in plasma glucose concentrations and insulin secretion correspondingly rising. The glucose tolerance test shows a delay in reaching peak glucose values and an increase in these values throughout the test despite significant increases in plasma insulin concentrations, which suggests relative insulin resistance. It has been speculated that these prolonged postprandial episodes of relative hyperglycaemia facilitate glucose transport to the fetus and may therefore contribute to the increased stores of glycogen and fat laid down at this time; however, there is as yet no evidence to support this.

There is evidence, however, that HPL or other growth-related hormones may contribute to the process by reducing peripheral insulin sensitivity as the peak in HPL concentrations corresponds to the greatest insulin responses. It has also been suggested that there may be alterations in the characteristics of insulin binding to its receptor.

Optimal blood glucose levels in the pregnant woman range between 4.4 and 5.5 mmol/L. Whereas in the non-pregnant woman signs of hypoglycaemia begin when the blood glucose level drops to approximately 2.2 mmol/L, in the pregnant woman hypoglycaemia is defined as a concentration below 3.3 mmol/L (O'Hare 1998, Reece & Homko 2001).

The so-called 'diabetogenic effect' of pregnancy, therefore, is a normal physiological adaptation that shifts maternal energy metabolism from carbohydrate to lipid oxidation. By using the fat stores laid down in the first half of pregnancy as the primary energy source, glucose is 'spared' for the growing fetus. As the nutritional demands of the fetus increase in the second half of pregnancy and insulin resistance increases, fat storage decreases as it is mobilised to provide the mother with extra energy supplies. Metabolically speaking, pregnant women live in a state of 'accelerated starvation'.

Theoretically, this mechanism of accelerated fat metabolism and ketone body formation should protect mother and fetus during prolonged starvation, fasting or hard physical exercise (Reece & Homko 2001) (see Ch. 19). However, it is recommended that pregnant women neither fast, skip meals nor restrict carbohydrate intake. Maternal blood glucose levels are of critical importance for fetal well-being and prolonged fasting in pregnancy produces a more intense ketonaemia, which may be dangerous to fetal health (Cunningham et al 1997).

Although Muslim women are exempt from fasting while pregnant, those who wish to fast during Ramadan may do so under medical supervision if it occurs during the second trimester. Fasting during the first and third trimesters, however, is not recommended, the main danger to the fetus possibly being from dehydration rather than from malnutrition (Athar 1990). Interestingly, fasting during Ramadan has been shown not to affect the mean birthweight of babies at any stage of pregnancy. Mothers may report less fetal movement during the day but this is compensated for by increased activity at night as the fetal diurnal cycle changes with that of the mother (Sadiq 2000).

If carbohydrate and fat consumption in pregnancy is inadequate, the energy requirements of the mother will be met by the catabolism of protein stores. However, amino acids thus used for energy are not available for protein synthesis. The diabetogenic effect of HPL results in the mobilisation of lipids as free fatty acids, thereby making glucose and amino acids available to the fetus (Reece & Homko 2001).

Maternal plasma calcium concentration falls during pregnancy, primarily because of the decrease in serum albumin that is required for binding calcium. However, there is a substantial need for calcium to provide for the mineralisation of the fetal skeleton mostly during the third trimester; therefore more is absorbed from the upper gastrointestinal tract, less is excreted and there is little change in bone deposition. Marked alterations in vitamin D metabolism have been reported. Vitamin-D-binding protein, which transports vitamin D and its metabolites in the circulation, also increases two- to threefold during pregnancy under the influence of parathyroid hormone. This is probably the reason for the enhanced absorption of calcium. Calcium supplements are not generally necessary since the maternal skeleton acts as a calcium reservoir. The only exception may be in teenage pregnancy when the mother herself is still growing (Campbell-Brown & Hytten 1998, Hosking 1998). Advice to supplement the diet with extra calcium in order to reduce leg cramp in pregnancy appears to have been based on tradition as the evidence to date based on randomised trials is weak and seems to depend on the placebo effect (Young & Jewell 2002a).

Maternal weight

Weight gain during pregnancy comprises the products of conception (fetus, placenta, and amniotic fluid), and hypertrophy of several maternal tissues (uterus, breasts, blood, fat stores, and extracellular and extravascular fluid). Protein is laid down predominantly in the fetus, but also in the uterus, blood, placenta and breasts. In contrast, fat is deposited mainly in maternal adipose tissue, particularly in the gluteal and upper thigh regions, with the fetus the only other major site of importance (Prentice et al 1996) (Table 13.3).

Fetal weight gain is slow in the first half of pregnancy and increases more rapidly in the second 20 weeks. The increase in placental weight is the opposite, being more rapid in the first half of pregnancy. Amniotic fluid increases rapidly from the 10th week, from 300 ml at 20 weeks, to a peak of 1000 ml at 35 weeks, after which it declines slightly. The weight of the uterus is more rapid in the first 20 weeks. The weight of breasts and blood volume increases steadily throughout pregnancy. Most of the fat gained is deposited in the first 30 weeks. Most of the fluid is retained in the first 30 weeks, but even in the absence

Table 13.3 Distribution of average increase in weight in pregnancy, showing relative proportions of protein and fat

Site	Wt (kg)	Protein (%)	Fat (%)
Fetus	3.2	44	15
Placenta	0.6	10	
Amniotic fluid	0.8		
Uterus	0.9	17	
Breasts	0.4	8	
Blood	1.5	14	
Water	2.6		
Adipose tissue	2.5		85
Total	12.5		

of clinical oedema 2 to 3 litres of extracellular fluid are retained in the last 10 weeks (Prentice et al 1996).

An optimal weight gain for an average pregnancy is 12.5 kg, 9 kg of which is gained in the last 20 weeks. This is associated with the lowest risk of complications during pregnancy and labour and of low birthweight babies (Llewellyn-Jones 1999).

Many factors influence weight gain. The degree of oedema, metabolic rate, dietary intake, vomiting or diarrhoea, smoking, amount of amniotic fluid and size of the fetus must all be taken into account. Maternal age, prepregnancy body size, parity, race–ethnicity, hypertension and diabetes also influence the pattern of maternal weight gain (Abrams et al 1995).

Appropriate weight gain for each individual woman is now based on the prepregnancy body mass index (BMI), which reflects the mother's weight-to-height ratio (see Ch. 12). In general, optimal growth of the unborn baby occurs if women with a low prepregnancy BMI (< 20) gain more weight and women with a high BMI (> 27) gain less weight than women who enter pregnancy with a healthy body weight (BMI between 20 and 25) (Health Canada 1999). In the UK there are no official weight gain recommendations for different populations, whereas in the USA and Canada there are different recommendations for women who enter pregnancy underweight, normal weight or overweight, and for teenagers and some ethnic groups. In well-nourished women of normal pre-pregnant BMI with uncomplicated pregnancies resulting in normal birthweight babies, average gestational weight gains are between 11 and 16 kg, but the variability is very large (Goldberg 2000).

Skeletal changes

During pregnancy, relaxation of the pelvic joints probably results from hormonal changes (Cunningham et al 1997). Oestrogen, progesterone and relaxin all appear to be implicated. Oestrogen is responsible for making connective tissue more pliable, causing the joint capsules to relax and making the pelvic joints mobile (Miller & Hanretty 1997). Progesterone has the effect of relaxing or weakening the pelvic ligaments (Musumeci & Villa 1994). However, it is the effects of relaxin that have stimulated the most interest in recent years. Relaxin regulates collagen and softens pelvic joints and ligaments in preparation for delivery (Kristiansson et al 1996). This allows some expansion of the pelvic cavity during descent of the fetal head in labour (Symonds & Symonds 1998). However, the increase in diameter of the pelvic outlet occurs only if the sacrum is allowed to rotate posteriorly. Relaxation of the symphysis pubis commences during the first half of pregnancy and increases in the last 3 months. The increase in width of the symphysis pubis, which has been associated with severe pelvic pain, occurs more in multiparous than in primigravid women, and returns to normal soon after birth (Cunningham et al 1997). The role of relaxin in causing pelvic pain is, however, inconclusive (Bjorklund et al 2000).

Posture usually alters to compensate for the enlarging uterus, particularly if abdominal muscle tone is poor. A progressive lordosis shifts the woman's centre of gravity back over her legs. There is also increased mobility of the sacroiliac and sacrococcygeal joints which may contribute to the alteration in maternal posture leading to low back pain in late pregnancy, particularly in the multiparous woman. In late pregnancy aching, numbness and weakness are occasionally experienced in the arms, possibly as a result of the marked lordosis, with anterior flexion of the neck and slumping of the shoulder girdle, which in turn put traction on the ulnar and median nerves (Cunningham et al 1997). The muscles of the abdominal wall may stretch and lose some tone, further aggravating back pain (Lowdermilk et al 1999) (see Ch. 15).

Skin changes

From the 3rd month until term, some degree of skin darkening is observed in 90% of all pregnant women.

This was previously thought to be due to a rise in melanocyte-stimulating hormone (MSH). However, oestrogen and progesterone are also reported to have melanocyte-stimulating effects and are now considered to be a more likely cause of skin pigmentation. Hyperpigmentation is more marked in dark-skinned women and is more pronounced in areas such as the areolae, perineum and umbilicus and in areas prone to friction such as the axillae and inner thighs (Cunningham et al 1997).

The pigmented linea alba, now called the *linea nigra*, runs from the os pubis to above the umbilicus. This line lies over the midline of the rectus muscles where occasionally *diastasis recti abdominis* occurs (see Ch. 15). Pigmentation of the face, which affects at least half of all pregnant women, is called *chloasma* or *melasma*, or 'mask of pregnancy'. Melasma is caused by melanin deposition into epidermal or dermal macrophages. Epidermal melanosis usually regresses postpartum but dermal melanosis may persist for up to 10 years in one-third of women. Oral contraceptives may aggravate melasma and should be avoided in susceptible women (Cunningham et al 1997). Chloasma can be minimised or prevented by avoiding sun exposure, and by the application of blanching creams containing hydroquinone, followed by high protection factor sun creams (Turner 2000).

As maternal size increases, stretching occurs in the collagen layer of the skin, particularly over the breasts, abdomen and thighs. In some women the areas of maximum stretch become thin and stretch marks, *striae gravidarum*, appear as red stripes changing to glistening, silvery white lines approximately 6 months after delivery (Cunningham et al 1997). Stretch marks are related to the increased production of adrenocortical hormones in pregnancy and to the stress on skin folds associated with expansion of the abdomen (Symonds & Symonds 1998). There is no evidence of benefit for the general use of creams to prevent stretch marks (Young & Jewell 2002b).

Although not common, itching of the skin in pregnancy (not due to liver disease) can be distressing. The latest evidence suggests that, in the absence of a rash, aspirin is effective but if there is a rash that chlorphenamine (chlorpheniramine) may be more effective (Young & Jewell 2002c).

The proportion of growing hairs to resting hairs is increased in pregnancy so the woman reaches the end of pregnancy with many overaged hairs. This ratio is reversed after delivery so that sometimes alarming amounts of hair are shed during brushing or washing, leading to the common anxiety that hair is coming out 'in handfuls' (de Sweit 1998a). Normal hair growth is usually restored by 6–12 months. Mild hirsutism is common during pregnancy, particularly on the face (Cunningham et al 1997).

A rise in temperature by 0.2–0.4°C occurs as a result of the effects of progesterone and to the increased basal metabolic rate (BMR). As a result, pregnant women 'feel the heat' and often sweat profusely, particularly in hot, humid climates. Peripheral vasodilation and acceleration of sweat gland activity help to dissipate the excess heat produced by maternal, placental and fetal metabolism (Lowdermilk et al 1999).

Angiomas or *vascular spiders* (minute red elevations on the skin of the face, neck, arms and chest) and *palmar erythema* (reddening of the palms) frequently occur, possibly as a result of the high levels of oestrogen. They are of no clinical significance, and disappear after pregnancy (Cunningham et al 1997).

Changes in the breasts

Owing to the increased blood supply, and stimulated by secretion of oestrogen and progesterone from both corpus luteum and placenta, major changes take place in the breasts during pregnancy, and new ducts and acini cells are formed (Cunningham et al 1997) (Box 13.2). The greatest activity takes place in the first trimester, but proliferation continues throughout pregnancy (see Ch. 40).

Changes in the endocrine system

Endocrine changes in pregnancy are complex and understanding of them is incomplete. It is now clear that during pregnancy the intrauterine tissues can also produce many of the peptide and steroid hormones that are produced by the endocrine glands in the non-pregnant state. Many hormones exert their actions indirectly by interacting with cytokines and chemokines. During pregnancy these substances are substantially altered (Campbell & Lees 2000). Early effects of placental hormones are described in Chapter 9. Later physiological effects caused by hormones have been highlighted throughout this chapter as they impact on the various systems, and are now summarised.

Box 13.2 Breast changes in chronological order

3–4 weeks

Prickling, tingling sensation due to increased blood supply particularly around nipple.

6–8 weeks

Increase in size, painful, tense and nodular due to hypertrophy of the alveoli. Delicate, bluish surface veins become visible just beneath the skin.

8–12 weeks

Montgomery's tubercles become more prominent on the areola. These hypertrophic sebaceous glands secrete sebum, which keeps the nipple soft and supple. The pigmented area around the nipple (the primary areola) darkens and may enlarge and become more erectile.

16 weeks

Colostrum can be expressed. The secondary areola develops with further extension of the pigmented area that is often mottled in appearance.

Late pregnancy

Colostrum may leak from the breasts; progesterone causes the nipple to become more prominent and mobile.

Placental hormones

HCG is produced by the trophoblast, is detectable within maternal circulation within days of implantation and forms the basis for the pregnancy test. Its role in maintaining the function of the corpus luteum is complete when placental production of progesterone becomes dominant between 10 and 12 weeks' gestation, after which concentrations of HCG decline. It has been suggested that HCG may have a thyrotrophic function and that maternal TSH production may be suppressed during the first trimester when levels of HCG are maximal (Campbell & Lees 2000).

HPL is another peptide that probably has major effects on maternal production of prolactin and HCG. Like HCG, it is detected in the trophoblast as early as the 2nd or 3rd week after fertilisation of the ovum. The concentration in maternal plasma then steadily rises until 34–36 weeks, when it is approximately proportional to the placental mass. HPL may participate in a number of important metabolic processes including increasing maternal blood free fatty acids, glucose and insulin concentrations, and increasing lipolysis and insulin resistance. This impairs glucose uptake and gluconeogenesis resulting in enhanced glucose and amino acid availability for fetal uptake (Myatt 2001).

The major oestrogens in the urine of pregnant women are oestrone, oestradiol, and oestriol. Oestrone excretion increases 100-fold, whereas oestriol excretion increases 1000-fold. The ovary makes a minimal contribution to this increase as the placenta is the major source of oestrogen in pregnancy. The substrate for oestriol production comes from the fetal adrenal gland. Oestrone and oestradiol are synthesised by the syncytiotrophoblast. During pregnancy the high oestrogen concentrations stimulate the liver to produce serum cortisol, testosterone and thyroxine-binding proteins, and to increase the production of cholesterol. It also causes proliferation of the ductal system of the breast and stimulates secretion of prolactin by the pituitary gland. In addition, oestrogens facilitate growth of the uterus, its increasing blood flow and the onset of contractions at term. Urinary and plasma levels of oestriol increase progressively throughout pregnancy until 38 weeks' gestation, after which there is a slight fall owing to fetal adrenal suppression (Cunningham et al 1997).

Progesterone is synthesised within the syncytiotrophoblast very early in gestation; however, until 35 to 47 days' postovulation it needs to be supplemented with progesterone from the corpus luteum. Ninety per cent of this hormone is secreted into the maternal circulation, with the remaining 10% being secreted into the fetal circulation. Placental production of progesterone increases steadily throughout pregnancy until it reaches maximal levels around 38 weeks. Its main function is to maintain uterine quiescence but it also exerts effects on the smooth muscle of blood vessels, and urinary and gastrointestinal tracts (Campbell & Lees 2000).

Pituitary gland and its hormones

The pituitary gland enlarges during pregnancy owing to hypertrophy of the anterior lobe. The weight of the pituitary gland increases by 135% and could be responsible for compressing the optic chiasma, reducing visual fields and perhaps causing headaches. Visual changes during pregnancy are minimal, however. If such symptoms occur they should be investigated because occasionally in pregnancy there is rapid increase in the size of a prolactinoma.

Secretion of FSH and LH (see Ch. 9) is greatly inhibited during pregnancy by the negative feedback of progesterone and oestrogen. In contrast there is increased secretion of hormones by the pituitary gland. The anterior lobe secretes thyroid-stimulating hormone (TSH), ACTH, prolactin and MSH. The posterior lobe of the pituitary gland secretes oxytocin and vasopressin (antidiuretic hormone) (Beischer et al 1997).

Prolactin is essential for lactation and levels rise up to 20-fold during pregnancy and lactation. Its effect of producing milk is suppressed during pregnancy by high levels of oestrogen and progesterone. There is now clear evidence of intrauterine production of prolactin, especially from cells within the decidua (Campbell & Lees 2000).

The posterior pituitary gland releases oxytocin throughout pregnancy. Concentrations of oxytocin in the maternal circulation do not change significantly during pregnancy or prior to the onset of labour, but do rise late in the second stage of labour. There is, however, an increased uterine sensitivity to oxytocin during labour that is influenced by the ratio of oestrogen to progesterone. The pulsatile release produces more effective uterine contractions. Oxytocin is also important for successful lactation (Norwitz et al 2001) (see Ch. 40).

Thyroid function

Alterations in the structure and function of the thyroid gland cause many thyroid symptoms to be mimicked in pregnancy, resulting in diagnostic confusion in the interpretation of thyroid function tests. Overall control of the thyroid gland, however, is unaltered during normal pregnancy. There is a moderate increase in size early in pregnancy, but some researchers consider this occurs only in women who are relatively iodine deficient because it is not found in women from Iceland and The Netherlands where iodine intake is greater. There is a marked increase in thyroid-binding globulin,

and the bound forms of thyroxine (T_4) and tri-iodothyronine (T_3) peak at about 12 weeks' gestation, but the circulating concentrations of unbound (inactive) T_3 and T_4 are essentially unaltered. Similarly TSH shows no change in pregnancy. Thus there is no evidence to support the role of the thyroid gland in the increase in BMR, body temperature and heart rate in pregnancy. Much of the increase in oxygen consumption is the result of fetal metabolic activity. An index of free thyroxine is the best guide to thyroid function (Campbell & Lees 2000) (Table 13.4).

Adrenal glands

In early pregnancy the levels of ACTH are strikingly reduced, but from 3 months until term there is a significant rise along with the increase in serum concentrations of circulating free cortisol. The placenta and the trophoblast cells also produce corticotrophin releasing factor and ACTH. These hormones are important in relation to the priming of myometrial activity and may also influence the fetal adrenals. The raised levels of unbound cortisol are reflected in the excretion of double the amount of urinary cortisol and could be responsible for impaired carbohydrate metabolism, hypertension and the pseudo-Cushingoid features of pregnancy, but this remains controversial (Campbell & Lees 2000, Dunlop 1999).

From 15 weeks' gestation until the third trimester there is a 10-fold increase in the secretion of aldosterone and deoxycorticosterone by the maternal adrenal glands and also by fetal intrauterine tissues, which is stimulated to a certain extent by the acute rise in ACTH (Campbell & Lees 2000). This rise was formerly attributed entirely to progesterone; however, it is now clear that its main means of control is via the renin–angiotensin system (see Fig. 13.9) with involvement of factors such as atrial natriuretic peptide and angiotensins (Ramsay & Davison 1998).

Table 13.4 Normal levels for thyroid function test in pregnancy			
T4 (nmol/L)	T3 (nmol/L)	Thyroid-stimulating hormone (mU/L)	Free T4 (pmol/L)
55–144	0.9–2.8	0.35–5.0	9–26

Data from Greer et al 2001, p. 133.

Diagnosis of pregnancy

There are few experiences in the life of a woman that evoke such emotions of absolute joy or profound despair than that of pregnancy; therefore correct diagnosis is very important (Cunningham et al 1997). The woman herself often diagnoses pregnancy even before she has missed a period because she feels different. Breast changes (see Box 13.2), nausea, changes in food and drink preference, overwhelming tiredness, frequency of micturition and backache confirm her suspicion (Table 13.5) (Beischer et al 1997). The date of *quickening*, the first fluttering movements of the fetus felt by the mother, can be used to check the date of expected confinement. A primigravid woman feels it at 18–20 weeks, and a multigravid woman at 16–18 weeks (Miller & Hanretty 1997).

Table 13.5 Signs of pregnancy

Sign	Time of occurrence (gestational age)	Differential diagnosis
Possible (presumptive) signs		
Early breast changes (unreliable in multigravida)	3–4 weeks +	Contraceptive pill
Amenorrhoea	4 weeks +	Hormonal imbalance Emotional stress Illness
Morning sickness	4–14 weeks	Gastrointestinal disorders Pyrexial illness Cerebral irritation, etc.
Bladder irritability	6–12 weeks	Urinary tract infection Pelvic tumour
Quickening	16–20 weeks +	Intestinal movement, 'wind'
Probable signs		
Presence of human chorionic gonadotrophin (HCG) in:		
Blood	9–10 days	Hydatidiform mole
Urine	14 days	Choriocarcinoma
Softened isthmus (Hegar's sign)	6–12 weeks	
Blueing of vagina (Chadwick's sign)	8 weeks +	
Pulsation of fornices (Osiander's sign)	8 weeks +	Pelvic congestion
Uterine growth	8 weeks +	Tumours
Changes in skin pigmentation	8 weeks +	
Uterine soufflé	12–16 weeks	Increased blood flow to uterus as in large uterine myomas or ovarian tumours
Braxton Hicks contractions	16 weeks	
Ballottement of fetus	16–28 weeks	
Positive signs		
Visualisation of gestational sac by:		
Transvaginal ultrasound	4.5 weeks	
Transabdominal ultrasound	5.5 weeks	
Visualisation of heart pulsation by:		
Transvaginal ultrasound	5 weeks	
Transabdominal ultrasound	6 weeks	
Fetal heart sounds by:		
Doppler	11–12 weeks	
Fetal stethoscope	20 weeks +	No alternative diagnosis
Fetal movements:		
Palpable	22 weeks +	
Visible	Late pregnancy	
Fetal parts palpated	24 weeks +	
Visualisation of fetus by:		
X-ray	16 weeks +	

Other methods of ascertaining pregnancy and estimating early gestational age involve the observation of certain characteristics, but as these are not associated exclusively with pregnancy they cannot be considered positive signs. Furthermore the development of quick and sensitive laboratory tests for pregnancy have rendered them obsolete.

Hegar's sign. This is a bimanual examination for assessing the softening and compressibility of the isthmus between the 6th and 12th weeks of pregnancy. It is difficult to elicit and could be mistaken for pelvic congestion by an inexperienced examiner (Lowdermilk et al 1999).

Chadwick's sign. This is the dark purplish discoloration and congestion of the vaginal membrane, caused by increased vascularity. It could be mistaken for any condition that causes pelvic congestion (Cunningham et al 1997).

Osiander's sign. This is an increased pulsation of blood in the uterine arteries, felt with the fingers in the lateral vaginal fornices (Beischer et al 1997).

X-rays are not used nowadays to diagnose pregnancy because of the dangers of irradiation to the fetus. However, this does not preclude X-rays from being performed if clinically indicated, the radiation exposure to the fetus from a chest X-ray being the same as that from a one-way transatlantic flight (Girling 2000).

Using transvaginal ultrasound, the gestational sac can be visualised at 4.5 weeks and heart pulsation can be seen at 5 weeks, providing conclusive evidence when early diagnosis is necessary. Using transabdominal ultrasound, visualisation of gestational sac and heart pulsation is possible 1 week later (Smith & Smith 2002). Doppler can detect the fetal heart at 11–12 weeks gestation (Burnett 2001). The palpation of fetal parts and fetal movements from about 22 weeks are good positive signs of pregnancy (Lowdermilk et al 1999) (see Table 13.5).

All biochemical pregnancy tests depend on the detection of human chorionic gonadotrophin (hCG) produced by the trophoblast. Production of hCG begins on the day of implantation and can be detected in blood as early as 6 days after conception, and in urine 26 days after conception. Many different pregnancy tests are available, but the most popular over-the-counter home pregnancy test is the *enzyme-linked immunosorbent assay* (ELISA). The test can detect very low levels of HCG in the urine. The woman usually applies a morning specimen of urine to a strip and she can read the result within 5 minutes. The test kits come with instructions for the collection of the specimen, the testing procedure and the reading of the results (Lowdermilk et al 1999).

REFERENCES

Abrams B, Carmichael S, Selvin S 1995 Factors associated with the pattern of maternal weight gain during pregnancy. Obstetrics and Gynaecology 86(2):170–176

Athar S 1990 Medical aspects of Islamic fasting. Midwives Chronicle 103(1227):106

Baylis C, Davison J 1998 The urinary system. In: Chamberlain G, Broughton Pipkin F (eds) Clinical physiology in obstetrics. Blackwell Science, Oxford, p 264–268, 281–289

Beischer N, Mackay E, Colditz P 1997 Obstetrics and the newborn, 3rd British edn. W B Saunders, London, p 23, 54, 324, 378

Bennett W, Cowan B 2001 Uterus from birth to maturity. In Seifer D, Samuels P, Kniss D (eds) The physiologic basis of gynecology and obstetrics. Lippincott Williams & Wilkins, Philadelphia, p 208

Bjorklund K, Bergstrom S, Nordstrom M, Ulmsten U 2000 Symphyseal distension in relation to serum relaxin levels and pelvic pain in pregnancy. Acta Obstetricia et Gynecologica Scandinavica 79(4):269–275

Blackburn S, Loper D 1992 Maternal, fetal and neonatal physiology – a clinical perspective. W B Saunders, London, p 111, 207

Burnett A 2001 Clinical obstetrics and gynaecology. Blackwell Science, Oxford, p 48, 74–75, 254

Calder A 1999 Normal labour. In: Edmonds K (ed) Dewhurst's textbook of obstetrics and gynaecology for postgraduates, 6th edn. Blackwell Science, Oxford, p 246

Campbell S, Lees C (eds) 2000 Obstetrics by ten teachers. Oxford University Press, New York, p 47–59, 107, 109, 150, 169, 177, 259

Campbell-Brown M, Hytten F 1998 Nutrition. In: Chamberlain G, Broughton Pipkin F (eds) Clinical physiology in obstetrics. Blackwell Science, Oxford, p 169–177

Cardozo L, Gleeson C 1997 Pregnancy, childbirth and continence. British Journal of Midwifery 5(5):277–281

Chamberlain G, Dewhurst J, Harvey D 1991 Obstetrics, 2nd edn. Gower Medical Publishing, London, p 30

Ciliberto C F, Marx G F 1998 Physiological changes associated with pregnancy. Issue 9, article 2, p 2–3 Online. Available: www.nda.ox.ac.uk/wfsa/html/u09/u09_003.htm

Coad J, Dunstall M 2001 Anatomy and physiology for midwives. Harcourt, London, p 119, 208–226

Coustan D 1995 Maternal physiology. In: Coustan D, Haning R, Singer D (eds) Human reproduction – growth and development. Little, Brown & Company, London, p 163, 181

Cunningham F, MacDonald P, Gant N et al 1997 William's obstetrics, 20th edn. Prentice Hall, London, p 22, 25, 43–49, 61, 142, 178–263, 1154–1164, 1273–1274, 1999

de Sweit M 1998a The cardiovascular system. In: Chamberlain G, Broughton Pipkin F (eds) Clinical physiology in obstetrics. Blackwell Science, Oxford, p 33–61

de Sweit M 1998b The respiratory system. In: Chamberlain G, Broughton Pipkin F (eds) Clinical physiology in obstetrics. Blackwell Science, Oxford, p 114–115

Dunlop W 1999 Normal pregnancy: physiology and endocrinology. In: Edmonds K (ed) Dewhurst's textbook of obstetrics and gynaecology for postgraduates, 6th edn. Blackwell Science, Oxford, p 79–88

Edmonds D 1999 Miscellaneous disorders in pregnancy. In: Edmonds K (ed) Dewhurst's textbook of obstetrics and gynaecology for postgraduates, 6th edn. Blackwell Science, Oxford, p 238–239

Girling J 2000 Physical adaptations to pregnancy. In: Page L, Percival P (eds) The new midwifery. Churchill Livingstone, Edinburgh, p 325

Girling J 2001 Physiology of pregnancy. Obstetrics, anaesthesia and intensive care medicine, p 167–170. Medicine Publishing Company, Abingdon, Oxon, Online. Available: www.medicinepublishing.com/girl_ 1–4

Goldberg G 2000 Nutrition in pregnancy. Nutrition in Practice 1(2):4. Online. Available: www.sugar-bureau.co.uk/BULLETINS/bulletinsN8.htm

Greer I, Cameron I, Kitchener H, Prentice A 2001 Mosby's Colour atlas and text of obstetrics and gynaecology. Mosby, Edinburgh, p 133

Health Canada 1999 Family-Centred Maternity and Newborn Care: National Guidelines. Canadian Government Publishing Directorate, Ottawa, ch 4, p21. Online. Available:www.hc-sc.gc.ca/hppb/childhoodyouth/cyfh/pdf/fcmc/fcmc04.pdf.

Hinchliff S, Montague S, Watson R (eds) 1996 Physiology for nursing practice, 2nd edn. Baillière Tindall, London, p 226

Hosking D 1998 Calcium metabolism. In: Chamberlain G, Broughton Pipkin F (eds) Clinical physiology in obstetrics. Blackwell Science, Oxford, p 212

Johnson M, Everitt B 2000 Essential reproduction. Blackwell Science, Oxford, p 189–191

Kristiansson P, Svardsudd K, von Schoultz B 1996 Serum relaxin, symphyseal pain, and back pain during pregnancy. American Journal of Obstetrics and Gynaecology 175(5):1342–1347

Letsky E 1998 The haematological system. In: Chamberlain G, Broughton Pipkin F (eds) Clinical physiology in obstetrics. Blackwell Science, Oxford, p 71–79

Levy D, Williams O, Magides A, Reilly C 1994 Gastric emptying is delayed at 8 to 12 weeks' gestation. British Journal of Anaesthesia 73(2):237–238

Llewellyn-Jones D 1999 Fundamentals of obstetrics and gynaecology, 7th edn. Mosby, London, p 31–35, 57–59, 130

Lowdermilk D, Perry S, Bobak I 1999 Maternity nursing, 5th edn. Mosby, London, p 123, 188–200

McFadyen I 1995 Maternal physiology in pregnancy. In: Chamberlain G (ed) Turnbull's obstetrics, 2nd edn. Churchill Livingstone, Edinburgh, ch 7

MacFie A, Magides A, Richmond N, Reilly C 1991 Gastric emptying in pregnancy. British Journal of Anaesthesia 67:54–57

MacGillivray I, Rose G, Rowe B (1969) Blood pressure survey in pregnancy. Clinical Science 37:395

Maltby J 2000 Pre-operative fasting guidelines. Issue 12, article 2, p 2. Online. Available: www.nda.ox.ac.uk/wfsa/html/u12/u1202_02.htm#dela

Miller A, Hanretty K 1997 Obstetrics illustrated, 5th edn. Churchill Livingstone, Edinburgh, p 34–35, 59–60

Musumeci R, Villa E 1994 Symphysis pubis separation during vaginal delivery with epidural anaesthesia. Case report. Regional Anaesthesia 19(4):289–291

Myatt L 2001 Placental physiology. In: Seifer D, Samuels P, Kniss D (eds.) The physiologic basis of gynecology and obstetrics. Lippincott Williams & Wilkins, Philadelphia, p 387

Neilson J 2002 Symphysis–fundal height measurement in pregnancy (Cochrane review). In: The Cochrane Library, Issue 1. Update Software, Oxford. Online. Available: www.update-software.com

Neuberg R (1995) Obstetrics – a practical manual. Oxford University Press, Oxford, p 4

Norwitz E, Robinson J, Repke J 2001 The initiation and management of normal labour. In: Seifer D, Samuels P, Kniss D (eds) The physiologic basis of gynecology and obstetrics. Lippincott Williams & Wilkins, Philadelphia, p 416–419

O'Hare J 1998 Carbohydrate metabolism. In: Chamberlain G, Broughton Pipkin F (eds) Clinical physiology in obstetrics. Blackwell Science, Oxford, p 193, 200

Pollard I 1994 Guide to reproduction: special issues and human concerns. Cambridge University Press, Cambridge, p 167

Prentice A, Spaaij C, Goldberg G et al 1996 Energy requirements of pregnant women and lactating women. European Journal of Clinical Nutrition 50 (Suppl 1): S82–S111

Ramsay I, Davison R 1998 The adrenal gland. In: Chamberlain G, Broughton Pipkin F (eds) Clinical physiology in obstetrics. Blackwell Science, Oxford, p 387–388

Ramsay M, James D, Steer P et al (eds) 2000 Normal values in pregnancy, 2nd edn. Harcourt, London, p 21–22

Reece E, Homko C 2001 Metabolism of maternal fuels in pregnancy. In Seifer D, Samuels P, Kniss D (eds) The physiologic basis of gynecology and obstetrics. Lippincott Williams & Wilkins, Philadelphia, p 502–510

Reiss R 2001 Intrauterine growth restriction. In: Seifer D, Samuels P, Kniss D (eds) The physiologic basis of gynecology and obstetrics. Lippincott Williams & Wilkins, Philadelphia, p 516

Reynolds F 1998 Pharmacokinetics. In: Chamberlain G, Broughton Pipkin F (eds) Clinical physiology in obstetrics. Blackwell Science, Oxford, p 243

Robson S, Hunter S, Boys R, Dunlop W 1989 Serial study of factors influencing changes in cardiac output during human pregnancy. American Journal of Physiology 256:1061–1065

Sadiq A 2000 Managing the fasting patient: sacred ritual, modern challenges, p 5. Online. Available: www.primarycareonline.co.uk/humaneffect/muslim/chap6.htm

Shah S, Nathan L, Singh R et al 2001 E2 and not P4 increases NO release from NANC nerves of the gastrointestinal tract: implications in pregnancy. American Journal of Physiology – Regulatory, Integrative and Comparative Physiology 250(5):R1546–R1554

Smith N, Smith P 2002 Obstetric ultrasound made easy. Churchill Livingstone, Edinburgh

Steer P, Johnson M 1998 The genital system. In: Chamberlain G, Broughton Pipkin F (eds) Clinical physiology in obstetrics. Blackwell Science, Oxford, p 316, 324

Steer P, Alam M, Wadsworth J, Welch A 1995 Relation between maternal haemoglobin concentration and birth weight in different ethnic groups. British Medical Journal 310:489–491

Steinfeld J, Wax J 2001 Maternal physiologic adaptations to pregnancy. In: Seifer D, Samuels P, Kniss D (eds) The physiologic basis of gynecology and obstetrics. Lippincott Williams & Wilkins, Philadelphia, p 365–371

Symonds E, Symonds I 1998 Essential obstetrics and gynaecology, 3rd edn. Churchill Livingstone, Edinburgh, p 26–31, 130

Turner A 2000 The mask of pregnancy: causes and treatment of chloasma. British Journal of Midwifery 8(9):594

Verrals S 1993 Anatomy and physiology applied to obstetrics, 3rd edn. Churchill Livingstone, Edinburgh, p 119

Young G, Jewell D 2002a Interventions for leg cramps in pregnancy (Cochrane review). In: The Cochrane Library, Issue 1. Update Software, Oxford. Online. Available: www.update-software.com

Young G, Jewell D 2002b Creams for preventing stretch marks in pregnancy (Cochrane review). In: The Cochrane Library, Issue 1. Update Software, Oxford. Online. Available: www.update-software.com

Young G, Jewell D 2002c Antihistamines versus aspirin for itching in late pregnancy (Cochrane review). In: The Cochrane Library, Issue 1. Update Software Oxford. Online. Available: www.update-software.com

FURTHER READING

Blackburn S, Loper D 1992 Maternal, fetal and neonatal physiology – a clinical perspective. W B Saunders, London.

Written primarily for advanced clinical practice nurses in maternal, perinatal and neonatal nursing in the USA, this textbook is an excellent foundation reference for midwives. It brings together detailed information on normal physiological adaptation in pregnancy, labour and the puerperium, with emphasis on the interrelationships between mother, fetus and neonate. It provides the scientific basis and rationale underpinning the assessment and management of women in both low and high risk categories, and examines the clinical implications of these physiological adaptations.

Chamberlain G, Broughton Pipkin F (eds) 1998 Clinical physiology in obstetrics. Blackwell Science, Oxford

This textbook aims to provide an in-depth understanding of the physiological background of the changes in pregnancy, with particular emphasis on how these changes can be confused with pathological processes. It presents detailed reviews of research studies relating to each body system and concludes each discussion with an analysis of the findings from a clinical perspective.

Coad J, Dunstall M 2001 Anatomy and physiology for midwives. Harcourt, London.

Written for midwives and student midwives this textbook provides a thorough review of anatomy and physiology applicable to midwifery from first principles through to current research, with the primary aim being to integrate theory with practice. The chapters are arranged according to body systems or stages of the childbearing process, and all contain learning objectives, case studies, excellent illustrations, key points, and 'application to practice' boxes.

Edmonds K 1999 Dewhurst's textbook of obstetrics and gynaecology for postgraduates, 6th edn. Blackwell Science, Oxford

Highly qualified and experienced contributors wrote this textbook as a postgraduate text for obstetricians and gynaecologists. Detailed reviews are presented of research findings to date, with special emphasis on the clinical application of these findings within obstetrics.

Ramsay M, James D, Steer P et al (eds) 2000 Normal values in pregnancy, 2nd edn. Harcourt, London.

This invaluable reference text provides a comprehensive range of physical and laboratory values based on studies identifying normal levels for mother and fetus, with a commentary on the maternal and fetal physiology that leads to the changes in these values throughout pregnancy.

Stables D 1999 Physiology in childbearing with anatomy and related biosciences. Baillière Tindall, Edinburgh

This textbook provides midwives and student midwives with a very comprehensive overview of the physiology of pregnancy and childbearing, and a sound evidence base on which decisions for practice can be made. Of particular relevance is the section relating to pregnancy, in which the altered normal physiology of pregnancy is discussed in depth under the chapter headings of each body system.

Wylie L 2000 Essential anatomy and physiology in maternity care. Churchill Livingstone, Edinburgh

This textbook has been specially written for student midwives. Each chapter applies basic anatomy and physiology of the different systems directly to the changing physiology of childbirth. Clinical issues are presented providing the student with a good foundation for the provision of evidence-based midwifery practice.

14 Parent Education: a New Dimension

Karen Blakey

CHAPTER CONTENTS

The midwife is in a unique position to educate and empower women through the phases of childbirth in order for them to achieve a healthy pregnancy with the optimum outcome of a healthy baby. Education for childbirth is an area that is likely to be new for many women and their partners. The preparation and education for childbirth begin at the first meeting and continues throughout all the childbirth process until care is transferred to the health visitor. This means that the midwife is the prime educator in all aspects of childbirth and therefore she is in a unique position to be able to guide, assist and empower these prospective parents to become competent parents. The intention of this chapter is to enable readers to be more confident in their abilities to teach parent education either on a one-to-one basis or when facilitating a parent education session for a group of prospective parents.

The chapter aims to:

- provide an insight into the origins of parent education

- define the midwife's role in parent education

- consider some of the more common disorders of pregnancy and offer midwifery advice on how to cope with them

- address the factors that affect teaching and learning

- analyse how parent education is taught

- consider the needs of special groups and whether these needs are being met

- explore the future role of midwives as educators.

The origins of parent education

The concept of educating women about the process of childbirth is not new. The origins of health education began as far back as 1851 when the Sanitary Association was formed to teach the laws of health to the poor in the communities. This was followed 10 years later by the Ladies Sanitary Association whose mission was to teach mothers about health aspects of baby care (Baly 1980). The mothers they were trying to educate and help did not receive these women kindly, they were seen as interfering busybodies. The Industrial Revolution was a landmark, and not a particularly positive one, in changing the way middle class women mothered their children. As the husbands of these women became more prosperous they expected their wives to stay at home and supervise the smooth running of the household. This led to the women being separated from their female network of relatives and friends where much health education, particularly in relation to childbirth, was passed on. They no longer saw babies being born in the home and so subsequently lacked opportunities to help in the care of the newborn. Nannies and housekeepers were often employed, which further separated women from caring for their own children and hence led to the failure of knowledge and skills being passed on to the next generation.

It was very different in the working class societies. Women still had this involvement in childbirth as they helped each other through the childbirth process and then offered each other support in the postnatal period (Nolan 1997). In these areas there was more of a community spirit where women helped to care and support other women. Before the First World War, and in some areas until the mid 1930s, the majority of working class women in Britain were attended in childbirth by a woman who lived within the community and was known as the 'handywoman' (Leap & Hunter 1993). These handywomen would provide care for the women during labour and birth and continue this support during the postnatal period. Within their duties would be included such activities as cooking and cleaning as well as supporting the new mother in caring for her baby. Doctors rarely attended women in labour unless there was a complication that the handywoman could not deal with. This was because doctors required payment for their visits and the women were poor and therefore could not afford the services of a medical practitioner. It can be seen that, from those early beginnings as the handywoman (who in time through education and legislation became the midwife), midwifery was entrenched within the community setting and viewed women from the holistic perspective, including emotional, psychological, social and financial perspectives and providing care for women according to their needs, as suggested by Crichton (1997).

Society during the twentieth century has changed significantly. The extended family network is less evident today, the nuclear family being more the norm. The introduction of contraception and its free availability have meant that fertility can be controlled. Women are now in a position of choice and control in terms of deciding the number of children they wish to have and at what stages in their lives they wish to have them. The large families that once were the norm in Western society are less common in today's society. These changes have also meant that the support network that was so readily available is no longer a nearby presence. This is why the midwife is nowadays recognised as the prime educator of women and their families in relation to the childbirth process. Education is a substantial part of the midwife's role as laid down within the Midwife's code of practice (UKCC 1998). This role is one that is often undervalued and underutilised by clients, health professionals and those who hold the purse strings in terms of allocation of resources. However, it is a role that is vital if couples are to be equipped for the challenges of modern day parenting.

It has been stated by Spiby et al (1999) that the aim of antenatal education is to 'provide information about the childbirth process and choices available for labour, infant feeding options, and opportunity to meet other women in the same situation which will facilitate the forming of new relationships and supportive networks' (p. 389). These authors suggest that childbirth educators need to move away from that prescriptive narrow approach and widen the arena to include more on postnatal and baby care aspects and also include emotional and psychological issues, including issues of role and relationship changes. These aspects will be returned to later on in this chapter.

Empowering women through education

Midwifery care has traditionally been linked with the drive to empower women (McLoughlin 2000) in order for them to be able to make informed choices over the type of care they wish to receive. This, Collington (1998) would argue, is the purpose of educating parents regarding the childbirth process. It is the midwife who is predominantly caring for the women who are undergoing a normal pregnancy, labour and puerperium and it is therefore the midwife who is the best professional to educate and empower them. The midwife's role as a health educator is evident in all the phases of the childbirth process, from preconception care advice (Dignan 2000) (see Ch. 12), screening procedures, aspects of labour and the teaching of baby care skills in the postnatal period. The ability of the midwife to foster confidence in new parents so that they become competent parents can be very rewarding for the midwife. Becoming parents is a life-changing event, including adjustments to new roles as a couple as well as adapting to parenthood. Midwives are in a unique position to help facilitate this transition.

Common disorders of pregnancy and the role of the midwife in education

Every pregnancy is a unique experience for that woman and each pregnancy that the woman experiences will be new and uniquely different. This is why it is so important that the midwife has a knowledge and understanding of the common disorders of pregnancy in order to advise the woman on strategies that will help her to cope with the condition and minimise the effects she experiences. Although such disorders are often termed 'minor disorders', they are far from minor for the woman who is experiencing them and the midwife must remember this. It is also important that the midwife recognises when a common disorder of pregnancy becomes a medical disorder of pregnancy for which the woman must be referred to the appropriate medical practitioner. Davis (1996) has stated that the majority of discomforts experienced during pregnancy can be related to either hormonal changes or the physical changes related to the growing uterus.

The midwife is the key person educating the woman about these common disorders of pregnancy and the booking interview, which in the majority of instances is conducted within the home environment, is where this advice can be given. The midwife's knowledge of these common disorders of pregnancy and the recognition of when they become a medical disorder is vital in initiating the most appropriate management for the woman. There is an abundance of literature available with regard to the use of complementary and alternative medicine (CAM) (see Ch. 49) for alleviating symptoms caused by these common disorders of pregnancy. It is important that the midwife advises the woman to seek advice from a registered practitioner prior to commencing any medication.

Nausea and vomiting

Nausea and vomiting are said to affect over 50% of pregnancies (Snell et al 1998). Their exact cause is not truly explained but is thought to be a combination of hormonal changes, psychological adjustments and neurological factors (Nagendran & Nagendran 1990). The midwife may suggest such remedies as eating a dry biscuit or cracker with a drink before rising in the morning, avoidance of spicy or pungent odours and eating little and often. Eating small frequent meals will help to maintain the body's blood sugar levels and having small amounts of fluid between meals will help to maintain hydration. Other remedies suggested have been the use of neurological devices, which transmit electrical stimulation via the wrist, and are thought to trigger sensory and neurological impulses that control vomiting (Evans et al 1993). The use of complementary therapies, such as acupuncture, has been suggested by Stone (1993) and homeopathic and herbal remedies as suggested by Newman et al (1993) may also be of benefit in minimising the discomfort of this condition. Nausea and vomiting generally improve around the 16th week of pregnancy, but until that time may cause such debilitation for the woman as to affect her daily life (O'Brien & Naber 1992).

A small proportion of those women, 0.3 to 2%, will develop a more serious condition know as hyperemesis gravidarum (Eliakim et al 2000), which requires urgent referral to a doctor. A study was undertaken by Signorello et al (1998) to investigate the effect of prepregnancy dietary fat intake on severe hyperemesis.

They concluded that a high total fat intake, and particularly one high in saturated fat, increased the risk of severe hyperemesis. This study would suggest that a well-balanced diet containing all the required food groups in adequate proportions prior to conception could reduce the incidence of this disorder.

Breast changes

Often changes in the breast are one of the first alterations that the woman notices in relation to her pregnancy. The breasts often become tender and feel fuller because of hormonal changes. The levels of oestrogen increase, which is instrumental in laying down fat stores in preparation for breastfeeding. The vascular circulation is increased and the nipples become larger and the areola more deeply pigmented. It is at the booking interview that the promotion of breastfeeding can be initiated (see Ch. 40).

Backache and ligament pain

Backache is a common disorder that is not restricted to a particular trimester but may span all three trimesters and continue into the postnatal period. Obviously women who experience backache for whatever reason prepregnancy are at an increased risk of suffering from this condition during their pregnancy; that is why it is important to distinguish the backache of pregnancy from a predisposing back condition. During pregnancy a woman's body undergoes many changes and backache can ensue from the growing uterus causing a change in posture and the influence of the hormone relaxin on ligaments. There are simple steps that the midwife can advise the woman to take in order to alleviate the discomfort, such as to maintain good posture, to adopt the appropriate position when lifting either small children or heavy objects and to avoid standing for prolonged periods of time. Instruction in pelvic exercises (see Ch. 15) may also be beneficial, along with the wearing of a supporting maternity girdle (Davis 1996). A woman who has a healthy diet and takes regular exercise such as walking or swimming will do much to minimise this condition.

The growth of the uterus as pregnancy progresses causes stretching of the supporting ligaments in which the woman may experience sharp painful spasms called 'ligament pain'. Again advice can be given on avoidance of stretching, taking a warm bath and massaging the area; these will do much to alleviate the symptoms.

Leg cramp

Cramp, which is a sudden gripping contraction of the calf muscle, frequently occurs during the third trimester of pregnancy. It is usual for the woman to be woken during the night and to be left with a painful calf the following day. The cause is thought to be a lowered serum ionised calcium level and increased level of phosphates (Davis 1996). In a study by Valbo & Bohmer (1999), 120 women were sent a questionnaire 3 days postdelivery to assess the extent to which they had suffered leg cramps during pregnancy. The results revealed that 45% had suffered leg cramps during pregnancy, 54% of the women had suffered the condition after the 25th week of pregnancy, and 76% of the women had experienced the symptoms twice a week or less, which demonstrates that leg cramps are a common disorder of pregnancy. To minimise the risk of night cramps the midwife may advise the woman to do some leg-stretching exercises before retiring to bed. A dietary adjustment in which the woman reduces her intake of milk, soft drinks and processed foods may help to reduce the occurrence of leg cramps. When the woman is troubled by cramps then she should be advised to flex the foot in the opposite direction.

Headache

Frequently women complain of headaches during pregnancy and there are many reasons put forward as to why these should occur, such as hormonal changes, eye strain, sinusitis, fatigue and emotional changes (Peterson & Scotland 1994). Whatever the cause it is important that the midwife is aware of the nature of these headaches and can give advice on how to alleviate them. Headaches can occur at any stage of gestation, but should they occur during the third trimester together with an increase in blood pressure or proteinurea, or both, then medical aid should be sought urgently (see Ch. 20).

Fatigue

Fatigue is a condition that affects the woman not only during pregnancy but also during the postnatal period

(Lee 1999). During the postnatal period it can be attributed to the stress of labour and the physical demands of caring for a new baby, which will include disturbed sleep patterns. Fatigue that occurs during the first trimester can be attributed to hormonal changes and the organogenesis that is taking place. These factors cause the woman to have feelings of overwhelming sleepiness. This situation does resolve during the second trimester only to reoccur during the third trimester. During the third trimester the fatigue can be related to the increase in weight, making mobility difficult and the increase in metabolic demands of the body in preparation for labour and preparation for breastfeeding.

Constipation

Constipation can be a very distressing and uncomfortable condition and the midwife should be able to advise women on how to avoid, and measures to deal with, this common complaint. There are several factors that predispose to the condition (see Ch. 13). The woman may also be prescribed oral iron therapy for anaemia, which is a common cause of constipation (Hardman et al 1996). A diet that is rich in fibre will help to prevent the condition and will also help in resolving it. A two-centre study by Anderson (1984) that included pregnant women from Israel and England demonstrated that 11% and 38% respectively of women in these countries identified themselves as being constipated. The lower rate in women from Israel is thought to be due to the higher amounts of fresh fruit and vegetables in their diet. It is important that the woman also has an adequate fluid intake, which will keep the stools soft and easy to pass. The midwife should enquire about any changes in the frequency and consistency of the woman's bowel movements and offer advice accordingly. If constipation persists then haemorrhoids may develop, caused by straining at defecation, which can subsequently cause particular difficulties during the birth process. Haemorrhoids can be particularly painful and may bleed, therefore avoidance of this condition should be the aim of the management of constipation.

Emotional factors

Emotional instability is common during pregnancy. It is due to many factors. There are the hormonal changes, which influence how the woman feels and reacts to situations, but there is also the physical discomfort of some of the common disorders of pregnancy to contend with. It is important that the midwife is able to reassure the woman and her family that the situation is fairly common and normal. However, it is important that the midwife is aware of any stressful life event, other than the pregnancy, that may be causing the situation. Such life events as moving house, death of a close family member or the breakdown of the relationship occurring antenatally may also affect the woman in the postnatal period and predispose to postnatal depression (see Ch. 35).

Education from conception through to birth and beyond

The first meeting with the midwife

Education begins at the first meeting between the woman, and often her partner, and the midwife. Ideally this should be preconception but in practice it is often at the booking interview (see Ch. 16). It is most often the couples in the higher socioeconomic groups who are aware of the benefits of preconception care advice and who avail themselves of this service, but, as Dignan (2000) states, it is the couples in the lower socioeconomic groups who would benefit the most from this information. The midwife's role in providing preconception care advice can be the start of the educational process for the prospective parents in their journey to parenthood.

Because of the changes in delivery of care brought about by the Changing Childbirth report (DoH 1993) there has been an increase in the number of women who have their booking interview in their own homes. This allows for a mutually agreeable time to be set in order for the midwife and the woman/couple to make this initial meeting – one where time is given to forming and developing a relationship that will last beyond the baby's birth. The home is a conducive environment for the booking interview to take place because the woman will be relaxed and feel at ease and she also has some control over the situation because the midwife is a visitor in the home. Time is allowed for the woman/couple to ask questions and discuss any anxieties that there may be. The midwife also has more time to devote to explaining the options of care available to the woman, the screening tests available and their implications and the value of attending parent education classes. The booking interview is an ideal opportunity to educate the woman/couple on lifestyle issues that may be relevant, such as reducing alcohol intake, smoking cessation and nutritional advice. This is perhaps the time when the prospective parents are at their most receptive because their desire to have a healthy baby may be instrumental in taking on board these positive lifestyle changes with benefit to all. There is a lot of information exchanged during the booking interview and therefore it is easy to see why women feel overwhelmed by it all. This is why it may be necessary to revisit certain aspects at subsequent meetings to reinforce the health education message and also it gives the woman/couple time to digest the information and formulate any questions. This type of one-to-one interaction between the midwife and the woman/couple is a valuable exchange of information and one that is frequently entered into. Every time the midwife engages in conversation with the woman/couple about matters relating to childbirth then parent education is taking place, even though perhaps this interaction is less recognised as parent education than the more formalised classes. In order to meet the needs of clients a more flexible approach in terms of content delivery and method needs to be adopted, along with client participation.

Parent education classes

Parent education classes can either be NHS funded or privately run classes by such organisations as the National Childbirth Trust (NCT). The woman/couple have a choice over which classes to attend, or indeed they may decide to attend both because there are differences in the way both are organised. Whichever type of classes the prospective parents decide to attend, the midwife/childbirth educator must be aware of factors that may affect the way parent education is received. It is essential to be aware of factors that inhibit learning and those that promote learning. One of the most important aspects to consider when organising classes is the environment in which they will be conducted. The midwife can be instrumental in providing good learning opportunities for the prospective parents, which will enhance their learning.

The environment

The midwife should ensure that the environment is comfortable in terms of heating, space and appropriate equipment and that refreshments are made available. It must be acknowledged that not all venues are suitable as a good learning environment but the midwife has to try to adapt the situation in order to facilitate a good learning opportunity. The size and shape of the room used for parent education obviously cannot be changed but the midwife, with her knowledge of what makes a good learning environment, can make certain changes in order to improve the situation. The way the seating is arranged is important as this will encourage or discourage dialogue between all parties present. Parent education classes are run on an informal basis and therefore it is important that the seating arrangements are conducive to facilitate interaction between every participant. Seating arranged in a horseshoe shape allows every individual to be seen by the others and therefore communication, both verbal and non-verbal, is encouraged. With a large class, however, it may be more appropriate, particularly if the midwife/childbirth educator wishes to involve the participants in group work activities, to arrange the seating in smaller clusters (Curzon 1991). This would allow group work to be done within the individual groups, but subsequent presentation of the material would be made to the group as a whole.

Motivation

Motivation to learn plays a key role in the learning process and no one is more likely to be well motivated than prospective parents. However, it is well recognised that anxiety can inhibit the learning process and if the parents are overly worried then new learning of either knowledge or a skill will be impeded. Tiredness, pain, hunger and feeling unwell, suggests Hinchliff (1999), may have a negative effect upon learning; these are facts the midwife needs to keep in mind when planning the parent education programme.

Hinchliff (1999) has also identified that motivation may either be intrinsic or extrinsic, but often there is overlap of both. By this she means that there are factors inherent within individuals that encourage motivation, but also there are factors impinging from outside influences that the individual has little or no control over.

Maslow (1987), a psychologist, identified five levels of intrinsic motivation. Knowledge of these five levels can help midwives to understand why parent education sessions might be more or less effective for different women and their partners in the group:

1. *Physiological* – this relates to having an environment that is conducive to learning. Attention must be paid to such aspects as warmth of the building, the noise level, the degree of privacy and the décor. Consideration should be given to the provision of refreshments.

2. *Safety* – people need to feel that they are in a safe environment and be comfortable with the people they are with. This will encourage dialogue between all participants.

3. *Social* – the social aspects of intrinsic motivation relates to the group's dynamics and an acceptance of each of its members.

4. *Self-esteem* – this relates to mutual respect between the individuals attending parent education sessions and this would also include the midwife.

5. *Self-actualisation* – when all the stages above have been achieved then couples will be able to maximise their full potential as parents.

How prospective parents learn and the sources of information used

The phrase 'evidence-based practice' is one that is frequently quoted and means that all practice should be based on the best evidence available. As Kelly (1998) states, it is essential that midwife educators provide information to prospective parents that reflects the culture of today's society. In the past there was a tendency for midwives to paint an unrealistic picture of parenthood and therefore couples were ill prepared for the realities of family life. It has been noted that often women get their sources of information about childbirth issues from family and friends as their main resource. This has its obvious drawbacks, as the information passed down like this by word of mouth may not be accurate or current. Another readily available source is many magazines available on the market that address childbirth and parenting issues. The problem with media publicity is that it frequently portrays a rosy picture of parenthood. This leads parents to have unrealistic expectations of their baby and of themselves as parents, which will leave the parents feeling a loss of confidence and self-esteem when they fall short of the ideal (see Ch. 35). A third and widely used source of information is the internet; people can access a variety of websites and glean a lot of valuable information if they have this facility.

It is important that the information the midwife presents during the parent education sessions is based on research evidence, but conveyed in a way that the client group understands. Because of all the sources of literature available to prospective parents they will often have some knowledge of the topic areas chosen. Again, this is where the midwife's communication skills are important for translating the evidence into understandable language in order for the prospective parents to be fully informed.

How that information is conveyed is also an important factor in people's learning. People learn and assimilate information in a variety of ways. According to Hinchliff (1999) there are two methods of teaching: the formal method, which is preplanned and organised, and the informal method, which arises out of spontaneous discussions. The formal method is perhaps more appropriate to a group session, particularly if the group have set their own agenda of topics they wish to be covered. This setting of an agenda of topics means that the midwife will have prepared the relevant information and decided on the best method of delivering that information to the client group. The informal method arises when something is taught spontaneously, such as teaching a new mother how to put a nappy on a baby or discussing terms and phrases written on client's notes that they do not understand. Both of these approaches have their value in terms of delivering parent education advice when applied appropriately to the information or skill required.

In a group setting, such as parent education classes, a lecture-style approach is not the most appropriate method of conveying information. Group settings allow for small group discussions to identify the level of knowledge that the class has and the midwife can then build upon that knowledge. This is termed '*brainstorming*'. It relies, however, on all the participants feeling comfortable enough with each other to voice what they feel may be relevant information. Approaching relevant topics in this way means that knowledge is not assumed and that the lowest level of knowledge is started at and built on so that no participants are left with gaps in their knowledge. All ideas are pooled together, which means that the group members have contributed to the whole process. This helps to build the group members' confidence both with themselves and with each other. Abbott & McMahon's (1993) model of brainstorming has four phases, and within each phase the ideas and concepts develop to make the whole.

Buzz groups may prove to be useful with certain topics, such as pain relief in labour. This is a large topic but can be broken into smaller parts. Each small group could discuss what knowledge they already have on one method of pain relief and then the groups would discuss and share the information within the larger group. The midwife would then be in a position to build upon the information that the groups had presented and the group would have a comprehensive knowledge of the methods of pain relief available at their local maternity units. It is the expertise of the midwife as an educator that will allow facilitation of the group and smooth running of the classes. Time must also be allowed for women/couples to ask questions and this may mean that they wish to see the midwife in private at the end of the classes. This is often related to queries that they may have relating to information written on their handheld notes.

Audio-visual aids. The use of audio-visual aids in order to enhance learning can be advantageous, particularly when covering aspects such as positions in labour or how to position the baby for breastfeeding. The use of overhead transparencies may not be entirely appropriate for a group such as those attending parent education classes. The use of card games makes learning fun but also helps elicit people's fears and anxieties about issues surrounding childbirth, such as fear of coping with the contractions or fear of not being able to cope with the new baby. In this way card games may be a good teaching method to use. These types of learning strategies allow people to voice their concerns in a controlled environment and within the safety of a like-minded group of individuals. The use of a video to reinforce information previously given is very useful, but care must be taken that it is not used for the whole session as interest can be lost.

Practical demonstrations. It may be appropriate during a session on breastfeeding for a mother who is successfully breastfeeding her baby to provide a practical demonstration. It is practical situations such as these that, due to the changes within the family, are no longer learned within the family environment. These types of situations will also allow new mothers to express how becoming a parent has affected them and their partner and present the realities of the new and demanding role.

Handouts and leaflets. It may be appropriate after sessions that have been presented more formally that information is reinforced by the use of handouts and/or leaflets. This allows the participants to take information away with them to read at a later date. The use of MIDIRS information leaflets may be of value in order to enhance and support the information that the midwife presents. These leaflets are all based on current research evidence that has been peer reviewed by specialists and provide a comprehensive reference list.

Designing parent education programmes

There has been much debate over the years regarding the topics that are covered in parent education classes and it would appear that some have changed very little. Despite the changes in society, the couple's expectations of parenting and the employment changes, which may affect the timing of women returning to work, appear not to have been considered. There are certain core topics that are likely to be requested but there are other topics that might not be included unless couples are given the opportunity to ask for them. Nolan (1997) undertook a study to establish what topics parents would like included during the education classes in order to establish how the classes could best meet their needs. The participants were all first time prospective parents. It was interesting to discover that postnatal topics were identified as frequently as labour topics. It has always been a commonly held belief that women/couples cannot see beyond labour and therefore there is no point in including these aspects of postnatal care. However, it would appear from this study that that is a misconception and perhaps one that requires urgent rectification. One of the suggestions from the study was that the participants should set their own agenda and the way the sessions would meet the needs of that particular group. It could be argued that it is very difficult to prepare couples for childbirth and parenting because no birth is the same and no couples are the same, but what parent education aims to do is prepare them for an experience that is unique to them.

There are certain topics that prospective parents need to be informed about, such as nutritional information, methods of pain relief that are available, both non-pharmacological and pharmacological, and recognition of when labour may have commenced. It seems impractical to demonstrate how to bath a baby, with a doll, in a clinic setting. It would be far more relevant and meaningful to bath the couple's baby within the home environment. This would demonstrate how babies could be quite slippery when wet and that they move and cry, something that dolls do not do. This is a realistic situation and one in which the equipment used is the baby's own. It could be argued that a baby could be used in parent education classes to demonstrate how to bath a baby correctly. However, many of the settings used for classes are clinic buildings, which are not ideal in terms of heating, and to subject a new baby to being unclothed and bathed and then for it to have to go out into what may be a cold environment seems inappropriate.

The midwife, in allowing the participants to set the agenda for the sessions that they feel they require instruction in, knows that the topics identified will be of importance to the clients. By encouraging the participants to set the agenda she could be said to be entering into a learning contract with them. It is important that the midwife makes it clear that the topics identified are not set in tablets of stone and that further topics can be added if necessary. It is important also that the midwife uses effective communication skills in order to break down any barriers that there might be between them so that the learning is effective (Childs 1997).

The changing role from that of a couple to that of parents is one that perhaps there is least preparation for. Yet it is a time when there is great anxiety and the transition to parenthood may not always be smooth. It has been documented over the years by several authors (Curry 1983, McKim et al 1995, Sheenhan 1981) that new mothers often forget what has been told to them during the antenatal period and feel anxious and lack confidence in caring for their new baby. The lack of information regarding baby care skills, disturbed sleep patterns and such like was acknowledged as a deficit within the structure of traditional parent education classes.

Aspects of education include a range of skill-based activities, from bathing a baby to information on contraception. Parent education has been criticised for being too medically focused in the information given with regard to such aspects as the process of labour and the options available in terms of pain relief. There should be more of an emphasis on the psychological adaptation to parenthood or the realities of caring for a new baby. Nolan's (1997) study of couples attending parent education classes confirmed that new parents would have welcomed more information and preparation for the realities of becoming parents, whereas midwives focused on preparing prospective parents for the labour and birth of their baby. The changing roles new parents have to adopt may prove to be very frightening, with the realisation of the degree of responsibility that caring for a new life brings. The organising and facilitating of parent education classes that meet all the needs of the community client group that they service will do much to promote and enhance positive parenting.

Not all midwives feel prepared to facilitate parenthood education classes despite the fact that many have now undertaken courses on teaching and assessing in clinical practice or its equivalent. It is perhaps fair to say that these courses equip them to teach students more effectively than a group of prospective parents. It is largely because of lack of confidence in speaking to a group of prospective parents that midwives may shy away from this important role. Confidence will be gained only by undertaking parent education along side a midwife who is experienced at facilitating this type of group education. It has been acknowledged by Underdown (unpublished BEd dissertation, 1997) that most midwives seem to learn parent education skills from their enthusiastic peers.

Parent education seems to have evolved from two roots (Williams & Booth 1980). First, women were given instructions on hygiene and baby care in an attempt to improve perinatal and maternal mortality. Secondly, they were given training in alleviating pain by a theoretical and practical preparation for labour by a childbirth trainer who was deemed to be the expert. All these education sessions amounted to the women being spoken to and not listened to. The content of the classes was medically driven, with an absence of the emotional, social and psychological aspects of childbirth. This is not to say that such parent education classes were not good – they were – but the progress that has been made within this field of health care should be recognised and acknowledged. Pregnancy and childbirth are increasingly viewed from a holistic concept, which includes the emotional, social and psychological effects of childbirth and parenting. Coombes & Schonveld (1992, cited in Deane-Gray 1997) undertook a critique of parent education and presented several identified gaps within the structure and quality of education offered. They found that the educational quality was poor, the programme was medically driven, special groups such as teenagers were not catered for and there was a lack of interdisciplinary cooperation. More recently there has been a change in the format and content of parent education classes. The report Changing Childbirth (DoH 1993) may have influenced the way parent education is delivered.

Within this report there was a re-emphasis on the provision of antenatal and postnatal care within the community setting and an acknowledgement that women should have continuity of carer and choice over aspects of their care. In order that the maternity services can strive towards achieving these aims it must start with good working relations between the midwife and the GP in order that women may receive adequate advice prior to their first antenatal appointment (McGinley 2000). New mothers have cited lack of support from midwives, particularly in the postnatal period, where improvements in service provision can be made (McGinley 2000). The postnatal period has been termed the Cinderella of the maternity services (Ball 1982), yet it is the most worrying of times for new parents and one in which the midwife's role as an educator can provide so much advice and support that would be truly appreciated. The re-emergence of the midwife's public health role and extension of the postnatal visiting period up to 6 weeks will do much to aid the transition of parents into their new role.

Factors to be considered in the transition to parenthood

The length of time a mother stays in hospital after her baby's birth has been reduced in recent years. The length of time that the community midwife visits may also have been reduced, along with the introduction of selective visiting. With the changes in social structures that have taken place, new mothers/parents may now have little educational support to help them into their new role. More time needs to be devoted to issues that occur in the postnatal period and the midwife is the prime professional who is in a position to deliver this information.

Fathers and working mothers

Among the many changes occurring over the years is the way fathers are now involved during the childbirth and child-rearing process. Thomas & Upton (2000) have suggested that it is the changes in society and the changing roles of both men and women that have brought about the increased involvement of men in this process. The changes within society, and particularly within the family structure from the extended family network to the nuclear family, have perhaps had the most profound effect upon men becoming more involved in the process. Increasingly men are attending childbirth preparation classes, with an attendance rate of 97% in the 1990s as compared with only 5% in the 1950s. Women's roles have also changed quite significantly within society, education and the employment market. Women are less willing or able to stay at home and care for the baby full time but want to be active contributors to the economy and therefore part of the workforce. Women who do stay at home to care for their babies and children often feel that they are not viewed as contributing to the welfare of society in the same light as women who undertake paid work outside the home. One could argue quite the reverse, however, because women who do stay at home and care for their baby or children are providing a stable environment for children to grow up in and are teaching them many skills. Women are also pursuing their educational needs far more that they used to. There has been a gradual breakdown of barriers between educational subjects that were either male or female dominated. This has meant that there are more opportunities open to women in different areas of the employment market. Women are returning to work sooner than the mothers of a generation ago. Although the facility for the mother to have 12 months' maternity leave is an option available to many women, this obviously depends upon whether financial resources will allow them to do so. A possible consequence of the woman returning to work is that the father may have to assume more responsibility for the care of the baby; or the couple might even decide that it will be the father who will provide the majority of the child care.

Gallaway et al (1997) conducted a study to examine the views and experiences of new fathers concerning the role that parent education classes had played in their transition to fatherhood. Eighteen men took part in the study, which consisted of a semistructured taped interview, and all the participants attended either NCT or NHS classes, or both. The study findings were that the men attended in order to support their wives or partners and did not expect to gain anything for themselves. On the whole the results showed that men were satisfied with the content of the classes, which provided them with information on labour and birth, and they found the role-play situations to be of value. According to Taylor (1985), in the United States of America there are some men-only classes, which are very well received. In contrast, only nine of the men in Gallaway et al's study (1997) stated that they would be interested in men-only classes if they were available to them. In Sweden it is most unusual for first time prospective fathers not to attend parent education classes, particularly in view of the legislation regarding paternity leave (Hallgren et al 1998). It has been recognised that, due to the changes within Sweden's society, there needs to be education for childbirth and beyond. Education generally starts when the woman is 20 weeks' pregnant and continues until the baby is 1 year old. It may be difficult to maintain attendance for that length of time; however Hallgren et al do not state how regularly the classes meet, which may be a very influential factor in determining attendance rates.

Social and economic deprivation

There has been much written about social class differences when accessing health care needs (Davey et al 1995, Graham 1987, Townsend et al 1990, Wilkinson 1986, 1996). The Black report (Townsend & Davidson 1982) highlighted quite clearly that the lower social classes live in the poorer areas, are less well educated and suffer more ill health. It was also clear from the report that in such areas there are fewer resources to improve the lives of these already disadvantaged groups. A study undertaken by Cliff & Deery (1997) set out to investigate patterns of attendance and non-attendance at antenatal classes for first time mothers. There were 50 women included in the study: 29 categorised

as middle class and 21 as working class. The method consisted of an initial questionnaire followed by an in-depth interview 4 weeks later in the woman's own home. The study's findings were that it was not only social difference that was a factor in non-attendance; more significant was the age of the woman and her marital status. The study clearly identified that it was predominantly the young, single and working class women who did not attend parent education class and that the social class factor was not the sole reason for non-attendance, although the women did feel threatened by their social class status.

Women have reported their lack of attendance at classes as being due to practical difficulties. There is still evidence that classes are not organised to suit the needs of the clients that they are there to help. Some women in Cliff & Deery's study (1997) stated that the classes were on the same day as their antenatal appointment so they would rather keep the clinic appointment and miss the parent education class. Women are now working longer into their pregnancy in order that they may have more time off after the birth. Provided that the pregnancy is normal and the woman feels well then there should not be a problem; however, time should be afforded these women to attend antenatal and parent education classes within their working day as is their right. It must be recognised that the day and time of parent education classes will not suit every woman/couple; however, if the day and time can be arranged to suit the majority then this is one way of attempting to increase the attendance at the classes.

Minority ethnic groups

Women from minority ethic groups do not regularly attend parent education classes. It could be argued that they are more likely to have a more supportive family network and therefore they learn their parenting skills within their own family unit. This might not be the case, however, and also family members may not always provide the most current and up-to-date practice. A study by Walker & Pollard (1995) to find out the reasons why Asian women did not attend parent education classes was undertaken in Bradford. Among the reasons women cited were that other family members would teach them how to care for their baby, they were anxious about attending the classes, domestic commitments took priority and they needed to be accompanied by another family member. In order to get the parent education message across the authors produced a video, which provided the information that the women would have received in the classes. The video covered topics such as pregnancy and antenatal care, coping with labour, caesarean section, breastfeeding and how to care for a new baby. The videos were produced in two different languages, Urdu and Bengali, in order to meet the needs of the women in that community. They proved to be a great success and the authors hoped to produce the video in other languages and to cover other topics. Perhaps in order to meet the needs of minority groups midwives need to look at how best to deliver parent education programmes to meet those groups with specialised needs.

Teenage mothers

Another group of women who have special needs in terms of the maternity service are teenagers. The United Kingdom has the highest rate of teenage pregnancy in Europe (Social Exclusion Unit 1999). The government has recognised the failures of the Health of the Nation report (DoH 1992) in relation to reducing unintended conceptions in these young women by 50% by the year 2000. Unfortunately there has been no significant decline in the figures, which is why the Labour Government commissioned the Social Exclusion Unit's report in 1999. The report identified teenage pregnancy as having many negative effects upon the young woman and her subsequent baby. First, teenagers are disadvantaged in terms of education because they are less inclined to return to full-time education in order to complete their studies (Hobcraft & Keirnan 1999). This also affects their chances of obtaining full-time employment in a reasonable status job that offers future prospects. It has also been identified that these young women are more at risk from such complications as anaemia, pregnancy-induced hypertension and prolonged labour (Irvine et al 1997). The baby is at greater risk of being of low birthweight (Botting et al 1998) and there is a higher perinatal mortality rate (Fraser et al 1995). It has to be said that these complications do not occur to every teenager who is pregnant or her subsequent child as many do achieve a healthy pregnancy and outcome. Many do progress to being competent mothers and do fulfil their desired goals in life despite their untimely conception. However, there are a significant number of young women who do suffer adversely either physically, educationally, emotionally or psychologically. It is with this special group that the midwife has a vital and ongoing role to play.

There are many maternity units now who have instigated teenage antenatal clinics with many running parent education classes alongside them. The introduction of the Sure Start initiative (see Ch. 50) by the government in 1999 has meant that there are now many midwives specifically identified to work with this vulnerable group of pregnant young women (Sure Start Unit 1999). It is in these situations that the midwife as a parent educator can help to develop the young woman's self-confidence and self-esteem. It is important that these are developed in order that she feels able to learn all the new skills and knowledge required in order for her to become a competent mother. It is by encouraging these young women in their ability to care for the new baby that their confidence in other areas of their lives will develop, which will benefit themselves and ultimately their baby.

Conclusion

It is clear from the evidence presented that the content and delivery of many parent education classes needs to change. The midwife is the lead professional in normal midwifery and in educating for parenthood. The educational role of the midwife is integrated into every aspect of her work and enters into every communication with the prospective parents. There need to be special classes that will meet the needs of specially identified groups, such as minority ethnic groups of women and young teenage women. It can be seen from the evidence stated previously that these special groups would benefit from providing education in various formats, such as video presentations in the home or health centres and in the first language of the ethnic minorities, or providing teen-only antenatal and parent education classes. Specially identified midwives, perhaps from the Sure Start initiative, would be ideally placed to provide this service because often these special groups of women are from the lower socioeconomic groups and live in the more deprived areas. It is the present government's plan to improve the health of childbearing women and their families through the Sure Start initiative, so again the midwife is ideally placed to take this initiative forward through education and be instrumental in improving the communities' health.

It is important to consider the day and the time of classes because in Cliff & Deery's (1997) study there appeared to be a clash between the time of the parent education class and the antenatal clinic appointment. Women opted to attend the antenatal class in preference to the parent education class. With a little communication and organisation situations like this would be avoided.

The format and content of the classes need to be addressed because classes have been accused of being too medically focused. Involving the participants in the decision-making process (DoH 1993) and the content of parent education classes and having a flexible approach to the session will ensure that the group's needs are met and that a good relationship is formed with the midwife. Encouraging women and their partners to set the agenda will address the needs of that particular group and therefore more participation will be achieved. The midwife must recognise that many prospective parents can be quite knowledgeable in aspects of childbirth education and therefore to facilitate group discussions and build upon that knowledge is a good foundation. The content of the classes needs to address the changes that have occurred within today's society. There are core topics that women/couples will want to know about, such as signs of onset of labour and methods of pain relief, but there are also topics that clearly need to be included such as adjustment to parenthood and the realities of parenting. Midwives have been blamed in the past for painting too rosy a picture of parenthood and therefore parents have unrealistic expectations of their baby and of themselves as parents. This can further undermine new parents who are struggling with the realities of parenting. More time should be devoted to the period after the birth and a more realistic but not negative view of the realities of being parents should be given. These aspects can then be revisited during the postnatal period when the midwife is visiting the new family at home.

The psychological adaptation to parenthood is an aspect that can be discussed in the postnatal period and each mother/couple should have their own worries and fears addressed. This may be a more realistic time to elicit how the mother/couple feel as new parents. The changing roles for the couple and the added responsibility of caring for a new life is both exciting and frightening and again the individual anxieties of mother/couples can be addressed in the postnatal period. The ability of the midwife to continue parent education through until care is transferred to the health visitor will prove to be valuable to the parents and rewarding to the midwife.

The way forward

In looking at the history of midwifery it is easy to see where the notion of the midwife in the public health arena stems from. Midwives have always made an enormous contribution to improving public health, not only in terms of reducing maternal and infant mortality and morbidity but in educating and assisting mothers and families to achieve a lifelong pattern of optimum well-being (Allison 1992). In fact the public health role of the midwife was recognised by Daphne Olorenshaw in 1943 when she stated that 'midwifery was the oldest branch of public health' (p. 310). From this it would appear that continuity of care is not a new concept but rather an old one that got lost along the way (Allison 1992).

The public health role has evolved from the days when its priority was public sanitation, but this is not to belittle its beginnings but to acknowledge its early contributions to improving the health of communities. In more recent times there has been a bigger emphasis on health education and health promotion strategies in order to encourage individuals to adopt healthier lifestyles (Kaufmann 2000).

There are now national policies in place to expand the role of health professionals within the field of public health. The Acheson report (1998) recommended that high priority should be given to the health of families with children and particularly to improving health and reducing inequalities in women of childbearing age, expectant mothers and young children. The government's strategy for strengthening the family extends the role of the midwife in several areas, such as parent education and increased postnatal support. New initiatives such as Sure Start, which aims to help families in deprived areas, have been introduced. In many areas midwives are involved in these projects and are working hard within that role to improve the detection rates of postnatal depression, improve breastfeeding rates, continue parent education programmes and offer support for isolated mothers.

There are many activities that come under the public health umbrella, but the ones that are pertinent to midwifery practice are parent education, health-promoting services, social policy measures and empowerment strategies – all of which should address the wider determinants of health. Public health education, by the very nature of what public health stands for, takes education to families and communities in order to educate and improve health matters. The very essence of midwifery is to promote long term health for women and babies (RCM 2001) and there are many ways that this aim can be achieved. Midwives are the prime carers who advise on the screening tests that are available, give advice on nutrition, exercise and other lifestyle issues, promote and encourage breastfeeding and inform and advise on the various phases of the childbirth process.

It has long since been recognised that antenatal and postnatal care should be provided within the community setting and that women should have continuity of care and choice within aspects of their care (DoH 1993). The postnatal period is the time when new parents are learning their newly acquired role and this transition to parenthood can be a time of great anxiety; at this time the midwife is able to give much advice and support to educate parents and lessen their anxiety.

A woman will often suffer ill health after childbirth with conditions such as anaemia, urinary incontinence, backache and tiredness (McGinley 2000) and would welcome the opportunity to discuss these often embarrassing conditions with the person who she has come to know and respect, her midwife. The postnatal period is the time when the relationship with the midwife is firmly established and there is respect and cooperation between the midwife and the mother. It is perhaps at this crucial time that it would be valuable both to the new parents and to the midwife to extend the postnatal visiting time to the time around the postnatal examination, which is generally 6 weeks after the birth. This would allow the continuity of care from the midwife, who is perhaps the best-placed person to assess how the new mother is adjusting to her demanding but rewarding role. The value to the mother is that the trusted relationship she has formed with the midwife continues and this then allows for continued advice and the development of baby care skills. The value to the midwife is that she can assess how the new mother is adapting to such aspects of care as breastfeeding and also the midwife is best able to identify those mothers who are at risk from postnatal depression (McGinley 2000).

In preparing the next generation of parents, midwives must take account of the changes within society, education, employment and the roles that men and women now adopt. Targeting parent education sessions to meet the needs of differing client groups and giving participants ownership of the content is in line with the midwifery philosophy of care being woman focused and family centred. It is essential as midwives that we do not lose sight of our important educational role because it is through this vital aspect that we can contribute to the improved health of the community we serve and empower women for childbirth and motherhood.

REFERENCES

Abbott F, McMahon R 1993 Teaching healthcare workers: a practical guide, 2nd edn. Macmillan, London

Acheson D (Chair) 1998 Independent inquiry into inequalities in health. Stationery Office, London

Allison J 1992 Midwives step out of the shadows. Midwives Chronicle and Nursing Notes July: 167–174

Anderson A S 1984 Constipation during pregnancy: incidence and methods used in its treatment in a group of Cambridgeshire women. Health Visitor 12:363–364

Ball J M 1982 Stress and the postnatal care of women. Nursing Times Nov 10:1904–1907

Baly M E 1980 Nursing and social change, 2nd edn. Heinemann Medical, London

Botting B, Rosato M, Wood R 1998 Teenage mothers and the health of their children. Population Trends 93

Childs D 1997 Psychology and the teacher, 5th edn. Holt, Reinehart and Winston, London

Cliff D, Deery R 1997 Too much like school: social class, age, marital status and attendance/non-attendance at antenatal classes. Midwifery 13:139–145

Collington V 1998 Do women share midwives' views of their educational role? British Journal of Midwifery 6(9):556–563

Coombes G, Schonveld D 1992 Life will never be the same again: a review of antenatal and postnatal education. Health Education Authority London Department of Health, 1993 cited in Deane-Gray T 1997 What is wrong with sitting by Nelly? Midwifery Matters 75(winter):16–18

Crichton M A 1997 Assessment of needs model in midwifery care. British Journal of Midwifery 5(6):330–333

Curry M 1983 Variables related to adaptation to motherhood in normal primiparous women. Journal of Obstetrics, Gynaecology and Neonatal Nursing 12(2):115–121

Curzon L B 1991 Teaching in further education: an outline of principles and practice, 4th edn. Cassell, London

Davey B, Gray A, Seale C (eds) 1995 Health and disease. Open University Press, Buckingham

Davis D 1996 The discomforts of pregnancy. Journal of Obstetrics, Gynaecology and Neonatal Nursing 25(1):73–81

Deane-Gray T 1997 What is wrong with sitting by Nelly? Midwifery Matters 75(winter):16–18

Dignan K 2000 Pre-conception care, Chapter 3. In: Kerr J (ed) Community health promotion: challenges for practice. Baillière Tindall, London, p 51–64

DoH (Department of Health) 1992 The health of the nation. HMSO, London

DoH (Department of Health) 1993 Changing childbirth: report of the Expert Maternity Group. HMSO, London

Eliakim R, Abulafia O, Sherer D M 2000 Hyperemesis gravidarum: a current review. American Journal of Perinatology 17(4):207–218

Evans A T, Samuels S N, Marshall C, Bertolucci L E 1993 Suppression of pregnancy-induced nausea and vomiting with sensory afferent stimulation. Journal of Reproductive Medicine 38:603–606

Fraser A M, Brockert J E, Ward R H 1995 Association of young maternal age with adverse reproductive outcomes. New England Medical Journal 332:1113–1117

Gallaway D, Svensson J, Clune L 1997 What do men think of antenatal classes? International Journal of Childbirth Education 12(2):38–41

Graham H 1987 Women's smoking and family health. Social Science and Medicine 1:47–56

Hallgren A, Kihlgren M, Forslin L, Norberg A 1998 Swedish fathers' involvement in and experiences of childbirth preparation and childbirth. Midwifery 10:6–15

Hardman J G, Limbird L E, Molinoff P B, Rudon R W, Gilman A G (eds) 1996 The pharmacological basis of therapeutics, 9th edn. McGraw-Hill, New York. Cited in Broussard B S 1998 The constipation assessment scale for pregnancy. Journal of Obstetrics, Gynaecology and Neonatal Nursing 27(3):297–301

Hinchliff S 1999 The practitioner as a teacher, 2nd edn. Baillière Tindall, London

Hobcraft J, Keirnan K 1999 Childhood and poverty, early motherhood and adult social exclusion. Analysis for the Social Exclusion Unit, CASE paper 28. London School of Economics, London. Cited in Kaufmann T 2001 Teenage pregnancy: how can we help? RCM Midwives Journal 4(10):322–333

Irvine H, Bradley T, Cupples M, Boohan M 1997 The implications of teenage pregnancy and motherhood for primary health care: unresolved issues. British Journal of General Practice 47:323–326

Kaufmann T 2000 Public health: the next step in woman-centred care. Midwives Journal January 3(1):26–27

Kelly S 1998 Parent education survey. RCM Midwives Journal 1(1):23–25

Leap N, Hunter B 1993 The midwife's tale. Scarlet Press, London

Lee K 1999 Longitudinal changes in fatigue and energy during pregnancy and the postpartum period. Journal of Obstetrics, Gynaecology and Neonatal Nursing 28(2):183–191

McGinley M 2000 The public health agenda: what does it mean for midwives? Practising Midwife 3(8):4–5

McKim E, Kenner C, Flandermeyer A et al (1995) The transition to home for mothers of healthy and initially ill newborn babies. Midwifery 11:184–194

McLoughlin A 2000 Empowerment and childbirth, Chapter 4. In: Kerr J (ed) Community health promotion: challenges for practice. Baillière Tindall, London, p 65 81

Maslow A 1987 Motivation and personality advice. Harper & Row, London

Nagendran T, Nagendran S 1990 Mechanism and treatment of nausea and vomiting. Alabama Medicine. Journal of MASA 60:12–16

Newman V, Fullerton J T, Anderson P O 1993 Clinical advances in the management of severe nausea and vomiting during pregnancy. Journal of Obstetrics, Gynaecology and Neonatal Nursing 22:483–490

Nolan M L 1997 Antenatal education: failing to educate for parenthood. British Journal of Midwifery 5(1):21–26

O'Brien B, Naber S 1992 Nausea and vomiting during pregnancy: effects on the quality of women's lives. Birth 19:138–143

Olorenshaw D 1943 The place of midwifery in the health services of the future. Nursing Mirror August 14:310. Cited in Allison J 1992 Midwives step out of the shadows. Midwives Chronicle and Nursing Notes July:167–174

Peterson L, Scotland N 1994 Your body, your feelings. Lamaze Parents' Magazine 1:14–20

RCM (Royal College of Midwives) 2001 Position paper. The midwife's role in public health. Midwives Journal 4(7):222–223

Sheehan F 1981 Assessing postpartum adjustment: a pilot study. Journal of Obstetrics, Gynaecology and Neonatal Nursing

Signorello L B, Harlow B L, Wang S, Erick M A 1998 Saturated fat intake and the risk of severe hyperemesis gravidarum. Epidemiology 9(6):636–640

Snell L H, Haughey B P, Buck G, Marecki M A 1998 Metabolic crisis: hyperemesis gravidarum. Journal of Perinatal and Neonatal Nursing 12(2):26–37

Social Exclusion Unit 1999 Teenage pregnancy. Report No. Cmnd 4342. Stationery Office, London

Spiby H, Henderson B, Slade P, Escott D, Fraser R B 1999 Strategies for coping with labour: does antenatal education translate into practice? Journal of Advanced Nursing 29(2):388–394

Stone C 1993 Acupressure wristbands for the nausea of pregnancy. Nurse Practitioner 18:15–23

Sure Start Unit 1999 Sure Start: a guide for second wave programmes. DfEE, Nottingham

Taylor A 1985 Antenatal classes and the consumers: mothers' and fathers' views. Health Education News 44(2):79–82

Thomas S G, Upton D 2000 Expectant fathers' attitudes towards pregnancy. British Journal of Midwifery 8(4):218–221

Townsend P, Davidson N 1982 Inequalities in health: the Black report. Penguin, Harmondsworth

Townsend P, Davidson N, Whitehead M 1990 The Black report and the health divide, 2nd edn. Penguin, Harmondsworth

UKCC (United Kingdom Central Council for Nursing, Midwifery and Health Visiting) 1998 Midwives rules and code of practice. UKCC, London

Underdown A 1997 An investigation into the learning environment and educational techniques used by health professionals in childbirth and parenting classes, BEd dissertation, University of Hertfordshire

Valbo A, Bohmer T 1999 Leg cramps in pregnancy – how common are they? Tidsskrift for Den Norske Laegeforening 119(11):1589–1590

Walker J, Pollard L 1995 Parent education for Asian mothers. Modern Midwife September:22–23

Wilkinson R (ed) 1986 Class and health: research and longitudinal data. Tavistock, London

Wilkinson R (ed) 1996 Unhealthy societies: the afflictions of inequality. Routledge, London

Williams M, Booth D 1980 Antenatal education: guidelines for teachers, 2nd edn. Churchill Livingstone, Edinburgh

FURTHER READING

Crafter H 1997 Health promotion in midwifery: principles and practice. Arnold, London

This is a useful book written by a midwife for midwives.

USEFUL ADDRESS

MIDIRS and the NHS Centre for Review and
Dissemination
PO Box 669
Bristol
BS99 5FG

15

Special Exercises for Pregnancy, Labour and the Puerperium

Eileen Brayshaw

CHAPTER CONTENTS

Specific exercises and postures can help the pregnant woman to adapt to the physical changes in her body during the childbearing year. They will help to ease the minor aches and pains during pregnancy and may also help to prevent longer term postpartum problems. In addition, coping skills such as relaxation, positioning and breathing awareness will provide the mother and her partner with the practical means of managing labour. If practised during pregnancy, the knowledge of these skills will increase the confidence of both partners.

The chapter aims to:

- give midwives an insight into the teaching of physical skills

- provide practical information about exercise, relaxation and beathing for pregnancy, labour and the puerperium

- discuss the role of exercise in relieving aches and pains

- consider basic back care in pregnancy and postpartum.

The information given is relevant for group practice or use on a one-to-one basis and includes advice for the whole of the childbearing year.

Introduction

A women's health physiotherapist is the ideal choice to teach the physical skills required for parenthood. However, in areas where there is no physiotherapist available, midwives may find themselves responsible for physical preparation as well as parent education in antenatal classes or on a one-to-one basis.

Preparation for parenthood classes provide the opportunity for talks, exercise and discussion sessions with a combined approach from midwives, physiotherapists, health visitors and other health care professionals. They should aim to create a learning environment with a relaxed atmosphere, where parents-to-be can enjoy developing a confidence to cope with pregnancy, labour, delivery and the early postnatal days. Specific therapeutic aims of physical preparation include the prevention or relief of common discomforts such as backache, the promotion of a speedy postnatal recovery and the prevention of future gynaecological and orthopaedic problems. Exercise sessions should be designed to stimulate interest in the physical changes occurring, to promote body awareness and to facilitate physical and mental relaxation. Classes held early in pregnancy allow for advice and discussion relating to rest and work activities, anticipated postural changes and relief of common discomforts. Sessions covering relaxation, positions for labour and postnatal exercises are probably more appropriate during the third trimester of pregnancy.

Moderate exercise during pregnancy has many advantages including improved cardiovascular fitness, limited weight gain, an improved attitude and mental state, an easier and less complicated birth and a speedy postnatal recovery (Clapp 2000). Yeo at al (2000) state that exercise in pregnancy may lower diastolic blood pressure, and Hartmann & Bung (1999) believe it may prevent gestational diabetes. The risk of preterm labour may be reduced in nulliparous women who exercise regularly (MacPhail et al 2000). Clapp (2000) also maintains that there are fetal benefits from maternal exercise in pregnancy including decreased growth of the fat organ, improved stress tolerance and advanced neurobehavioural maturation.

Walking. Walking in the fresh air remains the most natural and simplest form of exercise and should be encouraged whenever possible.

Cycling. Cycling is another popular form of exercise that allows for good mobility of the lower limbs with the body weight supported. It is an easy way to travel, although short rather than long distances are preferable and steep hills should be avoided.

Swimming. Swimming is excellent exercise as water relieves the effects of gravity on the body, and muscles can be strengthened and the flexibility of joints retained without undue fatigue. However, it is important to avoid diving during pregnancy and also more strenuous strokes such as crawl or butterfly. Breast stroke is usually the most popular but has a tendency to aggravate backache. Leisurely back stroke with gentle supporting arm movements is often comfortable.

Aquanatal classes. In many areas there are antenatal classes at local swimming pools. Exercise in water raises the plasma beta endorphin levels significantly (McMurray et al 1990) and has a beneficial effect on the respiratory, cardiovascular and musculoskeletal systems. Hartmann & Bung (1999) state that aquatic exercise can be highly recommended because of its beneficial effects as long as potential dangers and contraindications are observed. If the classes are well designed and carefully supervised by a suitably qualified professional following set guidelines (ACPWH 1995), they are an excellent and very enjoyable way of keeping fit.

Aerobic exercise classes. Many midwives have undergone training in exercise to music for ante- and postnatal groups. These sessions can be fun as well as providing aerobic exercise. Exercise teachers, running aerobic classes for pregnancy and postpartum in leisure centres, should have undertaken additional training and assessment to teach ante- and postnatal women.

Pilates. Pilates is a scheme of exercises that offers both mental and physical training. It targets the deep postural muscles necessary to develop core stability and postural alignment and works to develop balance, centring, posture, abdominal and back strength. Classes are held in leisure centres for all age groups. The concentration on transversus and pelvic floor strengthening makes it an ideal preparation for labour and postnatal recovery if the exercises are especially adapted for pregnancy by a specialist teacher. A Pilates in pregnancy video (Jackson 2001) will allow women who cannot get to classes to exercise in their own homes.

Energetic and competitive sports. Activities such as squash, high impact aerobics, horse riding, jogging and skiing are best avoided during pregnancy and it is not the time to take up new sports. Strenuous keep-fit exercises such as sit-ups and double-leg-lifts should *never* be performed as these may cause ligamentous strain and consequent back problems. For the same reason, pregnant women should avoid lifting heavy weights or objects.

Postural changes in pregnancy

Accompanying the gradual gain in weight in pregnancy and its centralising redistribution there is a hormonal influence on ligamentous structures (see Ch. 13). Both of these factors alter the posture of the pregnant woman (Fig. 15.1) and her self-image. The body's centre of gravity moves forwards and, when combined with stretching of weak abdominal muscles, this often leads to a subsequent hollowing of the lumbar spine with a rounding of the shoulders and poking chin. There is a tendency for the back muscles to shorten as the abdominal muscles stretch causing a muscle imbalance around the pelvis and extra strain placed on the ligaments. The result is backache, which is usually of sacroiliac or lumbar origin, and the possibility of long term back problems if the muscle balance and pelvic stability are not restored postnatally. Postural re-education, including correction of the 'pelvic tilt', should be taught, preferably with the benefit of a full-length mirror. The theme of back care must be developed with advice relating to comfortable positions when sitting, standing and lying, general mobility and how to lift correctly.

Back care

Sitting. The pregnant woman should choose a comfortable chair that supports both back and thighs. She should sit well back and if necessary place a small cushion or folded towel behind the lumbar spine for additional comfort. Equal weight should be placed on each of her buttocks to prevent strain on the pelvic ligaments. The seat height should allow the feet to rest on the floor, or a small footstool or cushion may be placed under the feet to raise them slightly (Fig. 15.2). If she is relaxing in an easy chair, the head can be supported and the legs elevated slightly on a stool. The legs should not be crossed.

Standing. The posture should be as tall as possible with both the abdomen and buttocks tucked in; women should try to imagine being pulled up from the top and back of the head. Weight must be evenly distributed on both legs, to prevent undue strain on the pelvic ligaments, and spread between the heels and balls of the feet. High heels will throw the balance of the pregnant woman too far forward and are best discarded in favour of a medium- or low-heeled shoe that also gives support. Shoulders that are relaxed and down help to prevent thoracic aches.

Lying. Equal pressures on all parts of the body will lead to a good posture in lying with no undue strain on any one area. Lying flat on the back must be discouraged because of the danger of supine hypotension due to pressure from the gravid uterus on the inferior

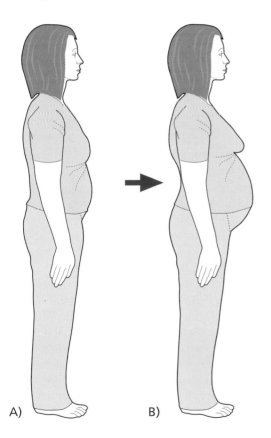

Fig. 15.1 (A) Posture in early pregnancy. (B) Posture in later pregnancy – note the increased lordosis.

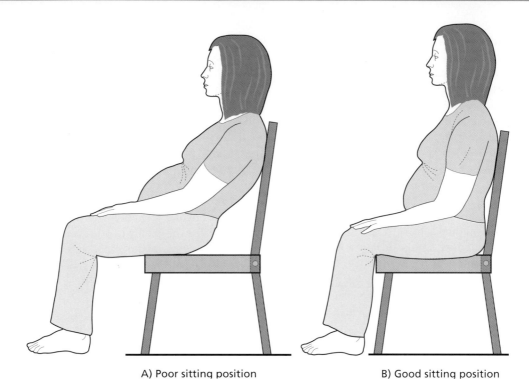

A) Poor sitting position   B) Good sitting position

Fig. 15.2 (A) Poor sitting posture. (B) Good sitting posture.

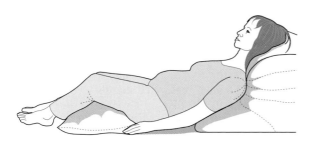

Fig. 15.3 Half back-lying supported with pillows.

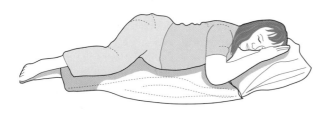

Fig. 15.4 Side-lying supported with pillows.

vena cava (see Ch. 13): three or four pillows or a wedge or beanbag will raise the head and shoulders sufficiently to avoid that risk (Fig. 15.3). This may be more comfortable with a pillow placed under the thighs to reduce the tension behind the knees. Side-lying in the coma position with pillows under the top forearm and knee is usually a comfortable position in pregnancy but is not advised if the woman is suffering from any pelvic discomfort. Instead, side-lying with the top leg supported by the underneath leg but separated by a pillow will be more comfortable (Fig. 15.4).

The woman should get up from lying by bending the knees, rolling on to one side then using the arms to push up into a sitting or kneeling position. This will prevent strain on both the back and the abdominal muscles.

Household activities. Discussion needs to take place on the way in which the woman does her housework. Many tasks such as ironing or preparing food can be undertaken in a sitting position instead of standing. Working surfaces at the correct height or the use of a high stool will avoid the need to stoop and the subsequent backache that a stooping posture can bring about. Making beds or cleaning the bath in a kneeling position prevents lumbar strain.

Work activities. Women should be encouraged to make sure their seating is suitable particularly if sitting for any length of time. Placing a small cushion or folded towel in the lower back will encourage a good posture, and regular change of task and alteration of positions are beneficial. If the woman's work involves constant standing she should ensure she sits at regular break-times and practises foot and leg exercises whenever the opportunity arises.

Lifting heavy or awkward objects. This should be avoided during pregnancy if at all possible. If lifting is unavoidable, then the object or toddler must be held close to the body with the knees bent and the back kept straight (Fig. 15.5). That way the strain is taken by the thigh muscles, not those of the back. All twisting movements whilst lifting are dangerous and must not be performed.

Relief of aches and pains

Back and pelvic pain

This is a common problem during pregnancy. Mantle et al (1977) and Ostgaard (1997) quoted that 50% of pregnant women surveyed in Britain and Scandinavia reported significant backache, and Bullock-Saxton (1998) found that 70% of women in Australia experienced back pain at some stage of their pregnancy. Backache can be eased by encouraging good posture and the practice of the transversus exercise and pelvic-tilting exercise in standing, sitting and lying positions (see p. 233–234). Women complaining of severe pain involving more than one area of the pelvis (*pelvic arthropathy*) should be referred to a women's health physiotherapist for assessment, advice and possible manipulation. Sciatica-like pain may be relieved by lying on the side away from the discomfort so that the affected leg is uppermost. Pillows should be placed strategically to support the whole limb. Symphysis pubis dysfunction (SPD), formerly known as diastasis of the symphysis pubis, is covered in Chapter 18. Midwives should be aware of necessary precautions and positions to be aware of in relation to labour.

Cramp

Prevention of cramp is helped by practising foot and leg exercises. To relieve sudden cramp in the calf muscles whilst in the sitting position, the woman should hold the knee straight and stretch the calf muscles by

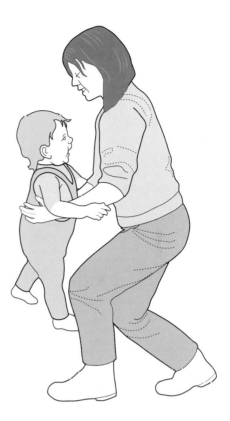

Fig. 15.5 Correct lifting.

pulling the foot upwards (dorsiflexing) at the same time. Alternatively, standing firmly on the affected leg and striding forwards with the other leg will stretch the calf muscles and solve the problem.

Rib stitch or discomfort

Discomfort around the rib cage can often be relieved by adopting a good posture, or by specifically stretching one or both arms upwards, depending on which side the pain is present.

Preparing to teach antenatal exercises

Before teaching exercises it is essential to understand the simple anatomy and functions of the muscles involved, in order to be able to select and/or adapt appropriate exercises in different circumstances.

Anatomy of the anterior wall abdominal musculature

The anterior abdominal wall consists of four pairs of muscles, namely: rectus abdominis, obliquus externus (external oblique), obliquus internus (internal oblique) and transversus abdominis.

Rectus abdominis (Fig. 15.6)

This pair of muscles runs vertically one on either side of the midline from the symphysis pubis to the xiphisternum. Each muscle arises by two tendons and fibres pass upwards to the xiphoid process and the costal cartilages of the fifth, sixth and seventh ribs. Three transverse tendinous intersections are present in the rectus muscles (recti), one at the level of the xiphoid process, one at the level of the umbilicus and the third lying approximately midway between the previous two. The recti are separated in the midline by a tendinous raphe running from the symphysis to the xiphoid process and known as the *linea alba*.

External oblique (Fig. 15.7)

The external oblique muscles are situated on the anterolateral aspect of each side of the abdominal wall and are the most superficial of the flat abdominal muscles. The main anterior fibres run obliquely in a downwards and medial direction from the outer borders and costal cartilages of the lower ribs and insert by an *aponeurosis* (a flat tendon composed of layers of collagen fibres) into the linea alba. The aponeurosis forms the anterior part of the rectus sheath as it passes anterior to the rectus abdominis. The most lateral of the external oblique muscle fibres pass from the lower four ribs almost vertically down to insert as the inguinal ligament.

Internal oblique (Fig. 15.8)

The internal oblique muscles form the middle layer of the flat abdominals with the majority of the fibres running obliquely upwards and laterally at right angles to those of the external obliques. The lower anterior fibres arise from the inguinal ligament and iliac crest and run almost transversely to insert into the crest of the pubis, pectineal line and, by an aponeurosis, into the linea alba. The most posterior fibres run vertically upwards to insert in the lower ribs. The upper anterior fibres arise from the iliac crest and travel in an upwards and medial direction to insert into the linea alba via an aponeurosis. The lateral fibres of the internal oblique are attached to the iliac crest and thoracolumbar fascia and pass upwards and medially to insert into the lower ribs and, by an aponeurosis, into the linea alba.

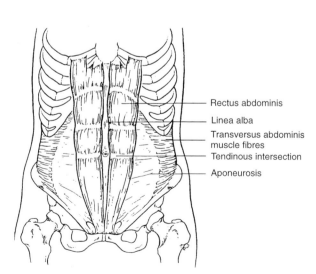

Rectus abdominis
Linea alba
Transversus abdominis muscle fibres
Tendinous intersection
Aponeurosis

Fig. 15.6 Rectus abdominis. (Reproduced from Brayshaw & Wright 1994 by kind permission.)

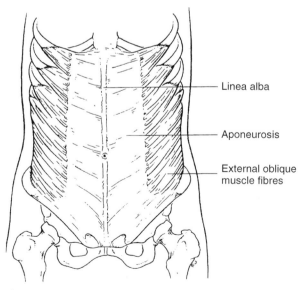

Linea alba
Aponeurosis
External oblique muscle fibres

Fig. 15.7 External oblique. (Reproduced from Brayshaw & Wright 1994 by kind permission.)

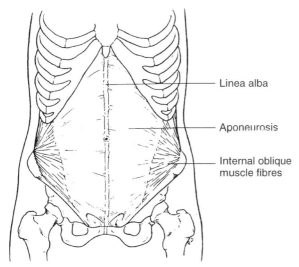

Fig. 15.8 Internal oblique. (Reproduced from Brayshaw & Wright 1994 by kind permission.)

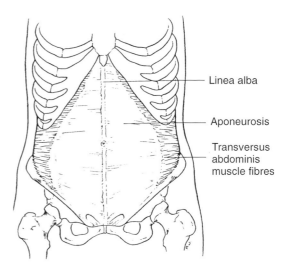

Fig. 15.9 Transversus abdominis. (Reproduced from Brayshaw & Wright 1994 by kind permission.)

Transversus abdominis (Fig. 15.9)

This pair of muscles is the deepest of the abdominal muscle sheets with fibres running transversely from the lateral one-third of the inguinal ligament, the anterior two-thirds of the inner lip of the iliac crest, the thoracolumbar fascia and the inner surfaces of the costal cartilages of the lower six ribs. Most of the fibres run transversely to form a broad aponeurosis inserting into the linea alba. The fibres from the inguinal ligament curve down to join with the inferior fibres of the internal oblique to form the conjoint tendon. The transversus muscles are the most important in relation to pregnancy and the prevention of back problems as they are responsible for the stability of the pelvis, which is essential for correct posture and prevention of long term back problems. Because of their attachment to the lumbar fascia the transversus muscles complete the deep layer of the abdominal corset.

Rectus sheath

The aponeuroses of the oblique and transverse abdominals form the rectus sheath. Anteriorly, the aponeurosis of the external oblique muscle passes in front of the rectus belly. The aponeurosis of the internal oblique muscle divides at the lateral border of the rectus muscle, with the anterior part fusing with the aponeurosis of the external oblique, whilst the posterior part runs behind the rectus belly and fuses with the aponeurosis

of the transversus muscle. The aponeuroses from each side fuse in the midline at the linea alba.

Linea alba

The linea alba lies between the medial borders of the rectus bellies and is formed by the interlacing fibres of the aponeuroses of the external and internal oblique and transversus muscles. As the rectus muscle bellies are closer together below the umbilicus, the linea alba is narrower below and wider above the umbilicus. Above the umbilicus, it may be seen as a shallow groove in fit persons. It is attached to the pubis and the xiphisternum and adjacent ribs. The linea alba is composed of collagen fibres that are under hormonal influence during pregnancy.

Actions of the abdominal muscles

Rectus abdominis

This flexes the vertebral column by bringing the thorax and pelvis closer together anteriorly. The rectus abdominis is assisted by the external and internal obliques and psoas major and minor and works with the other abdominal muscles to raise intra-abdominal pressure. Bilateral weakness of the rectus abdominis will cause decreased ability to flex the lumbar spine. Posterior pelvic tilt will be much more difficult to perform, as will head and shoulder raising in the supine position.

The difficulty in tilting the pelvis posteriorly will result in an increased lumbar lordosis with associated postural problems.

External oblique

The lateral fibres of the external oblique muscle on one side work with the lateral fibres of the internal oblique muscle on the same side to flex the trunk sideways, approximating the pelvis and thorax laterally at that side. The anterior fibres of both sides contract together with the recti to tilt the pelvis posteriorly. The posterior fibres together with the recti flex the trunk. Contracting unilaterally, the external oblique muscle works together with the anterior fibres of the internal oblique muscle of the opposite side to rotate the vertebral column.

Internal oblique

The lower anterior fibres of the internal oblique muscles work with the transversus abdominis to compress and support the lower abdominal viscera. The upper anterior fibres of both internal obliques contract to flex the spine, support and compress the abdominal viscera, depress the thorax and assist in respiration. Contracting unilaterally, the upper anterior fibres of the oblique muscle work with the anterior fibres of the external oblique muscle of the opposite side to rotate the vertebral column. The lateral fibres of the internal oblique muscle on one side work with the lateral fibres of the external oblique muscle on the same side to flex the trunk sideways. They also assist in rotation of the spine.

Transversus abdominis

The transversus muscles compress the abdominal viscera, giving support similar to a girdle. They also help to stabilise the linea alba during lateral trunk flexion. The transversus are postural muscles that work with and assist the pelvic floor muscles to function efficiently (Sapsford et al 2001). Weakness of these muscles contributes to a protruding abdominal wall and separation of the rectus muscles. Research has shown that it is the transversus muscles that are responsible for the stability of the spine and their weakness causes muscular imbalance and pelvic instability leading to back problems and pain (Hodges & Richardson 1996, Richardson & Jull 1995).

Combined actions

The combined actions of all four pairs of abdominal muscles can be related to the function of raising intra-abdominal pressure. If the diaphragm is lowered and remains active, the resultant increase in intra-abdominal pressure brings about downward expulsive actions such as defecation, micturition, and parturition if in conjunction with the relaxation of the pelvic floor. If the diaphragm is relaxed then the increased intra-abdominal pressure can bring about upward expulsive actions (e.g. sneezing, coughing and vomiting). Together with the diaphragm, the abdominal muscles provide a muscular corset keeping the viscera in place.

Influence of pregnancy on the abdominal corset

During pregnancy, the hormones relaxin and progesterone affect the collagen fibres in the fascia, tendons, aponeuroses and linea alba causing these tissues to become more elastic and less supportive (Ostgaard 1997). In exercising, it is important to remember the abdominal muscle attachments so that rotation exercises are not encouraged. This is because these exercises could cause a pulling action on the linea alba and separate it and the rectus muscle bellies lying within the rectus sheath, resulting in diastasis of the rectus muscles (diastasis recti) (Noble 1995).

The antenatal exercises

The positions that pregnant women adopt for exercises should be carefully considered. Women should not be asked to lie flat in the later second and third trimesters because of the danger of supine hypotension (Revelli et al 1992). Instead, a half-lying position with the back raised to an angle of approximately 35° can be used. Foot and leg exercises and pelvic tilting can be performed in sitting or half-lying positions, whereas transversus and pelvic floor exercises can be carried out in any position. *Remember that, before asking a group to exercise on the floor, the correct way of getting down and up again must be demonstrated* (see 'Lying' p. 233).

Muscles of good tone are more elastic and will regain their former length more efficiently and more quickly after being stretched than muscles of poor tone. Exercising the abdominal muscles antenatally

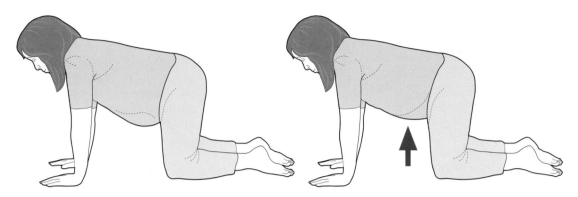

Fig. 15.10 Transversus exercise.

will ensure a speedy return to normal postnatally, effective pushing in labour and the lessening of backache in pregnancy. An important function of the abdominal muscles is the control of pelvic tilt. As the ligaments around the pelvis stretch and no longer give such firm support to the joints, the muscles become the second line of defence, helping to prevent an exaggerated pelvic tilt and unnecessary strain on the pelvic ligaments. It must be remembered that overstretched ligaments and weakened abdominal muscles during pregnancy can lead to chronic skeletal problems postnatally (Hodges & Richardson 1996) as well as backache antenatally. To prevent this and to maintain good abdominal tone, exercises for the transversus muscles (transversus exercise) and rectus muscles (pelvic tilting) are taught.

Exercises that involve the oblique abdominal muscles should be avoided in later pregnancy because these muscles are inserted into the linea alba (see p. 236–237). If twisting movements are performed, there is the danger that the shearing effect may pull the linea alba and the rectus muscle bellies apart (Noble 1995). If this occurs, the condition is known as diastasis recti and is more often diagnosed postnatally.

Transversus exercise

* Sit comfortably or kneel on all fours with a level spine. Breathe in and out, then gently pull in the lower part of the abdomen below the umbilicus keeping the spine still and breathing normally (Fig. 15.10). Hold for up to 10 seconds then relax gently. Repeat up to 10 times.

This exercise tones the deep transverse abdominal muscles, which are the main postural support of the spine, and will help to prevent backache in the future (Hodges & Richardson 1996). When mastered, this simple exercise can be practised in any position and whilst doing other activities. The transversus muscles should be tensed when standing for any length of time and before moving and handling objects.

Pelvic tilting or rocking

* Do this in a half-lying position, well supported with pillows, knees bent and feet flat. Place one hand under the small of the back and the other on top of the abdomen. Tighten the abdominals and buttocks, and press the small of the back down on to the underneath hand (Fig. 15.11). Breathe normally, hold for up to 10 seconds then relax. Repeat up to 10 times. Pelvic tilting can also be performed sitting, standing or kneeling.

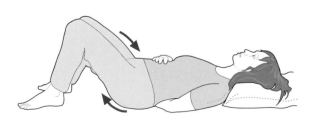

Fig. 15.11 Pelvic-tilting exercise.

Pelvic floor exercise

A great strain is put on the *pelvic floor* during pregnancy because of hormonal influence on the pelvic floor fascia, the weight of the developing fetus and the altered pelvic posture. It is important, therefore, to teach pregnant women pelvic floor exercises ante-natally in order to maintain the tone of the muscles so they retain their functions. The muscles will also relax during parturition and regain their former strength quickly during the puerperium (for anatomy and functions see Ch. 7).

All women should be able to perform the following simple exercise, which can be practised anywhere and at any time.

- Sit, stand or half-lie with legs slightly apart. Close and draw up around the back passage as though preventing a bowel action then repeat around the front two passages as though preventing the flow of urine. Draw up inside and hold for as long as possible, up to 10 seconds, breathing normally, then relax. Repeat up to 10 times.

This exercise will build up the endurance of the postural slow twitch fibres in the pelvic floor but the exercise can also be performed quickly for up to 10 times without holding the contraction. This works the fast twitch fibres which are needed to work quickly to prevent leakage (e.g. when coughing). All women should practise this exercise very regularly antenatally, particularly after emptying the bladder. For those with diminished pelvic floor awareness, attempting to 'stop midstream' occasionally or 'gripping' on to an imaginary tampon that is slipping out may assist the ability to contract the correct muscles.

Foot and leg exercises

The circulation during pregnancy, particularly the venous return, is sluggish and this can lead to problems such as cramp, varicose veins and oedema. To help to prevent these the following simple exercises and advice will improve the circulation.

- Sit or half-lie with legs supported. Bend and stretch the ankles at least 12 times. Circle both feet at the ankle at least 20 times in each direction. Brace both knees, hold for a count of four, then relax. Repeat 12 times.

These exercises should be performed before getting up from resting, last thing at night and several times during the day. Women should be discouraged from standing unnecessarily and encouraged to put their feet up whenever possible. Crossing the legs at the knee or ankle will impede circulation further. If varicose veins or oedema are present, support tights may be prescribed with the appropriate advice to put them on before allowing the legs to drop over the edge of the bed.

Breathing awareness

It is important to be aware of one's own natural breathing rhythm so variations can be recognised if they occur.

- Sit comfortably with eyes closed. 'Listen in' to your breathing, concentrating especially on the outward breath, recognising the short pause before the inward breath naturally follows. Keep the movement fairly low down in the chest and be aware of your own breathing rate whilst resting.

A few deeper breaths occasionally will help the venous return and aid the oxygen supply to both the pregnant woman and her fetus, but only three or four deep breaths should be taken at a time as hyperventilation is more likely during pregnancy (Bush 1992).

Teaching exercises

Anyone who is teaching exercises to others must first be proficient at performing those particular exercises herself. Next the instructor must familiarise herself with instructions describing the execution of the exercise and practise teaching two or three colleagues or family members before introducing the teaching to a larger group. It is important to describe or demonstrate fully and to give appropriate additional information that makes the topic more interesting and relevant (Brayshaw & Wright 1994). When planning to teach specific exercises, such as foot and leg exercises, think in the way shown in Box 15.1.

Stress, relaxation and respiration

The normal stresses of everyday life often lead to a build-up of tension within the body. If anxiety, fear or

---

Box 15.1 Teaching foot and leg exercises

Why the exercise is relevant

- During pregnancy, circulatory changes occur that may lead to cramp, oedema or varicose veins.

What we hope to achieve

- Improvement in circulation and prevention or alleviation of cramp, oedema and varicose veins.

How

- Bend and stretch the ankles.
- Circle feet at the ankles.
- Brace knees and let go.
- Repeat several times.

When

- Several times per day and always before getting up from resting and last thing at night.

Additional information

- Avoid long periods of standing, which may increase oedema, but encourage walking.
- Discourage sitting or lying with legs crossed, which can impede the circulation.
- Describe how to relieve cramp.
- Advise on correct use of support tights.
- Stress the importance of supporting footwear of sensible height.
- Advise sitting with feet elevated whenever possible and heels higher than hips if oedema is present.

- frowning face
- tense jaw
- hunched shoulders
- elbows bent and close to sides
- fingers gripping or tapping
- trunk bent forward
- legs crossed
- feet pulled up or tapping.

When tension increases, breathing often becomes shallow and rapid, or when severe, breath holding may feature. The higher the stress level, the greater the degree of postural change that will be evident. Mental tension often leads to physical tension and a vicious circle is established. Ideas about relaxation have been developed and exchanged over many years but today it is generally recognised that simply saying 'relax' is a negative instruction and does not readily bring results for most individuals. Muscles can work singly but usually they work in groups and when any group of muscles is working, the opposite group relaxes. This is a physiological fact and is known as *reciprocal inhibition* or *reciprocal relaxation*. Try the following example:

- Concentrate on your right hand.
- Stretch your fingers really long. Hold for a moment. (This is tightening the muscles on the back of your hand and wrist.)
- Now stop stretching and feel the ease not only in the muscles you were stretching but in the palm of your hand and fingers.

Reciprocal relaxation ensures that, when following a series of instructions for the whole body, one will be able to bring release of tension and relaxation to all areas.

Planning a scheme of relaxation

To be effective, relaxation must be practised regularly and it is important to develop a theme running through classes and to encourage daily practice at home. The environment should be relatively peaceful with no irritating distractions such as the telephone. An adequate supply of mats, blankets and pillows is essential. Participants should be encouraged to wear loose, comfortable clothing, to remove shoes and spectacles and then choose a comfortable position in which to relax. This could be side-lying, half back-lying or sitting with supporting pillows strategically placed.

pain are present the body may unconsciously adopt a posture that is extreme. Relaxation is concerned with reducing body tension to a minimum and once learned can be used whenever increased tension is a problem. It can be particularly useful during pregnancy and labour and the early postnatal days. Women who have had a previous preterm baby had larger newborns and longer gestations when they practised relaxation in subsequent pregnancies (Janke 1999).

Tension manifests itself with muscle tightening and shows in the following ways:

Physiological relaxation

This technique (Box 15.2) consists of a series of instructions and movements that help the body to move away from the posture caused by tension and so achieve a position of comfort, ease and relaxation. Following each individual instruction and movement, any tension in that part of the body will disappear.

When group participants are fluent in the practice of relaxation there is no need to go through the whole checklist of instructions every time. Gradually shorten the list of instructions given and work towards the situation where relaxation can be achieved almost spontaneously. The shoulders, arms and hands are usually the first areas to respond to stress and the following can be practised and used during contractions:

- shoulders down
- arms and hands comfortably supported
- easy breathing and *sigh out slowly*.

Box 15.2 Physiological relaxation technique

For each part of the body where tension manifests itself there is a threefold instruction:

- an order to the reciprocal muscle group to work strongly
- a command to that muscle group to stop working
- a direction to the brain to recognise the new position of ease and to remember it.

As with exercises, the teacher of relaxation techniques must first practise them herself and become familiar with the instructions before teaching others.

- Lie down comfortably on a firm surface with pillows supporting your head and thighs (see Fig. 15.3) or sit in a suitable chair, with head, shoulders, arms and thighs supported.

- **Shoulders**. Pull your shoulders towards your feet – stop pulling – concentrate on this new position of ease – your shoulders are relaxed and down.

- **Arms**. Push your elbows slightly out from your body as though straightening the elbows – stop pushing, think about this position – your arms are relaxed and comfortably supported.

- **Hands**. Let them rest on your tummy or thighs or the supporting surface – stretch the fingers really long and straight – stop stretching – feel the new position – comfortably supported and relaxed.

- **Hips**. Tighten your buttocks and press your knees out sideways – stop tightening, register this comfortable position – your hips are relaxed.

- **Knees**. Move your knees slightly – stop moving them – feel the comfort you have created in your knees and thighs.

- **Feet**. Press your feet down – away from your face – stop pressing – you now have comfortably relaxed feet.

- **Body**. Press your body into the support, such as the floor, bed or chair – stop pressing – be aware of comfort and relaxation in your trunk.

- **Head**. Press your head into the support, that is, the pillow or chair – now stop pressing – notice how this movement has relaxed your neck and shoulders.

- **Face**. Close your eyes if you want to. Drop your lower jaw slightly so that your teeth are not touching. Make sure that your tongue is resting comfortably in the lower jaw and not stuck to the roof of your mouth. Imagine that someone is smoothing away the frown lines from your forehead.

- **Breathing**. Give a big sigh out and continue to breathe gently, keeping the movement fairly low down in the chest; be aware of the outward breath. Your body is now in a position of ease and is as relaxed as is possible in that position and you are breathing at your normal resting rate.

- Never get up in a hurry after a spell of relaxation. Instead, gently exercise the hands and feet to stir the circulation and slowly roll over on to one side, getting up in the correct way.

- Relaxation can be adapted and used as labour progresses by combining the most comfortable positions with easy breathing in the lower part of the chest (breathing awareness).

This can be practised for the approximate duration of a contraction with concentration on easy breathing, which helps to achieve comfort and relaxation.

Respiration

Respiration is affected by stress and adapted breathing is one of the easiest ways of assisting relaxation. Breathing can be used to increase the depth of relaxation by varying its speed; slower breathing leads to deeper relaxation. Natural rhythmic breathing must not be confused with specific unnatural levels or rates of breathing, which research has proved to be harmful to both mother and fetus (Bush 1992, Caldeyro-Barcia 1979). Women in labour frequently breathe very rapidly at the peak of a contraction but should be encouraged not to do so. Persistent rapid breathing or breath holding is usually a sign of panic.

Very slow deep breathing can cause hyperventilation, which produces tingling in the fingers and may proceed to carpopedal spasm and even tetany. Rapid shallow breathing or panting is only tracheal and can lead to hypoventilation with subsequent oxygen deprivation. During pregnancy, labour and delivery, emphasis should be placed on easy, rhythmic breathing and on avoiding very deep breathing, shallow panting or long periods of breath holding.

Labour

It is important to stress to the parents-to-be the importance of working together with the midwife. The need for relaxation and breathing techniques should be stressed together with how and when they can be used. As individuals, we appear to experience discomfort and pain to varying degrees but with good training it is possible to raise the individual's threshold of tolerance. It must be remembered that continual support and reminding will be necessary as labour progresses, if the breathing and relaxation techniques are to achieve their maximum potential.

Early first stage of labour

A woman in labour should be encouraged to keep mobile and active if there are no complications. She should be advised to try alternative positions of ease as alteration of position leads to productive uterine contractions (Roberts et al 1983). When discomfort increases, the woman should be encouraged to stay relaxed and concentrate on rhythmical easy breathing during contractions.

Coping with early first stage of labour

The following positions of ease may help during the early stages of labour and can be discussed and practised in the antenatal period:

- sitting against a table and relaxing forwards so that shoulders, arms and head are supported
- standing, leaning backwards against the wall of the room
- kneeling on all fours
- kneeling on the floor and leaning forwards on to a chair
- leaning forward against a partner
- sitting astride an armless chair with arms supported on the chair back and body relaxing forwards
- the birthing room will have additional aids (e.g. rocking chair, large ball, mat).

Pelvic rocking in any of these positions may be helpful. Deep massage of the lower back or gentle stroking of the abdomen soothes many women and can be taught to the partner at couples' classes.

Later first stage of labour

As labour progresses it becomes more difficult to find a comfortable position and frequent changes may be necessary. Many women, however, are content to sit back against pillows on the bed at this stage and concentrate on relaxation and breathing. As each contraction builds up, the speed and depth of breathing sometimes alter but mothers must be encouraged to keep it as natural and easy as possible. They may find that 'sighing out slowly' (SOS) helps to avoid panic breathing and also relaxes physical tension especially in the shoulders.

The emotional aspects of the end of the first stage of labour will be explained to couples antenatally and coping strategies need to be discussed. With a premature urge to push, an interrupted out-breath can be introduced (that is, two shorter out-breaths followed by a longer out-breath). This is often known as 'pant, pant, blow' or 'puff, puff, blow' breathing and it prevents the diaphragm from fixing and the subsequent increase in intra-abdominal pressure. An alteration in position will take away some of the urge to push, for example side-lying or prone-kneeling with the forehead resting on the hands.

Second stage of labour

Positions for the second stage will depend on individual choice, method of pain relief and obstetric factors, but mothers should give some thought to the alternatives available in their delivery suite. These may include:

- side-lying
- kneeling and leaning forwards facing the backrest of the bed with pillows placed for comfort or facing the partner for support
- kneeling on all fours
- squatting on the bed or floor
- supported squatting with the partner holding from behind
- sitting fairly upright against the backrest with knees bent and feet resting on the bed.

A review of trials comparing positions for the second stage of labour concluded that there are several possible benefits for an upright posture including reduction in assisted deliveries, episiotomies, second degree perineal tears, severe pain and abnormal fetal heart rate patterns. However, a slightly increased blood loss was reported in upright positions (Gupta & Nikodem 2000).

If there is any pain in the area of the symphysis pubis, which may lead to SPD, undue abduction of the hips must be avoided during labour and delivery. Prone-kneeling or side-lying would be the most suitable positions for delivery (Fry 1999).

As the contraction starts, the mother is reminded to breathe in and out gently. When the urge to push becomes overwhelming she will bear down, keeping the pelvic floor relaxed. Breath holding for longer than a few seconds should not be encouraged because of the danger of fetal hypoxia in an already compromised baby (Caldeyro-Barcia 1979). To prevent pushing whilst the head is delivered, deep panting may be useful.

Postnatal exercises

These should be started as soon after birth as possible in order to improve circulation, strengthen pelvic floor and abdominal muscles and prevent transient and long term problems.

Circulatory exercises

Foot and leg exercises as described in the antenatal section must be performed very frequently in the immediate postnatal period to improve circulation and reduce oedema. Early ambulation will help prevent deep vein thrombosis (DVT). If oedema is present the woman's legs may be slightly elevated.

Pelvic floor exercises

The pelvic floor muscles have been under strain during pregnancy and stretched during delivery and it may be both difficult and painful to contract these muscles postnatally. Mothers should be encouraged to try the exercise as often as possible in order to regain full bladder control, prevent prolapse and ensure normal sexual satisfaction for both partners in the future. The exercise can be linked to and performed during everyday activities such as feeding, bathing, nappy changing and after each bladder emptying. The contraction, as described in the antenatal section, should be held for up to 10 seconds if possible before relaxing, and repeated up to 10 times at any one session, whilst breathing normally throughout. When this has been mastered, mothers should follow a pattern of 10 slow contractions then 10 quick ones without holding the contraction. This programme will strengthen both the slow twitch muscle fibres, which can contract over a long period of time, and the fast twitch muscle fibres, which produce a quick powerful contraction of the pelvic floor (Gilpin et al 1989). Mørkved & Bø (2000) found that the benefits from postpartum pelvic floor muscle training are still present 1 year after delivery. If mothers find the pelvic floor exercise difficult at first, then performing the transversus exercise at the same time will help the activation of the pelvic floor (Sapsford et al 2001).

Mothers should be encouraged to test their pelvic floor muscles after 2–3 months. With a full bladder they should be able to jump up and down with legs apart and cough deeply without leaking urine. If there is leakage, then the exercise must be continued several times a day for a further month and the test repeated. If leakage still occurs, the mother should report back to her GP for a physiotherapy or gynaecological referral.

Bump et al (1991) showed that only 49% of women who thought they were performing pelvic floor contractions were doing so correctly. Furthermore, 25% were performing the exercise in such a way that could potentially encourage incontinence. Bø et al (1998) concluded that pelvic floor exercises must be taught thoroughly to be effective. Even if there is no leakage on testing, every woman should exercise her pelvic floor muscles regularly to prevent continence problems.

Abdominal exercises

The deep muscles need to regain tone as soon as possible after delivery in order to protect the spine, prevent back problems and help the mother regain her 'former figure'.

Transversus exercise

This very easy exercise described on page 239 will strengthen the deep transverse muscles, which are the main support for the spine and play a large part in preventing long term back problems (Richardson & Jull 1995). The exercise should not be performed in the prone-kneeling position postpartum until all bleeding has ceased so as to reduce the remote possibility of an air embolus being introduced to the placental site (Horsley 1998). Instead it can be done in prone-lying, supine, side-lying, sitting and standing positions and should be encouraged during activities with the baby, especially any lifting. The toning of the transversus muscles will also assist the performance of the pelvic floor muscles whilst they are weak and the two exercises can be performed together.

Pelvic tilting

Pelvic tilting as described in the antenatal exercise section will tone up the straight abdominal (rectus abdominis) muscles and, if performed in a rhythmical action, will ease any postural backache that may occur in the first few days of the puerperium. This exercise can now be done in supine-lying as well as side-lying, sitting and standing positions.

Pelvic tilting and head lifting may be performed only if there is no diastasis and no peaking of the abdominal muscles on lifting the head.

Rectus check

After 48 hours the rectus muscles should be checked for any undue diastasis which may have occurred antenatally or sometimes during labour (Fig. 15.12). A gap of two fingers' width at this stage is considered normal and the mother may progress to exercising the oblique abdominal muscles. However, if the gap is more than two fingers' width and 'peaking' of the abdominals is visible on lifting the head, then only the transversus and pelvic-tilting exercises should be performed very regularly until the gap reduces. A women's health physiotherapist should assess any woman found to have a gap of more than three fingers' width to advise on a regimen of progressive exercises to avoid future back problems. These women will also require abdominal support in the form of a 'tubigrip' from the xiphisternum to below the buttocks. Support throughout subsequent pregnancies is also advised to help protect the rectus muscles.

Knee rolling

This exercise will strengthen the oblique abdominal muscles, but may be performed only if there is no undue separation of the rectus muscles on the rectus check.

- In a back-lying position with knees bent, pull in the abdomen and roll both knees to one side as far as is comfortable, keeping the shoulders flat. Return the knees to an upright position and relax the abdomen. Pull in the abdomen again and roll both knees to the other side. This exercise can be performed up to 10 times.

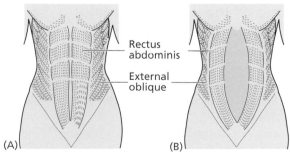

(A)　(B)

Fig. 15.12 (A) Rectus muscles before pregnancy. (B) Diastasis of rectus muscles after delivery.

Exercises following caesarean section

Foot and leg exercises as described earlier should be started as soon as possible, especially after epidural anaesthesia, as distal circulation will be especially sluggish. These may be followed by not more than four deep breaths to ensure full expansion of the lungs and pumping action on the inferior vena cava. If a general anaesthetic has been given, the mother may need to be taught how to clear secretions by coughing in a sitting position with the sutures supported by both hands or a pillow. Deep breathing and huffing will help to loosen the secretions.

The transversus exercise should be started whenever the mother feels comfortable in any position except prone kneeling. Pelvic tilting and very gentle modified knee rolling will ease the flatulence that many mothers experience.

Pelvic floor exercises are still important following a caesarean section even though one recent research study has shown that women in this group are less likely to suffer stress incontinence (Wilson et al 1996).

It will not be possible to check for separation of the recti before 5–6 days postpartum so exercises for the oblique muscles should be delayed until after that time and when the mother feels up to it.

Adequate rest is essential postnatally to allow the tissues to regain their normal function. After a caesarean section the woman has not only given birth but has also undergone major surgery, yet she still has to cope with her baby. The midwife must take every opportunity to remind relatives of the need to help with chores and the organisation of rest periods for the mother.

Care of the back postnatally

It may take up to 6 months before the ligaments completely resume their normal functions (Polden & Mantle 1990) so it is vital that mothers receive advice on back care in relation to everyday activities at this time.

When feeding, the mother should sit back in a chair, well supported, with the baby raised up on pillows to prevent a slouched forward position. Nappy changing and bathing are best carried out at waist level or with the mother kneeling at a surface of coffee-table height.

Lifting should be avoided if at all possible but if unavoidable the object should be as light as possible and kept close to the body whilst engaging the transversus and the pelvic floor muscles. All-purpose baby chairs are heavy and are best carried by holding them underneath and close to the body instead of by the carrying handle, which puts a strain on one side of the body especially when the ligaments are still lax. Whenever possible, the chair should be carried empty and placed in the position required before the baby is put in it.

Baby slings should be comfortable and not cause an arched back. The weight should be well supported and the mother should use her transversus and pelvic floor muscles to give a good posture and prevent backache.

Resuming sporting activities

The postnatal exercises shown above are safe and effective and need to be practised regularly and increased gradually. Brayshaw & Wright (1996) illustrate further postnatal exercises that are a natural progression before resuming more strenuous prepregnancy activities. The video Pilates in pregnancy (Jackson 2001) introduces gentle exercises for the first 6 weeks postpartum, which can then be followed by the exercises for pre/early pregnancy on the same video.

Walking, cycling and swimming will increase general fitness but more strenuous keep-fit exercises, aerobics and competitive sports are best left until 10–12 weeks after delivery and then resumed only after ensuring that the pelvic floor muscles are functioning effectively. *Double-leg-lifts* (Fig. 15.13) *and sit-ups should never be performed.*

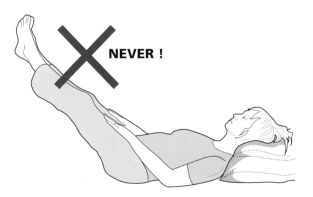

Fig. 15.13 Never attempt double-leg-lifts.

Immediate postnatal problems

Symphysis pubis dysfunction (SPD)

This condition may be present in late pregnancy, occur during labour or appear after delivery (Fry 1999). If the pain is severe, indicating complete separation of the pubic joint, then complete bedrest with some support around the level of the pubis is advised. The woman must be instructed to press her knees together when moving in bed. She should be encouraged to perform the transversus and pelvic-tilting exercises plus circulatory exercises whilst she is resting. The women's health physiotherapist may provide therapeutic ultrasound, TENS or ice to relieve local pain. Mobilisation of the woman should progress gently, and only when the acute pain has subsided (see Ch. 18 and the guidelines issued by ACPWH (2000)).

Diastasis recti

If, after performing the rectus check, it is found that the woman's rectus muscles are more than two fingers' width apart, the only exercises she should be prescribed are transversus and pelvic tilting (see p. 239). The pelvic tilting can be performed with the woman's own hands crossed over the abdomen to support the muscles and draw them towards the midline.

Painful perineum

To reduce pain, advice on positioning should be given plus analgesia and local pain-relieving agencies such as cold gel packs, therapeutic ultrasound or pulsed electromagnetic energy. These latter two may be administered only by a physiotherapist. If using a gel pack, the woman will be most comfortable in a side-lying position and should be reminded not to sit on the gel pack as the pressure would impede her circulation. When the pain is less, pelvic floor exercises should be encouraged with the aim of increasing the local circulation and easing the weight off the painful area.

Incontinence

The most common type of postnatal incontinence is stress incontinence. In a study of 1600 postpartum women it was discovered that 34% suffered from urinary incontinence 3 months after giving birth (Wilson et al 1996). This figure is substantiated by a report from Mørkved & Bø (1999) who stated that 38% of women complained of incontinence 2 months after delivery. Pelvic floor exercises will help to rehabilitate the pelvic floor, but the woman should be advised to seek a referral to a women's health physiotherapist if the problem persists. Mørkved & Bø (2000) found that specially designed postpartum pelvic floor muscle training was effective in the prevention and treatment of stress urinary incontinence.

Backache

Early postnatal backache is usually postural and can be relieved by warmth and pelvic-tilting exercises. However, a woman with persistent and severe back pain should be referred for physiotherapy.

Coccydynia

An acutely painful coccyx is incapacitating for a new mother. Pillows may be placed strategically to give some relief in sitting and advice on alternative positions for feeding should be given. A women's health physiotherapist can administer therapeutic ultrasound or pulsed electromagnetic energy with beneficial effects, or may manipulate a persistently displaced coccyx.

Conclusion

During pregnancy, labour and the puerperium, midwives and other health care professionals have many opportunities to influence parents-to-be, incorporating a sensible approach to exercise within the broader sphere of healthy routines for all family members. Relaxation, walking, cycling, swimming and other forms of exercise should be encouraged as part of a general lifestyle. Specific exercises for strengthening the pelvic floor and abdominal muscles, especially the transversus, or relieving aches and pains (e.g. cramp or backache), will have relevance far beyond the months of childbearing. Parents-to-be are an extremely receptive audience. These opportunities to develop both specific and general health care measures should not be missed.

REFERENCES

ACPWH (Association of Chartered Physiotherapists in Women's Health) 1995 Aquanatal guidelines. Chartered Society of Physiotherapy, London

ACPWH (Association of Chartered Physiotherapists in Women's Health) 2000 Guidelines for symphysis pubis dysfunction. Chartered Society of Physiotherapy, London

Bø K, Larsen S, Oseid S et al 1998 Knowledge about and ability to perform correct pelvic muscle exercise in women with urinary stress incontinence. Neurology and Urodynamics 7(3):261–262

Brayshaw E, Wright P 1994 Teaching physical skills for the childbearing year. Books for Midwives Press, Hale, Cheshire

Brayshaw E, Wright P 1996 Relaxation and exercise for the childbearing year. Books for Midwives Press, Hale, Cheshire

Bullock-Saxton J E 1998 Back pain in pregnancy: a retrospective study. Australian Physiotherapy Association National Conference, Canberra, p 84–91

Bump R C, Hurt W H, Fanti J A, Wyman J F 1991 Assessment of Kegel muscle exercise performance after brief verbal instruction. American Journal of Obstetrics and Gynecology 165:322–329

Bush A 1992 Cardiopulmonary effects of pregnancy and labour. Journal of the Association of Chartered Physiotherapists in Obstetrics and Gynaecology 71:3–4

Caldeyro-Barcia R 1979 The influence of maternal bearing-down efforts during second stage on fetal well-being. Birth and Family Journal 6:17–22

Clapp J F III 2000 Exercise during pregnancy. A clinical update. Clinical Sports Medicine 19(2):273–286

Fry D 1999 Perinatal symphysis pubis dysfunction: a review of the literature. Journal of the Association of Chartered Physiotherapists in Women's Health 85:11–18

Gilpin S A, Gosling J A, Smith A R B, Warrell D W 1989 The pathogenesis of genitourinary prolapse and stress incontinence of urine. A histological and histochemical study. British Journal of Obstetrics and Gynaecology 96:15–23

Gupta J K, Nikodem V C 2000 Woman's position during second stage of labour. Cochrane Database Systematic Review 2:CD002006

Hartmann S, Bung P 1999 Physical exercise during pregnancy – physiological considerations and recommendations. Journal of Perinatal Medicine 27(3):204–215

Hodges P, Richardson C A 1996 Inefficient muscular stabilization of the lumbar spine associated with low back pain. Spine 21(22):2640–2650

Horsley K 1998 Fitness in the child-bearing year. In: Spasford R, Bullock-Saxton J, Markwell S (eds) Women's health. A textbook for physiotherapists. W B Saunders, London, ch 16, p 185

Jackson L 2001 Pilates for pregnancy (video). Enhance Productions, 8 Raby Park, Wetherby

Janke J 1999 The effect of relaxation therapy on preterm labor outcomes. Journal of Obstetrics and Gynaecology Neonatal Nursing 28(3):255–263

MacPhail A, Davies G A, Victory R, Wolfe L A 2000 Maximal exercise testing in late gestation: fetal responses. Obstetrics and Gynecology 96(4):565–570

McMurray R G, Berry M J, Katz V 1990 The beta endorphin responses of pregnant women during aerobic exercise in the water. Medicine and Science in Sports and Exercise 22(3):298–301

Mantle M J, Greenwood R M, Currey H L F 1977 Backache in pregnancy. Rheumatological Rehabilitation 16:95–110

Mørkved S, Bø K 1999 Prevalence of urinary incontinence during pregnancy and postpartum. International Urogynecology Journal 10:394–398

Mørkved S, Bø K 2000 Effect of postpartum pelvic floor muscle training in prevention and treatment of urinary incontinence: a one-year follow up. British Journal of Obstetrics and Gynaecology 107(8):1022–1028

Noble E 1995 Essential exercises for the childbearing year, 4th edn. New Life Images, Harwich MA

Ostgaard H C 1997 Lumbar back and posterior pelvic pain in pregnancy. In: Vleeming A, Mooney V, Dorman T, Sniders C, Stoeckart R (eds) Movement, stability and low back pain. Churchill Livingstone, Edinburgh, ch. 33, p 411–420

Polden M, Mantle J 1990 Physiotherapy in obstetrics and gynaecology. Butherworth-Heinemann, London

Revelli A, Durando A, Massobrio M 1992 Exercise and pregnancy: a review of maternal and fetal effects. Obstetrical and Gynaecological Survey 47(6):355–367

Richardson C A, Jull G A 1995 Muscle control – pain control. What exercises would you prescribe? Manual Therapy 1:2–10

Roberts J E, Mendez-Bauer C, Wodell D A 1983 The effects of maternal position on uterine contractility and efficiency. Birth 10:243–249

Sapsford R R, Hodges P W, Richardson C A, Cooper D H, Markwell S J, Jull G A 2001 Co-activation of the abdominal and pelvic floor muscles during voluntary exercises. Neurology and Urodynamics 20:31–42

Wilson P D, Herbison P W, Herbison G P 1996 Obstetric practice and the prevalence of urinary incontinence three months after delivery. British Journal of Obstetrics and Gynaecology 103:154–161

Yeo S, Steele N M, Chang M C, Leclair S M, Ronis D L, Hayashi R 2000 Effect of exercise on blood pressure in pregnant women with a high risk of gestational hypertensive disorders. Journal of Reproductive Medicine 45(4):293–298

FURTHER READING

Brayshaw E 2003 Exercises for pregnancy and childbirth: guide for educators. Books for Midwives Press, Oxford

This up-to-date book is written by a women's health physiotherapist in answer to requests from midwives and health visitors. Easy to follow, it covers the teaching of ante- and postnatal exercises and coping strategies for labour. It includes relative anatomy and physiology, TENS in labour, musculoskeletal problems and alternative approaches to fitness.

Brayshaw E, Wright P 1996 Relaxation and exercise for the childbearing year. Books for Midwives Press, Hale, Cheshire

This book was written for parents-to-be and describes the antenatal and postnatal exercises and coping strategies for labour which would be taught by a women's health physiotherapist at antenatal classes.

Campion M J 1990 The baby challenge: a handbook on pregnancy for women with a physical disability. Routledge, London

A book highlighting the problems faced during pregnancy, labour and the postnatal period by women with special physical needs.

Mitchell L 1987 Simple relaxation. John Murray, London

This book discusses the causes and results of stress in all aspects of life. It introduces the application of the physiological reciprocal relaxation technique, which Laura Mitchell perfected in the 1980s and which is still widely taught in antenatal classes today for use in pregnancy, labour and postpartum.

Polden M, Mantle J 1990 Physiotherapy in obstetrics and gynaecology. Butterworth-Heinemann, London

A textbook written for physiotherapists which includes the anatomy and physiology of pregnancy, labour and postpartum, gynaecological conditions, surgery and incontinence.

Sapsford R, Bullock-Saxton J, Markwell S 1998 Women's health. A textbook for physiotherapists. W B Saunders, London

This is a comprehensive textbook for women's health physiotherapists with 36 chapters covering all aspects of women's health from adolescence, through the childbearing year to the mature woman.

LEAFLETS

ACPWH 2001 Fit for pregnancy
ACPWH 2001 Fit for birth
ACPWH 2001 Fit for motherhood
ACPWH 2001 Promoting continence with physiotherapy
ACPWH 2000 Symphysis pubis dysfunction guidelines

ACPWH 1995 Aquanatal guidelines
ACPWH 2002 Mitchell method of simple physiological relaxation (revised)
(The above are available from the ACPWH leaflet secretary, c/o the Chartered Society of Physiotherapy, Bedford Row, London WC1R 4ED.)

VIDEOTAPES

Ashton J, Conley R, Polden M 1991 BBC pregnancy and postnatal exercise. BBC Publications, London
Gaskell J, Jennings M 1991 Y plan before and after pregnancy. Central YMCA, London

Jackson L 2001 Pilates in pregnancy. Enhance Productions, 8 Raby Park, Wetherby

16 Antenatal Care

Anne Viccars

CHAPTER CONTENTS

Antenatal care refers to the care that is given to a pregnant woman from the time that conception is confirmed until the beginning of labour. The midwife will provide a woman-centred approach to the care of the woman and her family by sharing information with the woman to facilitate her to make informed choices about her care.

The chapter aims to:

- explore the role of the midwife in providing woman-centred care, which addresses her physical, psychological and sociological needs

- discuss the initial assessment visit, defining its objectives and considering the significance of the different components of the history taken by the midwife

- describe the physical examination and psychological support of the woman at the initial assessment and during subsequent visits

- explore the midwife's role in carrying out an abdominal examination to monitor the growth of the fetus, its position and heart rate and facilitate maternal–infant attachment

- emphasise the contribution of skilled communication to sensitive and effective antenatal care.

Introduction

The pattern of antenatal care was not challenged for over 50 years (MoH 1929). It followed a traditional pattern consisting of monthly visits until 28 weeks' gestation, fortnightly visits until 36 weeks and weekly visits until the birth of the baby. This pattern was questioned by Hall et al (1980) whose retrospective analysis demonstrated that the expectations of antenatal care might not be met. They found that conditions requiring hospitalisation, including pre-eclampsia, were neither prevented nor detected by antenatal care; and intrauterine growth restriction was overdiagnosed. A more flexible approach to both the timing of visits and place of consultation has been incorporated into midwifery practice in more recent years (Clement et al 1999, Jewell et al 2000, Sikorski et al 1996). This has been in an attempt to improve maternal satisfaction by the provision of holistic, individualised care and organisational change in the pattern of care (DoH 1993). Sikorski et al (1996) conducted a randomised controlled trial with low risk pregnant women to compare the acceptability and effectiveness of a reduced antenatal visit schedule of six to seven routine visits with the traditional 13 routine visits. The results showed no differences in clinical outcome between the two groups, but twice as many women in the reduced-visit group were dissatisfied with the frequency of attendance compared with women who received the full range of visits. A substantial number of women in both groups felt that the gaps in their care were too long, with women in the reduced-visit group feeling less remembered from one visit to the next. The need to provide a more individualised, flexible approach to care with increased psychosocial support for those pregnant women who needed it was one of the main conclusions of this study.

Traditional visiting versus flexible visiting was studied in 11 primary care centres with 609 women (Jewell et al 2000). Comparing the two groups, no difference was found either in attitudes to pregnancy and motherhood or in women urgently reporting antenatal problems. However, women in the flexible care group would like to have been seen more often, although they liked the choices associated with the individualised approach to planning visits (Jewell et al 2000). Rates of obstetric complications did not differ between groups (Jewell et al 2000). Villar & Khan-Neelofur (2001), who reviewed randomised controlled trials involving 25 000 women, support this finding. Evidence supports the view that perinatal outcomes are not adversely affected by a reduction in visits (Jewell et al 2000, Villar & Khan-Neelofur 2001).

Oakley et al (1990) explored how antenatal care could be tailored to meet the needs of particular women. A randomised controlled trial looked at the effect of providing social support to women who had previously had one or more babies with a birthweight less than 2500 g. Women who had an increased likelihood of being socially disadvantaged in pregnancy were identified and a research midwife gave additional support to the 'intervention' group of women. The midwife visited this group of women a minimum of three times during their pregnancy. She could be contacted by telephone 24 hours a day, gave practical advice and information, made referrals to other health care professionals as necessary but did not give any clinical care.

Women and babies in the intervention group experienced improved outcomes in several ways compared with the control group. There were fewer admissions to hospital during pregnancy and fewer very low birthweight babies, with babies generally needing less neonatal intensive care and mothers also reporting that their babies appeared healthier in the first few weeks of life.

A year later, women felt less anxious about their babies and more positive about motherhood. In 1996 Oakley et al looked at the same group of women, and the psychological and health benefits in the intervention group had continued, compared with women in the control group. Recent government-led initiatives such as Sure Start demonstrate support for Oakley's work; these have been developed throughout the UK, and over 128 projects have evolved since its inception, with plans for 500 projects by 2004 (Sure Start 2001) (see Ch. 50).

Aim of antenatal care

The aim is to monitor the progress of pregnancy in order to support maternal health and normal fetal development. It is essential that the midwife critically evaluates the physical, psychological and sociological effects of pregnancy on the woman and her family. The midwife achieves this by:

* developing a partnership with the woman
* providing a holistic approach to the woman's care that meets her individual needs
* promoting an awareness of the public health issues for the woman and her family
* exchanging information with the woman and her family and enabling them to make informed choices about pregnancy and birth
* being an advocate for the woman and her family during her pregnancy, supporting her right to

choose care that is appropriate for her own needs and those of her family

- recognising complications of pregnancy and appropriately referring women within the multidisciplinary team
- facilitating the woman and her family in their preparations to meet the demands of birth, and making a birth plan
- facilitating the woman to make an informed choice about methods of infant feeding and giving appropriate and sensitive advice to support her decision
- offering education for parenthood within a planned programme or on an individual basis.
- working in partnership with other pertinent organisations.

Optimal antenatal care can be achieved only if the service is flexible enough to be driven by the demands of pregnant women. Women now have greater expectations, improved education, information and choice, and have therefore taken control over their fertility. Women meet demands of work, family and children, which can be stressors affecting the pregnancy. Education from health professionals, schools, the media, television and lay childbirth organisations give contrasting views about the normality of pregnancy and childbirth. Families are encouraged to participate fully in decision making and to expect emotional satisfaction from the childbearing experience.

In order to respect the diversity of women, midwives should be approachable, flexible and adapt to meet individual needs. Midwives provide the infrastructure for antenatal care within an environment of trust and safety. This should provide women with evidence-based information upon which they can make informed choices (see Ch. 3). Five steps that help to integrate sensitivity and evidence for practice are (Page 2000, p. 10):

- 'finding out what is important to the woman and her family
- using information from the clinical examination
- seeking and assessing evidence to inform decisions
- talking it through
- reflecting on outcomes, feelings and consequences.'

This method of incorporating the individual needs of the woman with sources of evidence will facilitate optimum antenatal care. The midwife has a role as counsellor and mediator and may need to utilise skills to deal with conflict or communication difficulties. She has a principal role in referring the family to appropriate professional or lay organisations.

A birth plan can be instrumental in assisting the woman towards having the birth experience of her choice. Birth plans are most effective if they are written with the midwife sharing information to enable the woman to make plans that reflect current practice and care. Some women feel empowered by having a birth plan, but this is not the case for all women (Moore & Hopper 1995).

Studies have shown that if women carry their own maternity records it enhances their satisfaction with antenatal care (Webster et al 1996) and their feeling of control during pregnancy (Elbourne et al 1987, Homer et al 1999). If women have access to their own notes this can improve communication between women and health professionals, and midwives should try to use language that is easily understood by women to alleviate anxiety. The national maternity record, developed to standardise the collection and utilisation of information in pregnancy, is still not being utilised by all NHS Trusts in the UK.

The initial assessment (booking visit)

The purpose of this visit is to introduce the woman to the maternity service. Information will be shared between the woman and midwife in order to discuss, plan and implement care for the duration of the pregnancy, the birth and postnatally.

Although it is helpful to use a prepared list to ascertain salient information, it is important not to read out a list of questions. It is more effective to integrate questions into the discussion or conversation in a systematic way. Midwives often record information on to a computer; it is, however, important to acknowledge the woman during this recording process and make her feel valued and supported. Methven (1990) suggests that the first visit at home is important to communicate information and promote discussion (see Ch. 14).

The earlier the first contact is made with the midwife, the more appropriate and valuable the advice given relating to nutrition and care of the developing fetal organs, which are almost completely formed by 12 weeks' gestation. Medical conditions, infections, smoking, alcohol or drug taking may all have a profound and detrimental effect on the fetus during this time.

Early pregnancy may leave the mother feeling exhausted, nauseous and overwhelmed about the changes occurring in her body. Women are encouraged to access their midwife through their local health centre on confirmation or suspicion of a positive pregnancy test and should be facilitated to do this. They do not require referral from a GP.

Referral may be made to a physician or obstetrician if there are known medical or psychological problems that could impact on the pregnancy, or if the pregnancy could adversely affect the condition. It is important for the midwife to maintain continuity with the woman even if she is not providing total care during the pregnancy; she can act as an advocate for the woman to enhance care given (e.g. by accompanying her to consultant appointments). It is also important for the midwife to comprehend and promote normality within the context of high risk care.

Models of midwifery care

Women can choose from a variety of midwifery care options. However, there may be restrictions resulting from resource allocation to some of these depending on where the woman lives and what services are offered locally. Options for place of birth include the home, a birth centre, peripheral unit, or a tertiary hospital.

The majority of women receive antenatal care in the community, either in their own home or at a local clinic. Hospital-based clinics are available for women who receive care from an obstetrician or physician in addition to their midwife. Women who have risk factors identified or who develop complications during pregnancy will usually plan for a hospital birth.

Introduction to the midwifery service

The woman's first introduction to midwifery care is crucial in forming her initial impressions of the maternity service. A friendly, professional approach will enable the development of a partnership between the woman and the midwife. The initial visit focuses on the exchange of information (Box 16.1). This helps the midwife and the woman to get to know each other,

---

Box 16.1 Objectives for the initial assessment

- To assess levels of health by taking a detailed history and to offer appropriate screening tests
- To ascertain baseline recordings of blood pressure, urinalysis, blood values, uterine growth and fetal development to be used as a standard for comparison as the pregnancy progresses
- To identify risk factors by taking accurate details of past and present midwifery, obstetric, medical, family and personal history
- To provide an opportunity for the woman and her family to express and discuss any concerns they might have about the current pregnancy and previous pregnancy loss, labour, birth or puerperium
- To give public health advice and that pertaining to pregnancy in order to maintain the health of the mother and the healthy development of the fetus
- To build the foundation for a trusting relationship in which the woman and midwife are partners in care

---

ideally within the woman's own environment. The midwife may meet other members of the family and in this way gain a more holistic view of the woman's needs. None the less, the midwife will also recognise that there are occasions when the woman may need to spend time with her to facilitate discussion, which she may not feel able to have in the presence of family members. For example, it is important for the midwife to recognise her own attitudes to culture and religion and to accept individual differences that may conflict with these (Schott & Henley 1996). Receiving antenatal care from a midwife in an unknown or unfamiliar environment may be the first time some women have experiences outside their own community (Schott & Henley 1996) (see Ch. 2).

Communication

The midwife requires many skills to achieve optimal antenatal care, fundamentally the ability to communicate effectively. The World Health Organization

(WHO 1985) recommended that 'The training of health care professionals should include communication techniques in order to promote sensitive exchange of information between members of the health team and the pregnant woman and her family'. The 'Changing Childbirth' report 8 years later still emphasised these basic principles of care as a means of achieving increased satisfaction for women in pregnancy and childbirth (DoH 1993).

Listening skills involve attending to or focusing on what the woman is saying, considering the words, phrases and general content of what is said (Morrison & Burnard 1997). The fluency, timing, volume and pitch of the woman's voice all impact on how the midwife listens to her (Morrison & Burnard 1997). In addition, non-verbal responses, including facial expression, body position, eye contact, proximity to the midwife and touch, will affect the flow of information between woman and midwife.

The midwife can promote communication with the woman during discussion by gentle questioning, open-ended statements and reflecting back key words from what is said to encourage and facilitate exploration of what is being said (Stein-Parbury 1993). Communication encompasses writing accurate, comprehensive and contemporaneous records of information given and received and the plan of care that has been agreed (UKCC 1998a). This is essential when there is shared care within the multidisciplinary team, as well as to ensure that the woman understands the records she holds.

First impressions

A midwife can gain much from the initial observation and assessment of a woman at the start of their first meeting. A long wait or the prospect of an assessment that she has undergone in other pregnancies may have made her anxious, irritable or angry. She may be distressed at the failure of contraception; unresolved anger may lead to unresponsive behaviour. The assessment should be carried out sensitively, enabling the woman to express her concerns about this or previous experiences of pregnancy or birth.

Observation of physical characteristics is also important. Posture and gait can indicate back problems or previous trauma to the pelvis. The woman may be lethargic, which could be an indication of extreme tiredness, anaemia, malnutrition or depression.

Social history

It is important to assess the response of the whole family to the pregnancy. An additional child may mean overcrowding in the home or even the threat of eviction. A woman may doubt her ability to care for other children during the pregnancy, birth or afterwards; teenage children may find it difficult to accept the prospect of a new baby into the family. The woman may be a teenager, still under her parents' care and there may be issues of how much support they can offer their daughter during pregnancy and following the birth. Alternatively, parents may disassociate themselves from their daughter at this time (see Ch. 2).

The current government is committed to improving health and reducing health inequalities in pregnant women and their young children (see Chs 2 and 50). The midwife may, in partnership with the woman, advocate referral to a social worker who has a role in alleviating some of these difficulties or to other multi-professional agencies where assistance can be obtained.

General health

General health should be discussed and good habits reinforced, giving further advice when required. Exercise puts added demands on the cardiovascular and respiratory systems. However, usual exercise should be continued (see Ch. 15).

Smoking. Women may be ready to cut down or give up smoking, thinking about it, or not yet ready (Prochaska 1992). They often need a motivator in order to change; this may be their unborn baby, their own health, longevity, finance, wanting to see their grandchildren or any other factor. The midwife has a duty to help women set goals throughout their pregnancy and help them to cut down their smoking, ideally giving up. Strategies to help women cut down, such as making their home/car smoke free, doing something else, delaying having a cigarette, or drinking water, can be helpful. Babies born to women who smoke are frequently smaller (see Ch. 41), they frequently have respiratory problems at birth and in their first year; there are also higher rates of prematurity, stillbirth and low birthweight (Floyd et al 1993, Li & Windsor 1993). There is furthermore an increased risk of asthma and otitis media in these babies (Nafstad et al 1996). For women who are more addicted, start smoking earlier in the day, stop last thing at night or desperately feel the need to smoke, the midwife should offer referral to appropriate organisations such as the NHS Quit Smoking line (DoH 1999a). The woman, her partner and other family members should be informed about the direct and passive effects of smoking on the baby. Cigarette smoking in pregnancy increases the risk of babies dying from sudden infant death syndrome (Blair et al 1996). In women who smoke 20 cigarettes per day, the baby has a 15 times greater risk of dying from sudden infant death syndrome (SIDS) than a baby of a non-smoker (Mitchell et al 1997).

Alcohol. Alcohol abuse is less common but can affect the baby (see Ch. 47). There is no conclusive evidence of adverse effects on the fetus at a consumption level below 10 units per week; however, it is recommended that women do not exceed one to two units once or twice a week (RCOG 2000).

Menstrual history

An accurate menstrual history is taken to determine the expected date of delivery (EDD). This will enable the midwife to predict a birth date and subsequently calculate gestational age at any point in the pregnancy. Abdominal assessment of uterine size can be made in conjunction with gestational age during the antenatal consultation. The midwife has a role in helping the woman to understand that an EDD is 1 day within a 5 week time frame during which her baby is term, and may be born.

The EDD is calculated by adding 9 calendar months and 7 days to the date of the 1st day of the woman's last menstrual period. This method assumes that:

- the woman takes regular note of regularity and length of time between periods
- conception occurred 14 days after the 1st day of the last period; this is true only if the woman has a regular 28 day cycle
- the last period of bleeding was true menstruation; implantation of the ovum may cause slight bleeding.

The duration of pregnancy based on Naegele's rule suggests that the duration of a pregnancy is 280 days. However, it is useful to consider that if the woman has a 35 day cycle then 7 days should be added to the EDD owing to the long second menstrual phase; if her cycle is less than 28 days then the appropriate number of days is subtracted (see Ch. 9).

Controversy exists over the suitability of applying Naegele's rule to determine EDD. Predicted dates of delivery were studied in over 14 000 women with a reliable date of LMP (by average length of pregnancy, 280 or 282 days) (Nguyen et al 1999). They found the average discrepancies between date of delivery predicted from the bi-parietal diameter, or BPD (on ultrasound in the second trimester) were 7.96 and 8.63 days respectively. The error of the LMP method alone was reduced significantly by adding 282 days to the LMP instead of 280 days. This method would reduce the incidence of post-term pregnancy; however, the authors concluded that use of BPD alone is superior to the use of LMP, but if LMP is the only predictor available then 282 days should be added to the LMP. These findings support the work of Tunon et al (1996) who found that if LMP and ultrasound differ by less than 8 days then neither method could more accurately predict EDD. However, as the difference in gestational age between the two methods increases, ultrasound becomes the more accurate method for predicting the EDD. These findings do depend on the availability of and accessibility to an experienced ultrasonographer, however, and the woman's consent to have an ultrasound scan. Ultrasound before 15 weeks confirms the EDD; the 18–22 week scan identifies abnormalities. Women should be given information about ultrasound to help them make an informed choice about the screening test (MIDIRS and NHS Centre for Research and Dissemination 1999).

If the woman has taken oral contraceptives within the previous 3 months, this may also confuse estimation of dates because breakthrough bleeding and anovular cycles lead to inaccuracies. Some women become pregnant with an intrauterine contraceptive device (IUCD) still in place. Although the pregnancy is likely to continue normally, the position of the IUCD may be determined using ultrasound techniques.

Obstetric history

Past childbearing experiences have an important part to play in predicting the possible outcome of the current pregnancy. In order to give a summary of a woman's childbearing history, the descriptive terms *gravida* and *para* are used. 'Gravid' means 'pregnant', gravida means 'a pregnant woman', and a subsequent number indicates the number of times she has been

Box 16.2 Factors that may require additional antenatal surveillance or advice

Initial assessment

- Age less than 18 years or over 35 years
- Grande multiparity (more than four previous births)
- Vaginal bleeding at any time during pregnancy
- Unknown or uncertain expected date of delivery

Past obstetric history

- Stillbirth or neonatal death
- Baby small or large for gestational age
- Congenital abnormality
- Rhesus isoimmunisation
- Pregnancy-induced hypertension
- Two or more terminations of pregnancy
- Two or more spontaneous abortions
- Previous preterm labour
- Cervical cerclage in past or present pregnancy
- Previous caesarean section or uterine surgery
- Ante- or postpartum haemorrhage
- Precipitate labour
- Multiple pregnancy

Maternal health

- Previous history of deep vein thrombosis or pulmonary embolism
- Chronic illness
- Hypertension
- History of infertility
- Uterine anomaly including fibroids
- Smoking
- Family history of diabetes
- Alcohol or drug taking
- Psychological or psychiatric disorders

Examination at the initial assessment

- Blood pressure 140/90 or above
- Maternal obesity or underweight according to BMI
- Maternal height of 150 cm (5 feet) or less
- Cardiac murmur detected
- Other pelvic mass detected
- Rhesus negative blood group
- Blood disorders

pregnant regardless of outcome. 'Para' means 'having given birth'; a woman's parity refers to the number of times that she has given birth to a child, live or still-born, excluding abortions. A *grande multigravida* is a woman who has been pregnant five times or more irrespective of outcome. A *grande multipara* is a woman who has given birth five times or more.

Pregnancy-induced hypertension is more than twice as common in a first pregnancy (primigravida) than in multiparas (Hallak 1999). The incidence is, however, higher in women over 35 years of age (where it may be superimposed over chronic hypertension) and in women who have experienced it in a first pregnancy (Campbell et al 1985). It is also a risk factor in multi-gravidas who have a new partner (Dekker et al 1998) (see Ch. 20).

Previous termination of pregnancy is usually discussed although it may cause the woman embarrassment or distress. A sympathetic non-judgmental approach is required in order to elicit information and encourage the woman to talk freely about her feelings. Sometimes feelings are not expressed or resolved at the time of the miscarriage or termination. The interruption of the pregnancy may have affected the way in which the woman accepted it at the time, perhaps grieving the loss of hopes and expectations of a pregnancy (Rafael-Leff 1991). This may lead to the suppression of feelings, which could interfere with emotional adjustment to the present pregnancy. In rare cases techniques employed in termination may affect the viability of subsequent pregnancies. Dilatation and curettage could contribute to cervical incompetence (see Ch. 17). Any form of abortion occurring in a Rhesus negative woman requires prophylactic administration of anti-D immunoglobulin to reduce the risk of Rhesus incompatibility in a subsequent pregnancy (see Fig. 46.7, p. 870).

Confidential information may be recorded in a clinic-held summary of the pregnancy and not in the woman's handheld record if she requests this. Repeated spontaneous abortion (miscarriage) may indicate such conditions as genetic abnormality, hormonal imbalance or incompetent cervix. Diagnosis of the cause often depends on the time at which the abortion occurred. Screening or treatment may be necessary in the present pregnancy. The woman may also be more anxious about the pregnancy and will usually be relieved when it progresses past the date of previous miscarriages. Minor disturbances in pregnancy may be exacerbated and preoccupation with the pregnancy may lead to other psychological, social or physical problems. She is likely to feel reassured if she hears the fetal heart or sees the image on an ultrasound scan.

For completeness of the history, reference to old case notes should be made in case the pregnant woman has not recalled all the relevant information. A risk assessment should be carried out based on the woman's obstetric and medical history and current pregnancy. This will enable the midwife and woman to discuss the progress of her pregnancy and identify other health professionals who may need to be involved. If risk factors such as those listed in Box 16.2 are identified, they can help to determine the frequency of antenatal visits and alert staff to appropriate screening techniques. This should follow an individualised approach, using Page's five steps (Page 2000). The location of antenatal care will be determined by the availability of support services, senior obstetric staff and experienced midwives. Place of birth will also be influenced by the risk assessment but in all cases the ultimate decision is taken by the mother who should make an informed choice.

Medical history

During pregnancy both the mother and the fetus may be affected by a medical condition, or a medical condition may be altered by the pregnancy; if untreated there may be serious consequences for the woman's health.

- Urinary stasis and reflux occur during pregnancy. A urinary tract infection (UTI) can easily develop into pyelonephritis, which, untreated, may lead to kidney damage and cause preterm labour (Romero et al 1989). Between 30 and 50% of women with asymptomatic bacteriuria will develop pyelonephritis if it is untreated (Romero et al 1989).
- Pregnancy predisposes to deep vein thrombosis and thus pulmonary embolism. Women of increasing parity and maternal age, those who are obese and those with a history of thromboembolic disorders are most at risk (de Swiet 1999).
- Essential hypertension predisposes to pregnancy-induced hypertension (PIH), which can result in reduced placental function, intrauterine growth restriction, abruptio placenta, fetal compromise or death (Hallak 1999). Effects on the mother include congestive heart failure, intracerebral haemorrhage, acute renal failure, disseminated intravascular coagulation (DIC) or death as a result of any of the above (Hallak 1999, see Ch. 20)
- Other conditions including asthma, epilepsy, infections and psychiatric disorders may require drug treatment, which may adversely affect fetal development (see Ch. 48). Major medical complications such as diabetes and cardiac conditions require the involvement and support of a medical specialist (see Ch. 19).

Family history

Certain conditions are genetic in origin, others are familial or related to ethnicity, and some are associated with the physical or social environment in which the family lives. Evidence shows that there is a higher mortality rate in babies born to mothers of Pakistan or Caribbean origin (DOH 1999b). Bundey et al (1991) showed that the perinatal mortality rate of Pakistani infants was more than double that of Europeans, although there was a relationship between lower social class and this group. There was evidence of a high rate of consanguinity within the Pakistani families. Genetic disease in the baby is much more likely to occur if his biological parents are close relatives such as first cousins (Stoltenberg et al 1998).

Diabetes, although not genetically inherited, leads to a predisposition in other family members, particularly if they become pregnant or obese. Hypertension also has a familial component and multiple pregnancy has a higher incidence in certain families. Some conditions such as sickle cell anaemia and thalassaemia are more common in particular races.

Physical examination

Prior to conducting the physical examination of a pregnant woman, her consent and comfort are primary considerations. Sophisticated biochemical assessments and ultrasound investigations can enhance clinical observations.

Although women are not routinely measured to determine their height, short stature is associated with some complications of pregnancy and birth, for example shoulder dystocia (Olugibile & Mascarenhas 2000). The relationship between shoe size and pelvic capacity remains controversial (Frame et al 1985, Mahmood et al 1988). A woman who is short in stature may come from an ethnic group that is usually smaller than a Western woman; however, the size of the fetus is usually in proportion to the size of the woman's pelvis. It is therefore important to look holistically at the woman and her family and assess fetal growth and development by the recognised markers in conjunction with this knowledge.

Weight

Women with a BMI in the obese range are more at risk of complications of pregnancy (see Ch. 12). These may include gestational diabetes, PIH and shoulder dystocia. There may also be difficulty in palpating the fetal parts and defining presentation, position or engagement of the fetus.

All women should be weighed or asked for a pre-pregnant weight at booking, but if it is within the normal BMI range there is insufficient evidence to suggest that routine weighing is a good predictor of fetal growth (Hytten 1990). Overweight or underweight women should be carefully monitored and offered nutritional counselling (Boyle 1995).

Blood pressure

Blood pressure is taken in order to ascertain normality and provide a baseline reading for comparison throughout pregnancy. The systolic recording may be falsely elevated if a woman is nervous or anxious; long waiting times can cause additional stress. A full bladder can also cause an increase in blood pressure. Blood pressure should be checked with the woman relaxed. The woman should be comfortably seated or resting in a lateral position on the couch for the blood pressure to be taken. Brachial artery pressure is highest when sitting and lower when in the recumbent position. An adequate blood pressure is required to maintain placental perfusion but a systolic blood pressure of 140 mmHg or diastolic pressure of 90 mmHg at booking is indicative of hypertension and will need careful monitoring during pregnancy with both midwife and obstetrician support.

Until recently the Korotkoff 4 (K4) sound (muffled, fading sound) has been recorded as the diastolic pressure in pregnant women in the belief that the K5 (absence of sound) is not always present (Herbert & Alison 1996). However, in a recent study involving 85 pregnant women to compare the accuracy of recording K4 compared with K5, K4 was heard in fewer than half of measurements compared with K5, which was identified in all measurements. Listening for K5 in pregnancy was therefore recommended except in the rare cases when it is absent (Shennan et al 1996). A randomised trial with 220 women in 1998 concluded that the universal adoption of K5 should be considered, it found using this instead of K4 did not result in any adverse outcomes for the women or their babies and in no case was K5 registered as 0 mmHg. Steps that can be taken to increase accuracy of blood pressure measurement and recording are listed in Box 16.3.

Box 16.3 Factors that increase accuracy of blood pressure measurement and recording (Bisson et al 1990)

- A regularly serviced sphygmomanometer (conventional mercury sphygmomanometer is the most reliable, see Lewis & Drife 2001, p. 76)
- The correct width of cuff should be chosen for the woman
- The radial pulse should be estimated and the cuff pumped up 30 mmHg above this level before ausculating the brachial pulse
- Blood pressure should be recorded to the nearest 2 mmHg
- The woman should be relaxed and comfortable

Urinalysis

Urinalysis is performed at every visit to exclude abnormality (Way 2000). The woman can be shown how to test her own urine and encouraged to test it at subsequent visits. At the first visit a midstream specimen may be sent to the laboratory for culture to exclude asymptomatic bacteruria. This condition exists when a culture is grown of a specific bacterium that exceeds 10^6 organisms per millilitre of urine. As it is asymptomatic the woman is unaware of disease. Pyelonephritis can readily develop from it because of the changes in the renal tract during pregnancy.

Other possible findings during subsequent routine urinalysis include:

- ketones due to fat breakdown to provide glucose, caused by unmet fetal demands that may be due to vomiting, hyperemesis, starvation or excessive exercise
- glucose caused by higher circulating blood levels, reduced renal threshold or disease
- protein due to contamination by vaginal leucorrhoea, or disease such as urinary tract infection or hypertensive disorders of pregnancy.

(See Chapters 18 and 19 for further information.)

Blood tests in pregnancy

The midwife should explain why blood tests are carried out at the booking visit (UKCC 1998b). Women should be facilitated by the midwife to make an informed choice about the tests that are available. The midwife should be fully aware of the difference between screening and diagnostic tests, and their accuracy, and discuss these options with women. Blood tests taken at the initial assessment include the following:

ABO blood group and Rhesus (Rh) factor. Antibody screening is performed followed by titration if present. Normal follow-up of a woman whose blood group is Rh negative will include further blood samples at 28, 32, 36 and 40 weeks to ensure that the pregnancy is not stimulating antibody activity. Rhesus negative women who have threatened miscarriage, amniocentesis or any other uterine trauma should be given anti-D gammaglobulin within a few days of the event. If the titration demonstrates a rising antibody response then more frequent assessment will be made in order to plan management by a specialist in Rhesus disease (see Ch. 46).

Full blood count. This is taken to observe the woman's general blood picture, and includes:

Haemoglobin (Hb) estimations (see Ch. 13 for normal values). If the mean cell volume (MCV) is found to be low on the full blood count result, serum ferritin levels are also taken in order to assess the adequacy of iron stores. Haemoglobin estimation is repeated at 28–32 weeks when the physiological effects of haemodilution are becoming more apparent and sometimes at 36 weeks if levels were low and treatment has been commenced. Iron supplementation is not considered necessary in women who are taking adequate dietary iron and who have a normal Hb and MCV at the initial assessment. The decision to use supplements should be made on an individual basis and include clear information about dietary iron sources. Woman who are vegetarian, fasting for cultural reasons or have an aversion to some foods may be able to absorb sufficient iron to meet their own and their baby's needs given good information. Gastrointestinal upsets are common as a result of oral iron and many women find the tablets unpleasant. However, frequent conceptions and breastfeeding may deplete iron stores and necessitate replacement. Maximum absorption of iron in meat or green leafy vegetables will be achieved by consuming vitamin C at the same time and avoiding caffeine. The intestinal mucosa have a limited ability to absorb iron and when this is exceeded extra iron is excreted in the stools. Folic acid should be taken preconception and for the first 12 weeks of pregnancy to reduce the risk of spina bifida (McLeod et al 1996).

Venereal Disease Research Laboratory (VDRL) test. This is performed for syphilis. Not all positive results indicate active syphilis. Early testing will allow a woman to be treated in order to prevent infection of the fetus (see Ch. 21).

HIV antibodies. Routine screening to detect HIV infection is recommended in pregnancy given that pretest discussion is carried out (Ades et al 1999). Current evidence suggests that treatment in pregnancy is beneficial in reducing vertical transmission to the fetus (Nichol 1998). There are many views as to the ethical issues involved in screening. It is important to gain informed consent for any blood tests undertaken and offer appropriate counselling before and after the screening is carried out.

Rubella immune status. This is determined by measuring the rubella antibody titre. Women who are not immune must be advised to avoid contact with anyone suffering from the disease and may wish to discuss termination of pregnancy if they have been exposed. The live vaccination is offered during the puerperium, and subsequent pregnancy must be avoided for at least 3 months.

Investigations for other blood disorders. These may be sought in women and their partners of some ethnic groups, for example for sickle cell disease or thalassaemia. If a woman either has or is a carrier of one of these diseases her partner's blood should also be tested. The couple will be offered genetic counselling and management during pregnancy will be explained (see Ch. 23).

Routine screening for hepatitis B. This is now recommended in order to reduce the risk of perinatal transmission and the subsequent associated morbidity and mortality in the infant.

Screening tests for cytomegalovirus and toxoplasmosis. These are not routinely done in pregnancy. Wallon et al (1999) reviewed the evidence for treating toxoplasmosis in pregnancy to reduce the risk of congenital toxoplasma in infants; there were no clear findings. Considering that screening is expensive, the effects of treatment and the impact of screening programmes have yet to be evaluated (Wallon et al 1999) (see Ch. 23).

The midwife's examination

The midwife's examination of the woman is performed by exchange of information between the woman and midwife and observation rather than physical examination. Communication has been shown to be most effective if the woman is sitting in a comfortable position feeling that she has the attention of the midwife. The woman needs to consent to the procedures and give informed consent for any physical examinations that the midwife wishes to carry out.

The midwife's general examination of the woman is holistic and should encompass her physical, social and psychological well-being. The usual social contact gives the midwife an opportunity to look at the woman's face and assess her health and general well-being. Sleeping patterns can be disrupted in pregnancy. Women frequently continue to work throughout pregnancy, therefore they are unlikely to be able to rest during the day and many need to go to

bed earlier to alleviate the tiredness (see Ch. 14). If at any time the midwife notices any sign of ill health she should discuss this with the woman, and advocate referral to the most appropriate health professional.

The midwife should facilitate discussion about infant feeding. Breastfeeding should be promoted in a sensitive manner and information given about the benefits to both mother and baby (see Ch. 40, RCM 2000, UKCC 1998b). Most women will not require an examination of their breasts. Current evidence does not support the benefits of nipple preparation (Alexander et al 1992). The midwife may also discuss the woman's experiences of breast changes so far in her pregnancy, and expected changes as pregnancy progresses.

Some women will appreciate information about the body changes taking place during pregnancy. Increasing abdominal size may be an acceptable body change but breast changes may not have been anticipated. For some women breast size and appearance are an important part of their body image (see Ch. 13). Partners may also be affected by the changes. The midwife can be influential in discussions with women who had not realised the extent to which pregnancy would change their body. Open and honest discussion between the woman and her partner may help to resolve anxieties. A good relationship in which the couple feels able to share anxieties and fears may minimise some of the difficulties in making the transition to motherhood.

Bladder and bowel function may be discussed; dietary advice may be necessary at this visit or later in the pregnancy with reference to how hormonal changes may alter normal bowel and kidney function.

Early referral within the multidisciplinary team will be necessary if treatment is required or problems identified. Vaginal discharge increases in pregnancy; the woman may discuss any increase or changes with the midwife. Once the woman has identified what is normal she will then be able to report any changes to the midwife during subsequent visits. If the discharge is itchy, causes soreness, is any colour other than creamy-white or has an offensive odour then infection is likely, and should be investigated further. Later in pregnancy the woman may report a change from leucorrhoea to a heavier mucous discharge. Mucoid loss is evidence of cervical changes and if it occurs before the 37th week may be an early sign of preterm labour.

The obstetrician will investigate vaginal bleeding during pregnancy; however, in early pregnancy spotting may occur at the time when menstruation would have been due. Early bleeding is not uncommon; the midwife should advise the woman to rest at this time and avoid sexual intercourse until the pregnancy is more stable. Ultrasound will help the obstetrician to confirm a diagnosis.

Abdominal examination. This should be performed at each antenatal visit (see below). At the initial assessment the midwife will observe for signs of pregnancy. It is unlikely that the uterus will be palpable abdominally before the 12th week of gestation. If it has previously been retroverted it may not be palpable until the 16th week.

Oedema. This is not likely to be in evidence during the initial assessment but may occur as the pregnancy progresses. Physiological oedema occurs after rising in the morning and worsens during the day; it is often associated with daily activities or hot weather. At visits later in pregnancy the midwife should observe for oedema and ask the woman about symptoms. Often the woman may notice that her rings feel tighter and her ankles are swollen. Pitting oedema in the lower limbs can be identified by applying gentle fingertip pressure over the tibial bone: a depression will remain when the finger is removed. If oedema reaches the knees, affects the face or is increasing in the fingers it may be indicative of PIH if other markers are also present.

Varicosities. These are more likely to occur during pregnancy and are a predisposing cause of deep vein thrombosis. The woman should be asked if she has any pain in her legs. Reddened areas on the calf may be due to varicosities, phlebitis or deep vein thrombosis. Areas that appear white as if deprived of blood could be caused by deep vein thrombosis. The woman should be asked to report any tenderness that she feels either during the examination or at any time during the pregnancy. Referral should be made to medical colleagues as appropriate (UKCC 1998b). Advice about support tights can be offered.

Medical examination

If the woman is seen by a GP instead of a midwife she may undergo a medical examination. Some doctors still perform this examination as they see it as an opportunity to examine the heart and lungs. A soft systolic murmur is often heard in pregnant women but all other abnormalities would be referred for the physician's opinion.

A vaginal examination is unnecessary in the initial assessment. A Papanicolaou smear is usually deferred until the puerperium.

Abdominal examination

The abdominal examination is carried out to establish and affirm that fetal growth is consistent with gestational age during the progression of pregnancy.

The specific aims are to:

- observe the signs of pregnancy
- assess fetal size and growth
- auscultate the fetal heart
- locate fetal parts
- detect any deviation from normal.

The examination can be worrying for women, and sensitive communication throughout the procedure is vital (Olsen 1999).

Preparation

The abdominal examination will be most effective if the woman is consistently in the same position at each antenatal check (Engstrom et al 1993). A study comparing supine, trunk elevation, knee flexion and trunk elevation with knee flexion found there were significant differences between each in estimating fundal height measurements (Engstrom et al 1993). A full bladder will make the examination uncomfortable; this can also make the measurement of fundal height less accurate. It is important that the midwife exposes only that area of the abdomen she needs to palpate, and covers the remainder of the woman to enhance privacy. The woman should be lying comfortably with her arms by her sides to relax the abdominal muscles. She should then sit up to discuss the findings with the midwife.

Method

Inspection

The size of the uterus is assessed approximately by observation. A full bladder, distended colon or obesity may give a false impression of fetal size, however. The shape of the uterus is longer than it is broad when the lie of the fetus is longitudinal, as occurs in the majority of cases. If the lie of the fetus is transverse, the uterus is low and broad.

The multiparous uterus may lack the snug ovoid shape of the primigravid uterus. Often it is possible to see the shape of the fetal back or limbs. If the fetus is in an occipitoposterior position a saucer-like depression may be seen at or below the umbilicus. The midwife may observe fetal movements, or they may be felt by the mother; this can help the midwife determine the position of the fetus. The umbilicus becomes less dimpled as pregnancy advances and may protrude slightly in later weeks. When the woman is standing, lightening may be evident (see Ch. 13).

Lax abdominal muscles in the multiparous woman may allow the uterus to sag forwards; this is known as *pendulous abdomen* or anterior obliquity of the uterus. In the primigravida it is a serious sign as it may be due to pelvic contraction.

Skin changes. Stretch marks from previous pregnancies appear silvery and recent ones appear pink. A *linea nigra* may be seen; this is a normal dark line of pigmentation running longitudinally in the centre of the abdomen below and sometimes above the umbilicus. Scars may indicate previous obstetric or abdominal surgery.

Palpation

The midwife's hands should be clean and warm; cold hands do not have the necessary acute sense of touch, they tend to induce contraction of the abdominal and uterine muscles and the woman may find palpation uncomfortable. Arms and hands should be relaxed and the pads, not the tips, of the fingers used with delicate precision. The hands are moved smoothly over the abdomen in a stroking motion in order to avoid causing contractions.

In order to determine the height of the fundus the midwife places her hand just below the xiphisternum. Pressing gently, she moves her hand down the abdomen until she feels the curved upper border of the fundus, noting the number of fingerbreadths that can be accommodated between the two (Fig. 16.1). Alternatively, the distance between the fundus and the symphysis pubis can be determined with a tape measure, although current research has shown that there is still insufficient evidence to evaluate this method fully (Neilson 2001). Measurements can be recorded in the pregnancy record or plotted on a chart that gives average findings for gestational age: a symphysis–fundal

height chart (Gardosi & Francis 1999). The height of the fundus correlates well with gestational age, especially during the earlier weeks of pregnancy. For example, the uterine size is approximately 22–24 weeks' gestation if the fundus of the uterus can be felt at the umbilicus (Fig. 16.2).

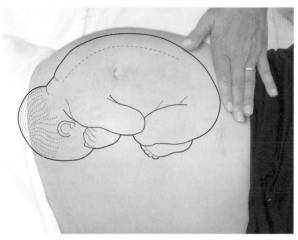

Fig. 16.1 Assessing the fundal height in fingerbreadths below the xiphisternum.

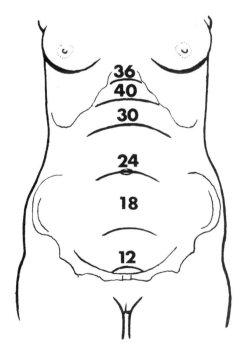

Fig. 16.2 Growth of the uterus, showing the fundal heights at various weeks of pregnancy.

Clinically assessing the uterine size to compare it with gestation does not always produce an accurate result because the size and number of fetuses and the amount of amniotic fluid vary. Variations in maternal size and parity may also affect the estimation. If the uterus is unduly big the fetus may be large, but multiple pregnancy or polyhydramnios may be suspected. When the uterus is smaller than expected the LMP date may be incorrect, or the fetus may be small for gestational age.

Pelvic palpation. Pelvic palpation can cause contractions of the uterus therefore it is often carried out before fundal and lateral palpation to make the findings easier to determine. However, some would argue that it should be carried out last. Pelvic palpation will identify the pole of the fetus in the pelvis; it should not cause discomfort to the woman.

The midwife should ask the woman to bend her knees slightly in order to relax the abdominal muscles and also suggest that she breathe steadily; relaxation may be helped if she sighs out slowly. The sides of the uterus just below umbilical level are grasped snugly between the palms of the hands with the fingers held close together, and pointing downwards and inwards (Fig. 16.3).

If the head is presenting, a hard mass with a distinctive round, smooth surface will be felt. The midwife should also estimate how much of the fetal head is palpable above the pelvic brim to determine engagement. The two-handed technique appears to be the most comfortable for the woman and gives the most information. Pawlik's manoeuvre is sometimes used to judge the size, flexion and mobility of the head but the midwife must be careful not to apply undue pressure. It should be used only if absolutely necessary. The midwife grasps the lower pole of the uterus between her fingers and thumb, which should be spread wide enough apart to accommodate the fetal head (Fig. 16.4). There is no research evidence to support one method over the other.

Lateral palpation. This is used to locate the fetal back in order to determine position. The hands are placed on either side of the uterus at the level of the umbilicus (Fig. 16.5). Gentle pressure is applied with alternate hands in order to detect which side of the uterus offers the greater resistance. More detailed information is obtained by feeling along the length of each side with the fingers. This can be done by sliding the hands down the abdomen while feeling the sides

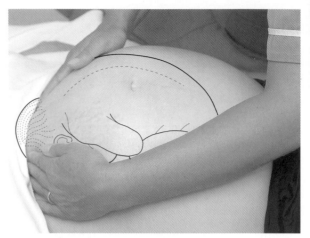

Fig. 16.3 Pelvic palpation. The fingers are directed inwards and downwards.

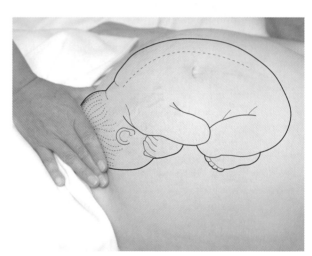

Fig. 16.4 Pawlik's manoeuvre. The lower pole of the uterus is grasped with the right hand, the midwife facing the woman's head.

of the uterus alternately. Some midwives prefer to steady the uterus with one hand and, using a rotary movement of the opposite hand, to map out the back as a continuous smooth resistant mass from the breech down to the neck; on the other side the same movement reveals the limbs as small parts that slip about under the examining fingers.

'Walking' the fingertips of both hands over the abdomen from one side to the other is an excellent method of locating the back (Fig. 16.6). The fingers

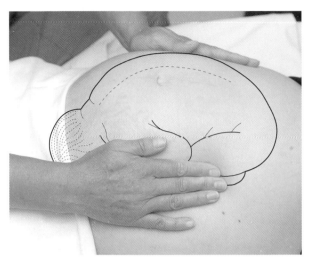

Fig. 16.5 Lateral palpation. Hands placed at umbilical level on either side of the uterus. Pressure is applied alternately with each hand.

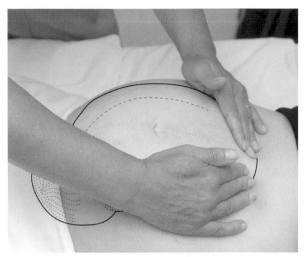

Fig. 16.7 Fundal palpation. Palms of hands on either side of the fundus, fingers held close together palpate the upper pole of the uterus.

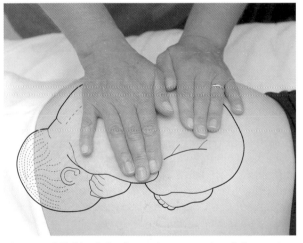

Fig. 16.6 'Walking' the fingertips across the abdomen to locate the position of the fetal back.

should be dipped into the abdominal wall deeply. The firm back can be distinguished from the fluctuating amniotic fluid and the receding knobbly small parts. To make the back more prominent, fundal pressure can be applied with one hand and the other used to 'walk' over the abdomen. Palpating from the neck upwards and inwards can locate the anterior shoulder.

Fundal palpation. This determines the presence of the breech or the head. This information will help to diagnose the lie and presentation of the fetus. Watching the woman's reaction to the procedure, the midwife lays both hands on the sides of the fundus, fingers held close together and curving round the upper border of the uterus. Gentle yet deliberate pressure is applied using the palmar surfaces of the fingers to determine the soft consistency and indefinite outline that denotes the breech. Sometimes the buttocks feel rather firm but they are not as hard, smooth or well defined as the head. With a gliding movement the fingertips are separated slightly in order to grasp the fetal mass, which may be in the centre or deflected to one side, to assess its size and mobility. The breech cannot be moved independently of the body as can the head (Fig. 16.7).

The head is much more distinctive in outline than the breech, being hard and round; it can be balloted (moved from one hand to the other) between the fingertips of the two hands because of the free movement of the neck.

Auscultation

Listening to the fetal heart is an important part of the process. Like all heartbeats it is a double sound, but more rapid than the adult heart. A Pinard's fetal stethoscope will enable the midwife to hear the fetal heart directly and determine that it is fetal and not maternal. The stethoscope is placed on the mother's abdomen, at right angles to it over the fetal back (Fig. 16.8). The ear must be in close, firm contact with the stethoscope but the hand should not touch it while listening because then extraneous sounds are produced. The stethoscope should be moved about until the point of maximum intensity is located where the fetal heart is heard most clearly. The midwife should count the beats per minute, which should be in the range of 110–160 (NICE 2001). The midwife should take the woman's pulse at the same time as listening to the fetal heart to enable her to distinguish between the two. In addition, ultrasound equipment (e.g. a sonicaid or Doppler) can be used for this purpose so that the woman may also hear the fetal heartbeat. However, use of a Pinard's stethoscope will enable the midwife to hear the actual heartbeat and not the reflected soundwaves produced from the ultrasound equipment.

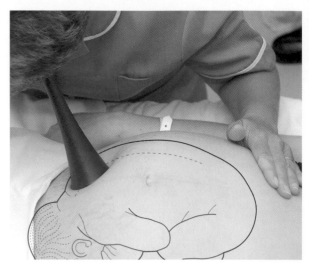

Fig. 16.8 Auscultation of the fetal heart. Vertex right occipitoanterior.

Findings

The findings from the abdominal palpation should be considered as part of the holistic picture of the pregnant woman. The midwife assesses all the information which she has gathered from inspection, palpation and auscultation and critically evaluates the well-being of the mother and the fetus. Deviation from the expected growth and development should be referred to the obstetrician. Concerns about this screening process may also be discussed within the interprofessional team.

Gestational age

During pregnancy the uterus is expected to grow at a predicted rate and in early pregnancy uterine size will usually equate with the gestation estimated by dates (see Fig. 16.2). Later in pregnancy, increasing uterine size gives evidence of continuing fetal growth but is less reliable as an indicator of gestational age.

Multiple pregnancy increases the overall uterine size and should be diagnosed by 24 weeks' gestation. In a singleton pregnancy the fundus reaches the umbilicus at 22–24 weeks and the xiphisternum at 36 weeks. In the last month of pregnancy lightening occurs as the fetus sinks down into the lower pole of the uterus. The uterus becomes broader and the fundus lower. In the primigravida strong, supportive abdominal muscles encourage the fetal head to enter the brim of the pelvis.

Lie

The lie of the fetus is the relationship between the long axis of the fetus and the long axis of the uterus (Figs 16.9–16.13). In the majority of cases the lie is *longitudinal* owing to the ovoid shape of the uterus; the remainder are oblique or transverse. *Oblique lie*, when the fetus lies diagonally across the long axis of the uterus, must be distinguished from *obliquity of the uterus*, when the whole uterus is tilted to one side (usually the right) and the fetus lies longitudinally within it. When the lie is *transverse* the fetus lies at right angles across the long axis of the uterus. This is often visible on inspection of the abdomen.

Attitude

Attitude is the relationship of the fetal head and limbs to its trunk. The attitude should be one of flexion. The fetus is curled up with chin on chest, arms and legs flexed, forming a snug, compact mass, which utilises the space in the uterine cavity most effectively. If the fetal head is flexed the smallest diameters will be presenting and, with efficient uterine action, the labour will be most effective.

Presentation

Presentation refers to the part of the fetus that lies at the pelvic brim or in the lower pole of the uterus.

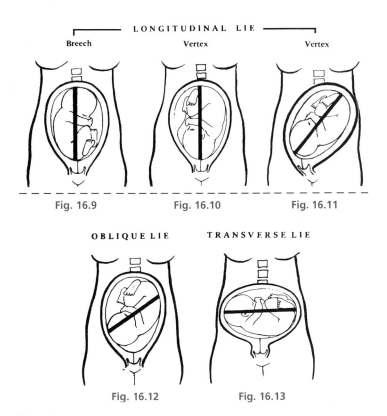

LONGITUDINAL LIE

Breech   Vertex   Vertex

Fig. 16.9   Fig. 16.10   Fig. 16.11

OBLIQUE LIE   TRANSVERSE LIE

Fig. 16.12   Fig. 16.13

Figs 16.9–16.13 The lie of the fetus.
Figures 16.9, 16.10, and 16.11 depict the longitudinal lie. Confusion sometimes exists regarding Figure 16.11, which gives the impression of an oblique lie, but the fetus is longitudinal in relation to the uterus and merely moving the uterus abdominally rectifies the presumed obliquity.
Figure 16.12 shows an oblique lie because the long axis of the fetus is oblique in relation to the uterus.
Figure 16.13 shows the true transverse lie with shoulder presentation.

Presentations can be *vertex, breech, shoulder, face* or *brow* (Figs 16.14–16.19). Vertex, face and brow are all head or cephalic presentations. When the head is flexed the vertex presents; when it is fully extended the face presents and when partially extended the brow presents (Figs 16.20–16.23). It is more common for the head to present because the bulky breech finds more space in the fundus, which is the widest diameter of the uterus, and the head lies in the narrower lower pole. The muscle tone of the fetus also plays a part in maintaining its flexion and consequently its vertex presentation.

Denominator

'Denominate' means 'to give a name to'; the denominator is the name of the part of the presentation, which is used when referring to fetal position. Each presentation has a different denominator and these are as follows:

- in the vertex presentation it is the occiput
- in the breech presentation it is the sacrum
- in the face presentation it is the mentum.

Although the shoulder presentation is said to have the acromion process as its denominator, in practice the dorsum is used to describe the position. In the brow presentation no denominator is used.

Position

The position is the relationship between the denominator of the presentation and six points on the pelvic brim (Fig. 16.24). In addition, the denominator may

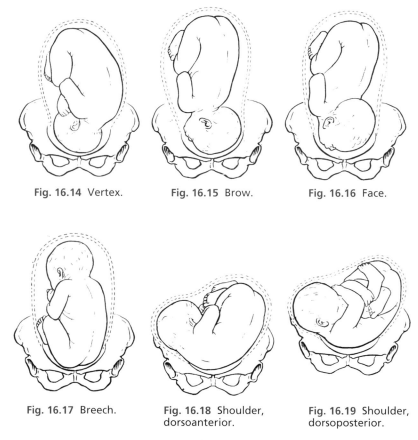

Fig. 16.14 Vertex.   Fig. 16.15 Brow.   Fig. 16.16 Face.

Fig. 16.17 Breech.   Fig. 16.18 Shoulder,   Fig. 16.19 Shoulder,
                            dorsoanterior.   dorsoposterior.

Figs 16.14–16.19 The five presentations.

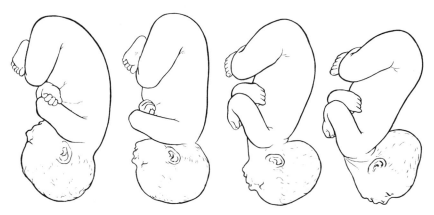

Fig. 16.20 Vertex   Fig. 16.21 Vertex   Fig. 16.22 Brow.   Fig. 16.23 Face.
(well-flexed head).   (deflexed head).

Figs 16.20–16.23 Varieties of cephalic or head presentation.

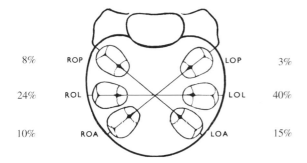

Fig. 16.24 Diagrammatic representation of the six vertex positions and their relative frequency: LOA = left occipitoanterior; LOL = left occipitolateral; LOP = left occipitoposterior; ROA = right occipitoanterior; ROL = right occipitolateral; ROP = right occipitoposterior.

be found in the midline either anteriorly or posteriorly, especially late in labour. This position is often transient and is described as *direct anterior* or *direct posterior*.

Anterior positions are more favourable than posterior positions because when the fetal back is in front it conforms to the concavity of the mother's abdominal wall and can therefore flex more easily. When the back is flexed the head also tends to flex and a smaller diameter presents to the pelvic brim. There is also more room in the anterior part of the pelvic brim for the broad biparietal diameter of the head.

The positions in a vertex presentation are summarised in Box 16.4.

Engagement

Engagement is said to have occurred when the widest presenting transverse diameter has passed through the brim of the pelvis. In cephalic presentations this is the biparietal diameter and in breech presentations the bitrochanteric diameter. Engagement demonstrates that the maternal pelvis is likely to be adequate for the size of the fetus and that the baby will birth vaginally.

In a primigravid woman the head normally engages at any time from about 36 weeks of pregnancy, but in a multipara this may not occur until after the onset of labour. When the vertex presents and the head is engaged the following will be evident on clinical examination.

- only two- to three-fifths of the fetal head is palpable above the pelvic brim (Fig. 16.31)
- the head is not mobile.

Box 16.4 Positions in a vertex presentation

Left occipitoanterior (LOA) The occiput points to the left iliopectineal eminence; the sagittal suture is in the right oblique diameter of the pelvis (Fig. 16.25).

Right occipitoanterior (ROA) The occiput points to the right iliopectineal eminence; the sagittal suture is in the left oblique diameter of the pelvis (Fig. 16.26).

Left occipitolateral (LOL) The occiput points to the left iliopectineal line midway between the iliopectineal eminence and the sacroiliac joint; the sagittal suture is in the transverse diameter of the pelvis (Fig. 16.27).

Right occipitolateral (ROL) The occiput points to the right iliopectineal line midway between the iliopectineal eminence and the sacroiliac joint; the sagittal suture is in the transverse diameter of the pelvis (Fig. 16.28).

Left occipitoposterior (LOP) The occiput points to the left sacroiliac joint; the sagittal suture is in the left oblique diameter of the pelvis (Fig. 16.29).

Right occipitoposterior (ROP) The occiput points to the right sacroiliac joint; the sagittal suture is in the right oblique diameter of the pelvis (Fig. 16.30).

Direct occipitoanterior (DOA) The occiput points to the symphysis pubis; the sagittal suture is in the anteroposterior diameter of the pelvis.

Direct occipitoposterior (DOP) The occiput points to the sacrum; the sagittal suture is in the anteroposterior diameter of the pelvis.

In breech and face presentations the positions are described in a similar way using the appropriate denominator.

On rare occasions the head is not palpable abdominally because it has descended deeply into the pelvis. If the head is not engaged, the findings are as follows:

- more than half of the head is palpable above the brim
- the head may be high and freely movable (ballotable) or partly settled in the pelvic brim and consequently immobile.

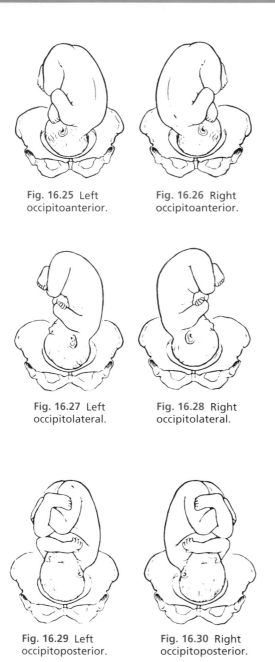

Fig. 16.25 Left occipitoanterior.

Fig. 16.26 Right occipitoanterior.

Fig. 16.27 Left occipitolateral.

Fig. 16.28 Right occipitolateral.

Fig. 16.29 Left occipitoposterior.

Fig. 16.30 Right occipitoposterior.

Figs 16.25–16.30 Six positions in vertex presentation.

the midwife should assess the woman as usual and monitor the progress of her pregnancy. Roshanfekr et al (1999) found that 86% of nulliparous women with a non-engaged head at the onset of active labour proceeded to have a vaginal birth.

Assessment of pelvic capacity

The size of the obstetric conjugate can be estimated by measuring the diagonal conjugate per vaginam. However, this is rarely carried out. A pelvic assessment may be carried out as part of labour care, if the presenting part has not engaged. If the presenting part is engaged, it would not be necessary to measure the obstetric conjugate. These assessments are of little use in the antenatal period because until labour commences it is still unknown whether the fetal head will engage. Retrospective ultrasound can be performed to measure pelvic size by pelvimetry, information which can be utilised in future pregnancies.

In the multigravid woman engagement often does not occur until labour has commenced. If, during palpation, it is thought that the fetus is much larger than previous vaginally delivered babies, further investigations may be warranted. It is usual to avoid diagnosing cephalopelvic disproportion until either X-ray evidence is unequivocal or after the onset of labour. The reason for this is that the force of labour contractions encourage flexion and moulding of the fetal head and the relaxed ligaments of the pelvis allow the joints to give. This may be sufficient to allow engagement and descent. Other causes of a non-engaged head at term include:

- occipitoposterior position
- full bladder
- wrongly calculated gestational age
- polyhydramnios
- placenta praevia or other space-occupying lesion
- multiple pregnancy
- pelvic brim inclination of more than 80° as occurs in a high assimilation pelvis.

Presenting part

The presenting part of the fetus is the part that lies over the cervical os during labour and on which the caput succedaneum forms. It should not be confused with presentation.

If the head does not engage in a primigravid woman at term, there is a possibility of a malposition or cephalopelvic disproportion. Referral to an obstetrician should be made. However, until labour commences,

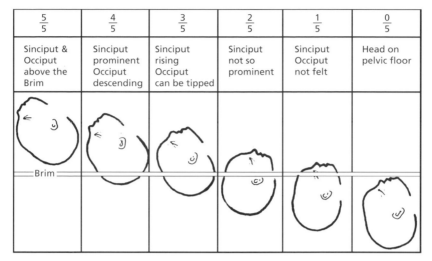

$\frac{5}{5}$	$\frac{4}{5}$	$\frac{3}{5}$	$\frac{2}{5}$	$\frac{1}{5}$	$\frac{0}{5}$
Sinciput & Occiput above the Brim	Sinciput prominent Occiput descending	Sinciput rising Occiput can be tipped	Sinciput not so prominent	Sinciput Occiput not felt	Head on pelvic floor

Fig. 16.31 Descent of the fetal head estimated in fifths palpable above the pelvic brim.

Ongoing antenatal care

The information gathered during the antenatal visits will enable the midwife and pregnant woman to determine the appropriate pattern of antenatal care (see Ch. 3 for models of midwifery care). The timing and number of visits will vary according to individual need and changes should be made as circumstances dictate (e.g. Box 16.5).

Indicators of fetal well-being

These include:

- increasing maternal weight in association with increasing uterine size compatible with the gestational age of the fetus
- fetal movements that follow a regular pattern from the time when they are first felt
- fetal heart rate that should be between 110 and 160 beats per minute during auscultation.

Eliciting information about recent fetal movement will reassure the mother. Patterns of fetal movements are a reliable sign of fetal well-being; evidence of at least 10 movements a day is considered usual. The midwife would, however, expect that these movements had occurred within a 12 hour period. The period of observation usually starts at 9 a.m. but fetal activity is often greatest during the late evening. If this is normal for an individual fetus then a period of

---

Box 16.5 Risk factors that may arise during pregnancy

- Fetal movement pattern reduced or changed
- Hb lower than 10 g/dl
- Poor weight gain, weight loss
- Proteinuria, glycosuria, bacilluria
- BP systolic of or above 140 mmHg, diastolic of or above 90 mmHg, or 15 mmHg or more above booking diastolic
- Uterus large or small for gestational age
- Excess or decreased liquor
- Malpresentation
- Head not engaged in primigravid woman at term
- Any vaginal, cervical or uterine bleeding
- Premature labour
- Infection
- Any chronic or acute illness or disease in the woman
- Relevant sociological or psychological factors

---

observation should be identified that includes the time during which the fetus is most active. The same time period should be used each day to allow for comparison. If the fetus is taking progressively longer each day to achieve 10 movements, this may be an indication of fetal compromise. The woman should urgently contact a fetal assessment unit or labour ward if these criteria have not been met. An assessment and a cardiotocograph (CTG) can be carried out to review the health of the fetus at that time. Subsequently, a plan can be made for follow-up care. Although there may be changes to fetal movement patterns prior to labour, due to reduced space, fetal activity should continue throughout pregnancy and labour.

Preparation for labour

During the latter weeks of pregnancy, plans for labour and birth will be a focus of discussion. Most hospitals provide a list of items that they require women to bring with them into hospital for themselves and their baby. If the woman has planned a home birth, she is visited by her midwife to make final arrangements for the birth. In both cases it is important to ensure that women know whom to contact if they need advice about the commencement of labour or have other related concerns.

The midwife will discuss the process of labour with the woman and her family. The focus on the positive progress of labour and birth, centring around normality, is a priority but if there is a need to change plans during labour then women and their families should be facilitated by the midwife to make an informed choice. Flexibility and adaptability should be built into the labour and birth plans to ensure a holistic approach is adopted and the woman's needs are met. Parents' wishes should be recorded in the pregnancy labour notes in addition to discussions about care, which take place between the woman, her family, the midwife and other health professionals who are involved antenatally.

REFERENCES

Ades A, Sculpher M, Gibb D et al 1999 Cost effectiveness analysis of antenatal HIV screening in United Kingdom. British Medical Journal 319(7219):1230–1234

Alexander J M, Grant A M, Campbell M J 1992 Randomised controlled trial of breast shells and Hoffman's exercises for inverted and non-protractile nipples. British Medical Journal 304(6833):1030–1032

Bisson D L, Golding I, MacGillivray P et al 1990 Blood pressure lability. Contemporary Reviews in Obstetrics and Gynaecology 2:11–15

Blair P, Bensley D, Smith I, Bacon C, Taylor E 1996 Smoking and the sudden infant death syndrome: results from 1993–5 case-control study for confidential enquiry into stillbirths and deaths in infancy. British Medical Journal 313:195–198

Boyle M 1995 Antenatal investigations. Books for Midwives Press, Hale, Cheshire

Bundey S, Alan H 1991 Why do UK born Pakistani babies have high perinatal and neonatal mortality rates? Paediatrica Perinatal Epidemiology 5(1):101–114

Campbell D M, Macgillivray I, Carr-Hill R 1985 Pre-eclampsia in second pregnancy. British Journal of Obstetrics and Gynaecology 92:131–140

Clement S, Candy B, Sikorski J et al 1999 Does reducing the frequency of routine antenatal visits have long term effects? Follow up of participants in a randomised controlled trial. British Journal of Obstetrics and Gynaecology 106(4):367–370

Dekker G A, Robillard P Y, Hulsey T C 1998 Immune maladaptation in the etiology of preeclampsia: a review of corroborative epidemiologic studies. Obstetrical and Gynecological Survey 53(6):377–382

de Swiet 1999 In: James D, Steer Wiener C, Gonik B (eds) High risk pregnancy, 2nd edn. W B Saunders, London

DoH (Department of Health) 1993 Changing childbirth: report of the expert maternity group. HMSO, London

DoH (Department of Health) 1999a New national helpline to be launched for pregnant mums who want to quit smoking. Tessa Jowell unveils further major step in the Government's strategy to cut smoking. DoH, London, 9 March 1999

DoH (Department of Health) 1999b Our healthier nation: reducing health inequalities: an action report. DoH, London

Elbourne D, Richardson M, Chalmers I et al 1987 The Newbury maternity care study: a randomised controlled trial to assess a policy of women holding their own obstetric records. British Journal of Obstetrics and Gynaecology 94(7):612–619

Engstrom J, Piscioneri L, Low L 1993 Fundal height measurement part 3 – the effect of maternal position on fundal height measurements. Journal of Nurse-Midwifery 38(1):23–27

Floyd R, Rimer B et al 1993 A review of smoking in pregnancy: effects on pregnancy outcomes and cessation efforts. Annual Review of Public Health 14:379–411

Frame S, Moore J, Peters A et al 1985 Maternal height as a predictor of pelvic disproportion: an assessment. British Journal of Obstetrics and Gynaecology 92:1239–1245

Gardosi J, Francis A 1999 Controlled trial of fundal height measurement plotted on customised antenatal growth charts. British Journal of Obstetrics and Gynaecology 106(4):309–317

Hall M H, Cheng P K, MacGillivray I 1980 Is routine antenatal care worth while? Lancet ii:78–80

Hallak M 1999 Hypertension in pregnancy. In: James D, Steer Weiner C, Gonik B (eds) High risk pregnancy management options, 2nd edn. W B Saunders, London

Herbert R A, Alison J A 1996 Cardiovascular function. In: Hinchliff S M, Montague S E, Watson R (eds) Physiology for nursing practice, 2nd edn. Baillière Tindall, London

Homer C, Davis G, Everitt L 1999 The introduction of a woman-held record into a hospital antenatal clinic: the bring your own records study. Australian and New Zealand Journal of Obstetrics and Gynaecology 39(1):54–57

Hytten F 1990 Is it important or even useful to measure weight gain in pregnancy? Midwifery 6(1):28–32

Jewell D, Sharp D, Sanders J et al 2000 A randomised controlled trial of flexibility in routine antenatal care. British Journal of Obstetrics and Gynaecology 107(10):1241–1247

Lewis G, Drife J (eds) 2001 Why mothers die 1997–1999. The fifth report of the confidential enquiries into maternal deaths in the United Kingdom. RCOG Press, London

Li C, Windsor R 1993 The impact on infant birthweight and gestational age of cotinine-validated smoking reduction in pregnancy. Journal of the American Medical Association 269:1519–1524

McLeod S, Gillies A, Carter Y, Wilson S 1996 Folic acid: an essential ingredient for making babies? British Journal of Midwifery 4(8):404–406

Mahmood T A, Campbell D M, Wilson A W 1988 Maternal height, shoe size and outcome of labour in white primigravidas: a prospective study. British Medical Journal 297:515–517

Methven R C 1990 The antenatal booking interview. In: Alexander J, Levy V, Roch S (eds) Midwifery care. Antenatal care – a research-based approach. Macmillan, Basingstoke, pp 42–57

MIDIRS and NHS Centre for Research and Dissemination 1999 Ultrasound in pregnancy: should you have one? MIDIRS, Bristol

Mitchell E, Tuohy P et al 1997 Risk factors for sudden infant death syndrome following the prevention campaign in New Zealand: a prospective study. Pediatrics 100:835–840

MoH (Ministry of Health) 1929 Maternal mortality in childbirth. Antenatal clinics: their conduct and scope. HMSO, London

Moore M, Hopper U 1995 Do birth plans empower women? Evaluation of a hospital birth plan. Birth 22(1):29–36

Morrison P, Burnard P 1997 Caring and communicating. Macmillan Press, London

Naftstad P, Jakola J et al 1996 Breastfeeding, maternal smoking and lower respiratory tract infections. European Respiratory Journal 9(12):2623–2629

Neilson J P 2001 Symphysis-fundal height measurement in pregnancy. (Date of most recent substantive amendment: 29 November 1997.) In: The Cochrane Library. Update Software, Oxford, issue 3

Nguyen T, Larsen T, Enghollm G et al (1999) Evaluation of ultrasound-estimated date of delivery in 17 450 spontaneous singleton births: do we need to modify Naegele's rule? Ultrasound in Obstetrics and Gynecology 14(1):223–228

NICE (National Institute for Clinical Excellence) 2001 www.nice.org.uk

Nicholl A 1998 Antenatal screening for HIV in the UK: what is to be done? Journal of Medical Screening 5(4):170–171

Oakley A, Rajan L, Grant A 1990 Social support and pregnancy outcome. British Journal of Obstetrics and Gynaecology 97:155–162

Oakley A, Hickey D, Rajan L 1996 Social support in pregnancy: does it have long term effects? Journal of Reproductive and Infant Psychology 14:7–22

Olsen K 1999 Now just pop up here dear … revisiting the art of antenatal abdominal palpation. Practising Midwife 2(9):13–15

Olugibile A, Mascarenhas L 2000 Review of shoulder dystocia at the Birmingham Women's Hospital. Journal of Obstetrics and Gynaecology 20(3):367–370

Page L 2000 The new midwifery science and sensitivity in practice. Churchill Livingstone, London, p 10

Prochaska J 1992 What causes people to change from unhealthy to health enhancing behaviour? In: Heller T, Bailey L, Patison S (eds) Preventing cancers. Open University Press, Buckingham, p 147–153

Rafael-Leff J 1991 Psychological processes of childbearing. Chapman & Hall, London

RCOG (Royal College of Obstetricians and Gynaecologists) 2000 Alcohol consumption in pregnancy. RCOG, London, 8 September

Romero R, Oyarzun E, Maxor M et al 1989 Meta-analysis of the relationship between asymptomatic bacteriuria and preterm delivery/low birth weight. Obstetrics and Gynaecology 73:576–582

Roshanfekı D, Blakemore K J, Lee J et al 1999 Station at onset of active labor in nulliparous patients and risk of cesarean delivery. Obstetrics and Gynecology 93(3):329–331

Schott J, Henley A 1996 Culture, religion and childbearing in a multiracial society. Butterworth Heinemann, London

Shennan A, Gupta M, Halligan A, Taylor D J, de Swiet M 1996 Lack of reproducibility in pregnancy of Korotkoff phase IV as measured by mercury sphygmomanometry. Lancet 347:139–142

Sikorski J, Wilson J, Clement S, Das S, Smeeton N 1996 A randomised controlled trial comparing two schedules of antenatal visits: the antenatal care project. British Medical Journal 312:546–553

Stein-Parbury 1993 Patient and person developing interpersonal skills in nursing. Churchill Livingstone, Edinburgh

Stoltenburg C, Magnus P, Lie R et al 1998 Influence of consanguinity and maternal education on risk of stillbirth and infant death in Norway, 1967–1993. American Journal of Epidemiology 148(5):452–459

Sure Start 2001 Online. Available: www.surestart.gov.uk

Tunon K, Eik-Nes S, Grottum P 1996 A comparison between ultrasound and a reliable last menstrual period as predictors of the day of delivery in 15 000 examinations. Ultrasound in Obstetrics and Gynaecology 8:178–185

UKCC (United Kingdom Central Council for Nursing Midwifery and Health Visiting 1998a) Guidelines for records and record keeping. UKCC, London (reprinted NMC 2002)

UKCC (United Kingdom Central Council for Nursing Midwifery and Health Visiting 1998b) Midwives rules and code of practice. UKCC, London

Villar J, Khan-Neelofur D 2001 Patterns of routine antenatal care for low-risk pregnancy (Date of most recent amendment 19 May 1999.) In: The Cochrane Library. Update Software, Oxford; Issue 3

Wallon M, Liou C, Garner P et al 1999 Congenital toxoplasmosis: systematic review of evidence of efficacy of treatment in pregnancy. British Medical Journal 318(7197):1511–1514

Way S 2000 Core skills for caring and assessment. Books for Midwives Press, Manchester

Webster J, Forbes K, Foster S et al 1996 Sharing antenatal care: client satisfaction and use of the 'patient-held record'. Australian and New Zealand Journal of Obstetrics and Gynaecology 35(1):11–14

WHO (World Health Organization) 1985 Appropriate technology for birth. Lancet 2:436–437

USEFUL ADDRESSES

Association for Improvements in Maternity Services (AIMS)
www.aims.org.uk

Maternity Alliance
www.maternityalliance.co.uk

Quitline:
www.quit.org.uk
helpline: 0800 002200/0800 1699169 (pregnancy quitline)

17 Abnormalities of Early Pregnancy

Christine Shiers

This chapter deals with conditions that occur within the first 20 weeks of pregnancy. Many of these are potentially life threatening for the mother, so recognition and prompt treatment are vital for her well-being.

The chapter aims to:

- consider the three main categories of loss in early pregnancy – spontaneous abortion, induced abortion and ectopic pregnancy

- describe hydatidiform mole, which occurs much less frequently but still accounts for the loss of a pregnancy

- emphasise the need for midwives to be able to offer support and care for mothers early in pregnancy

- discuss conditions such as hyperemesis gravidarum and fibroids, which affect a smaller number of women but can each cause considerable discomfort during pregnancy.

Mothers are encouraged by midwives to seek their professional advice as early as possible in pregnancy. Increased knowledge and understanding of the abnormalities that can occur in early pregnancy will help to improve the quality of midwifery care offered to the mothers at this time.

Bleeding in pregnancy

Vaginal bleeding during pregnancy is abnormal. It is a cause of concern to mothers, particularly those who have had a previous experience of fetal loss. Any reports of bleeding should be viewed seriously by the midwife. If the woman presents with a history of bleeding in the current pregnancy it is important to establish when it occurred. How much blood was lost, the colour of the loss and whether it was associated with any pain should be noted. If the symptoms have subsided it is important to advise the mother to report any recurrence.

Assessment of fetal condition will depend on gestation. Ultrasound scanning can confirm viability of the pregnancy before heart sounds are audible or movements felt. In the second trimester the use of ultrasound equipment can elicit the heart sounds, and note of fetal movements may also be made.

Implantation bleeding

As the trophoblast erodes the endometrial epithelium and the blastocyst implants, a small vaginal blood loss may be apparent to the woman. It occurs around the time of expected menstruation, and may be mistaken for a period, although lighter. It is of significance if the estimated date of delivery is to be calculated from menstrual history.

Cervical eversion

This condition is commonly and erroneously known as a cervical erosion. The cervix is lined with two distinct cell types. Columnar epithelium lines the cervical canal, reaching the external os. The structure changes abruptly and stratified squamous epithelial cells cover the vaginal aspect of the cervix, and continue along the vagina itself (Fig. 17.1).

High levels of oestrogen cause proliferation of columnar epithelial cells, found in the cervical canal. These occupy a wider area, including the vaginal aspect of the cervix, encroaching on the squamous epithelial cells (metaplasia). The junction between is everted into the vagina. This eversion, or *ectropion* as it is correctly described, is a physiological response to the hormonal changes in pregnancy. Hyperactivity of the endocervical cells increases the quantity of vaginal discharge. As the cells are vascular it may cause intermittent bloodstained loss, or spontaneous bleeding.

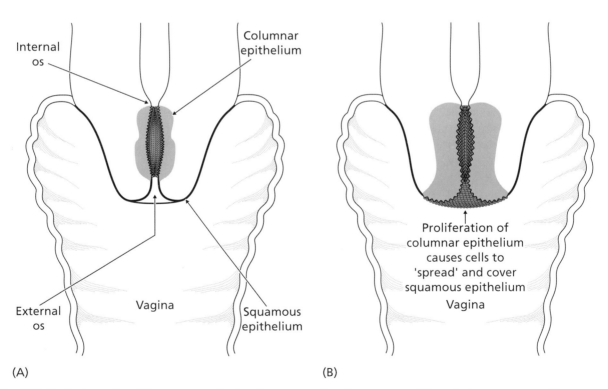

Fig. 17.1 Cervical eversion: (A) columnar epithelium becomes profuse in pregnancy; (B) cervical eversion caused by growth of columnar epithelial cells; the cervix appears reddened.

Bleeding following sexual intercourse is common with eversion. The eversion will usually disappear during the puerperium. Normally, eversion requires no treatment in pregnancy.

Cervical polyps

Small, vascular pedunculated growths attached to the cervix may bleed during pregnancy. They can be visualised on speculum examination and no treatment is required during pregnancy, unless bleeding is profuse or a cervical smear suggests malignancy.

Carcinoma of the cervix

The incidence of cancer in pregnancy is 1 in 6000 live births (Lewis & Drife 2001). Carcinoma of the cervix is the most frequently diagnosed cancer in pregnancy. It is a treatable condition if detected early and 80% of cases detected in pregnancy are diagnosed in the first or second trimester. After breast cancer, it is the commonest carcinoma in women worldwide, and a major contributor to mortality in women in developing countries. Statistics for the European Union (EU) show the United Kingdom as having the second highest incidence of cervical cancer (Ferlay et al 1999).

Cervical intraepithelial neoplasia (CIN) is the precursor to invasive cancer of the cervix. If the condition is detected at this stage, treatment can be given and the cytology reverts to normal. The principal screening test used is the Papanicolaou smear (Pap smear).

Risk factors

Human papillomavirus (HPV) infection. These are a small group of viruses transmitted primarily through genital–genital sexual contact. There are many types of HPV virus that are broadly classified as low or high risk depending on their association with cancer in the genital tract. High risk HPV types are present in almost all women with cervical cancer (IARC 1995, Lehtinen et al 1996) but it should be noted that not all women with these viruses develop cervical cancer. They also cause genital warts, and are a common viral infection. HPV type 16 is the main organism linked to the development of cervical cancer and persistent infection with the virus may contribute to the development of carcinoma (Schlecht et al 2001).

Sexual behaviour. Women who become sexually active at an early age, have many sexual partners and who have unprotected sex will have an increased risk of getting HPV infection. Women whose partners have had many partners are also at risk. It should be noted that the incidence of cervical cancer in lesbian women is lower than in the general female population but there is no research to measure risk in this specific group. HPV can be transmitted from woman to woman as it is spread by touch and contact. Lesbians who have had unprotected heterosexual intercourse at any time may also have been exposed to the HPV so could develop cervical carcinoma.

Smoking. Women who smoke are twice as likely to develop cervical cancer than those who do not smoke. It is thought that the link between smoking and cervical cancer may be through a weakening of the immune system thus lowering the body's ability to eliminate HPV. Another possibility is that the harmful substances present in tobacco damage the deoxyribonucleic acid (DNA) of cells in the cervix and may contribute to the development of cervical cancer. The size of the lesion is associated with the duration and quantity of cigarettes smoked (Deacon et al 2000).

Pregnancy. Woman with a late first pregnancy have a lower risk than those with an early pregnancy; the risk rises with parity (Kjellberg et al 2000).

Social class. Women in manual social classes are at higher risk than those in non-manual social classes (Brown et al 1997).

Cervical smear tests. Sexually active women should have a cervical smear every 5 years. Fifty per cent of new cases of cervical cancer in the UK occur in women who have never had a smear test. UK screening programmes call women aged between 20 and 64 for a cervical smear at least once every 5 years.

Types

There are two main types of cervical cancer:

Squamous cell carcinoma. Squamous cell carcinoma is the most common, accounting for around 90% of all cancers of the cervix. They arise from squamous cells in the cervix and screening tests detect abnormalities in the squamous cells (Jones et al 1996).

Adenocarcinoma. These are rare, accounting for around 10% of cervical cancers. Adenocarcinoma is, however, increasing but diagnosis is problematic as the cells are to be found within the cervical canal. In very rare cases, cervical cancers may have features of both cell types (Cancer Research Campaign 2001).

Clinical signs

Bleeding is the most common symptom, with vaginal discharge being the next most common. As symptoms may be mistakenly diagnosed as symptoms of pregnancy there may be delay in diagnosis.

Investigation

A Papanicolaou smear test (Box 17.1) will detect atypical cells on the surface of the cervix, or within the endocervix. When changes are detected a repeat smear test followed by colposcopy is indicated. Colposcopy allows the cervix to be visualised with a powerful light source and examined microscopically to reveal the extent of the lesion. Abnormality or CIN can be detected as visible changes on the cervix. Biopsies can be taken to reveal the extent of the lesion.

As with any investigation, the mother and her partner should be fully informed about any tests and treatments that are offered. She should be aware of when and from whom results will be available. Adequate

---

> **Box 17.1** Papanicolaou smear test
>
> - The test allows identification and treatment of premalignant changes to cervical cells and detection of cervical cancer.
> - Early diagnosis of cervical cancer increases the long term survival rates.
> - The Pap smear is a painless investigation in which the cervix is visualised using a speculum. Shaped spatulas are used to remove a layer of cells from the cervix and the area of the vagina surrounding the cervix. The area includes the squamocolumnar junction.
> - National guidelines in the UK recommend that all personnel carrying out smear tests be properly trained. All results should be available within 6 weeks of the smear being taken and 80% of women should have results within 4 weeks.
> - Lack of information, embarrassment, fear of pain during the test and fear of the results have been cited as reasons for women failing to attend appointments for the screening test.

---

time should be made to ensure that the results are discussed in a non-hurried manner. A positive test result following a smear test will cause anxiety to the mother and her family and it is important that accurate information is available along with supportive counselling.

Treatment

Treatment depends on the stage of the disease and gestation. Laser treatment or cryotherapy following colposcopy can be carried out on an outpatient basis and will result in the destruction of the abnormal area of cells.

Cone biopsy under general anaesthesia involves excision of cervical tissue and is both a diagnostic tool and a treatment but may increase the risk to the mother. The cervix is highly vascular in pregnancy and the risk of haemorrhage is high, as is the possibility of causing the mother to miscarry. Delaying treatment until the end of pregnancy is an option for women who are found to have early changes in cervical cytology.

If the changes to the cervix are advanced and diagnosis is made in the first or second trimester, the mother may have to make a choice as to whether to terminate the pregnancy in order to undergo treatment. If diagnosis is made later in pregnancy, a decision to deliver the fetus may be taken to allow the mother to commence treatment.

Midwives have a role in explaining the value of regular smear tests to mothers. National guidelines in the UK recommend that every woman between the ages of 20 and 64 has a cervical smear test every 5 years. Where there is no evidence of a recent smear having been carried out, it may be appropriate for a smear to be taken during pregnancy. Simple explanations about the procedure can help overcome anxieties about the smear test. Cervical screening may be carried out at the 6 week postnatal examination. Women should be encouraged to continue to attend for regular cervical smear tests on completion of their pregnancy. Midwives acting as advocates for disadvantaged mothers should be aware that women who are at risk include those with learning disabilities, for whom assumptions of celibacy may be made. This group of women are vulnerable through sexual activity, sexual abuse and smoking and should be included in any screening programmes (NHSCSP 2000).

Spontaneous miscarriage

Spontaneous miscarriage is defined as the involuntary loss of the products of conception prior to 24 weeks' gestation. In the United Kingdom the fetus is said to be viable or capable of sustaining life outside of the uterus from 24 weeks' gestation. The term 'miscarriage' is commonly used in preference to the term abortion. The majority of miscarriages occur in the first trimester, or within the first 12 weeks of pregnancy, and are classed as early miscarriage; those occurring after the 13th week are known as late miscarriage. Midwives, general practitioners and clients should have direct access to Early Pregnancy Assessment Units (EPAU) to avoid unnecessary delays and distress. EPAU have the advantage over accident and emergency departments as they can provide ultrasound scans to confirm diagnosis, have access to laboratory facilities and have staff who are experienced in both physical and psychological care for mothers experiencing early pregnancy loss (Bradley & Hamilton-Fairley 1998).

Incidence

Fifteen per cent of all confirmed pregnancies are said to result in a miscarriage, the majority of which happen in the first trimester; 1–2% spontaneous miscarriages occur after the 13th week (Regan 1997).

Aetiology

The causes of miscarriage in most instances remain unknown, but may include the following:

Fetal causes. Where a cause is determined, 50% of miscarriages are due to chromosomal abnormalities of the conceptus. Genetic and structural abnormalities are also said to cause pregnancy loss.

Maternal causes. Spontaneous early pregnancy loss has been attributed to the following maternal influences:

- *Maternal age* – the risk increases with advancing maternal age.
- *Structural abnormalities of the genital tract* – these include retroversion of uterus, bicornuate uterus and fibroids.
- *Infections* – these include rubella, listeria and chlamydia.

- *Maternal diseases* – management and control of medical conditions such as diabetes, renal disease and thyroid dysfunction have reduced the risk of miscarriage in affected women. Where these conditions are not well controlled the risk of miscarriage remains (Regan & Rai 2000).
- *Environmental factors* – excessive consumption of alcohol and coffee along with cigarette smoking, including passive exposure to cigarette smoke, have been found to increase the risk of miscarriage. Exposure to organic solvents increases the likelihood of fetal malformation and miscarriage.

Previous obstetric history is a predictor of spontaneous miscarriage (Regan et al 1989). Multigravidae are significantly more at risk than primigravidae, with miscarriage in the previous pregnancy being a prime indicator of risk.

There are a number of types of spontaneous miscarriage (Fig. 17.2):

- threatened
- inevitable
- incomplete
- complete
- silent or delayed
- septic abortion.

In first trimester miscarriage, the embryo or fetus succumbs prior to the miscarriage. Later losses may involve a fetus who is still alive. As with any condition the symptoms may vary between individuals. The principles are described here but midwives should be aware of the range of signs and symptoms that may present (Table 17.1).

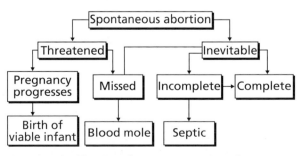

Fig. 17.2 Classification of spontaneous miscarriage.

Table 17.1 Signs of miscarriage

Signs and symptoms	Threatened miscarriage	Inevitable miscarriage	Incomplete miscarriage	Complete miscarriage	Delayed miscarriage	Septic miscarriage
Pain	Variable	Severe/rhythmical	Severe	Diminishing/none	None	Severe/variable
Bleeding	Scanty	Heavy/clots	Heavy profuse	Minimal/none	Some spotting possible Brown loss	Variable May smell offensive
Cervical os	Closed	Open	Open	Closed	Closed	Open
Uterus (if palpable)	Soft, no tenderness	Tender, may be smaller than expected	Tender/painful	Firm contracted	Smaller than expected	Bulky/tender/painful
Additional signs and symptoms			Tissue present in cervix Shock			Maternal pyrexia

Threatened miscarriage

As any vaginal bleeding in pregnancy is abnormal, so any vaginal blood loss in early pregnancy should be thought of as a threatened miscarriage until shown otherwise. In a threatened miscarriage, blood loss may be scanty, with or without low backache and cramp-like pains. The pain may resemble dysmenorrhoea or period pains (Moulder 2001). The cervix remains closed and the uterus soft, with no tenderness when palpated. The symptoms may continue over a period of time. The presence of a fetal heartbeat in conjunction with a closed cervical os is often reassuring; 70–80% of all mothers diagnosed as having a threatened miscarriage in the first trimester continue with their pregnancies to term.

Traditionally mothers have been advised to rest, but there is a lack of research evidence to suggest this as effective in preventing miscarriage. If the bleeding settles and the pregnancy continues, subsequent management should take account of the possibility of intrauterine growth retardation, due to poor placental function. There is also an increased risk of a preterm labour.

If the loss persists, the pain may become rhythmical and the uterus contracts to expel its contents as the miscarriage becomes inevitable.

Inevitable miscarriage

Management may require hospital admission and this should be to a dedicated EPAU if available or to a ward where staff are practised in caring for mothers having a miscarriage. A urine sample is taken for a pregnancy test and baseline observations of pulse and blood pressure and general well-being are noted. Blood should be taken to confirm Rhesus factor, if not already known.

Initial medical assessment ought to be carried out within locally agreed time limits, ideally within 1 hour of arrival. The use of transvaginal ultrasound is specific in detecting retained products and its use can prevent mothers having to undergo repeated vaginal examinations to confirm diagnosis. Vaginal bleeding may be heavy, with clots or gestational sac containing the embryo or fetus. The uterus, if palpable, may be smaller than expected. The membranes can rupture at this time, and amniotic fluid will be seen. The cervix dilates and tissue or clots may be seen in the vagina, or protruding through the os. Blood loss may be excessive and oxytocin 20 units intravenously can be given, or ergometrine 0.5 mg intravenously or intramuscularly, to control haemorrhage. The presence of a positive pregnancy test, pain, distress and heavy bleeding would normally indicate the need for surgical curettage but medical and expectant management are being used as alternative methods of treatment.

In some cases of spontaneous miscarriage the mother may present in a state of shock that is out of proportion to the revealed blood loss. This is caused by products of conception becoming trapped in the cervix and will resolve with their removal.

Mothers experiencing a miscarriage may be totally overwhelmed by the symptoms and distressed by the blood loss, pain and sense of loss. The pain during miscarriage may be as intense as any during labour. Adequate analgesia should be available and the mother's privacy and dignity protected. The woman and partner need to be kept informed of what is happening. Depending on gestation, an identifiable body or complete embryo may be lost. In some cases nothing is identifiable. The couple need to be prepared for these eventualities (Moulder 2001).

Cases of sporadic spontaneous miscarriage in the second trimester may result in the birth of a live baby. Rapid assessment of the baby at birth is required as, depending on gestation and place of birth, the baby may be capable of breathing and survive, albeit for a short time. In this event, midwives should acknowledge signs of life, inform the parents and obtain assistance from a paediatrician. Immediate transfer to a neonatal intensive care unit may be required if it appears that the baby is viable. Alternatively the baby may be given to the woman to hold. In the event of a live birth the midwife is obliged to notify that birth, and if the baby dies the death is also registered.

Incomplete miscarriage

In incomplete miscarriage, remnants of placenta remain within the uterine cavity contributing to bleeding that may be heavy and profuse. Intravenous or intramuscular ergometrine 0.5 mg may be given to control the loss. Evacuation to remove retained tissue should be under general anaesthetic, once the mother is in a stable condition. Visual estimation of blood loss is generally inaccurate, with underestimation of as much as 50% reported, and treatment of hypovolaemia may be required prior to anaesthesia. Use of vacuum aspiration is recommended in preference to sharp curettage (Forna & Gülmezoglu 2001). In uncomplicated cases surgical curettage may be avoided as tissue can be reabsorbed and bleeding is minimal.

Incomplete miscarriage contributes to the mortality and morbidity of women worldwide and vacuum aspiration may not be available to some women in developing countries, but it is seen by the WHO as an essential tool in the prevention of trauma and infection in childbearing women.

Complete miscarriage

Here the conceptus, placenta and membranes are expelled completely from the uterus. The pain stops, and signs of pregnancy regress. The uterus is firmly contracted on palpation, and an empty cavity is seen on ultrasound examination. No further medical intervention is required, although support through the aftermath of pregnancy loss should be available. Mothers should be advised to seek advice if bleeding recurs or a pyrexia develops.

Silent or delayed miscarriage (early fetal demise)

This term applies when the embryo dies, despite the presence of a viable placenta, and the sac is retained as the cervix remains closed. Embryo death usually occurs before 8 weeks' gestation but the mother's body does not recognise its demise. A brown loss originating from the degeneration of placental tissue may present, and threatened miscarriage be suspected. Women report a reduction then cessation of the symptoms of pregnancy. Uterine growth stops and diagnosis is confirmed by ultrasound scan.

Treatment of a delayed miscarriage may be medical through the administration of prostaglandins alone (RCOG 2001), or evacuation of the uterus under general anaesthetic. During the operation, the cervical canal is gently dilated to allow a small curette to be introduced into the uterine cavity. The curette is used to remove any retained products. Prostaglandins, inserted vaginally, make the cervix favourable prior to surgery. This avoids trauma to the cervix caused by forcible dilatation, and reduces the risk of cervical incompetence in subsequent pregnancies. There is a risk of hypofibrinogenaemia when the fetus has been retained for some weeks (see Ch. 18).

The term 'blighted ovum' should no longer be used to describe this condition.

Septic abortion

This condition is most commonly a complication of induced abortion or incomplete miscarriage, and is due to ascending infection. In addition to the signs of miscarriage, the mother complains of feeling unwell and may have a headache, nausea and be pyrexial. It may present as either a localised infection in the uterine tubes and the uterine cavity, or as generalised septicaemia with peritonitis.

Blood culture and vaginal swabs should be taken to identify the cause of the infection and intravenous antibiotics administered commencing with both broad spectrum antibiotics and one effective against anaerobic infection.

Sequelae to early pregnancy loss

Following a miscarriage the degree of support required from midwives will vary according to the individual and locality. The effect of the loss of a baby should not be underestimated by professionals, who may see it as a routine clinical situation (Cecil & Slade 1996). Community midwives may be involved in support and care for women following early miscarriage, working alongside the general practitioner. Increased use of early pregnancy units in hospitals means that nurses specialising in this area of care may also be involved. Where a mother has a late miscarriage, care on a gynaecology unit or delivery suite is possible depending on local practices.

All staff should pay particular attention to avoid medical jargon that cannot be understood by the client. Language should be appropriate, avoiding terms such as 'products' or 'scrape', recognising that most women will be grieving for the lost baby (Moulder 2001). Interpreters trained in bereavement support should be available to enable staff overcome problems communicating to parents where there is no common language. Facilities should also be accessible for visually or hearing-impaired parents to have information communicated effectively to them (Kohner 1995).

Feelings of failure and inadequacies may be expressed by the mother, as she blames herself, or some action, for the loss of her child. She may also be afraid that she is incapable of bearing children (Iles 1989). Regardless of gestation, the parents may want to see and hold the baby. Some parents may want to see the loss when there is no body and should be given the opportunity to do so. Creation of memories are important for the grieving process, and midwives can assist by taking photographs of the baby for the parents, and by providing a letter or certificate to confirm the loss. Photographs can be retained on file should the parents not wish them at this point. Parents should be able to name their baby if they so wish and should be enabled to talk about their loss in a safe and supportive environment (see Ch. 37).

Parents need information on how the remains will be disposed. All hospitals and maternity units should have guidance for parents, and staff who are knowledgeable in the local procedures. Written information should be available explaining the choices available and parents should be given adequate time to decide on events. Up to 6 weeks is recommended (Moulder 2001).

Under 24 weeks' gestation the baby is not registrable in the UK, therefore is not legally required to be buried or cremated but nevertheless respectful disposal is paramount. At no time should any fetal remains be included with hospital clinical waste. Parents may wish to take the remains home; burial in a garden is not precluded in this instance. If cremation is considered then midwives should be aware that the size of the fetus may result in few if any ashes.

Full written consent must be given by the mother for postmortem or any other investigations involving fetal tissue (DoH et al 2001). Follow-up after miscarriage is needed, with parents able to receive further information about their loss and be offered advice regarding future pregnancies.

A summary of key points relating to spontaneous miscarriage is given in Box 17.2.

Induced abortion

Termination of pregnancy before 24 weeks' gestation is legal in the UK within the terms of current legislation. Amendments to the Abortion Act 1967 came into force in 1991; these made the termination of pregnancy legal in certain circumstances after 24 weeks.

Midwives will primarily be caring for mothers for whom termination of pregnancy is an option they are considering as a result of the antenatal screening or diagnostic tests offered. The aim of these investigations is to detect specific fetal abnormalities. The family need to be given accurate, factual information

> **Box 17.2** Summary of key points on spontaneous miscarriage
>
> - The term 'miscarriage' is used to describe spontaneous loss of pregnancy before 24 weeks.
> - Terms that perpetuate the notion of failure or convey negative connotations should be avoided.
> - Grieving is an essential part of the recovery process following miscarriage.
> - Bedrest will not prevent miscarriage.
> - Blood loss and pain associated with miscarriage can be profuse and profound, and overwhelming for the mother.

about the investigations and the possible anomaly as well as the options available in their local area to enable an informed choice to be made about termination (see Ch. 23).

All women who are opting to terminate a pregnancy need adequate support and counselling, both before and after the procedure. Social, medical and psychological factors all contribute to the decision.

There are four identified areas that allow grounds for ending a pregnancy before 24 weeks' gestation. Two medical practitioners are required to certify that one or more of the following apply:

1. Continuation of the pregnancy would involve risk greater than if the pregnancy were terminated, of injury to the physical or mental health of the pregnant woman or any existing children of her family.

2. Termination is necessary to prevent grave permanent injury to the physical or mental health of the woman.

3. The continuation of the pregnancy would involve risk to the life of the pregnant woman, greater than if the pregnancy were terminated.

4. There is substantial risk that if the child were born it would suffer such physical or mental abnormalities as to be seriously handicapped (Abortion Act 1967, as amended by Human Fertilisation and Embryology Act 1990).

After 24 weeks, termination of pregnancy is permitted under the above Acts where the woman's life is at risk or where, as in Clause 4 of the Act, there is a substantial risk of the child being born seriously physically or mentally disabled.

Methods

Abortion can be carried out in the first trimester, using vacuum aspiration, dilatation and evacuation under general anaesthetic. Medical methods using mifepristone and prostaglandin are licensed for use up to the 63rd day from the first day of a woman's last menstrual period. Mifepristone is an antiprogesterone compound that blocks the action of progesterone, a hormone essential for the maintenance of the pregnancy. It is taken orally, on licensed premises, in the presence of a doctor or nurse. By blocking progesterone with mifepristone the sensitivity of the uterus to prostaglandin rises. A low dose vaginal prostaglandin pessary is inserted to effect the termination (RCOG 2000).

In the second trimester, medical methods are used. Extrauterine prostaglandin, accompanied by large doses of oxytocin, produces uterine contractions. The mother experiences labour pains and the process may be protracted. Prophylactic antibiotics may be given following termination and for non-sensitised Rhesus negative women, anti-D immunoglobulin is recommended.

The mother needs to be cared for in a single room, her privacy being protected at all times. She should be offered information about the process so she is aware of what is happening. Adequate analgesia should be available and supportive staff identified to care for the mother and her family throughout the procedure (Kohner 1995). It may be appropriate for the named midwife to care for the mother during her termination.

Legal abortion should not result in a live birth and feticide may be carried out as part of or prior to the procedure. Amendments in 1991 to the Abortion Act 1967 allowed for the reduction of multiple pregnancies where one or more of the fetuses, but not all, may be terminated (Paintain 1994).

International perspective

Induced abortion contributes to the worldwide maternal mortality statistics. In the developing world, unsafe abortion is one of the five main causes of direct maternal death (WHO 1997). Infection is a possible consequence of any abortion but is more common following an induced abortion. Septic abortion remains a major complication of an illegal abortion or one carried out in non-sterile conditions.

Maternal mortality

Early pregnancy mortality figures for the triennium 1997–1999 include two deaths following spontaneous miscarriage, and two following induced abortion. Maternal deaths in the UK following miscarriage and termination have declined but the Confidential Enquiry into Maternal Deaths (CEMD) stressed the need to be vigilant for signs of infection, as sepsis continues to be a key contributor to the mortality associated with early pregnancy loss worldwide (Lewis & Drife 2001).

Ethical issues

Within the terms of the Abortion Act 1967, if an individual has a conscientious objection then he or she is not required to assist with abortion. A midwife would normally be required to notify her manager of such an objection before any care was expected. The Act requires practitioners, however, to provide care to prevent harm to the pregnant woman so the exception to this would be in the event of an emergency when conscientious objection does not preclude the midwife from involvement. The midwife otherwise has a duty of care to mothers for whom she is the named midwife. Midwifery practice may involve assisting with blood tests or amniocentesis, the results of which could lead to a termination. The duty of care and exercise of professional accountability means that mothers should be given the necessary information and advice. Professional guidelines require the midwife to care for clients in a non-judgmental manner. This applies when caring for a mother terminating a current pregnancy or a mother who has undergone termination in a previous pregnancy.

Recurrent miscarriage

Recurrent miscarriage is defined as the loss of three or more consecutive pregnancies. This is a problem that affects 1% of all women, and the risk of further abortion increases with each pregnancy lost (Stirrat 1990a).

The incidence of recurrent miscarriage suggests that there are significant underlying causes and the loss of the pregnancy is not chance. Factors associated with recurrent miscarriage include:

1. **Genetic causes.** The parental karyotype is abnormal; the most common abnormality is translocation.
2. **Immunological factors.** Women with a history of recurrent pregnancy loss have been found to lack an IgG-blocking agent. In a normal pregnancy IgG coats the fetal antigens and prevents rejection of the fetus.
3. **Hypersecretion of LH.** This may act on the oocyte causing it to age, or on the endometrium resulting in errors in implantation. Mothers with polycystic ovaries have reduced fertility, and an increased risk of early pregnancy loss (Regan & Rai 2000).
4. **Infection.** The role of infection in recurrent early pregnancy failure is unclear. Alteration of the normal vaginal flora may contribute to recurrent miscarriage when loss or reduced levels of lactobacilli occur with the condition bacterial vaginosis. Presence of this in the first trimester has been found to increase the risk of second trimester miscarriage and preterm labour (Hay et al 1994, Kurki et al 1992). *Toxoplasma gondii*, listeria and cytomegalovirus are infective agents associated with pregnancy loss, but their action in recurrent loss remains uncertain (Regan & Rai 2000, Stirrat 1990b).
5. **Structural anomalies.** Both uterine abnormalities and cervical incompetence have been attributed as causes of recurrent loss, although it is thought that too much emphasis has been given to their contribution (Rai et al 1996, Stirrat 1990b).

In many cases no causative factor is identified. Women should be referred to specialist clinics, where a screening service is available, thus enabling a probable cause to be identified (RCOG 1999a).

Cervical incompetence

Cervical incompetence describes painless dilatation of the cervix in the second or early third trimester, allowing bulging membranes through the cervical os into the vagina. Miscarriage or preterm birth may occur if the membranes rupture.

Cervical incompetence recurs in subsequent pregnancies. The causes are unclear although trauma to the cervix during dilatation and curettage or induced abortion appear to contribute to the risk. Cone biopsy or congenital weakness of the cervix may also be possible causes.

Treatment for subsequent pregnancies is by cervical cerclage, and is carried out after the risk of early miscarriage is thought to be over. At 14 weeks' gestation a non-absorbable, purse-string suture is inserted at the level of the internal os. This remains in situ until 38 weeks or the onset of labour, when it is removed.

The use of the term 'cervical incompetence' is now questioned because of the negative context it engenders. Language used by professionals has changed in recent years, taking account of the feelings of failure that result.

Ectopic pregnancy

An ectopic pregnancy is one where implantation occurs at a site other than the uterine cavity. Sites can include uterine tube, ovary, cervix and the abdomen (Fig. 17.3).

The incidence of ectopic pregnancies is an estimated 1.5% of all pregnancies. In the 2001 report by the CEMD, ectopic pregnancy accounted for 11.1 deaths per 1000 pregnancies in UK (Lewis & Drife 2001). Thirteen deaths were due to ectopic pregnancy: 12 tubal in origin, and 1 cervical pregnancy; substandard care contributed to the mortality, with the initial diagnosis being missed. The previous report had documented 12 maternal deaths in the UK and substandard care was also a factor (DoH et al 1998).

Women require prompt, appropriate treatment for this life threatening condition. Midwives need to consider the possibility of ectopic pregnancy being responsible for unexplained abdominal pain and bleeding in early pregnancy.

Tubal pregnancy

In tubal pregnancy, implantation can occur at any point along the tube, although the ampulla is the most common site. The isthmus is next in frequency, and the interstitial portion least common.

Risk factors for ectopic pregnancy

Any of the following alterations of the normal function of the uterine tube in transporting the gametes contributes to the risk of ectopic pregnancy:

- previous ectopic pregnancy
- previous surgery on the uterine tube
- exposure to diethylstilboestrol in utero
- congenital abnormalities of the tube
- previous infection including chlamydia, gonorrhoea and pelvic inflammatory disease
- use of intrauterine contraceptive devices
- assisted reproductive techniques.

Physiology of tubal pregnancy

In uterine pregnancy the blastocyst embeds in the decidua and the trophoblast erodes the maternal tissue anchoring the developing embryo. In tubal cyesis, the blastocyst rapidly erodes the epithelium and becomes attached to the muscle layer. It grows and expands within the wall, distending the tube. Maternal vessels are exposed and the pressure caused by the resultant blood flow can destroy the embryo.

The uterus increases in size, and changes associated with early pregnancy occur in the body. Degrees of change take place within the endometrium, under the influence of hormones. Vaginal bleeding associated with ectopic pregnancy is derived from degeneration of the decidua, which is passed in fragments, or as a decidual cast.

Outcomes of tubal pregnancy (Fig. 17.4)

1. *Tubal abortion* – the developing conceptus separates and is expelled through the fimbriated end of the uterine tube. This outcome is more common with ampullary implantation.

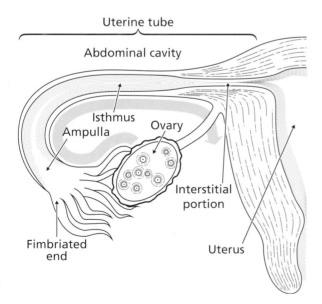

Fig. 17.3 Sites of implantation in ectopic pregnancy.

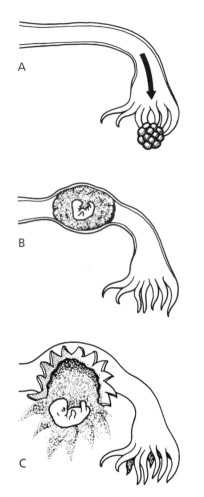

Fig. 17.4 Possible outcomes of tubal pregnancy: (A) tubal abortion; (B) tubal mole; (C) tubal rupture.

2. *Tubal mole* – bleeding around the embryo results in its death. The blood clots around the conceptus, enclosing it. Products are retained in the tube, and may need to be removed.

3. *Tubal rupture* – the wall is distended by the pregnancy and penetrated by the trophoblast to such an extent that it ruptures. This can be gradual or occur as an acute episode.

4. *Abdominal pregnancy*.

5. *Maternal death*.

Clinical presentation (Box 17.3)

Tubal pregnancy rarely remains asymptomatic beyond 8 weeks. It can be difficult to diagnose, but delay may

---

> **Box 17.3** Signs of ectopic pregnancy
>
> **Typical signs**
> - Localised/abdominal pain
> - Amenorrhoea
> - Vaginal bleeding or spotting
>
> **Atypical signs**
> - Shoulder pain
> - Abdominal distension
> - Nausea, vomiting
> - Dizziness, fainting
> - Apyrexia

endanger the life of the woman. Suspicion of ectopic pregnancy requires prompt hospital referral.

The mother may present with a history of amenorrhoea, followed by some vaginal spotting. This precedes the onset of abdominal pain, often localised in nature, described as sharp and stabbing. The mother complains of dizziness and nausea and can have shoulder pain, which is indicative of bleeding into the peritoneal cavity. Pelvic pain is severe. Acute symptoms are the result of tubal rupture, and relate to the degree of haemorrhage there has been.

Atypical signs can delay diagnosis and cause life-threatening deterioration of the woman's condition. Unexplained abdominal pain may be caused by bleeding into the peritoneal cavity. This causes abdominal distension, and pleuritic chest pain may be a sign of diaphragmatic irritation. Vomiting with or without diarrhoea are recorded as presenting symptoms of women who died as a result of failure to diagnose ectopic pregnancy (Lewis & Drife 2001).

Ultrasound enables an accurate diagnosis of tubal pregnancy, making management more proactive. Vaginal ultrasound combined with the use of sensitive blood and urine tests, which detect the presence of HCG, help to ensure diagnosis is made earlier and reduce risk of rupture (Ankum 2000, Lewis & Drife 2001).

If the tube ruptures, shock may ensue; therefore resuscitation followed by laparotomy is needed. The mother should be offered follow-up support and information regarding subsequent pregnancies. As with any loss during pregnancy, the midwife should be sensitive to her client's need to grieve.

Abdominal pregnancy

Abdominal pregnancy is rare. Fetal development may take place in the abdominal cavity and follows early rupture or abortion of a tubal pregnancy. The placenta remains attached to the uterine tube, but expands and attaches to neighbouring organs. The fetus develops within the peritoneal cavity but rarely survives. Infection can develop, causing peritonitis and septicaemia.

In very rare cases, abdominal pregnancy proceeds to term. On palpation the lie may be persistently abnormal and fetal parts readily felt. Reports describe the uterus as being enlarged, owing to hormonal activity, and felt separately from the fetus. A clear plan of care is required with a multiprofessional team drawn from all relevant health care professionals aware of their roles and requirements. Delivery is by laparotomy, with individual surgeons assessing the dangers involved with the separation and delivery of the placenta. Separation may be followed by major haemorrhage that is uncontrollable. Leaving the placenta in situ may result in infection but is considered to be the safer option.

The baby may be found to have compression deformities due to oligohydramnios.

Cervical pregnancy

This is also extremely rare, but potentially fatal owing to massive haemorrhage (Lewis & Drife 2001).

Ectopic pregnancy and maternal mortality

In the Confidential Enquiry into Maternal Deaths (Lewis & Drife 2001) for the triennium 1997–1999 there were 13 direct maternal deaths due to ectopic pregnancy, eight of these being associated with substandard care. Early diagnosis is essential, and facilities to make an accurate diagnosis should be widely available. This includes direct access to EPAUs where prompt diagnosis can be facilitated. Midwives encourage mothers to seek their advice as early as possible in pregnancy and could be the professional called on in the first instance. Midwives need to know of the facilities for early pregnancy screening in their area.

Accurate, comprehensive booking information may highlight those at risk of ectopic pregnancy. Women

---

> **Box 17.4** Summary of key points on ectopic pregnancy
>
> - Ectopic pregnancy is a significant cause of maternal death.
> - Women need prompt diagnosis and treatment.
> - Ectopic pregnancy should be suspected if women of childbearing age present with abdominal pain and amenorrhoea.
> - Information about ectopic pregnancy should be widely available and accessible to all social and cultural groups.

presenting with unexplained abdominal or gastrointestinal symptoms, including pain, diarrhoea and vomiting, may have an ectopic pregnancy and this should be excluded. As with any sensitive issue, clients should have the opportunity to be alone with the midwife (or other health professional) so any information disclosed remains confidential.

Fatalities occur amongst socially disadvantaged and socially excluded women, and those for whom English is not their native language. Failure to communicate and relate effectively for a variety of reasons can result in delay in diagnosis and that delay may be significant in terms of recovery. Comprehensive assessment of needs must take account of social circumstances and care planned accordingly. Multiagency referral may be needed.

A summary of key points relating to ectopic pregnancy is given in Box 17.4.

Gestational trophoblastic disease

Gestational trophoblastic disease is a general term covering both the benign hydatidiform mole and choriocarcinoma, which is malignant. A third condition, placental site trophoblastic tumour, exists but is outside the remit of this chapter.

Hydatidiform mole

Hydatidiform mole applies to a gross malformation of the trophoblast in which the chorionic villi proliferate and become avascular. They are found in the cavity of the uterus and, very rarely, within the uterine tube.

The incidence of hydatidiform mole in the United Kingdom is 1.54 in 1000 pregnancies (RCOG 1999b). The risk rises to 1 in 76 where the mother has previously had a molar pregnancy (Newlands et al 2001). Maternal age is a consistent risk factor, increasing for women under 20 and over 40 years of age, and for women of Asian origin (Bagshawe et al 1986, Newlands et al 2001). As this condition can lead to the development of cancer, accurate diagnosis, treatment and follow-up are essential.

For the midwife whose client is diagnosed as having a molar pregnancy it is important to recognise her psychological and physical needs, as she will grieve for the loss of her pregnancy, and the baby. Although the condition is curable, stress will inevitably affect the mother and her family while coming to terms with a potentially life-threatening condition. Advice and counselling on subsequent pregnancies will be required.

Two forms of mole have been identified, one of which carries an increased risk of the mother subsequently developing choriocarcinoma (Lawler et al 1991).

Complete hydatidiform mole

This type of mole contains no evidence of embryo, cord or membranes. Death occurs prior to the development of the placental circulation (Szulman 1988). The chorionic villi alter to form clear, hydropic vesicles, which hang in clusters from small pedicles, giving the appearance of a bunch of grapes. The size of vesicles varies, from being barely visible to a few centimetres in diameter. Hyperplasia affects the syncytiotrophoblast and the cytotrophoblast layers. The mass occupies the uterine cavity and can be large enough to mimic an advanced gestation.

In normal pregnancy the trophoblast erodes the decidua to anchor the conceptus, and this ability means that the developing mole is more than capable of penetrating beyond the site of implantation. The myometrium can be involved and, more rarely, the veins. Rupture of the uterus with massive haemorrhage is a possible outcome.

Complete moles usually have 46 chromosomes of paternal origin only. A haploid sperm fertilises a so-called empty egg, the maternal chromosomes being lost (Lawler et al 1991). The paternal chromosomes alone duplicate. Choriocarcinoma can develop from this type (Newlands et al 2001).

Partial mole

Evidence of an embryo, fetus or amniotic sac may be found, as death occurs around the 8th or 9th week. Hyperplasia of the trophoblast is confined to the single syncytiotrophoblast layer and is less widespread than in complete moles. Chromosome analysis will usually show this to be triploid, with 69 chromosomes – that is, three sets of chromosomes, one maternal and two paternal. It can be difficult to differentiate on histology between a partial mole and a silent miscarriage. This has a clinical significance because, although the risk to the mother of developing choriocarcinoma from a partial mole is slight, follow-up is still essential (RCOG 1999b).

Clinical features

Symptoms vary, according to the type of mole developing. Exaggerated signs of pregnancy, appearing by 6–8 weeks, are characteristic of complete hydatidiform mole. For partial mole the signs may be less obvious.

Bleeding or a bloodstained vaginal discharge after a period of amenorrhoea is the commonest symptom that may present as the first sign of abnormality. Rupture of a vesicle may result in a light pink or brown vaginal discharge. The vesicles can then detach and be passed vaginally allowing diagnosis, if not already suspected, to be made.

Anaemia as a result of the gradual loss of blood can be a problem. Medical intervention may be needed where excessive nausea and vomiting, due to high levels of HCG, result in the mother requiring treatment for hyperemesis gravidarum. Hyperthyroidism has been detected in cases of molar pregnancy and requires to be treated prior to evacuation of the mole (Goldstein & Berkowitz 1994). Pre-eclampsia developing early in pregnancy is suggestive of the presence of a hydatidiform mole.

On examination, the uterine size exceeds that expected for gestation. On palpation, the uterus feels 'doughy' or elastic, and it does not contract. Mothers with a partial mole may not show signs of increased growth. No fetal parts or movements are felt and the fetal heart is not heard, although this may be in keeping with expected findings, depending on gestation. Diagnosis is confirmed by ultrasound scan and serum HCG levels.

Treatment

The aim of treatment is to remove all trophoblast tissue. In some cases the hydatidiform mole aborts spontaneously. Where this does not occur, vacuum aspiration or dilatation and curettage is necessary. Spontaneous expulsion of the mole carries less risk of malignant change.

All women who have been treated for hydatidiform mole in the UK are recorded on a central register. In the majority of cases, removal of the mole results in resolution of the condition. In about 10%, however, the trophoblast tissue does not die off completely. For this reason and because of the possibility of developing a malignancy, women confirmed as having a complete mole require follow-up over a 2 year period. Following treatment, surveillance of urinary levels of HCG should demonstrate a reduction of level, with a return to normal after 6–8 weeks; rising levels are suggestive of recurrence (Newlands et al 2001).

Pregnancy should be avoided during the follow-up period. Intrauterine contraceptive devices are contraindicated because of risks of perforation and infection and hormonal methods of contraception are not prescribed until levels of HCG have returned to normal (RCOG 1999b).

The midwife can provide support and explanations of the importance of this protracted period of screening. An understanding of the condition should help the midwife to plan care in subsequent pregnancies.

Choriocarcinoma

Choriocarcinoma is a malignant neoplasm, which can develop as a consequence of a molar pregnancy. The growth actively invades the myometrium, putting the mother at risk of severe haemorrhage in the first instance. The mother is also at risk of developing lung, hepatic and cerebral metastases if the neoplasm goes undetected.

Choriocarcinoma can also occur after a normal term gestation, ectopic pregnancy or a termination of pregnancy.

Administration of anti-D immunoglobulin in early pregnancy

Anti-D immunoglobulin was introduced to reduce the risk of isoimmunisation in Rhesus negative women (see Ch. 46). It has been demonstrated that significant fetomaternal haemorrhage can occur following early pregnancy loss. Anti-D 250 IU is the normal dose given before 20 weeks' gestation. Women who have an ectopic pregnancy should have their blood group identified, and it is recommended that anti-D is given if this is found to be Rhesus negative. Retrospective analysis has shown that women in this group are particularly at risk of sensitisation.

Women who are Rhesus negative and have had evacuation of a hydatidiform mole should also have anti-D administered (NBTSIWP 1991).

Retroversion of the uterus

When the long axis of the uterus is directed backwards during pregnancy, the uterus is said to be retroverted. In most cases it corrects spontaneously, the uterus rising out of the pelvis into the abdomen as pregnancy progresses, causing no further problems.

Incarceration of the retroverted gravid uterus

If the retroverted uterus fails to rise out of the pelvic cavity by the 14th week, it is said to be incarcerated. The growing uterus is confined within the pelvis, beneath the sacral promontory. Pressure causes abdominal discomfort, and a feeling of pelvic fullness, low abdominal or back pain. Frequency of micturition, dysuria and paradoxical incontinence are the result of the urethra being elongated as the cervix is increasingly displaced. Compression of the bladder neck leads to urinary retention. Urinary stasis can result in infections developing, including pyelonephritis (Myers & Scotti 1995). The mother may also complain of rectal pressure and constipation with impacted faeces.

On examination, the bladder will be palpable abdominally. The fetal heart may be difficult to auscultate if the bowel is full. As this is regarded as a deviation from normal the midwife may seek advice from an obstetrician or an experienced midwife while assessing the mother's condition (UKCC 1998). Sound clinical judgement should be demonstrated and care documented to show clear decision making. Demonstrating effective clinical practice the midwife should explain, and gain consent for catheterisation to relieve the retention of urine. An indwelling catheter is used to keep the bladder empty, enabling the uterus to rise out of the pelvis.

Anterior wall sacculation occurs in extreme cases when the uterus remains entrapped. The lower portion of the uterus continues to expand and extend, forming a pouch to accommodate the fetus. Uterine rupture can result, and bladder rupture due to overextension, or from necrosis of the bladder wall during manual correction, has been reported.

Fibroids (leiomyomas)

These are firm, benign tumours of muscular and fibrous tissue, ranging in size from the very small to very large. The incidence of detectable fibroids in pregnancy is 1%, the lowest risk being in Caucasian women, but risk increases in Afro-Caribbean women and women over 35 years old (Lumsden & Wallace 1998).

Types of fibroid

Intramural. The commonest type, these are embedded in the uterus separated from the myometrium by a capsule of connective tissue, causing enlargement of the non-pregnant uterus.

Subserosal. These lie below the perimetrium, and may be irregular in shape. Subserosal fibroids can become pedunculated.

Submucosal. These are found within the endometrium, or decidua. Difficult to detect on examination, these can cause bleeding, and become both infected and necrotic.

Effect of pregnancy on fibroids

Ultrasound monitoring of fibroids has demonstrated that they do not significantly increase in size during pregnancy (Aharoni et al 1988, Davis et al 1990). Any increase in size is limited; most change occurs in the first 10 weeks of pregnancy (Exacoustos & Rosati 1993). The same factors that influence uterine growth were thought to affect the fibroid, the walls of the fibroid containing hormone receptors. The fibroid does, however, become more vascular and oedematous, making it softer and more difficult to detect on palpation.

Effect of fibroids on pregnancy

Early pregnancy loss is associated with submucosal fibroids (Benson et al 2001). Lesser effects include mild abdominal pain that resolves without treatment (Aharoni et al 1988). Lower segment or cervical fibroids may be felt on vaginal examination. Outcome of pregnancy is dependent on the position of the fibroid, and in some situations obstruction may occur. Fibroids located in the lower segment or on the cervix can prevent descent of the fetal head, causing malpresentation and obstructed labour. Caesarean section is more likely to be necessary where the fibroid is situated in the lower segment (Vergani et al 1994). Severe postpartum haemorrhage may be caused if the fibroids prevent the complete separation of the placenta, or contraction of the uterus. In anticipation of this, blood should be available for urgent cross-matching. Removal of fibroids during caesarean section can also result in excessive haemorrhage, so these should be noted but left in situ (Hutton 1999).

Red degeneration of fibroids

Degeneration of a fibroid occurs if a rapidly growing fibroid exceeds the available blood supply. The central core necroses, and bleeding occurs into the middle. The tumour takes on a reddish appearance. The mother experiences severe abdominal pain that is acute in nature (Katz et al 1989), the affected area is tender on palpation, and she may also have a low grade pyrexia. Other causes of pain need to be excluded – typically, appendicitis or placental abruption need to be considered.

Referral for ultrasound scan aids differential diagnosis of the pain, as the relationship between the placental site and the focus of pain can be established. The degeneration can be seen clearly on ultrasound. The pain is normally relieved by rest and analgesia; no other treatment is required (Lumsden & Wallace 1998).

Hyperemesis gravidarum

Excessive nausea and vomiting that start between 4 and 10 weeks' gestation, and resolve before 20 weeks, requiring intervention are known as hyperemesis gravidarum. Affecting 0.3–3% of all pregnant women, this is associated with dehydration, electrolyte imbalance and weight loss of up to 10% of prepregnant weight and should not be confused with the common symptoms of nausea and vomiting of pregnancy that are self-limiting (Eliakim et al 2000).

The aetiology of hyperemesis is uncertain, with multi-factorial causes such as endocrine, gastrointestinal and psychological factors proposed. Rising levels of oestrogen and HCG appear to be significant. Hyperemesis occurs more often where mothers have a multiple pregnancy, or a hydatidiform mole, both of which are associated with increased hormone levels. Simultaneous occurrence of hyperthyroidism and hyperemesis suggests transient thyroid dysfunction as a possible cause (Crump & Aten 1992). Infection with *Helicobacter pylori*, the organism implicated in gastric ulcers, may also contribute (Frigo et al 1998). Women with a previous history of hyperemesis are likely to experience it in subsequent pregnancies (Snell et al 1998).

The impact of nausea and vomiting on the woman and her daily life should not be underestimated. The midwife should enquire of all women attending for early antenatal care whether they are experiencing nausea or vomiting. Causes of vomiting not due to pregnancy, such as thyroid problems, urinary tract infection or gastroenteritis, need to be excluded. Diagnosis is made where there is a history of persistent, severe nausea and vomiting in early pregnancy. A mother suspected of suffering from hyperemesis presents as being unable to retain food or fluids. She may have lost weight, and be distressed and debilitated by her symptoms. The woman requires admission to hospital for assessment, and management of symptoms.

A history of the frequency and severity of the bouts of vomiting is taken. The mother's appearance is noted, including any dryness or inelasticity of the skin. In severe cases jaundice may be apparent. This indicates hepatic involvement, the cause of which is unclear. Additional signs of dehydration such as rapid pulse, low blood pressure and dry furred tongue may be seen. The mother's breath may smell of acetone, a sign of ketosis. Ptyalism may occur, contributing to the dehydration, but may not be a cause of complaint as the mother is retching and vomiting (Abell & Riely 1992).

Elevated haematocrit, alterations in electrolyte levels and ketonuria are associated with dehydration. Hypovolaemia and electrolyte imbalance are corrected by intravenous infusion. Vitamin supplements can be given parenterally, particularly where hyperemesis has been prolonged. Initially nothing is given by mouth, to allow time for the vomiting to be controlled. Gradual introduction of fluids and diet as her condition improves is closely monitored.

The mother should be encouraged to rest and may be cared for in a single room. The distress caused by repeated vomiting can be marked. Some women may be prescribed a mild sedative if they appear agitated. Small palatable meals on a regular basis help to encourage the mother to regain her appetite.

The use of antiemetics in pregnancy received widespread publicity when links were found between thalidomide and severe malformations of children born to mothers who had taken the drug for morning sickness. Currently antihistamines are the recommended pharmacological treatment for nausea and vomiting, no antiemetic being approved for treatment.

If hyperemesis is left untreated the mother's condition worsens. Wernicke's encephalopathy is a complication associated with a lack of vitamin B_1 (thiamine). Hepatic and renal involvement lead to coma and death. Termination of pregnancy may reverse the condition and has a place in preventing maternal mortality. Hyperemesis persisting into the third trimester should be further investigated as it may be symptomatic of serious illness such as acute fatty liver of pregnancy (Lewis & Drife 2001).

Box 17.5 is a summary of key points relating to abnormalities of early pregnancy.

Box 17.5 Summary of key points on abnormalities of early pregnancy

- Clinical care for conditions cited in this chapter will be provided, in many instances, outside of the maternity unit.

- Mothers need information to ensure they can make informed choices about care, and consent to treatment offered.

- Midwives need to be aware of conditions that may be life threatening, recognise a deviation from normal and seek appropriate advise and assistance.

- Midwives may not care for mothers in the acute stages of the conditions in this chapter, but may be key to the support and care provided for the mothers and their families at a later point.

REFERENCES

Abell T L, Riely C A 1992 Hyperemesis gravidarum. Gastroenterology Clinics of North America 21(4):835–847

Abortion Act 1967 HMSO, London

Aharoni A, Reiter A, Golan D, Paltiely Y, Sharf M 1988 Patterns of growth of uterine leiomyomas during pregnancy. A prospective longitudinal study. British Journal of Obstetrics and Gynaecology 95:510–513

Ankum A 2000 Diagnosing suspected ectopic pregnancy. British Medical Journal 321:1235–1236

Bagshawe K D, Dent J, Webb J 1986 Hydatidiform mole in England and Wales 1973–83. Lancet ii:673–675

Benson C B, Chow J S, Chang-Lee W, Hill J A, Doubilet P M 2001 Outcome of pregnancies in women with uterine leiomyomas identified by sonography in the first trimester. Journal of Clinical Ultrasound 29(5):261–264

Bradley E, Hamilton-Fairley D 1998 Managing miscarriage in early pregnancy assessment units. Hospital Medicine 59(6):451–456

Brown J, Harding S, Bethune A, Rosato M 1997 Incidence of health of the nation cancers by social class. Population Trends 90 (Winter 1997):40–47

Cancer Research Campaign 2001 Types of cervical cancer. Online. Available: http://www.cancerhelp.org.uk/help/default.asp?page=2758 8/12/01

Cecil R, Slade P 1996 Miscarriage. In: Niven C, Walker A (eds) Conception, pregnancy and birth. Butterworth Heinemann, Oxford, vol 2, ch 7, p 89

Crump W J, Aten L A 1992 Hyperemesis, hyperthyroidism or both? Journal of Family Practice 35(4):450–456

Davis J L, Ray-Mazumder S, Hobel C J, Baley K, Sassoon D 1990 Uterine leiomyomas in pregnancy: a prospective study. Obstetrics and Gynaecology 75(1):41–44

Deacon J M, Evans C D, Yule R et al 2000 Sexual behaviour and smoking as determinants of cervical HPV infection and of CIN3 among those infected: a case–control study nested within the Manchester cohort. British Journal of Cancer 83(11):1565–1572

DoH (Department of Health), Welsh Office, Scottish Home and Health Department, Department of Health and Social Services, Northern Ireland 1998 Why mothers die. Report on Confidential Enquiries into Maternal Deaths in the United Kingdom 1994–1996. Stationery Office, London

DoH (Department of Health), Department for Education and Employment, Home Office 2001 The removal, retention and use of human organs and tissue from post-mortem examination. Advice from the Chief Medical Officer. Stationery Office, London

Eliakim R, Abulafia O, Sherer D M 2000 Hyperemesis: a current review. American Journal of Perinatology 17(4):207–218

Exacoustos C, Rosati P 1993 Ultrasound diagnosis of uterine myomas and complications in pregnancy. Obstetrics and Gynecology 82(1):97–101

Ferlay F, Bray R, Sankila D, Parkin M 1999 EUCAN cancer incidence, mortality and prevalence in the European Union 1997, version 4.0. IARC CancerBase no. 4. IARC Press, Lyon. Limited version online. Available: http://www-dep.iarc.fr/eucan/eucan.htm 8/12/01

Forna F, Gülmezoglu A M 2001 Surgical procedures to evacuate incomplete abortion (Cochrane review). In: The Cochrane Library, Issue 3. Update Software, Oxford

Frigo P, Lang C, Reisenberger K, Kolbl H, Hirschl A M 1998 Hyperemesis gravidarum associated with Helicobacter pylori seropositivity. Obstetrics and Gynecology 91(4):615–617

Goldstein D P, Berkowitz R S 1994 Current management of complete and partial molar pregnancy. Journal of Reproductive Medicine 39(3):139–146

Hay P E, Lamont R F, Taylor-Robinson D, Morgan D J, Ison C, Pearson J 1994 Abnormal bacterial colonisation of the genital tract and subsequent pre-term delivery and late miscarriage. British Medical Journal 308:295–298

Human Fertilisation and Embryology Act 1990 HMSO, London

Hutton J 1999 Gynecological disease. In: James D K, Steer P J, Weiner C P, Gonik B (eds) High risk pregnancy management options, 2nd edn. W B Saunders, Edinburgh, ch 52, p 938

IARC (International Agency for Research on Cancer) 1995 Human papillomaviruses monographs on the evaluation of carcinogenic risks to humans, vol 64. IARC, Lyon, France

Iles S 1989 The loss of early pregnancy. Clinical Obstetrics and Gynaecology 3(4):769–791

Jones W B, Shingleton H M, Russell A et al 1996 Cervical carcinoma in pregnancy. A national patterns of care study of the American College of Surgeons. Cancer 77:1479–1488

Katz V L, Dotters D J, Droegemueller W 1989 Complications of uterine leiomyomas in pregnancy. Obstetrics and Gynecology 73(4):593–596

Kjellberg L, Hallmans G, Ahren A M et al 2000 Smoking, diet, pregnancy and oral contraceptive use as risk factors for cervical intra-epithelial neoplasia in relation to human papillomavirus infection. British Journal of Cancer 82(7):1332–1338

Kohner N 1995 Pregnancy loss and the death of a baby. Guidelines for professionals. SANDS, London

Kurki T, Sivonen A, Renkonen O-V, Savia E, Ylikorkala O 1992 Bacterial vaginosis in early pregnancy and pregnancy outcome. Obstetrics and Gynecology 80(2):173–177

Lawler S D, Fisher R A, Dent J 1991 A prospective genetic study of complete and partial hydatidiform moles. American Journal of Obstetrics and Gynecology 164(5):1270–1277

Lehtinen M, Dillner J, Knekt P et al 1996 Serologically diagnosed infection with human papillomavirus type 16 and risk for subsequent development of cervical carcinoma: nested case control study. British Medical Journal 312:537–539

Lewis G, Drife J (eds) 2001 Why mothers die. The fifth report of the Confidential Enquiries into Maternal Deaths in the UK 1997–1999. RCOG Press, London

Lumsden M A, Wallace E M 1998 Clinical presentation of uterine fibroids. Bailliéres Clinical Obstetrics and Gynaecology 12(2):177–195

Moulder C 2001 Miscarriage women's experiences and need, revised edn. Routledge, London

Myers D L, Scotti R J 1995 Acute urinary retention and the incarcerated, retroverted, gravid uterus. A case report. Journal of Reproductive Medicine 40:487–490

NBTSIWP (National Blood Transfusion Service Immunoglobulin Working Party) 1991 Recommendations for the use of anti-D immunoglobulin. Prescribers Journal 31:137–145

Newlands E S, Seckl S J, Boultbee J E, Fisher R A, Paradinas F J 2001 Gestational trophoblastic tumours. Information for medics. Hydatidiform Mole and Choriocarcinoma UK Information and Support Service. Online. Available: http://www.hmole-chorio.org.uk 19 December 2001

NHSCSP (National Health Service Cancer Screening Programme) 2000 Good practice in breast and cervical screening for women with learning disabilities. NHSCSP, Sheffield

Paintain D 1994 Induced abortion. In: Clements R V (ed) Safe practice in obstetrics and gynaecology. A medico-legal handbook. Churchill Livingstone, Edinburgh, ch 28, p 355

Rai R, Clifford K, Regan L 1996 The modern preventative treatment of recurrent miscarriage. British Journal of Obstetrics and Gynaecology 103:106–110

RCOG (Royal College of Obstetricians and Gynaecologists) 1999a The management of recurrent miscarriage, evidence based guidelines. Online. Available: http://www.rcog.org.uk/guidelines/recurrent.html 9/4/01

RCOG (Royal College of Obstetricians and Gynaecologists) 1999b The management of gestational trophoblastic disease, evidence based guidelines. Online. Available: http://www.rcog.org.uk/guidelines/guideline18.html 9/4/01

RCOG (Royal College of Obstetricians and Gynaecologists) 2000 The care of women requesting termination, evidence based guideline number 7. RCOG, London

RCOG (Royal College of Obstetricians and Gynaecologists 2001 Management of early pregnancy loss, evidence based guidelines. Online. Available: http://www.rcog.org.uk/guidelines/guideline25.html 9/4/01

Regan L 1997 Sporadic and recurrent miscarriage. In: Grudzinskas J G, O'Brien P M S (eds) Problems in early pregnancy advances in diagnosis and management. RCOG Press, London, ch 3, p 31–52

Regan L, Rai R 2000 Epidemiology and the medical causes of miscarriage. Best Practice and Research in Clinical Obstetrics and Gynaecology 14(5):839–854

Regan L, Braude P R, Trembath P L 1989 Influence of past reproductive performance on risk of spontaneous abortion. British Medical Journal 229:541–545

Schlecht N F, Kulaga S, Robitaille J et al 2001 Persistent human papillomavirus as a predictor of cervical intraepithelial neoplasia. Journal of the American Medical Association 286(24):3106–3114

Snell L H, Haughey B P, Buck G, Marecki M A 1998 Metabolic crisis: hyperemesis gravidarum. Journal of Perinatal and Neonatal Nursing 12(2):26–37

Stirrat G M 1990a Recurrent miscarriage I: definition and epidemiology. Lancet 336:673–675

Stirrat G M 1990b Recurrent miscarriage II: clinical associations, causes and management. Lancet 336:728–733

Szulman A E 1988 The biology of trophoblastic disease: complete and partial hydatidiform moles. In: Beard R W, Sharp F (eds) Early pregnancy loss, mechanisms and treatment. Springer-Verlag, London, p 309–316

UKCC (United Kingdom Central Council for Nursing, Midwifery and Health Visiting) 1998 The midwives rules and code of practice. UKCC, London

Vergani P, Ghidini A, Strobelt N et al 1994 Do uterine leiomyomas influence pregnancy outcome? American Journal of Perinatology 11(5):356–358

WHO (World Health Organisation) 1997 Unsafe abortion: Global and regional estimates of incidence of mortality due to unsafe abortion with a history of available country data, 3rd edn. WHO, Geneva

FURTHER READING

Moulder C 2001 Miscarriage: women's experiences and need. Revised edn. Routledge, London

This book explores the issues surrounding early pregnancy loss from the mother's perspective. It is based on the author's research, and includes guidelines for professional practice.

Wickham S 2000 Midwives and anti-D enabling choice. Practising Midwife 3(10):11–12

Brief journal article, reminding midwives of the need for mothers to be able to give informed consent to having anti-D, which is a blood product.

18 Problems of Pregnancy

Helen Crafter

CHAPTER CONTENTS

Problems of pregnancy range from the mildly irritating to life-threatening conditions. Fortunately the life-threatening ones are rare because of improvements to the general health of the population, improved social circumstances and lower parity. However, as women delay childbearing (an increasing phenomenon in the developed world) they become more at risk of disorders associated with increasing age, such as malignancy, placenta praevia and problems associated with obesity. Regular antenatal checks beginning early in pregnancy are undoubtedly valuable. They help to prevent many complications and their ensuing problems, contribute to timely diagnosis and treatment, and enable women to form relationships with midwives, obstetricians and other health professionals who become involved with them in striving to achieve the best possible pregnancy outcomes.

The chapter aims to:

- provide an overview of problems of pregnancy
- describe the role of the midwife in relation to the identification, assessment and management of the more common disorders of pregnancy
- consider the needs of both parents for continuing support and reassurance when a disorder has been diagnosed.

The midwife's role

The midwife's role in relation to the problems associated with pregnancy is clear. At initial and subsequent encounters with the pregnant woman it is essential that an accurate health history is obtained. General and specific physical examinations must be carried out and the results meticulously recorded. The examination and recordings give direction towards future referral and management. Although the elements of antenatal care are routine for the midwife they will be very individual for the mother in her care.

Where the midwife detects a deviation from the norm in the health of the mother or fetus, she must refer that woman to a registered medical practitioner (UKCC 1998). The midwife will continue to offer the woman care and support throughout her pregnancy and beyond. The woman who develops problems during her pregnancy is no less in need of the midwife's skilled attention; indeed, her condition and psychological state may be considerably improved by the midwife's continued presence and support.

Abdominal pain in pregnancy

Abdominal pain is a common complaint in pregnancy. It is probably suffered by all women at some stage, and therefore presents a problem for the midwife of how to distinguish between the physiologically normal (e.g. mild indigestion or muscle stretching), the pathological but not dangerous (e.g. degeneration of a fibroid) and the dangerously pathological requiring immediate referral to the appropriate medical practitioner for urgent treatment (e.g. ectopic pregnancy or appendicitis).

The midwife should take a detailed history and perform a physical examination in order to reach a decision about whether to refer the woman. Treatment will depend on the cause (Box 18.1) and the maternal and fetal conditions.

Many of the pregnancy-specific causes of abdominal pain in pregnancy listed in Box 18.1 are dealt with in this and other chapters. For many of these conditions abdominal pain is one of many, and not necessarily an overriding, symptom. However, an observant midwife may be crucial to a safe pregnancy outcome for a woman presenting with abdominal pain.

Uterine fibroid degeneration

The problems experienced in early pregnancy, as outlined in Chapter 17, may continue throughout the pregnancy as the muscle fibres continue to become hypertrophic and the fibroid (myoma) enlarges. Approximately 10% of women with uterine fibroids will experience acute pain, as fibroids situated within the myometrium may receive a diminished blood supply

---

Box 18.1 Causes of abdominal pain in pregnancy (Mahomed 1999)

Pregnancy-specific causes

- Physiological
  - Heartburn, excessive vomiting, constipation
  - Round ligament pain
  - Severe uterine torsion
  - Braxton–Hicks contractions
  - Miscellaneous discomfort in late pregnancy

- Pathological
  - Ectopic pregnancy
  - Miscarriage
  - Uterine fibroids
  - Placental abruption
  - Preterm labour
  - Severe pre-eclampsia
  - Uterine rupture

Incidental causes

- Common pathology
  - Appendicitis
  - Intestinal obstruction
  - Cholecystitis
  - Inflammatory bowel disease
  - Peptic ulcer
  - Renal disease
  - Ovarian pathology e.g. torsion
  - Acute pancreatitis
  - Urinary tract infection
  - Malaria
  - Tuberculosis (may be associated with HIV infection)

- Rare pathology
  - Rectus haematoma
  - Sickle cell crisis
  - Porphyria
  - Arteriovenous haemorrhage
  - Malignant disease

---

and, as the pregnancy progresses, there may be central core necrosis.

If the fibroid or fibroids were not diagnosed prior to pregnancy or in its early stages, diagnosis can be made at any stage by ultrasound, especially if a fibroid is seen where the pain is located. Often fibroids are easily palpable. The pain usually subsides within 4 to 7 days with adequate explanation to the woman, rest and analgesia. The pregnancy will usually progress to term. However, the pain is often recurrent, especially if more than one fibroid is present.

Occasionally, enlargement of the fibroid may impede the progress of labour. Rupture of the uterus at the affected site is a possibility that should always be considered when caring for the woman in labour.

Severe uterine torsion

As it grows during pregnancy, the uterus usually rotates to the right by no more than 40°. On rare occasions, the uterus rotates by more than 90° and this may cause abdominal pain in the latter half of pregnancy. There is almost always a predisposing factor in such cases of acute torsion, the most common being fibroid, congenital malformation of the uterus, adnexal mass or a history of pelvic surgery (Mahomed 1999).

The condition is usually managed conservatively by bedrest, altering the maternal position to correct the torsion spontaneously. Analgesia may be required and if administered then the well-being of both mother and fetus should be monitored, as in rare severe cases the mother can become shocked and the fetus deprived of oxygen. In such cases a laparotomy will need to be performed as it is difficult to make a clear diagnosis without surgical evidence. Delivery by caesarean section may be performed, either preceded or followed by manipulation of the uterus.

Symphysis pubis dysfunction (diastasis symphysis pubis)

Symphysis pubis dysfunction is characterised by abnormal relaxation of the ligaments supporting the pubic joint (see Ch. 15). This is brought about by high levels of pregnancy hormones, particularly relaxin. The result of the relaxation is increased mobility of the joint; the pubic bones move up and down alternately as the woman walks. Strain on the sacroiliac joints may also occur, particularly in grande multiparae. The woman will complain of pain in the pubic region, and also of backache, at any time from the 28th week of pregnancy. Pain may be experienced in the abdominal muscles owing to an attempt to stabilise the bones by muscular action. On examination, the mother will complain of tenderness over the symphysis pubis. She may be extremely debilitated by the condition.

The midwife should note whether there is any history of pelvic fractures that may be aggravated by the pregnancy. Otherwise the midwife should explain to the mother the cause of this condition and advise her that as much rest as possible will be beneficial, especially as the pregnancy advances and abdominal distension increases. The woman should also aim to reduce non-essential weightbearing activities and avoid straddle movements, which abduct the hips, for instance squatting (Fry et al 1997). A supportive panty girdle or 'tubigrip' and comfortable shoes may also help when the woman is up and about.

The midwife should notify the doctor of this condition and of the advice which she has given. Advice and treatment from an obstetric physiotherapist will be of great help to the woman. In severe cases, bedrest may be necessary on a firm mattress.

The ligaments should slowly return to normal following delivery. However, the woman should be informed during pregnancy that the pain and discomfort may last for some time after the birth, to give her the opportunity to make appropriate arrangements. Postnatal physiotherapy will aid the strengthening and stabilisation of the joint.

Antepartum haemorrhage (APH)

Bleeding from the genital tract in late pregnancy, after the 24th week of gestation and before the onset of labour, is referred to as an antepartum haemorrhage. This may place the life of the mother and unborn child at risk.

Effect on the fetus

Fetal mortality and morbidity are increased as a result of severe vaginal bleeding in pregnancy. Stillbirth or neonatal death may occur. Premature placental separation and consequent hypoxia may result in severe neurological damage in the baby (Manolitsas et al 1994).

Effect on the mother

If bleeding is severe, it may be accompanied by shock and disseminated intravascular coagulation (DIC; see Blood coagulation failure). The mother may die or be left with permanent ill health. These events are infrequently seen by practitioners in the UK.

Types of APH

If bleeding from local lesions of the genital tract *(incidental causes)* is excluded, Konje & Taylor (1999) state that vaginal bleeding in late pregnancy is confined to placental separation due to *placenta praevia* or *placental abruption* (Table 18.1).

Initial appraisal of a woman with APH

When a woman first loses blood from the vagina during pregnancy, she has little idea of the cause and will find the episode frightening and disturbing. She may call the midwife or present herself at hospital. Her first need is for a feeling that someone capable is in control of the situation. She will fear that she is losing her baby; her partner may fear for the lives of both mother and child. The midwife's role at this stage is to be supportive and ascertain as much detail as possible of the history and the circumstances surrounding the blood loss. This will assist both in assessing the woman's condition and in making a diagnosis. However, the midwife will also be aware that APH is unpredictable and the woman's condition can deteriorate rapidly at any time; she must therefore make a rapid decision about the urgency of need of a medical or paramedic presence, or both, often at the same time as observing and talking to the woman and her partner.

Sometimes, bleeding that the woman had presumed to be from the vagina will in fact be from haemorrhoids. The midwife should consider this differential diagnosis and confirm or exclude this as soon as possible by careful questioning and examination.

Assessment of physical condition

Maternal condition. The first priority is the wellbeing of the mother. The midwife should look for any pallor or breathlessness, which may indicate shock. She also assesses the woman's emotional state as she greets her and begins to ask for a history of events. She must generate the trust of both partners and remain calm.

Observation of pulse rate, respiratory rate, blood pressure and temperature will be made and recorded. The midwife must assess the amount of blood lost in order to ensure adequate fluid replacement. She will discuss with the couple how much has been lost earlier

Table 18.1 Causes of bleeding in late pregnancy (Konje & Taylor 1999)

Cause	Incidence (%)	
Placenta praevia	31.0	
Abruption	22.0	
'Unclassified bleeding'	47.0	
Marginal		60.0
Show		20.0
Cervicitis		8.0
Trauma		5.0
Vulvovaginal varicosities		2.0
Genital tumours		0.5
Genital infections		0.5
Haematuria		0.5
Vasa praevia		0.5
Other		0.5

Note: Konje & Taylor do not explain the lost 2.5% of 'unclassified bleeding'.

and should ask to see all soiled articles, retaining them for the doctor's inspection.

A gentle abdominal examination is made, observing for signs that the woman is going into labour. *On no account must any vaginal or rectal examination be made nor may an enema or suppository be given to a woman suffering from an APH, as these procedures could exacerbate the bleeding.*

Fetal condition. The mother should be asked if the baby has been moving as much as normal. The midwife must attempt to auscultate the fetal heart (see Fig. 16.8, p. 266) and may use ultrasound apparatus to obtain information.

Factors to aid differential diagnosis

The location of the placenta is perhaps the most critical piece of information that will be needed in order to make a correct diagnosis; initially the midwife will not usually have this fact at her disposal. However, if she is able to elicit the following information from her observations and talking to the woman and her partner then this will help her to arrive at a provisional diagnosis:

Pain. Did the pain precede bleeding and is it continuous or intermittent?

Onset of bleeding. Was this associated with any event such as coitus?

Amount of visible blood loss. Is there any reason to suspect that some blood has been retained in utero?

Colour of the blood. Is it bright red or darker in colour?

Degree of shock. Is this commensurate with the amount of blood visible or more severe?

Consistency of the abdomen. Is it soft or tense and board-like?

Tenderness of the abdomen. Does the mother resent abdominal palpation?

Lie, presentation and engagement. Are any of these abnormal when taking account of parity and gestation?

Audibility of the fetal heart. Is the fetal heart heard?

Ultrasound scan. Does a scan suggest that the placenta is in the lower uterine segment?

The relevance of the findings from these observations is further discussed in the context of the various causes of APH.

Supportive treatment

After emotional reassurance the first need is for restoration of physical condition if this is being compromised. This will necessitate fluid replacement first with a plasma expander and later with whole blood if necessary. If the mother is in severe pain she should be offered strong analgesia to help counteract shock. If the midwife is in attendance at home she must decide how best to arrange transfer to hospital. She may summon the emergency obstetric unit where this exists, or alternatively the ambulance service. If she carries intravenous equipment she can site an infusion. The obstetric registrar or paramedic will carry and infuse a plasma expander before transfer of the woman to hospital.

Subsequent management depends on the definite diagnosis.

Placenta praevia

In this condition the placenta is partially or wholly implanted in the lower uterine segment on either the anterior or posterior wall. The anterior location is less serious than the posterior.

The lower uterine segment grows and stretches progressively after the 12th week of pregnancy. In later weeks this may cause the placenta to separate and severe bleeding can occur. Bleeding is caused by shearing stress between the placental trophoblast and maternal venous blood sinuses. In some instances bleeding may be precipitated by coitus. Placenta praevia places the mother and fetus at high risk and it constitutes an obstetric emergency. Medical assistance is vital if the lives of the mother and fetus are to be saved. Women with suspected placenta praevia should be transferred to a consultant obstetric unit.

Degrees of placenta praevia

Type 1 placenta praevia. The majority of the placenta is in the upper uterine segment (Figs 18.1 and 18.5). Vaginal delivery is possible. Blood loss is usually mild and the mother and fetus remain in good condition.

Type 2 placenta praevia. The placenta is partially located in the lower segment near the internal cervical os (marginal placenta praevia) (Figs 18.2 and 18.6). Vaginal delivery is possible, particularly if the placenta is anterior. Blood loss is usually moderate, although the conditions of the mother and fetus can vary. Fetal hypoxia is more likely to be present than maternal shock.

Type 3 placenta praevia. The placenta is located over the internal cervical os but not centrally (Figs 18.3 and 18.7). Bleeding is likely to be severe, particularly when the lower segment stretches and the cervix begins to efface and dilate in late pregnancy. Vaginal delivery is inappropriate because the placenta precedes the fetus.

Type 4 placenta praevia. The placenta is located centrally over the internal cervical os (Figs 18.4 and 18.8) and torrential haemorrhage is very likely. Caesarean section is essential in order to save the lives of the mother and fetus.

Indications of placenta praevia

Bleeding from the vagina is the only sign and it is painless. The uterus is not tender or tense. The presence of placenta praevia should be considered when:

- the fetal head is not engaged in a primigravida (after 36 weeks)
- there is a malpresentation, especially breech
- the lie is oblique or transverse
- the lie is unstable, usually in a multigravida.

Localisation of the placenta using ultrasonic scanning will confirm the existence of placenta praevia and establish its degree.

It is noteworthy that the degree of placenta praevia does not necessarily correspond to the amount of bleeding. A type 4 placenta praevia may never bleed before elective caesarean section in late pregnancy or

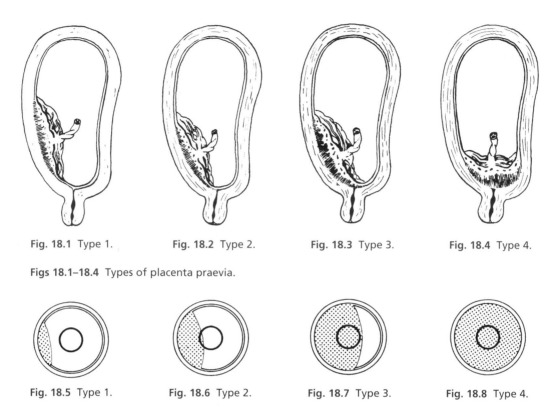

Fig. 18.1 Type 1.   Fig. 18.2 Type 2.   Fig. 18.3 Type 3.   Fig. 18.4 Type 4.

Figs 18.1–18.4 Types of placenta praevia.

Fig. 18.5 Type 1.   Fig. 18.6 Type 2.   Fig. 18.7 Type 3.   Fig. 18.8 Type 4.

Figs 18.5–18.8 Relation of placenta praevia to cervical os.

the onset of spontaneous labour; conversely, some women with placenta praevia type 1 may experience relatively heavy bleeding from early in their pregnancy.

Assessing the mother's condition

The amount of vaginal bleeding is variable; some mothers may have a history of a small repeated blood loss at intervals throughout pregnancy whereas others may have a sudden single episode of vaginal bleeding after the 20th week. However, severe haemorrhage occurs most frequently after the 34th week of pregnancy.

The haemorrhage may be mild, moderate or severe, is often not associated with any particular type of activity and may occur at rest. The colour of the blood is bright red, denoting fresh bleeding. The low placental location allows all of the lost blood to escape unimpeded and a retroplacental clot is not formed. For this reason pain is not a feature of placenta praevia.

General examination. If the haemorrhage is slight the woman's blood pressure, respiratory rate and pulse rate may be normal. In severe haemorrhage, however, the blood pressure will be low and the pulse rate raised owing to shock. The degree of shock correlates with the amount of blood lost from the vagina. Respirations are also rapid and the mother may have air hunger due to a reduction in the number of red blood cells in the circulation available for the uptake of oxygen. The mother's colour will be pale and her skin cold and moist.

Abdominal examination. The midwife may find that the lie of the fetus is oblique or transverse and the fetal head may be high in a primigravida near term. The uterine consistency is normal and pain is not experienced by the mother when her abdomen is palpated.

The midwife should not attempt to do a vaginal examination as this could precipitate a torrential haemorrhage and worsen the situation.

An attempt should be made to quantify the amount of blood lost and all blood-soaked material used by the mother should be saved. Although this will not provide an accurate estimation of the quantity, it may be a helpful clue in assessing fluid replacement.

Assessing the fetal condition

The mother should be asked whether fetal activity has been normal. She may be aware of diminution or cessation of fetal movements, which may occur if fetal hypoxia is severe. In some instances she may report that her fetal movements have been excessive, which is said to be another indication of severe fetal hypoxia.

The midwife should assess the fetal condition using an ultrasound fetal monitor such as a cardiotocograph (CTG) or handheld device. A Pinard fetal stethoscope may be used if these are not available. Fetal oxygenation depends upon the proportion of the placenta remaining attached. Fetal hypoxia is an emergency and medical assistance should be called urgently.

Management of placenta praevia

The management of placenta praevia depends on:

- the amount of bleeding
- the condition of mother and fetus
- the location of the placenta
- the stage of the pregnancy.

Conservative management. This is appropriate if bleeding is slight and the mother and fetus are well. The woman will be kept in hospital at rest until bleeding has stopped. A speculum examination will have ruled out incidental causes. Further bleeding is almost inevitable if the placenta encroaches into the lower segment; therefore it is usual to require the woman to remain in hospital for the rest of the pregnancy. Placental function is monitored by means of fetal kick charts and antenatal CTG. Ultrasound scans are repeated at intervals in order to observe the position of the placenta in relation to the cervical os as the lower segment grows. Fetal growth is also monitored as placental perfusion across the lower segment is less efficient than that in a fundally situated placenta, and intrauterine growth restriction may result.

A woman who is asked to stay in hospital for many weeks will have particular psychological and social needs. If she has other children, she will be anxious to know that good arrangements have been made for their care and they must be allowed to visit her frequently. She should be offered parent education and sometimes it may be possible to continue with a group she has been attending. Occupational therapy may help to alleviate the boredom often felt during long stay hospital admission. A visit to the Special Care Baby Unit, perhaps with her family, and answering any questions she has may also help to prepare her for the possibility of preterm delivery.

A decision will be made about how and when the woman will be delivered. If the woman does not have further severe bleeding she will be delivered when the fetus reaches maturity, vaginally if the placental location allows. Vaginal ultrasound allows for a more accurate estimation of placental site, on which the decision about mode of delivery will be based.

Vaginal delivery is usual with type 1 placenta praevia and possible with type 2, unless the placenta is situated immediately above the sacral promontory where it is vulnerable to pressure from an advancing fetal head and may impede descent. The degrees of placenta praevia that are amenable to vaginal delivery may be termed minor. Labour is likely to be induced from 37 weeks' gestation.

The midwife should be aware that, even if vaginal delivery is achieved, there remains a danger of postpartum haemorrhage. This is because the placenta has been situated in the lower segment where there is paucity of oblique muscle fibres and therefore the living ligature action will be poor.

Active management. Severe vaginal bleeding will necessitate immediate delivery by caesarean section regardless of the location of the placenta. This should take place in a unit with facilities for the appropriate care of the newborn, especially if the baby will be preterm.

Blood will be taken for a full blood count, crossmatching and clotting studies. An intravenous infusion will be in progress and several units of blood may need to be transfused quickly, with the woman's consent. In an emergency it may be necessary to give group O blood, if possible of the same Rhesus group as the mother.

An anaesthetist will be involved in the woman's care, assessing her fluid requirements and output and helping her to make a decision about the use of regional or general anaesthesia (if she is able). During the assessment and preparation for theatre the mother will be extremely anxious and the midwife must comfort and encourage her, giving her as much information as possible. The partner will also need to be supported, whether he is in the operating theatre or waits outside.

If the placenta is situated anteriorly in the uterus, this may complicate the surgical approach as it underlies the site of the normal incision. In major degrees of placenta praevia (types 3 and 4) caesarean section is required even if the fetus has died in utero. Such management aims to prevent torrential haemorrhage and possible maternal death.

Incidence

Placenta praevia occurring after 20 weeks' gestation complicates 3–6 of every 1000 pregnancies (Lockwood & Funai 1999). It is more common in multigravidae, with an incidence of 1 in 90 deliveries. (Placenta praevia rates rise in women with increasing age and increasing parity.) In primigravidae the incidence is 1 in 250 deliveries. Its aetiology is unknown, but a raised incidence is also seen in women who smoke and those who have had a previous caesarean section. The recurrence rate for women who have had a previous placenta praevia is in the order of 4–8%.

Complications include:

- maternal shock, resulting from blood loss and hypovolaemia
- anaesthetic and surgical complications, which are more common in women with major degrees of placenta praevia, and in those for whom preparation for surgery has been suboptimal (Lewis & Drife 2001)
- placenta accreta, in up to 15% of women with placenta praevia
- air embolism, an occasional occurrence when the sinuses in the placental bed have been broken
- postpartum haemorrhage: occasionally uncontrolled haemorrhage will continue, despite the administration of uterotonic drugs at delivery – even following the best efforts to control it, and a caesarean hysterectomy may be required to save the woman's life
- maternal death, a very rare outcome of this condition (Lewis & Drife 2001)

- fetal hypoxia and its sequelae due to placental separation
- fetal death, depending on gestation and amount of blood loss.

Placental abruption

Premature separation of a normally situated placenta occurring after the 22nd week of pregnancy is referred to as *placental abruption*. The aetiology of this type of haemorrhage is not always clear, but it is often associated with severe pre-eclampsia, although not chronic hypertension (Ananth et al 1997). Abruption can follow a sudden reduction in uterine size, for instance when the membranes rupture or after the birth of a first twin, and rarely is a result of direct trauma to the abdomen, perhaps through a road traffic accident (Reis et al 2000), seat-belt injury (Eckford et al 1995) or deliberate violence. All of these may partially dislodge the placenta. Abu-Heija et al (1998) found in their large case–control study of 18 256 women that high parity was a significant aetiological factor. Rasmussen et al (1999) found that caesarean section in the previous delivery increased the risk of placental abruption by 40%. There also appears to be a correlation between placental abruption and cigarette smoking (Andres 1996).

Interestingly, some researchers are starting to find links between pregnancy-induced hypertension, intrauterine growth restriction and preterm birth in that they may share a common early to mid-pregnancy aetiology of placental dysfunction, which may then manifest itself as placental abruption in the second half of pregnancy (Ananth & Wilcox 2001, Rasmussen et al 1999, 2000). This theory clearly needs to be tested in future research.

Unlike inevitable haemorrhage that is due to placenta praevia, placental abruption is an accidental occurrence of haemorrhage that occurs in 0.49–1.8% of all pregnancies (Konje & Taylor 1999). 'Accidental' in this context does not denote trauma.

Partial separation of the placenta causes bleeding from the maternal venous sinuses in the placental bed. Further bleeding continues to separate the placenta to a greater or lesser degree. If blood escapes from the placental site it separates the membranes from the uterine wall and drains through the vagina. Blood that is retained behind the placenta may be forced into the myometrium and it infiltrates between the muscle fibres of the uterus. This extravasation can cause marked damage and, if observed at operation, the uterus will appear bruised and oedematous. This is termed *Couvelaire uterus* or *uterine apoplexy*. There is no vaginal bleeding, but the mother will have all the signs and symptoms of hypovolaemic shock, caused by concealed bleeding into the muscle of the uterus. The concealed haemorrhage causes uterine enlargement and extreme pain.

A combination of these two situations where some of the blood drains via the vagina and some is retained behind the placenta is known as a mixed haemorrhage.

Types of placental abruption

The blood loss from a placental abruption may be defined as *revealed, concealed* or *mixed haemorrhage*, as described above. An alternative classification, based on the degree of separation and therefore related to the condition of the mother and baby, is of *mild, moderate* and *severe haemorrhage*. The midwife cannot rely on visible blood loss as a guide to the severity of the haemorrhage; on the contrary, the most severe haemorrhage is that which is totally concealed.

Assessing the mother's condition

There may be a history of pre-eclampsia. A recent history of headaches, nausea, vomiting, epigastric pain and visual disturbances may be a feature. Road traffic accidents are probably the most likely cause of trauma to the abdomen. Physical domestic violence should be considered by the midwife, which the woman may be too frightened to reveal (Bewley & Gibbs 2001). External cephalic version injudiciously performed may also result in placental separation. The midwife should be aware of the possibility of placental separation after the birth of a first twin or loss of copious amounts of amniotic fluid.

The mildest degrees of placental abruption are relatively pain free, although the mother may experience a slight localised pain. The blood loss is revealed. More severe degrees are associated with abdominal pain and the midwife should enquire about the time of onset and whether the bleeding (if any) began simultaneously or later.

General examination. The woman is likely to be anxious, experiencing abdominal pain, and her skin will be pale and moist if she is shocked. On clinical examination the mother may have obvious oedema of the face, fingers and pretibial area of the lower limbs due to pre-eclampsia.

The blood pressure and pulse should be taken immediately. A low blood pressure and raised pulse rate are signs of shock; if the mother has pregnancy-induced hypertension then the blood pressure may be within normal limits, having been raised prior to the haemorrhage. The respirations may be normal or rapid, and reduced oxygenation may lead to air hunger. The temperature will usually be normal but, as placental abruption may be caused by severe infection, it should be taken.

The amount of any visible blood loss should be estimated and its colour noted. Freshly lost blood is bright red; blood that has been retained in utero for any length of time changes to a brown colour.

Abdominal examination. Concealed haemorrhage may lead to uterine enlargement in excess of gestation. The uterus has a hard consistency and there is guarding on palpation of the abdomen. Palpation may be difficult and should not be attempted if the uterus is rigid and excessively painful. Fetal parts may not be palpable. In less severe cases palpation should be kept to a minimum in order to avoid further damage. The nature and location of the pain should be established.

The fetal heart is unlikely to be heard with a fetal stethoscope if there has been any concealed haemorrhage; an ultrasound scanner, CTG or hand-held device should be used. If the haemorrhage is severe, fetal death is a common outcome.

Assessing the fetal condition

The woman may be aware of a cessation of fetal movements. It is said that excessive fetal movements may also occur as a result of profound hypoxia. A CTG recording will give more complete information about fetal condition, as will an ultrasound scan of the heart chambers. Failure to elicit heart sounds with a Pinard stethoscope is not confirmation of fetal death.

The midwife should take care how she conveys information about the fetus to the mother. If the heart is inaudible on first examination, she should explain that a fetal monitor is needed to establish the condition of her baby. If fetal heart sounds can be detected with ultrasonic apparatus, this will be of great comfort to the mother. It is rarely, if ever, appropriate to attempt to conceal fetal death from the mother.

Management

Any woman with a history suggestive of placental abruption needs urgent medical attention. She should be transferred speedily to a consultant obstetric unit, preferably by the emergency obstetric service. The GP needs to be informed but the midwife remains responsible for ensuring that the woman is transferred to hospital (UKCC 1998). The midwife or a paramedic may site an intravenous cannula prior to transfer.

On arrival at the hospital the woman is admitted to the delivery suite and the registrar or consultant obstetrician is informed. The midwife should offer the woman comfort and encouragement by attending to her physical and emotional needs, including her need for information.

Pain exacerbates shock and must be alleviated. As it may be extreme, a suitable analgesic would be morphine 15 mg or pethidine 100–150 mg. If the woman has had a narcotic drug prior to admission, the midwife must alert those in attendance to the fact that analgesia has been given.

The acute pain of concealed haemorrhage from placental abruption is due to the extravasation of blood between the muscle fibres of the uterus. This must be differentiated from the pain of uterine contraction due to the onset of labour and from subcapsular liver haemorrhage as a result of pre-eclampsia. The nature of the pain should be discussed because labour may supervene following placental abruption.

Shock may be due to hypovolaemia, to extravasation and consequent pain or to consumptive coagulopathy. The latter is due to tissue damage and the liberation of thromboplastins into the circulation with resulting disseminated intravascular coagulation. (This is discussed later in this chapter.)

If blood is not available for immediate transfusion, hypovolaemia may be reduced by administering a suitable plasma expander. Letsky (1995) favours the use of Haemaccel, which does not interfere with platelet function or subsequent blood grouping and cross-matching of blood. It also helps to improve renal function. However, this is only a temporary palliative and blood transfusion must follow as quickly as possible.

The woman should rest on her side in order to prevent vena caval occlusion and aortic compression by the gravid uterus. If shock becomes severe and medical assistance cannot be immediately obtained, or intravenous access secured, placing the woman flat with a wedge, or in a semirecumbent position with the legs only raised will help to sustain the circulation to her upper body for a short period. However, under no circumstances should the foot of the bed be elevated as this will cause pooling of blood in the vagina and is unlikely to reduce shock.

Observations

Once the maternal and fetal conditions have been assessed, decisions will be made about management. If resuscitation of the woman is required her condition should be stabilised before surgery is undertaken. Likewise, if the woman and fetus are not in imminent danger (or the fetus has died) some time will elapse before surgery is considered, and at this time it is crucial that the midwife maintains continual and accurate observations.

The mother's blood pressure and pulse rate should be taken at frequent intervals, which will depend on the severity of her condition. If a pyrexia is present the temperature may be recorded every 1–2 hours; if the woman is not feverish, a 4-hourly recording is adequate. A central venous line is usually inserted in order to monitor the central venous pressure every 2 hours, or more frequently, as necessary (see Ch. 32). If the haemorrhage is not severe enough to warrant intravenous infusion, a cannula will be sited in case the haemorrhage suddenly worsens.

Urinary output is accurately assessed by the insertion of an indwelling catheter. Oliguria or anuria indicates suppression of renal function, which may persist until a postpartum diuresis occurs. The urine should be tested for the presence of protein, which may also be linked to pre-eclampsia. Fluid intake must also be recorded accurately and fluid balance assessed with the aid of the central venous pressure recordings.

Fundal height and abdominal girth may be measured at regular intervals. An increase indicates continued bleeding behind the placenta. If the fetus is alive, the fetal heart rate should be monitored continuously with the aid of a CTG.

Any deterioration in the maternal or fetal conditions must be reported immediately to the obstetrician.

Investigations

As soon as practicable following admission a full blood count, cross-match and clotting studies should be obtained. Blood samples may be needed at intervals in order to monitor the progress of the condition. If pre-eclampsia is suspected the relevant blood tests should also be ordered.

Management of different degrees of placental abruption

Mild separation of the placenta. In this case the placental separation and the haemorrhage are slight. Mother and fetus are in a stable condition. There is no indication of maternal shock and the fetus is alive with normal heart sounds. The consistency of the uterus is normal and there is no tenderness on abdominal palpation. It may be difficult to differentiate this condition from placenta praevia and from an incidental cause of vaginal bleeding.

An ultrasound scan can determine the placental location and identify any degree of concealed bleeding. Fetal condition should be continually assessed while bleeding persists by frequent, if not continuous, monitoring of the fetal heart rate. Subsequently CTG should be carried out once or twice daily because any degree of abruption by definition involves partial separation of the placenta.

If the woman is not in labour and the gestation is less than 37 weeks she may be cared for in an antenatal ward for a few days. She may then go home if there is no further bleeding and the placenta has been found to be in the upper uterine segment. Women who have passed the 37th week of pregnancy may be offered induction of labour, especially if there has been more than one episode of mild bleeding. Further heavy bleeding or evidence of fetal distress may indicate that a caesarean section is necessary.

It should also be noted that if the mother is already severely anaemic then even an apparently mild abruption should be dealt with with great caution.

Moderate separation of the placenta. This describes placental separation of about one-quarter. Up to 1000 ml of blood may be lost, some of which will escape from the vagina and some of which will be retained behind the placenta as a retroplacental clot or an extravasation into the uterine muscle. The mother will be shocked, with a raised pulse rate and a lowered blood pressure. There will be a degree of uterine tenderness and abdominal guarding. The fetus may be alive although hypoxic; intrauterine death is also a possibility.

The immediate aims of care are to reduce shock and to replace blood loss. Fluid replacement should be monitored with the aid of a central venous pressure line. The fetal condition should be assessed with continuous CTG if the fetus is alive, in which case immediate caesarean section may be indicated once the woman's condition is stabilised.

If the fetus is in good condition or has already died, vaginal birth may be contemplated. Such a delivery is advantageous because it enables the uterus to contract and control the bleeding. The spontaneous onset of labour frequently accompanies moderately severe placental abruption, but if it does not then amniotomy is usually sufficient to induce labour. Oxytocin may be used with great care if necessary. Delivery is often quite sudden after a short labour. The use of drugs to attempt to stop labour is usually inappropriate.

Moderate separation of the placenta may on occasion deteriorate into a more serious degree of separation.

Severe separation of the placenta. This is an acute obstetric emergency; at least two-thirds of the placenta has become detached and 2000 ml of blood or more are lost from the circulation. Most or all of the blood can be concealed behind the placenta. The woman will be severely shocked, perhaps to a degree far beyond what might be expected from the amount of visible blood loss. The blood pressure will be lowered; the reading may lie within the normal range owing to a preceding hypertension. The fetus will almost certainly be dead. The woman will have very severe abdominal pain with excruciating tenderness; the uterus has a board-like consistency.

Features associated with severe haemorrhage are coagulation defects, renal failure and pituitary failure. Treatment is the same as for moderate haemorrhage. Whole blood should be transfused rapidly and subsequent amounts calculated in accordance with the woman's central venous pressure. Labour may begin spontaneously in advance of amniotomy and the midwife should be alert for signs of uterine contraction causing periodic intensifying of the abdominal pain.

However, if bleeding continues or a compromised fetal heart rate is present, caesarean section may be required as soon as the woman's condition has been adequately stabilised. The woman requires constant explanation and psychological support, despite the fact that, because of her shocked condition, she may not be fully conscious. Pain relief must also be considered. The woman's partner will also be very concerned, and should not be forgotten in the rush to stabilise the woman's condition.

Care of the baby

Preparation should be made for an asphyxiated baby. The paediatrician must be present at the birth to resuscitate the infant. The baby may require neonatal intensive care following delivery and the staff of the neonatal unit will have been alerted. In addition to the insult of the haemorrhage, the baby may suffer from the effects of preterm delivery and the stay in the neonatal unit may be prolonged. A baby who is born in good condition will of course require minimal resuscitation and may be transferred to the postnatal ward together with the mother.

Psychological care

When a woman has a placental abruption she and her partner must be kept fully informed of what is happening at all times. The doctor should have a full and frank discussion with them about the events and the prognosis. The midwife should ensure that the partner is offered support and adequate explanation if the woman requires emergency surgery, or if her condition deteriorates suddenly. Whenever possible he should continue to be present and he may need another member of the family to share the burden.

If the fetus is alive, a midwife or nurse from the neonatal unit should visit the couple in order to introduce herself and explain where the baby will be cared for after delivery. The partner should be encouraged to visit the unit.

When the baby is born, if it is at all possible, the parents should be given a chance to see and handle their child before she or he is transferred to the neonatal unit. It is most helpful to have a photograph taken, which the mother can keep beside her, and the father should visit the baby at the earliest opportunity. Later the mother will be taken to see the baby, if necessary in her bed or in a wheelchair. As soon as she is able, she will be encouraged to participate in caring for her baby.

At a suitable time following her recovery, the mother must be invited to discuss the events and the prognosis for her baby. She may ask about the possibility of haemorrhage occurring in future pregnancies. There is some evidence that a previous abruption is a risk factor for abruption in the next pregnancy (Misra & Ananth 1999, Rasmussen et al 1997).

Complications

- DIC is a complication of moderate to severe placental abruption.
- Postpartum haemorrhage may occur as a result of the Couvelaire uterus and disseminated intravascular coagulation, or both. Intravenous ergometrine 0.5 mg is given at delivery as a prophylactic measure.
- Renal failure may occur as a result of hypovolaemia and consequent poor perfusion of the kidneys.
- Pituitary necrosis is another possible consequence of prolonged and severe hypotension (also known as Sheehan's syndrome; see medical texts for details of this rare condition).

Blood coagulation failure

Normal blood coagulation

Haemostasis refers to the arrest of bleeding, its function being to prevent loss of blood from the blood vessels. It depends on the mechanism of coagulation. This is counterbalanced by fibrinolysis which ensures that the blood vessels are reopened in order to maintain the patency of the circulation.

Blood clotting occurs in three main stages:

- When tissues are damaged and platelets break down, *thromboplastin* is released.
- In the presence of *calcium* ions, thromboplastin leads to the conversion of *prothrombin* into *thrombin*.
- Thrombin is a proteolytic (protein-splitting) enzyme that converts *fibrinogen* into *fibrin*.

Fibrin forms a network of long, sticky strands that entrap blood cells to establish a clot. The coagulated material contracts and exudes serum, which is plasma depleted of its clotting factors.

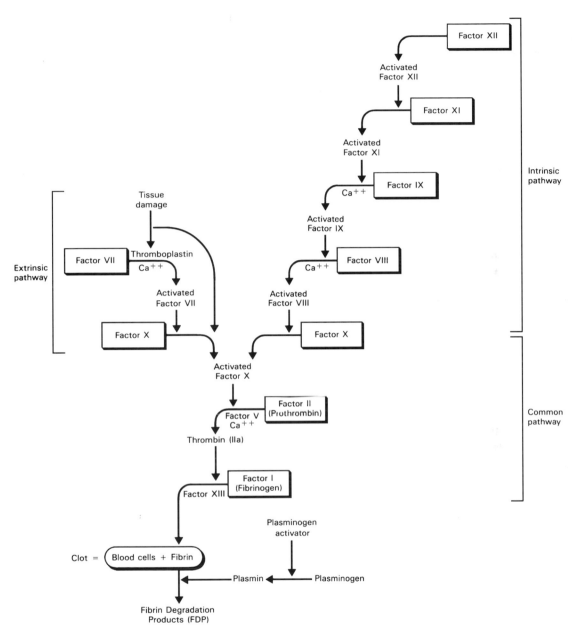

Fig. 18.9 The coagulation cascade.

This is the final part of a complex cascade of coagulation involving a large number of different clotting factors. These factors have been assigned numbers in order of their discovery and a summary of the process is shown in Figure 18.9.

It is equally important for a healthy person to maintain the blood as a fluid in order that it can circulate freely. The coagulation mechanism is normally held at bay by the presence of heparin, which is produced in the liver.

Fibrinolysis is the breakdown of fibrin and occurs as a response to the presence of clotted blood. Unless fibrinolysis takes place, coagulation will continue. It is achieved by the activation of a series of enzymes culminating in the proteolytic enzyme plasmin. This breaks down the fibrin in the clots and produces fibrin degradation products (FDPs).

Disseminated intravascular coagulation (DIC)

This is a situation of inappropriate coagulation within the blood vessels, which leads to the consumption of clotting factors. As a result clotting fails to occur at the bleeding site. DIC is rare when the fetus is alive and it usually starts to resolve when the baby is born (Enkin et al 2000).

Aetiology

DIC is never a primary disease – it always occurs as a response to another disease process. Such an event triggers widespread clotting with the formation of microthrombi throughout the circulation. Clotting factors are used up. The DIC triggers fibrinolysis and the production of FDPs. FDPs reduce the efficiency of normal clotting. A paradoxical feedback system is therefore set up, in which clotting is the primary problem, but haemorrhage the predominant clinical finding.

When DIC occurs during or after delivery, the reduced level of clotting factors and the presence of FDPs prevent normal haemostasis at the placental site. FDPs inhibit myometrial action and prevent the uterine muscle from constricting the blood vessels in the normal way. Torrential haemorrhage may be the outcome. Visible blood loss may be observed to remain uncoagulated for several minutes and even when clotting does occur, the clot is unstable.

Microthrombi may cause circulatory obstruction in the small blood vessels. The effects of this vary from cyanosis of fingers and toes to cerebrovascular accidents and failure of organs such as the liver and kidneys.

Events that trigger DIC

There are a number of obstetric events that may precipitate DIC:

- placental abruption
- intrauterine fetal death including delayed miscarriage
- amniotic fluid embolism
- intrauterine infection including septic abortion
- pre-eclampsia and eclampsia.

Each of these conditions is dealt with in the appropriate chapter and only those aspects relating to DIC are discussed here.

Placental abruption. Owing to the damage of tissue at the placental site large quantities of thromboplastin are released into the circulation and may cause DIC. If the placenta is delivered as soon as possible after the abruption the risk of DIC is reduced. (However, vaginal delivery where possible is often favoured over caesarean birth to reduce the risk of postpartum haemorrhage.)

Intrauterine fetal death. If a dead fetus is retained in utero for more than 3 or 4 weeks then thromboplastins are released from the dead fetal tissues. These enter the maternal circulation and deplete clotting factors. If labour does not follow fetal death spontaneously then it should be induced, with the woman's consent. If fetal death is known to have occurred some time previously, clotting studies should be performed prior to induction of labour; if DIC is diagnosed the appropriate medical action should be taken.

Amniotic fluid embolism. If death does not occur from maternal collapse, DIC may develop. Thromboplastin in the amniotic fluid is responsible for setting off the cascade of clotting.

Intrauterine infection. The causes of this include septic abortion, hydatidiform mole, placenta accreta and endometrial infection before or after delivery. DIC is caused by endotoxins entering the circulation and damaging the blood vessels. Therefore, as well as treating the DIC, the infection itself must be aggressively treated with antibiotics. It should be noted that if the woman develops haemolytic septicaemia any blood administered may be destroyed by the bacteria in the bloodstream. The baby may need treatment following delivery if the infection was antepartum. In postpartum infection any retained products must be evacuated from the uterus.

Pre-eclampsia and eclampsia. The occurrence of DIC with severe pre-eclampsia is fully dealt with in Chapter 20.

Management

The midwife should be aware of the conditions that may cause DIC. She should be alert for signs that clotting is abnormal and the assessment of the nature of the clot should be part of her routine observation during the third stage of labour. Oozing from a venepuncture site or bleeding from the mucous membrane of the mother's mouth and nose must be noted and reported. As well as a full blood count and blood grouping, the doctor will carry out clotting studies and also measure the levels of platelets, fibrinogen and FDPs.

Treatment involves the replacement of blood cells and clotting factors in order to restore equilibrium. This is usually done by the administration of fresh frozen plasma and platelet concentrates. Banked red cells will be transfused subsequently. The use of fresh whole blood is not now common, partly because the screening processes undertaken in the modern transfusion service can take up to 24 hours and the components are best given separately. In situations where the transfusion service is not so sophisticated, whole blood will be used.

Care by the midwife

DIC causes a frightening situation that demands speed both of recognition and of action. The midwife has to maintain her own calmness and clarity of thinking as well as helping the couple to deal with the situation in which they find themselves. Frequent and accurate observations must be maintained in order to monitor the woman's condition. Blood pressure, pulse rate and temperature are recorded. The general condition is noted. Fluid balance is monitored with vigilance for any sign of renal failure.

The father in particular is likely to be baffled by a sudden turn in events when previously all seemed to be under control. The midwife must make sure that someone is giving him appropriate attention and he will need to be kept informed of what is happening and be excluded as little as possible. The carers need to be aware that he may find it impossible to absorb all that he is told and he may require repeated explanations. He may be the best person to help the woman to understand. The death of the mother is a real possibility and this may be one of the rare situations when the midwife finds herself needing to minister to a grieving partner.

Hepatic disorders and jaundice in pregnancy

The metabolic changes in pregnancy influence hepatic function. These changes are brought about by the increased hormone levels. Some liver disorders are specific to pregnant women, and some pre-existing or coexisting disorders may complicate the pregnancy (Box 18.2).

Intrahepatic cholestasis of pregnancy (ICP)

This is an idiopathic condition that begins in pregnancy, usually in the third trimester but occasionally as early as the first trimester. It resolves spontaneously following delivery, but has a 60–80% recurrence rate in subsequent pregnancies (Walters 1999). The prevalence rate is 1–2 cases per 1000 pregnancies in low risk populations, but it is seen much more frequently in Scandinavia, Chile, Poland, Australia and China. Its cause is unknown although genetic, geographical and environmental factors would appear to be at play. Almes (1995), Davidson (1998) and Gaudet et al (2000) put forward a group of theories that suggest the biochemistry of bile metabolism is altered; this is possibly due to a genetic inherited hypersensitivity to oestrogens. A subsequent increase in serum bile acid levels then negatively affects placental blood flow, putting the fetus at risk. Disturbances in fetal steroid metabolism may also be implicated. It is not a life-threatening condition for the mother, but she is at increased risk of preterm labour, fetal compromise and meconium staining and her stillbirth risk is increased by 15% unless there is active management of her pregnancy.

Affected women will firstly start to notice pruritus at night, and may complain of fatigue and insomnia because of this. Two weeks later, 50% of women affected will develop mild jaundice, which will persist

---

Box 18.2 Hepatic disorders of pregnancy

Specific to pregnancy
- Intrahapatic cholestasis of pregnancy
- Acute fatty liver in pregnancy
- Pre-eclampsia and eclampsia (see Ch. 20)
- Severe hyperemesis gravidarum (see Ch. 17)

Pre- or coexisting in pregnancy
- Gall bladder disease
- Hepatitis

until the birth. Fever, abdominal discomfort and nausea and vomiting are not uncommon symptoms. Women may notice that their urine is darker and stools are paler than usual.

If this condition is suspected, blood will be tested for an increase in bile acids, serum alkaline phosphatase, bilirubin and transaminases. Hepatic viral studies, an ultrasound scan of the hepatobiliary tract and an autoantibody screen (for primary biliary cirrhosis) are also indicated as of value in excluding differential diagnoses. The woman will be prescribed local antipruritic agents, for instance antihistamines, and advised to keep any sores caused by scratching clean. Drugs such as phenobarbital, colestyramine and dexamethasone have disappointing results in controlling the condition and its symptoms (Walters 1999).

Because of concern about the implications of this condition for the fetus, the resultant jaundice and the severity of the itching, this woman will require sensitive psychological care. She will be prescribed a vitamin K supplement as her absorption will be poor (and the resulting hypoprothrombinaemia will predispose her to obstetric haemorrhage). Fetal well-being should be monitored, possibly by Doppler analysis of the umbilical artery blood flow, and elective delivery considered when the fetus is mature (usually at 35–38 weeks of gestation) or earlier if the fetal condition appears to be compromised by the intrauterine environment.

The woman can be advised that her pruritus will resolve within 3–14 days after the birth. She should be carefully monitored if she uses oral contraception in the future. The pruritus is often so severe and distressing that many women who have suffered from this condition will avoid future pregnancy.

Acute fatty liver of pregnancy (AFLP)

This is a rare condition of unknown aetiology with an incidence in various studies of between 1 in 6692 and 1 in 15 900 pregnancies (Samuels & Landon 1996). It is frequently fatal for the mother and baby unless there is a speedy diagnosis and the correct treatment is given.

Typically, an obese woman will present with vomiting and a headache in her third trimester. She will quickly complain of malaise and severe abdominal pain, followed by jaundice and drowsiness. Fagan (1995) comments that over 50% of these women have

symptoms of pre-eclampsia (hypertension and proteinuria), and so there is an inherent danger that the pre-eclampsia will mask the presentation of AFLP.

The condition is diagnosed by the clinical picture. The woman's liver is tender but not enlarged, and an ultrasound or computerised tomography (CT) scan of the liver demonstrates fatty infiltration. Liver biopsy is contraindicated owing to the risk of coagulopathy. The liver enzymes are moderately raised and the woman will also quickly show signs of renal failure and will become hypoglycaemic.

Management will firstly involve correcting any coagulopathy by measures such as infusing fresh frozen plasma. The woman must be delivered immediately. Caesarean section is said to have many advantages for the baby, but it is safest for the mother to deliver vaginally if this is possible. Epidural analgesia is contraindicated in all but the mildest cases owing to the coagulopathy problems, unless these have been corrected first.

Convalescence is prolonged but usually complete. In the few cases where further pregnancy has been undertaken and recorded in the medical literature, recurrence has been low.

Gall bladder disease

Pregnancy appears to increase the likelihood of gallstone formation but not the risk of developing acute cholecystitis. Diagnosis of gall bladder disease is made by listening to the woman's previous history or an ultrasound scan of the hepatobiliary tract, or both. She will require symptomatic treatment of the biliary colic by analgesia, hydration, nasogastric suction and antibiotics. Surgery should be avoided if at all possible.

Viral hepatitis (B)

Viral hepatitis is the most common cause of jaundice in pregnancy (Fagan 1995). Acute infection affects approximately 1 in 1000 pregnancies and has an incubation period of 1–6 months. Symptoms include nausea, vomiting, anorexia, pain over the liver, mild diarrhoea, jaundice lasting several weeks and malaise. Fever is rare and for many the disease is asymptomatic, or mimics mild influenza. Its main spread is by blood, blood products and sexual activity. The virus can also be transmitted across the placenta. Hepatitis B is more common in tropical and developing countries, especially where nutrition is poor and the use of barrier contraceptives is limited, but it is also a particular problem among injecting drug users who share needles in the Western world.

In healthy adults 90% of cases resolve completely within 6 months. In the remaining 10%, hepatitis B surface antigen (HBsAg) remains in the serum and the woman is considered to be a chronic carrier. Some of these will clear the antigen over the course of the next 6 months and the rest will develop chronic active hepatitis, and the symptoms described above will also continue. A few will develop hepatic failure, which can result in death unless liver transplantation is available (Box 18.3). If hepatitis B is transmitted from mother to fetus and immunisation does not prevent infection in the baby, the child will be at increased risk of liver cancer in later life (Yankowitz & Pastorek 1999). In pregnancy the risk is considered to be greater to the fetus than the mother through transplacental passage of the virus and particularly through blood and body fluids at birth.

Diagnosis is made from the woman's history of her symptoms and lifestyle. Serological studies will be performed, but it can be difficult to distinguish hepatitis B from other forms of viral hepatitis during the acute presentation, before antibodies have formed. Treatment is of the symptoms as they arise. Infection control measures should be instituted where the woman is considered to be infectious, and information not only about the disease, but also nutrition and sexual advice, should be offered. Liver function will be monitored and fetal condition assessed. Household contacts should be offered immunisation once their HBsAg seronegativity is established. Sexual partners should be traced and offered testing and vaccination. Postnatally the mother will be encouraged to accept vaccination for the baby. Advice about breastfeeding remains controversial.

Skin disorders

Many skin changes are noticed by pregnant women; most of these are so common as to be described as physiological.

Treatment of pre-existing skin disorders, such as eczema or psoriasis, should continue as required, bearing in mind that some topical agents should be used

> **Box 18.3** Pregnancy and liver transplantation
>
> There have now been a small number of pregnancies in women who have undergone liver transplantation before or during their pregnancy, many with sucessful outcomes. Although not desirable, liver transplantation in women of childbearing age is becoming increasingly common and such women now have the opportunity to consider having a family. However, the risks to pregnancy are great and these women require expert medical and midwifery care at a specialised centre equipped to deal with all of the complications, both of a physical and psychological nature, that such women may face.

with caution in pregnancy (such as steroid creams and applications containing nut oil derivatives).

Many women suffer from physiological pruritus in pregnancy, especially over the abdomen. Often reassurance, and the application of calamine lotion over the affected area, will suffice. However, for some women, pruritus with or without a rash will be a symptom of a more serious condition. Generalised pruritus should always be referred to a medical practitioner, as it may be a symptom of conditions such as intrahepatic cholestasis (see previous section), liver or thyroid disease, lymphoma or scabies.

Pemphigoid gestationis (herpes gestationis)

This is a disease specific to pregnancy that usually occurs in the mid-trimester and persists into the postnatal period, although sometimes it starts after the birth. It affects 1 in 50 000 pregnancies (Kennedy & Kyle 1999) and its aetiology is unknown; however, it is thought that the condition is initiated by a maternal autoimmune response to paternal antigens and persists under the influence of pregnancy hormones. Despite its name this skin condition is not related to the herpes virus – the misnomer came about in the nineteenth century when 'herpes' referred to skin blisters, rather than the virus.

The woman will complain of generalised itching and a burning sensation, and an erythematous rash will appear (see Plate 3). This is initially over the abdomen, but spreads to involve the remainder of the trunk and limbs. Blisters develop that may become infected and purulent, especially if the woman scratches.

The midwife should refer the woman to a medical practitioner and be supportive to her throughout her care. A skin biopsy may be needed to confirm the diagnosis. Topical or oral steroids may be prescribed depending on the severity of the disease. The lesions should be kept clean and may be covered to prevent the woman scratching. A diet high in vitamins should be encouraged. The woman will usually have her labour induced at about the 37th week of pregnancy as there is controversial evidence that there is a greater incidence of intrauterine growth restriction and raised infant mortality with the condition, which is suggestive of a link with placental insufficiency. The fetus may have a rash when born and will need paediatric examination for any skin lesions, although these are usually clinically mild.

Without excessive scratching or secondary infection, the woman's lesions will heal without scarring, although this may take some time and occasionally a few years. Once the condition has been activated by pregnancy, flare-ups may occur during menstruation, at ovulation or when the woman takes an oral contraceptive (Kennedy & Kyle 1999). The condition may recur in subsequent pregnancies, especially with the same partner.

Disorders of the amniotic fluid

Normal amniotic fluid increases in amount throughout pregnancy from a few millilitres until 38 weeks, when there is about a litre. After this it diminishes to approximately 800 ml at term. Amniotic fluid is not static; the water of which it is largely composed is changed every hour and the solutes are changed about every 3 hours.

There are two chief abnormalities of amniotic fluid: polyhydramnios (or hydramnios) and oligohydramnios.

Polyhydramnios

The amount of liquor present in a pregnancy is estimated by measuring 'pools' of liquor around the fetus with ultrasound scanning. The single deepest pool is measured to calculate the amniotic fluid volume (AFV). However, where possible a more accurate diagnosis may be gained by measuring the liquor in each of four quadrants around the fetus in order to establish an amniotic fluid index (AFI).

Polyhydramnios is said to be present when the AFV exceeds 8 cm, or the calculated AFI is more than 24 cm (Thompson et al 1998). Using these definitions, Thompson and colleagues report a prevalence of polyhydramnios of 0.15 and 0.36% respectively. Many et al (1995) categorise polyhydramnios into mild (AFI 25–30 cm), moderate (AFI 30.1–35 cm) or severe (AFI more than 35 cm).

Causes

These include:

- oesophageal atresia
- open neural tube defect
- multiple pregnancy, especially in the case of monozygotic twins
- maternal diabetes mellitus
- rarely, an association with Rhesus isoimmunisation
- chorioangioma, a rare tumour of the placenta
- in many cases, an unknown cause.

Types

Chronic polyhydramnios. This is gradual in onset, usually starting from about the 30th week of pregnancy. It is the most common type.

Acute polyhydramnios. This is very rare (see Plate 4). It usually occurs at about 20 weeks and comes on very suddenly. The uterus reaches the xiphisternum in about 3 or 4 days. It is frequently associated with monozygotic twins or severe fetal abnormality.

Recognition

The mother may complain of breathlessness and discomfort. If the polyhydramnios is acute in onset, she may have severe abdominal pain. The condition may cause exacerbation of symptoms associated with pregnancy such as indigestion, heartburn and constipation. Oedema and varicosities of the vulva and lower limbs may be present.

Abdominal examination. On inspection the uterus is larger than expected for the period of gestation and is globular in shape. The abdominal skin appears stretched and shiny with marked striae gravidarum and obvious superficial blood vessels.

On palpation the uterus feels tense and it is difficult to feel the fetal parts, but the fetus may be balloted between the two hands. A fluid thrill may be elicited by placing a hand on one side of the abdomen and tapping the other side with the fingers. A wave of fluid will move across from the side that is tapped and this is felt by the opposite examining hand. It may be helpful to measure the abdominal girth (Fig. 18.10), particularly in cases of acute polyhydramnios, in order to observe the rate of increase.

Auscultation of the fetal heart can be difficult if the quantity of fluid allows the fetus to move away from the stethoscope.

Ultrasonic scanning is used to confirm the diagnosis of polyhydramnios (Fig. 18.11). As well as calculating the AFV and AFI, and therefore the severity of the polyhydramnios, scanning may reveal a multiple pregnancy or fetal abnormality. X-ray examination is not often performed and the images are usually hazy where there is a large quantity of amniotic fluid.

Complications

These include:

- maternal ureteric obstruction
- increased fetal mobility leading to unstable lie and malpresentation
- cord presentation and prolapse
- prelabour (and often preterm) rupture of the membranes
- placental abruption when the membranes rupture
- preterm labour
- increased incidence of caesarean section
- postpartum haemorrhage
- raised perinatal mortality rate.

Management

The cause of the condition should be determined if possible. The woman may be admitted to a consultant obstetric unit. Subsequent care will depend on the condition of the woman and fetus, the cause and degree of the polyhydramnios and the stage of pregnancy. Diabetes mellitus will be managed as an entity; the polyhydramnios is managed much as in other cases. The presence of fetal abnormality will be taken

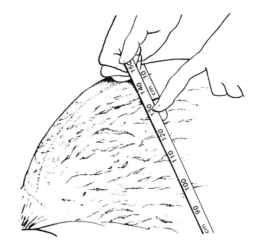

Fig. 18.10 Measuring abdominal girth in a case of polyhydramnios.

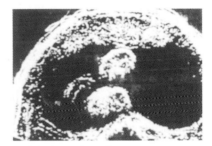

Fig. 18.11 Polyhydramnios: ultrasonogram.

into consideration in choosing the mode and timing of delivery. If gross abnormality is present, labour may be induced; if the fetus is suffering from an operable condition such as oesophageal atresia, it may be appropriate to arrange transfer to a neonatal surgical unit.

Mild asymptomatic polyhydramnios is managed expectantly. The woman is not usually admitted to hospital, but should be advised that if she suspects that her membranes have ruptured immediate admission is recommended. She should be encouraged to get adequate rest, and if she is working it may be helpful to discuss commencing maternity leave, although the physical nature of her job and the stress that may be engendered by stopping work should be assessed with the woman before making recommendations. She will require detailed explanation of the condition and support from her health professionals, but a recent study suggests that if the polyhydramnios is found to be idiopathic, as is more likely in mild asymptomatic cases, she can be reassured that fetal outcome is likely to be good (Panting-Kemp et al 1999).

Regular ultrasound scans will reveal whether or not the polyhydramnios is progressive. Many cases of idiopathic polyhydramnios resolve spontaneously as pregnancy progresses (Hendricks et al 1991).

For a woman with symptomatic polyhydramnios, an upright position will help to relieve any dyspnoea and she may be given antacids to relieve heartburn and nausea. If the discomfort from the swollen abdomen is severe then therapeutic amniocentesis, or amnioreduction, may be considered. However, this is not without risk, as infection may be introduced or the onset of labour provoked. No more than 500 ml should be withdrawn at any one time. It is at best a temporary relief as the fluid will rapidly accumulate again and the procedure may need to be repeated. Acute polyhydramnios managed by amnioreduction has a poor prognosis for the baby. The usual course of events is that the fluid continues to increase at an alarming rate, the membranes rupture spontaneously and the fetus or fetuses are born, grossly premature, in a river of amniotic fluid.

Administration of the drug indomethacin reduces fetal urine production and consequently amniotic fluid, but use of this drug is still in its experimental phase until the risks have been more fully ascertained.

The woman may need to have labour induced in late pregnancy if the symptoms become worse. The lie must be corrected if it is not longitudinal and the membranes will be ruptured cautiously, allowing the amniotic fluid to drain out slowly in order to avoid altering the lie and to prevent cord prolapse. Placental abruption is also a hazard if the uterus suddenly diminishes in size.

Labour is usually normal but the midwife should be prepared for the possibility of postpartum haemorrhage. The baby should be carefully examined for abnormalities and the patency of the oesophagus ascertained by passing a nasogastric tube.

Oligohydramnios

Oligohydramnios is an abnormally small amount of amniotic fluid. At term it may be 300–500 ml but amounts vary and it can be even less. When diagnosed in the first half of pregnancy it is often found to be associated with renal agenesis (absence of kidneys) or Potter's syndrome in which the baby also has pulmonary hypoplasia. When diagnosed at any time in pregnancy before 37 weeks it may be due to fetal abnormality or to preterm premature rupture of the membranes where the amniotic fluid fails to reaccumulate. The lack of amniotic fluid reduces the intrauterine space and over time will cause compression deformities. The baby has a squashed-looking face, flattening of the nose, micrognathia (a deformity of the jaw) and talipes. The skin is dry and leathery in appearance.

Oligohydramnios sometimes occurs in the post-term pregnancy and is believed to be linked with the development of placental insufficiency. As placental function reduces, so too does perfusion to the fetal organ systems including the kidneys. The decrease in fetal urine formation leads to oligohydramnios, as the major component of amniotic fluid is fetal urine.

Recognition

On inspection, the uterus may appear smaller than expected for the period of gestation. The mother who has had a previous normal pregnancy may have noticed a reduction in fetal movements. When the abdomen is palpated the uterus is small and compact and fetal parts are easily felt. Breech presentation is possible. Auscultation is normal.

Ultrasonic scanning will enable differentiation of oligohydramnios from intrauterine growth restriction (although both may occur together where there is placental insufficiency). Renal abnormality may be visible on the scan.

Management

The woman may be admitted to hospital. If the ultrasound scan demonstrates renal agenesis the baby will not survive. Liquor volume will also be estimated from the ultrasound scan, and if renal agenesis is not present them further investigations will include careful questioning of the woman to check the possibility of preterm rupture of the membranes. Placental function tests will also be performed.

Where fetal anomaly is not considered to be lethal, or the cause of the oligohydramnios is not known, prophylactic amnioinfusion with normal saline,

Ringer's lactate or 5% glucose may be performed in order to prevent compression deformities and hypoplastic lung disease, and prolong the pregnancy. Little evidence is available to determine the benefits and hazards of this intervention in mid-pregnancy. However, Pitt et al (2000) in a meta-analysis of randomised controlled trials concluded that prophylactic intrapartum amnioinfusion in women with oligohydramnios resulted in lower caesarean section rates and improved neonatal outcome. Early indications are that this is a useful intervention.

In cases of normal but prolonged pregnancy, where a woman does not wish to have her pregnancy induced, Chua & Arulkumaran (1999) suggest that it is useful to measure the AFI twice weekly, as fluid can reduce remarkably quickly and is highly suggestive of reduced placental function, and to perform a 20–40 minute fetal heart trace (non-stress test), although neither of these wholly guarantee fetal well-being. However, in 1995 Montan & Malcus demonstrated that the normal reduction in amniotic fluid in prolonged pregnancy (which they defined as 42 completed weeks of gestation) had no correlation with adverse fetal and neonatal outcome. Oligohydramnios in prolonged pregnancy is a poorly understood phenomenon, and its management therefore remains highly controversial.

In the case of a woman with oligohydramnios, labour may intervene or be induced because of the possibility of placental insufficiency. Epidural analgesia may be indicated because uterine contractions are often unusually painful with this condition. Impairment of placental circulation or cord compression may result in fetal hypoxia and therefore continuous fetal heart rate monitoring is desirable. In rare cases the membranes may adhere to the fetus. Also, if meconium is passed in utero it will be more concentrated and represent a greater danger to an asphyxiated baby during birth.

Preterm prelabour rupture of the membranes (PPROM)

This condition occurs before 37 completed weeks of gestation where rupture of the fetal membranes occurs without the onset of spontaneous uterine activity resulting in cervical dilatation. (Term prelabour rupture of the membranes is discussed in Ch. 29.)

PPROM affects 2% of pregnancies. Placental abruption is evident in 4–7% of women who present with PPROM. The condition has a 21–32% recurrence rate in subsequent pregnancies of affected women (Svigos et al 1999). It may be associated with cervical incompetence (although it is likely that uterine contractions accompany the rupture of membranes with this condition). There is a strong association between PPROM and maternal vaginal colonisation with potentially pathogenic microorganisms.

Risks of PPROM

These include:

- labour, which may intervene at any time, resulting in a preterm birth
- chorioamnionitis, which may be followed by fetal and maternal systemic infection if not treated promptly
- oligohydramnios if prolonged PPROM occurs, with associated fetal problems including pulmonary hypoplasia
- psychosocial problems resulting from uncertain fetal and neonatal outcome and long term hospitalisation
- cord prolapse
- malpresentation associated with prematurity
- primary antepartum haemorrhage.

Management

Because the pathophysiology of PPROM is still not fully understood, and trials into different management options have not been conclusive in their findings, contemporary management of the condition remains controversial.

Psychological consideration of the woman's, and her partner's, circumstances must always be considered with PPROM as it is known to be an extremely disturbing condition for parents, not least because causes and predictions of the outcome cannot be given. If PPROM is suspected, the woman will be admitted to the delivery suite where a careful history is taken and rupture of the membranes confirmed by a sterile speculum examination of any pooling of liquor in the posterior fornix of the vagina. Very wet sanitary towels over a 6 hour period will also offer a reasonably conclusive diagnosis if urine leakage has been excluded, but a positive nitrazine test should not be considered conclusive when it is the only sign (Svigos et al 1999). Where diagnosis is in doubt, a fetal fibronectin immunoenzyme test is useful in confirming rupture of the membranes.

Digital vaginal examination should be avoided to reduce the risk of introducing infection. Observations must also be made of the fetal condition from the fetal heart rate (an infected fetus may have a tachycardia) and maternal infection screen, temperature and pulse, uterine tenderness and any purulent or offensively smelling vaginal discharge. A decision on future management will then be made.

If the woman has a gestation of less than 32 weeks, the fetus appears to be uncompromised and APH and labour have been excluded, she will be managed expectantly. She is likely to be hospitalised and offered frequent ultrasound scans to check the growth of the fetus and the extent and complications of any oligohydramnios. She should be given corticosteroids as soon as PPROM is confirmed in case delivery occurs (Crowley 2001), and if labour intervenes then tocolytic drugs will be considered to prolong the pregnancy. Known vaginal infection should be treated with antibiotics and prophylactic antibiotics may also be offered to women without symptoms of infection. Although there is no proven benefit that giving antibiotics improves overall neonatal mortality and morbidity, they do appear to be effective in prolonging pregnancy and reducing maternal and neonatal infections morbidity (Kenyon & Boulvain 2001). Sometimes the leak will reseal (especially if it is a hindwater leak) and the pregnancy may proceed with no further complications (Svigos et al 1999). However, 'resealing' is said to occur in only 8% of cases of PPROM occurring in mid-trimester (Sciscione et al 2001). Serial amnioinfusion for otherwise normal pregnancies is an intervention that is gaining increasing interest at present; for instance Locatelli et al (2000) report improved perinatal outcomes where PPROM and oligohydramnios have occurred at less than 26 weeks of gestation. However, if the membranes rupture before 24 weeks of gestation the outlook is not good; the fetus is likely to succumb either to the problems caused by oligohydramnios or to those caused by preterm birth. The mother in such cases may be offered, and may accept termination of the pregnancy.

If the woman is more than 32 weeks' pregnant, the fetus appears to be compromised and APH or intervening labour is suspected or confirmed, active management will ensue. The method of delivery will be decided and induction of labour or caesarean section performed.

Malignant disease in pregnancy

It is estimated that 1 in 1000–1500 pregnancies are complicated by cancer (Munkarah & Morris 1999). The most common malignancies associated with pregnancy are, in descending frequency: cervix, breast, melanoma, ovary, thyroid, leukaemia, lymphoma and colorectum (Allen & Nisker 1986, quoted in Munkarah & Morris 1999). The incidence of cancer occurring alongside pregnancy increases as women delay childbearing (see Ch. 17 for cervical carcinoma). Pregnancy may adversely affect the course of the disease, and cancer in the mother can metastasise to the placenta and fetus, melanoma being the most likely to do so.

If cancer is discovered before pregnancy is embarked upon, it should be treated and followed up before pregnancy is attempted. Once successfully treated, and as long as the reproductive organs are not damaged, pregnancy is rarely contraindicated for medical reasons. However, cancer discovered during pregnancy leads to a host of management dilemmas. The options involve balancing the effects of the treatment, the disease and delivery on both the mother and her fetus.

If the woman is in early pregnancy her first dilemma may be whether or not to continue with the pregnancy. If she continues, the next dilemma will be whether to treat the disease during the pregnancy or wait until delivery, as both chemotherapy and radiation therapy may have toxic effects, particularly on the fetus. Surgery is the treatment least likely to affect the pregnancy adversely, particularly if it takes place in later pregnancy, but it may not be the treatment of first choice for the particular condition.

Elective preterm delivery is often favoured by medical practitioners involved in the woman's care and the woman herself, after which her condition can be assessed and more appropriate treatment of the disease administered.

Needless to say, the support of the midwife throughout pregnancy is likely to be crucial to the woman's psychological well-being.

Obesity or failure to gain weight in pregnancy

Although evidence exists to refute strongly the value of routine weighing of pregnant women in predicting various perinatal outcomes, surprisingly little is known about optimal weight gain and the effects of large and low weight gain in pregnancy. However, it is becoming increasingly clear that women who have a poor diet and their fetuses are at greater risk than well-nourished women (Dallison & Lobstein 1995).

Weight is no more than a very crude indicator of a woman's health status in pregnancy. However, the midwife's observation of a very obese woman, or a very thin one, should alert her to some of the risks such women may face during pregnancy and the longer term risks to both women and their children (see Ch. 12 for Quetelet index).

A woman who starts pregnancy while obese, or puts on an excessive amount of weight during pregnancy, appears to be at greater risk of hypertensive disturbances, including pregnancy-induced hypertension (see Ch. 20). She is also at greater risk of gestational diabetes (see Ch. 19) and both of these conditions make her more likely to be delivered by caesarean section. She is also at increased risk of urinary tract infection, uncertain fetal position, postpartum haemorrhage and thrombophlebitis. She is more likely to give birth to a baby who is either small or large for gestational age, although if her pregnancy has been otherwise uncomplicated she is not statistically at greater risk of shoulder dystocia (Wildschut 1999). There does not appear to be an association between maternal obesity and perinatal mortality. The woman is also more prone to wound infection following operative delivery. Obesity may also be associated with malnourishment from essential nutrient deficiency.

As well as excessive weight increase during pregnancy being a greater risk factor for the onset of hypertensive disorders, its sudden onset may signal occult oedema. If such weight gain is noted by the woman or the midwife it is prudent to take the woman's blood pressure and test her urine for protein.

Once oedema has been excluded, the midwife should make tactful attempts to discuss the woman's diet with her, when it becomes apparent that her weight may raise her risk of complications. It is debatable at what point the midwife should intervene with such a discussion. Ideally all women should be given the opportunity to discuss diet, as well as other general lifestyle factors, from as early on in their pregnancy as possible, or even before, and at regular intervals thereafter. Overweight women will often themselves express concerns to a friendly and generally supportive midwife and the midwife should be able to take such opportunities to discuss diet, nutrition, exercise and the reasons why excessive weight gain in pregnancy is undesirable. There is no advantage to dieting during pregnancy (and strict dieting may be dangerous), so sensible eating should be advocated. Referral to a dietician may be helpful.

Blood pressure measurements should always be taken accurately with a correctly sized cuff, and gestational diabetes and urinary tract infection screened for. Routine weighing is rarely of any practical benefit, and may only reduce a woman's self-esteem and make her dread her antenatal appointments. The midwife should also bear in mind that obesity can be a symptom of another disease, such as hypothyroidism, polycystic ovarian syndrome or Cushing's disease, and in such cases diet will have only a minimal effect on weight.

Conversely, the midwife may observe that a woman appears to be thin during her pregnancy and not laying down healthy fat stores. Detailed discussion should attempt to elicit the quality and quantity of the woman's diet and her weight pattern over previous years. Some women are naturally very slim and remain so because of genetic factors and a high metabolic rate, going on to produce a healthily sized infant. Of the rest, a medical disorder such as a malabsorption condition may be present, or starvation, if the woman has been living until recently in a country struck by famine.

The midwife needs to be aware that pregnant women can be afflicted by anorexia nervosa or bulimia, or both, often chronic conditions that may have been previously undetected despite their obsessive nature, or labelled 'dieting'.

Where a woman is suffering from nutritional deprivation she is at greater risk of anaemia, preterm birth and intrauterine growth restriction and its sequelae, including birth asphyxia and perinatal death. Bulimia may be wrongly diagnosed as hyperemesis gravidarum.

The midwife's role in the care of such women will depend on the cause. She should always involve the medical practitioner because of the risk of intrauterine growth restriction, and in cases with a medical cause. Where an eating disorder such as anorexia nervosa or bulimia is suspected, or admitted to, the involvement of a clinical psychologist or psychiatrist may be of value but, of course, the woman must be amenable to this. (It should also be said that if a midwife cares for a woman who has resolved a former eating disorder it would be most inappropriate to suggest that the woman requires psychiatric support in her pregnancy because of her history.) Dietary discussion and advice, including the use of supplements such as multivitamins and referral to a dietician, should be discussed with the woman. Quality of nutrition is as important, if not more so, than quantity. Where a woman is known to be suffering from an eating disorder, the importance of non-judgmental support from all of her carers cannot be overestimated in maintaining her well-being. As with the obese woman, some of the problem may lie with lowered self-esteem.

Problems associated with pregnancy following assisted conception

The rate of assisted conceptions has risen dramatically in the last few years, not least because of increasing understanding of the human reproductive cycle, its failings and technological advances that can correct childlessness from a variety of causes. Couples who achieve pregnancy following assisted conception may be at greater risk of complications during the pregnancy than those who conceive naturally, for a number of reasons.

The cause of the fertility problem may be a medical problem in itself that is aggravated by pregnancy, such as some forms of malignancy and their treatments. It is also known that with some forms of assisted conception there is an increased rate of multiple pregnancy, which will in turn increase the risk of pre-eclampsia, preterm labour and so on. Women who undergo assisted conception are by definition of an older age group, either having previously tried for some time to conceive a child naturally or having fertility problems because of their increased age. Increased maternal age has slight associations with multiple pregnancy and pre-eclampsia, and the older a woman is the more lifetime she has lived to develop a medical problem such as essential hypertension or diabetes mellitus, or a gynaecological problem such as fibroids.

The desire for a child by many couples will override potential risk to the woman and a couple may present a compelling case to the fertility clinic whose help they seek. Also, women who achieve pregnancy with medical assistance are more likely to be closely monitored, particularly with ultrasound scans and perhaps closer follow-up of otherwise mild symptoms. The couple themselves may feel greatly reassured to have their pregnancy the subject of such close medical scrutiny. However, the combination of the increased use of technology, and the stress engendered by searching for problems (which in today's open environment means explaining what each problem may entail) in a so-called 'precious pregnancy', can themselves invoke a perception of a more complicated pregnancy than may actually be the case.

Specific problems

These include:

- increased risk of ectopic pregnancy following assisted conception, especially ovulation induction and in vitro fertilisation and its derivatives, e.g. gamete intrafallopian transfer (GIFT) (Edwards & Brody 1995)
- multiple pregnancy and its sequelae – the biggest problem of assisted conception pregnancies being mediated by multiple birth and particularly problems of prematurity (Addor et al 1998)
- higher miscarriage rate, particularly if the woman has a condition such as 'incompetent' cervix or septate uterus which predisposes her to miscarriage; however, although early miscarriage rates appear to be higher in women with assisted conception, this is almost certainly because of a higher detection rate due to intensive monitoring of hormone levels and ultrasound scans from very early pregnancy, and heavy bleeding at the time the menstrual period was expected – normally a woman would not have been aware that she was pregnant

- more vaginal bleeding requiring hospital admission; Edwards & Brody (1995) also found that women with an assisted conception had a 3% placenta praevia rate as opposed to 1.4% seen in controls.

Interestingly, there does not appear to be a greater incidence of chromosomal abnormality following assisted conception.

REFERENCES

Abu-Heija A, Al-Chalabi H, El-Iloubani N 1998 Abruptio placentae: risk factors and perinatal outcome. Journal of Obstetrics and Gynaecology Research 24(2):141–144

Addor V, Santos-Eggimann B, Fawer C L et al 1998 Impact of fertility treatments on the health of newborns. Fertility and Sterility 69(2):210–215

Almes L T 1995 Intrahepatic cholestasis of pregnancy. Journal of the Society of Obstetricians and Gynaecologists of Canada 17(4):343–351

Ananth C V, Wilcox A J 2001 Placental abruption and perinatal mortality in the United States. American Journal of Epidemiology 153(4):332–337

Ananth C V, Savitz D A, Bowes W A et al 1997 Influence of hypertensive disorders and cigarette smoking on placental abruption and uterine bleeding during pregnancy. British Journal of Obstetrics and Gynaecology 104(5):572–578

Andres R L 1996 The association of cigarette smoking with placenta previa and abruptio placentae. Seminars in Perinatology 20(2):154–159

Beischer N A, Mackay E V, Colditz P B 1997 Obstetrics and the newborn, 3rd edn. W B Saunders, London

Bewley C, Gibbs A 2001 Domestic abuse and pregnancy. MIDIRS Midwifery Digest 11(2):183–187

Chua S, Arulkumaran S 1999 Prolonged pregnancy. In: James D K, Steer P J, Weiner C P, Gonik B (eds) High risk pregnancy management options. W B Saunders, London, p 1057–1070

Crowley P 2001 Prophylactic steroids for preterm birth. In: The Cochrane Database of Systematic Reviews. Update Software, Oxford, Issue 2

Dallison J, Lobstein T 1995 Poor expectations. NCH Action For Children, London

Davidson K M 1998 Intrahepatic cholestasis of pregnancy. Seminars in Perinatology 22(2):104–111

DoH et al (Department of Health, Welsh Office, Scottish Office Department of Health, Department of Health and Social Services, Northern Ireland) 1998 Why mothers die: Report on confidential enquiries into maternal deaths in the United Kingdom 1994–1996. Stationery Office, London

Eckford S D, Vyas S, Mills M S et al 1995 Delayed placental abruption after road traffic accident. Journal of Obstetrics and Gynaecology 15(3):186–187

Edwards R G, Brody S A 1995 Principles and practice of assisted human reproduction. W B Saunders, Philadelphia

Enkin M, Keirse M J N C, Neilson J et al 2000 A guide to effective care in pregnancy and labour. Oxford University Press, Oxford

Fagan E A 1995 Disorders of the liver, biliary system and pancreas. In: de Swiet M (ed) Medical disorders in obstetric practice. Blackwell Science, Oxford, p 321–378

Fry D, Hay-Smith J, Hough J, et al 1997 National Clinical Guideline for the care of women with symphysis pubis dysfunction. Midwives 110(1314):172–173

Gaudet R, Merviel P, Berkane N et al 2000 Fetal impact of cholestasis of pregnancy: experience at Tenon Hospital and literature review. Fetal Diagnosis and Therapy 15(4):191–197

Hendricks S K, Conway L, Wang K et al 1991 Diagnosis of polyhydramnios in early gestation: Indication for prenatal diagnosis? Prenatal Diagnosis 11(8):649–654

Kennedy C T C, Kyle P 1999 Skin disease. In: James D K, Steer P J, Weiner C P, Gonik B (eds) High risk pregnancy management options. W B Saunders, London, p 911–929

Kenyon S, Boulvain M 2001 Antibiotics for preterm premature rupture of membranes. In: The Cochrane Library. Update Software, Oxford, Issue 3

Konje J C, Taylor D J 1999 Bleeding in late pregnancy. In: James D K, Steer P J, Weiner C P, Gonik B (eds) High risk pregnancy management options. W B Saunders, London, p 111–128

Letsky E A 1995 Coagulation defects. In: de Swiet M (ed) Medical disorders in obstetric practice. Blackwell Science, Oxford, p 71–115

Lewis G, Drife J (eds) 2001 Why mothers die 1997–1999: The fifth report of the Confidential Enquiries into Maternal Deaths in the United Kingdom. RCOG Press, London

Locatelli A, Vergani P, Di Pirro G et al 2000 The role of amnioinfusion in the management of premature rupture of membranes at less than 26 weeks' gestation. American Journal of Obstetrics and Gynecology 183(4):878–882

Lockwood C J, Funai E F 1999 Placenta previa and related disorders. In: Queenan J T (ed) High-risk pregnancy. Blackwell Science, Massachusetts, p 466–474

Mahomed K 1999 Abdominal pain in pregnancy. In: James D K, Steer P J, Weiner C P, Gonik B (eds) High risk pregnancy management options. W B Saunders, London, p 983–998

Manolitsas T, Wein P, Beischer N A et al 1994 Value of cardiotocography in women with antepartum haemorrhage – is it too late for caesarean section when the cardiotocograph shows ominous features? Australian and New Zealand Journal of Obstetrics and Gynaecology 34(4):403–408

Many A, Hill L M, Lazebnik N et al 1995 The association between polyhydramnios and preterm delivery. Obstetrics and Gynaecology 86(3):389–391

Misra P, Ananth C V 1999 Risk factor profiles of placental abruption in first and second pregnancies; heterogeneous etiologies. Journal of Clinical Epidemiology 52(5):453–461

Montan S, Malcus P 1995 Amniotic fluid index in prolonged pregnancy: a cohort study. Journal of Maternal and Fetal Investigation 5(1):4–7

Munkarah A R, Morris R 1999 Malignant disease in pregnancy. In: James D K, Steer P J, Weiner C P, Gonik B (eds) High risk pregnancy management options. W B Saunders; London, p 945–958

Panting-Kemp A, Nguyen T, Chang E et al 1999 Idiopathic polyhydramnios and perinatal outcome. American Journal of Obstetrics and Gynecology 181(5) Part 1:1079–1082

Pitt C, Sanchez-Ramos L, Kaunitz A M et al 2000 Prophylactic amnioinfusion for intrapartum oligohydramnios: a meta-analysis of randomized controlled trials. Obstetrics and Gynecology 96(5):861–866

Rasmussen S, Irgens L M, Dalaker K 1997 The effect of the likelihood of further pregnancy of placental abruption and the rate of its reoccurence. British Journal of Obstetrics and Gynaecology 104(11):1292–1295

Rasmussen S, Irgens L M, Dalaker K 1999 A history of placental dysfunction and risk of placental abruption. Paediatric and Perinatal Epidemiology 13(1):9–21

Rasmussen S, Irgens L M, Dalaker K 2000 Outcome of pregnancies subsequent to placental abruption: a risk assessment. Acta Obstetrica et Gynecologica Scandinavica 79(6):495–501

Reis P M, Sander C M, Pearlman M D 2000 Abruptio placenta after auto accidents: a case–control study. Journal of Reproductive Medicine 45(1):6–10

Samuels P, Landon M B 1996 Hepatic disease. In: Gabbe S G, Niebyl J R, Simpson J L (eds) Obstetrics: normal and problem pregnancies. Churchill Livingstone, New York, p 1119–1133

Sciscione A C, Manley J S, Pollock M et al 2001 Intracervical fibrin sealants: a potential treatment for early preterm premature rupture of the membranes. American Journal of Obstetrics and Gynecology 184(3):368–373

Svigos J M, Robinson J S, Vigneswaran R 1999 Prelabour rupture of the membranes. In: James D K, Steer P J, Weiner C P, Gonik B (eds) High risk pregnancy management options. W B Saunders, London, p 1015–1024

Thompson O, Brown R, Gunnarson G et al 1998 Prevalence of polyhydramnios in the third trimester in a population screened by first and second trimester ultrasonography. Journal of Perinatal Medicine 26(5):371–377

UKCC (United Kingdom Central Council for Nursing, Midwifery and Health Visiting) 1998 Midwives rules and code of practice. UKCC, London

Walters B N J 1999 Hepatic and gastrointestinal disease. In: James D K, Steer P J, Weiner C P, Gonik B (eds) High risk pregnancy management options. W B Saunders, London, p 787–802

Wildschut H I J 1999 Maternal weight and weight gain. In: James D K, Steer P J, Weiner C P, Gonik B (eds) High risk pregnancy management options. W B Saunders, London, p 53–59

Yankowitz J, Pastorek II J G 1999 Maternal and fetal viral infection including listeriosis and toxoplasmosis. In: James D K, Steer P J, Weiner C P, Gonik B (eds) High risk pregnancy management options. W B Saunders, London, p 525–558

FURTHER READING

James D K, Steer P J, Weiner C P, Gonik B (eds) 1999 High risk pregnancy management options. W B Saunders, London

This is a large medical textbook that will be found in the reference section of good midwifery libraries. It covers practically all complications of pregnancy in depth and the contents are on the whole relevant to British obstetric practice.

Lewis G, Drife J (eds) 2001 Why mothers die 1997–1999. The fifth report of the Confidential Enquiries Into Maternal Deaths in the United Kingdom. RCOG Press, London. Online. Available: www.cemd.org.uk 2001

The Confidential Enquiries into Maternal Deaths have been running since 1952 in the current form and reports on every death of pregnant women and new mothers in the UK that is reported to the enquiry team. Each report covers a 3 year period. Although salutory and rather depressing reading, it is crucial that midwives access them and know why mothers die, and how their deaths can be prevented. The reports are stocked in every good midwifery library, and the present one is available online or through the RCOG bookshop.

19

Common Medical Disorders Associated with Pregnancy

Carmel Lloyd

CHAPTER CONTENTS

Pregnancy may be complicated by a variety of disorders and conditions that can profoundly affect the woman and her fetus. This chapter describes the most common cardiac, respiratory, renal, haematological, metabolic, neurological and autoimmune conditions that may complicate pregnancy.

The pathophysiology of these disorders may adversely affect the pregnancy. Similarly, the physiological changes occurring in pregnancy may modify the clinical course of these disorders and their management. These pregnancies are often regarded as high risk and a collaborative approach is recommended to ensure careful monitoring of both the pregnant woman and the fetus. Involvement of the woman and her family in decisions regarding her care engenders feelings of autonomy and control over a condition that has the potential to result in the medicalisation of childbirth.

Where there is chronic illness this can have profound effects on the physical, psychological, sexual and social aspects of women's lives. Midwives have a role in supporting women and their families, ensuring that the needs of the woman are met and that the pregnancy is treated as normal, so far as is possible.

The chapter aims to:

- outline the common medical disorders
- describe the effects of the different disorders on the woman and her fetus or neonate
- identify the treatment required and implications for midwifery care
- consider the midwifery care and support required by the client and her family during pregnancy, labour and the postnatal period.

Introduction

Medical disorders that predate pregnancy are important both because of the way that pregnancy affects them and because of the way in which the disorder, or the treatment, affects the pregnancy. They are also important for their social and psychological consequences. For example, a woman with anaemia not only has a medical problem but may become tired and depressed, she may find herself unable to cope with existing children and she may have to take time off from her employment. Her ideals about the place of confinement and the conduct of her labour may be compromised and the added anxiety of her medical condition may increase her need for pain-relieving drugs. Postnatally, the woman's lactation may suffer and her ability to enjoy her baby may be inhibited, which may predispose her to postnatal psychological problems. It can be seen that the woman's physical, social and psychological conditions are inseparable.

When the midwife is assessing the needs of the woman and her family and planning their care, this interplay of social, psychological and physical factors is important. If the medical problem is one that is likely to continue into the next pregnancy, the midwife can use the postnatal period to begin preconception care and advice. If the midwife can make the experience of this pregnancy a positive one, the woman will be encouraged to seek contact with the maternity services early in subsequent pregnancies, or even before.

Cardiac disease

In most pregnancies, heart disease is diagnosed before pregnancy. There is, however, a small but significant group of women who will present at an antenatal clinic with an undiagnosed heart condition. Although heart disease is an uncommon problem in pregnancy, complicating less than 1% of maternities, it continues to contribute significantly to maternal morbidity and mortality (Lewis & Drife 2001). Cardiac disease takes a variety of forms; those more likely to be seen in pregnancy are described below.

Rheumatic heart disease

The incidence of rheumatic heart disease (RHD) has declined progressively in the Western world but in the developing world it remains the most common cardiac problem. RHD causes inflammation and scarring of the heart valves and results in valve stenosis. The mitral valve is most often affected with stenosis, occurring in two-thirds of cases. This condition classically remains asymptomatic and is often diagnosed for the first time during pregnancy – particularly in immigrant or refugee women who have not had access to medical care. Most women with valvular heart disease can be managed medically with the use of drugs such as diuretics, beta blockers or digoxin. Those with more severe symptomatic disease may require surgical intervention such as balloon valvoplasty or valve replacement, although both of these procedures carry a degree of maternal and fetal mortality (Prasad & Ventura 2001).

Congenital heart disease

The most common congenital heart defects found in pregnancy are atrial septal defect (ASD), ventricular septal defect (VSD), patent ductus arteriosus (PDA), pulmonary stenosis, aortic stenosis and tetralogy of Fallot. The majority of these lesions will have been corrected surgically in childhood. Uncorrected cardiac lesions may give rise to pulmonary hypertension, cyanosis and severe left ventricular failure (McFall et al 1988).

Congenital heart conditions include:

Eisenmenger's syndrome. This is a condition caused by a right–left shunt of blood usually through a VSD, ASD or PDA. This results in an increase in the pulmonary blood flow, which over time leads to fibrosis and the development of pulmonary hypertension and cyanosis. Women with this condition are advised against pregnancy as maternal mortality lies in the region of 30%. The greatest risk to the fetus is prematurity but, because of the advances in neonatal care, the perinatal mortality rate is low (Yentis et al 1998).

Marfan's syndrome. This is caused by an autosomal dominant defect on chromosome 15. It is a connective tissue disease that affects the musculoskeletal system, the cardiovascular system and the eyes. The cardiovascular abnormalities are the most life threatening as the elastic fibres in the media of the blood vessels weaken. This results in dilatation of the ascending and descending aorta, which may be followed by dissection or rupture, or both. The mean age at which these events occur is 32 years and it often results in premature death. Pregnancy poses a significant risk because of the increased stress on the cardiovascular system; also there is a 50% chance of a child inheriting Marfan's syndrome if one parent is affected. Women and their partners should be counselled carefully regarding these potential outcomes before embarking on a pregnancy (Lipscomb et al 1997).

Ischaemic heart disease (IHD). This is an uncommon cardiac complication of pregnancy, but is becoming more frequent with increasing maternal age. Other risk factors include smoking, hypercholesterolaemia, obesity and drug misuse (Lewis & Drife 2001). A myocardial infarction is most likely to occur in the third trimester and peripartum period when the haemodynamic changes are having their maximum effect. The midwife is able to identify women who have risk factors associated with IHD and can encourage them to make lifestyle changes. Smoking cessation should be stressed and referral made to community smoking cessation programmes. Advice regarding diet and nutrition is appropriate in women with a high BMI (see Ch. 12) and referral to a dietician may be required.

Endocarditis. This is an inflammation of the heart usually involving the heart valves. It is caused by microorganisms such as bacteria and fungi. Streptococcal organisms are the most common cause and give rise to the subacute form of the disease. Acute endocarditis is due to more virulent organisms such as *Staphylococcus aureus*, *Streptococcus pneumoniae* and *Neisseria gonorrhoeae*. Women with valvular heart disease, prosthetic valves, a previous history of endocarditis and intravenous substance misusers are particularly vulnerable to this condition.

Peripartum cardiomyopathy. This is a relatively rare but potentially fatal disease; mortality rates range from 25 to 50% with a significant number of deaths occurring shortly after the onset of the signs and symptoms. Diagnosis is made within a specific period of time, occurring between the last month of pregnancy and the first 5 months postpartum. Commonly women have no previous history of heart disease and it has a higher incidence in older and multiparous women, those with multiple pregnancies and those complicated by hypertension. The inflammation and enlargement of the myocardium (cardiomegaly) give rise to left ventricular heart failure and thromboembolic complications. Management centres on relieving the symptoms of congestive heart failure with medication. As the cardiomegaly resolves there should be a corresponding improvement in the woman's condition but this process may take up to 6 months. Some women who are severely affected by peripartum cardiomyopathy will require a heart transplant (Futterman & Lemburg 2000).

Changes in cardiovascular dynamics during pregnancy

In normal pregnancy the haemodynamic profile alters in order to meet the increasing demands of the growing fetoplacental unit (see Ch. 13). Although this increases the workload of the heart quite significantly, normal, healthy pregnant women are able to adjust to these physiological changes quite easily. In women with coexisting heart disease, however, the added workload can precipitate complications. The haemodynamic changes commence early in pregnancy and gradually reach their maximum effect between 28 and 32 weeks. During labour there is a significant increase in cardiac output as a result of uterine contractions. In the 12–24 hours following birth there is further alteration with the shift of blood (approximately one litre) from the uterine to the systemic circulation. These three peak periods of cardiovascular stress are the most critical and life threatening for women with heart disease (Hunter & Robson 1992).

Recognition of cardiac compromise

The recognition of heart disease in pregnancy may be difficult as many of the symptoms of normal pregnancy resemble those of heart disease. The signs and symptoms of cardiac compromise include: fatigue, shortness of breath (dyspnoea), difficulty in breathing unless upright (orthopnoea), palpitations, bounding/collapsing pulse, chest pain, development of peripheral oedema, distended jugular veins and progressive limitation of physical activity

Symptoms of cardiac disease may be classified by the degree of compromise and can be determined by the utilisation of a classification system based on the signs and symptoms (Table 19.1).

Diagnosis

Along with the signs and symptoms, laboratory tests can assist with the diagnosis of cardiac disease and

Table 19.1 The New York Heart Association's functional classification of cardiac disease

Class	Definition
Class I	No limitation of physical activity. Ordinary activity does not cause undue fatigue, palpitations, dyspnoea or angina
Class II	Slight limitation of physical activity. Comfortable at rest. Ordinary physical activity results in fatigue, palpitations, dyspnoea or angina
Class III	Marked limitation of physical activity. Comfortable at rest. Less than ordinary physical activity results in fatigue, palpitations, dyspnoea or angina
Class IV	Inability to carry on any physical activity without discomfort. Symptoms of cardiac insufficiency or angina may be present even at rest, and are intensified by activity

(Comport & Seng 1997)

determine the type of lesion together with an assessment of current functional capacity. Tests include:

- full blood count
- electrocardiography
- chest radiograph to assess cardiac size and outline, pulmonary vasculature and lung fields (nowadays chest X-rays are considered safe in pregnancy and should always be performed in unwell pregnant women with chest pain (Lewis & Drife 2001))
- clotting studies
- echocardiography, which may be utilised where information is required with regard to the severity of the abnormality particularly when this is diagnosed for the first time in pregnancy.

Risks to mother and fetus

The majority of pregnancies complicated by maternal heart disease can be expected to have a favourable outcome for both mother and fetus. The risk for morbidity and mortality depends on three factors: (1) the nature of the cardiac lesion, (2) its affect on the functional capacity of the heart and (3) the development of pregnancy-related complications such as hypertensive disorders of pregnancy, infection, thrombosis and haemorrhage. Congestive heart failure precipitated by the altered haemodynamic state is a serious complication that may result in maternal death and can occur at any time during pregnancy (Lewis & Drife 2001). Fetal effects are the result of decreased systemic circulation or decreased oxygenation. If maternal circulation is compromised, there will be a reduction in the functional capacity of the heart and the uterine blood flow

will be affected. This can lead to spontaneous abortion, intrauterine growth retardation, fetal hypoxia and preterm birth. If maternal oxygenation is impaired, as in cyanotic heart disease or acute pulmonary oedema, fetal oxygenation will be impaired leading to severe fetal hypoxia, which may result in fetal loss. If either parent has a congenital heart defect this may be inherited by their offspring (Tan 1999).

Preconception care

Women with known heart disease should seek advice from a cardiologist and an obstetrician before becoming pregnant so that the risks of the condition can be discussed. General health advice can be given by a midwife with regard to diet, weight, exercise, rest, the prevention of anaemia and the avoidance of tobacco, drugs and alcohol.

Antenatal care

The symptoms of normal pregnancy together with the haemodynamic changes can mimic the signs and symptoms of heart disease for example: dypsnoea on exertion, orthopnoea, palpitations, dizziness, fainting, a bounding pulse, tachycardia, peripheral oedema, distended jugular veins and alterations in heart sounds. Maternal investigations should be carried out prior to and at the onset of pregnancy in order to gain baseline referral points.

Management. All pregnant women with heart disease should be managed in obstetric units with a multidisciplinary approach involving midwives, obstetricians, cardiologists and anaesthetists (Badawy

& El-Metwally 2001). During the antenatal period women with heart disease are often monitored more frequently than healthy, pregnant women. The aim is to maintain a steady haemodynamic state and prevent complications, as well as promote physical and psychological well-being. Visits to a joint clinic run by a cardiologist and obstetrician are usually every 2 weeks until 30 weeks' gestation and weekly thereafter until birth. At each visit functional grading is made according to the New York Heart Association classification (Table 19.1) and the severity of the heart lesion assessed by clinical examination.

Evaluation of fetal well-being will include:

- ultrasound examination to confirm gestational age and congenital abnormality
- assessment of fetal growth and amniotic fluid volume both clinically and by ultrasound
- monitoring the fetal heart rate by CTG
- measurement of fetal and maternal placental blood flow indices by Doppler ultrasonography.

Physical and psychological care. The midwife can give advice with regard to modifying and adjusting physical activity during pregnancy. Regardless of the cardiac classification level, all women with heart disease will require additional rest during pregnancy. Some women will need to commence maternity leave earlier than anticipated and may need assistance with claiming their maternity rights and benefits (see Ch. 50). In late pregnancy, women may require admission to hospital for rest and close monitoring. Psychological support by the midwife is important, particularly at times when there are complications that may require hospital admission. Consideration must also be given to the emotional stress that may be caused when women are separated from their children. Where possible, care in the community is preferable, although the importance of adequate rest should be emphasised.

Dietary advice. Women with heart disease require the same health and dietary advice as other women. The midwife should give guidance about what constitutes a well-balanced diet. Cholesterol, sodium-rich foods and salt should be restricted. Weight gain should be monitored in these women as excess weight gain will place additional strain on the heart. Compliance with taking iron and folic acid supplementation is important for preventing anaemia. The

woman may need to be referred to a dietician for nutritional advice in order to balance pregnancy requirements with the restrictions necessary for some women with more severe heart disease.

Prevention of infection. Infections often cause a pyrexia and tachycardia, which will increase the cardiac output and put an added strain on the heart. In addition the infective organism can cause further damage in women with heart lesions by causing endocarditis. The midwife needs to give advice to women about how she may identify respiratory, urinary and vaginal infections and the necessity of seeking treatment for these infections as quickly as possible. An early dental examination is important to detect and treat caries and gum disease, which will also precipitate endocarditis. Prophylactic antibiotic therapy is recommended for women who are at high risk of endocarditis (Endocarditis Working Party of the British Society of Antimicrobial Chemotherapy 1990). All invasive procedures should be carried out using a strict aseptic technique and the number of vaginal examinations in labour should be kept to a minimum.

Antithrombotic therapy. The hypercoagulable state in pregnancy increases the risk of thromboembolic disease in women who have arrhythmias, mitral valve stenosis or who have had cardiac valve replacements. Three types of valves are generally seen in pregnancy: mechanical, bioprosthetic (pork tissue) and homograft. Mechanical valves pose the greatest risk to mother and fetus and require therapeutic anticoagulation in pregnancy. Bioprosthetic values have good outcomes providing there is no structural deterioration. Homograft valves do not seem to be associated with any complications (Sadler et al 2000).

The treatment of women requiring antithrombotic therapy is controversial. Warfarin is commonly used in the non-pregnant state but is teratogenic when used in early pregnancy and is associated with a high fetal loss rate. It also predisposes the woman and her fetus to haemorrhage when used in the third trimester. The use of unfractionated heparin became the drug of choice in early and late pregnancy as it does not cross the placenta. However, prolonged maternal exposure can result in heparin-induced complications such as thrombocytopenia and osteoporosis. More recently, the use of subcutaneous low molecular weight heparins, such as enoxaparin, have been found to provide effective thromboprophylaxis with minimal side-effects (Ellison et al 2000). High thromboembolic support stockings should be worn if the woman is admitted to the antenatal ward for rest and assessment. They should also be worn during labour and in the immediate postnatal period.

Intrapartum care

The first stage of labour

In view of the increase in cardiac output during labour and immediately after the birth it is important to plan for and manage labour carefully. A coordinated team approach with good communication between the midwife, obstetrician, cardiologist, neonatologist, anaesthetist, the woman and her family is essential. Women with heart disease often have quite rapid, uncomplicated labours. Vaginal birth is preferred unless there is an obstetric indication for caesarean section. Optimal management involves monitoring the maternal condition closely; this will include the measurement of temperature, pulse, respiration, blood pressure and urine output. Pulse oximetry may be utilised to assess arterial haemoglobin saturation, which may be reduced in women with heart disease owing to disruption of normal gas exchange between the lungs and blood. If oxygen saturation levels fall below 92%, oxygen therapy will be required. The use of invasive haemodynamic studies may be required in women with moderate to severe heart disease, for example ECG monitoring and insertion of a central venous pressure (CVP) catheter. Blood and urine tests are utilised to determine the haematological and metabolic changes occurring during labour. There also needs to be a risk assessment for the stress of labour and the maintenance of an adequate blood volume (Edwards 1998).

Fluid balance. Women with significant heart disease require care concerning fluid balance in labour. Indiscriminate use of intravenous crystalloid fluids will lead to an increase in circulating blood volume, which women with heart disease will find difficult to cope with and they may easily develop pulmonary oedema.

Pain relief. The midwife should help the woman to use the techniques that she has learned for coping with stress, as she and her labour companion are likely to be very anxious. In the majority, an epidural would be the analgesia of choice, inserted by a skilled anaesthetist. It

is an effective form of analgesia that decreases cardiac output and heart rate. It causes peripheral vasodilatation and decreases venous return, which alleviates pulmonary congestion. Nitrous oxide and oxygen (Entonox) and pethidine are usually considered safe, but it is important to consult a doctor before administering any form of pain-relieving drug to a woman with a heart condition.

Positioning. Cardiac output is influenced by the position of the labouring woman. It is important to remember that women with heart disease are particularly sensitive to aortocaval compression by the gravid uterus in the supine position. This decreases the cardiac output by inhibiting venous return to the heart resulting in maternal hypotension and fetal bradycardia (Edwards 1998). It is preferable that all labouring women, as well as those with heart disease, adopt an upright or left lateral position and are encouraged by the midwife to find a position in labour that is comfortable.

Preterm labour. If a woman with heart disease should labour prematurely then beta sympathomimetic drugs widely used for the treatment of premature labours are contraindicated. The vasodilatory side-effects of these cause tachycardia, and an increase in the circulating blood volume and cardiac output. This may lead to the development of pulmonary oedema. In addition, these drugs have metabolic effects that may further impair myocardial function (Dabbs et al 1996).

Induction. The least stressful labour for a woman with cardiac disease will be spontaneous in onset; induction is considered safe only if the benefits outweigh the disadvantages. Prostaglandins should be used with caution as they are potent vasodilators and cause a marked increase in cardiac output. Oxytocin by intravenous infusion causes a degree of fluid retention and it is important for the midwife to keep a careful record of fluid balance if this is used. Caution is urged in the use of oxytocin (Lewis & Drife 2001, p. 153).

The second stage of labour

This should be short without undue exertion on the part of the mother. Prolonged pushing with held breath such as the Valsalva manoeuvre, which is undesirable for healthy women, may be dangerous for a woman with heart disease. It raises the intrathoracic pressure, pushes the blood out of the thorax and impedes venous return, with the result that cardiac output falls. The midwife should encourage the woman to breathe normally and follow her natural desire to push, giving several short pushes during each contraction. Forceps or ventouse may be used to shorten the second stage if the maternal condition deteriorates. Care should be taken when the woman is in the lithotomy position, where the lower part of the body is higher than trunk, as this produces a sudden increase in venous return to the heart, which may result in heart failure.

The third stage of labour

This is usually actively managed owing to the increased risk of postpartum haemorrhage (PPH). Oxytocin is the drug of choice but its use in the prevention of PPH must be balanced against the risk of oxytocin-induced hypotension and tachycardia in women with cardiovascular compromise (Lewis & Drife 2001). Administration should follow the guidance in the British National Formulary (BMA & RPS 2001) and when given as an intravenous bolus the drug should be given slowly in a dose that should not exceed 5 i.u. Ergot-containing preparations such as ergometrine are contraindicated as these act on smooth muscle and will have a direct effect on the heart as well as producing a tonic uterine contraction.

Postnatal care

During the first 48 hours following birth the heart must cope with the extra blood from the uterine circulation and it is important that the midwife monitors the woman's condition during this time. Close observation should identify early signs of infection, thrombosis or pulmonary oedema. Breastfeeding is not contraindicated as cardiac output is not affected by lactation although drug therapy for specific heart conditions may need to be reviewed for safety during breastfeeding. The midwife provides support with breast feeding similar to that with other women (see Ch. 40) and the importance of rest and an adequate diet whilst breastfeeding must be emphasised. Discharge planning is particularly important for women with heart disease. The midwife can evaluate the help and support that will be available in the home during the postnatal period. Relatives and friends often fulfil this need but community social

services can be approached if this is thought to be insufficient. The woman and her partner will need to discuss the implications of a future pregnancy with the cardiologist and obstetrician. Following this the midwife can provide advice to the woman and her partner about contraception.

Respiratory disorders

Asthma

Asthma is a common respiratory disorder with an incidence of 3% of the general population; it may complicate 0.4–1.3% of all pregnancies (Mabie 1996). Pregnancy does not consistently affect the maternal asthmatic status; some women experience no change in symptoms whereas others have a distinct worsening of the disease (James 2001). Women with severe disease and those who have poor control of asthma seem to have an increased incidence of adverse maternal and neonatal outcomes including preterm labour and birth, hypertensive disorders of pregnancy, babies small for gestational age, abruptio placentae, chorioamnionitis and caesarean birth (Demissie et al 1998, Liu et al 2001). Conversely, it has been suggested that controlled asthma is related to improved perinatal outcomes (Schatz 1999).

Antenatal care

At booking the midwife should be able to discuss with the woman the frequency and severity of her asthma, family history, any known asthma triggers and current treatment. Information about the interactions of pregnancy and asthma and how this may be managed is effectively provided through a multidisciplinary approach. The ideal is care provided jointly between the midwife, GP, chest physician and obstetrician in order that consistency in the management of care is communicated to all health professionals involved. The main anxiety for women and those providing care is generated by the use of medication and the fear that this may harm the fetus. To date all medications commonly used in the treatment of asthma, including systemic steroids, are considered safe and it is crucial that therapy is maintained during pregnancy in order to prevent deterioration of the condition and precipitate adverse pregnancy events. The principles of management do not differ from those adopted in the non-pregnant woman but will include fetal surveillance. The lynchpin of management is the use of peak expiratory flow rates (PEFR) to monitor the level of resistance in the airways caused by inflammation or bronchospasm, or both. A range of normal values can be predicted for each person according to sex, height and age. Knowledge of her usual PEFR and self-monitoring at home will enable an asthmatic to determine when to take or increase her medication and when to seek medical attention. Hospital admission is usually required if the PEFR is less than 50% of the normal value and the woman is too breathless to complete sentences. If during the pregnancy there are any difficulties in controlling the asthma the woman should be admitted to hospital. The British asthma management guidelines (BTS 1997) provide comprehensive multidisciplinary advice on best practice in asthma care.

Intrapartum care

An increase in cortisone and adrenaline (epinephrine) from the adrenal glands during labour is thought to prevent asthma attacks during labour (de Swiet 1995). If an asthma attack does occur, it should be treated with the same rapidity and medication as an attack outside of pregnancy. There are certain drugs that should be avoided in pregnancy and labour because of their bronchospasm action; these are intravenous, intra-amniotic and transcervical prostaglandins (Schatz 1999). Any woman who has received corticosteroids in pregnancy should have increased doses for the stress of labour and, normally, hydrocortisone 100 mg intramuscularly every 6 hours and for 24 hours after childbirth (Landon & Samuels 1996).

Postnatal care

Breastfeeding should be encouraged, particularly as it may protect infants from developing certain allergic conditions (Kelnar & Harvey 1995). None of the drugs used in the treatment of asthma is likely to be secreted in breastmilk in sufficient quantities to harm the neonate.

In conclusion, asthma is a common condition affecting many women in pregnancy. Although generally pregnancy is successful, good control of the woman's asthma will further improve the quality for the mother and inevitably the fetus. It is imperative

therefore that women and health professionals are aware of maintaining the treatment of asthma throughout pregnancy in order to prevent a potentially life-threatening exacerbation of the condition.

Cystic fibrosis

Cystic fibrosis (CF) is a genetic disorder found in caucasians that has an incidence of 1:2000 live births (Nakielna 1995). It is an autosomal recessive disorder affecting the exocrine glands that causes production of excess secretions with abnormal electrolyte concentrations, resulting in the obstruction of the ducts and glands. This affects the pancreas, sweat glands, and respiratory, digestive and reproductive tracts (Kent & Farquharson 1993). Pulmonary disease is the primary cause of morbidity and mortality associated with CF and accounts for 90% of fatalities (Ramsey 1995). Traditional treatments have included chest physiotherapy, antibiotics and pancreatic enzyme supplements. More recent developments include improved nutrition, use of DNase (a synthetic protein) to break down mucus and heart–lung transplantation. Future treatment is likely to include gene therapy whereby the faulty CF gene is replaced with a normal healthy one (Jaffe & Bush 1999). Owing to advances in the diagnosis and treatment of this disease, the life expectancy for a child with CF has steadily increased from an average of 8 years in 1970 to 30 years in 1998. A consequence of this is that there is an increasing number of women with CF becoming pregnant although fertility may be reduced, principally because of alteration in the chemical make-up of the cervical mucus (Bolyard 2001).

Prepregnancy care

When planning a pregnancy, a woman with CF and her partner should have genetic counselling. One in 25 people carry the defective gene and therefore if both parents are carriers there is a one in four chance that their children will have CF. Specific changes in respiratory, cardiac and pancreatic function as well as increased nutritional demands during pregnancy pose a serious health risk for many women with CF and should be assessed prior to pregnancy. As part of the counselling process the pregnancy outcome also needs to be discussed. Although pregnancy appears to be well tolerated in women with pre-existing mild pulmonary function, morbidity and mortality are increased in women with pancreatic insufficiency or moderate–severe lung disease, or both (Edenborough et al 2000). Significant deterioration in either pulmonary status or general health may result in a therapeutic termination or the spontaneous onset of preterm labour (Hilman et al 1996, Olson 1997).

Antenatal care

Once pregnancy is confirmed a multidisciplinary approach combining midwifery, obstetric, dietetic, medical, nursing and physiotherapy expertise is essential. Specific assessment during pregnancy includes pulmonary function tests, arterial blood gases, sputum culture, liver function tests, glucose tolerance test, chest radiogram, electrocardiogram, echocardiogram and monitoring of weight gain (Olson 1997). An essential component of CF care is the use of postural drainage techniques in order to keep the lungs clear of mucoid secretions. This becomes more difficult as the pregnancy progresses owing to the enlarging uterus and therefore alternative techniques need to be suggested by the physiotherapy team. An important part of maternity care is also the early recognition and prompt treatment of acute exacerbations of CF or pulmonary infections. Compliance with antibiotic therapy must be stressed as the potential risks to the fetus are outweighed by the risk of the mother developing a severe lung infection. In addition it is important to pay attention to nutrition and CF-related diabetes, the risks of which increase with age and are more likely to be problematic in pregnancy (Knox et al 1999). Poor maternal nutrition and deterioration in lung function will affect the supply of nutrients and oxygen to the fetus resulting in intrauterine growth restriction and preterm labour and birth.

Intrapartum care

During labour close monitoring of cardiorespiratory function will be required and an anaesthetist should be involved at an early stage. Fluid and electrolyte management requires careful attention as women with CF may easily become hypovolaemic from the loss of large quantities of sodium in sweat. Epidural analgesia is the recommended form of pain relief in labour and general anaesthesia should be avoided because of the potential risks from respiratory complications (Holdcroft & Thomas 2000).

Postnatal care

Women should be cared for in a high dependency unit and be closely monitored as studies have highlighted that cardiorespiratory function often deteriorates following birth (Hilman et al 1996). Sodium concentration in breastmilk has been found to be similar to women without CF and therefore breastfeeding is not contraindicated. However, in order for breastfeeding to be successful women need to be well nourished and maintain an adequate calorie intake (Kent & Farquharson 1993). Given that the incidence of CF is the UK's most common life-threatening inherited disease, it is recommended that universal neonatal testing is undertaken, a relatively cheap test that can be incorporated into the Guthrie test.

In summary, women with mild pulmonary disease and good nutritional status are expected to do well. In contrast, women with severe complications associated with their CF are likely to have a poor outcome and therefore should be advised against becoming pregnant. Midwives should also be aware that many women with CF have diabetes.

Pulmonary tuberculosis

Tuberculosis (TB) is caused by the tubercule bacillus, *Myobacterium tuberculosis*. The lungs are the organ most commonly affected, although it may involve any organ. It is transmitted through inhalation of infected airborne droplets from a person with active TB. It may also be contracted from infected cattle through the consumption of milk and dairy products that have not be pasteurised. The incidence of TB had been declining for decades until recently when the number of cases of TB began to rise. The largest percentage increase has occurred among people aged 25–44 years of age; therefore TB has become more prevalent in women of childbearing age (Vo et al 2000). A number of these women will first be diagnosed with TB infection during pregnancy; a prevalence of 143.3 per 100 000 deliveries was found by Llewelyn et al (2000) in their prospective study. All forms of TB are notifiable under the Public Health (Control of Disease) Act 1984 and therefore community nurses, midwives and health visitors are among the first to be involved in the prevention, screening and treatment of TB (JTC of the British Thoracic Society 2000). Contributory factors leading to the increasing incidence of this disease include: (1) women and children who have immigrated to the UK from areas where TB is endemic, principally South Asia and the Indian subcontinent, African countries especially Somalia, Russia, Eastern Europe and the Baltic states, (2) the development of multidrug-resistant organisms and (3) increases in adults and children who have become infected with HIV. The greatest percentage increase is seen in inner city areas where additional social factors such as poverty, homelessness, substance misuse, poor nutrition and crowded living conditions contribute to the transmission of the disease (Scowen 2001).

Effects on the woman

The onset of primary TB is often insidious and the symptoms are non-specific: fatigue, malaise, loss of appetite, loss of weight, alteration in bowel habit and low grade fever. These can be interpreted as usual symptoms occurring in pregnancy. The classic symptoms of chronic cough, night sweats, haemoptysis, dyspnoea and chest pain occur quite late in the disease process and are often absent when the TB is extrapulmonary. This leads to a delay in diagnosis, which is compounded by the reluctance of women to accept and doctors to perform chest X-rays in pregnancy. Microscopic examination and culture of sputum are also required to confirm the presence of mycobacterial infection and identify drug sensitivity (Ormerod 2001).

Management

All pregnant women with TB should be under the care of a physician who manages the clinical aspect of the woman's treatment and a specialist nurse with full training in the disease. It is also important that they work collaboratively with the midwife, GP and obstetrician to promote continuity of care. The key to a successful outcome is to ensure that the woman adheres to the prescribed treatment. Figueroa-Damian & Arredondo-Garcia (1998, 2001) found that maternal morbidity and mortality are significantly higher where active TB remains untreated and when treatment is started late in pregnancy. In addition, neonates of women with TB have a higher risk of prematurity and perinatal death and weigh less than 2500 g at birth.

The JTC (2000) and Bothamley (2001) recommend that standard antituberculous therapy should be used to treat TB in pregnancy. TB is treated in two phases. The first involves taking rifampacin, isoniazid and pyrizinamide daily for the first 2 months. In the second (continuation) phase, rifampicin and isoniazid are taken for a further 4 months. These drugs are considered to be safe and are not associated with human fetal malformations. Congenital deafness has been reported in infants with exposure to streptomycin in utero and therefore this antituberculous drug is best avoided in pregnancy. Part of the midwife's role during this time is to ensure that women are compliant with the drug therapy and understand the importance of adhering to the regimen in order to cure the disease and prevent the bacillus becoming resistant to the drugs. Care is planned individually so that those women at risk of non-adherence have thrice weekly directly observed therapy (DOTS) whereby health workers directly observe the woman taking her medicine and evaluate her progress. Other women will require minimum supervision and a monthly review will be sufficient to monitor progress (JTC 2000).

Attention should also be placed on rest, good nutrition and education with regard to preventing the spread of the disease. TB is usually rendered non-infectious by 2 weeks of treatment. Where possible the treatment is undertaken in the woman's home to disrupt the family unit as little as possible. Some women may require admission to hospital because of the severity of the illness, or adverse effects of drug therapy, for obstetric reasons such as the onset of labour, for social reasons or for further investigations. Assessment for the likelihood of infectiousness and multi-drug resistant tuberculosis should be made in order to determine the degree of barrier nursing required (JTC 2000).

Postnatal care

Following birth, babies born to mothers with infectious TB should be protected from the disease by the prophylactic use of isoniazid syrup 5 mg/kg/day for 6 weeks and then to be tuberculin tested. If negative, BCG vaccination should be given and drug therapy discontinued. If the tuberculin test is positive the baby should be assessed for congenital or perinatal infection and drug therapy continued if these are excluded (JTC 2000, Ormerod 2001). Antituberculous drugs are considered to be compatible with breastfeeding and breastfeeding is contraindicated only if the mother has active TB as the disease is transmitted through the breastmilk (Ormerod 2001).

Caring for a child at home makes great demands on the woman and extra help should be arranged if possible. Midwives should explain that poor nutrition, stress and overtiredness will encourage a recurrence of active disease. Family planning advice is an integral part of postnatal and preconception care and it is advisable for a woman with TB to avoid further pregnancies until the disease has been quiescent for at least 2 years. When choosing her method of family planning, the woman needs to be aware that rifampicin reduces the effectiveness of oral contraception (BMA and RPS 2001). Long term medical and social follow-up is necessary in order to monitor the progress of the disease and the response to treatment, also to provide help for the socially and economically disadvantaged.

Because of demographic changes, pregnancy and tuberculosis will be seen more frequently in future both in developing and developed countries, so the primary health care team needs to have a raised awareness of this disease. The outcome for both mother and fetus is improved by early diagnosis and effective treatment. Midwives are pivotal in ensuring compliance with drug therapy and providing general health education during pregnancy in order to reduce the incidence of TB in both the obstetric and the general population.

Renal disease

When considering renal disorders in pregnancy, a knowledge of the changes in renal physiology and function in healthy pregnancy is crucial (see Ch. 13). This will assist the midwife in understanding the impact of pregnancy on existing renal disease and the predisposition women have to develop urinary tract infections.

Asymptomatic bacteriuria

Urinary tract infections are common in pregnancy, *Escherichia coli* being the most common causative organism. All women should be screened for bacteriuria using a clean voided specimen of urine at their first antenatal visit. A diagnosis of asymptomatic bacteriuria (ASB) is made when there are more than 100 000 bacteria per millilitre of urine. ASB occurs in 2–10% of pregnant women as a result of the physiological changes in the urinary tract during pregnancy. If ASB is not identified and treated, 20–30% of these women will develop a symptomatic urinary tract infection such as cystitis or pyelonephritis. These infections represent a significant risk for both mother and fetus and there is evidence to suggest that they may play a role in the onset of preterm labour. It is therefore considered beneficial to treat ASB with antibiotics; women who develop recurrent urinary tract infections may require prophylactic antibiotic treatment (Smaill 2001).

Pyelonephritis

Acute pyelonephritis complicates nearly 1% of all pregnancies (Norman et al 2001). The woman who develops pyelonephritis usually feels extremely unwell. The signs and symptoms include: a pyrexia, which may reach 40°C, rigors, tachycardia, nausea and vomiting leading to dehydration. There is usually pain and tenderness over the loin area, which may be accompanied by muscle guarding. The pain tends to follow the path of the ureters and radiates down the suprapubic region. The woman may also complain of dysuria and frequency. Examination of the urine shows it to be cloudy and the infecting organism is often found to be *E. coli*.

Management

Women with acute pyelonephritis may develop significant complications such as preterm labour, transient renal failure, acute respiratory distress syndrome (ARDS), sepsis and shock (Gilstrap & Ramin 2001). Therefore, if a woman experiences any of the signs and symptoms of pyelonephritis she should be seen by a doctor immediately. A midstream specimen of urine (MSU) needs to be obtained and sent to a laboratory to test for culture and sensitivity. Admission to hospital is usual in order that intravenous antibiotics can be administered as soon as possible. Once the pyrexia settles oral antibiotics can be taken.

During the early stages of the illness the woman will feel quite ill and it is likely that she will remain in bed. Severe nausea and vomiting will lead to dehydration and intravenous fluids may be required. An accurate record of fluid balance is maintained in order to assess renal function. The midwife should provide general nursing care; this will include 4-hourly observation of temperature and pulse. It may be necessary to reduce the temperature by the use of tepid sponging and antipyretics. Uterine activity should be monitored to detect the onset of preterm labour. The midwife should also take steps to prevent the complications of immobility such as deep vein thrombosis; this requires the use of antithrombotic stockings and the doctor may prescribe low dose heparin therapy.

Antibiotic therapy is maintained for 10 days. Repeat cultures should be done 2 weeks after completion of the course of treatment and monthly until birth in order to ensure there is no recurrence. Follow-up excretion urography is often carried out 3 months postnatally as persistent or recurrent infection, with or without symptoms, may be associated with an abnormality of the renal tract.

Chronic renal disease

In order to determine the impact of pregnancy on a woman with chronic renal disease, the following factors need to be considered (Skaredorf & Besinger 1996):

- type of pre-existing renal disease
- general health status of the woman
- presence or absence of hypertension
- current renal function
- prepregnancy drug therapy.

If renal disease is under control the maternal and fetal outcome is usually good. In some instances renal function may deteriorate and the chance of pregnancy complications subsequently rises. If this is compounded by hypertension this will increase the glomerular capillary reserve and further decrease renal function. Renal disease combined with hypertension is associated with fetal growth restriction, preterm birth and increased perinatal mortality. Pregnant women with mild renal insufficiency (serum creatinine (Scr) < 125 µmol/L) have relatively few complications of pregnancy. Moderate or severe renal insufficiency (Scr 125–250 µmol/L) in pregnancy appears to accelerate the underlying disease and reduce fetal survival. Complications are frequent and include a rise in hypertension, high grade proteinuria (urinary excretion > 3 g in 24 h) and loss of renal function, which may persist up to 1 year following birth. Ten per cent of cases will progress to end-stage renal failure necessitating dialysis during or shortly after pregnancy; this is most likely to occur when the Scr is > 250 µmol/L at the beginning of pregnancy (Epstein 1996, Jones & Hayslett 1996).

Care and management

Assessment of renal function prior to conception is important in order to advise a couple appropriately on the risks of embarking on a pregnancy. The aim of pregnancy care in women with chronic renal disease is to prevent deterioration in renal function. This will necessitate more frequent attendance for antenatal care and close liaison between the midwife, obstetrician and nephrologist. Renal function can be assessed on a regular basis by measuring serum urate levels, serum electrolyte and urea, 24 hour creatinine clearance and serum creatinine. Urinalysis is undertaken to screen for glycosuria, proteinuria and haematuria. Regular urine cultures will detect the presence of urinary tract infection and advice should be given regarding the signs and symptoms so that women can seek medical attention and treatment early. The emergence and severity of hypertension and pre-eclampsia are monitored by recording blood pressure, undertaking urinalysis and utilising pre-eclampsia blood screening tests. A full blood count will detect anaemia as the production of erythropoietin is suppressed in chronic renal disease. Fetal surveillance includes fortnightly ultrasound scans from 24 weeks, Doppler flow studies and keeping of daily fetal activity charts. Admission to hospital is advised when there is evidence of fetal compromise, if renal function deteriorates and proteinuria increases or the blood pressure rises. If the maternal condition becomes life threatening, the risks and benefits of continuing with the pregnancy need to be discussed with the woman and her family.

Women on haemodialysis/peritoneal dialysis

Dialysis is the procedure performed to undertake the function of the kidneys when they are unable to do this because of either disease or injury. In haemodialysis the blood is shunted from the body via the major blood vessels in the arm, through a machine for filtration and then returned to the patient's circulation. In peritoneal dialysis the peritoneum acts as a diffusible membrane and, together with a dialysate solution infused into the peritoneal cavity, allows the transfer of electrolytes and the removal of waste products. Both procedures cause significant disruption to the person's lifestyle and the development of a number of complications particularly infection. Most women undergoing dialysis are infertile; however, those who conceive and continue a pregnancy on dialysis are at significant risk for adverse maternal and fetal outcomes. Some women who develop end-stage renal failure during pregnancy may also require dialysis. Pregnancy will increase the length and frequency of dialysis in these women in order to achieve a serum urea below 20 mmol/L. Higher levels are associated with an increased risk of fetal demise (Norman et al 2001). During dialysis it is important to prevent fluid overload and the development of hypertension, which will be influenced by other factors such as an imbalance of electrolytes. The anaemia of chronic renal disease is exacerbated and this may require erythropoietin (Epo) therapy and blood transfusions to resolve. Hypertension and superimposed pre-eclampsia are common maternal complications. Many pregnancies in dialysed patients end in early spontaneous abortion, therapeutic abortion and preterm birth with only 40–50% of pregnancies resulting in a successful outcome (Davison 2001).

Renal transplant

Renal transplantation reverses abnormal renal, endocrine and sexual functions and therefore women are likely to become pregnant following a renal transplant. Preconception advice is particularly important as the woman must be in optimal health before embarking on a pregnancy. It is also advisable for the woman to wait a minimum of 2 years before attempting pregnancy as this allows time for the success of the graft to be evaluated and pregnancy outcome is more likely to be successful (Davison 2001). During pregnancy, women are monitored closely by the multidisciplinary team and close liaison between the midwife, obstetrician and nephrologist is required. Clinic visits are likely to be more frequent, during which time renal function including urinalysis, blood pressure, haemoglobin levels and the status of the graft are assessed. Close monitoring of the fetus is also required to detect fetal growth restriction. Immunosuppressive therapy is usually continued during pregnancy although the effect on the pregnancy and the fetus is unknown

(Davison 2001). It is likely, however, to make the woman more vulnerable to infection. The newborn baby will also be more prone to infection as immunosuppressive therapy reduces the transmission of maternal antibodies to the fetus.

Kuvacic et al (2000) identify the following specific factors that appear to contribute to the higher rate of therapeutic and spontaneous abortion, preterm birth and low birthweight infants in pregnancies following renal transplant:

- transplant–pregnancy interval less than 2 years
- maternal hypertension
- elevated serum creatinine levels
- asymptomatic bacteriuria.

The anaemias

Anaemia is a reduction in the oxygen-carrying capacity of the blood; this may be caused by a decrease in red blood cell (RBC) production, or reduction in haemoglobin (Hb) content of the blood, or a combination of these. It is often defined by the decrease in Hb levels in the blood to below the normal range of 13.5 g/dl (men), 11.5 g/dl (women) and 11.0 g/dl (children) (Higgins 2001). The effect on the individual will depend on the severity of the anaemia and the degree to which the oxygen-carrying capacity of the blood is diminished. Signs and symptoms include pallor of the mucous membranes, fatigue, dizziness and fainting, headache, exertional shortness of breath, increased heart rate (tachycardia) and palpitations.

It is estimated that 18% of women in industralised countries are anaemic; in the developing world this figure rises to 56% and is a contributory factor to women developing health problems and dying during pregnancy and childbirth (WHO 1992). Iron deficiency anaemia in women is usually due to:

- reduced intake or absorption of iron; this includes dietary deficiency and gastrointestinal disturbances such as diarrhoea or hyperemesis
- excess demand such as frequent, numerous or multiple pregnancies
- chronic infection, particularly of the urinary tract
- acute or chronic blood loss, for example menorrhagia, bleeding haemorrhoids, or antepartum or postpartum haemorrhage.

In the developing world other common causes include hookworm infestation, infections such as amoebic dysentery, malaria due to *Plasmodium falciparum* and haemoglobinopathies.

In order to help prevent anaemia in pregnant women, midwives must understand not only the medical problem but also the social and demographic circumstances that give rise to it. The midwife should be able to identify the woman at risk of anaemia through clinical observation and by taking an accurate medical, obstetric and social history. This may reveal a preexisting problem or a woman whose racial origin or lifestyle predisposes her to anaemia.

When giving advice in early pregnancy regarding the dietary intake of iron, the midwife needs to take into consideration how the intake of iron may be affected by social, religious and cultural preferences. She also needs to explain how iron is absorbed and identify the optimal sources of iron (bioavailability). The absorption of iron is complex and tends to decrease during the first trimester and then rises throughout the remainder of the pregnancy and during the first months of the puerperium. Iron absorption is also influenced by the bioavailability of iron in the diet. Iron is most easily absorbed in the form found in red meat and wholegrain products such as wholemeal bread (haem iron). Where the diet is mainly vegetarian (non-haem), iron is of low bioavailability. Absorption of iron is inhibited by tea and coffee but enhanced by ascorbic acid, which is present in orange juice and fresh fruit (Bothwell 2000). It is estimated that a median amount of 840–1210 mg of iron needs to be absorbed over the course of the pregnancy (Beard 2000). The demand for absorbed iron increases from 0.8 mg/day in early pregnancy to 6 mg/day in late pregnancy owing to the increase in maternal Hb, and in oxygen consumption by both mother and fetus, fetal growth and deposition of iron, placental circulation, the replacement of daily loss through stools, urine and skin, the replacement of blood lost at birth and in the postnatal period and lactation (Bothwell 2000). WHO (1992) data on the prevalence of anaemia in women suggest that the normal dietary intakes of iron are insufficient to meet these requirements for the majority of women. The Centers for Disease Control in the US (1998) has identified that approximately 30% of women in the industrialised world will have depleted iron stores by the end of pregnancy and in some countries in the developing world this figure can rise to 80%.

Physiological anaemia of pregnancy

During pregnancy the maternal plasma volume gradually expands by 50%, or an increase of approximately 1200 ml by term. The total increase in RBCs is 25%, or approximately 300 ml. This relative haemodilution produces a fall in Hb concentration, which reaches a nadir during the second trimester in pregnancy and then rises again in the third trimester. These changes are not pathological but are considered to represent a physiological alteration of pregnancy necessary for the development of the fetus. Fetal outcomes appear to mirror this U-shaped curve, with an increased incidence of low birthweight and preterm birth in mothers who have either a very low or very high haemoglobin concentration (Rasmussen 2001). A low Hb level is likely to effect the ability of the maternal system to transfer sufficient oxygen and nutrients to the fetus. High Hb levels are considered to reflect poor plasma volume expansion as found in some pathological conditions such as pre-eclampsia (Yip 1996).

Iron deficiency anaemia

A low haemoglobin concentration only indicates anaemia is present; it does not reveal the cause. The red cell indices, the mean cell volume (MCV, i.e. the average volume occupied by the red cell, normal value 80–95 femtolitres) and the mean cell haemoglobin concentration (MCHC, which indicates how well filled with Hb the cells are, normal value 32–36 g/dl) are usually used to identify the cause of anaemia. Iron deficiency anaemia is microcytic (low MCV) and hypochromic (low MCHC). By the time the Hb falls, the iron stores will already be depleted. Lack of iron in the tissues can be demonstrated by measuring the serum iron levels; which will be reduced (normal value 10–30 µmol/L), and the total iron-binding capacity (TIBC), which will be raised (normal range 40–70 µmol/L). Total iron body stores can be estimated by measuring serum ferritin (normal range 10–300 µg/L); ferritin is the body's main iron storage protein. Serum ferritin levels fall in proportion to the decrease in iron stores and will show changes before the level of haemoglobin falls (Higgins 2001).

Assessing iron status in pregnancy can, however, be difficult. The haemodynamic changes associated with pregnancy (see Ch. 13) render the usual red cell indices used in laboratory investigations unreliable and serum ferritin levels can appear normal or raised in the presence of chronic inflammatory disease. A more reliable test in pregnancy may be to assess cellular iron status by measuring serum transferrin receptor (TfR) concentrations. The TfR concentrations remain normal in pregnancy unless tissue iron deficiency is present (Carriaga et al 1991).

Management

Decisions about whether to prescribe prophylactic iron supplements during pregnancy in order to maintain the Hb at 11 g/dl as recommended by WHO (1992), remain controversial. However, most authors who have contributed to the current debate (Beard 2000, Beaton 2000, Bothwell 2000, Rasmussen 2001, Scholl & Reilly 2000) agree on the following:

- It is recommended that iron status should ideally be assessed prior to pregnancy as iron deficiency in early pregnancy has the most significant effect on fetal growth. Letsky (2000) suggests that women with a serum ferritin of < 50 µg/L would require daily iron supplements and those with serum ferritin concentration of > 80 µg/L are unlikely to require iron supplements.
- It is advisable to prescribe supplements where there is an iron deficiency anaemia with a Hb of 9–10 g/dl. Although this degree of anaemia is not severe enough to have a detrimental effect on the mother or fetus, treatment does have long term benefits. It will provide the mother with adequate stores should she require an operative birth or have a postpartum haemorrhage and she will embark on her next pregnancy with better iron reserves. Whilst breastfeeding, the amount of iron the baby can store will be dependent on the maternal iron stores. This has a significant impact on neurological development and brain function during childhood.
- Women with adequate iron stores should not take iron supplements. High Hb levels are likely to make RBCs macrocytic and the blood more viscose. This will affect uteroplacental blood flow and decrease placental perfusion. High levels of iron have also been associated with free radical formation, causing

oxidative damage. Oxidative stress is thought to initiate various pathological processes such as cardiovascular disease, inflammatory diseases, immune function, cancer and pre-eclampsia (Walsh 1998).

Oral iron preparations given prophylactically consist of one of the iron salts, either alone or in combination with folic acid. WHO (1992) recommends that supplements of 30–60 mg/day should be given prophylactically and 120–240 mg/day in divided doses to those with iron deficiency anaemia. Common iron preparation include ferrous sulphate, 200 mg tablets containing 60 mg of available iron, and ferrous gluconate, 300 mg tablets containing 35 mg of available iron. There are gastrointestinal side-effects of oral iron therapy that women need to be aware of. These are largely dose related and include nausea, epigastric pain and constipation. These discomforts can be reduced by taking iron supplements after meals and delaying administration until the 16th week of pregnancy. Some women may find one form of iron salts more tolerable than another; slow release preparations, although more expensive, are relatively free from side-effects.

Iron can also be given intramuscularly or intravenously thereby bypassing the gastrointestinal tract. This can be beneficial in women who are unable to take, tolerate or absorb oral preparations. Intramuscular iron is given in the form of iron sorbitol. The injection should be given using a 'Z technique' deep in to the muscle to prevent staining and irritation at the injection site. Injections should not be given in conjunction with oral iron as this enhances the toxic effects such as headache, dizziness, nausea and vomiting.

Iron dextran is given as total dose intravenous infusion. The dosage is calculated by taking account of bodyweight and the Hb concentration deficit. Side-effects include allergic reaction, which may take the form of severe anaphylactic shock. The infusion should therefore be administered slowly and the woman observed closely for the first few minutes. Joint pain occurring within 24 hours of the infusion is not uncommon.

Oral, intramuscular and intravenous administrations of iron show similar rates of increase in the Hb concentration. An increase of 0.8 g/dl is usual irrespective of the route of administration. Blood transfusion is rarely used to treat iron deficiency anaemia in pregnancy. It may be considered where there is an inadequate amount of time to treat severe anaemia prior to birth.

In women with iron deficiency anaemia, oral iron supplementation should continue postnatally particularly if they are breastfeeding. Blood tests should be repeated at the 6 week postnatal check and further investigation undertaken should iron deficiency anaemia remain.

Folic acid deficiency anaemia

Folic acid is needed for the increased cell growth of both mother and fetus but there is a physiological decrease in serum folate levels in pregnancy. Anaemia is more likely to be found towards the end of pregnancy when the fetus is growing rapidly. It is also more common during winter when folic acid is more difficult to obtain and in areas of social, economic and nutritional deprivation. The MRC Vitamin Study Research Group (1991) found a positive correlation between folate deficiency and the development of neural tube defects in the fetus.

The cause of folic acid deficiency anaemia is primarily a reduced dietary intake or reduced absorption, or a combination of these. In some instances there may be excessive demand and loss of folic acid. In haemolytic anaemia there is an increased demand for the production of new red cells and consequently for folic acid. Multiple pregnancy also results in an increased demand. Some drugs may interfere with the utilisation of folic acid, for example anticonvulsants, sulphonamides and alcohol.

Investigation

The signs and symptoms are varied and may be mistaken as 'minor disorders of pregnancy' such as pallor, lassitude, weight loss, depression, nausea and vomiting, glossitis, gingivitis and diarrhoea. Examination of the red cell indices will reveal that the red cells are reduced in number but enlarged in size. This condition is termed *macrocytic* or *megaloblastic anaemia*. The MCV rises, the MCHC may remain the same but as there are fewer cells the Hb level falls.

Management

The risk of folic acid deficiency can be reduced by advising pregnant women on the correct selection and preparation of foods that are high in folic acid. Folic acid is found in leafy green vegetables such as brussels sprouts, broccoli and spinach but it is destroyed easily by prolonged boiling or steaming. Other sources include peanuts, chick peas, bananas and citrus fruits. It is also found in avocado pears, asparagus and mushrooms but these are expensive sources. Following the MRC trial in 1991, the DoH Expert Advisory Group recommended that all women of childbearing age should eat more folate-rich foods, eat food fortified with folic acid such as bread and cereals and take a folic acid supplement of 0.4 mg per day (DOH 1992). Some women require extra folate supplements from early pregnancy in order to prevent megaloblastic anaemia. The recommended daily supplement is 5–10 mg orally in the following circumstances (Letsky 2000):

- diagnosed folate deficiency
- malabsorption syndrome
- haemoglobinopathy
- epilepsy requiring anticonvulsant treatment
- multiparity
- multiple pregnancy
- adolescence.

Vitamin B_{12} deficiency anaemia

Deficiency of vitamin B_{12} also produces a megaloblastic anaemia. Vitamin B_{12} levels fall during pregnancy but anaemia is rare because the body draws on its stores. Deficiency is most likely in vegans, who eat no animal products at all, and should therefore take vitamin B_{12} supplements during pregnancy (Letsky 2000).

Haemoglobinopathies

This term describes inherited conditions where the haemoglobin is abnormal. Haemoglobin consists of a group of four molecules, each of which has a haem unit made up of an iron porphyrin complex and a protein or globin chain. The position of the amino acids in the globin chain determines the type of haemoglobin produced. Ninety-seven per cent of adult Hb (HbA) has two alpha and two beta chains; the remaining 3% is HbA_2 and is composed of two alpha and two delta chains. Fetal Hb (HbF) has two alpha and two gamma chains; by 6 months of age this has been replaced by adult haemoglobin. The type of globin chain is genetically determined. Defective genes lead to the formation of abnormal haemoglobin; this may be as a result of impaired globin synthesis (thalassaemia syndromes) or from structural abnormality of globin (haemoglobin variants such as sickle cell anaemia). These conditions prevail in certain geographical areas because the heterozygous (trait) form of thalassaemia and sickle cell offers some protection against malaria. It is found mainly in people whose families come from Africa, the West Indies, the Middle East, the eastern Mediterranean and Asia (Higgins 2000).

As these conditions are inherited, and in the homozygous form can be fatal, screening of the population at risk should be carried out. Blood is examined by electrophoresis, which detects the different types of haemoglobin. Prospective parents who are known to have (or carry genes for) abnormal haemoglobin need genetic counselling in order to help them make an informed decision before embarking on a pregnancy. All women in the at-risk population are screened in early pregnancy and, where possible, their partners. If both parents are carriers (i.e. heterozygous) there is a 1 in 4 chance that the fetus will be homozygous for the condition (Fig. 19.1). This raises considerable ethical and moral issues concerning screening of the fetus and possible termination of the pregnancy (Adams 1994).

Thalassaemia

This condition is most commonly found in people of Mediterranean, African, Middle and Far Eastern origin. The basic defect is a reduced rate of globin chain synthesis in adult haemoglobin. This leads to ineffective erythropoiesis and increased haemolysis with a resultant inadequate haemoglobin content. The red cell indices show a low Hb and MCHC level but raised serum iron level. Definitive diagnosis is obtained by electrophoresis. The severity of the condition depends on whether the abnormal genes are inherited from one parent or from both. There are also different types of thalassaemia depending on whether the alpha or beta globin chain synthesis is affected. Box 19.1 shows the number of abnormal genes in each type of thalassaemia.

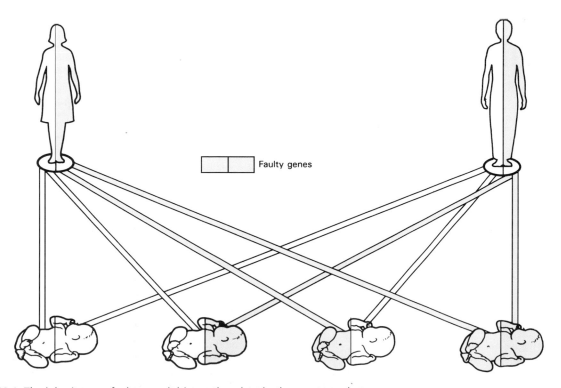

Faulty genes

Fig. 19.1 The inheritance of a haemoglobinopathy when both parents are heterozygous.

> **Box 19.1** Types of thalassaemia and their inheritance
>
> Alpha chains are formed by two genes from each parent.
> Beta chains are formed by one gene from each parent.
> Therefore:
>
> | | | |
> |---|---|---|
> | Alpha thalassaemia major | = | four defective alpha genes |
> | Alpha thalassaemia intermedia | = | three defective alpha genes |
> | Alpha thalassaemia minor | = | two or one defective alpha genes |
> | Beta thalassaemia major | = | two defective beta genes |
> | Beta thalassaemia minor | = | one defective beta gene |

Alpha thalassaemia major. This condition is more commonly found in Southeast Asia. The child inherits abnormal genes from both parents. Rapid red cell breakdown produces a severe anaemia, which is incompatible with extrauterine life.

Beta thalassaemia major. The defective genes present result in severe haemoglobin deficiency, which may result in cardiac failure and death in early childhood. In those that survive, the ineffective erythropoiesis and increased haemolysis cause hypersplenism. A splenectomy is often performed in order to increase RBC survival and reduce the need for frequent blood transfusions. Blood transfusions increase the possibility of survival to childbearing age although the constant breakdown of the RBCs from donated blood results in an accumulation of iron in the body. This is removed by an iron-chelating agent, desferrioxamine, in order to prevent toxicity. Despite this, iron overload is inevitable and results in hepatic, cardiac and endocrine disorders by 10–11 years of age. Bone marrow transplantation is the only treatment that can cure this condition. Until recently, the high mortality rate made pregnancy in transfusion-dependent thalassaemia rare. However, advances in paediatric and haematological management have resulted in good maternal and fetal outcomes in women with beta thalassaemia major (Tuck & Jensen 1998).

Alpha and beta thalassaemia minor. The heterozygous condition is the more common form of thalassaemia and produces an anaemia that is similar to iron deficiency in that the Hb, the MCV and the MCH are all lowered. A deficiency in iron is not, however, usually a problem because RBCs are broken down more rapidly than normal and the iron is stored for future use. In pregnancy, oral iron and folate supplements are necessary in order to maintain the iron stores. Parenteral iron should never be given. Blood transfusions may be required if the haemoglobin is thought to be inadequate for the stress of labour and blood loss at birth (Letsky 2000).

Sickle cell disorders

Sickle cell disorders are found most commonly in people of African or West Indian origin. In this condition defective genes produce abnormal haemoglobin beta chains; the resulting Hb is called HbS. In sickle cell anaemia (HbSS, or SCA) abnormal genes have been inherited from both parents, whereas in sickle cell trait (HbAS) only one abnormal gene has been inherited.

Sickle cell anaemia. Sickle cells have an increased fragility and shortened life span of 17 days, which results in chronic haemolytic anaemia and causes episodes of ischaemia and pain, known as *sickle cell crises*. Sickling crisis may occur whenever oxygen concentration is low. Precipitating factors that affect oxygen uptake include psychological stress, cold climate and extreme temperature changes, smoking-induced hypoxia, strenuous physical exertion and fatigue, respiratory disease, infection and pregnancy. When subjected to low oxygen tension, HbS contracts damaging the cell and causing it to assume a sickle shape. Damaged cells block capillaries and the resulting infarction leads to pain, affecting particularly the bones, joints and abdominal organs. The spleen may also be damaged, which affects the individual's ability to fight infection. Emboli may be thrown off into the circulation, which may cause a stroke and threaten life (Thomas 1997).

Maternal and fetal effects. There have been significant decreases in both maternal and perinatal mortality owing to improvements in the general medical and obstetric care of women with SCA and advancements in neonatology. Women with SCA are still at an increased risk for medical complications during pregnancy although overall pregnancy outcome is favourable. The maternal risks include antenatal and postnatal pain crisis, infections, pulmonary complications, anaemia, pre-eclampsia and caesarean section (Howard et al 1995, Seoud et al 1994, Sun et al 2001). Fetal and neonatal complications include preterm birth, being small for gestational age and neonatal jaundice (Brown et al 1994, Koshy 1995). Antenatal care aims to minimise these complications and comprises a multidisciplinary approach.

Antenatal care. All women in the at-risk population are screened in early pregnancy and where possible their partners. Those who are diagnosed as having SCA should be referred to a specialist sickle cell centre with trained haemoglobinopathy and genetic counsellors (Rochester-Peart 1997). If both partners carry genes for sickle cell disease there is a chance that the fetus will inherit the condition. Counselling will assist the parents in making an informed decision with regard to prenatal diagnosis and the future of the pregnancy.

Management. Monitoring of pregnancy is performed at frequent intervals and involves the midwife, obstetrician, haematologist and haemoglobinopathy specialists maintaining close liaison and discussion with the woman and her family. Midwives have an important role in providing information and education about SCA and how it affects pregnancy, particularly in emphasising the factors that may precipitate sickle crisis. Fluid intake should be well maintained to prevent dehydration and it is important to detect bacterial infections, particularly urinary tract and respiratory infections, at an early stage. Regular monitoring of the haemoglobin concentration is required throughout pregnancy; this is usually in the range of 6–9 g/dl. Good nutrition and taking folic acid supplements assist in maintaining a steady haematological state. The use of prophylactic blood transfusions to improve the outcome of pregnancy remains controversial. Mindful of the complications regarding blood transfusion in women with SCA (El-Shafei et al 1995, Howard et al 1995), most authors recommend a policy of transfusing only when indicated, for example in symptomatic anaemia, severe anaemia with a haematocrit less than 18%, sickle crisis, cardiac failure or prior to caesarean section (El-Shafei at al 1995, Koshy 1995, Rahimy et al 2000, Seoud et al 1994). Thirty-five to fifty per cent of women with SCA will experience sickle crisis during pregnancy, which requires hospital admission (Howard et al 1995, Rahimy et al 2000, Sun et al 2001). This is an extremely painful condition that is often poorly managed and undertreated by nursing, midwifery and medical staff (Alleyne & Thomas 1994). Larrabee & Cowan (1995), Howard et al (1995) and Gorman (1999) identify that effective management of sickle cell crisis can be achieved by:

- utilisation of pain assessment tools to determine severity of the pain
- administration of effective analgesia; rapid pain relief can be obtained by intravenous diamorphine followed by patient-controlled opioid analgesia; it may be necessary to supplement with regular doses of oral analgesia such as paracetamol or non-steroidal anti-inflammatory agents
- liaison with the acute pain management team to ensure adequate and continuing pain relief
- administration of intravenous fluids to correct dehydration and electrolyte imbalance caused by pyrexia, vomiting or diarrhoea
- pulse oximetry to assess oxygen saturation and the administration of oxygen therapy if indicated
- antibiotic treatment if infection is suspected
- assessment of haematological indices and liaison with the haematology department
- provision of social, psychological and physical support to alleviate symptoms associated with chronic pain.

Fetal assessment includes regular ultrasound scans to assess fetal growth. If growth restriction is identified then more intensive monitoring will be required utilising biophysical profiles and Doppler ultrasound.

Intrapartum care. During labour the midwife must ensure that the woman is kept well hydrated with intravenous fluids, and given prophylactic antibiotics, effective analgesia, preferably epidural, and oxygen therapy if needed. The fetus should be monitored closely for signs of distress.

Postnatal care. Prevention of puerperal sepsis is paramount; therefore antibiotic cover is continued throughout the postnatal period. Neonatal testing of all babies at risk must be undertaken by obtaining a cord blood sample at birth. The sickle cell test does not yield positive results until the age of 3–4 months as HbF recedes. A positive test does not distinguish between HbAS and SCA; therefore all children showing positive results should be investigated and followed up by the haematologist. In order to prevent the high incidence of infant mortality from sickle cell anaemia, early diagnosis combined with prophylaxis against infection, parental education and adequate follow-up are recommended.

Sickle cell trait. This is usually asymptomatic. The blood appears normal, although the sickle screening test is positive. There is no anaemia even under the additional stress of pregnancy.

Combinations of abnormal haemoglobins

Sickle cell haemoglobin C anaemia (HbSC). This is a mild variant of HbSS more commonly found in Ghanaians. It presents with normal or near-normal levels of Hb. Owing to its mildness, neither the woman nor the obstetrician is aware of its presence or its complications. Women with HbSC may have mild sickling episodes; therefore close supervision is required to avoid any stimulus to a crisis such as hypoxia, dehydration or trauma. This particularly applies immediately following childbirth. These women should be cared for during labour in the same way as those with HbSS.

Sickle cell disease may also be combined with beta thalassaemia.

Other rare inherited disorders

Glucose-6-phosphate dehydrogenase (G6PD) deficiency. This is found in Africa, Asia and Mediterranean countries. It is inherited through an X-linked gene and is therefore seen predominantly in males. G6PD is an enzyme necessary for the survival of the red cell. When it is deficient, RBCs are destroyed in the presence of certain substances. These include fava beans, sulphonamides, vitamin K analogues, salicylates and camphor (found in products such as Vicks VapoRub). Clinically G6PD deficiency takes two forms:

- jaundice in the neonatal period, usually occurring on the 2nd or 3rd day of life, reaching a maximum by the 6th day and subsiding by the end of the 1st week

- acute self-limiting haemolysis precipitated by contact with the substances listed above. This may be indirect contact via the placenta or breastmilk. Death from haemolysis is rare.

Spherocytosis. This is found in northern Europe. In this condition the red cells are spherical instead of biconcave and are easily destroyed. In this disease the abnormal gene is dominant. It may cause a haemolytic jaundice in the neonate.

Diabetes mellitus

Diabetes is the most common medical condition to affect pregnancy and occurs in approximately 4 per 1000 pregnancies in the UK (Maresh 1998). It complicates approximately 1% of all pregnancies in caucasian populations, but a higher percentage of pregnancies in other ethnic groups. Recent audits undertaken by Casson et al (1997), Hawthorne et al (1997) and Hadden et al (2001) identified persistently poorer outcomes in pregnant women with diabetes compared with the overall obstetric population. The aim of both the St Vincent declaration of the European Association for the Study of Diabetes and of the UK Task Force (SVD Working Party 1990) is to achieve a pregnancy outcome for the diabetic mother equal to that of a non-diabetic mother.

The term *'diabetes mellitus'* (DM) describes a metabolic disorder of multiple aetiology that affects the normal metabolism of carbohydrates, fats and protein. It is characterised by increasing levels of glucose in the blood (hyperglycaemia) and excretion of glucose in the urine (glycosuria) resulting from defects in insulin secretion, or insulin action, or both. The classic signs and symptoms are excessive thirst (polydipsia), excessive urinary excretion (polyuria) and unexplained weight loss. The long term effects of DM are reflected in the development of macrovascular and microvascular disease producing coronary heart disease, peripheral arterial disease, kidney disease (diabetic nephropathy), loss of vision (diabetic retinopathy) and nerve damage (diabetic neuropathy).

A normal fasting blood glucose of < 6.1 mmol/L is regulated by the pancreatic hormones insulin and glucagon. Following the ingestion of carbohydrates the rising blood glucose stimulates the pancreas to secrete insulin, which reduces blood glucose. Falling blood glucose levels induce glucagon production, which prevents further glucose reduction. The combined action of these two hormones maintains the blood glucose within normal limits.

Hyperglycaemia is usually the result of insulin deficiency or when there is a high secretion of hormones antagonistic to insulin action; severe hyperglycaemia (blood glucose > 25.0 mmol/L) may result in diabetic ketoacidosis, coma or death. *Hypoglycaemia* is defined as a blood glucose < 2.2 mmol/L. Symptoms of a falling blood glucose include tremor, sweating and tachycardia. Severe hypoglycaemia, particularly in neonates, can result in fits, coma and death. Repeated severe episodes of hypoglycaemia are associated with the risk of permanent brain damage (Higgins 2001).

Classification

Type 1 DM. This occurs when beta cells in the islets of Langerhans in the pancreas are destroyed, stopping insulin production. Insulin therapy is required in order to prevent the development of ketoacidosis, coma and death. It presents more commonly in childhood, but can occur at any age and in some cases is attributable to an autoimmune process (WHO 1999).

Type 2 DM. This results from a defect(s) in insulin action and insulin secretion and insulin therapy is not needed to survive. The risk of developing this type of DM increases with age, obesity and lack of physical activity. It occurs more frequently in women with prior gestational diabetes mellitus (see below) and in individuals with hypertension. Its frequency varies between different racial or ethnic groups and there is some suggestion of a genetic predisposition (WHO 1999).

Gestational diabetes mellitus (GDM). This is defined as carbohydrate intolerance resulting in hyperglycaemia of variable severity, with its onset or first recognition during pregnancy (WHO 1999).

Impaired glucose regulation. This includes *impaired glucose tolerance* (IGT) and *impaired fasting glycaemia* (IFG), which are metabolic states intermediate between normal glucose homeostasis and diabetes. IGT is categorised as carbohydrate metabolism resulting in slightly raised postmeal blood glucose levels of > 7.8 mmol/L. IFG refers to fasting glucose concentrations that are lower than those required to diagnose DM but higher than the 'normal' reference range (i.e. > 6.1 mmol/L but < 7.0 mmol/L). Individuals with

impaired glucose regulation are at increased risk of developing DM and cardiovascular disease (WHO 1999).

Diagnosis

WHO (1999) recommend the following criteria for diagnosing DM:

1. diabetes symptoms of increased thirst, increased urine volume, unexplained weight loss, plus
2. a random venous plasma glucose concentration > 11.1 mmol/L or,
   a fasting plasma concentration > 7.0 mmol/L or,
   a 2 hour plasma concentration > 11.1 mmol/L
   2 hours after 75 g anhydrous glucose in an oral glucose tolerance test (OGTT)
3. without symptoms, diagnosis should not be based on a single glucose determination but requires confirmatory plasma venous determination taken on another day
4. the OGTT should always be used to diagnose gestational diabetes mellitus and impaired glucose regulation.

Monitoring diabetes

The main objective of diabetic therapy is to maintain blood glucose levels as near to normal as possible and to reduce the risk of long term complications. Diabetics are therefore encouraged to monitor their blood glucose concentration regularly by obtaining a finger-prick sample of capillary blood and using reagent test strips (e.g. BM test) with or without a reflectance glucose meter. Blood glucose can also be estimated by testing urine for glucose using reagent strips, although this is less accurate than the blood test and not recommended in pregnancy. Long term blood glucose control can be determined by undertaking a laboratory test to measure glycosylated haemoglobin (HbA1c). Five to eight per cent of haemoglobin in the red blood cells carries a glucose molecule and is said to be glycosylated. The degree of haemoglobin glycosylation is dependent on the amount of glucose the red blood cells have been exposed to during their 120 day life. A random blood test measuring the percentage of haemoglobin that is glycosylated will reflect the average blood glucose during the preceding 1–2 months. The higher the HbA1c the poorer is the blood sugar control. Good diabetic control is defined as an HbA1c of < 6.5% (Higgins 2001).

Carbohydrate metabolism in pregnancy

Pregnancy is characterised by several factors that produce a diabeticogenetic state so that insulin and carbohydrate metabolism is altered in order to make glucose more readily available to the fetus. Increasing levels of oestrogen, progesterone and prolactin produce progressive hyperplasia of the pancreatic beta cells resulting in the secretion of 50% more insulin (hyperinsulinaemia) by the third trimester. However, progesterone, human placental lactogen and cortisol are insulin antagonists and reduce the effectiveness of insulin. This is considered to be a 'glucose-sparing mechanism', which enables large quantities of glucose to be taken up by the maternal circulation and transferred to the fetus via the placenta by a process known as 'facilitated diffusion'. After the placenta is delivered insulin resistance and requirements decrease rapidly and the prepregnancy sensitivity to insulin is restored (Holdcroft & Thomas 2000). Gestational diabetes is most likely to emerge during the third trimester when the extra demands on the pancreatic beta cells precipitate glucose intolerance. Women with DM do not have the capacity to increase insulin secretion in response to the altered carbohydrate metabolism in pregnancy and therefore glucose accumulates in the maternal and fetal system leading to significant morbidity and mortality.

Prepregnancy care

The risk of the development of congenital malformations increases significantly in women with DM. The malformations associated with diabetes – cardiac, neural tube defects and caudal regression syndrome – occur during the first trimester of pregnancy and are thought to be related to poor diabetic control at this time. It is important therefore that good metabolic control is established before pregnancy. Women should have access to a prepregnancy counselling service and ideally meet a diabetic specialist midwife before becoming pregnant (Jardine-Brown et al 1996). Assessment is made of current diabetic control aiming for premeal glucose levels of < 6 mmol/L and HbA1c of ≤ 7% (Diabetes UK 2000). Insulin dosage is reviewed and an explanation given of the adjustments that will be required during pregnancy. Women with type 2 DM on oral hypoglycaemics will need to transfer to insulin to prevent the possibility of teratogenesis. Pregnancy may lead to a deterioration of diabetes and for this reason the presence of renal, cardiovascular or retinal changes need to be assessed. Angiotensin-converting enzyme (ACE) inhibitors to control hypertension are widely used in women with diabetes. However, these drugs are contraindicated in pregnancy because of possible teratogenesis and therefore alternative therapy such as methyldopa or nifedipine needs to be considered. Diet, including weight control and folic acid supplementation, and general health measures, including checking rubella status and smoking cessation, need to be discussed in addition to giving advice regarding the effect of diabetes on pregnancy and of pregnancy on diabetes (Maresh 1998).

Antenatal care

Women and their partners should ideally be seen in a combined clinic by a team that includes a physician, an obstetrician with a special interest in diabetes in pregnancy, a specialist diabetes nurse, a specialist midwife and dietician. The woman is seen as often as required in order to maintain good diabetic control; this may entail fortnightly visits until 28 weeks' gestation and then weekly until term. Blood glucose levels should be monitored frequently (four times a day using a reflectance meter) and insulin levels adjusted to achieve premeal blood sugar levels of 5.0–6.0 mmol/L and postmeal levels of < 7.8 mmol/L. Additional estimations of blood glucose control such as monthly HbA1c measurements are also recommended (Jardine-Brown 1996, Diabetes UK 2000). Diabetic control is particularly difficult to maintain in early pregnancy owing to the effects of pregnancy on diabetes. This may be exacerbated by other pregnancy disorders such as nausea and vomiting. Women with DM are more likely to become hypoglycaemic at this time and loss of hypoglycaemic warning symptoms is common. Women and their relatives need to be warned of this and advice should be given regarding the recognition, management and treatment of hypoglycaemia. A glucagon kit should be supplied and her partner and relatives instructed on how to use it. Dietary advice and monitoring is continued throughout pregnancy as the need for carbohydrate increases as the fetus grows. A diet that is high in fibre is beneficial as carbohydrates are released slowly and therefore a more constant blood glucose level can be achieved. Glycosuria is common in pregnancy owing to the increased glomerular filtration rate and decreased renal threshold. Women with DM have a predisposition to urinary and vaginal infections during pregnancy; these should be discussed with the midwife so women can recognise the signs and symptoms and seek treatment as soon as possible.

Pre-existing vascular disease will increase the risk of a woman with DM developing hypertensive disorders in pregnancy and will cause a deterioration of diabetic retinopathy.

In view of the increased risk of congenital malformations, anomaly ultrasound screening should be offered at 20 weeks' gestation. It is also recommended that fetal echocardiography is undertaken at 20–22 weeks to detect cardiac abnormalities. Serum screening for Down syndrome is altered with maternal diabetes and care should be taken when interpreting the results.

Fetal growth must be observed carefully because of the risk of growth restriction due to maternal vascular disease, pre-eclampsia, or a combination of both. A baseline measurement of the fetal abdominal circumference is taken at 20 weeks. This is followed by serial measurements every 2-4 weeks commencing at 24 weeks. Serial ultrasound should also detect fetal macrosomia and whether polyhydramnios is present.

As far as possible the woman monitors her diabetes at home and diabetic care is provided on an outpatient basis. It is important that the midwife assesses the progress of the pregnancy in the normal way in order to detect any complications. Hospital admission may be required because of poor diabetic control, a destabilising illness or obstetric complications.

Intrapartum care

Ideally labour should be allowed to commence spontaneously at term for women with uncomplicated DM during pregnancy. Poor diabetic control or a deterioration in the maternal or fetal condition may necessitate earlier, planned birth. Induction of labour may also be considered where the fetus is judged to be macrosomic (Maresh 1998). Routine induction of labour at 37–38 weeks' gestation is no longer recommended as it does not reduce the perinatal mortality rate and is more likely to result in respiratory morbidity. It may also

contribute to the high caesarean section rate for diabetic pregnancies compared with normal pregnancies (Moran et al 2000). The St Vincent declaration states that caesarean sections are to be performed solely for obstetric indications. Fetal lungs mature more slowly when the mother is diabetic and it is important to take this into account if early induction of labour is planned. In addition, steroids such as dexamethasone, which may be used to aid lung maturation and surfactant production, will increase insulin requirements in women with DM.

The aim of intrapartum care is to maintain normoglycaemia in labour (i.e. < 7.0 mmol/L). Maternal hyperglycaemia leads to an increase in fetal insulin production, which will cause neonatal hypoglycaemia. The St Vincent declaration recommends that maternity units should aim to maintain a maternal blood glucose concentration of between 4 and 6 mmol/L. However, Moran et al (2000) found there to be a wide variation within UK maternity units with 15% of units aiming to maintain a concentration of 8.0 mmol/L or above. All units should have their own written guidelines for the management of diabetes in labour although regimens will vary. An example of such a regimen utilising a sliding scale of insulin dosage depending on the maternal blood glucose concentration is outlined in Figure 19.2.

Fetal distress is more common as placental blood flow is reduced and glycosylated haemoglobin decreases oxygen carriage in diabetic pregnancies. In addition, maternal ketoacidosis may result from dehydration and unstable diabetes. If the mother becomes acidotic, ketones will cross the placenta and affect the fetal acid–base status. Continuous electronic fetal monitoring is recommended and fetal blood sampling should be utilised if acidosis is suspected (Holdcroft & Thomas 2000). Adequate pain relief, such as epidural analgesia, assists in regulating the blood sugar levels and preventing the development of metabolic acidosis in women with DM. It is also useful if difficulties should arise with the birth of the shoulders or an operative birth is required.

Postpartum care

Immediately after the third stage of labour the insulin requirements will fall rapidly to prepregnancy levels. The insulin infusion rate should be reduced by at least 50%. Carbohydrate metabolism returns to normal

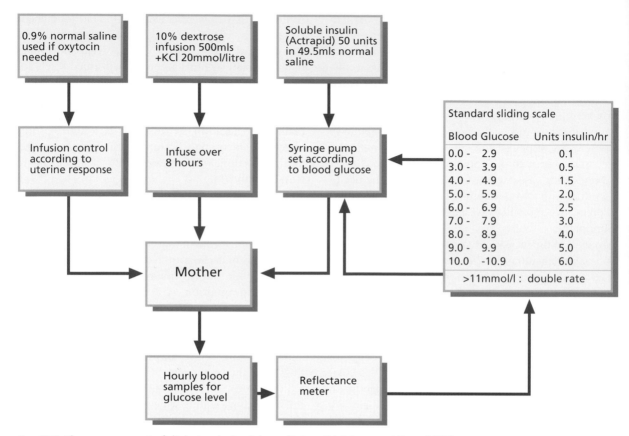

Fig. 19.2 The management of diabetes during labour (Baker, Edelstone and Kean 2000).

very quickly and women can resume their prepregnancy insulin regimen. Women with type 2 DM who were previously on oral hypoglycaemics or dietary control need to be reviewed prior to recommencing therapy. Monitoring of blood glucose levels should continue during this interim period. Breastfeeding should be encouraged in all women with diabetes. An additional carbohydrate intake of 40–50 g is recommended and insulin therapy may need to be adjusted accordingly. Operative birth, together with diabetes, predisposes these women to infection and delayed healing. The administration of antibiotics may be a useful preventative measure in this instance. All women should be offered contraceptive advice so that optimum metabolic control is achieved prior to planning the next pregnancy. The issues governing choice of contraception for women with DM are similar to those for non-diabetic women. All contraceptive methods are considered safe, acceptable and effective for diabetic women. Women with DM, gestational diabetes or IGT

should be reviewed at 6 weeks, ideally at a combined diabetes clinic or alternatively by their GP.

Neonatal care

The development of complications in the neonate is related to maternal hyperglycaemia during pregnancy leading to fetal hyperinsulinaemia. This will result in the following conditions: macrosomia, hypoglycaemia, polycythaemia and respiratory distress syndrome (Jones 2001).

Macrosomia. This is defined as a fetal birth weight > 4500 g. Maternal hyperglycaemia and consequently fetal hyperglycaemia induce fetal hyperinsulinaemia. This leads to an increase in the amount of fetal body fat and the enlargement of fetal organs such as the liver, heart, spleen, adrenals and the beta cells of the pancreas (beta cell hyperplasia). The increased fetal size may cause prolonged labour due to cephalopelvic disproportion. It also predisposes the infant to difficult deliveries, such as shoulder dystocia and birth injuries. As a consequence asphyxia is common and these infants are more likely than babies of normal weight to die from an intrapartum-related event (CESDI 1999).

Hypoglycaemia. Beta cell hyperplasia causes the baby to continue to produce more insulin than required for up to 24 hours following birth. The impaired metabolic response to this hyperinsulinaemia causes neonatal hypoglycaemia (blood glucose of < 1.9 mmol/L in the term infant). To prevent this complication the neonatal blood glucose needs to be assessed 1–2 hours after birth and then every 4–6 hours for the first 24–48 hours. Regular feeding is encouraged to maintain a blood glucose of at least 2 mmol/L.

Polycythaemia. Fetal hyperinsulinaemia during pregnancy also leads to an increase in red cell production resulting in polycythaemia (venous haematocrit > 65%). The rapid breakdown of the excess red blood cells combined with the relative immaturity of the liver in the newborn predisposes the baby to jaundice. This will be exacerbated if there is bruising as a result of birth trauma.

Respiratory distress syndrome. Hyperinsulinaemia is thought to impair the production of surfactant and delay lung maturation. Hence, babies born at term may display symptomatology of respiratory distress. Infants of diabetic mothers are not routinely admitted to a neonatal unit. A paediatrician should examine the baby carefully at birth, who should be allowed to stay with his mother unless there are medical complications as outlined above. Observations of temperature, apex beat and respirations and monitoring of blood sugar levels are important in the first 24–48 hours. Clinical signs together with symptomatology such as respiratory distress, apnoea or tachypnoea, cyanosis, jitteriness, irritability, seizures, feeding intolerance and temperature instability may all be indicative of respiratory distress syndrome, polycythaemia and hypoglycaemia, which will require further investigation and treatment in a neonatal unit (Jones 2001).

Gestational diabetes

The incidence of GDM varies widely across different ethnic groups. In Caucasians it is 1–2%, in Afro-Caribbeans 2–3% and in Asians 4–5% (Lowy 1997). An agreement as to what is considered a 'normal' blood glucose level in pregnancy and at what level maternal and fetal morbidity ensues remains illusive. Hence, the significance of GDM is difficult to determine (Mitchell 2001). The strongest evidence suggests that fetal macrosomia and caesarean section rates are increased. In the longer term there appears to be an association between raised glucose levels in utero and the development of obesity and diabetes in later life. There is also evidence to suggest that women who develop GDM are at risk of developing type 2 DM (Virjee et al 2001). Davey & Hamblin (2001) identify that some women are at high risk of developing GDM and there may be some benefit in selective screening for GDM in women where the following risk factors are identified:

- maternal age > 25 years
- DM affecting a first degree relative
- high risk racial heritage e.g. Asian–Indian, Middle Eastern, Afro-Caribbean
- BMI > 27 kg/m^2.

Diabetes UK (2000) also provides the following guidance with regard to screening for GDM with the proviso that these are likely to alter as new information becomes available.

1. urine should be tested for glucose at every antenatal visit
2. timed random laboratory plasma glucose measurements should be made whenever glycosuria (1+ or more) is detected, at the booking visit and 28 weeks' gestation
3. a 75 g 2 hour OGTT should be performed if the random blood glucose concentrations are ≥ 6.1 mmol/L in the fasting state or > 2 hours after food, or ≥ 7.0 mmol/L within 2 hours of food.

Diagnosis is based on the WHO (1999) recommendations; however, caution should be exercised if these occur in the third trimester when glucose tolerance is known to be impaired:

1. if the fasting venous plasma glucose is > 7.0 mmol/L, or
2. a fasting venous plasma glucose < 7.0 mmol/L and a plasma glucose of > 7.8 mmol/L 2 hours after a 75 g glucose load.

Treatment will depend on the blood glucose levels. The midwife should involve both the diabetic nurse specialist and dietician in dietary interventions to regulate carbohydrate intake and restrict fat and sugars. Advice regarding exercise in pregnancy will be of benefit and smoking cessation strategies may also need to be employed. Grossly abnormal results are likely to require insulin therapy. Blood glucose monitoring should continue on a regular basis throughout pregnancy in order to detect hyperglycaemia. Fetal macrosomia is the main complication and therefore fetal growth and well-being should be closely monitored for the remainder of the pregnancy. Decisions can then be made about the optimal mode and time of birth. Following birth the baby should be closely monitored for hypoglycaemia. If the woman is on insulin therapy this is withdrawn immediately after the birth of the baby. It is recommended that a postnatal OGTT is performed at 6 weeks; if the results are abnormal then appropriate referral should be made. Those with normal glucose levels require advice regarding the implications for future pregnancies and the development of type 1 or type 2 DM. If the woman adopts a healthy lifestyle and avoids obesity this risk may be reduced.

Epilepsy

The prevalence of epilepsy in the general population is 1 in 200 and it affects 0.3–0.5% of pregnant women (Donaldson 1995). Between 1997 and 1999, nine women died as a result of epilepsy (Lewis & Drife 2001). It is important therefore that midwives are aware of the complications that may occur and closely monitor women with epilepsy in order to reduce the risk of maternal death and fetal loss.

An epileptic seizure results from abnormal electrical activity in the brain, which is manifest by brief sensory, motor and autonomic dysfunction. These disturbances recur spontaneously and are classified according to the parts of the brain affected. Seizures may be described as *partial*, usually arising from the temporal or frontal lobe of the brain, or *generalised*, resulting from disturbances involving both halves of the brain. General seizures may be further classified as *absence seizures* (petit mal), *myoclonic seizures*, *tonic–clonic seizures* (grand mal), *atonic seizures* and *status epilepticus* (Appleton et al 1994).

The cause of epilepsy in most instances is unknown. There is some suggestion that there is a genetic component, which in certain circumstances predisposes an individual to epileptic seizures. In other cases an underlying cause such as hypoglycaemia, encephalitis, meningitis, cerebral hypoxia, toxicity from alcohol or drugs, or structural damage or abnormality of the brain may result in epilepsy. A number of 'trigger' factors have been identified that may precipitate an attack in those who have been diagnosed as epileptic; these include stress, alcohol, hyperventilation, hot/steamy environments, lack of sleep or physical exhaustion and exposure to strobe lighting (Coleman & Rund 1997).

Identification of the type of epilepsy is important in the treatment of epilepsy. The aim of treatment is to identify the cause of the seizure and provide appropriate therapy to prevent recurrence. The control of seizures can be achieved for the majority of people through the use of antiepileptic drugs (AED). Most of the drugs have side-effects, which include drowsiness, sedation, nausea and skin rashes. These are most notable when the drug is first taken or if the dosage is too high. The ideal treatment is a single AED prescribed at the lowest effective dose (Morrow 1996).

Prepregnancy care

Women on AEDs become folic acid deficient and may develop macrocytic anaemia. Folic acid deficiency has also been associated with neural tube defects and other congenital malformations such as orofacial clefts and congenital heart defects. There is a 1–2% risk of neural tube defects if a woman is taking sodium valproate (Epilim) or carbamazepine (Tegretol) in pregnancy. Of the other older AEDs, phenytoin gives rise to a combination of malformations termed 'fetal hydantoin syndrome', which comprises craniofacial dysmorphic features, digital defects, microcephaly and growth retardation. There are insufficient data with regard to the effects of the newer AEDs such as vigabatrin, lamotrigine, gabapentin, topiramate and tiagibine (Gilmour-White 2000).

Preconception advice is therefore essential for women with epilepsy. AED therapy may be withdrawn gradually prior to pregnancy in order to reduce the risk of teratogenicity where women (a) suffer from seizures that are unlikely to harm the fetus such as absence, partial or myoclonic seizures or (b) have been seizure free for over 2 years and a recurrence is unlikely (Coleman & Rund 1997). Folic acid supplementation (5 mg/day) should be commenced before pregnancy and continued throughout pregnancy to prevent congenital malformations and the development of anaemia (Rutherford & Rubin 1996).

Antenatal care

Antenatal care should be shared between the neurologist, the obstetrician and the midwife, preferably at a combined clinic as this maximises professional surveillance of the women's condition without the added stress of multiple hospital appointments (Lindsay 1990). Antenatal care should include a detailed anomaly scan at 18–22 weeks, which will detect any fetal abnormalities. Abnormalities are more common if anticonvulsant drugs are prescribed in high concentration and particularly if more than one is used. In spite of these potential problems most babies are unaffected and 90% are born normal (RCM/Joint Epilepsy Council of the UK and Ireland 1996). In general, women whose epilepsy is well controlled have few problems from their condition in pregnancy. Some women may experience an increase in seizures; this is often due to non-compliance with the drug regimen, sleep deprivation during pregnancy and the decline in plasma concentrations of the AED as the pregnancy progresses. Most of the complications in pregnancy are increased when the epilepsy is poorly controlled (Kilpatrick & Hopper 1993). Particular emphasis should also be placed on the first aid measures that should be adopted following an epileptic seizure in order to prevent aspiration, and the dangers of hot baths inducing fainting and consequent drowning (Lewiso & Drife 2001).

Intrapartum care

Care during labour and childbirth is not likely to be different from that of other mothers. Tonic–clonic seizures occur in only 1–2% of women during labour (Scottish Obstetric Guidelines & Audit Project 1997). Seizures are more likely to occur in conditions such as sleep deprivation, hypoglycaemia, anaemia, stress or hyperventilation – all of which may arise during labour. AEDs should therefore be maintained throughout labour and careful observation by the midwife

is required through labour and the early postnatal period.

Postnatal care

Midwives and other health professionals have an important role in the education of women and their families. Safety precautions in the home are important and should be discussed with the woman and her partner. The mother is given advice about how to minimise risks when feeding, bathing, changing and transporting the baby (Doran 2000). AED therapy should be reviewed 6 weeks postnatally and the dosage adjusted to prepregnancy levels. Future pregnancy plans should be discussed and appropriate contraceptive advice given. All methods of contraception are available to women with epilepsy. Oral contraceptives are less effective with some AEDs, namely phenytoin, phenobarbital, primidone and carbamazepine, as they induce hepatic enzymes which metabolise oestrogen faster. These women will require oral contraceptives with a higher dosage of oestrogen (i.e. > 50 mg oestrogen) (Gilmour-White 2000).

Effect of epilepsy on the fetus and neonate

According to Donaldson (1995), when status epilepticus occurs, one-third of mothers and half of the fetuses do not survive. Convulsive status epilepticus is a medical emergency. A single seizure may cause fetal morbidity from hypoxia or placental abruption. AEDs cross the placenta freely and decrease production of vitamin K leading to the risk of haemorrhagic disease of the newborn (HDN, see Ch. 46). This can be prevented by routine administration of vitamin K to the mother from 36 weeks' gestation and to the baby shortly after birth (Scottish Obstetric Guidelines & Audit Project 1997). The rate of clearance of AEDs varies according to the drug. Newborn infants may therefore suffer harmful effects from the AED level and, as a group, tend to be less efficient at feeding and gain weight more slowly. A minority will suffer withdrawal symptoms such as tremor, excitability and convulsions. AEDs pass into the breastmilk in relatively small quantities and therefore breastfeeding is recommended. Some AEDs such as phenobarbital, primidone or benzodiazepines may have a sedative effect, in which case bottle feeding or mixed feeding may be advised (Rutherford & Rubin 1996).

The majority of women with epilepsy will have uncomplicated pregnancies with normal deliveries and healthy children. There is a small group of women with epilepsy who will require careful monitoring from the midwife, obstetrician and neurologist in order to prevent significant morbidity/mortality in either the mother or fetus.

Autoimmune disease

Autoimmune disease arises from a disruption in the function of the immune system of the body, resulting in the production of antibodies against the body's own cells. Antigens normally present on the body's cells stimulate the development of autoantibodies, which, unable to distinguish the self antigens from non-self or foreign antigens, act against the body's cells to cause localised and systemic reactions. The cause of this condition is unknown but it is thought to be multifactorial with genetic, environmental, hormonal and viral influences. Many autoimmune diseases are more prevalent in women, particularly between puberty and and the menopause, which suggests that female hormonal factors may play a role. They broadly fall into two groups:

1. multisystem disease such as systemic lupus erythematosus (SLE)
2. tissue- or organ-specific disorders such as autoimmune thyroid disease.

These disorders are characterised by periods of remission interrupted by periods of crisis, which may require hospitalisation. This cyclical variation appears to be related to some external factors, for example excessive emotional stress. Treatment is aimed at lessening the severity of the symptoms rather than effecting a cure. Mild cases usually respond to anti-inflammatory drugs; more severe illnesses may require steroids or immunosuppressant therapy.

Systemic lupus erythematosus

SLE, or lupus, is an inflammatory disorder of the connective tissue, which forms the fibrous, elastic, fatty or cartilaginous matrix that connects and supports other tissues. It is a rare condition although the incidence has tripled over the past four decades. It is thought to affect less than 1 in 1000 people. It is nine times more common in women than men, and nine times more common in Afro-Caribbeans and Asians than in white people (Hay & Snaith 1995). Connective tissue is found throughout the body and in almost every organ; therefore SLE produces multisystem disorders affecting muscles, bone, skin, blood, eyes, nervous system, heart, lungs and kidneys.

The initial manifestation of SLE is often arthritis accompanied by fever, fatigue, malaise, weight loss, photosensitivity and anaemia. A wide range of skin lesions are seen and an erythematous facial 'butterfly' rash is characteristic of the disorder. Depending on the organs involved, inflammatory conditions such as pluritis, pericarditis, glomerulonephritis, neuritis and gastritis may arise. Renal disease and neurological abnormalities are the most serious manifestations of the disease (Hay & Snaith 1995). Most people with SLE have a normal life expectancy and serious complications are rare. Infection is the major cause of mortality at all stages of SLE; early deaths are usually due to active SLE and late deaths are attributed to thromboembolic disorders (Ruiz-Irastorza et al 2001).

Diagnosis

The diagnosis of SLE is based on a collection of the signs and symptoms particularly when joint pain, skin conditions and fatigue occur in combination or evolve over time. Blood tests are used to confirm the diagnosis and comprise full blood count, erythrocyte sedimentation rate (ESR) and testing for antinuclear antibody (ANA). There is often normochromic normocytic anaemia, the ESR is elevated even when the disease is in remission and more than 95% of people with SLE will have ANA. Antiphospholipid syndrome (APS) is found in conjunction with SLE in 30% of cases. A blood test will detect antiphospholipid antibodies (aPL), lupus anticoagulant and anticardiolipin antibodies (anti-Ro and anti-La) if APS is present. This will identify a group of people with SLE at particular risk of thromboembolic disorders and a high rate of fetal loss in pregnancy (Hay & Snaith 1995).

Effects of SLE on pregnancy

As SLE occurs primarily in women during their childbearing years it is likely to complicate pregnancy and it may arise for the first time in pregnancy. The effect of SLE on pregnancy is variable although most studies suggest that lupus flares (worsening of SLE symptoms) are common and may occur at any trimester of pregnancy and in the postpartum period. The frequency of the flares is, however, lower in women with mild and well-controlled disease. There is general agreement that, providing the disease is in remission at the time of conception, it is unlikely that it will become active during the course of the pregnancy. Women with SLE should be counselled about planning a pregnancy and the importance of being in remission for at least 6 months before conception. Exacerbation of SLE with major organ involvement (such as the kidneys and central nervous system) may occur in approximately 20% of cases (Classen et al 1998).

Overall pregnancies in SLE women have an increased incidence of adverse pregnancy outcome. Approximately one-third of pregnancies will result in fetal wastage owing to spontaneous abortion, therapeutic abortion, intrauterine death or stillbirth. Maternal renal disease and the presence of aPL have been found to be significant predictors of fetal loss (Rahman et al 1998). The rate of preterm birth and intrauterine growth restriction is closely related to the incidence of pre-eclampsia and many women with SLE give birth before 37 weeks (Yasmeen et al 2001).

Neonatal lupus syndrome is rare but may occur as a result of the transplacental passage of maternal anti-Ro/La antibodies. The neonate presents with a mild form of lupus that is transient and resolves when the antibodies are cleared in a few months following birth. The more severe form of the disease results in fetal anaemia, leucopenia and thrombocytopenia. The baby may also develop congenital heart block (CHB), which is permanent and carries significant mortality and morbidity (Classen et al 1998).

Antenatal care

A multidisciplinary approach is recommended and women should be referred as soon as possible to a centre that specialises in the care of people with lupus disorders. The frequency of antenatal visits is dependent on the severity of the disease, but women with SLE may have additional social and psychological needs requiring consistent midwifery care and support. Baseline haematological and immunological blood tests are performed at the first antenatal visit. A baseline 24 hour urine collection for creatinine clearance and total protein to assess renal function is also recommended.

An early first trimester scan is undertaken to confirm fetal viability and an anomaly scan is performed at 18–20 weeks. Women with SLE and APS are offered a fetal cardiac anomaly scan at 24 weeks' gestation and echocardiography to detect CHB.

In view of the high incidence of intrauterine fetal death, monitoring of fetal growth and well-being should begin at 28–32 weeks. This should include serial ultrasound examinations for fetal growth, placental size and quality and amniotic fluid volume, as well as CTG. Doppler flow studies are performed at 20 and 24 weeks and thereafter according to fetal growth and well-being (Lakasing & Khamashta 1997).

During pregnancy the aim is to control disease activity and achieve clinical remission whilst keeping drug therapy to a minimum (Georgiou et al 2000). Women who have a mild form of the disease or are in remission require minimal to no medication. Avoidance of emotional stress and the promotion of a healthy lifestyle may play a part in reducing the likelihood of flares or exacerbations of SLE arising during pregnancy. Alternative therapies and low impact exercise may be utilised by women to reduce the effects of pain, joint stiffness and fatigue (Classen et al 1998). If treatment is required simple analgesics such as paracetamol and co-dydramol are used for symptomatic relief. Mild flares with joint pain, skin lesions and fatigue respond well to low dose steroid therapy such as prednisone or prednisolone. Antimalarial drugs are effective as maintenance therapy in women with frequent flares and hydroxychloroquine is considered safe to use in pregnancy. Advanced renal disease requires immunosuppressants such as azathioprine (Mok & Wong 2001). Women with SLE and APS have associated recurrent miscarriage, thrombosis and thrombocytopenia and it is recommended that treatment with low dose aspirin (75 mg daily) and heparin (5000 u every 12 hours given subcutaneously) is commenced as soon as these women have a positive pregnancy test. This combination therapy has been found to promote successful embryonic implantation in the early stages of pregnancy and protect against thrombosis of the uteroplacental vasculature after successful implantation (Rai et al 1997).

Intrapartum care

The timing of childbirth in women with this condition depends on current activity of the disease and whether there are any complications present such as pre-eclampsia or renal disease. Birth should otherwise be at term. Generally, intrapartum care falls into the high risk category and a hospital protocol for the management of these women should be followed. Close liaison is required between all health care professionals involved: the midwife, obstetrician, rheumatologist, anaesthetist, paediatrician and haematologist. The woman and her family should continue to be involved in the decision-making process.

Women with SLE are particularly prone to infection, hypertension, thrombocytopenia and thromboembolic disorders. Careful hand washing, strict aseptic techniques with invasive procedures and limiting the number of vaginal examinations will reduce the risk of infection. Close monitoring of the maternal condition is required by the midwife, obstetrician and anaesthetist to evaluate cardiac, pulmonary and renal function. Blood tests should be undertaken to screen for haematological conditions, which may lead to clotting disorders. Comfort measures, nursing interventions and the use of TED stockings can reduce pressure sores and the development of deep vein thrombosis. Women who have been on long term steroid therapy will require parenteral steroid cover during labour (Classen et al 1998).

As SLE may compromise the uteroplacental circulation, continuous fetal monitoring in conjunction with fetal blood gas estimation is recommended.

Postpartum care

During the immediate postpartum period the midwife should observe closely for signs of SLE flares that may occur as a result of the stress of labour. In addition, she should watch for signs and symptoms of infection, pre-eclampsia, renal disease, thrombosis and neurological changes.

Careful consideration needs to be given to breastfeeding as most of the drugs used to treat SLE are excreted in breastmilk. Large doses of aspirin should be avoided and non-steroidal anti-inflammatory drugs (NSAIDs) are contraindicated when breastfeeding jaundiced neonates; paracetamol is the drug of choice for postpartum analgesia. Low dose steroids such as prednisone and prednisolone and the antimalarial hydroxychloroquine are considered safe to use when breastfeeding. Immunosuppressive therapy is contraindicated and should be avoided.

The midwife has a role in advising women with regard to her contraceptive options as the choice of contraceptives for a woman with SLE may be limited. Combined oral contraception increases the risk of hypertension, thrombosis and SLE flares. Low dose oestrogen combined pills may be considered in women with well-controlled SLE without a history of thromboembolic disease or APS. Intrauterine contraceptive devices are associated with an increased risk of infection in SLE women. Progestogens and barrier methods represent the safest options and may be suitable for those women where other methods are contraindicated (Mok & Wong 2001).

Thyroid disease

The thyroid gland secretes two iodine-containing hormones, *thyroxine* (T_4) and *tri-iodothyronine* (T_3) which are essential for normal body growth in infancy and childhood and affect the metabolic rate of the body. The thyroid gland also produces *calcitonin*, which is required for calcium metabolism. Production of the thyroid hormones depends on dietary consumption of iodine and calcium. After digestion and synthesis the thyroid hormones become bound to a transport protein called *thyroid-binding globulin* (TBG) and are stored within the thyroid. Stored thyroid hormone is capable of supplying the body with the required amount of hormone for 2–3 months. The production and release of the thyroid hormones, T_4 and T_3, is regulated by *thyroid-stimulating hormone* (TSH), which is secreted through a negative feedback mechanism by the anterior pituitary gland. When released into the circulation 99% of T_4 and T_3 are bound to plasma proteins and serve as a reservoir or store of thyroid hormones in the body. Less than 1% remain as 'free' (unbound to protein) T_4 and T_3, which can be utilised metabolically and act as indicators of the thyroid level in the body, stimulating the release of TSH when T_4 and T_3 levels fall (Diehl 1998). In pregnancy, hypothalamic and pituitary regulation maintain normal levels of TSH; however, thyroid function is affected by three factors that increase the basal metabolic rate by 20%:

1. Oestrogen stimulates the production of TBG, which binds more of the thyroid hormones resulting in a doubling of the total serum levels of T_4 and T_3.
2. Human chorionic gonadotrophin (HCG) secreted by the placenta appears to stimulate the thyroid gland directly as TSH levels fall in early pregnancy and then increase in the second and third trimesters, with a corresponding rise and then fall in the level of HCG. This overstimulation of the thyroid in early pregnancy may explain the hyperemesis of pregnancy (Goodwin & Mestman 1998).
3. A rise in the glomerular filtration rate in pregnancy leads to increased renal clearance of iodine, resulting in an increase in dietary iodine requirement.

Clinical assessment of thyroid dysfunction is difficult as pregnancy-related symptoms are similar to hyperthyroidism and hypothyroidism. Thyroid function can be assessed by biochemical tests that measure total T_4, free thyroxine (FT_4), total (T_3) and TSH. It is important to remember that thyroid function tests may appear abnormal in pregnancy despite normal activity of the thyroid gland (Higgins 2000).

Hyperthyroidism

Hyperthyroidism (also called thyrotoxicosis) occurs in 2 per 1000 pregnancies (Girling 1996). The most common cause of hyperthyroidism in pregnancy is *Graves' disease*, which is an autoimmune disorder that results in antibody activation of the thyroid gland. The gland becomes enlarged and secretes an increased amount of thyroid hormone. The metabolic processes of the body are accelerated resulting in fatigue, heat intolerance, palpitations, diarrhoea and mood lability. Clinical diagnosis may be difficult as the physiological signs and symptoms that pregnant women normally exhibit may mask this condition. The disease should be suspected in any woman who loses weight despite a good appetite. Other symptoms include an enlarged thyroid gland (goitre), exophthalmos, eyelid lag and persistent tachycardia (Mazzaferri 1997). A serious complication of untreated or poorly controlled hyperthyroidism is *thyroid storm*. This may occur spontaneously or be precipitated by infection or stress. It is characterised by signs and symptoms associated with a high metabolic rate: hyperthermia (temperature > 41°C) leading to dehydration, tachycardia, acute respiratory distress and cardiovascular collapse. This is a medical emergency requiring oxygen, cooling, hydration, antibiotics and drug therapy to stop the production and reduce the effect of thyroid hormone (Diehl 1998). Hyperthyroidism in pregnancy is associated with an increase in the incidence of pre-eclampsia, preterm birth, low birthweight and fetal death (Millar et al 1994).

Treatment

Treatment of hyperthyroidism is achieved through the use of antithyroid drugs. Propylthiouracil and carbimazole may be used in pregnancy. Propylthiouracil is the drug of choice as less of it crosses the placenta and only small amounts are found in breastmilk. The aim of management is to use the lowest dose possible as these drugs may cause goitre and hypothyroidism in the fetus (Mazzaferri 1997). During the antenatal period the pregnant woman should be seen monthly by the endocrinologist for clinical evaluation and monitoring of her thyroid levels. The midwife should be aware of factors that may precipitate thyroid storm, such as infection, the stress of labour and caesarean section.

Hypothyroidism

Hypothyroidism occurs as the result of decreased activity of the thyroid gland and occurs in 9 per 1000 pregnancies (Girling 1996). The most common cause of hypothyroidism in pregnancy is *autoimmune thyroiditis* (*Hashimoto's disease*). It may also be induced following treatment for Graves' disease. Slowing of the body's metabolic processes may occur giving rise to mental and physical lethargy, excessive weight gain, constipation, cold intolerance and dryness of the skin. However, the symptoms may be non-specific and the condition can be difficult to diagnose (Diehl 1998). Thyroid hormone is essential for human brain development and the fetus obtains its hormone almost entirely from its mother. Hypothyroidism in pregnancy will result in reduced availability of the hormone for fetal requirements resulting in subsequent poor neurological development (Haddow et al 1999).

Women should be encouraged to increase their dietary iodine intake during pregnancy and hypothyroidism should be treated with daily thyroxine. It is important to identify and treat hypothyroidism as early as possible; Haddow et al (1999) advocate screening all pregnant women at the first antenatal visit in the first trimester. Following birth, the neonate's thyroid status should be checked to identify whether neonatal hypothyroidism is present. There is no contraindication to breastfeeding but the dose of thyroxine may need adjustment postpartum because of maternal weight loss following childbirth.

Postpartum thyroiditis

This is an autoimmune disorder and is a form of Hashimoto's thyroiditis, which occurs in 5% of women during the first year following childbirth. It is a transient thyroid disorder, characterised by a period of mild hyperthyroidism occurring a few months after delivery and followed by a phase of hypothyroidism. In both phases the disorder presents with fatigue and a painless goitre; the condition may also mimic postpartum depression. Treatment is not required as recovery is usually spontaneous but the disorder tends to recur in subsequent pregnancies and may progress to permanent hypothyroidism (Mazzaferri 1997).

REFERENCES

Adams S 1994 Sickle cell disease: a case to answer? British Journal of Midwifery 2(10):475–478

Alleyne J, Thomas V J 1994 The management of sickle cell crisis pain as experienced by patients and care givers. Journal of Advanced Nursing 19(4):725–732

Appleton R, Baker G, Chadwick D et al 1994 Epilepsy, 4th edn. Martin Dunitz, London

Badawy A M, El-Metwally A G 2001 Cardiac disease during pregnancy: who will manage? Journal of Obstetrics and Gynaecology 21(1):36–38

Baker PN, Edelstone DI, Kean LH 2000 Saunders, Philadelphia

Beard J L 2000 Effectiveness and strategies of iron supplementation during pregnancy. American Journal of Clinical Nutrition 71:1288S–1294S

Beaton G H 2000 Iron needs during pregnancy: do we need to rethink out targets? American Journal of Clinical Nutrition 72:265S–271S

BMA and RPS (British Medical Association and Royal Pharmaceutical Society of Great Britain) 2001 British National Formulary 42. BMJ Books, London

Bolyard D R 2001 Sexuality and cystic fibrosis. Maternal–Child Nursing 26(1):39–41

Bothamley G 2001 Drug treatment for tuberculosis during pregnancy: safety considerations. Drug Safety 24(7):553–565

Bothwell T H 2000 Iron requirements in pregnancy and strategies to meet them. American Journal of Clinical Nutrition 72(1):257S–264S

Brown A K, Sleeper L A, Pegelow C H et al 1994 The influence of infant and maternal sickle cell disease on birth outcome and neonatal course. Archives of Paediatric and Adolescent Medicine 148(11):1156–1162

BTS (British Thoracic Society) 1997 The British guidelines on asthma management: 1995. Review and position statement. Thorax 52(2):suppl 1–21.

Carriaga M T, Skikne B S, Finley B et al 1991 Serum transferrin receptor for the detection of iron deficiency in pregnancy. American Journal of Clinical Nutrition 54:1077–1081

Casson I F, Clarke C A, Howard C V et al 1997 Outcomes of pregnancy in insulin dependent diabetic women: results of a 5 year population study. British Medical Journal 315:275–278

Centers for Disease Control & Prevention 1998 Recommendations to prevent or control iron deficiency in the US. MMWR 47:1–29

CESDI (Confidential Enquiry into Stilbirths and Deaths in Infancy) 1999 6th Annual report. Maternal and Child Health Research Consortium, London

Classen S R, Paulson P R, Zacharias S R 1998 Systemic lupus erythematosus: perinatal and neonatal implications. Journal of Obstetric, Gynaecological and Neonatal Nursing Sept/Oct:493–500

Coleman M T, Rund D A 1997 Nonobstetric conditions causing hypoxia during pregnancy: asthma and epilepsy. American Journal of Obstetrics and Gynecology 177(1):1–7

Comport L A, Seng J K 1997 Aortic stenosis in pregnancy: a case report. Journal of Obstetric, Gynaecological and Neonatal Nursing 26(1):67–77

Dabbs A D, Kraemer K L, Hoops S 1996 Pulmonary oedema associated with the treatment of preterm labor: what critical care nurses need to know. Critical Care Nurse 16:44–51

Davey R X, Hamblin P S 2001 Selective versus universal screening for gestational diabetes mellitus: an evaluation of predictive risk factors. Medical Journal of Australia 174:118–121

Davison J M 2001 Renal disorders in pregnancy. Current Opinion in Obstetrics and Gynaecology 13:109–114

Demissie K, Breckenridge M B, Roads C G 1998 Infant and maternal outcomes in the pregnancies of asthmatic women. American Journal of Respiratory Critical Care Medicine 158:1091–1095

de Swiet M (ed) 1995 Medical disorders in obstetric practice, 3rd edn. Blackwell Science Publications, Oxford

Diabetes UK 2000 Recommendations for the management of pregnant women with diabetes (including gestational diabetes). Diabetes UK, London

Diehl K 1998 Thyroid dysfunction in pregnancy. Journal of Perinatal and Neonatal Nursing 11(4):1–12

DOH (Department of Health), Scottish Office Home and Health Department, Welsh Office, Department of Health & Social Services, Northern Ireland 1992 Folic acid and the prevention of neural tube defects. Report from an expert advisory group. Health Publications Unit, Lancashire

Donaldson J 1995 Neurological disorders. In: de Swiet M (ed) Medical disorders in obstetric practice, 3rd edn. Blackwell Scientific, Oxford

Doran C 2000 Learning curve; managing epilepsy. Nursing Times 96(19):37–38

Edenborough F P, Stableforth D E, Webb A K et al 2000 The outcome of 72 pregnancies in 55 women with cystic fibrosis in the United Kingdom. British Journal of Obstetrics and Gynaecology 107(2):254–261

Edwards S 1998 Haemodynamic monitoring of the pregnant woman in intensive care. Nursing in Critical Care 3(3):112–121

Ellison J, Walker I D, Greer I A 2000 Antenatal use of enoparin for prevention and treatment of thromboembolism in pregnancy. British Journal of Obstetrics and Gynaecology 107:1116–1121

El-Shafei A M, Dhaliwal J K, Shandhu A K et al 1995 Indications for blood transfusion in pregnancy with sickle cell disease. Australian and New Zealand Journal of Obstetrics and Gynaecology 35(4):405–408

Endocarditis Working Party of the British Society of Antimicrobial Chemotherapy 1990 Antibiotic prophylaxis of infective endocarditis. Recommendations. Lancet 335:88–90

Epstein F H 1996 Pregnancy and renal disease. New England Journal of Medicine 335(4):277–278

Figueroa-Damian R, Arredondo-Garcia J L 1998 Pregnancy and tuberculosis: influence of treatment on perinatal outcome. American Journal of Perinatology 15(5):303–306

Figueroa-Damian R, Arredondo-Garcia J L 2001 Neonatal outcome of children born to women with tuberculosis. Archives of Medical Research 32(1):66–69

Futterman L G, Lemburg L 2000 Peripartum cardiomyopathy: an ominous complication of pregnancy. American Journal of Critical Care 9(5):362–366

Georgiou P E, Politi E N, Katsimbri P et al 2000 Outcome of lupus pregnancy: a controlled study. Rheumatology (Oxford) 39(9):1014–1019

Gilmour-White S 2000 Epilepsy. In: Lee A, Inch S, Linnigan D (eds) Therapeutics in pregnancy and lactation. Radcliffe Medical, Oxford

Gilstrap L C, Ramin S M 2001 Urinary tract infections during pregnancy. Obstetric and Gynaecology Clinics of North America 28(3):581–591

Girling J 1996 Thyroid disease in pregnancy. Maternal and Child Health 21(9):202–205

Goodwin T M, Mestman J 1998 Transient hyperthyroidism of hyperemesis gravidarum. Contemporary Obstetrics and Gynaecology 18(2):65–78

Gorman K 1999 Sickle cell disease. American Journal of Nursing 99(3):38–44

Hadden D R, Alexander A, McCance D R et al 2001 Obstetric and diabetic care for pregnancy in diabetic women: 10 years outcome analysis 1985–1995. Diabetes UK. Diabetic Medicine 18:546–553

Haddow J E, Palomaki G E, Allan W C et al 1999 Maternal thyroid deficiency during pregnancy and subsequent neuropsychological development of the child. New England Journal of Medicine 341(8):549–555

Hawthorne G, Robson S, Ryall E A et al 1997 Prospective population based survey of outcome of pregnancy in diabetic women: results on the Northern Diabetic Pregnancy Audit, 1994. British Medical Journal 315:279–281

Hay E M, Snaith M L 1995 ABC of rheumatology: systemic lupus erythematosus and lupus-like syndromes. British Medical Journal 310:1257–1261

Higgins C 2000 Understanding laboratory investigations. A text for nurses and healthcare professionals. Blackwell Science, Oxford

Higgins C 2001 Diagnosing diabetes: blood glucose and the role of the laboratory. British Journal of Nursing 10(4): 230–236

Hilman B C, Aitken M L, Constantinescu M 1996 Pregnancy in patients with cystic fibrosis. Clinics in Obstetrics and Gynaecology 39(1):70–86

Holdcroft A, Thomas T A 2000 Principles and practice of obstetric anaesthesia and analgesia. Blackwell Science, Oxford

Howard R J, Tuck S M, Pearson T C 1995 Pregnancy in sickle cell disease in the UK: results of a multicentre survey of the effect of prophylactic blood transfusion on maternal and fetal outcome. British Journal of Obstetrics and Gynaecology 102:947–951

Hunter S, Robson S C 1992 Adaptation of the maternal heart in pregnancy. British Heart Journal 68(6):540–543

Jaffe A, Bush A 1999 Cystic fibrosis: a management update. Prescribers Journal 39(2):91–96

James A W 2001 Asthma. Obstetrics and Gynecology Clinics of North America 28(2):305–320

Jardine-Brown C, Dawson A, Dodds R et al 1996 Report of the pregnancy and neonatal care group. Diabetic Medicine 13:S43–S53

JCT (Joint Tuberculosis Committee of the British Thoracic Society) 2000 Control and prevention of tuberculosis in the United Kingdom: Code of practice 2000. Thorax 55:887–901

Jones C 2001 Gestational diabetes and its impact on the neonate. Neonatal Network 20(6):17–23

Jones D C, Hayslett J P 1996 Outcome of pregnancy in women with moderate or severe renal insufficiency. New England Journal of Medicine 335:226–232

Kelnar C, Harvey D 1995 The sick newborn baby, 3rd edn. Baillière Tindall, London

Kent N E, Farquharson D F 1993 Cystic fibrosis in pregnancy. Canadian Medical Association Journal 149:512–516

Kilpatrick C J, Hopper J L 1993 The effect of pregnancy on the epilepsies: a study of 37 pregnancies. Australian and New Zealand Journal of Medicine 23(4):370–373

Knox A J, Petkova D, Johnson S 1999 Respiratory disease in pregnancy. Current Obstetrics and Gynaecology 9:69–74

Koshy M 1995 Sickle cell disease and pregnancy. Blood Review 9(3):157–164

Kuvacic I, Sprem M, Skrablin S et al 2000 Pregnancy outcome in renal transplant recipients. International Journal of Gynaecology and Obstetrics 70(3):313–317

Lakasing L, Khamashta M A 1997 Late pregnancy complications in systemic lupus erythematosus and antiphospholipid syndrome. British Journal of Hospital Medicine 58(5):211–213

Landon M B, Samuels P 1996 Cardiac and pulmonary disease. In: Gabbe S G, Niebyl J R, Simpson J L (eds) Obstetrics: normal and problem pregnancies, 3rd edn. Churchill Livingstone, New York

Larrabee K, Cowan M 1995 Clinical nursing management of sickle cell disease and trait during pregnancy. Journal of Perinatal and Neonatal Nursing 9(2):29–41

Letsky E A 2000 Anaemia. In: James D K, Steer P J, Weiner C P et al (eds) High risk pregnancy management options, 2nd edn. W B Saunders, Philadelphia

Lewis G, Drife J (eds) 2001 Why mothers die 1997–1999. The Confidential Enquiries into Maternal Deaths in the United Kingdom. RCOG Press, London

Lindsay P 1990 Epilepsy in pregnancy. Nursing Times 86(24):36–38

Lipscomb K J, Clayton Smith J, Clarke B et al 1997 Outcome of pregnancy in women with Marfan's syndrome. British Journal of Obstetrics and Gynaecology 104:201–206

Liu S, Wen S W, Demissie K et al 2001 Maternal asthma and pregnancy outcomes: a retrospective cohort study. American Journal of Obstetrics and Gynecology 184(2):90–96

Llewelyn M, Cropley I, Wilkinson R J et al 2000 Tuberculosis diagnosed during pregnancy: a prospective study from London. Thorax 55:129–132

Lowy C 1997 Diabetes and pregnancy. Medicine:25(7):57–58

Mabie W C 1996 Asthma in pregnancy. Clinics in Obstetrics and Gynaecology 39:56–69

McFall P B, Dornan J C, Lamki H 1988 Pregnancy complicated by maternal heart disease. A review of 519 women. British Journal of Obstetrics and Gynaecology 95:861–867

Maresh M 1998 Diabetes in pregnancy. In: Studd J (ed) Progress in Obstetrics and Gynaecology 13. Churchill Livingstone, Edinburgh

Mazzaferri E L 1997 Evaluation and management of common thyroid disorders in women. American Journal of Obstetrics and Gynecology 176(3):509–514

Millar L, Wing D, Leung A et al 1994 Low birth weight and preeclampsia in pregnancies complicated by hyperthyroidism. Obstetrics and Gynecology 84:946–949

Mitchell M 2001 Gestational diabetes: a controversial concept. British Journal of Midwifery 91:26–34

Mok C C, Wong R W S 2001 Pregnancy in systemic lupus erythematosus. Postgraduate Medical Journal 77:157–165

Moran P A, Aldrich C J, Gillmer D G 2000 Management of diabetic pregnancies in the United Kingdom. Journal of Obstetrics and Gynaecology 20(5):455–459

Morrow J L 1996 Epilepsy: treatment and prognosis. Medicine 24(6):65–68

MRC (Medical Research Council) Vitamin Study Research Group 1991 Prevention of neural tube defects: results of the Medical Research Council Vitamin Study. Lancet 338:131–137

Nakielna B E M 1995 Cystic fibrosis and pregnancy. Journal of the Society of Obstetricians and Gynaecologists of Canada 17(5):453–461

Norman J C, Davison J M, Lindheimer M D 2001 Renal disorders in pregnancy. Contemporary Clinical Gynaecology and Obstetrics 1:59–67

Olson G L 1997 Cystic fibrosis in pregnancy. Seminars in Perinatology 21(4):307–312

Ormerod P 2001 Tuberculosis in pregnancy and the puerperium. Thorax 56:494–499

Prasad A K, Ventura H O 2001 Valvular heart disease and pregnancy. Postgraduate Medicine 110(2):69–88

Public Health (Control of Disease) Act 1984. HMSO, London

Rahimy M C, Gangbo A, Adjou R et al 2000 Effect of active prenatal management on pregnancy outcome in sickle cell disease in an African setting. Blood 96(5):1685–1689

Rahman P, Gladman D D, Urowitz M B 1998 Clinical predictors of fetal outcome in systemic lupus erythematosus. Journal of Rheumatology 25(8):1526–1530

Rai R, Cohen H, Dave M et al 1997 Randomised controlled trial of aspirin and aspirin plus heparin in pregnant women with recurrent miscarriage associated with phospholipid antibodies or antiphospholipid antibodies. British Medical Journal 314(7076):191–208

Ramsey I D 1995 Thyroid disease. In: de Swiet M (ed) Medical disorders in obstetric practice, 3rd edn. Blackwell Science, London

Rasmussen K N 2001 Is there a causal relationship between iron deficiency or iron-deficiency anaemia and weight at birth, length of gestation and perinatal mortality? Journal of Nutrition Feb 131(25–2):590S–603S

RCM (Royal College of Midwives) The Joint Epilepsy Council of the UK and Ireland 1996 Guidelines for women with epilepsy. RCM, London

Rochester-Peart C 1997 Specialist nurse support for clients with blood disorders. Nursing Times 93(41):52–53

Ruiz-Irastorza G, Khamashta M A, Castellino G et al 2001 Systemic lupus erythematosus. Lancet 357:1027–1032

Rutherford J M, Rubin P C 1996 Management of epilepsy in pregnancy: therapeutic aspects. British Journal of Hospital Medicine 55(10):620–622

Sadler L, McCown L, White H et al 2000 Pregnancy outcomes and cardiac complications in women with mechanical, bioprosthetic and homograft valves. British Journal of Obstetrics and Gynaecology 107(2):245–253

Schatz M 1999 Asthma and pregnancy. Lancet 353:1202–1204

Scholl T, Reilly T 2000 Anaemia, iron and pregnancy outcome. Journal of Nutrition 130:443S–447S

Scottish Obstetric Guidelines and Audit Project 1997 The management of pregnancy in women with epilepsy. Scottish Programme for Clinical Effectiveness in Reproductive Health, Aberdeen

Scowen P 2001 Tuberculosis in the UK and worldwide: the current picture. Professional Care of Mother and Child 11(3):63–65

Seoud M A, Cantwell C, Nobles G et al 1994 Outcome of pregnancies complicated by sickle cell disease and sickle-C hemoglobinopathies. American Journal of Perinatology 11(3):187–191

Skaredoff M N, Besinger R E 1996 Renal disease. In: Datta S (ed) Anesthetic and obstetric management of high-risk pregnancy, 2nd edn. Mosby-Year Book, St Louis

Smaill F 2001 Antibiotics for asymptomatic bacteriuria in pregnancy (Cochrane review). Cochrane Database Systematic Review 2:CD000490

Sun P M, Wilburn W, Raynor B D et al 2001 Sickle cell disease in pregnancy: Twenty years of experience at Grady Memorial Hospital, Atlanta, Georgia. American Journal of Obstetrics and Gynecology 184(6): 1127–1130

SVD (Saint Vincent declaration) Working Party 1990 Diabetes care and research in Europe: the St Vincent declaration. Diabetic Medicine 7:360

Tan J 1999 Diagnosis of unsuspected heart disease in pregnancy. Contemporary Reviews in Obstetrics and Gynaecology 10(2):85–91

Thomas N 1997 Sickle cell disease. Nursing Standard 11(25):40–45

Tuck S M, Jensen C E 1998 Effects of major haemoglobinopathies on pregnancy. In: Bonnar J (ed) Recent advances in obstetrics and gynaecology. Churchill Livingstone, Edinburgh

Virjee S, Robinson S, Johnston D G 2001 Screening for diabetes in pregnancy. Journal of the Royal Society of Medicine 94:502–509

Vo Q T, Stettler W, Crowley K 2000 Pulmonary tuberculosis in pregnancy. Primary Care Update in Obstetrics and Gynaecology 7(6):244–249

Walsh S W 1998 Maternal–placental interactions of oxidative stress and antioxidants in pre-eclampsia. Seminars in Reproductive Endocrinology 6:93–104

WHO (World Health Organization) 1992 The prevalence of anaemia in women: a tabulation of available information, 2nd edn. WHO, Geneva

WHO (World Health Organization) 1999 Definition, diagnosis and classification of diabetes mellitus and its complications. Report of a WHO consultation. Part 1: diagnosis and classification of diabetes mellitus. WHO, Geneva

Yasmeen S, Wilkins E E, Field N T et al 2001 Pregnancy outcomes in women with systemic lupus erythematosus. Journal of Maternal Fetal Medicine 10(2):91–96

Yentis S M, Steer P J, Plaat F 1998 Eisenmenger's syndrome in pregnancy: maternal and fetal mortality in the 1990s. British Journal of Obstetrics and Gynaecology 105:921–922

Yip R 1996 Iron supplementation in pregnancy: is it effective? American Journal of Clinical Nutrition 63:853–855

FURTHER READING

Blackburn S T, Loper D L 2001 Maternal, fetal and neonatal physiology: a clinical perspective. W B Saunders, Philadelphia

Creasey R K, Resnik R 1999 Maternal–fetal medicine, 4th edn. W B Saunders, Philadelphia

Nelson Piercy C 2001 Handbook of obstetric medicine, 2nd edn. Martin Dunitz, London.

20

Hypertensive Disorders of Pregnancy

Carmel Lloyd

Hypertensive disease is a significant cause of maternal and fetal/neonatal morbidity and mortality. The triennial report of maternal deaths in the UK 1997–1999 (Lewis & Drife 2001) identified that the hypertensive disorders of pregnancy were the second most common cause of maternal death with 5.2 deaths per million maternities from pre-eclampsia and 2.4 per million maternities from eclampsia. Hypertension is the commonest medical condition encountered in pregnancy, complicating approximately 10% of all pregnancies. Careful observation of this condition worldwide has identified that the incidence varies with geographical location and race.

Cardiovascular alterations, which occur as a consequence of pregnancy, may induce hypertension in women who have been normotensive prior to pregnancy, or may aggravate existing hypertensive conditions. Hypertensive disorders include a variety of vascular disturbances such as gestational hypertension, pre-eclampsia, HELLP syndrome, eclampsia and chronic hypertension.

This chapter aims to:

- list the classifications for hypertensive disorders in pregnancy including the main differentiating characteristics

- describe the signs, symptoms and potential sequelae of the hypertensive disorders

- provide an overview of the medical and alternative therapeutic regimens that may be utilised in the treatment of hypertensive disorders

- identify the midwifery care and support required by a woman with a hypertensive disorder.

Definition and classification

The definition and classification of the hypertensive disorders are complex as the pathophysiology remains poorly understood and their clinical variation is extremely large (Chappell et al 1999). It is important to recognise the distinction between a woman whose hypertension antedates pregnancy (chronic hypertension) and one who develops an increased blood pressure during pregnancy (gestational hypertension). Recent work undertaken by the National High Blood Pressure Education Program Working Group on High Blood Pressure in Pregnancy (2000) describes five major categories of hypertension during pregnancy:

1. *Chronic hypertension* – this is known hypertension before pregnancy or a rise in blood pressure > 140/90 mmHg before 20 weeks' gestation, and persisting 6 weeks after delivery.
2. *Gestational hypertension* – this is the development of hypertension without other signs of pre-eclampsia. It is diagnosed when, after resting, the woman's blood pressure rises above 140/90 mmHg, on at least two occasions, no more than 1 week apart after the 20th week of pregnancy in a woman known to be normotensive. Hypertension that is diagnosed for the first time in pregnancy and that does not resolve postpartum is also classified as gestational hypertension.
3. *Pre-eclampsia* – this is diagnosed on the basis of hypertension with proteinuria, when proteinuria is measured as > 1+ on dipstick or > 0.3 g/L of protein in a random clean catch specimen or an excretion of 0.3 g protein/24 hours. In the absence of proteinuria, pre-eclampsia is suspected when hypertension is accompanied by symptoms including headache, blurred vision, abdominal/epigastric pain, or altered biochemistry, specifically low platelet counts and abnormal liver enzyme levels (i.e. of alanine aminotransferase (ALT), aspartate aminotransferase (AST) and gamma glutamyl transpeptidase (GGT)). These signs and symptoms, together with blood pressure > 160 mmHg systolic or > 110 mmHg diastolic and proteinuria of 2+ or 3+ on a dipstick, demonstrate the more severe form of the disease.
4. *Eclampsia* – this is defined as the new onset of convulsions during pregnancy or postpartum, unrelated to other cerebral pathological conditions, in a woman with pre-eclampsia.

5. *Pre-eclampsia superimposed on chronic hypertension* – this may occur in women with pre-existing hypertension (< 20 weeks' gestation) who develop:

- new proteinuria (> 0.3 g/24 hours)
- sudden increases in pre-existing hypertension and proteinuria
- thrombocytopenia (platelet count < 100×10^9/L)
- abnormal liver enzymes.

An incremental rise in blood pressure is not included in this classification system. However, the working group considered that women who have a rise of 30 mmHg systolic or 15 mmHg diastolic blood pressure require close observation especially if proteinuria and hyperuricaemia (raised uric acid level) are also present.

Aetiology

The placenta is generally considered to be the primary cause of the hypertensive disorders of pregnancy as following birth the disease regresses. Early studies by Roberts & Redman (1993) indicated that abnormal placentation may be one of the initial events in the disease process. In normal pregnancy placentation involves invasion of the decidua by the syncytiotrophoblast. During early pregnancy, the muscular walls and endothelium of the spiral arteries are eroded and replaced by trophoblast to ensure an optimum environment for the developing blastocyst. A second phase of this invasive process occurs between 16 and 20 weeks' gestation when the trophoblast erodes the myometrium of the spiral arteries. The loss of this musculoelastic tissue results in dilated vessels that are incapable of vasoconstriction; hence a system of low pressure and high blood flow into the placenta is produced with maximal placental perfusion (Sheppard & Bonnar 1989). In pre-eclampsia trophoblastic invasion of the spiral arteries is thought to be inhibited resulting in decreased placental perfusion, which may ultimately lead to early placental hypoxia.

Several epidemiological studies suggest that the abnormal placentation is caused by a genetically predetermined maternal immune response to fetal antigens, derived from the father, and expressed in normal placental tissue (Redman et al 1999, Robillard 2002). Additional evidence for the immune response theory includes the high incidence of hypertensive disease in primigravidae, decreased prevalence after long term exposure to the paternal sperm (Robillard et al 1994), increased inflammatory substances in the maternal circulation and pathological indications of organ rejection in placental tissues (Taylor 1997).

Abnormal placentation and reduced placental perfusion can also be seen in conditions with associated microvascular disease such as diabetes, hypertension or thrombophilia. It may in addition occur where there is a large placental mass such as in multiple pregnancy or gestational trophoblastic disease (hydatidiform mole). Women with these conditions are at an increased risk of developing pre-eclampsia (Roberts & Redman 1993).

The maternal immune response triggers the release of one or more factors that damage the endothelial cells. Endothelial cells form the endothelium, which lines the cardiovascular system and serous cavities of the body. These cells play an important role in regulating capillary transport, controlling plasma lipid contact and modulating vascular smooth muscle reactivity in response to various stimuli. They also synthesise several substances, two of which – prostacyclin and nitrous oxide – are mediators in vasodilation and inhibit platelet aggregation, thus preventing blood clot formation. Damage to the endothelial cells will:

- reduce the production of prostacyclin and nitrous oxide (Seligman et al 1994)
- increase vascular sensitivity to angiotension II (a substance that controls blood pressure and the excretion of salt and water from the body)
- activate the coagulation cascade and the production of thromboxane (Tx), a potent vasoconstrictor (Wang et al 1992)
- increase the production of lipid peroxides and decrease antioxidant production, known as 'oxidative stress' (Walsh 1998).

The combined effect of these events will cause vasospasm and increased blood pressure, abnormal coagulation and thrombosis and increased permeability of the endothelium leading to oedema, proteinuria and hypovolaemia. These are the characteristic features of pre-eclampsia, which become manifest throughout the body resulting in pathological changes consistent with a multisystem disorder.

Pathological changes

Blood. Hypertension together with endothelial cell damage affects capillary permeability. Plasma proteins leak from the damaged blood vessels causing a decrease in the plasma colloid pressure and an increase in oedema within the intracellular space. The reduced intravascular plasma volume causes hypovolaemia and haemoconcentration, which is reflected in an elevated haematocrit. In severe cases the lungs become congested with fluid and pulmonary oedema develops, oxygenation is impaired and cyanosis occurs. With vasoconstriction and disruption of the vascular endothelium the coagulation cascade is activated.

Coagulation system. Increased platelet consumption produces thrombocytopenia and may be responsible for the development of disseminated intravascular coagulation (DIC – comprising low platelets, prolonged prothrombin time and low fibrinogen levels). As the process progresses fibrin and platelets are deposited, which will occlude blood flow to many organs, particularly the kidneys, liver, brain and placenta.

Kidneys. In the kidney, hypertension leads to vasospasm of the afferent arterioles resulting in a decreased renal blood flow, which produces hypoxia and oedema of the endothelial cells of the glomerular capillaries. Glomeruloendotheliosis (glomerular endothelial damage) allows plasma proteins, mainly in the form of albumin, to filter into the urine, producing proteinuria. Renal damage is reflected by reduced creatinine clearance and increased serum creatinine and uric acid levels. Oliguria develops as the condition worsens signifying severe pre-eclampsia and kidney damage.

Liver. Vasoconstriction of the hepatic vascular bed will result in hypoxia and oedema of the liver cells. In severe cases oedematous swelling of the liver causes epigastric pain and can lead to intracapsular haemorrhages and, in very rare cases, rupture of the liver. Altered liver function is reflected by falling albumin levels and a rise in liver enzyme levels (Knapen et al 1999).

Brain. Hypertension, combined with cerebrovascular endothelial dysfunction, increases the permeability of the blood–brain barrier resulting in cerebral oedema and microhaemorrhaging. Clinically this is characterised by the onset of headaches, visual disturbances and convulsions. Where the mean arterial pressure (MAP – i.e. the systolic blood pressure plus twice the diastolic pressure divided by 3) exceeds 125 mmHg, the autoregulation of cerebral flow is disrupted resulting in cerebral vasospasm, cerebral oedema and blood clot formation. This is known as *hypertensive encephalopathy*, which if left untreated can progress to cerebral haemorrhage and death (Vaughan & Delanty 2000).

Fetoplacental unit. In the uterus, vasoconstriction caused by hypertension reduces the uterine blood flow and vascular lesions occur in the placental bed, which can result in placental abruption. Reduction in blood flow to the choriodecidual spaces diminishes the amount of oxygen that diffuses through the cells of the syncytiotrophoblast and cytotrophoblast into the fetal circulation within the placenta. The result is that the placental tissue becomes ischaemic, the capillaries in the chorionic villi thrombose and infarctions occur, leading to fetal growth restriction (Odegard et al 2000). Hormonal output is also impaired with reduced placental function and this has serious implications for the survival of the fetus. This combination of factors often results in preterm labour and birth.

The midwife's role in assessment and diagnosis

As the hypertensive disorders are unlikely to be prevented, early detection and appropriate management can minimise the severity of the condition (Dekker & Sibai 2001). A high standard of antenatal care will contribute to the maintenance of optimum health. The midwife is in a unique position to identify those women with a predisposition to pre-eclampsia. A comprehensive history taking at their first meeting will identify:

- adverse social circumstances or poverty which could prevent the woman from attending for regular antenatal care
- the mother's age and parity
- primipaternity and partner related factors
- a family history of hypertensive disorders
- a past history of pre-eclampsia
- the presence of underlying medical disorders for example, renal disease, diabetes, SLE and thromboembolic disorders.

On subsequent visits the midwife must take note of any further pregnancy associated risk factors such as multiple pregnancy. The two essential features of pre-eclampsia, hypertension and proteinuria, are assessed for at regular intervals throughout pregnancy. Diagnosis is usually based on the rise in blood pressure and the presence of proteinuria after 20 weeks' gestation.

Blood pressure measurement

In order to detect incipient increases in blood pressure, the midwife should take the mother's blood pressure early in pregnancy and compare this with all subsequent recordings, taking into account the normal pattern in pregnancy. It is important to consider several factors in assessing blood pressure.

Blood pressure machines should be calibrated for use in pregnancy and regularly maintained. Although mercury sphygmomanometry is still considered the gold standard for blood pressure measurement, the use of mercury has been banned in many centres for clinical purposes. This raises problems with regard to the accurate assessment of blood pressure in pregnancy. As yet automated devices have not been validated for use in pregnancy and the use of ambulatory blood pressure monitoring is still to be fully evaluated (Higgins & de Swiet 2001). In addition, automated blood pressure measuring devices such as the Dinamap can systematically underestimate blood pressure by at least 10 mmHg in pre-eclampsia (Pomini et al 2001).

Blood pressure should not be taken immediately after a woman has experienced anxiety, pain, a period of exercise or has smoked. A 10 minute rest period is recommended before measuring the blood pressure in these circumstances. The position of the person in whom the blood pressure is measured is important in pregnancy. The supine and right lateral positions are not recommended in view of the effect of the gravid uterus on venous return resulting in postural hypotension. Sitting or lying in the left lateral position with the sphygmomanometer cuff approximately level with the heart is recommended (Shennan & Halligan 1996). Blood pressure can be overestimated as a result of using a sphygmomanometer cuff of inadequate size relative to the arm circumference. The length of the bladder should be at least 80% of the arm circumference. Two cuffs should be available with inflation bladders of 35 cm for normal use and 42 cm for large arms (Petrie et al 1986).

The rounding off of the blood pressure measurements should be avoided and an attempt made to record the blood pressure as accurately as possible to the nearest 2 mmHg. The question of whether to use Korotkoff IV (muffling sound) or V (disappearance of sound) as a measure of the diastolic blood pressure remains controversial. Karotkoff V has been found to be easier to obtain, more reproducible and closer to the intra-arterial pressure (Rubin 1996); therefore this reading should be used unless the sound is near zero, in which case Karotkoff IV should be used instead (Shennan & Shennan 1996).

Urinalysis

Proteinuria in the absence of urinary tract infection is indicative of glomerular endotheliosis. The amount of protein in the urine is frequently taken as an index of the severity of pre-eclampsia. A significant increase in proteinuria coupled with diminished urinary output indicates renal impairment. Interobserver variation in the assessment of proteinuria and a high proportion of false positive and false negative results by dipstick analyses have been well documented (Kuo et al 1992). It is important therefore to follow the instructions provided with the dipsticks in order to reduce the likelihood of error. Studies show that in routine clinical practice 'nil' or 'trace' proteinuria will miss significant proteinuria in one out of eight hypertensive women. However, observers can achieve a positive predictive value of 92% for significant proteinuria (1 or 2+) (Meyer et al 1994). Vaginal discharge, blood, amniotic fluid and bacteria can contaminate the specimen and give a false positive reading. A 24 hour urine collection for total protein measurement will be required to be certain about the presence or absence of proteinuria and to provide an accurate quantitative assessment of protein loss. A finding of > 3 g/24 hours is considered to be indicative of mild–moderate pre-eclampsia, and > 5 g/24 hours is considered to be severe (Brown & Buddle 1995).

Oedema and excessive weight gain

These used to be included in the diagnostic criteria for pre-eclampsia but both are variable findings and nowadays are usually considered only when a diagnosis of pre-eclampsia has been made based on other criteria. Clinical oedema may be mild or severe in nature and the severity is related to the worsening of the pre-eclampsia. Oedema of the ankles in late pregnancy is a common occurrence. It is of a dependent nature, usually disappears overnight and is not significant in the absence of raised blood pressure and proteinuria. However, the sudden severe widespread appearance of oedema is suggestive of pre-eclampsia or some underlying pathology and further investigations are necessary. This oedema pits on pressure and may be found in non-dependent anatomical areas such as the face, hands, lower abdomen, vulval and sacral areas.

Laboratory tests

These now make a significant contribution to the assessment and diagnosis of pre-eclampsia particularly when the presentation is atypical and hypertension or proteinuria, or both, are absent. The expected normal blood values in pregnancy are outlined in Box 20.1. It is important to state that the data are limited and therefore the quoted normal range may vary (Girling et al 1997, Nelson-Piercy 2002, Ramsay et al 2000). The

---

Box 20.1 Normal blood values in pregnancy

Full blood count[a]

Haemoglobin	11.1–12 g/dl
Haematocrit	33–39%
Platelets	$150–400 \times 10^9$/L
Fibrinogen	3.63–4.23 g/L

Renal function[b]

Creatinine	44–73 μmol/L
Urate	2.4–4.2 mmol/L
Uric acid	0.14–0.38 mmol/L

Liver function[c]

ALT	10–30 i.u./L
AST	6–32 i.u./L
GGT	5–43 i.u./L
Albumin	28–35 g/L
Total protein	48–65 g/L

[a]Ramsay et al 2000; [b] Nelson-Piercy 2002; [c]Girling et al 1997, Ramsay et al 2000.

following alterations in the haematological and bio-chemical parameters are indicative of pre-eclampsia:

- increased haemoglobin and haematocrit levels
- thrombocytopenia
- prolonged clotting times
- raised serum creatinine and urea levels
- raised serum uric acid level
- abnormal liver function tests, particularly raised transaminases.

Symptoms may contribute to the diagnosis as described earlier, but these are rarely experienced by the woman until the disease has progressed to an advanced stage.

Care and management

The aim of care is to monitor the condition of the woman and her fetus and if possible to prevent the hypertensive disorder worsening by using appropriate interventions and treatment. The ultimate aim is to prolong the pregnancy until the fetus is sufficiently mature to survive, while safeguarding the mother's life. Numerous psychosocial implications are involved in caring for a woman who develops hypertensive dis-ease in pregnancy. The maternal and fetal condition, together with the plan of care, need to be discussed with the woman and her partner and family. Helping the woman and her partner to interpret the situation, in particular the prognosis for the pregnancy and the potential for perinatal loss, is an important considera-tion. The midwife should be sensitive to the needs of the family if the woman requires admission to hospi-tal, particularly if she is feeling well enough to be at home. She is likely to be anxious about the well-being of her children and visiting should be encouraged to allay her fears. The woman and her partner will be concerned for the current pregnancy; sensitive support and encouragement will be required of the midwife. The midwife is best suited for the psychological sup-port these women require and good communication with the multidisciplinary team involved in the care of the woman and her baby is essential (Stainton 1994).

Antenatal care

If the midwife diagnoses hypertension or pre-eclampsia during pregnancy, the woman should be referred to a doctor or directly to a maternity unit for assessment.

Gestational hypertension will require close monitoring and if pre-eclampsia develops then admission to hospital and more therapeutic interventions will be required. Care and management will vary depending on the degree of pre-eclampsia. Guidelines for the management of severe pre-eclampsia are identified in Lewis & Drife (2001) and where appropriate these have been incorporated below.

Rest. Women are advised to rest as much as possible and may be admitted to hospital to facilitate this; however, this has not been found to be cost effective and can be disruptive to family life. In addition Tuffnell et al (1992) found that inpatient care does not improve outcomes, nor does it prevent the develop-ment of proteinuria. They recommend attendance at a day assessment unit as a means of reducing the need for antenatal admissions and the number of medical interventions. It is preferable for the woman to rest at home and to have regular visits by the midwife or GP and in some instances this can be highly effective where there is the availability of distance monitoring. When proteinuria develops in addition to hyperten-sion the risks to the mother and fetus are considerably increased. Admission to hospital is requisite to monitor and evaluate the maternal and fetal condition.

Diet. There is little evidence to support dietary inter-vention for preventing or restricting the advance of pre-eclampsia. As for any pregnant woman a diet rich in protein, fibre and vitamins may be recommended. There is some evidence to suggest that prophylactic fish oil in pregnancy may act as an antiplatelet agent, thereby preventing hypertension and proteinuric pre-eclampsia (Roberts & Redman 1993). Calcium supplementation has also been investigated and appears to be beneficial for women at high risk of developing hypertension in pregnancy and in communities with low dietary cal-cium intake (Atallah et al 2002). A pilot study under-taken by Chappell et al (1999) suggests that the use of the antioxidant supplements vitamins C and E may be effective in decreasing oxidative stress and improving vascular endothelial function, thereby preventing or controlling the development of pre-eclampsia.

Weight gain. The efficacy of routine weighing during antenatal visits has been questioned and in many areas has now been abandoned as a form of antenatal screening for pre-eclampsia (Dawes et al 1992). However, weight gain may be useful for monitoring the progression of pre-eclampsia in conjunction with other parameters (Surratt 1993). The initial BMI (see Ch. 12) is considered a more useful predictor of hypertension in pregnancy, since this is higher in women developing hypertension (Masse et al 1993).

Blood pressure and urinalysis. The blood pressure is monitored daily at home or every 4 hours when in hospital. Urine should be tested for protein daily. If the woman or midwife identifies protein in a midstream specimen of urine a 24 hour urine collection is instigated in order to determine renal function. The level of protein indicates the degree of vascular damage. Reduced kidney perfusion is indicated by proteinuria, reduced creatinine clearance and increased serum creatinine and uric acid.

Abdominal examination is carried out daily. Any discomfort or tenderness should be recorded and reported immediately to the doctor as this may be a sign of placental abruption. Upper abdominal pain is highly significant and indicative of HELLP syndrome associated with fulminating (rapid onset) pre-eclampsia (Barry et al 1994).

Fetal assessment. It is advisable to undertake a biophysical profile in order to determine fetal health and well-being. This is done by the use of the following: kick charts, CTG monitoring, serial ultrasound scans to check for fetal growth, assessment of liquor volume and fetal breathing movements or Doppler flow studies, or both, to determine placental blood flow (see Ch. 23).

Laboratory studies. These include a full blood count, platelet count and clotting profile, urea and electrolytes, creatinine and liver function tests including albumin levels. In severe pre-eclampsia there should be blood samples taken every 12–24 hours (Lewis & Drife 2001).

Antihypertensive therapy. The use of antihypertensive therapy as prophylaxis is controversial as this shows no benefit in significantly prolonging pregnancy or improving maternal or fetal outcome. Its use is, however, advocated as short term therapy in order to prevent an increase in blood pressure and the development of severe hypertension, thereby reducing the risk to the mother of cerebral haemorrhage. Methyldopa is the most widely used drug in women with mild to moderate gestational hypertension and appears to be safe and effective for both mother and fetus. Beta blockers such as atenolol and labetalol are considered safe in pregnancy although their use over the long term is not recommended as they may cause

significant fetal growth restriction (Butters et al 1990, Pickles et al 1989). Nifedipine, a calcium channel blocker, is increasingly used to treat severe hypertension in pregnancy although its safety and efficacy are still to be fully evaluated (Smith et al 2000).

Antithrombotic agents. Early activation of the clotting system may contribute to the later pathology of pre-eclampsia, as a result the use of anticoagulants or antiplatelet agents has been considered for the prevention of pre-eclampsia and fetal growth restriction. Aspirin is thought to inhibit the production of the platelet-aggregating agent thromboxane A_2. The CLASP trial concluded that low dose aspirin might be beneficial for those women at high risk of early onset pre-eclampsia (CLASP Collaborative Group 1994). A large randomised trial undertaken by the ECPPA Collaborative Group (1996) found that aspirin may prevent a few preterm deliveries per 100 high risk women treated but no other benefits were identified. The conclusion from both trials is that the routine use of aspirin does not prevent pre-eclampsia or other hypertensive complications in pregnancy.

Intrapartum care

The midwife should remain with the woman throughout the course of labour as pre-eclampsia can suddenly worsen at any time. It is essential to monitor the maternal and fetal condition carefully. Marked deviations should be noted and medical assistance sought. The woman should be made as comfortable as possible, which will necessitate attention to general care. The woman with gestational or mild pre-eclampsia will require less intensive care than a women with severe eclampsia.

Vital signs. Blood pressure is measured half-hourly, 15–20 minutes in severe pre-eclampsia. Because of the potentially rapid haemodynamic changes in pre-eclampsia, a number of authors recommend the measurement of the MAP. As mentioned earlier this can be calculated manually or by the use of an automated blood pressure recorder such as the Dinamap. MAP reflects the systemic perfusion pressure, and therefore the degree of hypovolaemia, whereas manual measurement of diastolic pressure alone is a better indicator of the degree of hypertension (Churchill & Beevers 1999). Observation of the respiratory rate (> 14/min) will be complemented with pulse oximetry in severe pre-eclampsia; this is a non-invasive measure of the saturation of haemoglobin with oxygen and gives an indication of the degree of maternal hypoxia. Temperature should be recorded hourly. In severe pre-eclampsia, examination of the optic fundi can give an indication of cerebral oedema, and cerebral irritability can be assessed by the degree of hyperreflexia or the presence of clonus (less than three beats).

Fluid balance. The reduced intravascular compartment in pre-eclampsia together with poorly controlled fluid balance can result in circulatory overload, pulmonary oedema, adult respiratory distress syndrome and ultimately death (Lewis & Drife 2001). In severe pre-eclampsia a central venous pressure (CVP) line may be considered in order to monitor the fluid status more effectively. This is inserted and supervised by an anaesthetist and measurements are taken hourly. If the value is >10 mmHg then 20 mg furosemide (frusemide), a diuretic drug, should be considered. Intravenous fluids are administered using infusion pumps and the total recommended fluid intake in severe pre-eclampsia is 85 ml/h. Oxytocin should be administered with caution as it has an antidiuretic effect. Urinary output should be monitored closely and urinalysis undertaken every 4 hours to detect the presence of protein, ketones and glucose. In severe pre-eclampsia a urinary catheter should be in situ and urine output is measured hourly; a level > 30 ml/h reflects adequate renal function.

Plasma volume expansion. Although women with pre-eclampsia have oedema they are hypovolaemic. The blood volume is low, as shown by a high haemoglobin concentration and a high haematocrit level. This results in movement of fluid into the extravascular compartment causing oedema. The oedema initially occurs in dependent tissues, but as the disease progresses oedema occurs in the liver and brain giving rise to the symptoms described previously. In severe pre-eclampsia expansion of the blood volume may be required to improve the maternal systemic and uteroplacental circulation, thereby preventing hypoxia and reducing the effect of haemorrhage. Clear fluids will leak out and aggravate pre-existing oedema, therefore gelatin solutions such as Haemaccel and Gelofusin may be used. These solutions increase the colloid osmotic pressure and pull fluid back into the circulation, thereby reducing the oedema and increasing the blood volume. Where there is hypoalbuminaemia (low levels of albumin in the blood), oliguria (urine output < 100 ml in a consecutive 4 hour period) or a CVP value < 10 mmHg, the use of human albumin solution is recommended (Lewis & Drife 2001). This is more expensive than the gelatin products but has a higher molecular weight and is therefore likely to be retained in the intravascular compartment for longer.

Pain relief. Epidural analgesia may procure the best pain relief, reduce the blood pressure and facilitate rapid caesarean section should the need arise. It is important to ensure a normal clotting screen and a platelet count > 100×10^9/L prior to insertion of the epidural.

Fetal condition. The fetal heart rate should be monitored closely and deviations from the normal reported and acted on.

Birth plan. When the second stage commences, the obstetrician and paediatrician should be notified. The midwife will continue her care of the woman and will usually assist the woman to birth her baby. A short second stage may be prescribed depending on the maternal and fetal conditions; in this instance a ventouse extraction or forceps delivery will be performed by the obstetrician. If the maternal or fetal condition shows significant deterioration during the first stage of labour, a caesarean section will be undertaken. Oxytocin is the preferred agent for the management of the third stage of labour. Ergometrine and Syntometrine will cause peripheral vasoconstriction and increase hypertension and therefore should not normally be used in the presence of any degree of pre-eclampsia unless there is severe haemorrhage.

Postpartum care

The maternal condition should continue to be monitored at least every 4 hours for the next 24 hours following childbirth as there is still the potential danger of the mother developing eclampsia.

Signs of impending eclampsia

The signs and symptoms described in Box 20.2 will signal the onset of eclampsia. The midwife should be alert to any of these signs and summon medical assistance immediately. The aim of care at this time is to preclude death of the mother and fetus by controlling hypertension, inhibiting convulsions and preventing coma.

Box 20.2 Signs of impending eclampsia

- A sharp rise in blood pressure
- Diminished urinary output, which is due to acute vasospasm
- Increase in proteinuria
- Headache, which is usually severe, persistent and frontal in location
- Drowsiness or confusion due to cerebral oedema
- Visual disturbances, such as blurring of vision or flashing lights, due to retinal oedema
- Epigastric pain, which denotes liver oedema and impairment of liver function
- Nausea and vomiting

HELLP syndrome

The syndrome of haemolysis (H), elevated liver enzymes (EL) and low platelet count (LP) was first described by Weinstein in 1982 and is generally thought to represent a variant of the pre-eclampsia/eclampsia syndrome. Pregnancies complicated by this syndrome have been associated with significant maternal and perinatal morbidity and mortality. The incidence of the disease is reported as being 0.17–0.85% of all livebirths (Rath et al 2000). Serious maternal morbidity and mortality may result from DIC, acute renal failure, pulmonary oedema and subcapsular liver haematoma (Lewis & Drife 2001, Sibai et al 1993). Infants whose mothers have HELLP syndrome are often small for gestational age and are at risk of perinatal asphyxia (Harms et al 1995).

Clinical presentation

HELLP syndrome typically manifests itself between 32 and 34 weeks' gestation and 30% of cases will occur postpartum. The woman often complains of malaise, epigastric or right upper quadrant pain and nausea and vomiting; some will have nonspecific viral-syndrome-like symptoms. Hypertension and proteinuria may be absent or slightly abnormal (Rath et al 2000).

Diagnosis

Pregnant women presenting with the above symptoms should have a full blood count, platelet count and liver function tests irrespective of maternal blood pressure. Haemolysis with elevated lactate dehydrogenase (LDH) and raised bilirubin levels, low ($< 100 \times 10^9$/L) or falling platelets and elevated liver transaminases (AST, ALT and GGT) assist in confirming the diagnosis of HELLP syndrome (Knappen et al 1999).

Complications

Subcapsular haematoma or rupture of the liver, or both together, is a rare but potentially fatal complication of the HELLP syndrome. The condition usually presents with severe epigastric pain, which may persist for several hours. In addition women may complain of neck and shoulder pain. Radiographic imaging of the liver is required to assess the extent of the damage (Barton & Sibai 1996). Surgical intervention or liver transplantation, or both of these, will be required to prevent haemorrhagic shock and liver failure (Reck et al 2001).

Treatment

Women with the HELLP syndrome should be admitted to a consultant unit with intensive or high dependency care facilities available. In pregnancies less than 34 weeks' gestation conservative treatment using plasma volume expanders and antihypertensives may be considered (Visser & Wallenburg 1995). Stabilisation and significant improvement in the laboratory and clinical parameters of the HELLP syndrome may be seen in women who also receive high dose antenatal corticosteroids (Megann & Martin 2000, O'Brien at al 2000). In term pregnancies, or where there is a deteriorating maternal or fetal condition, immediate delivery is recommended (Curtain & Weinstein 1999).

Eclampsia

Eclampsia is rarely seen in developed countries today, especially if there are good facilities for antenatal care. The reported rate of eclampsia in Europe and other developed countries is 1 in 2000–3000 deliveries

(Mattar & Sibai 2000). In the UK it has an incidence of 4.9 per 10 000 maternities (Lewis & Drife 2001). In developing countries, the estimates vary from 1 in 100 to 1 in 700 deliveries (Duley 1994). Usually pre-eclampsia is diagnosed and treatment instituted to prevent eclampsia but occasionally pre-eclampsia is so rapid in onset and progress that eclampsia ensues before any action can be taken. In this situation pre-eclampsia is termed 'fulminating' (Katz et al 2000).

Eclampsia is associated with increased risks of maternal and perinatal morbidity and mortality (ETCG 1995). Significant maternal life-threatening complications as a result of eclampsia include pulmonary oedema, renal and hepatic failure, DIC, HELLP syndrome and brain haemorrhage.

A major problem for preventing and treating eclampsia is that the cause of the condition is unknown. There is a proposed link between the hypertension, which may not be extreme, and cerebral disease; Vaughan & Delanty (2000) identify the clinical similarities between eclampsia and hypertensive encephalopathy. A significant finding, however, is that hypertension is not necessarily a precursor to the onset of eclampsia but will almost always be evident following a seizure (Witlin et al 1999). Detecting and managing imminent eclampsia is also made more difficult in that, unlike other types of seizure, warning symptoms are not always present before onset of the convulsion.

Variations also exist according to the gestational period. In the UK, 44% of the seizures occur in the postnatal period, with 38% occurring antenatally and 18% occurring in the intrapartum period (Douglas & Redmond 1994).

In fulminating pre-eclampsia or eclampsia, delivery of the mother should take place as soon as possible once the condition has been stabilised by the following measures.

Care of a woman with eclampsia

The aims of immediate care are to:

- summon medical aid
- clear and maintain the mother's airway – this may be achieved by placing the mother in a semiprone position in order to facilitate the drainage of saliva and vomit
- administer oxygen and prevent severe hypoxia
- prevent the mother from being injured.

The midwife must remain with the mother constantly and provide assistance with medical treatment. In the first instance all effort is devoted to the preservation of the mother's life and the well-being of the baby is secondary. This may seem arbitrary, but if the mother dies then fetal death is inevitable. The woman will require intensive/high dependency care as she may remain comatosed for a time following the seizure or may be heavily sedated. Recordings should be carried out as previously mentioned for severe pre-eclampsia. The midwife must observe for periodic restlessness associated with uterine contraction, which indicates that labour has commenced. The woman's partner should be kept informed and the midwife will need to give emotional support through this unexpected and anxious time. It is usual to expedite delivery of the baby as soon as possible when eclampsia occurs. In this instance caesarean section is the usual mode of delivery. Treatment may be given as follows:

Anticonvulsant therapy. Discussion about the care of women with eclampsia has focused largely on the control of convulsions with various opinions as to the most appropriate anticonvulsant to use. Magnesium sulphate, diazepam and phenytoin were the most widely used anticonvulsants for the management of eclampsia. The rationale for their use was principally historical rather than scientific. Diazepam is used to control other types of seizures and has a sedative effect. Phenytoin is effective in controlling convulsions and has been advocated for eclampsia as there is no sedative effect. Magnesium sulphate is thought to aid vasodilatation thereby reducing cerebral ischaemia (Belfort & Moise 1992).

The findings from the Collaborative Eclampsia Trial provide evidence of the superiority of magnesium sulphate over diazepam and phenytoin in terms of preventing further seizures and possibly reducing the incidence of pneumonia, artificial ventilation and admission to intensive care (ETCG 1995). Magnesium sulphate is now the recommended drug of choice for routine anticonvulsant management of women with eclampsia rather than diazepam or phenytoin (ETCG 1995, Lewis & Drife 2001). Results from the MAGPIE Trial (MAGnesium sulphate for the Prevention of Eclampsia) also clearly demonstrate that magnesium sulphate is effective in reducing the risk of eclampsia for women with pre-eclampsia (Magpie Trial Collaborative Group 2002). Magnesium sulphate is administered intravenously according to a protocol.

The Confidential Enquiries into Maternal Deaths (Lewis & Drife 2001) recommend that a loading dose of 4 g is given over 5–10 minutes intravenously followed by a maintenance dose of 5 g/500 ml normal saline given as an intravenous infusion at a rate of 1–2 g/h until 24 hours following delivery or the last seizure. Recurrent seizures should be treated with a further bolus of 2 g. Magnesium sulphate can be toxic and therefore the deep tendon reflexes should be monitored hourly. The respiratory rate and oxygen saturation levels are measured hourly and should remain > 14/min and > 95% respectively. In women with oliguria, serum magnesium levels should be monitored and maintained within the therapeutic range (2–4 mmol/L). Calcium gluconate is the antidote for magnesium toxicity and should be readily available.

Treatment of hypertension. Severe hypertension is defined as greater than 160/110 mmHg or a mean arterial pressure > 125 mmHg. Intravenous hydralazine is the most useful agent to gain control of the blood pressure quickly; 5 mg should be administered slowly and the blood pressure measured at 5 minute intervals until the diastolic pressure reaches 90 mmHg. The diastolic blood pressure may be maintained at this level by titrating an intravenous infusion of hydralazine against the blood pressure. Labetelol may be used in preference to hydralazine, in which case 20 mg is given intravenously followed at 10-minute intervals by 40 mg, 80 mg and 80 mg up to a cumulative dose of 300 mg (Lewis & Drife 2001, p. 92).

Fluid balance. Care must be taken not to overload the maternal system with intravenous fluids as discussed in the management of pre-eclampsia.

Anaesthesia. Use of anaesthesia in eclampsia is difficult as the condition of women with eclampsia varies considerably. Both general and regional (epidural/ spinal) anaesthesia carry a degree of risk in the eclamptic woman. In general, epidural is preferred in eclamptic women who are conscious, haemodynamically stable and cooperative (Moodley et al 2001).

Postnatal care. As soon as the baby is born, the partner should be encouraged to hold him and accompany him to the neonatal intensive care unit where he will be cared for. It is important that the partner has early interaction with the baby so that an account can be given of the baby's progress from the time of birth. Likewise, the midwife should liaise with the neonatal unit staff and explain the treatment given to the baby and the likely prognosis. A photograph is taken of the baby so that the mother can see him as soon as she recovers. As almost half of eclamptic fits occur following childbirth (Lewis & Drife 2001) intensive surveillance of the woman is required in a high dependency or intensive care unit. Parameters to monitor are: a return to normal blood pressure, an increase in urine output, a reduction in oedema and a return to normal laboratory indices. Thromboelastic stockings should be worn to prevent deep vein thrombosis. All the usual postpartum care is given and as soon as the mother's condition permits she should be taken in her bed or a chair to see her baby. Alternatively, if the baby's condition is good, he may be returned to his mother.

Future care and management following hypertensive disease

There is no indication that the hypertensive disorders of pregnancy cause later hypertensive disease but it can bring to the fore an inherent disposition towards hypertension. Women with a history of severe pre-eclampsia before 32 weeks' gestation have a 5% risk of recurrence by this gestational age and a 15% risk of recurrence overall (Mattar & Sibai 2000). There is also evidence that the risk of recurrence may be higher if the pregnancy is with a new partner (Robillard et al 1994).

Usually the blood pressure returns to normal within several weeks but the proteinuria may persist for a longer period. Six months after delivery, the mother is examined by the obstetrician and if all is well she will be discharged and advised to seek advice as soon as a subsequent pregnancy occurs. Referral to voluntary organisations such as Action on Pre-eclampsia (see Useful address, p. 371) may provide additional information, advice and support following a pregnancy complicated by hypertensive disorders.

The mother may have very little recollection of the birth and the events surrounding it if she was unconscious or heavily sedated at the time. It is essential that the midwife enquire further if a mother gives no clear history of a previous birth or if she says that she was ill. It is advisable to obtain the previous case notes where possible. In this way good care can be provided and prophylactic management established where indicated.

Chronic hypertension

Chronic hypertension has two possible causes:

1. It may be a long term problem, present before the beginning of the pregnancy, for example essential hypertension, which accounts for 5% of the cases of hypertension in pregnancy.
2. It may be secondary to existing medical problems such as:
   - renal disease
   - SLE
   - coarctation of the aorta
   - Cushing's syndrome
   - phaeochromocytoma, which is a rare but dangerous tumour of the adrenal medulla.

Diagnosis

Consistent blood pressure recordings of 140/90 mmHg or more, on two occasions more than 24 hours apart during the first 20 weeks of pregnancy, suggest that the hypertension is a chronic problem and unrelated to the pregnancy. The diagnosis may be difficult to make because of the changes seen with blood pressure in pregnancy. This is a particular problem in women who present late in their pregnancy with no baseline blood pressure measurement. In addition, Sibai (1996) found that women with chronic hypertension show greater decreases in their blood pressure during pregnancy than do normotensive women. Hence the chronic hypertension may be missed unless the woman is seen prior to or in early pregnancy.

Investigation

When taking a history the midwife may identify potential or existing problems, which may include a known medical condition. Women with chronic hypertension tend to be older, parous and have a family or personal history of hypertension.

Accurate measurement of blood pressure is important and the midwife needs to consider the guidelines mentioned earlier. Serial blood pressure recordings should be made in order to determine the true pattern as even normotensive women show occasional peaks.

The doctor's physical examination of the woman may reveal the long term effects of hypertension such as retinopathy, ischaemic heart disease and renal damage.

Renal function tests may be performed; however, it is important to realise the extent to which the alterations in the physiological norms may affect clinical interpretation in pregnancy. Blood urate levels may help to differentiate between chronic hypertension and pre-eclampsia; they do not rise in the former as they do in the latter.

Admission to a hospital or day assessment unit for initial assessment may be necessary. The midwife can enquire about the woman's social background and investigate her physiological needs, offering her support as necessary.

Complications

The perinatal outcome in mild chronic hypertension is good. However, the perinatal morbidity and mortality are increased in those women who develop severe chronic hypertension or superimposed pre-eclampsia. Other complications are independent of pregnancy and include renal failure and cerebral haemorrhage. In 1–2% of cases hypertensive encephalopathy may develop if the blood pressure suddenly rises above 250/150 mmHg (Sibai 1996). Maternal mortality is high if phaeochromocytoma is left untreated.

Management

Mild chronic hypertension

This is defined as a systolic blood pressure of < 160 mmHg and a diastolic blood pressure of < 110 mmHg. The woman is unlikely to need antenatal admission to hospital and may be cared for in the community by the midwife and the general practitioner. The woman's condition should be carefully monitored in order to identify any pre-eclampsia that develops.

Severe chronic hypertension

The systolic blood pressure is > 160 mmHg and the diastolic blood pressure is > 110 mmHg. Ideally the woman will be cared for by the obstetric team in conjunction with the physician. Frequent antenatal visits are recommended in order to monitor the maternal condition. This includes blood pressure monitoring, urinalysis to detect proteinuria and blood tests to measure the haematocrit and renal function.

Antihypertensive drug therapy is used in order to prevent maternal complications but has no proven benefit for the fetus, nor in the prognosis of the pre-eclamptic process. The most commonly used agent is methyldopa 1–4 g/day in divided doses. It has a sedative effect lasting 2–3 days and is generally considered safe for mother and fetus. Other drugs in common usage include labetalol, nifedipine and oral hydralazine. Sedative drugs may be given to reduce anxiety and help the woman to rest. The midwife may do much to settle anxiety by the use of counselling skills and by mobilising resources to meet social needs if required. In the rare event of a phaeochromocytoma being present, the blood pressure will be treated with appropriate antihypertensive drugs during the pregnancy and the tumour resected postnatally.

Monitoring of fetal well-being and of placental function should be carried out assiduously because of the risk of fetal compromise. This would include using serial growth scans and placental blood flow studies by Doppler ultrasound (see Ch. 23). If the maternal or fetal condition causes concern, the woman will be admitted to hospital. The timing of the birth is planned according to the needs of mother and fetus. If early delivery is deemed necessary, induction of labour is preferred to caesarean section.

Renal function should be reassessed postnatally and the woman is seen by the physician with a view to long term management of persistent hypertension. Antihypertensive therapy may be required. These drugs are excreted in breastmilk but Sibai (1996) suggests there are no short term adverse effects on the infant exposed to methyldopa, hydralazine or beta blockers. The midwife who is advising the woman on family planning should be aware of the hypertensive effect of the combined oral contraceptive pill.

REFERENCES

Atallah A N, Hofmeyr G J, Duley L 2002 Calcium supplementation during pregnancy for preventing hypertensive disorders and related problems (Cochrane review). Cochrane Database Systematic Review 1:CD001059

Barry C, Fox R, Stirrat G 1994 Upper abdominal pain in pregnancy may indicate pre-eclampsia. Student British Medical Journal 308(2):1562–1563

Barton J R, Sibai B M 1996 Hepatic imaging in HELLP syndrome (haemolysis, elevated liver enzymes, and low platelet count). American Journal of Obstetrics and Gynecology 174(6):1820–1827

Belfort M A, Moise K J 1992 Effect of magnesium sulfate on brain blood flow in preeclampsia: a randomised placebo-controlled study. American Journal of Obstetrics and Gynecology 167:661–666

Brown M A, Buddle M L 1995 Inadequacy of dipstick proteinuria in hypertensive pregnancy. Australian and New Zealand Journal of Obstetrics and Gynaecology 35(4):366–369

Butters L, Kennedy S, Rubin P C 1990 Atenolol in essential hypertension during pregnancy. British Medical Journal 301:587–589

Chappell L, Poulton L, Halligan A et al 1999 Lack of consistency in research papers over the definition of pre-eclampsia. British Journal of Obstetrics and Gynaecology 106:983–985

Churchill D, Beevers D G 1999 Hypertension in pregnancy. BMJ Books, London

CLASP (Collaborative Low-dose Aspirin Study in Pregnancy) Collaborative Group 1994 CLASP: a randomised trial of low-dose aspirin for the prevention and treatment of pre-eclampsia among 9364 pregnant women. Lancet 343:619–629

Curtain W M, Weinstein L 1999 A review of HELLP syndrome. Journal of Perinatology 19(2):138–143

Dawes M G, Green J, Ashurst H 1992 Routine weighing in pregnancy. British Medical Journal 304:487–489

Dekker G, Sibai B 2001 Primary, secondary and tertiary prevention of pre-eclampsia. Lancet 357:209–215

Douglas K A, Redman C W 1994 Eclampsia in the United Kingdom. British Medical Journal 309:1395–1400

Duley L 1994 Maternal mortality and eclampsia: the eclampsia trial. MIDIRS Midwifery Digest 4(2):176–178

ECPPA (Estudo Colaborativo para Prevencao da Pre-eclampsia com Aspirina) Collaborative Group 1996 ECPPA: randomised trial of low-dose aspirin for the prevention of maternal and fetal complications in high-risk pregnant women. British Journal of Obstetrics and Gynaecology 103:39–47

ETCG (Eclampsia Trial Collaborative Group) 1995 Which anticonvulsant for women with eclampsia? Evidence from the Collaborative Eclampsia Trial. Lancet 345:1455–1463

Girling J C, Dow E, Smith J H 1997 Liver function tests in pre-eclampsia: importance of comparison with a reference range derived for normal pregnancy. British Journal of Obstetrics and Gynaecology 104:246–250

Harms K, Rath W, Herting E 1995 Maternal haemolysis, elevated liver enzymes, low platelet count, and neonatal outcome. American Journal of Perinatology 12(1):1–6

Higgins J R, de Sweit M 2001 Blood-pressure measurement and classification in pregnancy. Lancet 357:131–135

Katz V L, Farmer R, Kuller J A 2000 Preeclampsia into eclampsia: toward a new paradigm. American Journal of Obstetrics and Gynecology 182(6):1389–1396

Knapen M F C M, Peters W H M, Steegers E A P 1999 Liver function tests in pregnancies complicated by hypertensive disorders of pregnancy or the HELLP syndrome. Contemporary Reviews in Obstetrics and Gynaecology 10(2):105–112

Kuo V S, Koumantakis G, Gallery E D 1992 Proteinuria and its assessment in normal and hypertensive pregnancy. American Journal of Obstetrics and Gynaecology 167(3):723–728

Lewis G, Drife J (eds) 2001 Why mothers die 1997–1999. The Confidential Enquiries into Maternal Deaths in the United Kingdom. RCOG Press, London

Magpie Trial Collaborative Group 2002 Do women with pre-eclampsia, and their babies, benefit from magnesium sulphate? The Magpie Trial: a randomised placebo-controlled trial. Lancet 359:1877–1890

Masse J, Forest J-C, Moutquin J-M et al 1993 A prospective study of several biological markers for early prediction of the development of pre-eclampsia. American Journal of Obstetrics and Gynecology 169:501–508

Mattar F, Sibai B M 2000 Eclampsia VIII. Risk factors for maternal morbidity. American Journal of Obstetrics and Gynecology 182(2):307–312

Megann E F, Martin J N 2000 Critical care of HELLP syndrome with corticosteroids. American Journal of Perinatology 17(8):417–422

Meyer N L, Mercer B M, Friedman S A et al 1994 Urinary dipstick protein: a poor predictor of absent or severe proteinuria. American Journal of Obstetrics and Gynecology 170:137–141

Moodley J, Jjuuko G, Rout C 2001 Epidural compared with general anaesthesia for caesarean delivery in conscious women with eclampsia. British Journal of Obstetrics and Gynaecology 108(4):378–382

National High Blood Pressure Education Program Working Group on High Blood Pressure in Pregnancy 2000 Report of the National High Blood Pressure Education Program Working Group on high blood pressure in pregnancy. American Journal of Obstetrics and Gynecology 183:S1–S22

Nelson-Piercy C 2002 Handbook of obstetric medicine, 2nd edn. Martin Dunitz, London

O'Brien J M, Milligan D A, Barton J R 2000 Impact of high-dose corticosteroid therapy for patients with HELLP (haemolysis, elevated liver enzymes and low platelet count) syndrome. American Journal of Obstetrics and Gynecology 183(4):921–924

Odegard R A, Vatten L J, Nilsen S T 2000 Risk factors and clinical manifestations of pre-eclampsia. British Journal of Obstetrics and Gynaecology 107(11):1410–1416

Petrie J C, O'Brien E T, Littler W A et al 1986 Recommendations on blood pressure measurement. British Medical Journal 293:611–615

Pickles C J, Symonds E M, Broughton Pipkin F 1989 The fetal outcome in a randomized double-blind controlled trial of labetalol versus placebo in pregnancy-induced hypertension. British Journal of Obstetrics and Gynaecology 96:38–43

Pomini F, Scavo M, Ferrazzani S et al 2001 There is poor agreement between manual auscultatory and automated oscillometric methods for the measurement of blood pressure in normotensive women. Journal of Maternal Fetal Medicine 10(6):398–403

Ramsay M M, James D K, Steer P J, Weiner C P, Gonik B (eds) 2000 Normal values in pregnancy. W B Saunders, London

Rath W, Faridi A, Dudenhausen J W 2000 HELLP syndrome. Journal of Perinatal Medicine 28(4):249–260

Reck T, Bussenius-Kammerer M, Ott R et al 2001 Surgical treatment of HELLP syndrome-associated liver rupture – an update. European Journal of Obstetric Gynaecological Reproductive Biology 99(1):57–65

Redman C W G, Sacks G P, Sargent I L 1999 Pre-eclampsia: an excessive maternal inflammatory response to pregnancy. American Journal of Obstetrics and Gynecology 180(2):499–506

Roberts J M, Redman C W G 1993 Pre-eclampsia: more than pregnancy-induced hypertension. Lancet 341(June 5):1447–1451

Robillard P Y 2002 Interest in preeclampsia for researchers in reproduction. Journal of Reproductive Immunology 53(1):279–287

Robillard P-Y, Hulsey T C, Perianin J et al 1994 Association of pregnancy-induced hypertension with duration of sexual cohabitation before conception. Lancet 344:973–975

Rubin P 1996 Measuring diastolic blood pressure in pregnancy. British Medical Journal 313:4–5

Seligman S, Buyon J, Clancy R et al 1994 The role of nitric oxide in the pathenogenesis of preeclampsia. American Journal of Obstetrics and Gynecology 171:944–948

Shennan A, Halligan A 1996 Blood pressure measurement in pregnancy: room for improvement. Maternal and Child Health 21(3):55–59

Shennan C, Shennan A 1996 Blood pressure in pregnancy: the need for accurate measurement. British Journal of Medicine 4(2):102–108

Sheppard B L, Bonnar J 1989 The maternal blood supply to the placenta. In: Studd J (ed) Progress in Obstetrics and Gynaecology, vol 7. Churchill Livingstone, Edinburgh

Sibai B M 1996 Hypertension in pregnancy. In: Gabbe S G, Niebyl J R, Simpson J L (eds) Obstetrics: normal and problem pregnancies 3rd edn. Churchill Livingstone, New York

Sibai B M, Ramadan M K, Usta I 1993 Maternal morbidity and mortality in 442 pregnancies with haemolysis, elevated liver enzymes, and low platelets (HELLP syndrome). American Journal of Obstetrics and Gynecology 169(4):1000–1006

Smith P, Anthony J, Johanson R 2000 Nifedipine in pregnancy. British Journal of Obstetrics and Gynaecology 107:299–307

Stainton M 1994 Supporting family functioning during a high-risk pregnancy. Maternal Child Nursing 19:24–28

Surratt N 1993 Severe preeclampsia: implications for critical-care obstetric nursing. Journal of Obstetric, Gynaecological and Neonatal Nursing 22(6):500–507

Taylor R N 1997 Review: immunobiology of preeclampsia. American Journal of Reproductive Immunology 37:79–86

Tufnell D J, Lilford R J, Buchan P C 1992 Randomised controlled trial of day care for hypertension in pregnancy. Lancet 339(8787):224–227

Vaughan C J, Delanty N 2000 Hypertensive emergencies. Lancet 356:411–417

Visser W, Wallenburg H C S 1995 Temporising management of severe pre-eclampsia with and without the HELLP syndrome. British Journal of Obstetrics and Gynaecology 102(2):111–117

Walsh S W 1998 Maternal–placental interactions of oxidative stress and antioxidants in preeclampsia. Seminars in Reproductive Endocrinology 16(1):93–104

Wang Y, Walsh S W, Kay HH 1992 Placental lipid peroxides and thromboxane are increased and prostacyclin is decreased in women with pre-eclampsia. American Journal of Obstetrics and Gynecology 167:946–949

Weinstein L 1982 Syndrome of haemolysis, elevated liver enzymes and low platelet count: a severe consequence of hypertension in pregnancy. American Journal of Obstetrics and Gynecology 142:159–167

Witlin A G, Saade G R, Mattar F et al 1999 Risks factors for abruptio placentae and eclampsia: analysis of 445 consecutively managed women with severe preeclampsia and eclampsia. American Journal of Obstetrics and Gynecology 180:1322–1329

USEFUL ADDRESS

Action on Pre-eclampsia (APEC)
33–35 College Road
Harrow
Middlesex HA1 1EJ

21

Sexually Transmissible and Reproductive Tract Infections in Pregnancy

Susan Dapaah   Victor E. Dapaah

This chapter focuses on sexually transmissible and reproductive tract infections and pregnancy. Specialist detail on these infections and the wider issues surrounding their transmission, diagnosis and management can be obtained from other sources such as Homes et al (1999). Treatment regimens are mentioned but specific drug dosages have intentionally not been included. It is advised that these be obtained from regularly updated pharmaceutical publications.

The chapter aims to:

• consider the implications facing health care professionals regarding the rising trends of sexually transmissible infections

• describe the features of the main sexually transmissible and reproductive tract infections

• discuss the significance of these infections in relation to pregnancy and midwifery practice

Genitourinary medicine (GUM) clinics specialise in the holistic management of individuals with many of the infections discussed. Midwives need to be aware of these services so that interprofessional working is facilitated and women are referred appropriately for treatment.

Trends in sexual health

The rates of sexually transmitted infections (STIs) in the UK have risen sharply since 1995 and the number of new episodes seen at GUM clinics now stands at over a million a year. The highest rates of STIs are found in women, gay men, teenagers, young adults and black and minority ethnic groups (DoH 2001). Females account for most cases of uncomplicated chlamydia and first attack herpes and males account for most cases of primary and secondary syphilis and uncomplicated gonorrhoea. The number of cases of first attack wart virus is slightly higher in males than females (PHLS 2001).

Prior to 1995, the number of diagnoses of acute STIs had been stable or in decline (PHLS et al 2000). It is possible that this was due to modified sexual behaviour to the HIV epidemic. The factors responsible for such high present rates may include improved detection, poor control of infections, increasing unsafe sexual practice, changing sexual behaviour and declining levels of awareness of HIV and AIDS among young people. However, it is possible that, as well as increased transmission, factors such as improved acceptability of GUM clinic services coupled with greater public and professional awareness have contributed to the rise in acute STI diagnoses (PHLS et al 2000).

Recent trends of particular concern are the high rates and increase in STI diagnoses found in the 16 to 24 year age group. The highest rates of gonorrhoea and chlamydia are found in women aged 16 to 19 and men aged 20 to 24. Young people are particularly at risk from STIs as they are more likely to have high numbers of sexual partners, partner change and unprotected sexual intercourse (Johnson et al 1994). Young women may also be vulnerable to sexual exploitation and coercion through lack of skills and confidence to negotiate safer sex. The inconsistent use of barrier contraception and the tendency to have older male partners who have a relatively high rate of partner change may be contributory factors to the high incidence of STIs and teenage pregnancy (PHLS et al 2000).

GUM clinics are a vital source of data for the surveillance of STIs and sexual health in the UK. Other health services that contribute to sexual health include family planning, gynaecology and antenatal clinics, general practice, prison health services and schools. Unless patients are referred to a GUM clinic the statistics are not recorded. The total number of STI diagnoses is therefore likely to be underestimated. In addition, many infections are often asymptomatic and are consequently not diagnosed. Some individuals may not access sexual health services (PHLS et al 2000). It is estimated that, in the UK, 30 000 people are living with HIV, of which a third are undiagnosed (DoH 2001).

The national strategy for sexual health and HIV

Sexually transmitted diseases are an important cause of morbidity and mortality throughout the world. In the UK, in response to the rising prevalence of STIs and of HIV, the Government launched a 10 year national strategy (DoH 2001).

The aims of the strategy are to:

- reduce the transmission of HIV and STIs
- reduce the prevalence of undiagnosed HIV and STIs
- reduce unintended pregnancy rates
- improve health and social care for people living with HIV
- reduce the stigma associated with HIV and STIs.

Public health

Health professionals are expected to play their part in promoting public health and midwives already make a substantial contribution by giving information and advice on screening and testing (RCM 2001). It is important that all midwives understand this role and contribute to its development and enhancement by involvement in public health activities and strategies.

Multidisciplinary team work

The diagnosis, treatment and care of women with STIs during pregnancy present an opportunity for a range of health professionals to work together collaboratively to cater for individual needs, improve pregnancy outcomes and lower maternal and neonatal morbidity and mortality. Joint management between an obstetrician and a GUM physician during pregnancy is essential for women with infections that are serious, life threatening, or both, such as HIV; in addition, a paediatrician is required in the care and management of the neonate infected through vertical transmission. The midwife plays a vital role in caring for the mother and her family in the provision of individualised care throughout pregnancy, labour and the puerperium and especially in health education and promotion. The psychological aspects of some STIs will require the expertise of specially trained counsellors. This is particularly important for those diagnosed with an STI during pregnancy and those who will have the extra burden of worrying about the welfare of their babies.

Confidentiality

Confidentiality is an important principle that binds all health care professionals, and is vital in the promotion of mutual trust, respect and effective partnerships. It is important for midwives to assure clients that sensitive information will not be disclosed to others without their prior knowledge or permission. The maintenance of confidentiality in relation to STIs, particularly HIV, is a common source of worry for individuals with these infections. Midwives should discuss such concerns with clients and ensure that such information is protected and not recorded in documents to which other people may have access, such as patient-held records. Many people may be involved in the care of women during the course of pregnancy. These numbers should if possible be kept to a minimum so that the likelihood of an inadvertent breach of confidentiality is reduced. An accepted principle in health care is that information should be divulged only on a 'need to know basis' (Harpwood 1996).

Infections of the vagina and vulva

There are three main types of vaginal and vulval infections: trichomoniasis, bacterial vaginosis and candidiasis.

Trichomoniasis

Trichomoniasis is almost exclusively sexually transmissible. It is caused by infection with the parasite *Trichomonas vaginalis*, a round or oval flagellated protozoan. Common symptoms include vaginal discharge, vulval pruritus and inflammation, although 10–50% of women are asymptomatic. Vaginal discharge is present in up to 70% of cases and may vary in consistency from thin and scanty to profuse and thick. A classic frothy yellow-green discharge occurs in 10–30% of women. Dyspareunia, mild dysuria and lower abdominal pain may also be experienced (Ackers 2000).

Trichomoniasis in pregnancy

Trichomoniasis has been linked with a small risk of preterm delivery and low birth weight, and an increase in the risk of HIV via sexual intercourse (Ackers 2000, Cotch et al 1997). Trichomoniasis may be acquired perinatally and occurs in about 5% of babies born to infected mothers (Sherrard 2001).

Diagnosis and treatment

In women, 95% of cases can be diagnosed by cultures and 40–80% of cases by microscopic examination of a wet-film or acridine-orange-stained slide from the posterior fornix.

A Cochrane systematic review of interventions for treating trichomoniasis in women concluded that treatment with nitroimidazoles is effective (Forna & Gülmezoglu 2001). The recommended treatment is metronidazole daily for 5–7 days or in a single dose. Although contraindicated, meta-analyses have concluded that there is no evidence of teratogenicity from its use in women during the first trimester of pregnancy. Clotrimazole pessaries daily for 7 days can be used in early pregnancy. High single dose regimens should be avoided during pregnancy and breastfeeding. It is usual to treat the partner(s) and advise against sexual intercourse until the treatment is completed. In addition, patients should be advised not to take alcohol during the treatment and for at least 48 hours afterwards as this may cause nausea and vomiting.

Bacterial vaginosis (BV)

BV is the most common cause of vaginal discharge in women of childbearing age. It can arise and remit spontaneously in sexually active and non-sexually active women. It often coexists with other sexually transmitted infections. It is more common in black women than white, those with an intrauterine contraceptive device and those who smoke (Hay 2001). The incidence of BV is high in women with pelvic inflammatory disease (PID) and some populations of women undergoing elective termination of pregnancy (TOP). It is also associated with post-TOP endometritis.

In this condition the normal lactobacilli-predominant vaginal flora are replaced with a number of anaerobic bacteria including *Gardnerella vaginalis*, *Prevotella* species, *Mobiluncus* species and *Mycoplasma hominis* (Sonnex 1997). The vaginal epithelium is not inflamed, hence the term 'vaginosis' rather than 'vaginitis'. The main symptom is a malodorous and greyish watery vaginal discharge, although approximately 50% of women are asymptomatic. The odour is usually more pronounced following sexual intercourse owing to the release of amines by the alkaline semen (Sonnex 1997). Vulval irritation may occur in about one-third of women.

Bacterial vaginosis in pregnancy

BV is present in up to 20% of women during pregnancy, although the majority of these cases will be asymptomatic (Brocklehurst et al 2001). There is substantial evidence that BV during pregnancy is associated with preterm delivery (Hillier et al 1995). Other adverse outcomes include late miscarriage, low birth weight, preterm premature rupture of membranes, intra-amniotic infection and postpartum endometritis (Hay 2001).

Diagnosis and treatment

A diagnosis of BV is confirmed if three of the following criteria are present:

1. a thin, white to grey, homogenous discharge
2. 'clue cells' on microscopy (squamous epithelial cells covered with adherent bacteria)
3. a vaginal pH of > 4.7
4. the release of a fishy odour when adding potassium hydroxide to a sample of the discharge.

A Gram-stained vaginal smear is another diagnostic technique.

A Cochrane systematic review assessing the effects of antibiotic treatment of BV in pregnancy concluded that antibiotic therapy was highly effective at eradicating infection and improved the outcome of pregnancy for women with a past history of preterm delivery (Brocklehurst et al 2001). The treatment regimen is the same as for trichomoniasis. Alternative treatments include oral clindamycin, intravaginal clindamycin cream or metronidazole gel. All these treatments have been shown in controlled trials to achieve cure rates of 70–80% after 4 weeks, but recurrences of infection are common. Women should be advised to avoid vaginal douching, use of shower gel and use of antiseptic agents or shampoo in the bath (Hay 2001). The routine screening and treatment of partners is not indicated.

Candidiasis

Candidiasis is a common cause of vulvitis, vaginitis and vaginal discharge. The causative organism is usually *Candida albicans*, a fungal parasite. It is a commensal and is found in the flora of the mouth, gastrointestinal tract and vagina. Colonisation of the vagina and vulva may be introduced from the lower intestinal tract or through sexual intercourse. During the reproductive years 10–20% of women may harbour *Candida* species but remain asymptomatic and do not require treatment. Predisposing factors that encourage *C. albicans* to convert from a commensal to a parasitic role include:

- local changes to the vaginal immunity (e.g. vaginal douches)
- immunosuppressant disease or treatment (e.g. AIDS, chemotherapy)
- drug therapy (e.g. antibiotics)
- endocrine disease (e.g. diabetes mellitus)
- physiological changes (e.g. pregnancy)
- miscellaneous disorders (e.g. iron deficiency).

The signs and symptoms of candidiasis include intense vulval pruritus and soreness and often a thick, white curdy discharge, although this is not always present. On examination the vulva, vagina and cervix may be erythematous and oedematous, and white plaques will be noted. Dyspareunia is a common complaint.

Candidiasis in pregnancy

Vaginal candidiasis is found 2–10 times more frequently in pregnant than in non-pregnant women and it is more difficult to eradicate. Candidal colonisation rates rise from less than 10% of pregnant women in the first trimester to over 50% in the third trimester (Wang & Smaill 1989).

Diagnosis and treatment

Vaginal culture is the most sensitive method currently available for detecting candida cells. Candidiasis is treated primarily with antifungal pessaries or cream inserted high into the vagina at night. Preparations that may be given include clotrimazole pessaries, nystatin pessaries or gel, or oral fluconazole (Diflucan). Diflucan is available from chemists without a prescription but this form of treatment has not been tested in pregnancy and it cannot be assumed to be safe. It should also be used with caution whilst breastfeeding owing to toxic effects in high doses.

A Cochrane systematic review of topical treatments for vaginal candidiasis in pregnancy concluded that topical imidazole drugs are more effective than nystatin when treating vaginal candidiasis in pregnancy, that single dose treatments are less effective than 3 or 4 day treatments and that treatment lasting for 4 days is less effective than treatment for 7 days (Young & Jewell 2001).

Recurrence is common. This may be due to resistant cases or failure to complete the treatment. It is usual to treat the partner and advise against sexual intercourse until the treatment is completed. It is helpful to advise on general and genital hygiene but vaginal douches or irritants such as perfumed products should be avoided. Washing and wiping should always be from front to back. The wearing of tight-fitting synthetic clothing should be discouraged.

Bacterial infections

Chlamydia

Chlamydia trachomatis is an intracellular bacterium. It is the most common cause of sexually transmitted bacterial infection and a leading cause of PID. Serotypes D to K are sexually transmitted and are important causes of morbidity in both sexes. Serotypes A, B and C cause trachoma and blindness and serotypes L1 to L3 cause the genital disease lymphogranuloma venerium.

Chlamydial infection is asymptomatic in approximately 80% of cases. Some women may have a purulent vaginal discharge, postcoital or intermenstrual bleeding, lower abdominal pain, mucopurulent cervicitis and/or contact bleeding. Chlamydial infection of the cervix is found in 15–30% of women attending GUM clinics, and concurrently in 35–40% of women with gonorrhoea (Schachter et al 1998). Specific high risk groups include women aged less than 25, those with a new sexual partner or more than one sexual partner in recent years, those not using barrier contraception, those using oral contraception and those presenting for termination of pregnancy (Horner & Caul 2001). Chlamydial infection has been estimated to account for 40% of ectopic pregnancies (DoH 1998).

Chlamydia in pregnancy

Infection rates of *C. trachomatis* in pregnancy range from 2 to 30%. It can cause amnionitis and postpartum endometritis. Its role in preterm rupture of membranes, preterm delivery and neonatal death is not clear. Although some studies have reported an association (Martin et al 1982), others have had no confirmation of differences in controlled trials (Sweet et al 1987). It is not certain either that *C. trachomatis* can cause spontaneous abortion.

Fetal and neonatal infections

Although intrauterine infection can probably occur, the major risk to the infant is from passing through an infected cervix during delivery. Up to 70% of babies born to mothers with chlamydial infection will become infected, with 30–40% developing conjunctivitis and 10–20% a characteristic pneumonia (Schachter et al 1998). Ophthalmia neonatorum of chlamydial aetiology is more common than that of gonococcal aetiology. In practice, the conditions are indistinguishable and may occur together, with 50% of gonococcal ophthalmia being concurrently infected with *C. trachomatis*. The incubation period of chlamydial ophthalmia is 6–21 days, compared with 48 hours for gonococcal ophthalmia. Chlamydial pneumonia usually occurs between the 4th and 11th week of life. It affects about half the babies who develop conjunctivitis but is not always preceded by it. It is thought that children affected by chlamydial pneumonia are more likely to develop obstructive lung disease and asthma than are those who have had pneumonia due to other causes. The pharynx, middle ear, rectum and vagina are also targets for infection, with a delay of up to 7 months before cultures become positive. There would seem to be little doubt that screening in pregnancy can be justified on the grounds of preventing neonatal morbidity.

Diagnosis and treatment

Nucleic acid amplification (NAA) techniques have revolutionised the diagnosis of *C. trachomatis*. There are four commercially available NAA tests that are based on:

- polymerase chain reaction (PCR)
- ligase chain reaction (LCR)
- transcription-mediated amplification (TMA)
- strand displacement assay (SDA).

These tests are highly sensitive and specific but studies in pregnancy are awaited. The sensitivity of LCR for chlamydial detection is thought to exceed by far that of older methods. The enzyme immunoassays (EIAs) that have been widely used up to now are 55–65% sensitive compared with 90–95% for NAAs.

Serological tests have no place in the routine diagnosis of acute chlamydial genital infection owing to their low sensitivity and specificity. The DoH (1998) recommended that NAA tests should be used to screen women for genital chlamydial infection.

Genital chlamydial infections are sensitive to three classes of antibiotics. These are the tetracyclines, the macrolides (e.g. erythromycin) and the fluorinated quinolones, especially ofloxacin. The tetracyclines and the fluoroquinolones are currently contraindicated in pregnancy. Erythromycin has long been the preferred treatment for cervical chlamydial infection despite its gastrointestinal effects, which may affect compliance (Oriel & Ridgway 1980). Erythromycin is also used for chlamydial infections in infants, young children and pregnant and lactating women (Taylor-Robinson et al 2000). Single dose azithromycin is expensive but gaining favour because of its effectiveness, low incidence of adverse gastrointestinal effects and enhanced compliance. The high effectiveness and tolerance of azithromycin in pregnancy have been reported (Miller 1995).

Gonorrhoea

Gonorrhoea is caused by *Neisseria gonorrhoeae*, a Gram negative diplococcus. Transmission is by sexual contact. This organism adheres to mucous membranes and has a preference for columnar rather than squamous epithelium. The primary sites of infection are therefore the mucous membranes of the urethra, endocervix, rectum, pharynx and conjunctiva. Gonorrhoea may coexist with other genital mucosal pathogens, notably *T. vaginalis*, *C. albicans* and *C. trachomatis*. Up to 80% of cases of PID in women under the age of 26 years are caused by *N. gonorrhoeae* or *C. trachomatis*, or both (Weström 2000). The sequelae of PID include infertility, ectopic pregnancy and chronic pelvic pain. Although uncommon, gonorrhoea may also cause disseminated systemic disease and arthritis.

The most common symptom is an increased or altered vaginal discharge although up to 50% of women are asymptomatic. Lower abdominal pain, dysuria, intermenstrual uterine bleeding and menorrhagia may also be experienced, ranging in intensity from minimal to severe.

Gonorrhoea in pregnancy

The incidence of gonorrhoea in pregnancy is low and ranges from 1 to 5% (Wang & Smaill 1989). However, there is strong evidence that maternal gonococcal infection is detrimental to pregnancy. It has been associated with spontaneous abortion, very low birth weight, prelabour rupture of the membranes, chorioamnionitis, preterm delivery, and postpartum endometritis and pelvic sepsis, which may be severe (Brocklehurst 2001, Temmerman et al 1992).

Fetal and neonatal infections

N. gonorrhoeae can be transmitted from the mother's genital tract to the newborn during birth, or occasionally in utero when there is prolonged rupture of the membranes. The risk of transmission from an infected mother is between 30 and 47% and usually manifests as gonococcal ophthalmia neonatorum, a notifiable condition. A profuse, purulent discharge is usually evident within a few days of birth. It can be diagnosed by microscopy and culture of an eye swab. The eyes may be cleaned with saline but systemic antibiotics are required. If left untreated the condition will eventually lead to blindness, and occasionally the neonate may develop further infection such as gonococcal arthritis.

Diagnosis and treatment

Culture on antibiotic-containing medium has long been considered to be the 'gold standard' for detecting *N. gonorrhoeae*. The sensitivity is almost 100% in specialised clinics, but isolation rates are lower in non-specialised settings. Other methods include EIAs, immunofluorescence and DNA probes (Barlow 2000).

A Cochrane systematic review of interventions for treating gonorrhoea in pregnancy concluded that the well-established antibiotic regimen of penicillin and probenicid remains effective. Oral, single dose preparations are now most commonly given. In the case of penicillin allergy or penicillin-resistant organisms, spectinomycin or ceftriaxone are also effective (Brocklehurst 2001).

Syphilis

Syphilis is caused by the bacterium *Treponema pallidum*, a spiral organism (spirochaete), and is usually acquired by sexual contact. It can also be congenitally transmitted. It is a complex systemic disease that can involve virtually any organ in the body. Syphilis in pregnancy and congenital syphilis are rare in the UK but remain a major cause of fetal and neonatal loss in many developing countries, particularly parts of Africa (Brocklehurst 1999).

Acquired syphilis is divided into the following stages (Adler 1998):

Early infectious:

- *primary* – 9–90 days after exposure (mean 21 days)
- *secondary* – 6 weeks–6 months after exposure (4–8 weeks after primary lesion)
- *latent (early)* – 2 years after exposure.

Late non-infectious:

- *latent (late)* – ≥ 2 years after exposure with no symptoms or signs
- *neurosyphilis, cardiovascular syphilis, gummatous syphilis* – 3–20 years after exposure.

Syphilis in pregnancy

Untreated syphilis in pregnancy may result in spontaneous abortion, preterm birth, stillbirths, neonatal deaths and significant infant or later morbidity, although this is dependent on the stage of infection in the mother. Vertical transmission may occur at any time during pregnancy, but is more likely if the mother has primary, secondary or early latent syphilis owing to the considerable numbers of organisms present in the circulation during these stages (Adler 1998). The infection does not usually occur before the 4th month of pregnancy because treponemes from the maternal circulation are unable to pass through the Langhan's cell layer of the early placenta. Once this layer begins to atrophy during the 4th month of pregnancy, the fetus is exposed to the first risk of infection, although this is most likely after the 6th month when complete atrophy has taken place (Ingall et al 1990). A pregnant woman found to have early syphilis is likely to be suffering from early infectious syphilis and early treatment prevents most cases of congenital syphilis (Connor & Nicoll 1998). In pregnant women with untreated early syphilis, up to one-third of cases will result in stillbirth and 70–100% of infants will be infected (Goh 2001).

Congenital syphilis

The prevalence of congenital syphilis in the UK is estimated to be about 70 per million deliveries (Newell 2001). It is classified into early, latent and late stages and the clinical picture varies depending on the stage (see Ch. 46). Approximately two-thirds of live-born infected infants do not have any signs or symptoms at birth, but they present over the following weeks, months or years. Lesions develop only after the 4th month when immunological competence becomes established (Wright & Csonka 2000). Serology at birth is unreliable owing to passive transfer from the mother and the treponemal-specific IgM test is prone to false positive and negative results.

Diagnosis and treatment

Women in the UK are screened for syphilis at antenatal booking and treated if needed. However, this does not detect women who acquire the infection during pregnancy, or women who are incubating syphilis at the time of serological testing (Connor & Nicoll 1998). A range of serological tests is used for screening:

- Venereal Diseases Research Laboratory (VDRL)
- rapid plasma reagin test (RPR)
- *Treponema pallidum* haemagglutination assay (TPHA)
- *Treponema pallidum* particle agglutination assay (TPPA)
- fluorescent treponemal antibody absorption test (FTA-abs)
- treponemal EIA.

If syphilis is suspected on the basis of clinical findings, dark-field microscopic examination or fluorescent antibody staining of a specimen taken from a lesion should be undertaken (see Plate 5) (Goh 2001).

A Cochrane systematic review of antibiotics for syphilis diagnosed during pregnancy determined that the preferred treatment is intramuscular penicillin (Walker 2001). In the case of penicillin allergy, the alternative is erythromycin as tetracycline is contraindicated in pregnancy. However, the poor placental transfer of erythromycin does not reliably cure the fetus and as a precaution the baby may be given a course of penicillin at birth (Adler 1998).

Patients should be warned of possible reactions to treatment with penicillin. The Jarisch–Herxheimer reaction is an acute febrile illness that is common in the treatment of primary and secondary syphilis. It is thought to be due to the release of endotoxin-like substances when large numbers of *T. pallidum* are killed by antibiotics. Headache, myalgia, chills and rigors may occur 4–12 hours after the first injection of penicillin (Wright & Csonka 2000). In pregnancy it may cause fetal distress and preterm labour (Adler 1998). Even if the mother has had an adequate course of penicillin during pregnancy it is recommended that the baby be examined and have serological tests performed. They should also be performed at 6 weeks and 3 months of age, as time must be allowed for the passively transmitted maternal antibodies to disappear (Adler 1998). It is debatable whether or not treatment is required in subsequent pregnancies. It is possible that even after treatment some treponemes may persist in the body and give rise to transplacental transfer. However, Adler (1998) suggests that, if the woman has already been followed up for 2 years after treatment and discharged as cured, serological tests should be performed on the baby at 3 months of age.

The low incidence of syphilis nationally has caused health care professionals to question the need for continued antenatal syphilis screening. The overall prevalence of syphilis among pregnant women in the UK is 0.06 per 1000 live births (Connor & Nicoll 1998). However, routine surveillance from GUM clinics does not include information on pregnancy, therefore this is likely to be underestimated. The rates of infectious syphilis in England and Wales have increased substantially since 1995 in 16 to 24-year-old females (PHLS et al 2000). Despite the low prevalence of syphilis in pregnancy the policy of routine universal screening is thought to remain a cost-effective approach (Welch 1998).

Group B streptococcus (GBS)

GBS (*Streptococcus agalactiae*) is a Gram positive bacterium that naturally colonises the body. It is harboured primarily in the gastrointestinal tract with approximately 30% of adults asymptomatically carrying the organism at any one time. It also colonises the vagina in up to 25% of women (Feldman 2001). Carriage increases with sexual activity and is highest in women attending GUM clinics (Eykyn 2000).

Group B streptococcus in pregnancy

In pregnant women colonised with GBS, high risk factors associated with vertical transmission include: preterm delivery, prolonged rupture of membranes, maternal pyrexia during labour, GBS cultured in a urine sample, known carriage of GBS or a history of a GBS infection in a previous pregnancy (Feldman 2001,

Smaill 2001). GBS is able to infiltrate the amniotic cavity, whether or not the membranes are intact, and infects the fetus through the lung epithelium. Postpartum endometritis and postcaesarean wound infection may also occur in the mother.

Fetal and neonatal infections

GBS is the commonest cause of overwhelming sepsis in newborns during the first days of life, occurring at a rate of approximately 1–2 per 1000 live births (Blumberg & Feldman 1996). The respiratory infection rapidly progresses to sepsis and shock and causes significant morbidity and mortality. GBS infection in the neonate may be early onset, in which case the infection starts in utero, or late onset, which usually presents between 7 days and 3 months of age (Eykyn 2000). Ninety per cent of neonatal infections are early onset, of which 70% are symptomatic at birth.

Diagnosis and treatment

Vaginal and rectal swabs can detect colonisation with GBS, although higher rates are detected with a special enrichment culture medium. Pregnant women in the UK are not routinely screened for this organism, unlike in the USA where GBS is a much more serious problem. However, the degree of colonisation is extremely variable and the tendency for recolonisation after treatment makes control difficult. Swabs taken late in pregnancy at around 35 weeks are effective in predicting whether or not GBS will be carried during labour (Yancey et al 1996).

Intrapartum antimicrobial prophylaxis has been studied extensively in the USA. A Cochrane systematic review concluded that intrapartum antibiotic treatment of women colonised with GBS appears to reduce neonatal infection (Smaill 2001). The usual regimen is intravenous ampicillin during labour. Alternatives include benzyl penicillin or erythromycin.

Viral infections

Genital warts

Genital warts are caused by the human papillomavirus (HPV) types 6 and 11. Transmission is most often by sexual contact, although infants and young children may develop laryngeal papillomas after being infected from maternal genital warts at delivery (Adler 1998).

Diagnoses of first attack genital warts have risen substantially in the UK over the past 10 years, with the highest rates seen in females aged between 16 and 24 years (PHLS et al 2000). Genital warts may cause some physical discomfort, but they are also disfiguring and psychologically distressing, which some patients feel is the worst aspect of the disease (Clarke et al 1996).

In pregnancy they may dramatically increase in size and appear like cauliflower-like masses (see Plate 6), although they usually diminish in size following delivery. Occasionally they can obstruct a vaginal delivery therefore a caesarean section would be indicated.

Genital warts are difficult and time consuming to treat. They are usually treated initially with locally applied caustic agents such as podophyllum. However, this is contraindicated in pregnancy because of possible teratogenic effects. It is recommended that no treatment be offered during pregnancy, although there are alternatives such as trichloroacetic acid, cryotherapy or electrocautery (Adler 1998). Women presenting with genital warts should be fully investigated to exclude other sexually transmitted infections. In addition, colposcopy should be performed to exclude flat warts on the cervix. Most genital warts are benign, but cervical intraepithelial neoplasia is strongly associated with HPV types 16, 18, 31, 33 and 35, therefore an annual cervical smear is recommended (Adler 1998).

Hepatitis B virus (HBV)

HBV infection is a major public health problem worldwide and is an important cause of morbidity and mortality from acute infection and chronic sequelae that include chronic active hepatitis, cirrhosis and primary liver cancer (Zuckerman & Zuckerman 2000). HBV can be transmitted sexually or parenterally through infected blood or blood products. Body fluids such as saliva, menstrual and vaginal discharges, serous exudates, seminal fluid and breastmilk have been implicated in the spread of infection, but infectivity is largely related to blood and body fluids contaminated with blood. It can be transmitted by means of unsterilised equipment such as may occur in injecting drug-users sharing needles and syringes, tattooing or acupuncture, or as a consequence of needle-stick injury in health care workers (Brook 2001). Vertical transmission is a major mode of transmission occurring most frequently perinatally. Acute HBV infection during pregnancy is associated with an increased rate of spontaneous abortion and preterm labour (Medhat et al 1993).

There are usually two phases of symptoms: the prodromal phase characterised by flu-like symptoms, followed by the icteric phase characterised by jaundice, anorexia, nausea and fatigue. The infection may be asymptomatic in 10–50% of adults in the acute phase and in virtually all infants and children. If chronic infection occurs there are often no physical signs but there may be signs of chronic liver disease.

In the acute early phase the hepatitis B surface antigen (HBsAg, formally called Australia antigen) is produced by the infected hepatocytes and appears in the sera of most patients. The presence of the hepatitis Be antigen (HBeAg) in the serum indicates viral activity, which can persist over days or weeks. IgM and IgG type antibodies to the core antigen develop. IgG antibodies may be detectable for many years after recovery. As the infection resolves, HBeAg becomes undetectable, and once cleared the antibody to the surface antigen component, anti-HBs, appears indicating immunity. If HBsAg remains detectable for more than 6 months the patient is usually referred to as a hepatitis B virus carrier. This affects 5–10% of adults and up to 90% of infants infected perinatally. Only about 1 in 1000 of the population carry the virus in the UK (Adler 1998).

All pregnant women should be offered antenatal screening for HBV and babies born to infected mothers should be vaccinated (NHS Executive 1998). The injections should be administered at birth and at 1 and 6 months respectively. In addition, the babies of mothers who have become infected with HBV during pregnancy and those who do not have anti-HBe antibodies should also receive hepatitis B specific immunoglobulin (HBIg) at birth. This should be injected at a different site to the vaccine (the anterolateral thigh is the preferred site in infants). This confers immediate immunity and reduces vertical transmission by 90%. Infected mothers should continue to breast feed as there is no additional risk of transmission (Brook 2001).

Hepatitis C virus (HCV)

HCV infection is another type of viral hepatitis that occurs throughout the world. The principal route of transmission is by percutaneous inoculation, blood and blood products. The prevalence varies in the UK from 0.06% in blood donors to over 60% in intravenous drug users (Brook 2001). Until the screening of blood donors was introduced in the UK in 1991, hepatitis C accounted for the vast majority of non-A, non-B post-transfusion hepatitis (Zuckerman & Zuckerman 2000). The incidence of transmission by sexual contact is low (Weller & Gilson 1998). Vertical transmission is low, occurring at 5% or less, but higher rates are seen if the mother is HIV and HCV positive. At present, there is no known way of reducing the risk of vertical transmission. There is no firm evidence that breastfeeding constitutes additional risk of transmission unless the mother is symptomatic with a high viral load (Brook 2001).

Herpes simplex virus (HSV)

There are two types of HSV: HSV-1 and HSV-2. HSV-1 causes the majority of orolabial infections, and is often acquired during childhood through direct physical contact with oral secretions. HSV-2 is the most common cause of genital herpes and is sexually transmitted via genital secretions. Infections may be primary or non-primary. Once infected, the virus remains in the individual for life, causing recurrent infection. Prior infection with HSV-1 modifies the clinical manifestations of first infection by HSV-2 (Langenberg et al 1999). The incidence of HSV infection depends on factors such as age, duration of sexual activity, number of sexual partners, socioeconomic status, previous genital infections and race (Mertz et al 1992).

In adults, HSV infection may be asymptomatic, but painful, vesicular or ulcerative lesions of the skin and mucous membranes occur frequently (see Plate 7). Dysuria and vaginal or urethral discharge may also occur (Barton et al 2001). There may be systemic symptoms of fever and myalgia. Symptoms are more common in primary infection.

Genital herpes infection

This is defined as:

- *First episode primary infection* – first infection with either HSV-1 or HSV-2 in an individual with no pre-existing antibodies to either type. The local symptoms tend to be severe and lesions may last for 2–3 weeks.

- *First episode non-primary infection* – first infection with either HSV-1 or HSV-2 in an individual with pre-existing circulating antibodies to the other type.
- *Recurrent infection* – recurrence of clinical symptoms due to reactivation of pre-existent HSV-1 or HSV-2 infection after a period of latency.

Herpes simplex virus in pregnancy

The most important complication of HSV infection in pregnancy is neonatal herpes, a rare but potentially very serious condition. Congenital infection, a consequence of primary infection early in pregnancy, can cause severe abnormalities that in the absence of vesicles are difficult to distinguish from similar syndromes caused by rubella, toxoplasmosis or cytomegalovirus (see Ch. 46). The risk of neonatal infection is about 40% with active primary infection, but less than 8% with recurrent infections at the time of delivery and rare with asymptomatic shedding (Kurtz 2000).

Diagnosis

Viral cultures from open lesions are one of the best methods of diagnosing infection but they have a significant false negative rate. Culture levels are normally available within 48–96 hours (Kurtz 2000). Serological tests that demonstrate rising titres of HSV antibodies can be used for the diagnosis of primary infections only by confirming seroconversion. The presence of antibody titre in an initial specimen or the presence of a typical lesion is suggestive of non-primary first episode or recurrent disease. These tests cannot reliably distinguish between HSV-1 and HSV-2 except by using HSV-type specific glycoprotein G as the antigen.

PCR and hybridisation methods are increasingly available. Studies have demonstrated the greater sensitivity of PCR compared with viral culture in the detection of genital HSV (Ryncarz et al 1999). PCR is likely to be more widely used in the diagnosis of genital HSV in the future.

Management of herpes simplex virus infection in pregnancy

The treatment and management of genital HSV infection include antiviral therapy, saline bathing, analgesia and topical anaesthetic gels.

Primary infection acquired during the first or second trimester should be treated with oral or intravenous antiviral therapy depending on the clinical condition. Acyclovir reduces viral shedding, reduces pain and promotes the healing of lesions. It is not licensed for use in pregnancy but there is substantial clinical experience supporting its safety (Barton et al 2001). The recommended dose is the same as for non-pregnant adults, but higher doses may be required for immunocompromised women. Continuous acyclovir in the last 4 weeks of pregnancy reduces the risk of clinical recurrence at term and delivery by caesarean section (Scott et al 1996). In the third trimester, women with active genital lesions after 34 weeks should be delivered by caesarean section, as the risk of viral shedding and vertical transmission is high. Recurrent HSV infection during pregnancy is also treated with acyclovir. Caesarean section is not indicated unless genital lesions or prodromal symptoms of an impending outbreak such as vulval pain or burning are present.

Cytomegalovirus (CMV)

Cytomegalovirus is a member of the herpes virus family. It is so named because it has the effect of enlarging the cells that it infects. Seroepidemiological studies show that CMV infection is common. About 60% of women of childbearing age in developed countries show evidence of past infection, and virtually 100% of those brought up in developing countries (Griffiths & Baboonian 1984).

Most CMV infections are subclinical. However, the clinical manifestations of CMV infection vary with age, route of transmission and the immune competence of the subject. Primary infection may cause generally mild mononucleosis-type symptoms such as malaise, myalgia and fever in immunocompetent adults, whereas it is particularly pathogenic among immunosuppressed individuals, recipients of organ transplants, premature infants and patients with AIDS (Stagno 2000). Recurrent CMV infections do not usually have any recognisable clinical abnormalities.

Cytomegalovirus infection in pregnancy

Several studies have shown that primary infection occurs in all trimesters with about 37% of neonates being born with congenital infection. It is unclear why in the remaining cases the primary infection does not cross the placenta, but since the majority of infected neonates do not develop disease the risk of a woman

with primary infection having a baby damaged by congenital CMV is only about 7% (Griffiths 2001). It has thus been proposed that maternal primary infection on its own is not a sufficient criterion to recommend TOP (Griffiths & Baboonian 1984).

Women already immune to CMV before pregnancy can still deliver a baby with congenital CMV infection (Rutter et al 1985). In such cases it is not possible to distinguish between the type of recurrent infection but it is more likely due to reactivation of maternal latent CMV rather than reinfection from a common source such as the father.

The incidence of vertical transmission with recurrent infections may vary between 0.15% and 1.5% of seropositive women depending on prevalence. This would suggest that circulation of CMV in a community is a risk factor not just for primary infection during pregnancy but also for recurrent maternal infection (Griffiths 2001).

Fetal and neonatal infections

CMV is the most common intrauterine infection affecting from 0.4 to 2.3% of all live births. Unlike rubella, which has a teratogenic effect, CMV allows fetal organs to develop normally but causes disease by the secondary destruction of the cells. Up to 18% of infants born to mothers with primary infection may be symptomatic at birth. The prognosis is thus poor. More than 90% of all symptomatic patients develop sensorineural hearing loss, mental retardation, chorioretinitis and other more subtle complications in later years (Fowler et al 1992; Stagno et al 1986). In infants with subclinical infection the outlook is much better, but 5–15% will develop some sequelae that are generally less severe than in infants with symptomatic infection at birth. Most symptomatic congenital infections and those resulting in sequelae are the result of primary infection acquired during gestation (10–25%) rather than recurrent infections in pregnant women (0–2%) (Stagno 2000).

Perinatal infections result from exposure to CMV in the maternal genital tract at delivery or to breastmilk. They usually occur in the presence of maternally derived, passively acquired antibody. The majority of infants are asymptomatic but occasionally perinatally acquired infection is associated with pneumonitis in preterm and sick full-term infants, neurological sequelae and psychomotor retardation (see Ch. 46).

Diagnosis and treatment

CMV infections can be diagnosed by direct methods such as viral cultures (from urine, saliva, breastmilk, cervical secretions, biopsy and autopsy specimens), PCR and antigen detection. Viraemia suggests active disease and a worse prognosis whether the infection is primary, recurrent or unknown. Direct methods cannot distinguish between primary and recurrent infections. The best way of distinguishing congenital from perinatal CMV infection is by isolating the virus during the first 2 weeks of life from urine or saliva.

Primary infection is confirmed by seroconversion or simultaneous detection of IgG and IgM antibodies. IgG antibodies persist for life and rising titres may follow primary or recurrent infections. IgM antibodies can be demonstrated transiently (4–16 weeks) during the acute phase of symptomatic or asymptomatic primary infection in adults. Other methods include radioimmunoassay, enzyme immunoassay and IgM-capture radioimmunoassay.

Ganciclovir and foscarnet have been used with encouraging results in life threatening CMV infections in immunocompromised hosts. Both drugs are, however, extensively toxic (Stagno 2000). Other measures such as the use of CMV-free blood and blood products, and where possible the use of organs from CMV-free donors, are important ways of preventing CMV infection and disease in non-immune patients.

Human immunodeficiency virus (HIV)

There are two types of HIV: HIV-1 and HIV-2. HIV-1 is the cause of the worldwide spread of AIDS, whereas HIV-2 is largely confined to West Africa. The three principal means of HIV transmission are by blood or blood products, sexual contact and passage from mother to child.

Two to six weeks after exposure to HIV, 50–70% of those infected develop a transient non-specific illness (sometimes called seroconversion illness) with fever, myalgia, malaise, lymphadenopathy and pharyngitis (Luzzi et al 2000). Over 50% develop a rash. Oral and genital ulcers have also been reported. The illness begins abruptly and usually lasts for 1–2 weeks but could be more protracted. Seroconversion is usually followed by an asymptomatic period lasting on average 10 years without antiretroviral therapy. However, although the infection is latent clinically, there is intense viral and lymphocyte turnover with worsening immunodeficiency. Approximately one-third of patients will experience persistent generalised lymphadenopathy. The average time for progression from HIV to AIDS (acquired immunodeficiency syndrome) is about 10 years.

HIV in pregnancy

HIV-1 infection has become an important and common complication of pregnancy. An estimated 600 000 children become infected worldwide each year. Almost all these children are infected from their mothers. Ninety per cent of all these infections occur in sub-Saharan Africa. HIV infection during pregnancy appears to be associated with poor pregnancy outcomes. A systematic review of the literature produced conflicting results, but it seems that there is an increase in the risk of stillbirth, preterm delivery and intrauterine growth retardation (Brocklehurst & French 1998).

The most serious effect of HIV-1 infection during pregnancy is vertical transmission. This can occur during pregnancy, in the intrapartum period or postnatally (Newell et al 1997). In non-breastfed infants, up to 75% of transmission is thought to occur in late pregnancy and the period covering the labour and delivery. Transmission is influenced by a number of factors. The maternal plasma viral load is most important. A strong association between viral load and risk of transmission was observed in Thailand for both in utero and intrapartum transmission (Shaffer et al 1999). The level of virus shed in cervical and vaginal secretions may also be a factor for perinatal HIV-1 transmission.

HIV-1 DNA is present in breastmilk and so postnatal transmission can occur during breastfeeding. This type of transmission was first described in women newly infected after delivery through blood transfusion or heterosexual exposure (Ziegler et al 1985). Breastfed children have a higher risk of mother-to-child transmission than those who have never been breastfed, and prospective follow-up of children born to HIV-1-infected mothers has shown that some infants become infected postnatally after loss of maternal antibodies (Datta et al 1992, Lepage et al 1992).

Avoidance of breastfeeding by HIV-1-infected women is therefore recommended if safe and affordable alternatives are available. However, it is possible that in many developing countries the high expense and rates of infant morbidity and mortality associated with alternative feeding methods outweigh the benefits of reduced vertical transmission. Although breastfeeding has been estimated to double the risk of vertical transmission (Dunn et al 1992), the exact risk and timing of transmission attributable to breastfeeding remains unclear. Nduati et al (2000) estimated that the rate of breastmilk transmission of HIV 1 in their randomised clinical trial was 16.2%, and that, although children continued to acquire HIV-1 infection throughout their exposure to breastmilk, they suggested that most transmission occurs during the first few months. Early cessation of breastfeeding would therefore prevent some infections.

The rate of mother-to-child transmission of HIV in the absence of any treatment intervention varies from 14% to 48% in different settings (Fowler 1997, Wiktor et al 1997). Other factors have been associated with an increased risk of transmission including advanced clinical HIV disease, impaired maternal immunocompetence, maternal nutritional status, resistant viral strains, vaginal delivery, prolonged rupture of membranes, invasive obstetric procedures, the presence of maternal ulcerative genital infection, recreational drug use during pregnancy, prematurity and low birth weight.

A systematic review of the literature suggested that pregnancy might have a small but detrimental effect on the progression of HIV infection (French & Brocklehurst 1998). However, the immunosuppressant effect of pregnancy may cause problems with opportunistic infections, together with their diagnosis, as symptoms common during pregnancy may confuse the clinical picture (Mercey et al 1997). Breathlessness, tiredness and nausea, which are non-specific symptoms relatively common in pregnancy, may mask a serious problem resulting in a delay in its detection and treatment, thus highlighting the importance of knowledge of HIV status in pregnancy.

Diagnosis

Acute infection is accompanied by the development of serum antibodies in the case of core and surface proteins of the virus in 2–6 weeks. Over 90% of seroconversions occur within 3 months of infection. In a minority of cases seroconversion may be delayed to more than 6 months, therefore negative diagnostic tests need to be repeated 3 months after possible exposure and after 6–9 months where there has been a high risk of transmission. Following seroconversion, antibody persists indefinitely in the serum and forms a highly specific test for HIV infection. One or more EIA directed towards HIV-1 and HIV-2 are used as the initial screening tests.

Positive screening tests are confirmed by serum titre tests, a Western blot or immunofluorescence assay.

Primary infection in the neonatal period poses problems in the laboratory diagnosis of HIV. Tests for antibodies need to be repeated at intervals. However, rapid diagnosis during the early stages of infection, when anti-HIV antibodies may be absent, may be provided by detecting HIV viraemia using tests for HIV RNA or DNA (by PCR), p24 antigen or viral culture assays. These allow confirmation of HIV infection in 95% of infected infants by 1 month of age.

Management of HIV in pregnancy

In contrast to the increased mother-to-child transmission in developing countries, perinatal HIV infection has been reduced in many developed countries as a result of measures including counselling, testing, antiretroviral treatment and infant formula feeding.

A clinical trial in the USA and France showed that zidovudine given orally to HIV-1-infected pregnant women starting at 14–34 weeks' gestation, intravenously during labour and orally to babies for 6 weeks, in the absence of breastfeeding, lowered the risk of perinatal HIV-1 transmission by two-thirds (Connor et al 1996, Sperling et al 1996). This regimen was adopted in the USA and western Europe but not in most developing countries because of its complexity and cost. So far there has been no evidence that high doses of zidovudine lead to teratogenicity or short term adverse effects in the human fetus or newborn.

As well as the long course zidovudine regimens, long course combination antiretroviral therapy throughout pregnancy and short course zidovudine regimens have been reported (Shaffer et al 1999, Silverman et al 1998). Shorter drug regimens in pregnancy would be more feasible in resource-poor settings.

During labour and delivery, measures can be taken to avoid situations known to predispose to vertical transmission of HIV. Amniotomy is contraindicated and labour should be augmented if contractions are either weak or absent to avoid a prolonged membrane-rupture–delivery interval. Invasive techniques such as direct cardiotocograph (CTG) monitoring through scalp clips and fetal blood sampling should be avoided and the restrictive use of episiotomy is recommended. Instrumental delivery should be avoided to minimise abrasions to both mother and baby. It must be acknowledged that clinical management decisions must be made on an individual basis following an appraisal of the benefits and risks of prevailing circumstances.

Important evidence on the efficacy of elective caesarean section in the reduction of vertical transmission of HIV-1 infection is now available. The European Mode of Delivery Collaboration (1999) showed that elective caesarean section reduced the likelihood of vertical transmission by some 50%. breastfeeding should be avoided and the midwife has an important duty to provide each woman with information about the risks of breastfeeding and help her to make an individual decision (DoH 1999a).

HIV antibody testing and counselling in pregnancy

In August 1999, the DoH introduced an initiative to offer and recommend an HIV test to all pregnant women as part of their routine care by the end of 2000 (DoH 1999b). This was based on the results of the unlinked anonymous HIV-testing programmes in 1997, which found evidence of 265 births to HIV-infected women, 70% of whom would be unaware of having the infection (Communicable Disease Surveillance Centre et al 1999).

Outside London, most results have shown the prevalence of HIV among childbearing women to be low, at around 1 per 10 000 (DoH 1995). In Dundee and Edinburgh the prevalence is higher, at 1–2 per 1000, but this is mostly associated with injecting drug users (Goldberg et al 1996).

Substantial improvements have been achieved. In the first half of 2000, two-thirds of HIV positive pregnant women across England and Wales were diagnosed antenatally. The uptake of antenatal HIV testing is encouraging, with two-thirds of women having the test (PHLS 2001). However, cases remain concentrated in London, and in the rest of England half of HIV-infected mothers remain unaware of their infection when they give birth. It is estimated that there were approximately 380 births to HIV positive women in 1999 (PHLS 2001).

Pre- and post-test counselling is vitally important and should be undertaken by specialist counsellors or midwives who have received appropriate training (RCM 1998). Issues for discussion include the client's risk of HIV infection, the likelihood and meaning of positive, negative and indeterminate results, confidentiality and the difference between HIV (the virus) and AIDS (the clinical condition). Antenatal HIV antibody testing should be voluntary and subject to explicit informed consent.

Post-test counselling will involve the giving of positive, negative or indeterminate results. The impact that the diagnosis of HIV may have on a pregnant woman must be appreciated. It is important that adequate time is allowed to handle emotional distress and provide an opportunity for questions. Issues for discussion include the natural history of the infection, treatment options and safe sex to avoid transmission to an HIV negative partner(s) and acquisition of other STIs. A range of psychological and social problems such as depression, rejection by hostile family and friends and loss of employment may be encountered. About a third of all patients who are told of their HIV positivity experience a short-lived grief reaction (Adler 1998).

The diagnosis should be confirmed by a second test (Intercollegiate Working Party for Enhancing Voluntary Confidential HIV Testing in Pregnancy 1998) and an immediate referral should be made for specialist medical assessment. An important consideration for the woman is whether or not to continue with the pregnancy. The woman should be given relevant and up-to-date information about HIV and pregnancy and supported to reach an informed decision.

Conclusion

The morbidity and mortality associated with STIs are considerable and are a major health problem worldwide. The control of STIs represents a serious challenge to all health professionals. Health education of the public and health care workers about the transmission of STIs, sexual behaviour and attitudes and safe sexual practice is a primary prevention strategy. The accurate diagnosis and effective treatment of infections, together with the tracing and treatment of sexual contacts, form important aspects of management.

It is impossible to know whether or not clients possess any blood-borne pathogens, therefore universal precautions should be applied to the care of all clients whenever contact with body fluids is anticipated (Centers for Disease Control 1988). In midwifery practice these will include blood, amniotic fluid, cervical secretions and cerebrospinal fluid. Midwives should also be aware of COSHH (Control of Substances Hazardous to Health) regulations (HSE 1994) and local infection control policies and procedures.

REFERENCES

Ackers J P 2000 Trichomoniasis. In: Ledingham J G G, Warrell D A (eds) Concise Oxford textbook of medicine. Oxford University Press, Oxford, p 1774–1775

Adler M W (ed) 1998 ABC of sexually transmitted diseases, 4th edn. BMJ Books, London

Barlow D 2000 Neisseria gonorrhoeae. In: Ledingham J G G, Warrell D A (eds) Concise Oxford textbook of medicine. Oxford University Press, Oxford, p 1599–1602

Barton S, Brown D, Cowan F M et al 2001 National guideline for the management of genital herpes. Online. Available: http://www.agum.org.uk

Blumberg R M, Feldman R G 1996 Neonatal group B streptococcal infection. Current Paediatrics 6:34–37

Brocklehurst P 1999 Update on the treatment of sexually transmitted infections in pregnancy – 1. International Journal of STD and AIDS 10:571–580

Brocklehurst P 2001 Interventions for treating gonorrhoea in pregnancy (Cochrane review). In: The Cochrane Library, Issue 3. Update Software, Oxford

Brocklehurst P, French R 1998 The association between maternal HIV infection and perinatal outcome: a systematic review of the literature and meta-analysis. British Journal of Obstetrics and Gynaecology 105:836–848

Brocklehurst P, Hannah M, McDonald H 2001 Interventions for treating bacterial vaginosis in pregnancy (Cochrane review). In: The Cochrane library, Issue 3. Update Software, Oxford

Brook G 2001 National guideline on the management of the viral hepatitides A, B & C. Online. Available: http://www.agum.org.uk

Centers for Disease Control 1988 Universal precautions for prevention of transmission of human immunodeficiency virus, hepatitis B virus and other blood borne pathogens in health care settings. Morbidity and Mortality Weekly Report 37:377–388

Clarke P, Charles E, Cototti D N et al 1996 The psychosocial impact of human papillomavirus infection: implications for health care providers. International Journal of STD and AIDS 7:197–200

Communicable Disease Surveillance Centre, Scottish Centre for Infection and Environmental Health, Institute of Child Health (London) and Oxford Haemophilia Centre 1999 AIDS and HIV-1 infection in the United Kingdom: monthly report (HIV infection in pregnant women giving birth in the UK – levels of infection and of infection and proportions diagnosed). Communicable Disease Report 9:45–48

Connor N, Nicoll A 1998 Report to the National Screening Committee, antenatal syphilis screening in the UK: a systematic review and national options appraisal with recommendations. STD Section of the PHLS AIDS and STD Centre at the CDSC. Online. Available: www.phls.org.uk/publications/pdf/syphil1.pdf

Connor E M, Sperling R S, Gelber R et al 1996 Reduction of maternal–infant transmission of human immunodeficiency virus type 1 with zidovudine treatment. British Medical Journal 331:1173–1180

Cotch M, Pastorek J, Nugent R et al 1997 Trichomonas vaginalis associated with low birth weight and preterm delivery. Sexually Transmissible Disease 24:353–359

Datta P, Embree J, Kreiss J et al 1992 Resumption of breastfeeding in later childhood: a risk factor for mother to child human deficiency virus type 1 transmission. Pediatric Infectious Disease Journal 11:974–976

DoH (Department of Health) 1995 Unlinked anonymous HIV seroprevalence monitoring in England and Wales. HMSO, London

DoH (Department of Health) 1998 Report on the Chief Medical Officer's Expert Advisory Group on Chlamydia trachomatis. HMSO, London

DoH (Department of Health) 1999a HIV and infant feeding: Guidance from the UK Chief Medical Officers' Expert Advisory Group on AIDS. HMSO, London

DoH (Department of Health) 1999b Reducing mother to baby transmission of HIV. NHS Executive, London (HSC 1999/183)

DoH (Department of Health) 2001 The national strategy for sexual health and HIV. HMSO, London

Dunn D T, Newell M L, Ades A E et al 1992 Risk of human immunodeficiency virus type 1 transmission through breastfeeding. Lancet 340:585–588

European Mode of Delivery Collaboration 1999 Elective caesarean-section versus vaginal delivery in prevention of vertical HIV-1 transmission: a randomised clinical trial. Lancet 353:1035–1039

Eykyn S J 2000 Streptococci and enterococci. In: Ledingham J G G, Warrell D A (eds) Concise Oxford textbook of medicine. Oxford University Press, Oxford, p 1577–1582

Feldman R G 2001 Group B streptococcus prevention of infection in the newborn. Practising Midwife 4:16–18

Forna F, Gülmezoglu A M 2001 Interventions for treating trichomoniasis in women (Cochrane review). In: The Cochrane Library, Issue 3. Update Software, Oxford

Fowler K B, Stagno S, Pass R F et al 1992 The outcome of congenital cytomegalovirus infection in relation to maternal antibody status. New England Journal of Medicine 326:663–667

Fowler M G 1997 Update: transmission of HIV-1 from mother to child. Current Opinion in Obstetrics and Gynecology 9:343–348

French R, Brocklehurst P 1998 The effect of pregnancy on survival in women infected with HIV: a systematic review of the literature and meta-analysis. British Journal of Obstetrics and Gynaecology 105:827–835

Goh B 2001 National guidelines on the management of early syphilis. Online. Available: http://www.agum.org.uk

Goldberg D, Davis B, Allardice G et al 1996 Monitoring the spread of HIV and AIDS in Scotland. Scottish Medical Journal 5:131–138

Griffiths P D 2001 Cytomegalovirus infection in pregnancy. In: MacLean A, Regan L, Carrington D (eds) Infection and pregnancy. RCOG Press, London, p 207–216

Griffiths P D, Baboonian C 1984 A prospective study of primary cytomegalovirus infection during pregnancy: final report. British Journal of Obstetrics and Gynaecology 91:307–315

Harpwood V 1996 Legal issues in obstetrics. Dartmouth Publishing, Aldershot, p 1–28

Hay P 2001 National guideline for the management of bacterial vaginosis. Online. Available: http://www.agum.org.uk

Hillier S L, Nugent R P, Eschenbach D A et al 1995 Association between bacterial vaginosis and preterm delivery of a low birth-weight infant. New England Journal of Medicine 333:1737–1742

Homes K K, Sparling P F, Mårdh P A et al 1999 Sexually transmitted diseases, 3rd edn. McGraw-Hill, New York

Horner P, Caul E O 2001 Clinical effectiveness guideline for the management of Chlamydia trachomatis genital tract infection. Online. Available: http://www.agum.org.uk

HSE (Health and Safety Executive) 1994 Control of Substances Hazardous to Health regulations and the management of health and safety at work regulations. HMSO, London

Ingall D, Dobson S R M, Musher D M 1990 Congenital syphilis. In: Remington J S, Klein J D (eds) Infectious diseases of the fetus and newborn infant. W B Saunders, Philadelphia, p 367–394

Intercollegiate Working Party for Enhancing Voluntary Confidential HIV Testing in Pregnancy 1998 Reducing mother to child transmission of HIV infection in the United Kingdom: recommendations of an intercollegiate working party for enhancing voluntary, confidential HIV testing in pregnancy. Royal College of Paediatrics and Child Health, London

Johnson A, Wadsworth J, Wellings K et al 1994 Sexual attitudes and lifestyles. Blackwell Scientific Publications, Oxford

Kurtz J B 2000 Herpes simplex virus infection. In: Ledingham J G G, Warrell D A (eds) Concise Oxford textbook of medicine. Oxford University Press, Oxford, p 1497–1501

Langenberg A G, Corey L, Ashley R L et al 1999 A prospective study of new infections with herpes simplex virus type 1 and type 2. Chiron HSV vaccine study group. New England Journal of Medicine 341:1432–1438

Lepage P, Van de Pere P, Simonon A et al 1992 Transient seroreversion in children born to HIV-1 infected mothers. Pediatric Infectious Disease Journal 11:892–894

Luzzi G A, Weiss R A, Conlon C P 2000 HIV infection and AIDS. In: Ledingham J G G, Warrell D A (eds) Concise Oxford textbook of medicine. Oxford University Press, Oxford, p 1557–1574

Martin D H, Koutsky L, Eschenbach D A et al 1982 Prematurity and perinatal mortality in pregnancies complicated by maternal Chlamydia trachomatis infections. Journal of the American Medical Association 247:1585–1588

Medhat A, el-Sharkawy M M, Shaaban M M et al 1993 Acute viral hepatitis in pregnancy. International Journal of Gynecology and Obstetrics 40:25–31

Mercey D, Bewley S, Brocklehurst P 1997 A guide to HIV infection and childbearing, 2nd edn. Avert, Horsham

Mertz G, Benedetti J, Ashley R et al 1992 Risk factors for the sexual transmission of genital herpes. Annals of Internal Medicine 116:197–202

Miller J M 1995 Efficacy and tolerance of single dose azithromycin for the treatment of chlamydial cervicitis during pregnancy. Infectious Disease in Obstetrics and Gynecology 3:189–192

Nduati R, John G, Mbori-Ngacha D et al 2000 Effect of breastfeeding and formula feeding on transmission of HIV-1: a randomized clinical trial. Journal of the American Medical Association 283:1167–1174

Newell M L 2001 Antenatal screening for infections. In: MacLean A, Regan L, Carrington D (eds) Infection and pregnancy. RCOG Press, London, p 16–25

Newell M L, Gray G, Bryson Y 1997 Prevention of mother-to-child transmission of HIV-1 infection. AIDS 11:S165–172

NHS Executive 1998 Screening of pregnant women for hepatitis B and immunisation of babies at risk. HSC(98)127. HMSO, London

Oriel J D, Ridgway G L 1980 Comparison of erythromycin and oxytetracycline for the treatment of cervical infection by Chlamydia trachomatis. Journal of Infection 2:259–262

PHLS (Public Health Laboratory Service) 2001 Sexually transmitted infections. Data on STIs in the United Kingdom (1995 to 2000). Online. Available: http://www.phls.co.uk

PHLS (Public Health Laboratory Service), DHSS&PS and the Scottish ISD(D)5 Collaborative Group 2000 Trends in sexually transmitted infections in the United Kingdom 1990–1999. PHLS, London

RCM (Royal College of Midwives) 1998 HIV & AIDS. Position paper 16a. RCM, London

RCM (Royal College of Midwives) 2001 The midwife's role in public health. Position paper 24. RCM, London

Rutter D, Griffiths P, Trompeter R S 1985 Cytomegalic inclusion disease after recurrent maternal infection. Lancet i:1182

Ryncarz A J, Goddard J, Wald A et al 1999 Development of a high-throughput quantitative assay for detecting herpes simplex virus DNA in clinical samples. Journal of Clinical Microbiology 37:1941–1947

Schachter J, Ridgway G L, Collier L 1998 Chlamydia diseases. In: Hausler W J, Sussman M (eds) Topley and Wilson's microbiology and microbial infections, vol 3. Arnold, London, p 977–994

Scott L L, Sanchez P J, Jackson G L et al 1996 Acyclovir suppression to prevent cesarean delivery after first-episode genital herpes. Obstetrics and Gynecology 87:69–73

Shaffer N, Chuachoowong R, Mock P A et al 1999 Short-course zidovudine for perinatal HIV-1 transmission in Bangkok, Thailand: a randomised controlled trial. Bangkok Collaborative Perinatal HIV Transmission Study Group. Lancet 353:773–780

Sherrard J 2001 National guideline on the management of *Trichomonas vaginalis*. Online. Available: http://www.agum.org.uk

Silverman N S, Watts D H, Hitti J et al 1998 Initial multicenter experience with double nucleoside therapy from human immunodeficiency virus infection during pregnancy. Infectious Disease in Obstetrics and Gynecology 6:237–243

Smaill F 2001 Intrapartum antibiotics for Group B streptococcal colonisation (Cochrane review). In: The Cochrane Library, Issue 3. Update Software, Oxford

Sonnex C 1997 Diagnosis and management of bacterial vaginosis. Trends in Urology, Gynaecology and Sexual Health 10(2):33–38

Sperling R S, Shapiro E D, Coombs R W et al 1996 Maternal viral load, zidovudine treatment, and the risk of transmission of human immunodeficiency virus type 1 from mother to infant. New England Journal of Medicine 335:1621–1629

Stagno S 2000 Cytomegalovirus. In: Ledingham J G G, Warrell D A (eds) Concise Oxford textbook of medicine. Oxford University Press, Oxford, p 1509–1511

Stagno S, Robert F, Pass M D et al 1986 Primary cytomegalovirus infection in pregnancy. Journal of the American Medical Association 256:1904–1908

Sweet R L, Lander D, Walker C et al 1987 *Chlamydia trachomatis* infection and pregnancy outcome. American Journal of Obstetrics and Gynecology 156:824–833

Taylor-Robinson D, Mabey D C W, Treharne J D 2000 Chlamydial infections. In: Ledingham J G G, Warrel D A (eds) Concise Oxford textbook of medicine. Oxford University Press, Oxford, p 1705–1711

Temmerman M, Plummer F A, Kiragu D et al 1992 Gonorrhoea in pregnancy. Journal of Obstetrics and Gynecology 12:162–166

Walker G J A 2001 Antibiotics for syphilis diagnosed during pregnancy (Cochrane review). In: The Cochrane Library, Issue 3. Update Software, Oxford

Wang E, Smaill F 1989 Infection in pregnancy. In: Chalmers I, Enkin M, Keirse M (eds) Effective care in pregnancy and childbirth. Oxford University Press, Oxford, p 534–564

Welch J 1998 Antenatal screening for syphilis: still important in preventing disease. British Medical Journal 317:1605–1606

Weller I V D, Gilson R J C 1998 Viral hepatitis. In: Adler M W (ed) ABC of sexually transmitted diseases, 4th edn. BMJ books, London, p 28–32

Weström L 2000 Pelvic inflammatory disease. In: Ledingham J G G, Warrell D A (eds) Concise Oxford textbook of medicine. Oxford University Press, Oxford, p 1847–1849

Wiktor S Z, Ekpini E, Nduati R W 1997 Prevention of mother-to-child transmission of HIV-1 in Africa. AIDS 11 (suppl B):S70–87

Wright D J M, Csonka G W 2000 Syphilis. In: Ledingham J G G, Warrell D A (eds) Concise Oxford textbook of medicine. Oxford University Press, Oxford, p 1680–1686

Yancey M K, Schuchat A, Brown L K 1996 The accuracy of late antenatal screening cultures in predicting genital group B streptococcal colonization at delivery. Obstetrics and Gynecology 88:811–815

Young G L, Jewell D 2001 Topical treatment for vaginal candidiasis in pregnancy (Cochrane review). In: The Cochrane Library, Issue 3. Update Software, Oxford

Ziegler J B, Cooper D A, Johnson R O et al 1985 Postnatal transmission of AIDS-associated retrovirus from mother to infant. Lancet 1:896–898

Zuckerman J N, Zuckerman A J 2000 Hepatitis viruses and TT virus. In: Ledingham J G G, Warrell D A (eds) Concise Oxford textbook of medicine. Oxford University Press, Oxford, p 1551–1557

FURTHER READING

This chapter has concentrated on sexually transmissible infections in pregnancy. The reader is directed to the following texts for more general detail about the presentation, diagnosis, treatment and management of these infections:

Adler M W (ed) 1998 ABC of sexually transmitted diseases, 4th edn. BMJ Books, London

Homes K K, Sparling P F, Mårdh P A et al 1999 Sexually transmitted diseases, 3rd edn. McGraw-Hill, New York

22 Multiple Pregnancy

Margie Davies

The term 'multiple pregnancy' is used to describe the development of more than one fetus in utero at the same time. Families expecting a multiple birth have different health needs, requiring extra practical support and understanding throughout pregnancy, the postnatal period and the early years. Information and support from well-informed health care professionals from the time that the multiple pregnancy is diagnosed will help to prepare the parents and avoid potential problems.

The chapter aims to:

- describe how types of multiple pregnancy may be distinguished

- consider the diagnosis and management of twin pregnancy and labour and the care of the mother and babies after birth

- give an overview of the problems particularly associated with twins and higher order births and the fetal anomalies unique to the twinning process

- explain the special needs of the parents and identify the sources of help available.

Incidence

The incidence of multiple births in the UK continues to rise; in 2000 there were 9578 sets of twins born, that is 1 in 71 maternities, or 14.67 per 1000 (Table 22.1). In the 1940s and 1950s the incidence was similar at 1 in 80 but then fell to 1 in 104 in 1979 (Fig. 22.1). The full explanation for the fall is unknown, although smaller families and the earlier completion of families were contributing factors. The current rise is almost entirely due to the increased use of various kinds of treatments for infertility involving ovulation induction.

Table 22.1 Multiple birth rates per 1000 maternities 1989–2000

	1989	1990	1991	1992	1993	1994	1995	1996	1997	1998	1999	2000
England and Wales	11.40	11.60	12.10	12.50	12.80	13.20	14.10	13.80	14.50	14.40	14.46	14.68
Northern Ireland	10.9	10.3	12.3	10.5	11.7	13.0	14.1	13.3	13.7	13.3	14.95	14.98
Scotland	11.0	11.4	11.0	12.6	12.5	13.0	14.2	14.1	13.8	14.6	13.72	14.39
Whole of UK	11.30	11.60	12.00	12.40	12.70	13.20	14.10	13.80	14.40	14.40	14.42	14.67

Sources: Office of National Statistics London, General Register Office Northern Ireland, General Register Office Scotland.
NB: Figures include live and stillbirths.

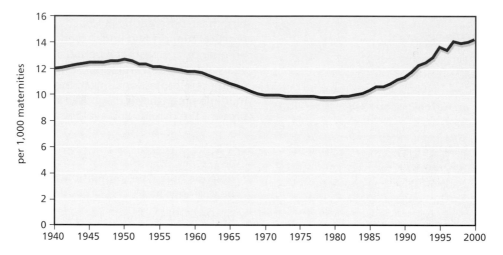

Fig. 22.1 Twinning rates in England and Wales 1940–2000. (Data from Office of National Statistics.)

The number of triplets has more than trebled in the last 15 years (Botting et al 1990); this is due to the rise in infertility treatments such as IVF and ovulation-stimulating drugs, like clomifene citrate and gonadotrophins. In 2000 there were 285 sets of triplets and 5 sets of quadruplets born in the UK. The increase in triplets and higher order multiples puts a considerable burden on the families, the health services and society (Mugford & Henderson 1995).

In other parts of the world the incidences are different: in West Africa they are much higher and in Japan much lower. Triplets in the UK occur in about 1 in 3000 pregnancies and quadruplets once in every 700 000.

Naturally occurring quadruplets and more are rare, but when IVF treatments were first introduced with no limit on the number of embryos that could be replaced the incidence of quintuplets, sextuplets and septuplets increased. Survival rates in such pregnancies, however, were poor.

The Human Fertilisation and Embryology Authority (HFEA) Act 1990 requires all centres providing IVF, using donated gametes (egg and sperm) in treatment, storing gametes and using human embryos in research to be licensed by the HFEA. In 1998/9, 1756 sets of twin births and 235 triplets resulted from IVF (HFEA 2000). The HFEA code of practice states that in normal circumstances only two embryos should be replaced, but there is now discussion on whether this number should be reduced to one only.

Twin pregnancy

Types of twin pregnancy

Twins will be either *monozygotic* (MZ) or *dizygotic* (DZ). Monozygotic or uniovular twins are also referred to as 'identical twins'. They develop from the fusion of one ovum and one spermatozoon, which after

Table 22.2 Relationship between zygosity and chorionicity

Dichorionic	Monochorionic
Two placentae (may be fused) Two chorions Two amnions	One placenta One chorion Two amnions (one amnion in monoamniotic twins is very rare)
These twins can be either dizygotic or monozygotic	These twins can only be monozygotic

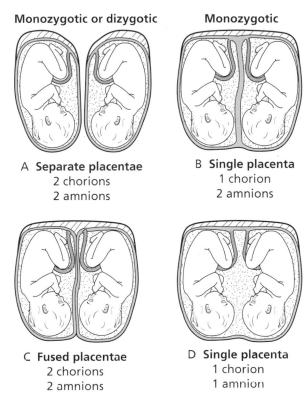

Fig. 22.2 Placentation of twins. (After Bryan 1984, with permission of Edward Arnold.)

fertilisation splits into two. These twins will be of the same sex and have the same genes, blood groups and physical features such as eye and hair colour, ear shapes and palm creases. However, they may be of different sizes and sometimes have different personalities.

Dizygotic or binovular twins develop from two separate ova that are fertilised by two different spermatozoa, and are often referred to as 'non-identical twins'. They are no more alike than any brother or sister and can be of the same or different sex. Because in any pregnancy there is a 50:50 chance of a girl or boy, half of dizygotic twins will be boy–girl pairs. A quarter of dizygotic twins will be both boys and a quarter both girls. Of all twins born in the UK, two-thirds will be dizygotic and one-third monozygotic. Therefore approximately one-third of twins are girls, one-third boys and one-third girl–boy pairs.

Superfecundation is the term used when twins are conceived from sperm from different men if a woman has had more than one partner during a menstrual cycle. It is not known how often this happens, but if suspected then paternity can be checked by DNA testing (Terasaki et al 1978).

Superfetation is the term used for twins conceived as the result of two coital acts in different menstrual cycles. This is thought to be very rare (Rhine & Nance 1976).

Determination of zygosity and chorionicity

Midwives should understand the differences between the two terms (Table 22.2) and why it is important.

Determination of zygosity means determining whether or not the twins are identical. In about a third

of all twins born it will be obvious as the children will be of a different sex. Of the remaining same-sex twins, the zygosity will usually be apparent from physical features by the time they are 2 years old, though parents are not usually prepared to wait this long. At birth, identical twins tend to have a greater weight variation than non-identical ones. In approximately two-thirds of identical twins a monochorionic placenta will confirm monozygosity. If the babies have a single outer membrane, the chorion, they must be monozygotic (Fig. 22.2). In one-third of identical twins the placenta will have two chorions and two amnions, and either fused placentae (Fig. 22.2C) or two separate placentae (dichorionic) (Fig. 22.2A), which is indistinguishable from the situation in non-identical twins. This occurs when the fertilised ovum splits within the first 3 or 4 days after fertilisation and while it is still in the uterine tube. When these are seen on an early scan they appear as two separate placentae and are dichorionic diamniotic, exactly the same as non-identical twins. In about two-thirds of cases the division occurs up to approximately 10–12 days; these will be monochorionic, diamniotic (Fig. 22.2B). Monoamniotic twins occur in about 1% of cases when the embryo divides after 12 days (Fig. 22.2D).

Despite the well-established facts about placentation and zygosity, there is still misinformation given to parents who are told that if same-sex twins are dichorionic they must be non-identical, which of course is incorrect.

Chorionicity: why is it important to know?

This knowledge is important clinically because monochorionic twin pregnancies have a three to five times higher risk of perinatal mortality and morbidity than dichorionic twin pregnancies (Fisk & Bennett 1995).

Prenatally the chorionicity is determined by ultrasound examination. Preferably this should be performed during the first trimester as the differences between the two types of placentation are more pronounced. The chorions forming the septum between the amniotic sacs can be seen more clearly in the first trimester of pregnancy. If the septum has a mean thickness of 2.4 mm or more than it is usually a dichorionic twin pregnancy; if it is a thin septum with a mean thickness of 1.4 mm then it is more likely to be a monochorionic pregnancy (Winn et al 1989).

Another method of determining chorionicity is by studying the septum at its base, adjacent to the placenta. A tongue of placental tissue is seen ultrasonically between the two chorions and this is termed the 'twin peak' (Finberg 1992) or 'lambda sign' (Kurtz et al 1992).

Zygosity determination after birth

The most accurate method of determining zygosity is to compare DNA. DNA can be extracted from cells taken from a cheek swab from inside the mouth. Specific genetic markers extracted from different chromosomes are compared and the results are up to 99.99% accurate.

Zygosity determination should be routinely offered to all same-sex twins for the following reasons:

- Most parents will want to know whether or not their twins are identical, so they can answer the most commonly asked question 'are they identical?'; also as they get older the twins themselves usually want to know.
- If parents are considering further pregnancies they will want to know their likelihood of having twins again. DZ twins tend to run in families and the increased likelihood is approximately fivefold, usually on the female side though not in all cases. MZ twins do not run in families and the likelihood does not change (except in rare families who carry a dominant gene for monozygotic twinning). The chance of any fertile woman having MZ twins is 1 in 300.
- It will help the twins in establishing their sense of identity; it will influence their life and family relationships.
- The information is important for genetic reasons, not just with monogenic disorders but with any serious illness later in life.
- Twins are frequently asked to be involved in research where knowledge of zygosity is essential.

Diagnosis of twin pregnancy

This is usually through ultrasound examination and the diagnosis can be made as early as 6 weeks into the pregnancy, or later at the routine detailed structural scan between the 18th and 20th weeks. When booking a woman in the antenatal clinic a family history of twins should alert the midwife to the possibility of a multiple pregnancy. If the pregnancy is diagnosed at 6 weeks the woman should have the 'vanishing twin syndrome' explained to her (Landy & Nies 1995). Occasionally one fetus may die in the second trimester and become a fetus papyraceous (Fig. 22.3), which

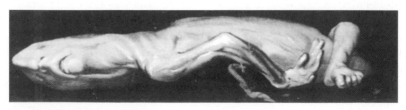

Fig. 22.3 Fetus papyraceous.

becomes embedded in the surface of the placenta and expelled with the placenta at delivery. This is very rare and probably occurs in 1 in 12 000 live births.

The news that a woman is expecting a multiple birth should be broken to the parents in a sensitive manner (Spillman 1985). As soon as a multiple pregnancy has been diagnosed the mother should be given relevant information about multiple pregnancy, including telephone numbers (see Parent education, also Useful addresses, p. 410). Many parents can spend weeks of unnecessary anxiety through ignorance of the help available (Spillman 1987).

Since the advent of routine ultrasound scanning it is very rare for a woman to get to delivery with undiagnosed twins, but this will not apply in areas where this technology is unavailable, or where the mother declines.

Abdominal examination

Inspection. On inspection, the size of the uterus may be larger than expected for the period of gestation, particularly after the 20th week. The uterus may look broad or round and fetal movements may be seen over a wide area, although the findings are not diagnostic of twins. Fresh striae gravidarum may be apparent. Up to twice the amount of amniotic fluid is normal in a twin pregnancy but polyhydramnios is not an uncommon complication of a twin pregnancy, particularly with monochorionic twins.

Palpation. On palpation the fundal height may be greater than expected for the period of gestation. The presence of two fetal poles (head or breech) in the fundus of the uterus may be revealed on palpation and multiple fetal limbs may also be palpable. The head may be small in relation to the size of the uterus and may suggest that the fetus is also small and that there may therefore be more than one present. Lateral palpation may reveal two fetal backs or limbs on both sides. Pelvic palpation may give findings similar to those on fundal palpation although one fetus may lie behind the other and make detection difficult. Location of three poles in total is diagnostic of at least two fetuses.

Auscultation. Hearing two fetal hearts is not diagnostic as one can often be heard over a wide area in a singleton pregnancy. If simultaneous comparison of the heart rates reveals a difference of at least 10 beats per minute, it may be assumed that two hearts are being heard.

The pregnancy

A multiple pregnancy tends to be shorter than a single pregnancy. The average gestation for twins is 37 weeks, for triplets 34 weeks, and for quadruplets 33 weeks.

Effects of pregnancy

Exacerbation of minor disorders. The presence of more than one fetus in utero and the higher levels of circulating hormones often exacerbate the common disorders of pregnancy. Sickness, nausea and heartburn may be more persistent and more troublesome than in a singleton pregnancy.

Anaemia. Iron deficiency and folic acid deficiency anaemias are common in twin pregnancies. Early growth and development of the uterus and its contents make greater demands on the maternal iron stores; in later pregnancy (after 28th week) fetal demands may lead to anaemia. However, recent research suggests that iron and folic acid supplements prescribed routinely are not necessary; only mothers with evidence of significant anaemia should be treated (MacGillivray 1991).

Polyhydramnios. This is also common and is particularly associated with monochorionic twins and with fetal abnormalities. Polyhydramnios will add to any discomfort that the woman is already experiencing. If acute polyhydramnios occurs it can lead to miscarriage or premature labour.

Pressure symptoms. The increased weight and size of the uterus and its contents may be troublesome. Impaired venous return from the lower limbs increases the tendency to varicose veins and oedema of the legs. Backache is common and the increased uterine size may also lead to marked dyspnoea and to indigestion.

Other. There can be an increase in complications of pregnancy (see Chs 18 and 20).

Antenatal screening

- Nuchal translucency for Down syndrome is accurate only if performed between 11 and 13 weeks.
- Serum screening is not usually performed in multiple pregnancy as results are too complex to interpret.
- Chorionic villus sampling (CVS) is not usually recommended in multiple pregnancy as loss rates are high.

- Amniocentesis can be performed in twin pregnancies, usually between 15 and 20 weeks. It should be performed in a specialist fetal medicine unit. Most obstetricians prefer to do a dual needle insertion so there is no chance of contamination between the two sacs.
- Chorionicity should be determined in the first trimester.
- All monozygotic twins should have echocardiography performed at approximately 20 weeks' gestation, as there is a much higher risk of cardiac anomalies in these babies. In the UK at present the incidence is 32 per 1000.

Ultrasound examination

- Monochorionic twin pregnancies should be scanned every 2 weeks from diagnosis to check for discordant fetal growth and signs of twin-to-twin transfusion syndrome (TTTS).
- Dichorionic twin pregnancies should be scanned at 20 weeks for anomalies, as with a singleton, and then usually ever 4 weeks.

Antenatal preparation

Early diagnosis of a twin pregnancy and of chorionicity is extremely important in order to prepare the parents by giving them the specialist support and advice they will need.

Parent education

When a multiple pregnancy is diagnosed, written information on multiple pregnancy should be given to the mother. This should also include contact phone numbers of local support organizations, of her local twins club, of national twin organizations (see Useful addresses, p. 410), and details of special antenatal and parent education classes that may be available. The news they are expecting twins or more may have come as a considerable shock to the parents and the midwife should give them the opportunity to discuss any worries or problems they may have. Two babies will add a considerable financial burden to any family's income, so the midwife should check whether they would like to be referred to a social worker.

Routine parent education classes should start earlier for twin mothers than for singleton mothers, ideally at 24–26 weeks' gestation or even earlier if a mother's work commitments allow. A specialist class for couples expecting a multiple birth should be offered at 28–30 weeks; usually one session is enough. In most hospitals these classes are held monthly, but a course of two or three held every 2 or 3 months may be preferred (Davies 1995). When planning these classes, contact with the local twins club can provide a valuable source of practical information. Mothers from the twins club are usually delighted to participate in the classes and talk on the more practical issues such as coping with two or more babies, equipment and breastfeeding (Denton & Bryan 1995).

Suggestions for class topics are listed in Box 22.1.

Preparation for breastfeeding

Mothers will inevitably give a lot of thought to how they are going to feed their babies, not only from the nutritional but also from the practical point of view, because it will take up a large amount of their time during the first 6 months. Mothers should be encouraged right from the beginning that it is not only possible to breastfeed two, and in some cases three, babies, but

---

Box 22.1 Topics for parent education classes

- Facts and figures on twins and twinning
- Diet and exercise
- Parental anxieties about obstetric complications
- Labour, pain relief and delivery
- Possibilities of premature labour and delivery and the outcome
- Visit to the neonatal unit
- Breastfeeding and bottle feeding
- Zygosity
- Equipment (prams and buggies, car seats, layette, etc.)
- Coping with newborn twins or more
- Development of twins including individuality and identity
- Sources of help

that it is the best way for her to feed her babies nutritionally and it can be a very rewarding experience for her as well (see Plates 8 and 9). Many sets of twins have been entirely breastfed, some beyond their first birthdays. Very few sets of triplets are totally breastfed (Fiducia 1995) but many manage to combine breast and bottle feeding very successfully.

Early in the antenatal period the mother should be given as much information and advice as possible about both breast and bottle feeding, so she can make an informed choice on how she wants to feed her babies. Both parents should have the opportunity to talk through any worries they have regarding feeding and should be encouraged to meet with another mother who is successfully breastfeeding her babies (Box 22.2). Introductions can usually be made through the local twins group.

Labour and delivery

Onset. The higher the number of fetuses the mother is carrying, the earlier the labour is likely to start. Term for twins is usually considered to be 37 weeks rather than 40, and approximately 30% of twins are born preterm, that is before 37 weeks' gestation. In addition to being preterm the babies may be small for gestational age and therefore prone to the associated complications of both conditions. If spontaneous labour begins very early, the chances of survival outside the uterus are small and the mother may be given drugs to inhibit uterine activity. Intravenous salbutamol and sulindac tablets are the drugs most commonly used.

Box 22.2 Support needed by the breastfeeding mother of twins or more

- Consistent professional advice
- Reassurance of her ability to produce enough milk to satisfy her babies
- Encouragement from professionals and family in her ability to cope with feeding two or more
- Support from her partner
- Help at home with household chores
- Help with older siblings
- A high calorie and high protein diet

Known causes of preterm labour must, if at all possible, be diagnosed and treated quickly, for example urinary tract infection should be treated with antibiotics.

It is very unusual for a twin pregnancy to last more than 40 weeks; many obstetricians advise induction of labour at 38 weeks. If the first twin is in a cephalic presentation, labour is usually allowed to continue normally to a vaginal birth, but if the first twin is presenting in any other way (Fig. 22.4), an elective caesarean section is usually recommended.

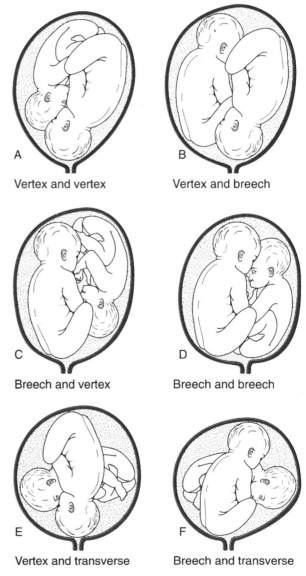

Fig. 22.4 Presentation of twins before delivery. (After Bryan 1984, with permission of Edward Arnold.)

A Vertex and vertex B Vertex and breech C Breech and vertex D Breech and breech E Vertex and transverse F Breech and transverse

Management of labour

During the antenatal classes the mother must be warned that a multiple birth is less common and, for educational purposes, a number of people may ask to observe the birth. If the mother has any objection to this, her wishes must be respected and a record made in her notes that she wants only those concerned with her care to be present.

Induction of labour usually occurs around 38 weeks' gestation. The presence of complications such as pregnancy-induced hypertension, intrauterine growth restriction or twin-to-twin transfusion syndrome may be reasons for earlier induction.

The majority of women expecting twins will go into labour spontaneously. Theoretically the duration of the first stage of labour should be no different from that of a single pregnancy. However, there is an increased incidence of dysfunctional labour in twin pregnancies, possibly because of overdistension of the uterus.

Labour in the mother of twins must be recognised as high risk and so continuous fetal heart monitoring of both babies is advocated. This can be achieved either with two external transducers or, once the membranes are ruptured, a scalp electrode on the presenting twin and an external transducer on the second. If a 'twin monitor' is available both heartbeats can be monitored simultaneously to give a more reliable reading. Uterine activity will also need to be monitored.

If cardiotocography is not available, use of the Doptone or Sonicaid may give more accurate recordings of the fetal heart rates than a fetal stethoscope. If the latter has to be used, two people must auscultate simultaneously so that fetal heart rates are counted over the same minute.

Whilst in labour the woman should be encouraged to adopt whichever position she finds most comfortable. A foam rubber wedge under the side of the mattress will help to prevent supine hypotensive syndrome by giving a lateral tilt. It may be preferable for her to adopt a semiprone position, well supported by pillows or a beanbag. A birthing chair or a reclining chair, if available, may be more comfortable than a delivery bed.

Regional epidural block provides excellent analgesia and, if necessary, allows easier instrumental deliveries and also manipulation of the second twin (Crawford 1978). The use of Entonox analgesia may be helpful, either before the epidural is in situ or during the second stage if the effect of the epidural is wearing off.

The woman should be encouraged to use whatever form of relaxation she finds helpful. If she chooses to use drugs only after other methods have failed, her wishes should be respected. The midwife should explain that, if complications arise, intervention and the use of drugs may be necessary. This should be discussed long before the onset of labour.

If fetal compromise occurs during labour, delivery will need to be expedited, usually by caesarean section. Action may also need to be taken if the mother's condition gives cause for concern.

If uterine activity is poor, the use of intravenous oxytocin may be required once the membranes have been ruptured. Artificial rupture of the membranes may be sufficient in its self to stimulate good uterine activity but may need to be used in conjunction with intravenous oxytocin. The cardiotocograph will give a good indication of the pattern of uterine activity, whether the labour is induced or spontaneous. The response of the fetal hearts to uterine contractions can be observed on the graph paper.

If the babies are expected to be premature, and of low birthweight or known to have any other problems, the neonatal unit must be informed that the woman is in labour so that they can make the necessary preparations to receive the babies. When the birth is imminent, the paediatric team should be summoned to be present when the babies are born.

Throughout labour the emotional as well as the general physical condition of the mother must be considered. She requires support from the midwife and may be apprehensive about the delivery. The presence of her partner or companion will be helpful to her, and the midwife should encourage her to ask questions and express her feelings.

Management of delivery

The onset of the second stage of labour should be confirmed by a vaginal examination. The obstetrician, paediatric team and anaesthetist should be present for the delivery because of the risk of complications.

If epidural analgesia has been used it may be 'topped up' prior to delivery. The possibility of emergency caesarean section is ever present and the operating theatre should be ready to receive the mother at short notice. Monitoring of both fetal hearts should continue until delivery. Provided that the first twin is presenting by the vertex, the delivery can be expected to proceed normally, as with a singleton pregnancy. When the first twin is born, the time of delivery and the sex are noted. This baby and cord must be labelled as 'twin one' immediately. The identity bracelets should be checked with the mother or father before they are applied to the infant's wrist and ankle. The baby may be put to the breast because suckling stimulates uterine contractions. If he requires active resuscitation, the paediatric team will take over his care once on the resuscitaire.

After the delivery of the first twin, abdominal palpation is made to ascertain the lie, presentation and position of the second twin and to auscultate the fetal heart. If the lie is not longitudinal, an attempt may be made to correct it by external cephalic version (see Ch. 30). If it is longitudinal, a vaginal examination is made to confirm the presentation. If the presenting part is not engaged it should be pushed into the pelvis by fundal pressure before the second sac of membranes is ruptured. The fetal heart should be auscultated again and a scalp electrode applied once the membranes are ruptured. If uterine activity does not recommence, intravenous oxytocin may be used to stimulate it.

When the presenting part becomes visible, the mother should be encouraged to push with contractions to deliver the second twin. The midwife should be aware that, owing to the reduced size of the placental site following the birth of the first twin, the second fetus may be somewhat deprived of oxygen. Delivery will proceed as normal if the presentation is vertex, but if the fetus presents by the breech the midwife may need to hand over the delivery to the doctor.

Delivery of the second twin should be completed within 45 minutes of the first twin as long as there are no signs of fetal distress in the second twin; if there are, the delivery must be expedited and the second twin is usually delivered by caesarean section. A uterotonic drug (usually syntocinon or syntometrine) is usually given intramuscularly or intravenously, depending on local policy, after the delivery of the anterior shoulder as with a singleton pregnancy. This baby and cord are labelled as 'twin two'. A note of the time of delivery and the sex of the child is made. The risk of asphyxia is greater for the second twin and the paediatric team may need to resuscitate this infant actively. He may need to be transferred to the neonatal unit immediately after delivery. He should, however, be shown to his mother prior to transfer and if at all possible she may cuddle him.

Once the uterotonic drug has taken effect, controlled cord traction is applied to both cords simultaneously and the placentae should be delivered without delay. Emptying the uterus enables bleeding to be controlled and postpartum haemorrhage prevented.

The placenta(e) should be examined and the number of amniotic sacs, chorions and placentae noted (see Fig. 22.2, p. 393). If the babies are of different sexes they are dizygotic. If the placenta is monochorionic they must be monozygotic. If they are of the same sex and the placenta is dichorionic then further tests will be needed (see above). Pathological examination of placenta and membranes may be needed to confirm chorionicity.

The umbilical cords should also be examined and the number of cord vessels and the presence of any abnormalities noted.

Complications associated with multiple pregnancy

The high perinatal mortality associated with twinning is largely due to complications of pregnancy, such as the premature onset of labour, intrauterine growth restriction and complications of delivery. The management of multiple pregnancy is concerned with the prevention, early detection and treatment of these complications.

Polyhydramnios

Acute polyhydramnios may occur as early as 18–20 weeks. It may be associated with fetal abnormality but it is more likely to be due to TTTS, which is also known as fetofetal transfusion syndrome (FFTS).

Twin-to-twin transfusion syndrome. This can be acute or chronic. The acute form usually occurs during labour and is the result of a blood transfusion from one fetus (donor) to the other (recipient) through vascular anastomosis in a monochorionic placenta. Both fetuses may die of cardiac failure if not treated immediately.

Chronic TTTS can occur in up to 35% of mono-chorionic twin pregnancies (Fisk 1995) and accounts for 15–17% of perinatal mortality in twins (Steinberg et al 1990). The placenta in TTTS transfuses blood from one twin fetus to the other. These cases are characterised by one or more deep unidirectional arterio-venous anastomoses. This results in anaemia and growth restriction in the donor twin (the term 'stuck twin' may be used) and polycythaemia with circulatory overload in the recipient twin (hydrops). The fetal and neonatal mortality is high but some infants may be saved by early diagnosis and prenatal treatment with either amnioreduction, which may have to be repeated regularly as fluid can reaccumulate rapidly, or laser coagulation of communicating placental vessels. Selective fetocide is sometimes considered.

The midwife should always be on the lookout for the mother who complains of a rapid increase in her abdominal girth in the second trimester, as well as a uterus that feels hard and uncomfortable continuously. This is due to polyhydramnios and if not treated as an obstetric emergency it will cause premature labour. This usually occurs in women who have a monochorionic pregnancy.

Fetal abnormality

This is particularly associated with monozygotic twins.

Conjoined twins. This extremely rare malformation of monozygotic twinning results from the incomplete division of the fertilised ovum; it occurs once in 50 000 births and over half the cases are stillborn. Delivery has to be by caesarean section. Separation of the babies is sometimes possible and will depend on how they are joined and which internal organs are involved. The site and extent of fusion of the fetuses are infinitely variable. Thoracopagus is the commonest form of fusion (over 70%) of cases. There is a high incidence of malformations not obviously associated with the site of junction. The feasibility of separating conjoined twins depends on the site and extent of fusion and the degree to which organs are shared (Creinin 1995). Many conjoined twins can now be successfully separated. Others pose major ethical dilemmas – particularly if one can be saved at the expense of the other (Mifflin 2001) (also see Ch. 4).

Acardiac twins (twin reversed arterial perfusion: TRAP). This occurs in about 1 in 30 000 deliveries. In acardia, one twin presents without a well-defined cardiac structure and is kept alive through placental anastomoses to the circulatory system of the viable fetus (Moore et al 1990).

Fetus-in-fetu (endoparasite). In fetus-in-fetu parts of a fetus may be lodged within another fetus; this can happen only in MZ twins (Eng et al 1989).

Malpresentations

Although the uterus is large and distended, the fetuses are less mobile than may be supposed. They can restrict each other's movements, which may result in malpresentations, particularly of the second twin. After delivery of the first twin, the presentation of the second twin may change.

Premature rupture of the membranes

Malpresentations due to polyhydramnios may predispose to preterm rupture of the membranes.

Prolapse of the cord

This, too, is associated with malpresentations and polyhydramnios and is more likely if there is a poorly fitting presenting part. The second twin is particularly at risk of cord prolapse.

Prolonged labour

Malpresentations are a poor stimulus to good uterine action and a distended uterus is likely to lead to poor uterine activity and consequently prolonged labour.

Monoamniotic twins

Approximately 1% of twins share the same sac. Monoamniotic twins risk cord entanglement with occlusion of the blood supply to one or both fetuses. Delivery usually is at around 32–34 weeks and by caesarean section.

Locked twins

This is a rare but serious complication of twin pregnancy. There are two types. One occurs when the first twin presents by the breech and the second by the vertex, the other when both are vertex presentations (Fig. 22.5). In both instances the head of the second twin prevents the continued descent of the first. Primigravida are more at risk than multiparous women (Khunda 1972).

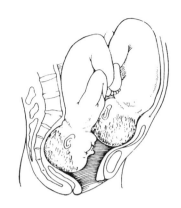 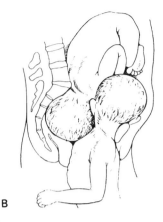

A   B

Fig. 22.5 Locked twins.

Delay in the birth of the second twin

After delivery of the first twin, uterine activity should recommence within 5 minutes. Delivery of the second twin is usually completed within 45 minutes of the first birth. In the past the delivery interval was limited to 30 minutes in an attempt to minimise complications such as cord prolapse, placental abruption and fetal compromise. With the introduction of fetal heart rate monitoring the interval time between babies is not so crucial as long as the fetal condition is monitored. Poor uterine action as a result of malpresentation may be the cause of delay. The risks of such delay are intrauterine hypoxia, birth asphyxia following premature separation of the placenta and sepsis as a result of ascending infection from the first umbilical, which lies outside the vulva. After delivery of the first twin the lower uterine segment begins to reform and the cervical canal may have to dilate fully again.

The midwife may need to 'rub up' a contraction and to put the first twin to the breast to stimulate uterine activity. If there appears to be an obstruction, medical aid is summoned and a caesarean section may be necessary. If there is no obstruction, oxytocin infusion may be commenced or forceps delivery considered.

Premature expulsion of the placenta

The placenta may be expelled before delivery of the second twin. In dichorionic twins with separate placentae, one placenta may be delivered separately; in monochorionic twins the shared placenta may be expelled. The risks of severe asphyxia and death of the second twin are the very high. Haemorrhage is also likely if one twin is retained in utero as this prevents adequate retraction of the placental site.

Postpartum haemorrhage

Poor uterine tone as a result of overdistension or hypotonic activity is likely to lead to postpartum haemorrhage.

Undiagnosed twins

The possibility of an unexpected undiagnosed second baby (though this is unlikely with ultrasound scanning) should be considered if the uterus appears larger than expected after delivery of the first baby or if the baby is surprisingly smaller than expected. If a uterotonic drug has been given after delivery of the anterior shoulder of the first baby, the second baby is in great danger and delivery should be expedited. He will require active resuscitation because of severe asphyxia. The midwife must break the news of undiagnosed twins gently to the parents. These parents will require special support and guidance during the postnatal period.

Delayed interval delivery of the second twin

There have been several reported cases where the first twin has been born, often quite very prematurely, and then there has been a long gap before labour recommences; it can be days or even weeks before the second twin is delivered. This opportunity can be used to give betamethasone to the mother in cases of immaturity of the lungs. Careful observations of the mother's condition must be made during this time for signs of infection and fetal distress. The mother will need support from the midwives to cope with her anxieties for her delivered premature baby, which may not survive, or time to grieve if the baby has died, as well as still being pregnant and her concerns for the outcome of her pregnancy.

Postnatal period

Care of the babies

Immediate care at delivery is the same as for a single baby. Maintenance of body temperature is vital, particularly if the babies are small; use of overhead heaters will help to prevent heat loss. Identification of the infants should be clear and the parents given the opportunity to check the identity bracelets and cuddle their babies. The infants may have to be admitted directly to the neonatal unit (NNU) from the labour ward, in which case the father should accompany them; otherwise they will be transferred to the postnatal ward with their mother if they are in good condition.

Temperature control

Maintenance of a thermoneutral environment is essential, particularly for infants in the neonatal unit. They may need to be nursed in incubators. American studies have shown that a sick baby can benefit from sharing the incubator with his twin (Hedberg Nyquist & Lutes 1998). Clothing should be light but warm and allow air to circulate. The babies' temperatures should be checked regularly and recorded. If they are below the normal range, rewarming is required.

Nutrition

Both babies may be breastfed either simultaneously or separately. The mother may choose to feed artificially but whatever her choice the midwife should support her. In the immediate postnatal days the mother may prefer to breastfeed the twins separately as this gives her time with each baby. If the babies are small for gestational age or preterm, the paediatricians may recommend that the babies be 'topped up' after a breastfeed. Expressed breastmilk is the best form of nutrition for these babies. If the babies are not able to suck adequately at the breast then the mother should be encouraged to express her milk regularly for her babies. If she does not have sufficient milk for them,

milk from a human milk bank can be used, which is much better for the preterm babies than formula milk (Lucas & Cole 1990) and reduces the risk of necrotising enterocolitis (NEC) (Beeby & Jeffrey 1992).

In the early postnatal days the mother may worry that her milk supply is inadequate for two babies and the midwife should reassure her that lactation responds to the demands made by the babies sucking at the breast. The more stimulation the breasts are given, the more plentiful is the milk supply. At feeding times the midwife must be with the mother to offer support and advice on positioning and fixing the babies (see Fig. 22.6), as well as encouraging her in her ability to breast feed two babies.

As the twin babies are both more likely to be preterm or small for gestational age, their ability to coordinate the sucking and swallowing reflexes may be poor. If so, they may need to be fed intravenously or by nasogastric tube, or cup fed (Lang 1995a,b), depending on their size and general condition. The mother should be encouraged to participate in whatever method is used. Careful monitoring of weight gain is required. Hypoglycaemia may occur and regular capillary blood glucose estimations may be needed.

Breastfeeding

The advantages of breastfeeding are the same as for single babies, but as twins have a higher tendency to be born prematurely and small for gestational age it is even more important that they should be breastfed. As well as the medical and nutritional reasons for it being better, there are the practical reasons too:

- It is cheaper, and breastmilk is available 24 hours a day at the correct temperature.
- There are no bottles to wash, no sterilising to organise or feeds to make up, all of which take time. Time is limited for a mother of twins in the early days.
- Twins can be breastfed together or separately. If the babies are to be fed together then the feeds will take only a little longer than with a single baby.

The mother must be encouraged to get everything organised before she starts feeding. The ideal place to sit is on either a bed or a sofa so there is room to put the babies down while organising pillows, etc. In the early days a mother may need to have someone to help position the babies. It is often easier to feed them separately in the very early days as well as giving the

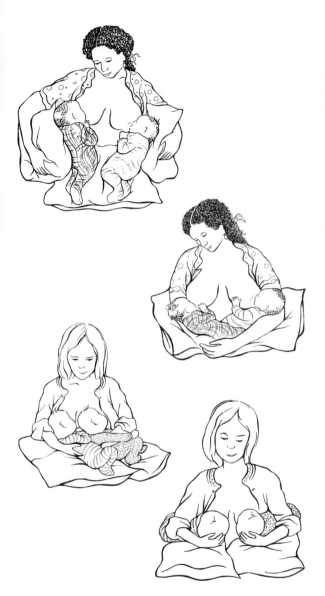

Fig. 22.6 Breastfeeding positions for twins (illustrator: Gillian Coupland).

mother a chance to get to know her babies individually. If she does feed this way to begin with, it is advisable to try to feed both together before being discharged from hospital, so that the midwife can stay with her throughout the entire feed, providing advice, support and another pair of hands.

Using pillows to support the babies, the mother is able to get herself into a comfortable sitting position (Fig. 22.6). She will need to have plenty of pillows so the weight of the babies is taken by the pillows and not by her arms as this will cause back pain.

Mothers of twins always complain that there is never enough time for cuddling; breastfeeding together is the only way for her to hold and feed both babies together at the same time.

The main advantage of bottle feeding is that someone else can always help, although this can be done by using expressed breastmilk.

Mother–baby relationships

Mothers who have a multiple birth often find it more difficult to bond with both babies equally. This is very common and they should be reassured that their feelings are not unusual and in a short time they will overcome these worries. If, for example, the babies are of markedly different sizes, a mother may favour one or the other, or if one baby is in the neonatal unit whilst the other is on the postnatal ward with her, she may find she bonds with the one on the ward much more quickly. In such cases the mother should be encouraged to spend as much time as practicable with the baby in the unit and to visit the NNU as soon as possible after the birth. If she has had an operative delivery she may find it difficult to care for two babies and extreme tiredness or anaemia will exacerbate the situation. She may have feelings of guilt if the birth and immediate postnatal period have not gone as she had expected. The midwife should be alert for such circumstances and help the mother to divide her attention between both babies and to give plenty of reassurance that she is not the first mother to feel like that.

Mother–partner relationships

A mother who has had twins or more will inevitably turn to her partner for help with the care of the babies, and in many families they all work well together in the care and upbringing of their children, despite the added strains and stresses a multiple birth puts on a family. But in some cases her partner may feel that she is devoting too much time to the babies and not enough to him, thus making him feel excluded, especially if when he comes home from work she is too exhausted to take any interest in him. The strain on any relationship when a new baby is born can be quite difficult for the couple to adjust to, but with a multiple birth it is even worse. The midwife should always encourage the father to be involved in the daily care of the babies, either in hospital or at home.

Care of the mother

Involution of the uterus will be slower because of its increased bulk. 'Afterpains' may be troublesome and analgesia should be offered. Some mothers may benefit from a night sedative and need adequate time to rest. A good diet is essential and if the mother is breast-feeding she requires a high protein, high calorie diet. It is quite common for breastfeeding mothers to feel hungry between meals and they should be encouraged to keep sensible snacks to hand for such times. A dietician may be able to offer help.

The physiotherapist or midwife should instruct the mother in her postnatal exercises (see Ch. 15).

The midwife must give the mother of twins extra support and help in caring for her babies as initially she may feel frightened or inadequate in what appears to her as the immensity of the task of coping with two or more babies. Teaching her simple parenting skills and encouraging her to carry them out with increasing assurance will build up her confidence.

The mother may feel 'in the way' if the babies are in the neonatal unit and require a lot of intensive care from the medical and nursing staff. She may also have feelings of guilt because of their prematurity and feel it was something she did or did not do that they were born early. In this situation she will need time to talk her feelings through. Whilst on the neonatal unit she should always be kept up to date with the care and condition of her infants. Most units now have a named nurse caring for each baby so parents know who to talk to. If one infant is very ill or dies, the mother will experience additional psychological problems.

It is very unusual for the babies to be discharged home from the NNU at different times but there are occasions when this happens. When it does, great demands are placed on the mother as she has to care for one baby at home and still visit the sick baby in hospital. Most units have a rooming-in policy so mothers can stay in the hospital with their babies for two or three nights before they are discharged home, to give them a chance to take over the total care of their babies and prepare them for coping at home. It is advisable for any new mother of twins or more to organise help at home for the first 2–3 weeks after discharge. Initially this may be in the form of her partner taking time off work. If relations or friends have offered to help, the mother should be sure to let them know what kind of help she is expecting from them before it is needed. If the parents are fortunate enough to be able to afford paid help then they can say exactly what it is they expect to be done. There is no statutory help available for twins or triplets in England and Wales. One excellent source of help that is free is nursery nurse students who in their final year need practical placements in families. Local colleges of further education will be able to put midwives or mothers in contact with the nearest college that runs these courses.

The community midwife will visit up to the 10th postnatal day, and can visit up to the 28th day if she considers it necessary. The health visitor should also visit at any time from the 11th day.

Once the mother is at home she must be encouraged to rest and catch up on her sleep during the day as much as possible, and eat a well-balanced diet in order to recover her strength and ability to cope with her family. Routine is the essence of coping with new babies and all mothers should be encouraged to establish one as soon as possible.

It may be wise to discourage visitors in the first week at home while the mother adjusts to the new circumstances. The father should be encouraged to help as much as possible.

Isolation can be a real problem for new mothers. The thought of getting two babies ready to go out can be quite fearful. In recent studies the incidence of postnatal depression has been shown to be significantly higher in twin mothers (Thorpe et al 1991). Stress, isolation and exhaustion are all significant precipitants of depression; mothers of twins are therefore bound to be more vulnerable.

Development of twins

Twins in most respects will do as well as a single baby, but the one area in which they can fall behind is language. With twins the mother tends to talk to both of them together in a threesome, so there is less one-to-one communication. Inevitably she will be much busier and the temptation to leave the twins to amuse themselves is much greater. Talking to each other they act as each other's role model for language (unlike the singleton baby, who has his mother). If one child speaks a word incorrectly the twin will copy it, reinforcing the mistake made. This is how the so-called 'secret language' of twins develops, otherwise known as 'cryptophasia' or 'idioglossia'. It is essential that each twin is spoken to individually as much as possible. Eye contact is vital in any relationship. If one twin is more responsive and makes eye contact more easily than the other, the mother may respond much more readily to this twin without realising it.

Identity and individuality

Parents of twins should be encouraged to think of their children as individuals. Ways to emphasise their individuality include choosing names that do not sound similar or rhyme, and avoiding the same first letter. Often parents feel a special pride in having twins and they want to preserve the twinship; this can be done by buying the same style of clothes, but in different colours. Relations and friends should have this explained to them before the babies are born. They will then not be offended if the mother does not dress them in identical outfits that they have been given. The distinction can start in the postnatal ward with differently coloured blankets, or different small soft toys. As they grow up, giving them different hair styles can make children look very different. People should be encouraged to refer to the children by name, or 'the girls' or 'boys' and not 'the twins'. At birthdays or Christmas, separate cards and different presents help to retain individuality. It takes a very dedicated mother to put on two separate parties but she should ensure that each child has an individual cake and 'happy birthday' song. The twins should be given the opportunity to spend time apart. Grandparents may find it daunting to be asked to look after both children, but would really enjoy just having one child, leaving the other at home with the mother to have special time alone with her.

Siblings of multiples

An elder brother or sister of twins may find their arrival very difficult, especially if he or she has had a number of years of undivided parental attention. Parents must be alert to the feelings of their other children and include them as much as possible in all activities with the twins. A single older sibling may see the parents as a pair, the twins as a pair, while he or she is on her own. It can be very helpful to find a 'special friend' for the older child, for instance a godparent, or teenager friend. It can be helpful if the parents arrange for the twins to have a present for the older child and also for the child to have a present to give to each of the twins. Two different small cuddly toys as the first presents the twins receive can become very special gifts.

Triplets and higher order births

The rapidly increasing number of surviving triplets and higher order births (Fig. 22.7) will produce many more families needing special advice and support from health care workers. The UK Triplet Study by Botting et al (1990) revealed that the problems these families face are even greater than were previously realised.

A woman expecting three or more babies is at risk of all the same complications as one expecting twins, but more so. She is more likely to have a period in hospital resting before the babies are born and they will almost certainly be delivered prematurely. Perinatal mortality rates are higher for triplets than twins and the incidence of cerebral palsy is also increased (Petterson et al 1990).

The mode of delivery for triplets or more is nearly always by caesarean section. The midwives must be prepared to receive several small babies within a very short time span. It is essential the paediatric team be present as expert care will be required. The special dangers associated with these births are asphyxia, intracranial injury and perinatal death.

The main difficulties the families experience are the insufficient practical and financial help and lack of awareness of their problems by professionals. All mothers of triplets or more must arrange for extra help at home before the babies are born. The emotional stress and anxiety of the birth, having babies in the NNU and the worries of coping with the babies when they go home will seem overwhelming if no arrangements for extra help have been made beforehand. A mother should never be expected to manage by herself. A study by the Australian Multiple Births Association (AMBA 1984) showed that it took 197.5 hours per week to care adequately for 6-month-old triplets and do the basic household tasks. Unfortunately

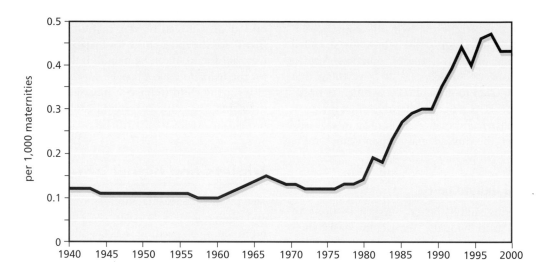

Fig. 22.7 Triplet rates England and Wales 1955–2000. (Data from Office of National Statistics.)

there are only 168 hours in a week, taking no account of the mother's need to sleep!

Taking triplets out for a walk or any expedition can need major organisation, even without the parents having to cope with uninvited comments from passers by. Midwives can help to educate the general public who may make these comments, some of which can be insensitive and hurtful, making inferences about fertility and the parents bringing extra work on themselves.

The midwife must ensure that the mother's health visitor and, if necessary, a social worker are involved in her care. If the family need extra outside help, the organisation of this must start before the babies are born. Applications to the council for rehousing may also be needed.

Disability and bereavement

Perinatal mortality and long term morbidity are both more common among multiple births than singletons. The perinatal mortality rate for twins is about four times that of singletons, and triplets 12 times (Fig. 22.8).

Where the parents lose both or all of their babies, their tragedy will be fully acknowledged by relatives, friends and carers. However, the grief of parents following the death of one of a multiple set is often underestimated. The specific problems they face are ill understood and their needs poorly met. It often feels 'easier' to concentrate on the survivor(s), thus denying

the parents essential time and space to grieve. All too often people say that they are lucky because they still have one healthy child (or more). No one ever says that to parents who lose one of their two or three singleton children (Bryan 1986). The conflicting emotions the parents will feel and the need to grieve for the child who has died, whilst wanting to rejoice at the birth of the healthy twin, can be confusing. Birthdays and anniversaries and the constant presence of the survivor(s) are all reminders of the dead child. The parents may need help in relating to the survivor(s). Addresses of organisations that offer such support should be made available to the parents. Where one or more of a multiple set is disabled it is often the healthy child who needs special attention. He may feel guilt that it was something he did that caused the twin's disability and may be resentful of the attention that the other one needs, or of the loss of twinship. Any of these may lead to emotional and behavioural problems if not addressed early on.

Embryo reduction

This is the reduction of an apparently healthy higher order multiple pregnancy down to two or even one embryo so the chances of survival are much higher. It may be offered to parents who have conceived triplets or more, whether spontaneously or as a result of infertility treatments, by the doctors who care for them.

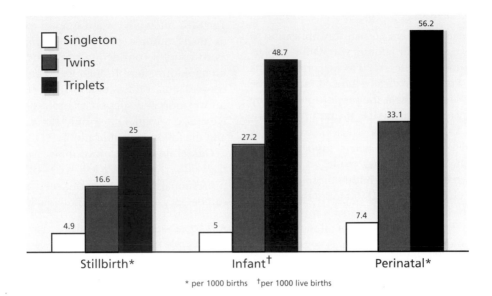

Fig. 22.8 Mortality rates in England and Wales in 2000 for multiple births. * = per 1000 births; † = per 1000 live births. (Data from Office for National Statistics.)

The procedure is usually carried out between the 10th and 12th week of the pregnancy. Various techniques may be used, either inserting a needle under ultrasound guidance via the vagina or, more commonly, through the abdominal wall into the fetal thorax. Potassium chloride is usually used, although some doctors prefer saline. Whichever technique is used, all embryos remain in the uterus until delivery. Usually the pregnancy is reduced to two embryos, but in some cases to three or even one (Bollen et al 1993). Any parents who have been offered this treatment must be given counselling, which should include:

- the advantages and disadvantages of reducing the pregnancy
- the risks of continuing with a higher multiple pregnancy
- the risks of embryo reduction
- the effects on the surviving children
- how the parents may feel afterwards
- help for the parents to reach the right decision for them
- organisations who can help them
- the offer of long term support if and when required.

Selective fetocide

This may be offered to parents with a multiple pregnancy, where one of the babies has a serious abnormality. The affected fetus is injected as described in embryo reduction, so allowing the healthy fetus to grow and develop normally. Counselling must again be offered to the parents on the lines shown above. The full impact of either of these procedures and their bereavement will often not be felt until the birth of their remaining baby (or babies) many weeks later. Moreover, unlike the termination of a single pregnancy, the parents will be more aware of what could have been as they watch the survivor(s) grow up. The midwife must always be aware of women who have undergone these procedures at other hospitals, as there may be very little documented in their own hospital's notes. When it comes to delivery she must be ready to offer the appropriate care and understanding of the parents' bereavement. The bereavement should be clearly indicated in the notes so it is not forgotten when the mother comes back for her postnatal check and for future pregnancies.

Sources of help

In the UK there is at present no statutory obligation to provide any extra help for families with twins, triplets or more. In some countries, such as Belgium, parents with triplets are automatically offered a full-time nanny for 3 years. In Britain the support provided by social services varies greatly so it is always advisable for families with triplets to apply. Health care workers should be prepared to write letters supporting any applications these families have made. In the UK a child allowance is paid to all children born. The first-born child receives at present £5.00 more than subsequent children. In multiple pregnancies it is only the firstborn child that receives the higher allowance.

Parents should be advised to contact organisations such as Home Start (see Useful addresses, p. 410), or the local colleges with nursery training courses, both of which are able to offer assistance in some cases.

Tamba (Twins and Multiple Births Association)

This is the umbrella organisation for the 250 or so local twins clubs throughout the country. The clubs are run by parents of twins and are the best source of practical advice and support for parents expecting twins.

They also run the following specialist groups: Supertwins (triplets or more), Single parent group, Bereavement group, Special needs group, Health and education group, Infertility group, Adoptive parents group, and Tamba Twinline, which is a national, confidential listening and information telephone service for all parents of twins, triplets and more. (See Useful addresses, p. 410).

The Multiple Births Foundation (MBF)

The MBF offers advice and support to families as soon as their multiple pregnancy is diagnosed, as well as to couples considering treatment for infertility. It offers information through its antenatal meetings for couples and professionals. The MBF also provides information and support to professionals through its education programme (study days, courses, lectures and the following publications.

Guidelines for Professionals. *Multiple births and their impact on families* is a series of publications for professionals. It comprises of a set of five books, which can be bought together or individually:

- Facts about multiple births
- Multiple pregnancy
- Bereavement
- Special needs in twins
- Twins and triplets: the first five years and beyond.

Other booklets available. These include:

- Multiple pregnancy and multiple birth – information for couples considering treatment for infertility
- Are they identical? – zygosity determination for twins, triplets and more
- Monochorionic twins – when twins share a placenta
- Preparing for twins and triplets
- Higher multiple pregnancies – fetal reduction
- Multiple pregnancy – selective fetocide
- Feeding twins or more
- When a twin or triplet dies
- How to get twins (or more) to sleep
- Individuality in twins.

(See Useful addresses, p. 410.)

REFERENCES

AMBA (Australian Multiple Births Association) 1984 Proposal submitted to the Federal Government concerning 'act of grace' payments for triplets and quad families. Coogee, Australia

Beeby P J, Jeffrey H 1992 Risk factors for necrotising enterocolitis: the influence of gestational age. Archives of Disease in Childhood 67:432–435

Bollen N, Campus M, Tournaye H 1993 Embryo reduction in triplet pregnancy after assisted procreation. A comparative study. Fertility and Sterility 60:504–509

Botting B, Macfarlane A J, Price F V 1990 Three four and more: a study of triplets and higher order births. HMSO, London

Bryan E M 1984 Twins in the family (a parents' guide). Constable, London

Bryan E M 1986 The death of a newborn twin. How can support for parents be improved? Acta Geneticae Medicae et Gemellologiae 5:166–170

Crawford J S 1978 Principles and practice of obstetric anaesthesia, 4th edn. Blackwell, Oxford, p 218

Creinin M 1995 Conjoined twins. In: Keith L G, Papiernik E, Keith D (eds) Multiple pregnancy, epidemiology, gestation and perinatal outcome. Parthenon, New York, ch 8, p 93–112

Davies M E 1995 Managing multiple births, supporting parents. Modern Midwife 5(11):10–14

Denton J, Bryan E M 1995 Prenatal preparation for parenting twins, triplets or more: the social aspect. In: Whittle M, Ward R H (eds) Multiple pregnancy. RCOG Press, London, ch 12, p 119

Eng H L, Chuang J H, Lee T Y 1989 Fetus-in-fetu, a case report and review of the literature. Journal of Pediatric Surgery 24:296–299

Fiducia A 1995 breastfeeding three babies at once. Twins, Triplets and More Magazine 6(3):10–11

Finberg H J 1992 The 'twin peak' sign: reliable evidence of dichorionic twinning. Journal of Ultrasound in Medicine 11:571–577

Fisk N 1995 The scientific basis of fetofetal transfusion syndrome and its treatment. In: Whittle M, Ward R H (eds) Multiple pregnancy. RCOG Press, London, ch 24, p 235

Fisk N, Bennett P 1995 Prenatal determination of chorionicity and zygosity. In: Whittle M, Ward R H (eds) Multiple pregnancy. RCOG Press, London, ch 6, p 56

Hedberg Nyquist K, Lutes L M 1998 Co-bedding twins: A developmentally supportive care strategy. Journal of Obstretrics, Gynecology and Neonatal Nursing 27(4):450–456

HFEA (Human Fertilisation and Embryology Authority) 2000 Annual report. HFEA, London

Human Fertilisation and Embryology Authority (HFEA) Act 1990 HMSO, London

Khunda S 1972 Locked twins. Obstetrics and Gynecology 39:453–459

Kurtz A B, Wapne R J, Mata J et al 1992 Twin pregnancies: accuracy of first trimester abdominal ultrasound in predicting chorionicity and amnionicity. Radiology 185:759–762

Landy H J, Nies B M 1995 The vanishing twin. In: Keith L, Papiernik E, Keith D, Luke B (eds) Multiple pregnancy, epidemiology, gestation and perinatal outcome. Parthenon, New York, ch 6, p 59

Lang S 1995a Cup feeding an alternative method of infant feeding. Archives of Disease in Childhood 71:365–369

Lang S 1995b Cup feeding alternate method. Midwives Chronicle 107:171–176

Lucas A, Cole T J 1990 breastmilk and neonatal necrotising enterocolitis. Lancet 336:1519–1523

MacGillivray I 1991 Obstetrical aspects of multiple births. In: Harvey D, Bryan E M (eds) The stress of multiple births. Multiple Births Foundation, London, p 11–21

Mifflin P C 2001 Jodie and Mary, ethical and legal implications of separating conjoined twins. Practising Midwife 4(7):48–49

Moore T R, Gale S, Benirschke K 1990 Perinatal outcome of forty nine pregnancies complicated by acardiac twinning. American Journal of Obstetrics and Gynecology 163:907–912

Mugford M, Henderson J 1995 Resource implications of multiple births. In: Humphrey Ward R, Whittle M (eds) Multiple pregnancy. RCOG Press, London, p 334–345

Patterson B, Stanley F, Henderson D 1990 Cerebral palsy in multiple births in Western Australia. American Journal of Medical Genetics 37:346–351

Rhine S A, Nance W E 1976 Familial twinning: case of superfetation in man. Acta Geneticae Medicae et Gemellologiae 25:66–69

Spillman J R 1985 'You have a little bonus my dear.' The effect on mothers of the diagnosis of multiple pregnancy. British Medical Ultrasound Society Bulletin 39:6–9

Spillman J R 1987 The emotional impact of multiple pregnancy: the midwives' role in supporting the family. Midwives Chronicle (March):58–62

Steinberg L H, Hurley V A, Desmedt E et al 1990 Acute polyhydramnios in twin pregnancies. Australia and New Zealand Journal of Obstetrics and Gynaecology 30:196–200

Terasaki P I, Gjertson D, Bernoco D et al 1978 Twins with two different fathers identified by HLN. New England Journal of Medicine 299:590–592

Thorpe K, Golding J, Magillivray I, Greenwood R 1991 Comparisons of prevalence of depression in mothers of twins and mothers of singletons. British Medical Journal 302:875–878

Winn H N, Gabrielli S, Reece E A et al 1989 Ultrasonographic criteria for the prenatal diagnosis of placental chorionicity in twin gestations. American Journal of Obstetrics and Gynecology 161:1540–1542

FURTHER READING

Bryan E M 1996 Twins, triplets and more: their nature, development and care, 2nd edn. Multiple Births Foundation, London

A paediatrician who is internationally renowned for her work with twins and more writes on many aspects of multiples from birth onwards; this is a must for parents and professionals.

Cooper C 1997 Twins and multiple births. Vermilion, London

A GP and mother of twins gives practical advice on coping with twins and more. Suitable for parents and professionals alike.

Lyons S 2001 Finding our way – life with triplets, quads and quins. A collection of experiences. Triplets, Quads and Quints Association, Mississanga, Ontario, Canada

Written by a group of Canadian parents who have had triplets and more giving a fantastic insight to life with higher order multiples, with comments and advice by medical professionals.

USEFUL ADDRESSES

Home Start
2 Salisbury Rd
Leicester LE1 7GR
Tel: 01162 339955

Multiple Births Foundation (MBF)
4th floor, Hammersmith House
Queen Charlottes and Chelsea Hospital
Du Cane Rd
London W12 0HS
Tel: 020 8383 3519
Fax: 020 8383 3041
email: mbf@hhnt.nhs.uk
www.multiplebirths.org.uk

Twins and Multiple Births Association (Tamba)
2 The Willows
Gardner Road
Guildford
GU1 4PG
Tel: 0870 770 3305
Tamba Twinline: 01732 868000

23

Specialised Fetal Investigations

Amanda Sullivan   Beverley Kirk

CHAPTER CONTENTS

Advances in technology mean that assessment of the fetus during pregnancy has become increasingly sophisticated and more widespread. For example, biochemical tests on maternal serum are commonly performed in order to identify which pregnancies carry a high risk of Down syndrome (trisomy 21) (Marteau 1993). Also, ultrasound scanning is continually being refined. More potential abnormalities are identified in the antenatal period. This increases the number of mothers who may be defined as at 'high risk' of having a fetal abnormality. The fact that childbirth among older mothers is becoming more prevalent (Langford 1992) also increases the proportion of expectant parents within a high risk category because some chromosomal abnormalities become more common with advancing maternal age.

Consequently, there are a number of factors that contribute to an ever-increasing emphasis on antenatal fetal assessments.

This chapter aims to explore:

- the psychological effects of fetal investigations
- the role of the midwife when caring for mothers considering or undergoing such tests
- effective information-giving techniques
- common screening and diagnostic procedures
- the use of new and emerging technologies.

Psychological aspects of prenatal testing

Pregnancy is a profound and life-changing event. During this time, the mother has to adapt physically, socially and psychologically to the forthcoming birth of her child. Many women feel more emotional than usual (Raphael-Leff 1991) and may have heightened levels of anxiety (e.g. Dragonas & Christodoulou 1998, Tindall 1997). As Hawkey (1998) states, the increasing availability of fetal investigations has been shown to cause women even greater anxiety and stress. Any feelings of excitement and anticipation can quickly change when the mother is introduced to the idea that she is 'at risk' of having a baby with a particular problem (Thomas 1998).

There is evidence that mothers over 35 years of age (with a higher risk of chromosomal abnormality) experience pregnancy in a way that is different to younger women. Older mothers are often more anxious and have fewer feelings of attachment to the fetus at 20 weeks of pregnancy (Berryman & Windridge 1995). Psychologists, sociologists and health professionals now generally accept the finding that high risk women delay attachment to the fetus until they receive reassuring test results. Rothman (1986) has classically termed this the 'tentative pregnancy', in a study of women undergoing amniocentesis.

Anxiety caused by consideration of possible fetal abnormality may be accompanied by moral or religious dilemmas. This is because parents may be faced with several difficult decisions. For instance, tests that can diagnose chromosomal or genetic abnormalities also carry a risk of procedure-induced miscarriage. Many parents agonise about whether to subject a potentially normal fetus to this risk in order to obtain this information. Parents may then need to consider whether they wish to terminate or continue with an affected pregnancy. Such dilemmas are an unfortunate but inevitable cost of the choices associated with the availability of some fetal investigations.

Despite this, there are important advantages to the acquisition of knowledge about the fetus before birth. First, the present consumerist society greatly values the freedom of individuals to choose. People are encouraged to accept some responsibility when making decisions about treatment options, in partnership with health care professionals. A second advantage is that reproductive autonomy may be increased. Women can choose for themselves whether they wish to embark upon the lifelong care of a child with special needs. This may be viewed as empowering and as a means of preventing later suffering and hardship for child and family alike.

In summary, prenatal testing is a two-edged sword. It enables midwives and doctors to give people choices that were unheard of in previous generations and that may prevent much suffering. However, in some circumstances they actually increase the amount of anxiety and psychological trauma experienced in pregnancy. The long term effects of such trauma on family dynamics are not currently understood.

The role of the midwife

Midwives need a broad knowledge of antenatal screening because they often have contact with women in early pregnancy. Some will develop a particular interest and expertise in this area, so that there is a line of referral for women whose needs are not met by routine services (Ferguson 2001). It will often be necessary for the midwife to present and discuss options with women, so that they can make a choice that best suits their circumstances and preferences. In order to do this, the midwife must strive to obtain informed consent *before* any tests are undertaken.

Andrews et al (1994) have described certain areas that need to be discussed. The main issues are presented in Box 23.1. It is also important that information is presented in a manner that is not coercive and is non-directive (Clarke 1994). However, women's needs are very individual. It may be argued that we should not impose unwanted choices and decision making on women who find this frightening and who would like some professional guidance (Cooper 2001). This is akin to the 'terrible question', whereby people ask 'what would you do in my position?' (Karp 1983).

In such circumstances, midwives should be very cautious about making recommendations. Instead, it

---

Box 23.1 Information required to obtain informed consent

- Purpose of the procedure
- All risks and benefits to be reasonably expected
- Details of all possible future treatments that could arise as a consequence of testing
- Disclosure of all appropriate techniques that may be advantageous
- The option of refusing any tests
- The offer to answer any queries

may be more appropriate to help mothers explore which potential consequences of testing would be most acceptable for them. Making a choice is often a balance, the best of a range of options. When the decision is difficult, it is inevitable that there may be some mixed feelings. The midwife can help the woman prepare for this.

Providing information and support

When discussing tests, it is important to understand the motivations and thought processes of pregnant women. The motivation for testing is often different for mother and practitioner. Whereas the medical indication for testing is to identify fetal anomalies, mothers commonly accept these tests in order to gain reassurance that their fetus is normal (Farrant 1985). Identification of potential abnormality often causes great shock and even panic, particularly if tests are perceived as routine (Robinson 2001).

It is also evident that, when feeling anxious or under stress, people are less able to remember the information portrayed (Ingram & Malcarne 1995). Parents may feel vulnerable and less able to ask questions. This may lead to dissatisfaction with the quality of communications with health carers. Since an unborn fetus is something of an enigma to parents, this may increase anxiety and sensitivity to real or imaginary cues. For example, professionals practising non-directive counselling may be perceived as evasive and as concealing bad news. One particular aspect of counselling that has been criticised by parents is the portrayal of risk estimates (Al-Jader et al 2000).

There is much evidence that people do not make consistent decisions about undertaking tests in pregnancy on the basis of the risk information received. For instance, a mother with a risk of Down syndrome of 1 : 200 may perceive herself to be at a very high risk and may request amniocentesis. However, others may view that same risk as very low. We do not fully understand the way in which parents interpret risk information, although it is clear that personal circumstances, preferences and beliefs are an integral part of this process. For this reason, it is vital that the midwife begins a consultation by investigating how mothers feel about testing and what they already know.

There are also common biases in the way people interpret risk information. The midwife should be aware of these in order to help parents choose the most appropriate course of action. For example, people tend to view an event as more likely if they can easily imagine or recall instances of it. This was clearly demonstrated in a study of estimates of lethal events (Lichenstein et al 1978). They found that murders were incorrectly judged to be more frequent than diabetes or gastric carcinoma. This may be due to the fact that murders are more commonly reported in the media than incidences of diabetes or gastric carcinoma.

The application of this to antenatal testing is that a mother whose friend or neighbour has a baby with Down syndrome may be sensitised to this possibility and overestimate the chances of it happening to her. In reality, her risk remains unchanged. Mothers who work with infirm people, or those with a disability, are most likely to seek prenatal diagnosis (Sjogren 1996). Perhaps these mothers are easily able to imagine the lifelong commitment of caring for a child with special needs. This common bias in risk perception is important because it means that some mothers may not easily be reassured by reiteration of the fact that the risk of abnormality may be comparatively rare.

The way in which the midwife tells a mother about risk will also greatly influence how that risk is perceived. For example, a mother who is told that her risk of a particular condition is 1 in 10 may be more alarmed than if she had been informed that there was a 90% chance of normality. This is known as the 'framing' effect (Kessler & Levine 1987). Examples of this effect are apparent in many advertisements. As such, the message is generally framed to focus on what we might gain from a particular purchase (e.g. status, sex appeal) and not what we might lose (e.g. the financial cost of the purchase, interest accrued on a loan). Where potential losses are included (such as the price), these are minimised and compared to the potential benefits or gains.

People vary considerably in the ways that they consider and understand risk, so it is important that this information is presented in a variety of ways. As such, a midwife discussing a 1 in 100 risk of a disorder should also point out the fact that 99% or 99 out of 100 similar people will not experience that disorder. This may help people cope when considering tests or when anxiously awaiting results.

There are other general considerations to take into account when providing information (Hunter 1994). These are described below.

- Be clear. Explain everything in terms that are not medical jargon or complex terminology.
- Be aware that people can remember only a limited amount of information at one time. Be simple, concise and to the point.
- Give important information first. This will then be remembered best.
- Group pieces of information into logical categories, such as treatment, prognosis and ways to cope.
- Information may be recalled more easily if it has been presented in several forms. For example, leaflets can be helpful after a consultation.
- Offer to answer any queries. Give contact numbers, in case people think of questions at a later date.
- Do not make assumptions about information requirements on the basis of social class, age or ethnic group.
- Repeat the information and ask people whether there is anything that remains unclear.

These general guidelines apply throughout the entire testing process. Unfortunately, midwives will be called upon to deliver bad news at some time. Such situations may include divulgence of a blood test result or identification of a problem with the baby after birth. If a test is undertaken in pregnancy, it is good practice to ensure that parents are clear about how, when and from whom they will be able to obtain the result. If possible, there should be some options available. Someone the parents already know should generally give bad news.

Sometimes, midwives will be faced with instances when they need to impart bad news without much time to plan (e.g. failure to hear the fetal heart). In such cases, the midwife will need to deal with the situation as sensitively as possible. However, if test results constitute bad news, the midwive should take time to think about how best to give this information to parents. Some general guidelines are as follows:

- Plan ahead, so that there is plenty of time available and that all information is to hand.
- Plan the main things you need to say.
- Invite friends or relatives to be involved if this is the mother's wish.
- The news should be given simply and clearly.
- Try to assess and match the mother's mood. Be empathetic and enquire about feelings if they are not expressed.

- Give people time to take in what has been said.
- Be honest and supportive.
- Repeat and summarise information you have given.
- Give all options for subsequent follow-up. This will be in conjunction with the multidisciplinary team.
- Keep full and accurate records of the discussion.
- Allow parents time to phone relatives, have a drink and sit in a quiet room after the discussion, unless they prefer to leave immediately.

Although obstetric colleagues are key to the diagnosis of fetal abnormalities and subsequent plan of care, there is a great need for midwives to be able to inform and support mothers through this process. It is only through collaborative, multidisciplinary working that all of the mother's needs can be met.

Termination of pregnancy for fetal abnormality

Testing for fetal anomaly is inherently different from many other assessments in pregnancy because there is often no treatment that can alter the prognosis. Sometimes, the only options are whether to continue with or terminate the pregnancy. This is a very traumatic decision for parents to make, particularly when there is some uncertainty about how severely affected their baby will be. For example, a diagnosis of Down syndrome does not inform us about the severity of learning difficulties or the medical problems that will be encountered. It can only tell us that the child will function within a wide spectrum of health and ability, previously identified in children with Down syndrome.

The midwife may need to spend a considerable amount of time supporting parents and facilitating difficult decisions regarding termination of pregnancy. It may be appropriate to reiterate prognostic information and to explore how parents feel they would cope with all possible scenarios. There are also charitable organisations, such as ARC (Antenatal Results and Choices), whom parents can contact at this time. This may give them the opportunity to talk to other parents who have faced similar situations. Likewise, parents may wish to speak to paediatricians who care for similar children. Other potentially helpful contacts are clinical genetic services and the chaplaincy.

Individual parents will be guided by their own moral and religious codes when making decisions about potential termination of pregnancy. There is also a legal framework, which governs clinical practice in this country. Before a termination can be induced, two doctors must give their written consent. They must agree that at least one of five clauses is fulfilled (HMSO 1991). These are presented in Box 23.2. Clause C is used when mothers seek terminations for 'social' reasons. In order for a mother to end her pregnancy on the grounds of fetal abnormality, Clause E must be satisfied. In practice, individual practitioners have interpreted the phrase 'seriously handicapped' in different ways. However, there is a general consensus that pregnancies with conditions such as Down syndrome (with varying degrees of impairment, but a reasonable life expectancy) can legally be terminated before the 24th week of pregnancy. Beyond this point, most obstetricians will consider termination of pregnancy only when it is clear that the baby would die in infancy or have considerable pain and suffering, or both.

Tests for fetal abnormality

Broadly speaking, there are two types of test for fetal anomaly. They are classified as screening or diagnostic tests. Each type has a specific purpose and particular advantages and disadvantages.

Screening for fetal abnormality

Screening tests aim to identify a proportion of individuals (often around 5% of a population) who have the highest chances of a named disorder. This makes it possible to target further investigations towards those with the best indication. Mothers who undergo screening tests will be classified as above or below an action limit, whereby they are recalled and offered follow-up procedures. Traditionally, this classification has been known as 'screen positive' or 'screen negative.' However, this terminology has caused problems with interpretation. As such, many mothers given a 'screen positive' result have assumed that there is a positive certainty that they have an affected pregnancy. Likewise, a 'screen negative' result has been interpreted as the exclusion of a problem. In fact, positive or negative in this context simply means that the chances of a problem are higher or lower than specified by an action limit. For this reason, screening results are now referred to as 'high(er) risk' or 'low(er) risk.'

It is also important to note that the action limit (or the dividing point between high and low risk) is usually defined in line with the level of resources available for follow-up procedures. There is no agreed scientific means of calculating what defines high risk. Consequently, some mothers within the low risk group will be sufficiently anxious to request follow-up, whereas some who are categorised as high risk will not wish to pursue subsequent investigations. Screening test results can sometimes herald a cascade of subsequent invasive diagnostic tests, which may be very frightening and distressing.

The performance of a screening test is defined in a number of ways:

> **Box 23.2** Legal clauses that must be fulfilled prior to termination of pregnancy
>
> A The continuance of the pregnancy would involve risk to the life of the pregnant woman greater than if the pregnancy were terminated
>
> B The termination is necessary to prevent grave permanent injury to the physical or mental health of the pregnant woman
>
> C The pregnancy has NOT exceeded its 24th week and that the continuance of the pregnancy would involve risk, greater than if the pregnancy were terminated, of injury to the physical or mental health of the pregnant woman
>
> D The pregnancy has NOT exceeded its 24th week and that the continuance of the pregnancy would involve risk, greater than if the pregnancy were terminated, of injury to the physical or mental health of any existing child(ren) of the family of the pregnant woman
>
> E There is a substantial risk that if the child were born it would suffer from such physical or mental abnormalities as to be seriously handicapped
>
> (HMSO 1991)

- *Detection rate/sensitivity* – this is the proportion of affected pregnancies that would be identified as high risk.
- *False positive rate* – this is the proportion of unaffected pregnancies with a high risk classification. The higher the specificity, the fewer are the false positives.
- *False negative rate* – this is the proportion of affected pregnancies that would not be identified as high risk. The higher the sensitivity, the fewer are the false negatives.

Diagnosis of fetal abnormality

Diagnostic tests are performed in order to confirm or disprove the presence of a particular abnormality. However, as stated, the diagnosis may not give certainty as to the severity of the disorder or the quality of life of a particular individual. Responses to a diagnosis will vary, according to cultural, social, moral and religious beliefs. Furthermore, we are not currently able to diagnose all fetal abnormalities and some will not be manifested until childhood or even adulthood.

The use of ultrasound in obstetrics

These days, most mothers undergo at least one ultrasound scan during pregnancy. This procedure can enable assessment and monitoring of many aspects of the pregnancy and is often presented as 'routine'. It can be used in order to screen for and to diagnose fetal abnormalities. Ultrasound works by transmitting sound at a very high pitch, via a probe, in a narrow beam. When the sound waves enter the body and encounter a structure, some of that sound is reflected back. The amount of sound reflected varies according to the type of tissue encountered. For example, fluid does not reflect sound and appears as a black image. Conversely, bone reflects a considerable amount of sound and appears as white or echogenic. Many structures appear as different shades of grey. Generally, pictures are transmitted in 'real time', which enables fetal movements to be seen.

Safety aspects of ultrasound

Ultrasound has been used as a diagnostic imaging tool since the 1950s, so we are now into the third generation of scanned babies. It seems reasonable to assume that any major adverse effects of this technology would have become apparent before now, but ultrasound should still be used with respect and only when there is good indication. For example, ultrasound waves have been shown to cause tissue heating, primarily within the first 40 seconds of exposure (Bosward et al 1993). There are also conflicting data regarding a possible association with low birth weight (Newnham et al 1993, Salvesen 1997), with dyslexia (Stark et al, 1984) and with non-right-handedness (Salvesen et al 1993). Ultrasound is a diagnostic tool, but diagnosis can only be as reliable as the expertise of the operator and the quality of the machine. As Wood (2000) states, abnormalities may be missed or incorrectly diagnosed if the operator is inexperienced or inadequately trained.

Women's experiences of ultrasound

In general, women experience ultrasound as a pleasurable opportunity to have visual access to their unborn baby (Sandelowski 1994). Parents have a profound curiosity about their baby and a scan can turn something nebulous into something which seems much more real as a living individual (Furness 1990). This can be particularly important for a woman's partner and family, who do not have the immediate physical experience of the pregnancy. Women tend to regard their scan as providing a general view of fetal well-being: the fact that the fetus is alive, growing and developing. However, this reassurance is temporary and begins to wear off after a few weeks (Clement et al 1998). Mothers may then seek other forms of reassurance (e.g. monitoring fetal movements, auscultation of the fetal heartbeat). This initial reassurance may also create an enthusiasm for scans when there is no clinical indication.

However, scans may also cause considerable anxiety, particularly if there is a suspected or actual problem with the fetus. There is evidence to suggest that women who miscarry after visualisation of the fetus on scan may feel a heightened sense of anguish because the fetus seemed more real. This may also be the case for parents considering termination of pregnancy on the grounds of fetal abnormality. However, others may view their scan as a treasured memory of the baby they lost (Black 1992).

The identification of fetal abnormality in the antenatal period has differing psychological effects for parents when the pregnancy is to continue. Some parents have reported feeling grateful that they were able to prepare for the birth of a handicapped child (Chitty et al 1996). However, others have reported feelings of wishing they had not known about their child's problems before birth because this created a powerful image of the fetus as a 'monster'. Some parents reported this to be far worse than the reality of caring for the baby after birth (Turner 1994). It is necessary for carers to be mindful of the powerful psychological effects ultrasound scans have on pregnant women and their families, if sensitive and appropriate care is to be given at this potentially distressing time.

The midwife's role concerning ultrasound scans

As for all procedures, mothers should be fully informed about the purpose of the scan. Information should be given about which conditions are being checked for and which problems the scan would be unable to detect. Because of the pleasurable aspect of seeing the fetus, ultrasound scans have traditionally been tests that mothers undertake willingly, without prior discussion and consideration of potential consequences. It is advisable to remind mothers gently of the medical indications for scans, so that they can decide whether or not they wish to undergo a procedure that may bring unwelcome news.

There is evidence that, although some mothers may find this information disturbing, most feel that this is outweighed by the positive aspects of seeing the baby and gaining reassurance (Oliver et al 1996). Indeed, extra information about the purpose of the scan has been shown to increase women's understanding and satisfaction with the amount of information received, whilst the proportion of women accepting a scan (99%) appears to remain unchanged (Thornton et al 1995).

The Royal College of Obstetricians and Gynaecologists recommends that, wherever scans are performed, a midwife or counsellor with a particular interest or expertise in the area should be available to discuss difficult news. Discussion about the implications of this should also take place with an obstetrician within one working day (RCOG 2000). Effective multidisciplinary team working and communication are therefore essential. It is also good practice for the midwife to liaise with the primary health care team, who would normally carry out the majority of antenatal care. With the increasing use of client-held records, mothers may have more opportunity to scrutinise the written results of their scan. Midwives may increasingly be called upon to explain and discuss these findings, both in hospital and in the community.

First trimester pregnancy scans

Many areas offer mothers a scan in early pregnancy, often around 12–14 weeks' gestation. The purpose of this is to establish:

- that the pregnancy is viable and intrauterine (not ectopic)
- gestational age
- fetal number (and chorionicity or amnionicity in multiple pregnancies)
- detection of gross fetal abnormalities, such as anencephaly (absence of the cranial vault, as shown in Figure 23.1).

There is evidence to suggest that at least one scan is beneficial, mainly in reducing the need to induce labour for postmaturity (Neilson 1999). A gestation sac can usually be visualised from 5 weeks' gestation

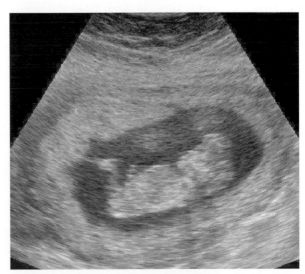

Fig. 23.1 Anencephaly. (Reproduced with permission of Nottingham City Hospital NHS Trust.)

and a small embryo from 6 weeks. Until 13 weeks, gestational age can be accurately assessed by crown–rump length (CRL) measurement. (This is the length of the fetus from the top of the head to the end of the sacrum.) This is demonstrated in Figure 23.2. Care must be taken to ensure that the fetus is not flexed at the time of measurement. If the mother is sure of her last menstrual period (LMP) and has a regular menstrual cycle, the expected date of delivery (EDD) is not generally altered unless the scan calculation of gestational age deviates by more than 1 week. Mothers are asked to attend with a full bladder, since this aids visualisation of the uterus at an early gestation.

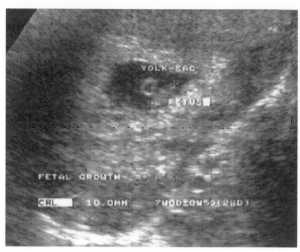

Fig. 23.2 Crown–rump length at 7 weeks' gestation. (Reproduced with permission of Nottingham City Hospital NHS Trust.)

Measurement of nuchal translucency at 10–14 weeks as a screen for Down syndrome

Additional information about the fetus can be gained by observation of the nuchal translucency (NT) at 10–14 weeks' gestation. This involves measuring the thickness of the subcutaneous collection of fluid at the back of the neck, as shown in Figure 23.3. During the last decade, a series of studies have reported that increased NT is associated with chromosomal abnormalities, as well as other structural and genetic disorders (Nicolaides et al 1999). Sometimes, this information is used as a basis upon which to screen for Down syndrome.

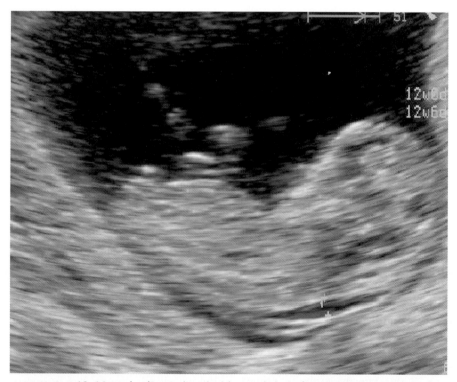

Fig. 23.3 NT measurement at 10–14 weeks. (Reproduced with permission of Nottingham City Hospital NHS Trust.)

Down syndrome is the most common cause of severe learning difficulty in children. In the absence of antenatal screening, around 1 in 700 births would be affected (Kennard et al 1995). Whilst some children with Down syndrome learn literacy skills and lead semi-independent lives, others remain completely dependent. Around one in three of these babies are born with a serious heart defect. The average life expectancy is around 60 years, although most people develop pathological changes in the brain (associated with Alzheimer's disease) after the age of 40 (Kingston 1994).

Antenatal screening for Down syndrome has been the subject of much controversy over the last decade, for a number of reasons. First, there are some moral objections to screening for this disorder and selectively terminating affected pregnancies. Secondly, counselling prior to screening is often inadequate. As Ward (2001) comments, many midwives do not currently have the time, knowledge or support to perform this task adequately. However, Down screening is an increasingly important aspect of antenatal care. In fact, the DoH recently announced that all pregnant women would be offered Down syndrome screening in some form by 2004. The Antenatal Sub-Group of the National Screening Committee have established a structure of screening coordinators based at regional and at local levels, to address the educational needs of health professionals and current inconsistencies in service provision. It is envisaged that these posts will gradually become effective over the next few years.

The incidence of Down syndrome increases with advancing maternal age. This is shown in Table 23.1. However, only 30% of affected babies are born to mothers over 35 years, so screening by maternal age alone would not result in a very high *detection rate*. Nicolaides et al (1999) found that the NT measurement, combined with maternal age risk, increases this detection rate to 80% (providing the scan is undertaken in centres with appropriately trained sonographers, using high quality equipment).

The main advantage of this test is that it offers an early way of assessing the mother's risk for Down syndrome. This can be particularly valuable for older mothers who may otherwise opt for a risky diagnostic first trimester procedure. In general, mothers greatly value the opportunity for early information about Down syndrome, so that they could consider the

Table 23.1 Estimated risk of having a Down syndrome birth according to maternal age at delivery (calculated using eight surveys)

Maternal age	Risk
15	1 : 1578
16	1 : 1572
17	1 : 1565
18	1 : 1556
19	1 : 1544
20	1 : 1528
21	1 : 1507
22	1 : 1481
23	1 : 1447
24	1 : 1404
25	1 : 1351
26	1 : 1286
27	1 : 1208
28	1 : 1119
29	1 : 1018
30	1 : 909
31	1 : 796
32	1 : 683
33	1 : 574
34	1 : 474
35	1 : 384
36	1 : 307
37	1 : 242
38	1 : 189
39	1 : 146
40	1 : 112
41	1 : 85
42	1 : 65
43	1 : 49
44	1 : 37
45	1 : 28
46	1 : 21
47	1 : 15
48	1 : 11
49	1 : 8
50	1 : 6

(From Cuckle et al 1987, with permission from Elsevier Science)

option of termination before they are visibly pregnant and can feel their baby's movements. Increased NT is also associated with other structural (mainly cardiac) and genetic syndromes, so increased pregnancy surveillance could be arranged. However, a disadvantage of this knowledge is that parents may suffer considerable anxiety until later scans offer some degree of reassurance.

Another potential disadvantage is that early identification of chromosomally abnormal pregnancies may mean that parents are faced with a decision about whether to terminate a pregnancy that may be destined to miscarry naturally. Approximately 40% of affected fetuses die between 12 weeks' gestation and term (Nicolaides et al 1999). Some parents may experience more feelings of guilt after a termination than they would have done had the pregnancy spontaneously miscarried.

Second trimester ultrasound scans

After 13 weeks of pregnancy, gestational age is primarily assessed using the biparietal diameter (BPD). This is the measurement between the two parietal eminences of the fetal skull. It is a very useful measurement during the second trimester, but becomes less accurate towards the end of pregnancy because the shape of the head may alter. Limbs are also measured, most notably the femur.

The detailed fetal anomaly scan

This scan is usually performed at 18–22 weeks of pregnancy, since visualisation of fetal anatomy is more difficult before that time (Drife & Donnai 1991). The purpose of this scan is to reassure the mother that the fetus has no obvious structural abnormalities. Detection rates vary considerably, but it is thought that around 50% of significant abnormalities are identified at this time (Boyd et al 1998). This is influenced by the expertise of the sonographer and quality of the equipment, however. There may also be technical difficulties, such as fetal position, multiple pregnancy or maternal obesity.

Also, some structural problems do not have associated sonographic signs. An example of this would be tracheo-oesophageal fistula (an opening between the trachea and the lower oesophagus). Moreover, some fetal abnormalities, such as hydrocephalus and bowel obstructions, may not appear until later in pregnancy. Diagnosis may therefore be missed. Average detection rates for some abnormalities are presented in Table 23.2. It is vital that mothers are fully aware of the precise purpose and limitations of the detailed scan. The structures to be examined during the detailed scan are presented in Box 23.3.

Markers for chromosomal abnormality

Markers are minor sonographic clue signs, which increase the chance that the fetus has a chromosomal abnormality (most are associated with Down syndrome). They are seen in many normal fetuses (at least 5%) and, when

---

Box 23.3 Features examined on detailed fetal ultrasound scans

- Spine
- Head shape and internal structures (cavum pellucidum, cerebellum, ventricular size at atrium < 10 mm)
- Abdominal shape and content – at level of the stomach
- Abdominal shape and content – at the level of kidneys and umbilicus
- Renal pelvis < 5 mm
- Longitudinal axis, abdominal–thoracic appearance (diaphragm/bladder)
- Thorax – at level of four chamber cardiac view
- Arms – three bones and hand
- Legs – three bones and foot
- Face and lips
- Cardiac outflow tracts

(RCOG 2000)

Table 23.2 Detection rates of fetal abnormalities, if present, on detailed ultrasound scan

Problem	Chance of being seen (%)
Spina bifida	90
Anencephaly	99
Hydrocephalus	60
Major congenital heart problems	25
Diaphragmatic hernia	60
Exomphalos/gastroschisis	90
Major kidney problems	85
Major limb abnormalities	90
Cerebral palsy	Never seen
Autism	Never seen
Down syndrome	May be associated with heart or bowel problems in about 40%

(From RCOG 2000, with permission)

---

isolated, are of dubious value (Whittle 1997). Examples of such markers include the following:

Choroid plexus cyst. This is collection of cerebrospinal fluid within the choroids plexi, from where cerebrospinal fluid is derived.

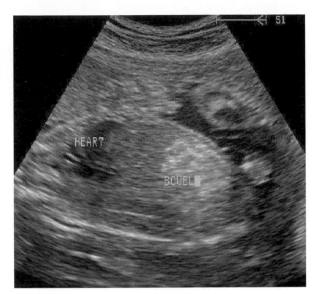

Fig. 23.4 Echogenic bowel. (Reproduced with permission of Nottingham City Hospital NHS Trust.)

Echogenic bowel. This is a bright appearance of the bowel, equivalent to the brightness of bone. It is also associated with intra-amniotic bleeding and fetal swallowing of bloodstained liquor (Fig. 23.4).

Nuchal fold >5 mm at 20 weeks' gestation. This is an increased thickness of fetal skin and fat at the back of the fetal neck. Subcutaneous fluid (NT) cannot usually be visualised after 14 weeks.

Echogenic foci in the heart. These are bright echoes from calcium deposits in the fetal heart, often the left ventricle. They do not affect cardiac function.

Dilated renal pelvis >5 mm. This may be due to slight backflow from the ureters and is more common in male fetuses.

Short femur. This is a shorter than average thigh bone, when compared with other fetal measurements.

Talipes. This is an abnormal angle between the leg and the foot. Most commonly, the foot points inwards and downwards. This is colloquially known as clubfoot.

Sandal gap. This is an exaggerated gap between the first and second toes.

The strength of association between each individual marker and Down syndrome varies considerably. As such, an increased nuchal fold increases the chances of an affected pregnancy by 10 times the background risk. Conversely, echogenic foci in the heart increase the chances only by a marginal factor of 1.2 (Snijders & Nicolaides 1996). When markers are identified, it is important to consider whether there are other risk factors, such as advancing maternal age or increased NT measurement at 10–14 weeks. The mother's aggregate risk for Down's can then be calculated, taking all these factors into account.

Advantages and disadvantages of fetal anomaly scans

Providing the sonographer has sufficient expertise, many lethal or severely disabling conditions can be detected during the 18–20 week scan. Although this means that parents may be faced with difficult and unexpected decisions, it may be that later psychological trauma and physical suffering can be prevented. Furthermore, many parents are offered reassurance that no obvious abnormalities were seen. There is also evidence that, for neonates requiring early surgical or paediatric interventions, prior knowledge of the abnormality allows a plan of care to be evolved in advance of the birth. The mother can then deliver in a unit with appropriate facilities. This has been shown to reduce morbidity in the cases of gastroschisis (an abdominal wall defect, adjacent to the umbilicus, allowing the intestines and other abdominal organs to protrude outside the body), cardiac abnormalities and intestinal obstruction (Chang et al 1991, Romero et al 1989).

However, there is also the potential for false positive findings that are not confirmed postnatally. In particular, markers for chromosomal abnormalities may cause considerable anxiety without having any clinical significance for the baby. Indeed, they may be regarded as variants of normal, particularly if the fetal chromosomes are proven to be normal.

There is also the problem of defining the prognosis for some recognisable abnormalities, as previously discussed. In summary, the 18–22 week scan appears to confer psychological and health improvement benefits in some cases, but also has the capacity to cause great anxiety and distress. Care must be taken to ensure that parents are fully informed of the purpose, benefits and limitations of ultrasound scans before they consent to this procedure. For a personal account of the psychological trauma experienced after an ultrasound scan, see the final section of this chapter.

Third trimester pregnancy scans

In general, late pregnancy scans are performed in response to a specific clinical need and not as a screen of the low risk pregnant population. However, fetal abnormalities may come to light or be reassessed at this time. Many late scans are performed as a means of monitoring fetal well-being, growth and development.

Fetal growth

Many scans are performed in order to detect instances when growth deviates from normal. Fetuses with excessive growth (*macrosomia*) have increased perinatal mortality and morbidity. There may be cephalopelvic disproportion or shoulder dystocia, with consequent birth asphyxia and trauma. In most cases, there is no apparent cause, but there is sometimes an association with maternal diabetes mellitus. Serial growth measurements are indicated in this latter group.

Fetuses may be small because they are preterm or because they are small for dates. Sometimes, these two problems overlap. In general, growth-restricted babies can be divided into two groups:

Symmetrical growth retardation. Most symmetrically small fetuses are entirely normal and may be genetically predetermined to be small. However, in some instances this may be caused by chromosomal abnormalities, infection or environmental factors such as maternal substance misuse.

Asymmetrical growth retardation. These fetuses have a head size appropriate for gestational age, but thin bodies. This is generally caused by placental insufficiency, whereby the placenta is unable to provide sufficient nourishment for the fetus. Glycogen stores in the liver are reduced, so there are less energy reserves for the fetus during labour. Asymmetrically growth-restricted fetuses are therefore more likely to suffer antenatal or perinatal asphyxia, or both. Other potential problems include hypoglycaemia, hypothermia and premature delivery.

In order to assess fetal growth, the gestational age must be accurately assessed on scan before 24 weeks. Women at high risk of having an abnormally grown fetus should have serial scans – often at 28, 32 and 36 weeks. Where there is a particular concern, growth may be measured every 2 weeks. The most important measurements are head circumference and abdominal circumference. In this way, trends in fetal growth can be assessed.

Doppler ultrasonography

In recent years, there have been major developments in the use of Doppler ultrasound techniques for the study of maternal and fetal circulation. Placental blood flow can be assessed using the Doppler shift (a change in the frequency of ultrasound wave reflection, according to the speed and direction of blood flow). Compromises in maternofetal circulation can then be identified. Abnormalities in Doppler measurements may be detected before growth becomes impaired and can be used as a prognostic indicator. This technique is now considered invaluable in high risk pregnancies (Trudinger 1999).

Biophysical profiling

Another ultrasound measure of fetal well-being is the fetal biophysical profile. This is used to determine whether there are signs of fetal hypoxia or compromised placental function, or both. A score is calculated on the basis of five criteria (Manning et al 1980). These are listed as follows:

- **Fetal breathing movements.** In the healthy fetus, breathing movements can be visualised in the third trimester of pregnancy. This helps develop respiratory muscles before birth. There should be at least 30 seconds of sustained fetal breathing movements in 30 minutes of observation.
- **Fetal movements.** Movement is often compromised in hypoxic fetuses. There should be three or more gross body movements in 30 minutes of observation. Simultaneous limb and trunk movements are counted as a single movement.
- **Fetal tone.** There should be at least one episode of motion of a limb from a position of flexion to extension and rapid return to flexion. Absence of fetal movement is counted as absence of fetal tone.
- **Fetal reactivity.** There should be two or more fetal heart accelerations of at least 15 beats per minute, within 40 minutes of observation. These should last at least 15 seconds and be associated with fetal movement. This may best be recorded on a fetal CTG.
- **Qualitative amniotic fluid volume.** There should be a pocket of amniotic fluid that measures at least 1 centimetre in two perpendicular planes. Placental

insufficiency often results in decreased renal perfusion in the fetus and reduced urinary output. Consequently, liquor volume can become reduced.

Findings from growth scans, biophysical profile scores and CTG recordings should be considered collectively, taking into account the full clinical picture and obstetric history.

Screening for fetal abnormality from maternal serum

Neural tube defect screening

Alpha fetoprotein (AFP) is present in fetal serum and amniotic fluid by 6 weeks' gestation. Thereafter, the levels alter according to gestation (Aitken & Crossley 1995). When the fetal neural tube does not fully close during organogenesis (resulting in spina bifida or anencephaly), AFP can escape in increased amounts. Therefore, when the fetus has an open neural tube defect, AFP levels are raised in maternal serum. A blood sample from the mother at 15–18 weeks' gestation has a detection rate of 98% (Aitken & Crossley 1995). Since the AFP level varies according to gestational age, it is important to assess the gestation accurately before results can be reliably interpreted.

Around 2% of mothers have a raised AFP level, but this is usually due to reasons other than fetal anomaly (Kennard et al 1995). Other reasons for raised AFP levels include multiple pregnancy, incorrect gestation and threatened miscarriage. These days, detailed ultrasound scanning is the main diagnostic tool for neural tube defects, so AFP screening is less useful. However, raised AFP levels can be predictive of intrauterine growth restriction and pre-eclampsia. Pregnancies with raised AFP levels are therefore considered to be high risk.

Down syndrome screening from maternal serum

A variety of biochemical markers in maternal serum have been used, in order to assess the risk of Down syndrome. The most common ones are AFP (reduced in many affected pregnancies), HCG (which is usually raised) and unconjugated estriol (uE_3, which is usually low). If all three markers are used, this is called the *triple test*. If only AFP and HCG are used, this is called the *double test*. Maternal blood is sampled at 15–18 weeks' gestation.

The levels of the biochemical markers are considered in conjunction with maternal age. A combined risk is then calculated. If this risk is greater than a specified limit (often 1 in 250), the mother is considered to be in a high risk group and is offered further diagnostic tests. On average, the detection rate for this test is 60%, with a false positive rate of 5% (Haddow & Palomaki 1999). This is better than the use of maternal age alone, but the test has some important limitations. To begin with, there is considerable overlap between the average levels of AFP in affected versus unaffected pregnancies. This is demonstrated in Figure 23.5 and results in difficulties in distinguishing between the two groups.

As for AFP alone, it is vital that the gestation is accurately assessed. Also, vaginal bleeding can alter the results by increasing AFP. Diabetic mothers may have reduced levels of all serum markers. These tend to be slightly high in Afro-Caribbean women. Since the incidence of Down syndrome is related to maternal age, this factor is included in the risk calculation. However, this method of analysis means that the detection rates and false positive rates vary considerably, according to the mother's age. This is presented in Table 23.3.

The increased probability of a high risk result among older mothers can cause much anxiety. It is

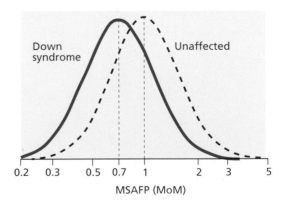

Fig. 23.5 Average values of AFP in normal and Down syndrome pregnancies. (From Haddow & Palomaki 1999, with permission of Harcourt.)

Table 23.3 Detection rates and false positive rates for the triple test (risk cut-off level 1 in 250)

Maternal age group (years)	Probability of a screen positive result	Detection rate (%)
Under 25	1 in 45	35
25–29	1 in 30	40
30–34	1 in 15	55
35–39	1 in 5	75
40–44	1 in 2	95
45 and over	>1 in 2	>99
All	1 in 20	60

(From Kennard et al 1995, reproduced with the permission of the Royal College of Midwives)

therefore important that mothers are aware of the chances of this happening before they consent to undergo the test. Mothers should also be aware that, in the event of a high risk result, they would be offered a diagnostic test with associated risk of miscarriage. Occasionally, parents may also be faced with unexpected decisions regarding termination of pregnancy.

Invasive diagnostic tests

If mothers are found to have an increased risk of chromosomal or genetic problems, they may wish to undergo a diagnostic procedure. The two most frequently used tests are chorionic villus sampling (CVS) and amniocentesis. They should be performed in specialist centres, by obstetricians with specific training and expertise. These tests provide the opportunity to examine the fetal karyotype (the number and structure of chromosomes, visible through a microscope during mitotic metaphase) or DNA analysis for particular gene mutations, or both.

Chorionic villus sampling

Chorionic villus sampling is the acquisition of chorionic villi (placental tissue) under continuous ultrasound guidance. Chorionic villi originate from the same cells as the fetus and therefore generally have the same genes and chromosomes. This may be performed at any stage after 10 weeks of pregnancy.

Access may be achieved transcervically (until 13 weeks' gestation) or via the transabdominal route. When CVS is performed *transcervically*, a catheter is introduced through the cervix and is guided into the chorion frondosum. Suction is then applied to an attached syringe and 10–40 mg of tissue are aspirated. This procedure is represented in Figure 23.6.

The *transabdominal* approach involves the insertion of a needle into the maternal abdomen. Under ultrasound guidance, the needle is pushed through the uterine wall and into placental tissue. Tissue is aspirated

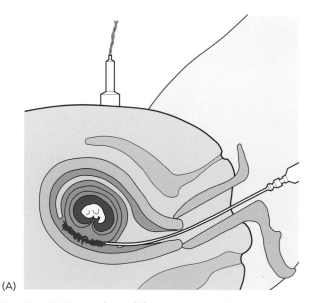

(A)

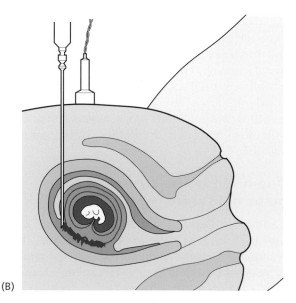

(B)

Fig. 23.6 CVS procedures: (A) transcervical catheter aspiration; (B) transabdominal puncture. (From Holzgreve et al 1999, with permission of Harcourt.)

via an attached syringe. Villi are carefully separated from maternal decidua under a dissection microscope, prior to cytogenetic (chromosome) analysis.

In general, there are two stages to the reporting of results. The direct preparation result is issued after 24–48 hours and gives a chromosome count (e.g. to test for Down syndrome). Cells are then cultured for 14–21 days, to confirm the direct results and to allow more detailed cytogenetic examination of the chromosome structure. DNA (for genetic) or biochemical (for metabolic) diagnoses can also be obtained from chorionic villi tissue.

The main advantage of CVS is that this is the earliest way mothers can obtain definitive information about the chromosomal/genetic status of the fetus. Mothers who are known carriers of particular disorders often have high recurrence risks and so are anxious until their results are known. If the news is not good and mothers wish to end their pregnancy, a surgical procedure can be performed. After 12–13 weeks, terminations are usually induced medically, in order to reduce the risk of causing cervical incompetence. This process of induction and vaginal delivery can be very distressing. Decisions about termination of pregnancy may also become more difficult as the pregnancy progresses, since the mother begins to feel fetal movements and becomes visibly pregnant. Most women considering diagnostic procedures prefer to have an early test (Abramsky & Rodeck 1991). The main disadvantage with CVS is the procedure-induced risk of miscarriage. This is 0.5–2%, depending upon the experience of the operator (National Electronic Library for Health 2001) and occurs because of infection or bleeding. Also, ambiguous results are obtained in 1% of samplings (Holzgreve et al 1999).

Early CVS has been associated with limb reduction abnormalities. However, a large WHO international trial found the incidence of these abnormalities to be equal to the background rate (6 per 10 000), providing CVS was performed after 10 weeks. If CVS is performed prior to this gestation (i.e. during organogenesis), there is a higher chance that it may be harmful. Consequently, the WHO recommends 10 weeks as the earliest safe gestation for the procedure (Froster & Jackson 1996). In general, if an experienced operator with sufficient counselling support performs CVS, it is an effective and safe means of gaining early information about the fetus.

Amniocentesis

This is usually performed after 15 weeks' gestation, since early amniocentesis has a higher loss rate than early CVS (Nicolaides et al 1994). The procedure involves transabdominal insertion of a fine needle into the amniotic fluid cavity, under continuous ultrasound guidance; 15 ml of amniotic fluid are aspirated. Cytogenetic, molecular (DNA) and biochemical analyses are possible. Amniocytes are often examined. These comprise cells that have been shed from several fetal sites, including skin, lungs and renal tract. The risk of procedure-induced miscarriage is 1% (National Electronic Library for Health 2001), although 2–3% of mothers have some leakage of amniotic fluid (Simpson et al 1981). Miscarriage is usually caused by infection or spontaneous rupture of the membranes at the puncture site.

Amniocentesis has traditionally been performed more commonly than CVS, mainly because more obstetricians had the required training. However, recent clinical governance initiatives have resulted in a move towards performing invasive procedures only in specialist centres. This is important because procedure loss rates are so dependent on the operator. In the second trimester of pregnancy, CVS and amniocentesis have similar risks and benefits. The miscarriage risks are comparable and, in most cases, both tests provide the required information.

Recent advances in cytogenetic techniques mean that mothers can obtain an initial set of results (usually for Down syndrome) and then a full culture result after 2–3 weeks. This involves the use of fluorescent in situ hybridisation (FISH), whereby a specific probe 'paints' the chromosomes to be examined. For example, for Down syndrome, the probe appears fluorescent under a microscope when in contact with chromosome 21. Cells are examined to determine whether there are two or three signals for this chromosome. Two is the normal count, whereas three indicates Down syndrome. Since many mothers undergo amniocentesis because of a high risk serum screening result or identification of markers on scan, they are very anxious to obtain quick results. For this reason, the use of FISH has greatly enhanced service delivery. For examples of cytogenetic analyses, see Figure 23.7 and Plate 10.

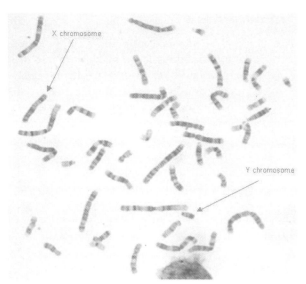

Fig. 23.7 Normal male chromosomes. (From Dept of Cytogenetics, Nottingham City Hospital NHS Trust, with permission.)

Fetal blood sampling

The use of this technique has declined in recent years because improved molecular and cytogenetic techniques allow more diagnoses to be made from chorionic villi or amniotic fluid. However, fetal blood may be advantageous when there are ambiguous findings from placental tissue. Also, when there is Rhesus isoimmunisation, it may be necessary to determine the fetal haemoglobin. When this is low, an intrauterine transfusion may be performed. Blood can be sampled from the umbilical cord or intrahepatic umbilical vein. The latter is less risky, as there are no umbilical arteries in close proximity. The loss rate also depends upon the gestation and condition of the fetus. In uncomplicated procedures after 20 weeks, the loss rate is around 1% (Holzgreve et al 1999).

New and emerging technologies

Magnetic resonance imaging

Magnetic resonance imaging (MRI) has been applied to examination of the fetus over the last two decades. This technique has not been widely applied because ultrasound can give similar diagnostic information at a lower cost. However, MRI may have a contribution to make, particularly when examining the brain. There is evidence that this may provide additional information and change the counselling and management for a significant number of pregnancies where brain abnormalities are suspected (Levine et al 1997). A further possible application is that MRI could offer an alternative to postmortem following termination or perinatal death. This may offer information to parents who decline postmortem because of its invasive nature (Editorial 1997). MRI may also be useful in providing serial brain images following asphyxia in the newborn. This may give us a better understanding of the evolution of brain injury (Maalouf et al 1998).

Fetal cells in the maternal circulation

There is presently much research into the use of fetal cells in maternal blood for genetic diagnosis. This would be helpful to mothers who want diagnostic information without the risk of procedure-induced miscarriage of a potentially normal fetus. Attention is currently focused on finding the best fetal cell type for analysis. There is also much research aiming to find the best techniques for isolating and enriching these cells for diagnosis.

Fetal cells are consistently detected in maternal serum by 10 weeks' gestation (Simpson & Elias 1999). The frequency of fetal cells in maternal blood may depend on cytogenetic status. It is thought that karyotypically abnormal pregnancies are more likely to have 'leaky' placentas, which allow more fetal cells to escape into the maternal circulation (Alter 1994). This finding may help the development of a non-invasive diagnostic technique.

One concern about the technique is that fetal cells may persist in fetal circulation from prior pregnancies. This may be significant if the mother has had a previous karyotypically abnormal pregnancy. Many such pregnancies miscarry early, so the mother may not be aware that this has happened. However, refinements in the particular type of cell to be targeted should minimise the risk of such an error occurring. It is not yet clear how this technology will be applied clinically. Certainly, a non-invasive method of diagnosis would be very attractive for mothers and clinicians alike. However, it may be that fetal cells in maternal blood can provide information only about the likelihood of a problem. In that case, it may be possible to use fetal cells only as an alternative screening test.

Fetal therapy

There are certain instances when therapeutic interventions may improve fetal prognoses. For instance, therapeutic amniocentesis may be performed to drain excess liquor. This may reduce the likelihood of preterm labour when the uterus is large-for-dates. Therapeutic amniocentesis is also sometimes performed in monochorionic twin pregnancies with twin-to-twin transfusion syndrome (discordant placental circulation and consequent discordant growth and liquor volume – if severe, this has a poor prognosis for both babies). Liquor is drained from the largest sac; this sometimes helps equal the pressures between the twins and allows both fetuses to grow satisfactorily.

Another treatment that is sometimes used is laser treatment to reduce pathological placental flow between the twins. Shunts can also be inserted into the fetus in order to drain pathological collections of fluid. These include ascites and renal obstruction (Freedman et al 1999). However, whilst there may be some improvement in outcome, much will depend on the underlying cause of the obstruction. This is often not known in the antenatal period.

Conclusion

A mother is now able to obtain a considerable amount of information about her unborn fetus. This may alter the experience of being pregnant, by increasing anxiety and delaying attachment. However, if mothers receive sufficient information and support, fetal investigations may increase autonomy and save long term suffering. It is necessary for the midwife to treat parents sensitively and honestly. This will help parents to cope with the choices and decisions created by the availability of antenatal fetal investigations. The profound psychological effects of ultrasound scans are vividly depicted by a mother in the following section: 'A testing time'.

A testing time

I was called upon some time ago to outline my experiences of antenatal investigations to a midwives' research group, I did this and thought at the time that I was bearing my soul to 200 people that I had never met before. I can only guess at the readership of this textbook and so with great trepidation I will attempt to give a taste of what antenatal investigations are like from the parents' side of the fence and hopefully 'bring alive' some of the traumas and dilemmas involved. The research, the facts, the paper evidence are there for all to see, whereas the emotions, considerations and 'angst' are less tangible; here is what it feels like to experience the process of diagnostic testing.

My husband and I knew early on in my pregnancy that I was expecting twins; having digested in some measure that awesome news, we nervously attended the hospital for my detailed scan. Everything seemed fine, the babies were assessed and all the checks made, except the position of the lower twin meant that the spine could not be seen clearly. We waited outside, I drank yet more water, though my bladder was bursting already, hoping that the baby would change position. We were euphoric, two baby girls on the way, how pleased our families would be, getting carried away we even started to consider possible names: Amy, Alice, Emily, Lucy … (see Figure 23.8).

We re-entered the room to continue the scan and amongst the, 'yes, that's fine, there's the other leg, etc.,' we detected a different intonation in the radiographer's voice as she said, 'Ah, echogenic foci, there's a small marker near the baby's heart, a calcium deposit. It's probably nothing, but I'll tell you about it anyway even though some radiographers would not even mention it. An echogenic focus is a soft indicator of Down syndrome.' The words hit us like a hammer; there was nothing remotely 'soft' about what we had just heard. In literally a few minutes and the length of a hospital corridor the effect of that discovery was to have a devastating impact on us and our families.

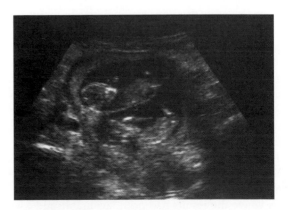

Fig. 23.8 The scan of the twins.

We were ushered to the other end of the corridor where the facts were explained to us. We were told percentage risk factors for women of a certain age and Down's, risk factors associated with amniocentesis; fact followed fact followed fact. That I was carrying twins complicated matters. Do we have both babies tested? How significantly does that increase the risk of miscarriage? What if one baby is fine and the other shows signs of abnormality? Would we be able to cope with a handicapped child? Can one baby be aborted? Question followed question followed question. We were given all the known evidence associated with our predicament and, whilst in our rational minds we understood the notion of professional ethics, we most desperately craved the one thing we could not have, a considered expert medical opinion. Fine we knew about all the research, but how could we, with so little medical knowledge or familiarity with such situations, even begin to make such a monumental decision?

The journey home was a silent one; to say that we hardly knew how we got from A to B is not to overstate our sense of confusion and trauma. My parents were in the middle of a meal when we arrived. Having delivered the news about two grand-daughters there followed the giant, 10 feet tall letters of BUT … The effect was instantaneous; not another bite was eaten.

There followed 3 days of complete bewilderment as we tried to cope with the dilemma we faced and the monstrous decisions we had to make. We considered a million times the avenues available and canvassed everyone's opinion: family, friends, work colleagues, my local midwife, my health visitor, people we knew in the medical profession. Despite comforting and reassuring words, no respite came as we were forced to acknowledge any decisions were going to be exclusively ours; how desperately we needed advice!

We decided to have the amniocentesis on one baby and even now, 2 years on, the reasons as to why we chose this option are not clear, just as they were not at the time. Intuition, selfishness, whim, we really did not know if we were doing the right thing. In our minds, facts and research belong in textbooks; we were people craving guidance.

Funnily enough I did not find the actual test too awful. As we waited our turn, a member of the consultant's team shared with us similar cases she had dealt with where the results had been favourable and I will never forget her words when she said, 'I've got a good feeling about this, I'm sure everything will be fine.' This was the most human of comments from a professional that we had the pleasure to hear; it truly was like manna from heaven. Of course we knew that she could not possibly anticipate the results of the test, but her words at least made us feel there was some hope. Over the next 2 weeks we were to cling to those words time and time and time again. As we left the unit we were told, 'give us a ring in a couple of weeks', and for what seemed like much longer than 2 weeks we were casually cast adrift to contemplate and imagine the results of the test.

Without wishing to jargonise or be drawn into using a cliché-ridden phrase, those 2 weeks were literally nightmarish. The comments people had made played over and over and over in our minds. 'I'll tell you this but it's probably nothing … echogenic-foci … soft indicator of Down's … I've got a good feeling about this …' We merely functioned at work, nothing more; our lives were on hold and we were both emotionally and physically drained. We shrank from conversation with others and between ourselves on occasions; we considered innumerable times the possible outcomes. We slept fitfully; one night I sat on the stairs sobbing as I contemplated death, funerals and the fact that our babies may never exist in our world. My own midwife made a poignant and frighteningly accurate comment when she said that I was 'mourning' my babies – she was right. I was numb, we both were!

When the day for the result finally arrived there was absolutely no possibility that I could have made the call to the hospital. My husband was to phone up and then relay the news to me at work, but there were safety measures! Bad news, no call, no test results, no call, this gave me a get-out and ensured that hope could live on. To say I shook as I took my husband's phone call is a massive understatement and upon hearing the good news I broke down, utterly and completely. The pent-up emotion of the previous 2 weeks poured out. That I hugged the headteacher, ignoring, forgetting or simply not caring about protocol, is an indication of the level of euphoria and relief I felt.

Our daughters were born on the 18th of January 1999, weighing in at 5 lbs 15 oz and 6 lb 11 oz (age 2¼ in Fig. 23.9).

Many, many issues were contemplated during this 'testing' experience – amongst them, can research be too advanced? A few years ago it is unlikely that such a marker would have been detected and a trouble-free pregnancy would have ensued! Most significantly the role of counselling and support offered to women undergoing diagnostic tests must be considered as a vital component in the whole process.

I do not know if I am a better or different person as a result of my experience of diagnostic testing. I do know, however, that it is forever etched in my mind and heart; talking and writing about it even now feels incredibly emotional, vivid and raw.

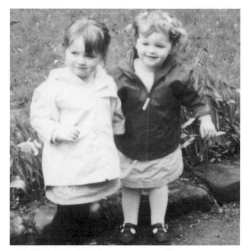

Fig. 23.9 The twins.

REFERENCES

Abramsky L, Rodeck C H 1991 Women's choices for fetal chromosome anomalies. Prenatal Diagnosis 11:23

Aitken D A, Crossley J A 1995 Prenatal screening – biochemical. In: Whittle M J, Connor J M (eds) Prenatal diagnosis in obstetric practice, 2nd edn. Blackwell Science, London, p 12–29

Al-Jader L N, Parry Langdon N, Smith R J 2000 Survey of attitudes of pregnant women towards Down syndrome screening. Prenatal Diagnosis 20:23–29

Alter E P 1994 Biology of erythropoiesis. In: Simpson J L, Elias S (eds) Fetal cells in maternal blood: prospects for non-invasive diagnosis. NY Academy of Science, New York, p 36–47

Andrews L, Fullerton J, Holtzman N, Motulsky A 1994 Assessing genetic risks. Implications for health and social policy. National Academy Press, Washington DC

Berryman J C, Windridge K C 1995 Motherhood after 35. A report of the Leicester motherhood project. Leicester University/Nestlé, England

Black R B 1992 Seeing the baby: the impact of ultrasound technology. Journal of Genetic Counselling 1:45–54

Bosward K L, Barnett S B, Wood A K et al 1993 Heating of guinea pig fetal brain during exposure to pulsed ultrasound. Ultrasound in Medicine and Biology 19(5):415–424

Boyd P A, Chamberlain P, Hicks N R 1998 Six-year experience of prenatal diagnosis in an unselected population in Oxford. Lancet 352:1577–1581

Chang A C, Huhta J C, Yoon G Y 1991 Diagnosis, transport and outcome in fetuses with left ventricular outflow tract obstruction. Journal of Thoracic and Cardiovascular Surgery 102:841–848

Chitty L, Barnes C A, Berry C 1996 Continuing with the pregnancy after a diagnosis of lethal abnormality. British Medical Journal 313:701–702

Clarke A 1994 Genetic counselling. Practice and principles. Routledge, London

Clement S, Wilson J, Sikorski 1998 Women's experiences of antenatal ultrasound scans. In: Clement S (ed) Psychological perspectives on pregnancy and childbirth. Churchill Livingstone, Edinburgh, p 117–132

Cooper T J 2001 Informed consent is a primary requisite of quality care. British Journal of Midwifery 9(1):42–45

Cuckle H S, Wald N J, Thompson S G 1987 Estimating a woman's risk of having a pregnancy associated with Down syndrome using her age and serum alpha feto-protein level. British Journal of Obstetrics and Gynaecology 94:387–402

Dragonas T, Christodoulou G N 1998 Prenatal care. Clinical Psychology Review 18(2):127–142

Drife J O, Donnai D 1991 Antenatal diagnosis of fetal abnormalities. Springer-Verlag, London

[Editorial] 1997 Postmortem perinatal examination: the role of magnetic resonance imaging. Ultrasound in Obstetrics and Gynaecology 145–147

Farrant W 1985 Who's for amniocentesis? The politics of prenatal screening. In: Homans H (ed) The sexual politics of prenatal screening. Gower Press, London

Ferguson P 2001 Skimming the surface: antenatal screening and testing. RCM Midwives Journal 4(8):262–264

Freedman A L, Johnson M P, Smith C A et al 1999 Long-term outcome in children after antenatal intervention for obstructive uropathies. Lancet 354:374–377

Froster U G, Jackson L 1996 Limb defects after chorionic villus sampling: results from an international registry, 1992–1994. Lancet 347:489–494

Furness M E 1990 Fetal ultrasound for entertainment? Medical Journal of Australia 153:371

Haddow J E, Palomaki G E 1999 Biochemical screening for neural tube defects and Down syndrome. In: Rodeck C H, Whittle M J (eds) Fetal medicine: basic science and clinical practice. Churchill Livingstone, Edinburgh, p 373–388

Hawkey M 1998 Psychological impacts on pregnancy: from hormones to genes. British Journal of Midwifery 6(5):310

HMSO 1991 Certificate A (form HSAI). Certificate to be completed before an abortion is performed under Section 1 of the Abortion Act 1967. HMSO, London

Holzgreve W, Tercanli S, Surbek D, Minig P 1999 Invasive diagnostic methods. In: Rodeck C H, Whittle M J (eds) Fetal medicine: basic science and clinical practice. Churchill Livingstone, Edinburgh, p 417–434

Hunter M 1994 Counselling in obstetrics and gynaecology. British Psychological Society Books, Leicester

Ingram R, Malcarne V 1995 Cognition in depression and anxiety. Same, different or a little of both. In: Craig K, Dobson K (eds) Anxiety and depression in adults and children. Sage, London, p 37–56

Karp L 1983 The terrible question. American Journal of Medical Genetics 23:359–362

Kennard A, Goodburn S, Golightly S et al 1995 Serum screening for Down syndrome. Royal College of Midwives Journal 108(1290):207–210

Kessler S, Levine E 1987 Psychological aspects of genetic counselling IV. The subjective assessment of probability. American Journal of Medical Genetics 28:361–370

Kingston H M 1994 ABC of clinical genetics. BMJ Publishing, London

Langford J 1992 Over 35 and at risk? New Generation 11(4):4–5

Levine D, Barnes P D, Madsen J R et al 1997 Fetal central nervous system anomalies: MR imaging augments sonographic diagnosis. Radiology 204(3):635–642

Lichenstein S, Slovic P, Fischhoff B et al 1978 Judged frequency of lethal events. Journal of Experimental Psychology: Human Learning and Memory 4:551–578

Maalouf E F, Counsell S, Battin M et al 1998 Magnetic resonance imaging of the neonatal brain. Hospital Medicine 59:41–45

Manning F A, Platt L D, Sipros L 1980 Antepartum fetal evaluation: development of a fetal biophysical profile. American Journal of Obstetrics and Gynaecology 136:787–795

Marteau T M 1993 Psychological consequences of screening for Down syndrome. Still being given too little attention. British Medical Journal 307:146–147

National Electronic Library for Health 2001 Down syndrome screening. Invasive diagnosis. Online. Available: www.nelh.nhs.uk/screening/

Neilson J P 1999 Ultrasound for fetal assessment in early pregnancy. Cochrane review. In: The Cochrane Library, Issue 3. Update Software, Oxford

Newnham J P, Evans S F, Mehael C A et al 1993 Effects of frequent ultrasound during pregnancy: a randomised controlled trial. Lancet 342:887–891

Nicolaides K, de Lourdes B M, Patel F, Snijders R 1994 Comparison of chorionic villus sampling and amniocentesis for fetal karyotyping at 10–13 weeks gestation. Lancet 344:435–439

Nicolaides K H, Souka A P, Noble P L 1999 Fetal nuchal translucency at 10–14 weeks of gestation. In: Rodeck C, Whittle M J (eds) Fetal medicine. Basic science and clinical practice. Churchill Livingstone, London, p 573–580

Oliver S, Rajan L, Turner H et al 1996 A pilot study of 'informed choice' leaflets on positions in labour and routine ultrasound. NHS Centre for Reviews and Dissemination, York

Raphael-Leff J 1991 Psychological processes of childbearing. Chapman & Hall, London

RCOG (Royal College of Obstetricians and Gynaecologists) 2000 Routine ultrasound screening in pregnancy. Protocol, standards and training. Supplement to ultrasound screening for fetal abnormalities report of the RCOG working party. RCOG, London

Robinson J 2001 Prenatal screening: a retrospective study. British Journal of Midwifery 9(7):412–417

Romero R, Ghidini A, Costigan K et al 1989 Prenatal diagnosis of duodenal atresia: does it make any difference? Obstetrics and Gynaecology 71:739–741

Rothman B 1986 The tentative pregnancy. How amniocentesis changes the experience of motherhood. Norton Paperbacks, New York

Salvesen K A 1997 Epidemiology of diagnostic ultrasound exposure during human pregnancies. BMUS Bulletin November:32–34

Salvesen K A, Vatten L J, Eik-Nes S H et al 1993 Routine ultrasonography in utero and subsequent handedness and neurological development. British Medical Journal 307:159–164

Sandelowski M 1994 Channel of desire: fetal ultrasonography in two-use contexts. Qualitative Health Research 4:262–280

Simpson J L, Elias S 1999 Fetal cells in the maternal circulation. In: Rodeck C H, Whittle M J (eds) Fetal medicine: basic science and clinical practice. Churchill Livingstone, Edinburgh, p 409–416

Simpson J L, Socol M I, Aladam S 1981 Normal fetal growth despite persistent amniotic fluid leakage after genetic amniocentesis. Prenatal Diagnosis 1:277

Sjogren B 1996 Psychological indications for prenatal diagnosis. Prenatal Diagnosis 16:449–454

Snijders R, Nicolaides K 1996 Ultrasound markers for fetal chromosomal defects. Parthenon, London

Stark C, Orleans M, Haverkamp A et al 1984 Short and long-term risks after exposure to diagnostic ultrasound in utero. Obstetrics and Gynaecology 63:194–200

Thomas B G 1998 The disempowering concept of risk. Practising Midwife 1(12):18–21

Thornton J G, Hewison J, Lilford R J et al 1995 A randomised trial of three methods of giving information about prenatal testing. British Medical Journal 311:1127–1130

Tindall N 1997 Psychology of childbearing. Midwifery practice guides 6. Books for Midwives Press, Hale, Cheshire

Trudinger B 1999 Doppler ultrasonography. In: Rodeck C H, Whittle M J (eds) Fetal medicine: basic science and clinical practice. Churchill Livingstone, Edinburgh, p 955–966

Turner L 1994 Problems surrounding late prenatal diagnosis. In: Abramsky L, Chapple J (eds) Prenatal diagnosis. The human side. Chapman & Hall, London

Ward P 2001 Antenatal screening: island to archipelago? Royal College of Midwives Journal 4(9):302–303

Whittle M J 1997 Ultrasonographic 'soft markers' of fetal chromosomal defects. (Editorial.) British Medical Journal 314:918

Wood P 2000 Safe and (ultra)sound – some aspects of ultrasound safety. Royal College of Midwives Journal 3(2):48–50

FURTHER READING

Hunter M 1994 Counselling in obstetrics and gynaecology. British Psychological Society Books, Leicester

This book provides practical guidelines for professionals dealing with sensitive issues.

Raphael-Leff J 1991 Psychological processes of childbearing. Chapman & Hall, New York

An in-depth exploration of the psychology of pregnancy, written by a practising psychoanalyst.

Rothman B 1986 The tentative pregnancy. How amniocentesis changes the experience of motherhood. Norton, New York

Although this text has been published for some time, it remains one of the key texts when considering the psychology of antenatal testing. The book contains many personal accounts from mothers undergoing tests and greatly assists the midwife's understanding of common feelings and emotions.

USEFUL ADDRESS

National Electronic Library for Health
www.nelh.nhs.uk/screening/
This website provides much information about screening, for professionals and the public. It gives up-to-date information about screening provision and changes in policy. This includes fetal, maternal and neonatal programmes.

4

Section 4
Labour

SECTION CONTENTS

24

The First Stage of Labour: Physiology and Early Care

Carol McCormick

CHAPTER CONTENTS

The transition from pregnancy to labour is a sequence of events that begins gradually. The first stage of labour, although difficult to diagnose, is usually recognised by the onset of regular uterine contractions and culminates in complete dilatation of the cervix.

The chapter aims to:

- encourage midwives to consider the onset and diagnosis of labour, and how it can be recognised by both the woman and the midwife

- describe some of the physical changes taking place as labour progresses

- reflect on interventions and timing of care in order to optimise the well being of the woman and her baby during the course of labour.

Changes during the last few weeks of pregnancy

The physiological transition from being a pregnant woman to becoming a mother means an enormous change for each woman both physically and psychologically. It is a time when every system in the body is affected and the experience, though unfortunately not joyous for all, represents a major occurrence in a woman's life.

During the last few weeks of pregnancy a number of changes may occur:

- Mood swings are common and a surge of energy may be experienced.
- Two to three weeks before the onset of labour the lower uterine segment expands and allows the fetal head to sink lower and it may engage in the pelvis, particularly in first time mothers. When this happens the fundus of the uterus descends and there is

more room for the lungs, breathing is easier, and the heart and stomach can function more easily. The woman experiences a relief, which is historically known as *lightening*. Under hormonal influence, the symphysis pubis widens and the pelvic floor becomes more relaxed and softened, allowing the uterus to descend further into the pelvis. There is engagement of the fetal head (Fig. 24.1).

- Walking may become more difficult for some women at the end of pregnancy because the symphysis pubis is more mobile and relaxation of the sacroiliac joints may give rise to backache. Conditions such as symphysis pubis dysfunction are increasingly being recognised and treated.
- Relief of pressure at the fundus results in an increase in pressure within the pelvis, which may be accounted for by the presence of the fetal head causing venous congestion of the whole pelvis. Vaginal secretions may also increase at this time. The presence of the fetal head in the pelvis can also give rise to frequency of micturition, urgency and some degree of stress incontinence.

In a healthy pregnancy the placenta nourishes and protects the growing fetus; the body of the uterus remains relaxed and the cervix closed (Fig. 24.2). As birth approaches the non-progressive Braxton Hicks contractions experienced during pregnancy alter and intensify to become the progressive form of labour. The cervix, which has remained firm and closed, becomes soft and dilatable. Accompanying the physical changes the woman may have feelings of great intensity varying from excited anticipation to fearful expectancy. The midwife and other supporters must exercise great sensitivity at this time in order to meet the specific needs and hopes of the woman.

Labour, purely in the physical sense, may be described as the process by which the fetus, placenta and membranes are expelled through the birth canal – but of course labour is much more than a purely physical event. What happens during labour can affect the relationship between mother and baby and can influence future pregnancies.

Normal labour occurs between 37 and 42 weeks' gestation, but, unlike other mammals, humans do not have a very precise gestation period (Kirkman 2001). Human gestation is said to be around 280 days, plus or minus 10 days. The World Health Organisation (WHO 1997) defines normal labour as low risk throughout, spontaneous in onset with the fetus presenting by the vertex, culminating in the mother and infant in good condition following birth. All definitions of labour appear to be purely physiological and do not encompass the psychological well-being of the parents.

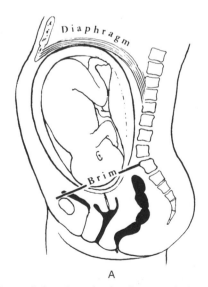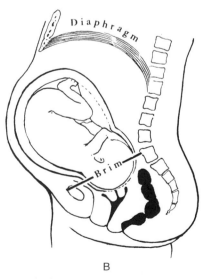

Fig. 24.1 (A) *Prior to lightening.* The fundus crowds the diaphragm. The lower uterine segment is not soft and has not stretched to accommodate the fetal head, which therefore remains high. The lower segment is `V' shaped. (B) *After lightening.* The fundus sinks below the diaphragm and breathing is easier. The lower segment is `U' shaped; it has softened and dilated so that the head sinks down into it and may partly enter the pelvic brim.

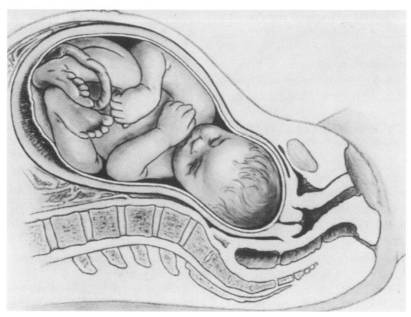

Fig. 24.2 Fetus in utero at the beginning of labour.

Once physiological labour commences its progress is measured by descent of the head and dilatation of the cervix. The expected rate of cervical dilatation in labour was based on work by Friedman during the 1950s, but more recent research demonstrates that the process of labour in terms of cervical dilatation should not be strictly timed and may last longer than some clinicians expect. The criteria for distinguishing normal labour from abnormal labour based on time limits needs revision (Albers 1999).

Traditionally three stages of labour are described: the first, second and third stage. But this is a rather pedantic view as labour is obviously a continuous process. There is increasing acknowledgement that there are not just three clear phases of normal labour. Sherblom Matteson (2001) gives a full description of this view of more than three stages to labour, along with not only the physical changes but the emotional effects observed in women at this time.

First stage

- The latent phase is prior to active first stage of labour and may last 6–8 hours in first time mothers when the cervix dilates from 0 cm to 3–4 cm dilated (Stables 1999) and the cervical canal shortens from 3 cm long to less than 0.5 cm long (Arulkumaran 1996).
- The active first stage is the time when the cervix undergoes more rapid dilatation. This begins when the cervix is 3–4 cm dilated and, in the presence of rhythmic contractions, is complete when the cervix is fully dilated (10 cm).
- The transitional phase is the stage of labour when the cervix is from around 8 centimetres dilated until it is fully dilated (or until the expulsive contractions during second stage are felt by the woman): there is often a brief lull in the intensity of uterine activity at this time (Sherblom Matteson 2001).

Second stage

- The second stage is that of expulsion of the fetus. It begins when the cervix is fully dilated and the woman feels the urge to expel the baby. It is complete when the baby is born.

Third stage

- The third stage is that of separation and expulsion of placenta and membranes; it also involves the control of bleeding. It lasts from the birth of the baby until the placenta and membranes have been expelled.

The onset of spontaneous normal labour

Women should have adequate information prior to labour to ensure comprehension of the changes labour will bring. This information is also needed to allow women to make their own choices based on good unbiased evidence. The complex physical, psychological and emotional experience of labour affects every woman differently and midwives must have sound knowledge as well as a range of different experiences to ensure the woman has some control over the birth of her baby. Women in labour should be encouraged to trust her own instincts, listen to their own body and verbalise feelings in order to get the help and support they need. Anxiety can increase the production of adrenaline (epinephrine), which inhibits uterine activity and may in turn prolong labour (Niven 1992, Seitchik 1987, Wuitchik et al 1989). The attitude of the midwife and the advice and guidance she gives during pregnancy influence the progress of labour and the attitudes of both the partners to each other and to their baby after it is born (Halldorsdottir & Karlsdottir 1996, Nolan 1995).

Recognition of the onset of normal spontaneous labour is not always easy. A woman may construe herself to be labouring, whereas sound midwifery judgement and understanding of the physiology of the first stage of labour may lead the midwife to the diagnosis of the latent phase of labour. Both the woman and midwife being aware of the latent phase of labour and allowing this time to pass with no intervention may prevent the medical diagnosis of 'poor progress' or 'failure to progress' later in labour. In a hospital setting, it is good practice not to commence the partogram until active labour has commenced.

Spurious labour

Many women experience contractions before the onset of labour; these may be painful and may even be regular for a time, causing a woman to think that labour has started. The two features of true labour that are absent here, are effacement and dilatation of the cervix (see below). It is important to note that the discomfort or even pain that the woman is conscious of is not false; the contractions she is experiencing are real but have not yet settled into the rhythmic pattern of 'true' labour and are not having an effect on the cervix.

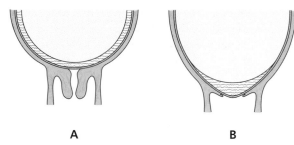

Fig. 24.3 (A) The cervix before effacement. (B) The cervix after effacement. The cervical canal is now part of the lower uterine segment.

Reassurance should be given; discussion of this potential situation earlier in the pregnancy will have allowed the woman and her partner to prepare for such a scenario.

Cervical effacement (taking up of the cervix)

Here the cervix is drawn up and gradually merges into the lower uterine segment (Fig. 24.3). In the primiparous woman this may result in complete effacement of the internal and external cervical os. But in the multiparous woman a perceptible canal may remain.

The onset of labour is determined by a complex interaction of maternal and fetal hormones and is not fully understood. It would appear to be multifactoral in origin, being a combination of hormonal and mechanical factors. Levels of maternal oestrogen rise sharply during the last weeks of pregnancy, resulting in changes that overcome the inhibiting effects of progesterone. High levels of oestrogens cause uterine muscle fibres to display oxytocic receptors and form gap junctions with each other. Oestrogen also stimulates the placenta to release prostaglandins that induce a production of enzymes that will digest collagen in the cervix, helping it to soften (Tortora & Grabowski 2000). The process is unclear but it is thought that both fetal and placental factors are involved. There is no clear evidence that concentrations of oestrogens and progesterone alter at the onset of labour, but the balance between them does facilitate myometrial activity.

Uterine activity may also result from mechanical stimulation of the uterus and cervix. This may be brought about by overstretching, as in the case of a multiple pregnancy, or pressure from a presenting part that is well applied to the cervix (Allman et al 1996, Beazley 1995).

The onset of labour is a process, not an event; therefore it is very difficult to pinpoint exactly when the painless (sometimes painful) contractions of prelabour develop into the progressive rhythmic contractions of established labour.

Diagnosing the onset of labour is extremely important since it is on the basis of this finding that decisions are made that will affect the management of labour (Gee & Olah 1993, O'Driscoll & Meagher 1993). It is part of the remit of the midwife to ensure that women have sufficient information to assist them to recognise the onset of true labour. Contact with the midwife should be made when regular, rhythmic, uterine contractions are experienced, and these are perceived by the woman as uncomfortable or painful.

When in labour, contractions will often be accompanied or preceded by a bloodstained mucoid 'show'. Occasionally the membranes will rupture; this should always be reported to the midwife, who will want to be assured that there are no changes in the fetal heart rate due to the rare complication of cord prolapse and that meconium is not present in the liquor.

Physiology of the first stage of labour

Duration

The length of labour varies widely and is influenced by parity, birth interval, psychological state, presentation and position of the fetus, maternal pelvic shape and size and the character of uterine contractions. By far the greater part of labour is taken up by the first stage; it is common to expect the active phase (see First stage, above) to be completed within 6–12 hours (Tortora & Grabowski 2000). Albers (1999) found the mean length of the active phase (4–10 cm dilated) was 7.7 hours in first time mothers (but up to 17.5 hours) and 5.6 hours in multiparous women (again up to 13.8 hours). On average the nulliparous woman will take longer than the parous woman, who one would expect to reach the second stage more quickly. In the individual case, however, averages can prove extremely misleading.

Uterine action

Fundal dominance (Fig. 24.4)

Each uterine contraction starts in the fundus near one of the cornua and spreads across and downwards. The contraction lasts longest in the fundus where it is also most intense, but the peak is reached simultaneously over the whole uterus and the contraction fades from all parts together. This pattern permits the cervix to dilate and the strongly contracting fundus to expel the fetus.

Polarity

Polarity is the term used to describe the neuromuscular harmony that prevails between the two poles or segments of the uterus throughout labour. During each uterine contraction these two poles act harmoniously. The upper pole contracts strongly and retracts to expel the fetus; the lower pole contracts slightly and dilates to allow expulsion to take place. If polarity is disorganised then the progress of labour is inhibited.

Contraction and retraction

Uterine muscle has a unique property. During labour the contraction does not pass off entirely, but muscle fibres retain some of the shortening of contraction instead of becoming completely relaxed (Fig. 24.5). This is termed *retraction*. It assists in the progressive expulsion of the fetus; the upper segment of the uterus becomes gradually shorter and thicker and its cavity diminishes.

Each labour is individual and does not always conform to expectations, but generally before labour becomes established these uterine contractions may occur every 15–20 minutes and may last for about 30 seconds. They are often fairly weak and may even be imperceptible to the mother. They usually occur with rhythmic regularity and the intervals between them gradually lessen; meanwhile the length and strength of the contractions gradually increase through the latent phase and into the active first stage. By the end of the first stage they occur at 2–3 minute intervals, last for 50–60 seconds and are very powerful.

Formation of upper and lower uterine segments

By the end of pregnancy the body of the uterus is described as having divided into two segments, which are anatomically distinct (Fig. 24.6). The upper uterine segment, having been formed from the body of the fundus, is mainly concerned with contraction and retraction; it is thick and muscular. The lower uterine segment is formed of the isthmus and the cervix, and is about 8–10 cm in length. The lower segment is pre-pared for distension and dilatation. Although there is no clear and strict division of these two segments, the muscle content reduces from the fundus to the cervix where it is thinner. When labour begins, the retracted longitudinal fibres in the upper segment pull on the lower segment causing it to stretch; this is aided by the force applied by the descending presenting part.

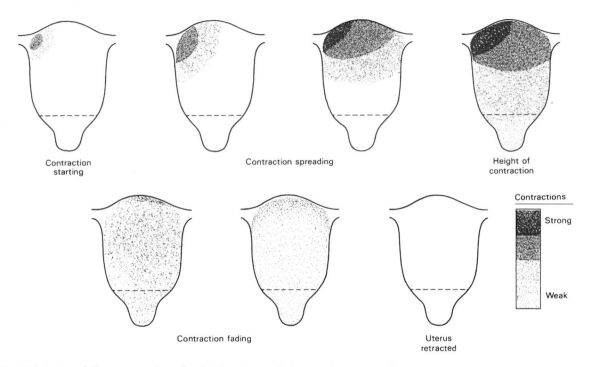

Fig. 24.4 Series of diagrams to show fundal dominance during uterine contractions.

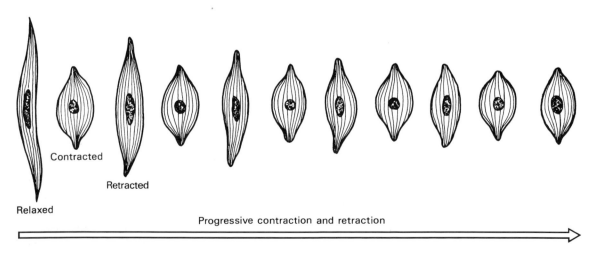

Fig. 24.5 Diagram to show how uterine muscle retains some shortening after each contraction.

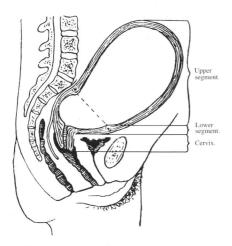

Fig. 24.6 Birth canal before labour begins.

The retraction ring

A ridge forms between the upper and lower uterine segments; this is known as the 'retraction', or 'Bandl's ring' (Fig. 24.7). It is customary to use the former term to describe the physiological retraction ring and to reserve the term 'Bandl's ring' for an exaggerated degree of the phenomenon that becomes visible above the symphysis in mechanically obstructed labour when the lower segment thins abnormally.

The physiological ring gradually rises as the upper uterine segment contracts and retracts and the lower uterine segment thins out to accommodate the descending fetus. Once the cervix is fully dilated and the fetus can leave the uterus, the retraction ring rises no further.

Cervical effacement

'Effacement' refers to the inclusion of the cervical canal into the lower uterine segment. According to conventional obstetric belief this process takes place from above downward; that is, the muscle fibres surrounding the internal os are drawn upwards by the retracted upper segment and the cervix merges into the lower uterine segment. The cervical canal widens at the level of the internal os whereas the condition of the external os remains unchanged (Cunningham et al 1989, O'Driscoll & Meagher 1993) (see Fig 24.3, p. 438).

However, an alternative mechanism of cervical effacement has been suggested, in which the tissues in the region of the external os are taken up first. By an outward unrolling movement, the cervix thins from the external os upwards, leaving the internal os to be affected last (Beazley 1995, Olah et al 1993).

Effacement may occur late in pregnancy, or it may not take place until labour begins. In the nulliparous woman the cervix will not usually dilate until effacement is complete, whereas in the parous woman effacement and dilatation may occur simultaneously and a small canal may be felt in early labour. This is often referred to by midwives as a 'multips os'.

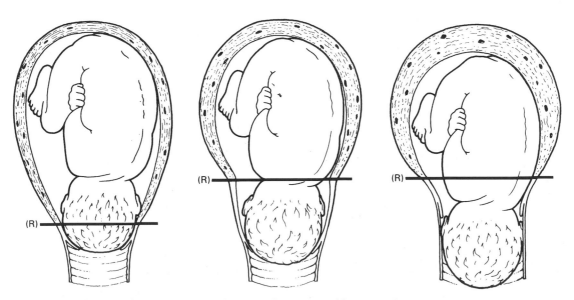

Fig. 24.7 Diagram showing the retraction ring between the upper and lower uterine segments.

Cervical dilatation

Dilatation of the cervix is the process of enlargement of the os uteri from a tightly closed aperture to an opening large enough to permit passage of the fetal head. Dilatation is measured in centimetres and full dilatation at term equates to about 10 cm.

Dilatation occurs as a result of uterine action and the counterpressure applied by either the intact bag of membranes or the presenting part, or both. A well-flexed fetal head closely applied to the cervix favours efficient dilatation. Pressure applied evenly to the cervix causes the uterine fundus to respond by contraction and retraction (Beazley & Lobb 1983, Ferguson 1941).

Show. As a result of the dilatation of the cervix, the operculum, which formed the cervical plug during pregnancy, is lost. The woman may see a bloodstained mucoid discharge a few hours before, or within a few hours after, labour starts. The blood comes from ruptured capillaries in the parietal decidua where the chorion has become detached from the dilating cervix. There should never be more than bloodstaining; frank fresh bleeding is not normal at this stage – though, as the first stage ends, during the transitional period there is often a small loss of bright red blood that heralds the second stage. Both are referred to as a 'show'.

Mechanical factors

Formation of the forewaters

As the lower uterine segment forms and stretches, the chorion becomes detached from it and the increased intrauterine pressure causes this loosened part of the sac of fluid to bulge downwards into the internal os, to the depth of 6–12 mm. The well-flexed head fits snugly into the cervix and cuts off the fluid in front of the head from that which surrounds the body. The former is known as the 'forewaters' and the latter the 'hindwaters'. In early labour it is often possible to feel intact forewaters bulging even when the hindwaters have ruptured, making ruptured membranes a difficult diagnosis at times.

The effect of separation of the forewaters prevents the pressure that is applied to the hindwaters during uterine contractions from being applied to the forewaters. This may help keep the membranes intact during the first stage of labour and be a natural defence against infection.

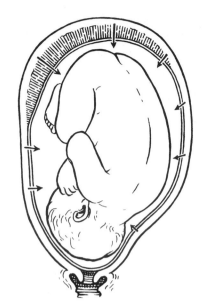

Fig. 24.8 General fluid pressure.

General fluid pressure (Fig. 24.8)

While the membranes remain intact, the pressure of the uterine contractions is exerted on the fluid and, as fluid is not compressible, the pressure is equalised throughout the uterus and over the fetal body; it is known as 'general fluid pressure'. When the membranes rupture and a quantity of fluid emerges, the placenta and umbilical cord are compressed between the uterine wall and the fetus during contractions and the oxygen supply to the fetus is diminished. Preserving the integrity of the membranes, therefore, optimises the oxygen supply to the fetus and also helps to prevent intrauterine and fetal infection, especially in longer labours.

Rupture of the membranes

The optimum physiological time for the membranes to rupture spontaneously is at the end of the first stage of labour after the cervix becomes fully dilated and no longer supports the bag of forewaters. The uterine contractions are also applying increasing force at this time.

Membranes may sometimes rupture days before labour begins or during the first stage. If for any reason there is a badly fitting presenting part and the forewaters are not cut off effectively then the membranes may rupture early. But in most cases there is no reason apparent for early spontaneous membrane rupture.

Occasionally the membranes do not rupture even in the second stage and appear at the vulva as a bulging sac covering the fetal head as it is born; this is known as the 'caul'.

Early rupture of membranes may lead to an increased incidence of variable decelerations on cardiotocograph (CTG), which may lead to an increase in caesarean section rate if fetal blood sampling is not available (Goffinet et al 1997). A large meta-analysis (Brissen-Carroll et al 1997) suggests that routine artificial rupture of membranes (ARM) may decrease the overall length of labour by 60–120 minutes. ARM does not reduce the overall caesarean section rate. It was concluded in this study that routine ARM should be reserved for women who are progressing slowly in labour or have abnormalities in the CTG. All women need to give consent for this intervention and the practitioner should have a positive indication for performing ARM, which should be recorded in the notes.

Fetal axis pressure (Fig. 24.9)

During each contraction the uterus rises forward and the force of the fundal contraction is transmitted to the upper pole of the fetus, down the long axis of the fetus and applied by the presenting part to the cervix. This is known as 'fetal axis pressure' and becomes much more significant after rupture of the membranes and during the second stage of labour.

Recognition of the first stage of labour

Ideally the woman should know her own midwife and be able to contact her when labour starts. Where this is not possible, it is crucial that the first meeting between the midwife, the labouring woman and her partner establishes a rapport, which sets the scene for the remainder of labour. If she is going to hospital the woman may worry about the reception she and her companion will receive and the attitude of the people attending her. In addition, an unfamiliar environment may provoke feelings of vulnerability and rob her of confidence. Comfortable surroundings, a welcoming manner and a midwife who greets the woman as an equal in a partnership will engender feelings of mutual respect, thus enabling the woman to relax and respond positively to the amazing forces of labour (Raphael-Leff 1993).

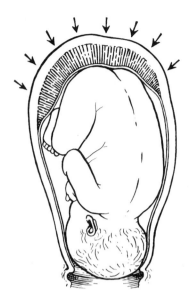

Fig. 24.9 Fetal axis pressure.

Recognition of labour by the woman

It is the woman herself who usually diagnoses the onset of normal labour and many women and their partners are apprehensive in case the labour is very quick, resulting in an unattended birth. Education during the prenatal period is important to enable the woman to recognise the beginning of labour and understand the latent phase.

Women should be aware of what a 'show' is like, and know that in late pregnancy vaginal secretions are increased but should not be blood stained. A 'show' in early labour or prior to the onset of labour is quite common. It is usually a pink or bloodstained jelly-like loss; labour may be imminent or under way. Women who are examined vaginally in late pregnancy should be made aware that there may be some slight blood loss after this procedure.

Braxton Hicks contractions are more noticeable in late pregnancy and some women experience them as painful. They are usually irregular or their regularity is not maintained for long spells of time. They seldom last more than 1 minute. In true labour, contractions exhibit a pattern of rhythm and regularity, usually increasing in length, strength and frequency as time goes on. When the woman first feels contractions she may be aware only of backache but if she places a hand on her abdomen she may perceive simultaneous hardening of the uterus. Contractions will often be short initially, lasting 30–40 seconds, and may be as much as half an hour apart. If the pregnancy is problem free, with a normal birth anticipated, the midwife should advise the woman to stay in her own surroundings, continue with her normal activities, to eat, be active and upright.

It is often difficult to be sure whether or not the membranes have ruptured spontaneously prior to labour or in early labour. The woman may be experiencing some degree of stress incontinence so she may be unsure if it is liquor or urine that she is passing. If there is any doubt, the woman should contact her midwife. The midwife may decide to pass a speculum and look for amniotic fluid in the vagina. Digital examination should be avoided if the woman is not in labour as it will increase the risk of ascending infection and chorioamnionitis.

Initial meeting with the midwife and care in labour

Communication

When a woman begins to labour she may have a mixture of emotions. Most women anticipate labour with a degree of excitement, anxiety, fear and hope. Many other emotions are influenced by cultural expectations and previous life experiences. The state of the woman's knowledge, her fears and expectations are also influenced by her companions during labour. By the time labour starts a decision will have been reached about where the woman plans to give birth. Some women may choose to give birth at home, some in hospital and some may wish to labour as long as possible at home but give birth in hospital. Whatever choice the woman makes, she must be the focus of the care, should be able to feel she is in control of what is happening to her and be able to make decisions about her care (DoH 1993).

Providing that there are no complications and labour is not well advanced, the woman may remain at home as long as she feels comfortable and confident. If labour is preterm, however, admission to hospital is always advised (see Ch. 25).

The initial examination will include details of when labour started, whether the membranes have ruptured and the frequency and strength of the contractions. The midwife should remember that the woman will be very conscious of her body and may therefore be unable to pay attention or respond while experiencing a contraction. Since the woman has embarked on an intensely energy-demanding process, inquiry should be made as to whether she has been deprived of sleep and also what food she has recently eaten. If still in early labour with a problem-free pregnancy she should be advised to eat or drink if she wishes and remain mobile, maybe to bathe if she would find this relaxing (Champion & McCormick 2002).

Thought should be given to the social circumstances, particularly the care of other children and whether a birthing partner is available and has been contacted.

Past history

Of particular relevance at the onset of labour are:

- the birth plan
- parity and age
- character and outcomes of previous labours
- weights and condition of previous babies
- if she has attended any specialist clinics
- any known problems – social or physical
- blood results including Rhesus isoimmunisation and haemoglobin.

Birth plan

Most women currently give birth in hospital. Admission to hospital of a woman in labour provides the opportunity for the midwife to discuss with each woman and her partner any plans that may have already been prepared by them. An outline may be present in the case notes, or the couple may bring a birth plan with them. Some women will not have prepared a birth plan and, if this is the case, the midwife can encourage the couple to consider any preferences that they may have. A birth plan simply means that a pregnant woman has (usually) written down, and may have discussed with her midwife, the kind of birth she would like. Frequently the partner is involved in this forward planning, which should be a flexible proposal that can be reviewed and revised during labour (DoH 1993). To welcome the woman who is being admitted in labour, to introduce oneself and to ascertain how she would like to be addressed should help the midwife establish a trusting relationship.

Whether or not they are already identified in a birth plan, she should explore the following issues:

- the woman's chosen birth companion
- her choice of clothes for labour
- ambulation
- pain relief
- position for labour and birth
- natural or managed third stage
- cutting the umbilical cord
- skin to skin contact and feeding the baby after birth.

The midwife should also offer to explain anything the woman or her partner wishes to know, and document all requests.

Midwife's initial physical examination of the mother

Prior to touching the woman a sound explanation of the proposed examination and their significance should be given. Verbal consent should be obtained and recorded in the notes. The midwife must be aware that a competent woman, with a capacity to make decisions, is within her rights to refuse any treatment regardless of the consequences to her and her unborn baby. She does *not* have to give a reason.

The woman is then asked to empty her bladder and a specimen of urine is tested for protein, glucose and ketones. Her temperature is taken. The pulse rate is counted, although not during a uterine contraction that increases the heart rate slightly. Blood pressure is also taken and recorded. The woman's hands and feet are usually examined for signs of oedema. Slight swelling of the feet and ankles is normal, but pretibial oedema or puffiness of the fingers or face is not.

A detailed abdominal examination as described in Chapter 16 should be carried out and recorded. Initial observations form a baseline for further examinations carried out throughout labour. The abdominal examination may be repeated at intervals in order to assess descent of the head. This is measured by the number of fifths palpable above the pelvic brim and should be recorded on the partogram.

Vaginal examination

A vaginal examination should always be preceded by an abdominal examination, an explanation and the obtaining of verbal consent from the woman. The woman's bladder should be empty as the head may be displaced by a full bladder as well as being very uncomfortable for the woman. With the combination of external and internal findings, the skilled midwife will have a very detailed picture of the labour and subsequent progress of labour.

Indications for vaginal examination

These are to:

- make a positive identification of presentation
- determine whether the head is engaged in case of doubt
- ascertain whether the forewaters have ruptured, or to rupture them artificially
- exclude cord prolapse after rupture of the forewaters, especially if there is an ill-fitting presenting part or the fetal heart rate changes
- assess progress or delay in labour
- confirm full dilatation of the cervix
- confirm the axis of the fetus and presentation of the second twin in multiple pregnancy, and if necessary in order to rupture the second amniotic sac.

The midwife should realise that a vaginal examination is not always the only way of obtaining this information and that careful, continuous observation of the labouring mother will enable her to avoid making unnecessary vaginal examinations, which should be kept to a miminum. Under no circumstances should a midwife make a vaginal examination if there is any frank bleeding unless the placenta is positively known to be in the upper uterine segment.

Method

A vaginal examination during labour is an aseptic procedure. The midwife should first explain the procedure carefully to the woman and give her an opportunity to ask questions. In order to obtain the most information, the woman is usually asked to lie on her back but the technique can be easily adapted to accommodate other positions that suit the woman better. During the examination the woman's dignity and privacy need to be considered; to avoid unnecessary exposure the woman can be asked to move and uncover herself when the midwife is ready to begin. It appears that there is no increased risk of infection to mothers and babies if the midwife does not swab the vulva with antiseptic solution or use sterile vaginal packs (McCormick 2001); what is important is using a good handwashing technique and wearing sterile gloves.

Findings

The midwife should observe the labia for any sign of varicosities, oedema or vulval warts or sores (see Ch. 21). She notes whether the perineum is scarred from a previous tear or episiotomy. Some cultures practise female genital mutilation (excision of the clitoris and the labia minora); scarring from this operation would be evident. The midwife should also note any discharge or bleeding from the vaginal orifice. If the membranes have ruptured the colour and odour of any amniotic fluid are noted. Offensive liquor suggests infection and green fluid indicates the presence of meconium, which may be a sign of fetal compromise or postmaturity.

Particularly in a multiparous woman, a cystocele may be found. A loaded rectum may also be felt through the posterior vaginal wall. If time allows, a suppository or microenema may be offered. Many women have some degree of loose bowels in early labour though, which reduces the need for enema or suppositories in most spontaneous labours.

As the examining fingers reach the end of the vagina they are turned so that their sensitive pads face upwards and come into contact with the cervix. Palpate around the fornices and sense the proximity of the presenting part of the fetus to the examining finger. The os uteri is located by gently sweeping the fingers from side to side. It will normally be situated centrally, but sometimes in early labour it will be very posterior. In the rare event of a sacculated retroverted gravid uterus the cervix may be located in an extreme anterior position.

The midwife must assess the length of the cervical canal. A long, tightly closed cervix indicates that labour has not yet started. The cervical canal may be partially or completely obliterated depending on the degree of effacement (see above). In a primigravida the cervix may be completely effaced but still closed; in this case it will be closely applied to the presenting part and can easily be confused with a completely dilated cervix until the small tell-tale depression in the centre is found.

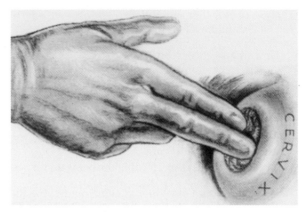

Fig. 24.10 Cervix 4 cm dilated.

The consistency of the cervix is noted. It should be soft, elastic and applied closely to the presenting part.

Dilatation of the cervix, that is the distance across the opening, is estimated in centimetres (Fig. 24.10); 10 cm dilatation equates to full dilatation (Fig. 24.11). In preterm labours the smaller fetal head will pass through the os at a smaller diameter. At the point where the maximum diameters of the fetal head have passed through the os, the cervix can no longer be felt.

The midwife should always take care to feel for the cervix in every direction as a lip of cervix frequently remains in one quarter only, usually anteriorly (see also Bishop score, Ch. 29).

Intact membranes can be felt through the dilating os. When felt between contractions they are slack but will become tense when the uterus contracts and the fluid behind them is then more readily appreciated. The consistency of the membranes can be likened to 'Cling film'. When the forewaters are very shallow it may be difficult to feel the membranes.

If the presenting part does not fit well, some of the fluid from the hindwaters escapes into the forewaters, causing the membranes to protrude through the cervix. This will be more exaggerated in obstructed labour. Bulging membranes are more likely to rupture early and in this case they will not be felt at all. Following rupture of the membranes the midwife needs to satisfy herself that the cord has not prolapsed by listening to the fetal heart through a contraction.

If the forewaters are felt following a leakage of amniotic fluid it may be supposed that the hindwaters have ruptured.

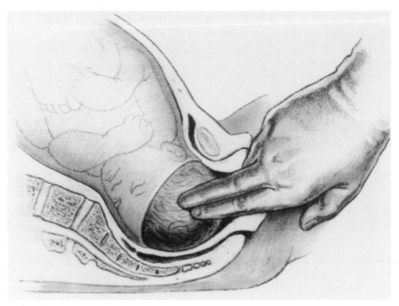

Fig. 24.11 Cervix fully dilated.

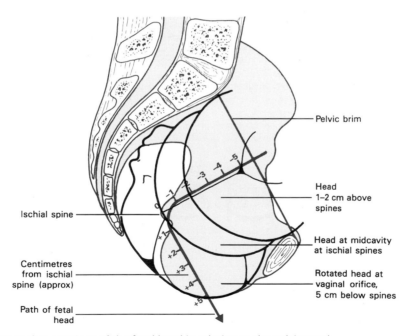

Fig. 24.12 Diagram to show stations of the fetal head in relation to the pelvic canal.

The presenting part is defined as the part of the fetus lying over the uterine os during labour. In order to assess the descent of the fetus in labour, the level of the presenting part is estimated in relation to the maternal ischial spines. The distance of the presenting part above or below the ischial spines is expressed in centimetres (Fig. 24.12). As a caput succedaneum (see Fig. 44.1, p. 826) may form over the presenting part, care must be taken to relate the bony part of the fetus to the ischial spines and not to the oedematous swelling. Moulding of the fetal skull can also result in the presenting part becoming lower without any appreciable advance of the head as a whole. The midwife must bear in mind that the fetus follows the curve of Carus (see Ch. 7) and it is impossible to judge the station precisely. The purpose of making this estimate is to assess progress and it is therefore valuable for the same person to make all the vaginal examinations on any particular mother.

In 96% of cases the vertex presents and is recognised by feeling the hard bones of the vault of the skull and the fontanelles and sutures in relation to the maternal pelvis. For details of the findings in face, brow, breech and shoulder presentations see Chapter 30.

By feeling the features of the presenting part, the midwife can deduce the position of the presentation. The vertex has the fewest diagnostic features but, being the most common presentation, is the one with which she must become most familiar.

Commonly, the first feature to be felt, even in early labour, is the sagittal suture. Its slope should be noted; most frequently it will be in the right or left oblique diameter of the maternal pelvis, or it may be transverse. Later it rotates into the anteroposterior diameter of the maternal pelvis (Fig. 24.13).

The sagittal suture should be followed with the finger until a fontanelle is reached. If the head is well flexed, this will be the posterior fontanelle, which is recognised because it is small and triangular with three sutures leaving it. The anterior fontanelle is diamond shaped, covered with membrane and with four sutures leaving it. The location of the fontanelle(s) in relation to the maternal pelvis will give information about the whereabouts of the fetal occiput.

Moulding (see Ch. 11). This can be judged by feeling the amount of overlapping of the skull bones; it can also give additional information as to position. The parietal bones override the occipital bone and the anterior parietal bone overrides the posterior.

An understanding of the mechanism of labour (see Ch. 27) will help the midwife to appreciate the significance of flexion, rotation and descent as determinants of progress in labour.

Although the capacity of the pelvis may have been assessed antenatally, the midwife should take the opportunity to assure herself of its adequacy as she completes her vaginal examination. She may be able to feel the ischial spines, which should be blunt, and note the size of the subpubic angle, which should be about 90° and accommodate the two examining fingers. Prominent ischial spines and a reduced subpubic angle are unfavourable features associated with the android pelvis.

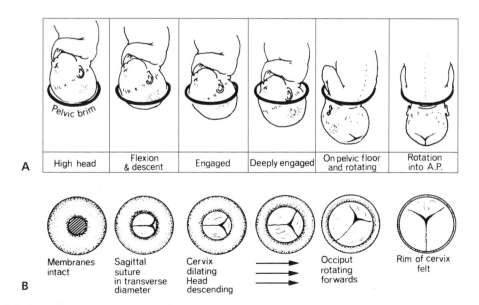

Fig. 24.13 (A) Diagrams showing descent of the fetal head through the pelvic brim. (B) Diagrams showing dilatation of the cervix and rotation of the fetal head as felt on vaginal examination.

Keeping the woman fully informed in labour shows sensitivity to her needs and is an essential, integral component of the support provided by the midwife.

Cleanliness and comfort

Bowel preparation

If there has been no bowel action for 24 hours or the rectum feels loaded on vaginal examination, the woman should be consulted and asked if she would like an enema or suppositories. This is never done as a routine procedure. A small, low volume disposable enema may be administered, or two glycerine suppositories. There is no evidence to suggest a full rectum causes delay in the progress of labour (Drayton 1990), but the woman may be embarrassed if she feels she is likely to pass faeces during labour.

Perineal shave

Routine perineal shaving has not been carried out in the UK for some years. Research has shown that perineal shaving is unnecessary and does not improve infection rates. Dislike of the procedure and abrasions sustained cause discomfort for many women and detract from the positive experience of labour (Drayton 1990).

Bath or shower

If a woman has had no access to a bath or shower at home she may wish to use these facilities on admission to the hospital. For women in normal labour a warm bath (or birthing pool) can be an effective form of pain relief that allows increased mobility with no increased incidence of adverse outcome for mother or baby (Alderdice et al 1995, Gilbert & Tookey 1999). The woman may choose to rest in the bath for a long time. The midwife should invite the mother who is mobile to have a bath or shower whenever she wishes during normal labour.

Clothing

It is entirely up to the individual woman what she wears in labour. If in hospital she may prefer to wear the loose gown offered or she may feel more comfortable wearing her own choice of clothing. As long as she is aware that the garment may become wet and bloodstained and that she may require more than one, there is no reason to restrict her choice.

Records

Midwifery is becoming increasing litigious. The midwife's record of labour is a legal document and must be kept meticulously. The records may be examined by any court for up to 25 years, they may go before the Nursing and Midwifery Council professional conduct or health committee, and will usually be examined in the audit process of statutory supervision or on behalf of the Clinical Negligence Scheme for Trusts. The Midwives rules and code of practice (UKCC 1998a) and Guidelines for records and record keeping (UKCC 1998b) both reiterate that records should be as contemporaneous as is reasonable, and must be authenticated with the midwife's full signature; it is good practice to print the author's name under the signature. A midwife must not destroy or arrange for destruction of these records and must be satisfied they are stored securely.

The records are created to give current comprehensive and concise information regarding the woman's observations, her physical, psychological and sociological state, and any problem that arises as well as the midwife's response to that problem, including any interventions. They are there to serve the interest of the woman and to demonstrate that the midwife has understood and carried out her duty of care as a reasonable midwife should.

An accurate record during labour provides the basis from which clinical improvements, progress or deterioration of the mother or fetus can be judged. For this reason the notes should be kept in chronological order.

The maternity record is shared between the midwife and the obstetrician. The obstetrician makes notes of his or her findings, timing of visits and any prescriptions made. The same standards apply to all practitioners. The midwife usually enters the summary of labour and initial details about the baby.

In recent years the partogram or partograph has been widely accepted as an effective means of recording the progress of labour. It is a chart on which the salient features of labour are entered in a graphic form and therefore provides the opportunity for early identification of deviations from normal. Figure 24.14 shows one example of a partogram, which is a visual means of recording all observations and includes a pictorial record of the rate of cervical dilatation. The charts are

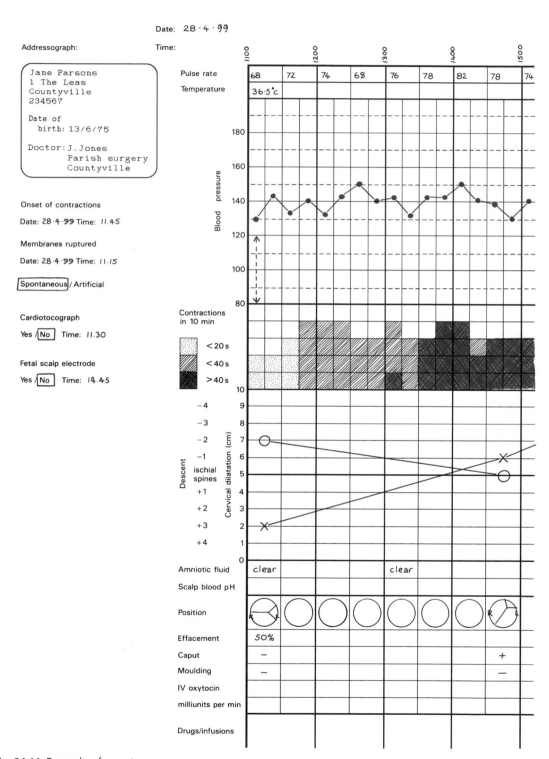

Fig. 24.14 Example of a partogram.

usually designed to allow for recordings at 15 minute intervals and include:

- fetal heart rate
- maternal temperature
- pulse
- blood pressure
- details of vaginal examinations
- strength of contractions
- frequency of contractions in terms of the number in 10 minutes
- fluid balance
- urine analysis
- drugs administered.

The cervicograph is the diagrammatic representation of the dilatation of the cervix charted against the hours in labour. Some studies have shown (Friedman & Sachtleben 1965, Pearson 1981) that the cervical dilatation time of normal labour has a characteristic sigmoid curve. This curve can be divided into two distinct parts – the latent phase and the active phase. The active phase has been said to proceed at a rate 0.5–1 cm an hour, but more recent work has challenged this rigid view (Albers 1999). The disadvantage of using such prescribed parameters of normal is the temptation to make all women fit predetermined criteria for normality. The rate of progress in labour must be considered in the context of the woman's total well-being and choice.

If it becomes necessary to confer with an obstetrician, paediatrician or other practitioner, the midwife records the times and the nature of the consultation, including whether the practitioner was informed, consulted or asked to be present.

Drug records

Midwives have an exemption from needing a prescription for specific drugs used for the care of women in normal labour (see Ch. 48). Even so, most NHS Trusts also have locally agreed patient group directions

---

Box 24.1 Key points for the first stage of labour

- Women should have adequate and unbiased information to make choices for their labour and birth including place of birth.
- Good communication and constant individualised care will improve outcomes of women and their babies.
- The midwife should assess the woman with a problem-free pregnancy at home to diagnose labour regardless of planned place of birth.
- Midwives should ensure women are aware of the latent phase of labour.
- Women in normal labour should remain mobile and in their own surroundings as long as possible when booked for hospital birth.
- Labour is a continuous process that may not always progress as obstetric curves currently suggest.
- It is the responsibility of the midwife to ensure all maternity records that she completes meet legal and professional standards.

---

to which the midwife should adhere; these usually guide the midwife as to which drugs are preferred and what doses and frequency are to be used within that Trust (UKCC 1998b). If the midwife is practising outside the area in which she has notified her intention to practise, she should consult the supervisor of midwives regarding any matters relating to the supply, administration, storage or surrender of controlled drugs or medicines.

As well as being entered on the partogram, doses of drugs are recorded on the prescription sheet, in the summary of labour and, in the case of controlled drugs, in the Controlled Drug Register.

Box 24.1 lists key points for care in the first stage of labour.

REFERENCES

Albers L L 1999 The duration of labor in healthy women. Journal of Perinatology 19(2):114–119

Alderdice F, Renfrew M, Marchant S et al 1995 Labour and birth in water in England and Wales. Report of a survey funded by the Department of Health into the safety of water birth. British Medical Journal 310(6983):837

Allman A C J, Genevier E S, Johnson M R, Steer P J 1996 Head to cervix force: an important physiological variable in labour. 1. The temporal relation between head to cervix force and intrauterine pressure during labour. British Journal of Obstetrics and Gynaecology 103:763–768

Arulkumaran S 1996 Poor progress in labour including augmentation, malpositions and malpresentations. In: James D, Steer P, Gonik B (eds) High risk pregnancy. W B Saunders, London, p 1063

Beazley J M 1995 Natural labour and its active management. In: Whitfield C (ed) Dewhurst's textbook of obstetrics and gynaecology for postgraduates, 5th edn. Blackwell Science, Oxford, ch 21

Beazley J M, Lobb M O 1983 Aspects of care in labour. Churchill Livingstone, New York

Brissen-Carroll G, Fraser W, Breart G, Krauss I, Thornton J 1997 The effect of routine early amniotomy on spontaneous labour: a meta analysis. The Cochrane Collaboration, Issue 4. Update Software, Oxford

Champion P, McCormick C 2002 Eating and drinking in labour: Books for Midwives, Oxford

Cunningham F G, MacDonald P C, Grant N F 1989 Williams obstetrics, 18th edn. Prentice-Hall, London

DoH (Department of Health) 1993 Changing childbirth: report of the expert maternity group (Chairman Lady Julia Cumberlege). HMSO, London

Drayton S 1990 Midwifery care in the first stage of labour. In: Alexander J, Levy V, Roch S (eds) Intrapartum care: a research based approach. Macmillan, Basingstoke

Ferguson J K 1941 A study of the motility of the intact uterus at term. Surgery, Gynecology and Obstetrics 73:359–366

Friedman E A, Sachtleben M R 1965 Station of the fetal presenting part. American Journal of Obstetrics and Gynecology 93(4):522–529

Gee H, Olah K S 1993 Failure to progress in labour. In: Studd J (ed) Progress in obstetrics and gynaecology. Churchill Livingstone, New York, vol 10, ch 10

Gilbert R E, Tookey P A 1999 Perinatal mortality and morbidity among babies delivered in water: surveillance study and postal survey. British Medical Journal 319(7208):483–487

Goffinet F, Fraser W, Marcoux S et al 1997 Early amniotomy increases the frequency of fetal heart rate abnormalities. British Journal of Obstetrics and Gynaecology 104:548–553

Halldorsdottir S, Karlsdottir S I 1996 Journeying through labour and delivery: perceptions of women who have given birth. Midwifery 12:48–61

Kirkman S 2001 The educational perspective. Practising Midwife 4(6):14

McCormick C 2001 Vulval preparation in labour: use of lotions or tap water. British Journal of Midwifery 9(7):453–455

Niven C 1992 Psychological care for families: before, during and after birth. Butterworth Heinemann, Oxford

Nolan M 1995 Supporting women in labour: the doula's role. Modern Midwife 5(3):12–15

O'Driscoll K, Meagher D 1993 Active management of labour, 3rd edn. Mosby, London

Olah K S, Brown J S, Gee H 1993 Cervical contractions: the response of the cervix to oxytocic stimulation in the latent phase of labour. British Journal of Obstetrics and Gynaecology 100:635–640

Pearson J 1981 Partography. Nursing Mirror (July 8):xxv–xxix

Raphael-Leff J 1993 Pregnancy: the inside story. Sheldon Press, London

Seitchik J 1987 The management of functional dystocia in the first stage of labour. Clinical Obstetrics and Gynecology 30(1):42–49

Sherblom Matteson P 2001 Women's health during the childbearing years: A community based approach. Mosby, New York, p 358–359

Stables D 1999 Physiology in childbearing. Baillière Tindall, London, p 450

Tortora G, Grabowski S 2000 Principles of anatomy and physiology, 9th edn. John Wiley, New York, p 1039–1040

UKCC (United Kingdom Central Council for Nursing Midwifery and Health Visiting) 1998a Midwives rules and code of practice. UKCC, London

UKCC (United Kingdom Central Council for Nursing Midwifery and Health Visiting) 1998b Guidelines for records and record keeping. UKCC, London

WHO (World Health Organization) Department of Reproductive Health and Research 1997 Care in normal labour. A practical guide. WHO, Geneva

Wuitchik M, Bakal D, Lipshitz J 1989 The clinical significance of pain and cognitive activity in latent labour. Obstetrics and Gynecology 73(1):25–41

FURTHER READING

Albers L L, Krulewitch C J, Lydon-Rochelle M T 1995 Maternal age and labor complications in healthy primigravidas at term. Journal of Nurse-Midwifery 40(1):4–12

Bastian H 1992 Confined, managed and delivered: the language of obstetrics. British Journal of Obstetrics and Gynaecology 99:92–93

Belbin A 1996 Power and choice in birthgiving: a case study. British Journal of Midwifery 4(5):264–267

Clinical Standards Advisory Group 1995 Women in normal labour: report of a CSAG committee on women in normal labour. HMSO, London

Dodds R, Goodman M, Tyler S (eds) 1996 Listen with mother (consulting users of maternity services). Books for Midwives Press, Hale, Cheshire

Nelki J, Bond L 1995 Positions in labour: a plea for flexibility. Modern Midwife (Feb):19–22

Philpott R H, Castle W M 1972 Cervicographs in the management of labour in primigravidae I. The alert line for detecting abnormal labour and II. The action line and treatment of abnormal labour. Journal of Obstetrics and Gynaecology of the British Commonwealth 79:592–598, 599–602

Tew M 1995 Safer childbirth?, 2nd edn. Chapman & Hall, London

25

The First Stage of Labour: Management

Carol McCormick

CHAPTER CONTENTS

Labour, the culmination of pregnancy, is an event with great psychological, social and emotional meaning for the mother and her family. In addition, many women experience stress and physical pain. The midwife as well as all other supporters should display tact and sensitivity, respect the needs of the individual and provide an environment within which each woman can labour and give birth with dignity, in a way that she chooses, having been given all the information necessary to make decisions.

Within the definition of a midwife (UKCC 1998, p. 25) it is stated she should '... be able to give care and advice to women during pregnancy, labour, and the postpartum period to conduct deliveries on her own responsibility and to care for the newborn and the infant. This care includes preventative measures, the detection of abnormality ... She has an important task in health counselling and education, not only for the woman but also within the family and the community.'

The chapter aims to:

- stress the importance of women's choice, control, comfort and companionship during labour

- describe the principles of consent and record keeping

- describe the process of monitoring, both the progress of labour and the condition of the mother and fetus

- briefly describe the current principles used in the management of preterm labour.

Communication and environment

Women may choose to give birth in their own home where they control the environment and feel comfortable in their own surroundings, or they may opt for a birth centre or hospital birth. The woman should make this decision herself only after full and unbiased discussion of her options and the associated outcomes. Her choice should be supported.

Currently in the UK most births occur in hospital; therefore the atmosphere and environment of hospital birthing rooms is important. Soft furnishings, the use of colour and the arrangement of furniture can help to soften a hospital atmosphere with its implications of sickness and institutional rules. The attitude of the staff, however, is much more important than physical surroundings. The Royal College of Obstetricians and Gynaecologists and the Royal College of Midwives in their joint report Towards safer childbirth (RCOG/ RCM 1999) make specific recommendations regarding making 'delivery' rooms more homely. This includes furnishings that allow women to adopt a variety of positions in labour, as well as the provision of dedicated bereavement rooms.

Labour ward staff having a shared philosophy and communicating well in multidisciplinary forums are helpful in improving the culture of busy labour wards. Improvement of multidisciplinary communication should be actively sought (Fraser et al 2000, Mackin & Sinclair 1998). Risk management issues and statutory supervision must be dealt with in a way that positively develops and supports staff. Good communication on labour wards between women and midwives, midwives and doctors, and doctors and women can have enormous impact (Brown & Lumley 1998). Communication is not only the content of what is said but includes non-verbal communication, written birth plans and involvement of the whole team in decision making. The 8th annual report from the Confidential Enquiry into Stillbirths and Deaths in Infancy (CESDI 2001) reiterated that all health care professionals involved in maternity care should be vigilant in identifying and communicating risk factors to specialist services, and that plans for both antenatal and intrapartum care should be made.

Prior to admission to the hospital the woman should have been given good information about the physical process of labour and should have considered what strategies she may use to cope during the birth. It is essential that the labouring woman is welcomed and encouraged to feel at ease, and most of all that the midwife spends time *actively listening* as the woman recounts the details of the onset of labour.

Emotional support

The midwife has a traditional and professional role to fulfil: of clinical assessment of the progress of labour and the physical status of mother and fetus. In addition, emotional support is provided by exercising skill in imparting confidence, expressing caring and dependability as well as being an advocate for the childbearing woman if needed. The midwife should display a tolerant non-judgmental attitude, ensuring that the woman is accepted whatever her reactions to labour may be. Women who feel in control of their own bodies, who retain control of their behaviour and who feel they have an active part in decision making have a more satisfactory birth experience (Green et al 1990, Lindow et al 1998, Wallace et al 1995).

Companion in labour

For more than 20 years research has consistently shown that continuous one-to-one support of a woman during labour creates a strong feeling of security and satisfaction as well as having a positive effect on outcomes (Ball 1994, Hodnett & Osborn 1989a,b, Langer et al 1998, Madi et al 1999). A meta-analysis by Hodnett (2001) demonstrates a number of benefits of one-to-one care for mothers and babies. These include reduction in pain relief, and in operative vaginal delivery and caesarean section as well as in length of labour; there were no harmful effects demonstrated.

The woman herself is central to all the decisions made about care during labour. Her chosen companion, whether sexual partner, friend or family member, should understand this. Ideally the companion should be involved in prelabour preparation and decision making, and have participated in compiling a birth plan and any contingency plans drawn up in the event of change.

Admission to hospital is always a traumatic experience and the company of a supportive companion can help reduce anxiety. During labour the companion can keep the woman company, walk with her if she is ambulant, especially in early labour, support her decisions about pain relief and encourage her with whatever she has chosen as her coping mechanism. Providing encouragement and reassurance that labour is progressing is also important, as is helping with physical comfort. In some areas a midwife will be able to remain with one woman through her entire labour but due to the unpredictable workloads on busy labour wards this is not always possible. Students can play an invaluable role in providing support.

The midwife should appreciate that the companion may also need direct support at times. This is particularly evident when a sudden emergency develops. If, for instance, a caesarean section becomes necessary, the midwife should delegate someone to keep the companion as informed as the woman wishes and ensure that he or she is not left feeling abandoned or uncared for.

Consent and information giving

Consent

Common law in the UK has developed rules that require patients to agree in meaningful terms to any recommended treatment. As Lord Donaldson has said (Re F 1990) 'The ability of the ordinary adult to exercise free choice in deciding whether to accept or refuse medical treatment … is a crucial factor in relation to all medical treatment.' It can therefore be concluded that patient autonomy is protected only when there is a meaningful choice made by the patient on the basis of adequate information and comprehension of that information.

The case of Re MB (1997) now clarifies, to some extent, the situation in court-ordered caesarean sections; in this, the principles of Sidaway v Bethlem Royal Hospital Governors & Ors (1985) were confirmed. Under common law a competent adult, including a competent pregnant woman, has the right to refuse medical treatment, however unreasonable this is deemed to be, even when the life of herself or her fetus is at risk. This is true whether the reason is rational or irrational, or even when there is no reason at all. The courts have no jurisdiction to declare non-consensual treatment of such women to be lawful. Only when a baby has been born does it acquire rights.

Capacity

A person lacks capacity if some impairment or disturbance of mental functioning renders that person unable to make a decision about treatment. This will occur when the person is unable to comprehend and retain the information material to the decision, or when the person is unable to retain information and weigh it in the balance as part of the process of arriving at a decision. Incompetence may be temporary, for instance if caused by shock, pain, fatigue, confusion, or panic induced by fear. If health care professionals fear a patient's decision-making (capacity) is impaired they should apply to the court. The Law Commission is keen to ensure that any decisions taken do not violate the European Convention on Human Rights. It is envisaged that, in the future, statutory protection will be given to the informal way decisions are currently made on behalf of incapacitated adults.

Midwives must provide support by giving information that ensures the woman understands events, feels free to ask questions and is aware of how labour is progressing. Before performing any examination verbal permission should be sought, and explanations should be given of what is about to be done and why. Following the procedure, the midwife provides feedback and verbal reinforcement; she then involves the woman in making further decisions about care. Relatives cannot give consent on behalf of a competent woman; it is the woman herself who needs to consent. It is an important principle that a midwife remembers no one else can consent on behalf of a competent adult.

Prevention of infection

Hospitals are notorious sources of infection, which can be resistant to antibiotic treatment. Effective cleaning will reduce the transfer of airborne organisms. A balance between encouraging visitors and accommodating lots of unnecessary people coming in and out of a birthing unit should be considered. Baths, sinks and toilets should be scrupulously cleaned and disinfected between users as necessary. Beds and rooms must also be cleaned thoroughly after use. It is part of ensuring a safe environment for the midwife to ensure that high standards of cleanliness are maintained even if she does not have managerial control over domestic services (Coombes 2001, DoH 2001).

Personal hygiene is important for both mothers and their attendants. The woman should be encouraged to bathe and wash as she wishes to maintain personal freshness and the midwife must wash her hands before and after examining the mother and wear gloves when handling used sanitary pads, bloodstained linen or body fluids.

Women with problems during pregnancy may be admitted to hospital for some time prior to labour; it should be possible to provide the woman with a quiet secure place to sleep as a tired, exhausted woman will have less resistance to combat infection. Some women will need very specialised care, especially women with any transmissible infection such as gastroenteritis, hepatitis or HIV infection.

Women with problem-free pregnancies and labours should be encouraged to stay in their own environment as long as possible, thus reducing the time spent in hospital. If a woman in normal labour is able to stay at home during the latent phase of labour this may also reduce the diagnosis of prolonged labour.

True prolonged labour increases the risk of infection and haemorrhage. Once the woman is admitted to hospital, invasive procedures should be kept to a minimum as an intact skin provides an excellent barrier to organisms and it is important to protect its integrity.

The fetal membranes should also be preserved intact unless there is a positive indication for their rupture that would outweigh the advantage of their protective functions (Clements 2001). Certain invasive techniques, such as the performance of vaginal examinations, may be deemed necessary during labour. However, the midwife should ensure that she has a sound reason before embarking on any procedure. Women whose labours are prolonged are at particular risk of infection and are often subjected to a number of invasive procedures including the administration of intravenous fluids, repeated vaginal examinations, epidural analgesia and fetal blood sampling.

Skin to skin contact

Wallace & Marshall (2001) found that skin-to-skin contact between mother and newborn baby facilitates the initiation of breastfeeding, helps neonatal thermoregulation and promotes maternal–infant attachment. Skin-to-skin contact may also ensure colonisation of the baby with the mother's own skin flora, for which the child will have some resistance.

There are cultural influences that may make implementation of skin-to-skin contact difficult. A mother may find it unacceptable to have a wet baby with some blood on it put straight on to her own skin at birth. In such a case the baby can be dried and cleaned prior to skin-to-skin contact. Hospitals working to adopt UNICEF's Baby Friendly best practice standards (see Ch. 54) must address the requirement that all mothers should be encouraged to hold their naked babies against their skin in a calm and unhurried environment after birth in order to encourage bonding, maintain warmth and initiate breastfeeding. Mothers should have the discussion during labour of what is the most acceptable way of achieving this. Skin-to-skin contact is also a remarkably potent reassurance for a baby against the amount of pain experienced during heel pricks if blood is needed from a newborn baby (Gray et al 2000).

Prelabour rupture of fetal membranes at term

Prelabour rupture of fetal membranes is often a difficult diagnosis. If there are no other signs of labour but the history of ruptured membranes is convincing or obvious liquor is draining then digital examination should be avoided owing to an increased risk of ascending infection. If the diagnosis is not obvious then one sterile speculum examination should be performed to try and visualise pooling of liquor in the posterior fornix; endocervical swabs may also be taken at this time.

For more than 20 years it has been established that 90–95% of women will labour spontaneously without any other intervention within 48 hours (Egan & O'Herlihy 1988). After 48 hours an obstetrician may consider augmentation of labour with vaginal prostaglandin or intravenous oxytocin. Women with prelabour ruptured membranes should have their temperature monitored and auscultation of the fetal heart to exclude a fetal tachycardia or other signs of fetal compromise associated with infection. This observation does not necessitate hospital admission in an otherwise uncomplicated pregnancy. In preterm pregnancies complicated by prelabour rupture of membranes the use of antibiotics (specifically erythromycin) reduces neonatal treatment and is associated with prolongation of pregnancy (Kenyon et al 2001).

Position and mobility

A prospective RCT (de Jong et al 1997) demonstrated that women who adopt an upright position during labour experience significantly less pain and suffer less perineal trauma. Lateral and posterior position of the fetal presenting parts may be associated with more painful, prolonged or obstructed labour and difficult birth. It is possible that maternal posture may influence fetal position (Hofmeyr & Kulier 2001).

Women should be encouraged to give birth in the position they find most comfortable. The benefits and risks of various labour and birthing positions need to be examined to ensure greater certainty. When methodologically stringent trials data are available, then women should be encouraged to use this information to make informed choices about the birth positions they might wish to assume. Midwives must be flexible in their approach to positions that women adopt as well as considering their own health, for example when assuming positions such as leaning to one side for sustained periods to assist women giving birth in a semi-sitting position on a labour ward bed.

Analgesia

Women should be aware of the advantages and disadvantages of all methods of analgesia available to them in their chosen birth environment. This is an essential part of antenatal education and the chosen method of analgesia may affect outcomes (see Ch. 26). Epidural analgesia gives the most effective pain relief in labour but is associated with increased rates of instrumental birth. The COMET study group (2001) reported a normal delivery rate of 35.1% with 'traditional epidural' and 42.7% with low dose (mobile) epidural.

Electronic fetal monitoring (EFM)

Electronic fetal monitoring (EFM) was introduced in the 1970s with the aim of reducing cerebral palsy. A reduction has not been demonstrated, however, and the rate of cerebral palsy remains 2–3 per 10 000 live births (Parkes et al 2001). What has been demonstrated by the use of continuous EFM is an increase in obstetric intervention.

The National Institute for Clinical Excellence (NICE 2001) has recommended that women with an uncomplicated pregnancy should not have EFM as a routine, but that intermittent auscultation with a Pinard stethoscope or handheld Doppler device should be the monitoring of choice. There is no evidence to support an admission CTG; it should therefore not be done as routine.

For women with problems in their pregnancy or other risk factors including the use of oxytocin, or epidural analgesia, EFM is appropriate.

The use of a CTG may appear to limit the choice of position. A telemetric apparatus allows the woman to walk around freely, provided that she remains within a given range. A conventional CTG does not necessarily confine the woman to bed but accurate external monitoring of uterine contractions may be difficult if she is very mobile.

Interpretation of CTG

Trusts should ensure that staff who are performing and interpreting CTG traces have received training and assessment of their skills to ensure these are up to date (NICE 2001). The Clinical Negligence Scheme for Trusts has also set a standard for 6 monthly updating.

Only four variables are considered when interpreting a CTG. These are the baseline rate, the baseline variability, whether accelerations are present and the presence or absence of decelerations. This makes a CTG interpretable into the three categories recommended by NICE (2001) (Fig. 25.1):

- normal
- suspicious
- pathological.

All areas that use EFM should have ready 24-hour access to fetal blood sampling facilities.

This is of course a rather simplistic view as the whole picture of labour must be taken into account, including the gestation, any complications, particularly if the baby is not well grown and is presumed to have less reserves, as well as the stage and length of that specific labour. These guidelines are an aid to clinical judgement with the exception of clearly pathological traces.

All CTG traces should be secured in the notes and kept for a minimum of 25 years along with all other maternity records.

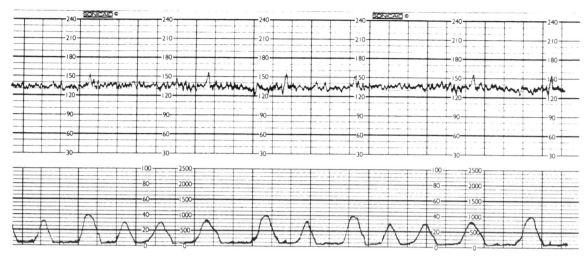

Fig. 25.1 Baseline variability: normal baseline rate.

Nutrition

Anecdotally there appears to be an inequity of care between the home and hospital environment. It seems that as care moves out of the policy-driven environment of the hospital towards the home so that policy seems to lose its power. For instance if there was a national policy stating that no woman was allowed to eat or drink in labour at home there would be a public outcry and we would be accused of violating human rights. Yet, it is acceptable to do exactly that in some hospitals.

The woman's need in labour is for energy and it is carbohydrate that will provide it. Low fat foods such as toast, breakfast cereal, yoghurt, fruit juice, tea, plain biscuits and clear broth are easily digested. Ice cream and jelly may also be refreshing. Fluids may be taken freely although women tend to reduce their drinking as labour progresses (Roberts & Ludka 1994).

Intake in normal labour

Opinions are divided and policies vary between hospitals. In many maternity units, there is little risk of a woman in normal labour needing a general anaesthetic. Some hospitals will allow such women to take a low fat, low residue diet according to appetite, in order to give her energy and ensure that she is not hungry. However, in some centres, women receive nothing to eat after labour is established and are allowed only ice chips to suck. The latter policy stems

from 'the widespread concern that eating and drinking during labour will put women at an increased and unacceptable risk of regurgitation and aspiration of gastric contents' (Johnson et al 1989, p. 827). Aspirated contents from the stomach may contain undigested food and predispose to airway obstruction. If the woman has been fasting, the strongly acidic gastric juice can cause a chemical pneumonitis if inhaled (Mendelson's syndrome). The cardiac sphincter, rendered less efficient by the effects of progesterone, allows a passive leak of stomach contents into the pharynx when loss of consciousness is induced with general anaesthesia. This, combined with the oedema of the pharynx so often present in pregnancy, makes intubation by the anaesthetist a difficult procedure. The answer clearly is to reduce the risk of general anaesthetic and use cricoid pressure during induction of such emergency anaesthetics (see Ch. 31).

Different foods and fluids empty from the stomach at different rates and gastric emptying is prolonged following the administration of narcotic analgesia. Johnson and colleagues point out that there is, however, 'no guarantee that withholding food and drink during labour will ensure that the stomach will be empty in the event that general anaesthesia should become necessary' (Johnson et al 1989, p. 829). In an effort to reduce gastric volume and decrease the gastric acidity of the labouring woman, prophylactic antacids may be administered (see Ch. 31). Newton & Beere

(1997) published a flow chart (Fig. 25.2) of Nottingham City Hospital's approach to eating and drinking in labour for women with problem-free pregnancies.

Glycogenic and fluid requirements

The vigorous muscle contractions of the uterus during labour demand a continuous supply of glucose. If this is not obtained from the diet, the body will start to metabolise protein and fat stores in an effort to provide glucose (gluconeogenesis) without which uterine muscle inertia will occur. This relatively inefficient method of producing glucose results in the occurrence of ketoacidosis. High concentrations of intravenous glucose may artificially increase fetal blood glucose levels, thereby causing fetal hyperinsulinism and resulting in hypoglycaemia of the neonate (Lowe & Reiss 1996, Steele 1995).

For women at increased risk of a general anaesthetic, giving small volumes of water or a weak fruit cordial may be acceptable. If the woman is permitted to follow her inclinations about drinking she is unlikely to become dehydrated. Simple measures such as brushing her teeth or using a mouthwash can help relieve the discomfort of a dry and uncomfortable mouth.

Bladder care

The woman should be encouraged to empty her bladder every 1–2 hours during labour. The midwife should not rely on the mother to request to use the toilet as the sensation of needing to micturate may be reduced, particularly if there is an effective epidural block in progress. If the woman is mobile she may visit the toilet. In women who suffer pregnancy complications with restricted fluids or an intravenous infusion the quantity of urine passed should be measured and a specimen obtained for testing. As urine in the bladder is a non-compressible mass it may interfere with descent of the presenting part or reduce the capacity of the uterus to contract, increasing the risk of postpartum haemorrhage.

A full bladder may also initially prevent the fetal head from entering the pelvic brim. In all cases of delay in labour the midwife should ascertain whether the bladder is full and encourage the woman to void regularly. If it is not possible for the woman to use the toilet the midwife should provide privacy and ensure maximum comfort by placing the bedpan on a stool or

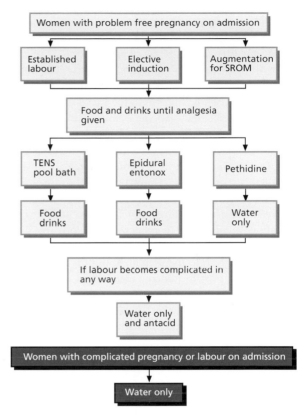

Nottingham City Hospital NHS Trust, Nottingham, UK 1999

Fig. 25.2 Flow chart for eating and drinking during labour in problem-free and complicated pregnancies. (From Newton & Beere 1997, with permission.)

chair or encouraging the woman to adopt a squatting position on the bed. The sound or feel of water can also help to trigger the micturition reflex. If the bladder is incompletely emptied or the woman is unable to void for some hours it may become necessary to pass a catheter.

Observations

The mother

Reaction to labour

As with other major life events, women vary in their reactions to labour. Some may view the contractions experienced as a positive, motivating, life-giving force. Others may feel them as pain and resist them. One woman may welcome the event with excitement because soon she will see her baby; another may be glad the pregnancy is over and with it the cumbersome ungainliness she experienced. However she views labour, the preparatory phase of pregnancy is at an end and within a relatively short period a baby will be born. There may be feelings of apprehension, fear and worry in case she does not conform to the social expectations of her culture. She may experience anxiety in case childbirth is painful and have concerns about her ability to control pain (Niven 1992). As labour progresses she may feel less confident in her ability to cope with the relentless nature of the contractions that control her body. The midwife, with her skillful observations, advice and assistance, can do much to help her. She can encourage and help the woman and when possible give her one-to-one care. Accurate and easy-to-understand information given to the woman about the progress of labour will provide encouragement. Consultation about methods of pain relief will increase feelings of being in control (Ball 1994, Lovell 1996). The management of pain is discussed in Chapter 26.

Pulse rate

The pulse rate is a good indicator of the general physical condition of the woman. If the rate increases to more than 100 beats per minute it may be indicative of anxiety, pain, infection, ketosis or haemorrhage. It is usual to record the pulse rate every 1–2 hours during early labour and every 30 minutes when labour is more advanced.

Temperature

This should remain within the normal range. Pyrexia is indicative of infection or ketosis, or may be associated with epidural analgesia. In normal labour the maternal temperature should be recorded at least every 4 hours.

Blood pressure

Blood pressure is measured every 2–4 hours unless it is abnormal, in which case more frequent recordings will be necessary depending on the individual situation. The blood pressure must also be monitored very closely following epidural or spinal anaesthetic (see Ch. 26). Hypotension may be caused by the supine position, shock or as a result of epidural anaesthesia.

In a woman who has had pre-eclampsia or essential hypertension during pregnancy, labour may further elevate a raised blood pressure.

Urinalysis

Urine passed during labour should be tested for glucose, ketones and protein. Ketones may occur as a result of starvation or maternal distress when all available energy has been utilised. A low level of ketones is very common during labour and thought not to be significant. Unless the non-diabetic mother has recently eaten a large quantity of carbohydrate or sugar, glucose is found in the urine only following intravenous administration of glucose.

A trace of protein may be a contaminant following rupture of the membranes or a sign of a urinary infection, but more significant proteinuria may indicate pre-eclampsia.

Fluid balance

A record should be kept of all urine passed to ensure that the bladder is being emptied. If an intravenous infusion is in progress, the fluids administered must be recorded accurately. It is particularly important to note how much fluid remains if a bag is changed when only partially used.

Abdominal examination

An initial abdominal examination is carried out when the midwife first examines the mother. This should be repeated at intervals throughout labour in order to assess the length, strength and frequency of contractions and the descent of the presenting part. The method is described in Chapter 16.

Contractions. The frequency, length and strength of the contractions should be noted. When a uterine contraction begins, it is painless for a number of seconds and painless again at the end. The midwife when feeling for contractions is aware of the beginning of the contraction before the woman feels it. This knowledge can be utilised when giving inhalational analgesia or using other coping mechanisms (see Ch. 26). The uterus should always feel softer between contractions. Contractions, which are unduly long or very strong and in quick succession give cause for concern as fetal hypoxia may develop. Hyperstimulation should be considered if oxytocin is being infused. It should be stopped if fetal compromise or hyperstimulation are apparent.

Descent of the presenting part. During the first stage of labour, descent can be followed almost entirely by abdominal palpation. It is usual to describe the level in terms of the fifths of the head, which can still be palpated above the brim (see Figs 16.31, p. 271 and 24.13, p. 448).

In the primiparous woman the fetal head is usually engaged before labour begins. If this is not the case, the level of the head must be estimated frequently by abdominal palpation in order to observe whether the head will pass through the brim with the aid of good contractions.

When the head is engaged, the occipital protuberance can be felt only with difficulty from above but the sinciput may still be palpable, owing to increased flexion of the head, until the occiput reaches the pelvic floor and rotates forwards.

Vaginal examination and progress in labour

Although it is not essential to examine the woman vaginally at frequent intervals, it may be useful to do so when progress is in doubt or another indication arises (see Ch. 24). The features that are indicative of progress are effacement and dilatation of the cervix, and descent, flexion and rotation of the fetal head. There do not appear to be many research-based recommendations on the timing and frequency of carrying out a vaginal examination in labour. As this intervention can be extremely distressing to some women, alternative methods of assessment should be considered (Nolan 2001); routine examinations in normal labour should be abandoned and an individualised approach taken. All examinations should be recorded on the labour record.

Effacement and dilatation of the cervix. In normal labour the primiparous cervix effaces before dilating, whereas in the parous woman these two events often occur simultaneously. The latent phase of labour is usually defined as up to 3–4 cm dilated (see Ch. 24). There is no agreed 'starting point' for the onset of labour. However, acknowledging the latent phase and not commencing a partogram too early will reduce the overdiagnosis of 'failure to progress' later in labour.

Progressive dilatation is monitored as labour continues and charted on either the partograph or the cervicograph. This will allow for early detection of abnormal progress and indicate when intervention is likely. The use of cervograms to monitor labour has limitations and must be understood and applied appropriately (Gee 2000) (see also Ch. 24).

Descent. When assessed vaginally, the level or station of the presenting part is estimated in relation to the ischial spines, which are fixed points at the outlet of the bony pelvis. During normal labour the head descends progressively. The midwife must be aware, while estimating whether the head is lower than previously, that marked moulding or a large caput will give a false impression of the level of the fetal head.

Flexion. In vertex presentations, progress depends partly on increased flexion. When the head is driven down on to the pelvic floor it encounters resistance: the lever principle causes the anterior part of the head to flex because there is less counterpressure. The midwife assesses flexion by the position of the sutures and fontanelles. If the head is fully flexed, the posterior fontanelle becomes almost central; if the head is deflexed, both anterior and posterior fontanelles may be palpable.

Rotation. Rotation is assessed by noting changes in the position of the fetus between one examination and the next. The sutures and fontanelles are palpated in order to determine position. Even if insufficient information is gained to make a definitive diagnosis, a record is made of what is felt and the findings will be evaluated with the abdominal findings at the time and compared with the findings of earlier or later vaginal examinations.

The fetus

Fetal condition during labour can be assessed by obtaining information about the fetal heart rate and patterns, the pH of the fetal blood and the amniotic fluid.

The fetal heart

The fetal heart rate may be assessed intermittently by a Pinard stethoscope or handheld Doppler device or continuously using EFM.

Intermittent monitoring. This term is used when the fetal heart is auscultated at intervals using a monaural fetal stethoscope (Pinard's) or a handheld Doppler device.

The rate of the fetal heart should be counted over a complete minute in order to listen for the beat-to-beat variation. The baseline rate should be between 110 and 160 beats per minute (b.p.m.). Doppler apparatus can be used throughout a contraction, but listening during a contraction with a monaural stethoscope

(Pinard) is uncomfortable for the woman and the fetal heart sounds may be inaudible. Using a Pinard the midwife can listen in to the fetal heart rate as the contraction is finishing to detect any slow recovery of the fetal heart rate back to the baseline. Normally the baseline rate is maintained during a contraction and immediately after it. However, in late labour some decelerations with contractions that recover quickly may be due to cord compression or compression of the fetal head and are normal. Variability of more than 5 b.p.m. should be maintained throughout labour. If decelerations are heard in the first stage of labour with a Pinard or Doppler instrument then electronic monitoring may be indicated to assess the extent of decelerations.

Continuous EFM. This depends on the use of electronic apparatus in the form of a fetal heart monitor. Continuous recording usually combines a fetal cardiograph and a maternal tocograph in a CTG apparatus. This presents a graphic record of the response of the fetal heart to uterine activity as well as information about its rate and variability.

An ultrasound transducer may be strapped to the abdomen at the point where the fetal heart is heard at maximum intensity. This method is less invasive than internal monitoring with a fetal scalp electrode attached to the fetal scalp, as it does not require rupture of the membranes. With modern monitors this external monitoring should be adequate in most labours that require electronic monitoring. In exceptional circumstances an electrode may be applied to the fetal scalp over a bone of the fetal skull, taking care to avoid the fontanelles. In order to achieve this the membranes must be ruptured and the cervix be at least 2–3 cm dilated. The electrode is connected to the CTG by electrical wiring. A small scalp wound is inevitable and is contraindicated in preterm (< 34 weeks' gestation) pregnancies, in women with known clotting disorders and in those with known bloodborne diseases.

Internal or external cardiography may be used in conjunction with telemetry to monitor the fetal heart when the mother wishes to move away from the machine. A portable battery-operated transmitter is carried about by the ambulant woman. The scalp electrode or transducer transmits the fetal heart recording by radio to the CTG where it is recorded on the readout chart. It is impossible to obtain a recording of uterine activity when the mother is walking about, but if she depresses a handheld button at the onset of each contraction the strip chart will be marked accordingly.

Findings. The CTG provides information on:

- baseline fetal heart rate
- baseline variability
- accelerations
- decelerations
- uterine activity.

Baseline fetal heart rate. This is the fetal heart rate between uterine contractions. A rate more rapid than 160 b.p.m. is termed *baseline tachycardia*; a rate slower than 110 b.p.m. is *baseline bradycardia*. Either may be indicative of fetal compromise due to a number of causes. If the baseline is outside the stated normal range then referral to an obstetrician is appropriate.

Baseline variability. Electrical activity in the fetal heart results in minute variations in the length of each beat. This causes the tracing to appear as a jagged rather than a smooth line (Fig. 25.3). The baseline rate should vary by at least 5 beats over a period of 1 minute. Loss of this variability (Fig. 25.4) may indicate fetal compromise. Reduced variability may be noted for a short period after the administration of maternal pethidine, which depresses the cardiac reflex centre in the fetal brain. Periods of 'fetal sleep' also cause a reduction in variability and commonly last for 20–30 minutes even in advanced labour (Gibb 1988, Lowe & Reiss 1996).

Response of the fetal heart to uterine contractions. The fetal heart rate will normally remain steady or accelerate during uterine contractions during the first stage of labour. In order to assess the significance of fetal heart rate decelerations accurately, their exact relationship to uterine contractions, size, shape and uniformity must be noted. Compression of the umbilical cord, or fetal head, will result in some decelerations particularly if the membranes are not intact. These would be early or variable decelerations lasting less than 3 minutes with good recovery to predeceleration rate.

A late or variable deceleration lasting longer than 3 minutes begins during or after a contraction reaches its nadir (lowest point) after the peak of the contraction and has not recovered by the time that the contraction has ended. Sometimes the deceleration has barely recovered by the onset of the next contraction. The *time lag* between the peak of the contraction and the nadir of the deceleration is more significant of severity than

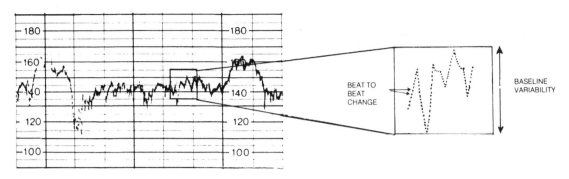

Fig. 25.3 Baseline variability.

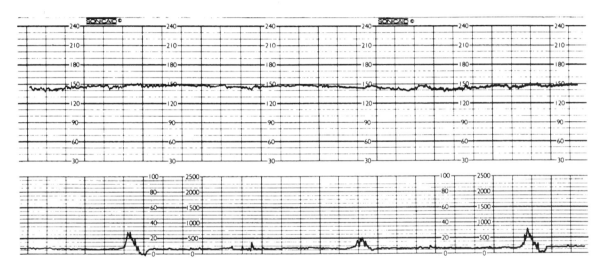

Fig. 25.4 Uncomplicated loss of baseline variability: normal rate, no decelerations.

the drop in the fetal heart rate. This is more sinister and would be classified as pathological. A midwife should refer this situation to an experienced obstetrician.

Fetal blood sampling

Units that use electronic fetal monitoring should have 24 hour access to fetal blood sampling (FBS) facilities. When the fetal heart rate pattern is suspicious or pathological and fetal acidosis is suspected then FBS should always be carried out (NICE 2001). The procedure should be carried out with the woman in the left lateral position as a lithotomy position is more distressing for both mother and fetus (Fig. 25.5). If imminent delivery is clearly indicated by a severely

pathological CTG then no time should be wasted performing an FBS. This would be the clinical decision of a senior obstetrician. A fetal blood sample result of 7.25 or below should be repeated usually within 30 minutes to an hour. An FBS below 7.20 indicates that the baby should be delivered.

Amniotic fluid

Amniotic fluid escapes from the uterus continuously following rupture of the membranes. This fluid should normally remain clear. If the fetus becomes hypoxic, meconium may be passed as hypoxia causes relaxation of the anal sphincter. The amniotic fluid becomes green as a result of meconium staining. Amniotic fluid that is a muddy yellow colour or is only slightly green may signify a previous event from which the fetus has recovered, but is common and of no significance in postdates babies.

If the breech is presenting and is compacted in the pelvis, the fetus may pass meconium because of the compression of the abdomen; a fetus presenting by the breech is also prone to fetal compromise and may pass meconium as a result of hypoxia.

In the rare case of a fetus that is severely affected by Rhesus isoimmunisation, the amniotic fluid may be golden-yellow owing to an excess of bilirubin.

Bleeding of sudden onset at the time of rupture of the membranes may be the result of ruptured vasa praevia and is an acute emergency (see Ch. 32).

Fetal compromise

'Fetal distress' is a term that should no longer be used. If the fetus suffers as a result of an intrapartum event resulting in oxygen deprivation then the following signs may be present:

- fetal tachycardia
- a pathological CTG and corresponding poor FBS result
- fetal bradycardia or a severe change in fetal heart rate or decelerations related to uterine contractions, or both
- passage of meconium-stained amniotic fluid.

Midwife's management of fetal compromise. If signs are apparent a midwife must call an appropriately trained obstetrician. If oxytocin is being administered, it should be stopped and the woman placed in a favourable position, usually on her left side. In cases of maternal oxygen lack, such as eclampsia or shock due to antepartum haemorrhage, oxygen may be given via a face mask. Prolonged oxygen administration will not benefit the fetus. The doctor may wish to take a sample of fetal blood for testing and arrangements should be made for this or delivery will be expedited depending on the clinical situation. In the first stage of labour this will necessitate caesarean section. In the second stage of labour a forceps delivery or ventouse extraction may be performed. In all cases of delivery following indications to expedite delivery, the presence of a paediatrician or appropriately trained practitioner is desirable (UKCC 1998).

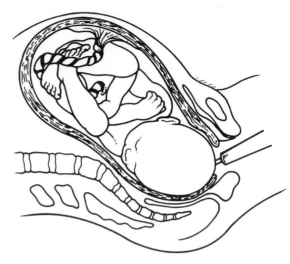

Fig. 25.5 Fetal blood sampling. Access to fetal scalp via amnioscope passed through the cervix.

Preterm labour

Preterm labour (for causes of this see Ch. 41) is defined as labour occurring before the 37th completed week of pregnancy, regardless of birthweight (WHO 1969). A fetus is legally viable from 24 weeks' gestation. If a fetus is expelled from the uterus prior to 24 weeks and shows no sign of life, it is classified in the UK as a miscarriage (abortion). The World Health Organisation recommends recording all deliveries of greater than 500 grams birthweight.

Preterm labour is associated with significant long term disability and morbidity. After 29–30 weeks' gestation the birthweight is a good predictor of survival. Prior to 29 weeks' gestation the birthweight, gender, multiple pregnancy and gestation are all considered in the equation of risks of morbidity and mortality. The incidence of preterm birth is increasing, but currently stands at around 8%, although with wide racial differences (Atalla et al 2000, p. 113).

Increased perinatal survival, which is attributed to increased neonatal intensive care facilities and appropriately trained personnel, has altered policies towards management of the woman in preterm labour. A woman who is at risk of delivering prematurely should be transferred to a unit with intensive neonatal facilities, preferably with the fetus in utero. Tocolytic drugs may be used in very early labour to delay delivery until transfer to such a unit. Antenatal administration of steroids has been shown to reduce the incidence of hyaline membrane disease, intraventricular haemorrhage and necrotising enterocolitis in fetuses of 26–34 weeks' gestation. Two doses given over 24 hours last for at least 7 days.

The 8th annual CESDI (2001) report on the project of 27/28 week gestation babies states that 88% of these survive – almost double that of 15 years previously.

Management of preterm labour

The gestation of the pregnancy in preterm labour influences the management. Generally, the earlier the gestational age the higher is the possibility of an infective cause, which is often followed by rapid labour and delivery. Caesarean section of cephalic preterm infants offers no reduction in fetal morbidity or trauma and is associated with its own morbidity. It is generally accepted that the mode of delivery of gestations less that 26 weeks does not alter the outcome. Prolonging pregnancies beyond 34 weeks does not improve neonatal outcomes; therefore no attempt is usually made to arrest labour if pregnancy has advanced to 34 weeks' gestation (Atalla et al 2000, p. 129).

Skilled care is required for the woman and the fetus during labour. The mother is faced with an unexpected emotional crisis because of the interruption of the normal progress of pregnancy. In extreme prematurity (22–25 weeks) a high perinatal mortality rate means the woman and her partner have to face the possibility of the death or disability of their baby. Full discussion regarding possible outcomes and whether or not to attempt resuscitation should be carried out with the senior clinicians involved in the care, and of course the parents. Continuous electronic heart rate monitoring is difficult to interpret at less than 30 weeks' gestation and should therefore be used and interpreted with caution. Baseline variability may be reduced on the CTG.

Records

The midwife and other practitioners have a legal and professional duty to keep clear and concise records of all events, of the woman's physical and psychological condition and of the condition of her fetus (see Ch. 24). Records must be legible in photocopiable ink; they must also be dated and signed. The purpose of records is to serve the interest of the woman, to demonstrate the chronology of events as well as all significant consultations, assessments, observations, decisions, interventions and outcomes.

A written individualised care plan should be recorded in labour following examination and consultation with the woman. This should attempt to follow the birth plan, which was devised in pregnancy. If the woman changes her mind as her labour progresses, or the situation changes, adjustments can be made. Whether or not a formal birth plan has been prepared, the midwife who is caring for the woman should communicate effectively with her, evaluate whether the labour is proceeding as expected and listen to her requests. A comprehensive record of the discussions that take place about changes in the plan or about proposed measures will ensure that the closest possible attention is paid to achieving the outcome that the parents are hoping for and will also provide an excellent documented history of the labour and improve communication.

Box 25.1 lists best practice points for this stage of labour.

Box 25.1 Best practice points

- Women should be well informed and choice offered on evidence-based information where possible.
- A competent woman can give or withhold consent for any procedure.
- Another adult cannot consent or withhold consent on behalf of a competent woman.
- Good communication between women, midwives and between professionals is a fundamental component of maternity services.
- The latent phase of labour should be more widely acknowledged in hospital settings.
- The use of strict time limits for first and second stage of labour should be reviewed in problem-free pregnancies.
- Good record keeping and care plans are an essential aspect of care.

REFERENCES

Atalla R, Kean L, McParland P 2000 Preterm labor and prelabor rupture of fetal membranes. In: Kean L, Baker P, Edlestone D (eds) Best practice in labour ward management. W B Saunders, London, p 113, 129

Ball J A 1994 Reactions to motherhood, 2nd edn. Books for Midwives Press, Hale, Cheshire

Brown S J, Lumley J 1998 Communication and decision-making in labour: do birth plans make a difference? Health Expectations 1(2):106–116

Clements C 2001 Amniotomy in spontaneous, uncomplicated labour at term. British Journal of Midwifery 9(10):629–634

CESDI (Confidential Enquiry into Stillbirths and Deaths in Infancy) 2001 8th annual report. Maternal and Child Health Research Consortium, London

Clinical Standards Advisory Group 1995 Women in normal labour: report of a CSAG committee on women in normal labour. HMSO, London

COMET (Comparative Obstetric Mobile Epidural Trial) Study Group UK 2001 Effect of low dose mobile versus traditional epidural techniques on mode of delivery: a randomized controlled trial. Lancet 358(9275):19–23

Coombes R 2001 Thoroughly modern matron. Nursing Times 97(15):10–11

de Jong P R, Johanson R B, Baxen P, Adrains V D, van der Westhusien S, Jones P W 1997 Randomised controlled trial comparing the upright and supine positions for second stage of labour. British Journal of Obstetrics and Gynaecology 104:567–571

DoH (Department of Health) 2001 Ward sisters to have greater control over cleaning standards: extra £30 m to drive up standards as part of biggest ever clean-up campaign. DoH, London, 17 January

Egan D, O'Herlihy C 1988 Expectant management of spontaneous rupture of membranes at term. Journal of Obstetrics and Gynaecology 8:243–247

Fraser D, Symonds M, Cullen L, Symonds I 2000 A university department merger of midwifery and obstetrics: a step on the journey to enhancing interprofessional learning. Medical Teacher 22(2):179–183

Gee H 2000 Abnormal patterns of labour and prolonged labour. In: Kean L H, Baker P, Edleston D I (eds) Best practice in labour ward management. W B Saunders, London

Gibb D 1988 A practical guide to labour management. Blackwell Scientific Publications, Oxford

Gray L, Watt L, Blass E M Skin-to-skin contact is analgesic in healthy newborns. Pediatrics 105(1) part 1:110–111

Green J M, Coupland V A, Kitzinger J V 1990 Expectations, experiences and psychological outcomes of childbirth: a prospective study of 825 women. Birth 17(1):15–24

Green J M, Coupland V A, Kitzinger J V 1998 Great expectations: a prospective study of women's expectations and experiences of childbirth, 2nd edn. Hale: Books for Midwives Press, Hale, Cheshire

Hodnett E D 2001 Caregiver support for women during childbirth. In: The Cochrane Library, Issue 3. Update Software, Oxford. (Date of most recent substantive amendment: 17 May 1999.)

Hodnett E D, Osborn R W 1989a Effects of continuous intrapartum professional support on childbirth outcomes. Research in Nursing and Health 12:289–297

Hodnett E D, Osborn R W 1989b A randomized trial of the effects of support during labor: mothers' views two to four weeks postpartum. Birth 16(4):177–183

Hofmeyr G, Kulier R 2001 Hands/knees posture in late pregnancy or labour for fetal malposition (lateral or posterior). In: The Cochrane Library, Issue 3. Update Software, Oxford. (Date of most recent substantive amendment: 9 November 1997)

Johnson C, Keirse M J N C, Enkin M, Chalmers I 1989 Nutrition and hydration in labour. In: Chalmers I, Enkin M, Keirse M J N C (eds) Effective care in pregnancy and childbirth. Oxford University Press, Oxford, vol 2, p 827–832

Kenyon S L, Taylor D J, Tarnow-Mordi W et al 2001 Broad-spectrum antibiotics for preterm, prelabour rupture of fetal membranes: the ORACLE I randomised trial. Lancet 357(9261):979–988

Langer A, Campero L, Garcia C et al 1998 Effects of psychosocial support during labour and childbirth on breastfeeding, medical interventions, and mothers' wellbeing in a Mexican public hospital: a randomised clinical trial. British Journal of Obstetrics and Gynaecology 105(10):1056–1063

Lindow S W, Hendricks M S, Thompson J W et al 1998 The effect of emotional support on maternal oxytocin levels in labouring women. European Journal of Obstetrics and Gynecology and Reproductive Biology 79(2):127–129

Lovell A 1996 Power and choice in birthgiving: some thoughts. British Journal of Midwifery 4(5):268–272

Lowe N K, Reiss R 1996 Parturition and fetal adaptation. Journal of Obstetric, Gynecological and Neonatal Nursing 25(4):339–349

Mackin P, Sinclair M 1998 Labour ward midwives' perceptions of stress. Journal of Advanced Nursing 27(5):986–991

Madi B C, Sandall J, Bennett R et al 1999 Effects of female relative support in labor: a randomized controlled trial. Birth 26(1):4–8

Newton C, Beere P 1997 Oral intake in labour: Nottingham's policy formulated and audited. British Journal of Midwifery 5(7)

NICE (National Institute for Clinical Excellence) 2001 The use of electronic fetal monitoring: the use and interpretation of cardiotocography in intrapartum fetal surveillance. NICE, London

Niven C 1992 Psychological care for families: before, during and after birth. Butterworth-Heinemann, Oxford

Nolan M 2001 Vaginal examinations in labour: expert view. Practising Midwife 4(6):22

O'Driscoll K, Meagher D 1993 Active management of labour, 3rd edn. Mosby, London

Parkes J, Dolk H, Hill N et al 2001 Cerebral palsy in Northern Ireland: 1981–93. Paediatric and Perinatal Epidemiology 15(3):278–286

RCOG/RCM (Royal College of Obstetricians and Gynaecologists/Royal Colleges of Midwives) 1999 Towards safer childbirth. RCOG/RCM, London

Re F [1990] 2 AC 1

Re MB [1997] The Times LR 18 April

Ritchie J W 1995 Fetal surveillance. In: Whitfield C (ed) Dewhurst's textbook of obstetrics and gynaecology for postgraduates, 5th edn. Blackwell Science, Oxford, ch 28

Roberts C C, Ludka L M 1994 Food for thought. Childbirth Instructor Magazine (Spring):25–29

Sidaway v Bethlem Royal Hospital Governors & Ors [1985] 1 All ER 643 (HL)

Steele R 1995 Midwifery care during the first stage of labour. In: Alexander J, Levy V, Roch S (eds) Aspects of midwifery practice: a research-based approach. Macmillan, Hampshire, vol 4, ch 2

UKCC (United Kingdom Central Council for Nursing Midwifery, and Health Visiting) 1998 Midwives rules and code of practice. UKCC, London

Umstad M, Permezel M, Pepperell R 1995 Litigation and the intrapartum cardiotocograph. British Journal of Obstetrics and Gynaecology 102:89–91

Walkinshaw S A 1995 Preterm labour and delivery of the preterm infant. In: Chamberlain G (ed) Turnbull's obstetrics, 2nd edn. Churchill Livingstone, New York, ch 33

Wallace H, Marshall D 2001 Skin-to-skin contact: benefits and difficulties. Practising Midwife 4(5):30–32

Wallace E M, Mackintosh C L, Brownlee M et al 1995 A study of midwife–medical staff interaction in a labour ward environment. Journal of Obstetrics and Gynaecology 15(3): 165–170

WHO (World Health Organisation) 1969 Prevention of Perinatal Morbidity and Mortality. Public Health Papers 42. WHO, Geneva

FURTHER READING

Graham H (ed) 2000 Understanding health inequalities. Open University Press, Buckingham

This book reiterates how midwifery has a huge public health agenda and highlights areas where better understanding of social disadvantage can help midwifery practice.

Kean L, Baker P, Edlestone D I (eds) 2000 Best practice in labour ward management. W B Saunders, London

This concise book is a guide to current best practice; it gives guidance on areas of labour that are likely to be scrutinised.

Kirkham M (ed) 2000 The midwife–mother relationship. Macmillan, Basingstoke

Communication issues can be reflected on whilst reading this book.

Kirkham M (ed) 2000 Developments in supervision. Books for Midwives Press, Manchester

This easy-to-read book gives good examples of how statutory supervision is changing for the benefits of midwives and women. It is a useful resource for both supervisors and supervisees.

Seymour J 2000 Childbirth and the law. Oxford University Press, Oxford

This helpful book will increase the student's understanding of the law in the UK and also offers practical scenarios.

Thomas A, Paranjothy S 2001 The National Sentinel Caesarean Section Audit. RCOG, London

This report contains data of 99% of all births during a 3 month period and offers a very informative snapshot of areas for debate.

26 Pain Relief and Comfort in Labour

Adela Hamilton

CHAPTER CONTENTS

This chapter will explore the variety of means used by the midwife to achieve, for each woman and her partner, a birth experience, that they can regard as positive.

This chapter aims to:

- present an overview of factors affecting women's perceptions of pain during labour
- discuss the physiology of pain with particular reference to the causes of pain in labour
- discuss how methods such as support and reassurance, encouragement, information giving and the provision of a relaxing environment can impact positively on birth experiences of women
- describe the strategies of pain relief that make use of the body's own control mechanisms
- consider the pharmacological methods of relieving pain in labour.

Definitions of pain

Pain is said to be 'a feeling of distress, suffering or agony caused by stimulation of specialised nerve endings' (O'Toole 1997). However, a definition more suited to midwifery would be that pain is 'a complex, personal, subjective, multifactorial phenomenon which is influenced by psychological, biological, sociocultural and economic factors' (Telfer 1997).

A variety of factors affect the intensity and amount of pain experienced by women in labour. These include:

- perceptions of pain
- tolerance of pain
- coping mechanisms
- individual meaning of pain
- expression of pain
- communication of pain
- cultural characteristics
- environment of pain – whether at hospital or at home, etc.

Factors influencing women's perceptions of pain

The biological, psychological, social, spiritual, cultural and educational dimensions of each woman have an impact on how they express themselves and, indeed, how they perceive pain during labour. The challenge for midwifery is to provide adequate and adapted care for each childbearing woman. The essence of midwifery is to be 'with woman', providing comfort in labour. Historically, the maintenance of health has been the role of women (Kitzinger 2000). Women have, throughout the ages, supported and helped each other during the process of birth. There is much literature to venerate the presence of the doula, midwife or friend of the birthing woman and the positive effect of the presence of this person on the outcome of labour. Much midwifery and medical research has indicated that the one-to-one support by a midwife in labour reduces the need for analgesia and improves the birth experience of the mother. It also shortens the length of the labour (Halldorsdottir & Karlsdottir 1996, Hodnett, 1995, Hodnett & Osborn 1989, Yerby 1996).

Some evidence still suggests that midwives continue to emphasise pharmacological methods and techniques to control pain in labour, rather than assisting women to use their own personal ability to cope with this (Niven, unpublished work, 1986). Odent (1984) has always defended a philosophy of natural childbirth, constantly believing in the aptitude and innate capability of the birthing woman. The midwife is a key figure in this process, supporting and assisting women through childbirth. Other reports reveal that there is little conformity between how women themselves perceive their pain relief and how this is viewed by the medical personnel, with medical staff finding that pain relief was sufficient for the woman, whereas women themselves stated that this was not so (Rajan 1993). Mander (1992) states that the pain itself and its severity, plus the side-effects of medication, make it difficult for the woman to maintain control during labour. Women then require care, support, attention and advice at this time. Concerns have been raised as to whether women in labour, or the technology that seems to be so conspicuous at this time, are the centre for attention and consideration of professionals (Deakin 2001, Gould 2000, Walsh 2000). Although there is much technology and many devices available to assist the birth process, the woman and her family must remain at the centre of attention of the midwife. Halldorsdottir & Karlsdottir (1996) state that a midwife who is involved in the woman's lived experience of giving birth is one who improves this experience for her.

Mobility and positioning in labour

Studies carried out on ambulation, mobility and positioning during labour agree that mobility during labour improves both the woman's experience and the outcome of labour (Deakin 2001, Downe et al 2001, Flynn et al 1978, Read et al 1981). In their studies, Flynn et al (1978) and Read et al (1981) found the following advantages:

- more effective uterine action
- shorter labour
- less oxytocin augmentation
- reduced need for pharmacological analgesia
- fewer operative deliveries
- lower incidence of fetal compromise.

It is also documented that recumbent positions result in supine hypotension, diminished uterine activity and a reduction in the dimensions of the pelvic outlet (Walsh 2000); de Jong et al (1997) state that women who take up an erect position during labour experience less pain, have significantly less perineal trauma and have fewer episiotomies.

Culture, movement and positioning

Kitzinger (2000) would go as far as pronouncing that 'birth is movement' (p. 749). Gould (2000) would agree, saying that movement is a significant characteristic of normal labour. Cultures where women are constrained and limited in their posture and positioning during labour are in fact the exception rather than the rule. Many cultures use movement, dance, physical contact and massage to encourage and sustain the process of labour. Writers now provide valuable reports and evidence of the engineering and movements made by some mothers in Africa, Japan and Fiji, which actually employ physiological responses of the woman. These include turning, moving and dancing.

These enhance the experience and facilitate the process of labour. There is much to be said for such an approach where the woman dictates the course of events and adapts to the activity of the uterus. This could well be considered to be an example of 'women-centred care'. One author also remarks how women move and swing their pelvis, thereby accommodating the passage of the fetal head through it (Kitzinger 2000). Walsh (2000) mentions that the compelling logic of gravity, meaning birthing in an upright position, should make us wonder how it has become routine practice to deliver in a semirecumbent position.

Walsh (2000) recommends that mobility in labour should be encouraged as it lessens the need for pharmacological analgesia. Many writers agree that midwives should adapt their role, attitude and care to each childbearing woman (Deakin 2001, Halldorsdottir & Karlsdottir 1996, Lundgren & Dahlberg 1998). Walsh (2000) remarks that there is much evidence to suggest that women are still being subjected to invasive procedures that invariably increase, not lessen, pain in labour – thereby failing to improve women's experience of childbirth.

The birth plan

The birth plan is a document that describes the woman's requests in relation to her antenatal, intrapartum and postnatal care. This may be adjusted and changed as necessary to meet the needs of the woman during the pregnancy, labour, birth and postpartum period. It is a valuable tool for midwives and facilitates the provision of holistic, individualised care. Many areas such as: personal choices, pain relief, methods of feeding, management of the third stage of labour and the giving of vitamin K to the neonate are discussed by the woman and the midwife. These requests are then written down and are kept in the handheld notes of the woman. It may also be useful to confirm the contents of the plan with the client as labour commences. It must also be made clear that these are the personal choices of the woman in labour, and may well change as labour progresses, the unpredictable nature of labour being as it is. It may be useful for providing an insight into how the woman has viewed her pain relief at the beginning of pregnancy, and on commencing labour. The midwife may use this information to tailor and plan suitable care for the woman.

Women's control of pain during labour

Pain control during labour is a very woman-centred concept. There is much evidence to suggest that women are not always more satisfied by a birth experience that is pain free (Fairlie et al 1999, Morgan et al 1982). Midwives are therefore required to give control of the pain to women rather than eradicating it (Mander 1992). The same author also states that a clear differentiation must be made between the traditional goal of pain relief and the control of pain in labour.

There is no evidence to suggest that information is of lesser importance to women of lower socioeconomic status. Midwives must also take into account that high expectations antenatally do not impact negatively on women's experience of birth (Green et al 1998). This evidence should be used by midwives to provide women-centred care, and, as Walsh states: 'Knowledge is power and a positive anticipation of birth is consistent with viewing it as a physiological … event' (Walsh 2000, p. 276).

The role of the midwife then is to encourage and assist women to 'anticipate positively' the birth of their baby. Two researchers in Japan revealed in their study on the intensity of memorised labour pain (Kabeyama & Miyoshi 2001) that 'Self-control is the most important predictor of satisfactory childbirth experience for mothers' (p. 51). They state that women who viewed labour as a challenge, in their attempt to control their breathing and relaxation, had much better outcomes. These active attitudes are supposed to reflect the positive attitudes to everything in daily life by the individual. The study goes on to say that not only does the removal of excessive fear and anxiety make a birth experience more satisfactory but that it also increases the mother's pride and self-confidence. A greater motivation for constructing good mother–baby relationships also comes about.

Pain perception and somatosensory sensation

Many writers and researchers now agree that emotions such as fear, confidence, and also cognition (i.e. the meaning or understanding of pain that an individual has), affect the person's perception of pain (Kitzinger

1996, Mander 1998). More than any other type of sensation, pain can be modified by past experience, anxiety, emotion and suggestion. Lack of food rest and sleep also impact on the woman's perception of pain. The midwife must take into account not only the level or extent of the pain, but also all other subjective or illusory aspects of this.

The physiology of pain

Pain stimulus and pain sensation

Pain is caused by a stimulus; this stimulus may cause, or be on the verge of causing, tissue damage. Pain sensation may therefore be distinguished from other sensations, although emotions such as fear and anxiety are also experienced at the same time, thereby affecting the person's perception of pain. It must also be remembered that a painful stimulus may also induce such changes by the sympathetic nervous system as increased heart rate, a rise in blood pressure, release of adrenaline (epinephrine) into the bloodstream and an increase in blood glucose levels. There is also a decrease in gastric motility and a reduction in the blood supply to the skin, causing sweating. Thus, stimuli that cause pain result in a *sensory* incident or occurrence.

Pain transmission

The pain pathway or ascending sensory tract originates in the sensory nerve endings at the site of trauma. The impulse travels along the sensory nerves to the dorsal root ganglion of the relevant spinal nerve and into the posterior horn of the spinal cord. This is known as the *first neuron*. The *second neuron* arises in the posterior horn, crosses over within the spinal cord (the sensory decussation) and transmits the impulse via the medulla oblongata, pons varolii and the midbrain to the thalamus. From here it travels along the *third neuron* to the sensory cortex (Fig. 26.1).

In cases of *acute pain*, sensations are transmitted along *A delta fibres*, which are large diameter nerve fibres. This type of pain is perceived as being a pricking pain that is readily localised by the sufferer. The pathway for *chronic pain* is slightly different, the nerve fibres involved being of smaller diameter, and are called *C fibres*. Chronic pain is often described as a burning pain that is difficult to localise.

Somatosensory function

'Somatic sensation' refers to the sensory function of the skin and body walls. This is moderated by a variety of somatic receptors. There are particular receptors for each sensation, such as heat, cold, touch, pressure, etc. On entering the central nervous system, the afferent nerve fibres from somatic receptors form synapses with interneurons that comprise the specific ascending pathways going to the somatosensory cortex via the brain stem and the thalamus.

An *afferent neuron*, with its receptor, makes up a sensory unit. Usually the peripheral end of an afferent neuron branches into many receptors. The receptors whose stimulation gives rise to pain are situated in the peripheries of small unmyelinated or slightly myelinated afferent neurons. These receptors are known as *nociceptors* because they detect injury (Noci: from Latin: harm, injury). The primary afferents coming from nociceptors form synapses with interneurons after entering the central nervous system. Substance P is a *neurotransmitter* that is liberated at some of these synapses when there is a pain impulse; it facilitates information about pain, which is transmitted to the higher centres.

The pain of labour (see Fig. 26.2 for pain pathways in labour) in transmitted by afferent or visceral sensory neurons, visceral pain being caused by the stretching or irritation of the viscera. Afferent neurons convey both autonomic sympathetic and parasympathetic fibres. Pain fibres from the skin and the viscera run adjacent to each other in the spinothalamic tract. Therefore pain from an internal organ, such as the uterus, may be perceived or felt as if it was coming from a skin area supplied by the same section or part of the spinal cord. Pain from the uterus may be perceived or felt in the back or the labia. When this sort of pain occurs or is experienced, it is commonly called *referred pain*.

One physiological explanation for the differing views, attitudes and perceptions of pain is that offered by Martini (2001, p. 93) who states that: 'Due to the facilitation that results from glutamate and substance P release, the level of pain experienced can be out of proportion to the amount of painful stimuli. This effect can be one reason why people differ so widely in their perception of pain associated with childbirth.'

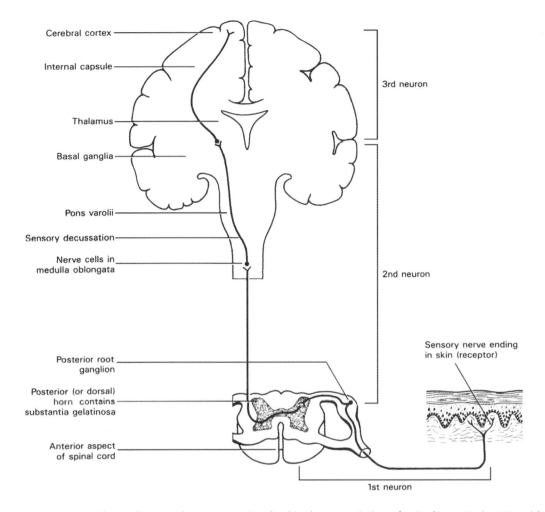

Fig. 26.1 The sensory pathway showing the structures involved in the appreciation of pain. (From Bevis 1984, with permission of Baillière Tindall.)

Endorphins and enkephalins

Endorphins are described as being opiate-like peptides, or *neuropeptides*, which are produced naturally by the body at neural synapses at various points in the central nervous system pathways. They modulate the transmission of pain perception in these areas. Endorphins are found in the limbic system, hypothalamus and reticular formation (Martini 2001). They bind to the presynaptic membrane, inhibiting the release of substance P. Therefore they inhibit the transmission of pain. *Enkephalins* are also neuropeptides; they have the ability to inhibit neurotransmitters along the pathway of pain transmission, thereby reducing it.

Theories of pain

Many theories of pain have been presented in the literature. These include specificity, pattern, affect and psychological/behavioural theory (Mander 1998). The most widely used and accepted theory is that of Melzack & Wall (1965). These researchers have established that gentle stimulation actually inhibits the sensation of pain (Mander 1998). Their *gate-control theory* states that a neural or spinal gating mechanism occurs in the substantia gelatinosa of the dorsal horns of the spinal cord. The nerve impulses received by nociceptors, the receptors for pain in the skin and tissue of the body, are affected by the gating mechanism. It is the

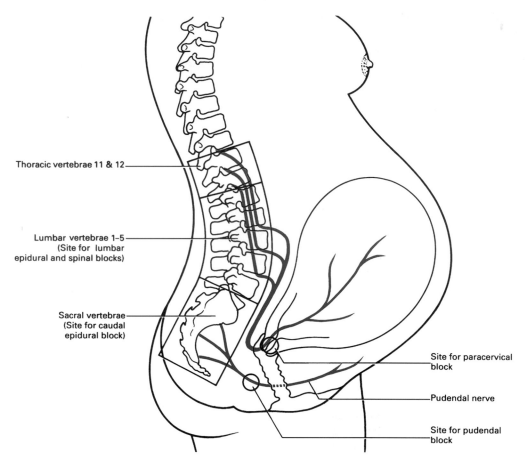

Thoracic vertebrae 11 & 12

Lumbar vertebrae 1–5
(Site for lumbar
epidural and spinal blocks)

Sacral vertebrae
(Site for caudal
epidural block)

Site for paracervical
block

Pudendal nerve

Site for pudendal
block

Fig. 26.2 Pain pathways in labour, showing the sites at which pain may be intercepted by local anaesthetic technique. (From Bevis 1984, with permission of Baillière Tindall.)

position of the gate that determines whether or not the nerve impulses travel freely to the medulla and the thalamus, thereby transmitting the sensory impulse or message, to the sensory cortex. If the gate is closed, there is little or no conduction. If the gate is open, the impulses and messages pass and are transmitted freely. Therefore, when the gate is open, pain and sensation is experienced.

Physiological responses to pain in labour

Several of the bodily systems are affected by labour. Pain of labour is associated with an *increased respiratory rate*. This may cause a decrease in the P_aCO_2 level, with a corresponding increase in the pH. The fetus is then affected and a subsequent drop in the fetal P_aCO_2 ensues. This may be suspected by the presence of late decelerations on the cardiotocograph. The acid–base equilibrium of the system may be altered by hyperventilation and breathing exercises. Alkalosis may then affect the diffusion of oxygen across the placenta, leading to fetal hypoxia.

Cardiac output increases during the first and second stages of labour. This can be by up to 20% and 50% respectively. The augmentation is caused by the return of uterine blood to the maternal circulation, about 250–300 ml with each contraction. Pain, apprehension and fear may cause a sympathetic response, thereby producing a greater cardiac output.

Both the above systems are affected by catecholamine release. Adrenaline (epinephrine), which comprises about 80% of this, has the effect of reducing the uterine blood flow. This may in turn lead to a reduction of uterine activity.

Non-pharmacological methods of pain control

Homeopathy

The aim of homeopathy is to reinforce the body's physiological response. It attempts to 'cure like with like' (Alexander et al 1990). Homeopathic remedies are prepared from plant extracts and from minerals. Professional advice is recommended during pregnancy as the holistic approach of this method entails a consideration of all the facets and the requirements of the individual. Castro (1992) recommends such solutions as Aconitum to relieve anxiety and Kali carbonicum to alleviate back pain during labour.

Hydrotherapy

Immersion in water during labour as a means of analgesia has been used for years (Forde et al 1999). Garland & Jones (1994) state that the effectiveness of hydrotherapy is due to two factors. Heat relieves muscle spasm, and therefore pain, and 'hydrokinesis' does away with the effects of gravity and also the discomfort and strain on the pelvis. Mander (1998) suggests that there is relatively little reliable and valid evidence to prove that bathing during labour increases maternal or neonatal infection. Other writers agree with this (Forde et al 1999, Waldenstrom & Nilsson 1992). Advantages such as less augmentation by oxytocics and a reduction of analgesia used were stated by several authors (Forde et al 1999, Mander 1998). Forde et al (1999) maintain that hydrotherapy has other benefits such as a reduction in the length of labour and a lower incidence of genital tract trauma. It is difficult to establish the evidence for hydrotherapy, because of the increase in pool births. However, these two – that is, hydrotherapy used as analgesia and birthing in the pool when the birth is carried out in water – are distinctly different.

Research by Moore (1997) has revealed that hydrotherapy during childbirth has the following outcomes:

- mothers require less augmentation of labour
- the mother's experience was positively affected by hydrotherapy
- the use of analgesia was consistently lower in this group
- the need for pethidine and Entonox was significantly reduced

One randomised controlled trial showed that pain increased less markedly in women who used hydrotherapy (Cammu et al 1994). Moore (1997) and Downe et al (2001) state that an aggressive and active approach to labour demands that all midwives question their actions and their attitude to this. They say that there is at present much intervention, not only of a surgical or medical nature.

Music therapy

There is little mention of this potentially very therapeutic stratagem. Most research has been carried out to examine its effect on chronic conditions (Zimmermann et al 1989) and also postoperatively (Locsin 1981). Mander (1998) suggests that there is need for more research in this area as women cannot be informed of the advantages of music therapy without sound evidence.

TENS

Transcutaneous electrical nerve stimulation (TENS) is a widely used, well-appreciated and an effective method of pain relief. This effectiveness is related to the action of TENS, which stimulates the production of natural endorphins and enkephalins and also its ability to impede incoming pain stimuli (Cluett 1994). One of its distinct advantages is that it includes the partner in the events surrounding the birth. Much documentary evidence suggests that when using TENS many husbands and birth partners feel able to assist and support their partner in labour and childbirth to a much greater degree. Walsh (1999) reports that partners feel a purposeful role. A reduction in the demand for pethidine was also found (Walsh 1999).

Technique

The apparatus consists of four electrodes and four flexes that connect these to the TENS unit, which has controls to alter the frequency and the intensity of the impulse. The electrodes are positioned at the level of T10 and L1 on the mother's back. These have been found to be effective for the control of pain during the first stage of labour (Johnson 1997). The other two electrodes are situated between S2 and S4 and provide control of pain during the second stage of labour. A boost control button conveys high intensity and high frequency patterns of stimulation of the dermatomes, thereby controlling pain during the uterine contraction and providing relief.

There are few contraindications to the utilisation of TENS in labour (Walsh 1999). There is a slight risk of interference with the fetal monitor. Skin allergies may also be caused by the electrodes or the tape used. Finally, clients who have pacemakers may not employ this mode of pain control.

TENS is often more effective when commenced in early labour, and this fact is upheld by the literature (Johnson 1997, Walsh 1999). Walsh (1999) and Cluett (1994) both agree that an important factor regarding TENS is that it is preferred by women. This is probably due to the fact that TENS enhances their control over the birth process.

TENS works by stimulating low threshold afferent fibres from, for example, the fibres of touch receptors. This then leads to inhibition of neurons in the pain pathways. As pathways activated by the touch receptors add a synaptic input into the pain pathways, people may rub or massage a painful area to relieve the pain; TENS functions in the same way.

The research on TENS recognises the lack of scientific evidence to substantiate the fact that women in labour do find the application of this method effective. The reality is that it is used in conjunction with other methods of pain relief, and this makes the method very difficult for researchers to verify (see Carrol et al 1997). There is, however, strong indication to substantiate the usefulness of TENS to women in labour. In one study by Johnson (1997), 71% of the respondents out of a population 10 077 stated having had either good or excellent pain relief from the TENS method. Although Johnson (1997) cautions against an oversimplistic interpretation of these results, as many of the participants used other methods of pain relief in conjunction with TENS, it can still be remarked that many women find TENS suitable, effective and beneficial.

Pharmacological methods of pain control

Opiate drugs

Opiate drugs are frequently used during childbirth because of their powerful analgesic properties. The action of these drugs lies in their ability to bind with receptor sites in the central nervous system. The receptor sites are mainly found in the substantia gelatinosa of the dorsal horn of the spinal cord. Others are located in the midbrain, thalamus and hypothalamus.

Three systemic opioids are commonly used for pain relief in labour. Pethidine (meperidine in the USA) is the most popular but some units prefer diamorphine or meptazinol (Meptid). All have similar pain-relieving properties but they also have side-effects. These include nausea, vomiting and drowsiness in the mother and depression of the baby's respiratory centre at birth. An antiemetic agent is sometimes given at the same time to reduce the nausea effect. According to a number of writers (e.g. Moore 1997, Ransjo-Arvidson et al 2001), opioids given to the mother in labour can make breast-feeding more difficult to establish as the baby tends to be sleepy. The side-effects are, however, variable and are influenced by maternal metabolism of drugs, the degree and speed of transfer of drugs and metabolites from maternal to fetal circulation and the ability of the fetus to process and excrete both. It is therefore important to ensure that the mother is fully informed antenatally so that she can make informed decisions about pain relief. A systematic review by Elbourne & Wiseman (2002) to compare different types of opioids concluded that no strong preference could be recommended and further better quality research is needed.

Pethidine

Pethidine is the most frequently used systemic narcotic analgesic. This is possibly because it is of low cost and midwives have been administering pethidine without a prescription for many years. It is a synthetic compound and acts on the receptors in the body. It is usually administered intramuscularly in doses of 50–150 mg (taking the size of the woman into account) and takes about 20 minutes to have an effect. Pethidine can be administered intravenously for a faster effect and some units use a machine to allow patient-controlled analgesia (PCA), but this is less common.

Pethidine delays stomach emptying and women may not use the birthing pool if they have been given an opiate drug. Some reports show that pethidine slows down the process of labour. Carson (1996) states that this may be due to the effect of opioids on the myometrium, relaxing it by their action on calcium ions, and also the effect of opioids on the hypothalamus, inhibiting the release of oxytocin from the posterior pituitary gland.

Diamorphine

Diamorphine has been found to provide effective analgesia for up to 4 hours in labour. It is also said to be more rapidly eliminated from maternal and neonatal plasma (Freeman et al 1982). Diamorphine is used far less commonly than other opiates in labour even though some claim it gives better pain relief and hence more comparative studies are needed (Fairlie et al 1999). It is possible that its lack of use in normal labour might be due to fears of the potentially addictive nature of diamorphine.

Meptazinol

Park & Fulton (1991) favoured the use of meptazinol as it is said to cause less respiratory depression in the neonate. It is usually given in doses of 100–150 mg intramuscularly. It is fast acting and is effective for about 4 hours. Meptazinol may be associated with an increased incidence of nausea and vomiting (Carson 1996). It has failed to replace pethidine in most maternity units.

Inhalation analgesia

Entonox is the most commonly used inhalation analgesia in labour. It is a premixed gas made up of 50% nitrous oxide and 50% oxygen. Nitrous oxide, like many other forms of analgesia, acts by limiting the neuronal and synaptic transmission within the central nervous system. The mixture is stable at normal temperature, but separates under the temperature of −7°C. In many large obstetric units the gas is piped, or alternatively is available in cylinders. Hospitals take responsibility for the safe storage of cylinders but in community practice midwives should store cylinders on their side, rather than upright. This is because nitrous oxide is heavier than oxygen and the horizontal position reduces the risk of delivering a severely hypoxic mixture. The cylinders must be brought into a warm room if they have been exposed to cold temperatures, and the gases remixed by inverting the cylinder at least three times before use.

Entonox apparatus is usually manufactured by the British Oxygen Company (BOC). Both the apparatus and the cylinder are made so that they do not fit on to other equipment. These fit together by a pin index system. The cylinder is blue with a blue and white shoulder. The one-way valve opens on inspiration and the mother needs to be adequately informed of the functioning of the apparatus, being advised that optimal analgesia is obtained by closely applying the lips around the mouthpiece or, in some cases, firmly applying the mask to the face (Fig. 26.3). Entonox takes effect within 20 seconds; it is therefore important that the woman uses it before a contraction. The maximum efficacy of the Entonox occurs after about 45–50 seconds and, if the timing is right, this should occur with the height of the contraction, providing maximum relief for the woman. This method of pain control is useful in that the woman is able to administer it herself. The effectiveness of it relies on the woman's prior instruction and ability to follow this (Mander 1998).

Some reports state that teratogenic and other side-effects exist among staff who are exposed to high levels of nitrous oxide (Ahlborg et al 1996). The main one of these is that of subfertility. Scavenging equipment, to extract expired gases, is recommended for all birthing rooms. Although there is some difficulty in finding evidence to support the efficacy of Entonox analgesia, Wraight (1993) claims that 85% of women voiced satisfaction with this method.

Regional (epidural) analgesia

More women are now requesting a pain-free labour and ask for epidural analgesia as soon as labour is established. Women who find alternative methods of pain relief inadequate once experiencing strong contractions might decide to request an epidural when labour is well advanced. This makes explanation of epidural analgesia antenatally even more important. The pain relief from an epidural is obtained by blocking the conduction of impulses along sensory nerves as they enter the spinal cord. When epidural block in labour was first introduced in the 1970s most attention

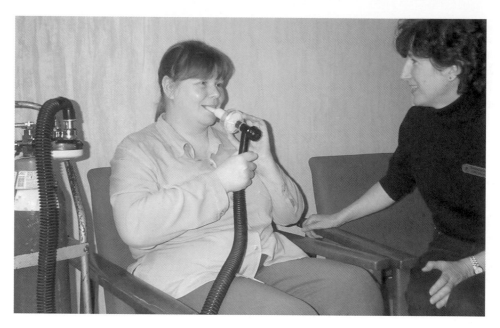

Fig. 26.3 Midwife explaining the use of Entonox apparatus. Note the mouthpiece and filter.

was focused on the technique and less on the problems it caused in relation to normal birth. In those early years, as well as providing the required sensory block, the blockade of motor and sympathetic nerves caused loss of bladder sensation and function, complete numbness of the legs, significant hypotension, relaxation of pelvic floor muscles and impairment of expulsive efforts in the second stage of labour.

When advising women about the advantages and disadvantages of epidural analgesia, it is important to use local evidence about availability and the procedure used so that women can make a realistic choice for their labour. Wide variations in the provision of an epidural service have been found (e.g. Mander (1995) reports epidural rates as high as 87% whereas Morgan (1993) reports a 14% rate), but in recent years a more equitable service has been available. Burnstein et al (1999) report that the ideal of providing an epidural service for all women who request it within a consultant unit is being achieved. The percentage of units providing a 24 hour epidural service has risen from 78% in 1991 to 90% in 1999. This study also confirms that the average epidural rate within UK obstetric units has increased to 24%. Almost half of the units indicate a rise in the uptake of epidural analgesia. However, there will always be a number of contraindications to the use of regional analgesia (Table 26.1).

Advantages and disadvantages of epidural analgesia

Goer (1995), Mander (1998) and Howell (2001; 2002) cite some of the advantages and disadvantages of epidural analgesia (Table 26.2). As well as the main advantage of epidural analgesia in labour – to eradicate pain (Howell & Chalmers 1992) – a further advantage is that it can be converted to anaesthesia (abolition of sensation) to facilitate operative delivery (see Ch. 31). However, even in normal labour, as well as blocking the pain impulses motor neurons are also affected causing varying degrees of immobility. The motor paralysis that used to be caused, and was disliked by women and midwives (Morgan & Kadim 1994), is being remedied by the use of low dose infusion epidurals or 'mobile' epidurals.

Preparation of the mother

The woman and her partner must have a clear explanation of the procedure and the woman's consent must be obtained. An intravenous infusion of crystalloid fluids is commenced prior to siting the epidural. The need for 'preloading' has reduced now that low dose epidural blockades are used, reducing the risk of hypotension. Frequently the mother is positioned in the left lateral for the procedure. This is partly because of the risk of supine hypotension and also because the

Table 26.1 Contraindications to regional analgesia, with associated risks

Contraindication	Risk
Uncorrected anticoagulation or coagulopathy	Vertebral canal haematoma
Local or systemic sepsis (pyrexia above 38°C not treated with antibiotics)	Vertebral canal abscess
Hypovolaemia or active haemorrhage	Cardiovascular collapse secondary to sympathetic blockade
Patient refusal	Legal action
Lack of sufficient trained midwives for continuous care and monitoring of mother and fetus for the duration of the epidural blockade	Maternal collapse, convulsion, respiratory arrest, fetal compromise

Table 26.2 Advantages and disadvantages of epidural

Disadvantages of epidural analgesia	Advantages of epidural analgesia
Ineffective blocks	Effective pain relief
More frequent monitoring of vital signs	The tendency to lower blood pressure can be an advantage in the case of PIH
Lengthens first stage of labour	If labour is prolonged, gives effective pain relief allowing mother to rest
Less able to adopt different birth positions	
Less sensation of expulsive efforts and lengthens second stage of labour; increase in instrumental vaginal delivery	Does not depress the respiratory centre of the fetus

mother may well be more comfortable in this position when in labour. Some anaesthetists may find it easier or may prefer to ask the mother to sit up and flex the spine, in an effort to separate the vertebrae, thus facilitating the management of the procedure. The position of the mother is very important for her and for the anaesthetist and this should be discussed and negotiated with her best interest in view. The fetal heart rate and the woman's blood pressure must be recorded throughout, especially in the case of pregnancy-induced hypertension, or in any case of suspicion of fetal compromise.

Epidural technique

A local anaesthetic is injected into the epidural space of the lumbar region, usually between vertebrae L1 and L2, or between L2 and L3, or between L3 and L4. The procedure is carried out by an experienced (obstetric) anaesthetist, under strict aseptic conditions. The usual aseptic technique is employed, the area disinfected and

the region draped. A small amount of local anaesthetic is used before inserting a Tuohy needle into the epidural space (Fig. 26.4). To locate the epidural space the anaesthetist advances the needle cautiously. The Tuohy needle, usually 16 g, is introduced little by little until the resistance of the ligamentum flavum is encountered. At this point a syringe is attached to the Tuohy needle, after removal of the stilette. The needle is then inserted further, cautiously, until it enters the epidural space. This is recognised by the loss of resistance when pressure is applied to the plunger of the syringe (loss of resistance to saline is sometimes preferred). It is particularly important that the woman keeps very still at this stage as the subarachnoid space is a few millimetres deeper. A slight movement by the woman could result in the Tuohy needle inadvertently puncturing the meninges and causing a 'dural tap'.

Once confident that the Tuohy needle is in the epidural space and there has been no leakage of blood or CSF, a catheter is threaded through the needle to

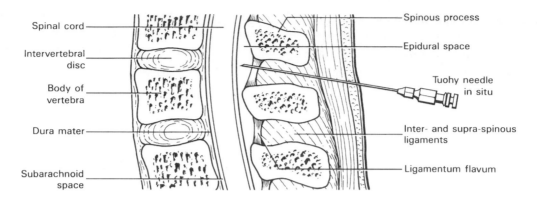

Fig. 26.4 Sagittal section of the lumbar spine with Tuohy needle in position.

facilitate bolus top-ups or a continuous infusion. A test dose of the local anaesthetic lidocaine (lignocaine), of about 4 ml, may then be given – although some anaesthetists prefer to inject the first dose of bupivacaine (Marcain) very slowly whilst observing for any adverse reactions. Continuous infusion of dilute bupivacaine and opioids (usually fentanyl) has permitted significant reductions in the amount of local anaesthetic used whilst ensuring rapid analgesia. A further advantage of this regimen lies in the mother's ability to move about and bear down in the second stage of labour because of the minimal motor block effect. The Comparative Obstetric Mobile Epidural Trial (COMET Study Group UK 2001) found that low dose infusion epidurals resulted in a lower incidence of instrumental vaginal deliveries compared with traditional bolus epidurals.

An antibacterial filter is attached to the end of the catheter. The catheter is then secured to the mother's back with strapping (ensuring that she is not allergic to plasters) and a syringe pump set up by the anaesthetist if there is to be a continuous infusion.

Observations and care by the midwife

After the administration of the first dose of bupivacaine and any subsequent top-up doses of local anaesthetic, the blood pressure and pulse should be measured and recorded every 5 minutes for 20–30 minutes and then every 30 minutes. The mother may sit up in bed once it has become established that her blood pressure is stable, but should be tilted to one side to prevent aortocaval compression.

Throughout labour the mother should be assisted to change her position regularly to avoid soft tissue damage. The fetal heart is usually monitored electronically. The mother may be unaware of a full bladder, so the midwife must ensure that the woman is encouraged to empty her bladder regularly. Similarly she will not feel uterine contractions, or a desire to bear down in the second stage of labour, so close observation is necessary. Uterine activity may be electronically monitored.

The spread of the block is checked regularly by the midwife. Units vary in whether they use a cold object or ethyl chloride spray to test the extent to which the mother has lost sensation; needles are no longer advocated for this purpose.

The epidural top-up

Midwives top up the epidural block by giving a further dose as prescribed by the anaesthetist. The prescription should indicate clearly the dosage and frequency of the drugs to be given, and the positioning of the woman. The midwife is personally responsible for ensuring that she is competent to carry out the procedure. The same observations are made as with the initial dose. The midwife should be aware of the possible complications and their immediate treatment. It is important to prevent aortocaval occlusion since this would compound the effects of any hypotension occurring as a result of the epidural block.

Complications of epidural analgesia

The use of low dose bupivacaine solutions for analgesia in labour has limited the risks of hypotension and local anaesthetic toxicity. The complications of epidurals may include:

- dural puncture and consequent headache
- total spinal: respiratory arrest
- local anaesthetic toxicity: cardiac arrest
- fetal compromise (resulting from hypotension or local analgesic toxicity)
- loss of bladder sensation (need for catheterisation)
- increased need for assisted vaginal birth
- neurological sequelae (serious damage extremely rare; weakness/sensory loss is uncommon but soon resolves).

For most women the side-effects following epidural are minimal and backache is more likely to be due to localised bruising and immobility than epidural analgesia. The increased use of epidural analgesia has in particular resulted in an increase in assisted vaginal birth (Goer 1995). According to Thorp et al (1993) intervention is much less likely to occur if the epidural has been sited after 5 cm of dilatation of the cervical os, but this view remains contentious. Thorp's study finding is, however, in keeping with the view of Sutton quoted in Nolan (1997), who puts forward the notion that the birth process necessitates the 'opening of the mother's back'. By this is meant the lifting up of the lower lumbar vertebrae and the sacrum to facilitate the passage and birth of the baby. It is argued that today's lifestyle, for example the way women sit with their legs crossed, and their knees higher than the pelvis, does not increase the available space for the fetus, therefore making it difficult for the head to enter the pelvis.

The fact that more forceps births are carried out if the cervical dilatation is less than 5 cm when the epidural is sited also supports the above view. If the head is engaged and below the ischial spines, the head is likely to be well flexed and satisfactory progress is made. The effect of the local anaesthetic reduces the muscle tone of the pelvic floor, which needs to remain firm to aid flexion and rotation of the fetal head, before allowing the fetal head to advance. The fetal head then, in the case of an epidural, may not fully flex and progression may be arrested. Intervention then follows.

Postdural puncture headaches and dural tap. If there has been a 'dural tap' during the procedure, women are likely to develop a severe postural headache caused by leakage of CSF. Headaches from a dural tap can also follow spinal anaesthesia for operative deliveries. However, needles used for deliberate spinal injection are much finer than Tuohy needles and the use of smaller gauge 'pencil point' needles has greatly reduced the leakage of CSF. Severe headache following a 'dural tap' is treated by epidural injection of 10–20 ml of maternal blood (a 'blood patch'), to seal the puncture and relieve the headache.

Hypotensive incident. Local analgesic affects the sympathetic nervous system by causing vasodilatation and a fall in blood pressure. For most women the fall is minimal. However, if the mother's systolic blood pressure falls below 75% of baseline (e.g. from 120 to 90 mmHg) she should be given oxygen and turned on her side while waiting for the anaesthetist. Hartmann's solution is normally infused rapidly if the blood pressure remains low. The lateral position should be assumed to prevent this happening. Adrenaline (epinephrine), a vasopressor, may be used if required to raise maternal blood pressure, increase cardiac output and the heart rate (Armand et al 1993).

Patchy blocks. The epidural may be more effective on one side or in certain areas of the woman's body. It may be extremely difficult for the anaesthetist to produce an even, effective block. The anaesthetist must be kept informed and will attempt to render the block more efficient, by resiting it, changing the position of the woman or injecting more local anaesthetic.

The responsibilities of the midwife

The midwife has an important enabling and facilitating role to help the woman maintain control of pain during childbirth. Careful administration of drugs and monitoring the effects of these is essential to the provision of quality care. Accurate and detailed records of all care given will provide a good basis from which proper decisions may be made concerning the progress and the needs of the woman.

REFERENCES

Ahlborg G, Axelsson J, Bodin L 1996 Shift work nitrous oxide exposure and subfertility among Swedish midwives. International Journal of Epidemiology 25(4):783–790

Al-Azzawi F 1990 A colour atlas of childbirth and obstetric techniques. Wolfe, London

Alexander J, Levy V, Roch S 1990 Intrapartum care: a research-based approach. MacMillan, London

Armand S, Tasson J, Talafre M L, Amiel-Tison C 1993 The effects of regional analgesia on the newborn. In: Reynolds F (ed) Effects on the baby of maternal analgesia and anaesthesia. W B Saunders, London

Beischer N A, Mackay E V, Colditz P B 1997 Obstetrics and the newborn: an illustrated textbook, 3rd edn. W B Saunders, London

Bevis R 1984 Anaesthesia in midwifery. Baillière Tindall, London

Burns E E, Blamey C, Lloyd A J 2000 Aromatherapy in childbirth: an effective approach to care. British Journal of Midwifery 8(10):639–643

Burnstein R, Buckland R, Pickett J A 1999 A survey of epidural analgesia for labour in the United Kingdom. Anaesthesia (54):634–640

Carrol D, Tramer M, McQuay H et al 1997 Transcutaneous electrical nerve stimulation in labour: a systematic review. British Journal of Obstetrics and Gynaecology 104:169–175

Carson R 1996 The administration of analgesics. Modern Midwife 12–16

Cammu H, van Clasen K, Wettere L et al 1994 'To bathe or not to bathe' during the first stage. Acta Obstetrica Gynaecologica Scandinavica 73(6):468

Castro M 1992 Homeopathy for mother and baby. McMillan, London

Cluett E 1994 Transcutaneous electrical nerve stimulation Analgesia in labour: a review of the TENS method. Professional Care of Mother and Child, March: 50–52

COMET (Comparative Obstetric Mobile Epidural Trial) Study Group UK 2001 Effect of low-dose mobile versus traditional epidural techniques on mode of delivery: a randomised controlled trial. Lancet 358:19–23

de Jong P, Johanson R, Baxen P, Adrians V, van der Westhuisen S, Jones P 1997 Randomised trial comparing the upright and supine positions for the second stage of labour. British Journal of Obstetrics and Gynaecology 104(5):567–571

Deakin B-A 2001 Alternative positions in labour and childbirth. British Journal of Midwifery 9(10):620–625

Downe S, McCormick C, Beech B L 2001 Labour interventions associated with normal birth. British Journal of Midwifery 9(10):602–606

Dunn C, Sleep J, Collett D 1995 Sensing an improvement: an experimental study to evaluate the use of aromatherapy, massage and periods of rest. Journal of Advanced Nursing 21(1):34–40

Elbourne D, Wiseman RA 2002 Types of intra-muscular opioids for maternal pain relief in labour (systematic review). Cochrane Pregnancy and Childbirth Group Database of Systematic Reviews, Issue 1. Update Software, Oxford

Fairlie F M, Marshall L, Walker J J, Elbourne D 1999 Intramuscular opioids for maternal pain relief in labour: a randomised controled trial comparing pethidine with diamorphine. British Journal of Obstetrics and Gynaecology (106):1181–1187

Flynn A M, Kelly J, Hollins G, Lynch P F 1978 Ambulation in labour. British Medical Journal (2):591–593

Forde C, Creighton S, Batty A, Hawdon J, Summers-Ma S, Ridgway G 1999 Labour and delivery in the birthing pool. British Journal of Midwifery 7(3):165–171

Freeman R M, Moreland T A, Blair A W 1982 Diamorphine, the obstetric analgesia: a neurobehavioural and pharmacokinetic study in the neonate. Journal of Obstetrics and Gynaecology (3):102–106

Garland D, Jones K 1994 Waterbirth, first stage immersion or non-immersion? British Journal of Midwifery 2(3):113–120

Gaylard D G, Carson R J, Reynolds F 1990 Effect of umbilical perfusate pH and controlled maternal hypotension on placental drug transfer in the rabbit. Anaesthesia and Analgesia (71):42–48

Goer H 1995 Obstetrical myths and research realities. A guide to the medical literature. Bergin & Garvey, London

Gould D 2000 Normal labour: a concept analysis. Journal of Advanced Nursing 31(2):418–427

Green J, Coupland B, Kitzinger J 1998 Great expectations: a prospective study of women's expectations and experiences of childbirth. Child Care and Development Group, Cambridge

Halldorsdottir S, Karlsdottir S I 1996 Journeying through labour and delivery: perceptions of women who have given birth. Midwifery (12):48–61

Henderson C, Jones K (eds) 1997 Essential midwifery. Mosby, London

Hodnett E D 1995 Support during childbirth in support from caregivers during childbirth. Cochrane Pregnancy and Childbirth Database, Issue 1. Update Software, Oxford

Hodnett E D, Osborn R W 1989 Effects of continuous intrapartum professional support on childbirth outcomes. Research in Nursing Health 12(5):289–297

House of Commons 1992 Health Committee Second Report, Maternity services. HMSO, London

Howell C J, Chalmers I 1992 A review of prospectively controlled comparisons of epidural with non-epidural forms of pain relief during labour. International Journal of Obstetrical Anaesthesia (1):93–110

Howell C J et al 2001 A randomized, controlled trial of epidural, compared with non-epidural analgesia in labour. British Journal of Obstetrics & Gynaecology 108:27–33

Howell C J 2002 Epidural versus non-epidural analgesia for pain relief in labour (Cochrane Review). In: The Cochrane Library, Issue 4 2002. Update Software, Oxford

Johnson M I 1997 Transcutaneous nerve stimulation in pain management. British Journal of Midwifery 5(7):400–405

Johnson R, Taylor W 2000 Skills for midwifery practice. Churchill Livingstone, London

Kabeyama K, Miyoshi M 2001 Longitudinal study of the intensity of memorized labour pain. International Journal of Nursing Practice (7):46–53

Kitzinger S 1987 Some women's experiences of epidurals: a descriptive study. National Childbirth Trust, London

Kitzinger S 2000 Some cultural perspectives of birth. British Journal of Midwifery 8(12):746–750

Locsin R G 1981 The effect of music on the pain of selected post-operative patients. Journal of Advanced Nursing 6(1):19–25

Lundgren I, Dahlberg K 1998 Women's experience of pain during childbirth. Midwifery 14:105–110

Mander R 1992 The control of pain in labour. Journal of Clinical Nursing 1(1):219–223

Mander R 1995 Forum on maternity and the newborn: pain in labour. Midwives 108(1289):180

Mander R 1998 Pain in childbearing and its control. Blackwell Science, London

Martini F H 2001 Fundamentals of anatomy and physiology, 5th edn. Prentice Hall, London

Melzack R, Wall P D 1965 Pain mechanisms: a new theory. Science 150(3699):971–979

Moore S 1997 Psychological support during labour. In: Henderson C, Jones K (eds) Essential midwifery. Mosby, London

Morgan B, Kadim M Y 1994 Mobile regional analgesia in labour. British Journal of Obstetrics and Gynaecology 101(10):839–841

Morgan B M 1993 Obstetrical anaesthesia. In: Chamberlain G, Wraight A, Steer P (eds) Pain and its relief in childbirth. Churchill Livingstone, Edinburgh

Morgan B M, Bulpitt C J, Clifton P, Lewis P J 1982 Analgesia and satisfaction in childbirth. Lancet ii:808–810

Morris P J 2001 Epidural analgesia: historical summary and present practice. British Journal of Midwifery 9(1):36–40

Nursing and Midwifery Council 2002 Code of professional conduct. NMC, London

O'Toole M 1997 Miller-Keane encyclopaedia and dictionary of medicine, nursing and allied health, 6th edn. W B Saunders, London

Odent M 1984 Birth reborn. Souvenir Press, London

Park G, Fulton B 1991 The management of acute pain. Oxford University Press, Oxford

Rajan L 1993 Perceptions of pain and pain relief in labour: the gulf between the experience and observation. Midwifery 9:136

Ransjo-Arvidson A-B, Matthieson A-S, Lilja G, Nissen E, Widstrom, A-M, Uvnas-Moberg K 2001 Maternal analgesia during labor disturbs newborn behavior: effects on breastfeeding, temperature and crying. Birth 28(1):5–11

Read J, Miller F, Paul R 1981 Randomised trial of ambulation versus oxytocin for labour enhancement: a preliminary report. American Journal of Obstetrics and Gynecology (139):669–672

Robinson J 1995 Use of heroin in labour. AIMS Journal 7(2):9–10

Steer P 1993 The methods of pain relief used. In: Chamberlain G, Wraight A, Steer P (eds) Pain and its relief in childbirth. Churchill Livingstone, Edinburgh

Telfer F M 1997 Relief of pain in labour. In: Sweet B R, Tiran D (eds) Mayes' midwifery, 12th edn. Baillière Tindall, London

Thorp J A et al 1993 The effect of intrapartum epidural analgesia on nulliparous labour: a randomised, controlled, prospective trial. American Journal of Obstetrics and Gynecology 169(4):851–8

Waldenstrom U, Nilsson C-A 1992 Warm tub bath after spontaneous rupture of membranes. Birth 19(2):57–63

Walsh D 1999 Transcutaneous electrical nerve stimulation. British Journal of Midwifery 7(9):580

Walsh D 2000 Evidence-based care series 1. Birth environment. British Journal of Midwifery 8(5):276–278

Wraight A 1993 Coping with pain In: Chamberlain G, Wraight A, Steer P (eds) Pain and its relief in childbirth. Churchill Livingstone, Edinburgh

Yerby M 1996 Managing pain in labour. Part 1: perceptions of pain. Modern Midwife, March:22–24

Zimmermann L, Pazehl B, Duncan K, Schmitz R 1989 Effects of music in patients who had chronic cancer pain. Western Journal of Nursing Research 11(3):298–309

USEFUL ADDRESS

A useful information leaflet for pregnant women has been produced by the Obstetric Anaesthetists Association and can be obtained through the secretariat: secretariat@oaa-anaes.ac.uk

27

Transition and the Second Stage of Labour

Soo Downe

When labour moves from the phase of dilatation to the phase of active maternal pushing, the whole tempo of activity changes. As the nature of her uterine activity changes, the mother's response to her labour often moves through confusion and loss of control to intense physical effort and exertion as her baby is finally pushed towards its birth. Both parents require stamina and courage, and confidence in the skill of the attendant midwife. Excitement and expectation mount as the birth becomes imminent. A happy outcome will depend upon mutual respect and trust between professionals and parents. A mother will never forget a midwife who positively supports her capacity to give birth to her baby.

The nature of normality in labour has been subject to debate for a number of years (Crawford 1983, Downe 1996, Gould 2000, Montgomery 1958). In the context of this debate, the chapter aims to:

- consider the nature of the transitional and second stage phases of labour

- describe the usual sequence of events during these stages

- summarise signs of transition and of the expulsive phase of labour

- discuss the care of the mother and her partner

- review the observations that should be carried out at this time.

The nature of transition and second stage phases of labour

There are a number of areas of controversy related to the second stage of labour. Box 27.1 lists some examples.

The second stage of labour has traditionally been regarded as the phase between full dilatation of the

Box 27.1 Examples of areas of controversy

- The need or otherwise for regular vaginal examinations to assess the progress of labour, and the onset of the anatomical second stage
- The nature of transition
- The nature and impact of the early pushing urge
- Pushing in the context of epidural analgesia
- The efficacy of signs such as the anal cleft line and the appearance of the rhomboid of Michaelas
- The significance of the tight nuchal cord at the time of birth
- The physiological limits to the length of second stage labour

cervical os and the birth of the baby. However, most midwives and labouring women are aware of a transitional period between the dilatation, or first stage of labour, and the time when active maternal pushing efforts begin. This period is typically characterised by maternal restlessness, discomfort, desire for pain relief, a sense that the process is neverending and demands to attendants to get the birth over as quickly as possible. A knowledge of the usual physiological processes of this phase, and of the mechanism of the birth, forms the basis for consideration of appropriate midwifery care in the context of an individual woman.

The physiological changes result from a continuation of the same forces that have been at work during the earlier hours of labour, but activity is accelerated once the cervix has become fully dilated. This acceleration, however, does not occur abruptly. Some women may experience the urge to push before the cervix is fully dilated, and others may have a lull in activity before the full expulsive nature of the second stage contractions becomes evident. This latter phenomenon is termed the *resting phase* of the second stage of labour. The onset of the second stage of labour is traditionally confirmed with a vaginal examination to check for full cervical dilatation. This examination is often undertaken in response to transitional maternal behaviours. An official finding of full cervical dilatation may therefore occur some time after this stage has in fact been reached.

Uterine action. Contractions become stronger and longer but may be less frequent, allowing both mother and fetus regular recovery periods. The membranes often rupture spontaneously towards the end of the first stage or during transition to the second stage. The consequent drainage of liquor allows the hard, round fetal head to be directly applied to the vaginal tissues. This pressure aids distension. Fetal axis pressure increases flexion of the head, which results in smaller presenting diameters, more rapid progress and less trauma to both mother and fetus. If the mother is upright during this time, these processes are optimised.

The contractions become expulsive as the fetus descends further into the vagina. Pressure from the presenting part stimulates nerve receptors in the pelvic floor (this is termed the 'Ferguson reflex') and the woman experiences the need to push. This reflex may initially be controlled to a limited extent but becomes increasingly compulsive, overwhelming and involuntary during each contraction. The mother's response is to employ her secondary powers of expulsion by contracting her abdominal muscles and diaphragm.

Soft tissue displacement. As the hard fetal head descends, the soft tissues of the pelvis become displaced. Anteriorly, the bladder is pushed upwards into the abdomen where it is at less risk of injury during fetal descent. This results in the stretching and thinning of the urethra so that its lumen is reduced. Posteriorly, the rectum becomes flattened into the sacral curve and the pressure of the advancing head expels any residual faecal matter. The levator ani muscles dilate, thin out and are displaced laterally, and the perineal body is flattened, stretched and thinned. The fetal head becomes visible at the vulva, advancing with each contraction and receding between contractions until crowning takes place. The head is then born. The shoulders and body follow with the next contraction, accompanied by a gush of amniotic fluid and sometimes of blood. The second stage culminates in the birth of the baby.

Recognition of the commencement of the second stage of labour

Progress from the first to the second stage is not always clinically apparent. Several of the signs are presumptive.

Presumptive signs and differential diagnoses

Expulsive uterine contractions. Although this is usually a sign that the cervix is fully dilated, it is possible for a woman to feel a strong desire to push before full dilatation occurs. Traditionally, it has been assumed that an early urge to push is pathological, and that it will lead to maternal exhaustion and/or cervical oedema or trauma. More recent research indicates that the early pushing urge may in fact be experienced by a significant minority of women, and some authors have suggested that, in certain circumstances, early pushing may be physiological (Enkin et al 2000, p. 290, Petersen and Besuner 1997, Roberts et al 1987). However, it is not clear whether these findings are influenced by factors such as maternal or fetal position, or parity, and there is not enough evidence to date to determine the optimal response to the early pushing urge. The midwife needs to work with each individual woman in the context of each labour to determine the best approach in that specific case.

Rupture of the forewaters. This may occur at any time during labour.

Dilatation and gaping of the anus. Deep engagement of the presenting part may produce this sign during the latter part of the first stage.

Anal cleft line. Some midwives have reported observing this line as a pigmented mark in the cleft of the buttocks that creeps up the anal cleft as the labour progresses (Hobbs 1998). The efficacy of this observation remains to be tested formally.

Appearance of the rhomboid of Michaelas. This phenomenon is sometimes noted when a woman is in a position where the back is visible. It presents as a dome-shaped curve in the lower back, and is held to indicate the posterior displacement of the sacrum and coccyx as the fetal occiput moves into the maternal sacral curve (Sutton & Scott 1996). This seems to lead the labouring woman to arch her back, push her buttocks forward, and throw her arms back to grasp any object she can find. Sutton & Scott hypothesise that this is a physiological response, since it causes a lengthening and straightening of the curve of Carus, optimising the fetal passage through the birth canal.

Upper abdominal pressure and epidural analgesia. It has been observed anecdotally that women who have an epidural in situ often have a sense of discomfort under the ribs as the fetus uncurls. This tends to coincide with full cervical dilatation. The efficacy of these observations in predicting the onset of the anatomical second stage of labour remains to be researched.

Show. This is the loss of bloodstained mucus, which often accompanies rapid dilatation towards the end of the first stage of labour. It must be distinguished from frank fresh blood loss caused by partial separation of the placenta, or that caused by ruptured vasa praevia.

Appearance of the presenting part. Although this is usually definitive, it is important to be aware that excessive moulding may result in the formation of a large caput succedaneum, which can protrude through the cervix prior to full dilatation. It is also important to be aware that, very occasionally, the presenting part may be visible at the perineum at the same time as a section of prolapsed undilated cervix. This is more common in women of high parity. Similarly a breech presentation may be visible when the cervix is only 7–8 cm dilated.

The appearance of any of these presumptive signs may indicate that the second stage of labour has been reached.

Confirmatory evidence

In many midwifery settings, it is held that a vaginal examination must be undertaken to confirm full dilatation of the cervix. This is both to ensure that a woman is not pushing too early and to provide a baseline for timing the length of the second stage of labour. However, there is an increasing movement in some maternity settings not to undertake vaginal examinations unless there are observable maternal or fetal signs, or both, that the labour is not progressing as anticipated. Although Enkin and colleagues note that vaginal assessment of cervical dilatation is currently largely unevaluated (Enkin et al 2000, p. 284), it is still expected by most midwives and obstetricians, as well as by many women. Whether the midwife undertakes an examination or not, she should record all the signs she observes and all the measurements she takes, and she should advise and support the birthing women on the basis of accurate observation and assessment of progress.

Two phases in progress have been recognised in some women. These are the *latent phase*, during which descent and rotation occur, and the *active phase*, with descent and the urge to push.

The latent phase

In some women, full cervical dilatation is recorded but the presenting part may not yet have reached the pelvic outlet. The soft tissues of the vagina and pelvic floor gradually stretch and thin under the pressure of the advancing fetal head. The woman may not experience a strong expulsive urge until the head has descended sufficiently to exert pressure on the rectum and perineal tissues. The head will then become visible. There is evidence from a study undertaken half a century ago that active pushing during the latent phase does not achieve much, apart from exhausting and discouraging the mother (Benyon 1990). More recent concerns over the impact of epidural analgesia on spontaneous birth have led to an increasing interest in the passive second stage of labour (Minato 2000). Passive descent of the fetus can continue with good midwifery support for the woman until the head is visible at the vulva, or until the mother feels a spontaneous desire to push.

Active phase

Once the fetal head is visible the woman will usually experience a compulsive urge to push.

The recognition of the two phases of descent is particularly important if an effective epidural is in progress as there is little benefit in encouraging active pushing until the head has descended and rotated as far as possible.

Duration of the second stage

Once a woman has reached the transition stage of labour, she should not be left without a midwife in attendance. Accurate observation of progress and of maternal responses is vital, for the unexpected can always happen. The time taken to complete the second stage will vary considerably. There is no good evidence about the absolute time limits of physiological labour. Officially sanctioned limits have changed over the years (Downe 1996). Recent research has indicated that some mothers and babies who labour for at least twice as long as the traditional limits do well (Albers 1999). In the presence of regular contractions, maternal and fetal well-being and progressive descent, the considerable variation between women in their duration of labour is probably physiological. Although many maternity units do currently impose routine limits of the second stage beyond which medical help should be called, these are not based on good evidence (Enkin et al 2000, p. 293).

Maternal response to transition and the second stage

Pushing

The urge to push may come before the vertex is visible. Traditionally, in order to conserve maternal effort and allow the vaginal tissues to stretch passively, the mother is encouraged to avoid active pushing at this stage. Techniques for doing this include finding her a comfortable position, often the left lateral, using controlled breathing, inhaling Entonox, or even advising narcotic or epidural pain relief. However, as noted above, this practice is currently under scrutiny (Enkin et al 2000, p. 290, Petersen & Besuner 1997, Roberts et al 1987).

It is now accepted that managed active pushing accompanied by breath holding (the *Valsalva maneouvre*) has adverse consequences (Aldrich et al 1995, Enkin et al 2000, pp. 290–291). Whenever active pushing commences, the woman should be encouraged to follow her own inclinations in relation to expulsive effort. Few women need instruction on how to push unless they are using epidural analgesia; the desire is so overwhelming that the response becomes involuntary and compelling. The pushing effort will be regulated in response to the varying intensity of the contractions. Most women fall into their own rhythm after the first few exertions. The mother is therefore the best judge of when and how to push. This usually results in maximum pressure being exerted at the height of a contraction, which allows the vaginal muscles to become taut and prevents bladder supports and the transverse cervical ligaments from being pushed down in front of the fetus's head. It is believed that this may help to prevent prolapse and urinary incontinence in later life, although this belief has not been formally tested (Benyon 1990).

Some mothers vocalise loudly as they push. This may help a woman to cope with the contractions and she should feel free to express herself in this way. The midwife's gentle reassurance and praise will help to boost confidence, enabling the mother to assert her own control over events. The atmosphere should be calm and the pace unhurried.

Position

There is evidence to suggest that if the mother lies flat on her back then vena caval compression is increased, resulting in hypotension. This can lead to reduced placental perfusion and diminished fetal oxygenation (Humphrey et al 1974, Kurz et al 1982). The efficiency of uterine contractions may also be reduced. It may also be difficult for a mother to direct her pushing efficiently unless she is well supported. The semirecumbent or supported sitting position, with the thighs abducted, is the posture most commonly used in Western cultures (Fig. 27.1). Although dorsal positions afford the midwife good access and a clear view of the perineum, the mother's weight is on her sacrum, which directs the coccyx forwards and reduces the pelvic outlet. In addition, the midwife needs to bend forward and laterally to support the birth, which may lead to injury.

Squatting, kneeling, all fours or standing. In Western countries these positions have been encouraged only in recent years. In cultures where women follow their own inclinations, the majority choose to adopt a variation or combination of these postures (Gupta & Nikodem 2000). Radiological evidence demonstrates an average increase of 1 cm in the transverse diameter and 2 cm in the anteroposterior diameter of the pelvic outlet when the squatting position is adopted. This produces a 28% increase in the overall area of the outlet compared with the supine position, resulting in obvious benefit to the progress and ease of birth (Russell 1969).

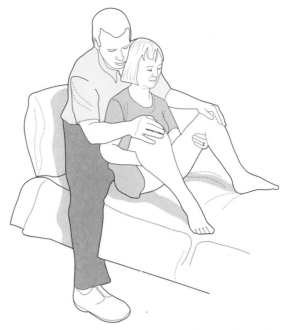

Fig. 27.1 Supported sitting position. (After Simkin et al, with permission of Blackwell Science.)

Left lateral position. This is a traditional position, although it is not widely used in current practice. The perineum can be clearly viewed and uterine action is effective but an assistant may be required to support the right thigh, which may not be ergonomic. It is an alternative position for women who find it difficult to abduct their hips.

Upright positions. A review of studies examining upright versus recumbent positions during the second stage of labour showed there were clear advantages for women in adopting an upright position (Gupta & Nikodem 2001). Women who were upright experienced less discomfort and backache, less difficulty in bearing down, fewer abnormal births and less perineal or vaginal trauma and vulval oedema compared with women who gave birth in a recumbent position. The only apparent disadvantage of upright positions is that there was an increased risk of blood loss. However, the experimental group included women who used birthing chairs, a technique known to be associated with increased blood loss (Stewart & Spiby 1989, Turner et al 1986); it is not clear whether this risk extends to all upright positions. More women who gave birth in upright positions expressed a positive response about the position.

The position the mother may choose to adopt is dictated by several factors:

- *The mother's instinctive preference* – this should always be a primary consideration.
- *The environment* – this should be such that the woman is not constrained by lack of privacy or lack of supports such as cushions and chairs from adopting her preferred position. In a hospital environment, it may help to move the labour bed from its traditional place in the middle of the room, and to place other supports such as cushions and birth balls in the room so that the mother is free to roam from one to another as the labour dictates. Low lighting and music of her choice may help the woman to see the room as a safe and secure place to give birth. Minimising unnecessary intrusion by other members of staff is essential.
- *The midwife's confidence* – a real understanding of the mechanism of labour should enable the midwife to adapt to any position that the woman wishes to adopt. It is important, however, that midwives recognise the need to ensure that their posture is not exerting undue strain on them and especially on their backs. One way of minimising this is to encourage more upright positions for the woman, and particularly to refrain from placing the woman in a low supported sitting position with her feet resting on the midwife's hip. Minimising vaginal examination in labour will also reduce the risk of back injury to the midwife. It is particularly important to minimise examinations where the woman is on the bed and the midwife has to bend laterally. If the woman has an epidural in situ, it is essential that help is called when the women needs to be moved and that ergonomic lifting positions are used.
- *The maternal and fetal condition* – if the mother has had pethidine or an epidural, or if there is any concern about the well-being of either the woman or her fetus, then a need for more frequent or continuous monitoring may limit the choices available to her. However, there are often creative solutions to these situations, and good midwifery care involves finding these solutions where possible (Downe 1999).

Whichever positions the mother moves to as her labour progresses, she is most likely to trust a midwife who supports her freedom of choice and active participation in her labour. Flexibility is the keynote. Positive and dramatic effects can be achieved by encouraging the mother to change and adapt her position in response to the way her body feels.

The mechanism of normal labour

As the fetus descends, soft tissue and bony structures exert pressures that lead to descent through the birth canal by a series of movements. Collectively, these movements are called the *mechanism of labour*. During vaginal birth, the fetal presentation, position, and size will govern the exact mechanism as the fetus responds to external pressures.

Knowledge and recognition of the normal mechanism enables the midwife to anticipate the next step in the process of descent, which in turn will dictate her response to the birth as it progresses. Her understanding and constant monitoring of these movements ensure that normal progress is recognised, that the woman and fetus have a positive experience of birth and that early assistance can be sought should any unresolvable problems occur. Principles common to all mechanisms are:

- descent takes place
- whichever part leads and first meets the resistance of the pelvic floor will rotate forwards until it comes under the symphysis pubis
- whatever emerges from the pelvis will pivot around the pubic bone.

It should be noted that, although the mechanism set out below is the most common, not all fetuses presenting in a certain position will follow it exactly. It is therefore a basis for assessing each unique labour, rather than an invariant template.

During the mechanism of normal labour the fetus turns slightly to take advantage of the widest available space in each plane of the pelvis. The widest diameter of the pelvic brim is the transverse; at the pelvic outlet the greatest space lies in the anteroposterior diameter.

At the onset of labour, the commonest presentation is the vertex and the most common position either left or right occipitoanterior; therefore it is this mechanism that will be described. When these conditions are met, the way that the fetus is normally situated can be described as follows:

- the lie is longitudinal
- the presentation is cephalic
- the position is right or left occipitoanterior
- the attitude is one of good flexion
- the denominator is the occiput
- the presenting part is the posterior part of the anterior parietal bone.

Main movements

Descent. Descent of the fetal head into the pelvis often begins before the onset of labour. The fetus of a nulliparous woman usually descends into the pelvis during the latter weeks of pregnancy. In multigravid women the muscle tone is often more lax and therefore engagement may not occur until labour actually begins. Throughout the first stage of labour the contraction and retraction of the uterine muscles allow less room in the uterus, exerting pressure on the fetus to descend. Following rupture of the forewaters and the exertion of maternal effort, progress speeds up.

Flexion. This increases throughout labour. The fetal spine is attached nearer the posterior part of the skull; pressure exerted down the fetal axis will be more forcibly transmitted to the occiput than to the sinciput. The effect is to increase flexion, resulting in smaller presenting diameters, which will negotiate the pelvis more easily. At the onset of labour the suboccipitofrontal diameter, which is on average approximately 10 cm, is presenting; with greater flexion the suboccipitobregmatic diameter presents, which is on average approximately 9.5 cm. The occiput becomes the leading part.

Internal rotation of the head. During a contraction the leading part is pushed downwards on to the pelvic floor. The resistance of this muscular diaphragm brings about rotation. As the contraction fades, the pelvic floor rebounds causing the occiput to glide forwards. Resistance is therefore an important determinant of rotation. This explains why rotation is often delayed following epidural analgesia, which causes relaxation of the pelvic floor muscles. The slope of the pelvic floor determines the direction of rotation. The muscles are hammock shaped and slope down anteriorly, so whichever part of the fetus first meets the lateral half of this slope will be directed forwards and towards the centre. In a well-flexed vertex presentation the occiput leads and meets the pelvic floor first and

rotates anteriorly through one-eighth of a circle. This causes a slight twist in the neck of the fetus as the head is no longer in direct alignment with the shoulders. The anteroposterior diameter of the head now lies in the widest (anteroposterior) diameter of the pelvic outlet (Fig. 27.2). The occiput slips beneath the subpubic arch and crowning occurs when the head no longer recedes between contractions and the widest transverse diameter (biparietal) is born. If flexion is maintained, the suboccipitobregmatic diameter, usually approximately 9.5 cm, distends the vaginal orifice.

Extension of the head. Once crowning has occurred the fetal head can extend, pivoting on the suboccipital region around the pubic bone. This releases the sinciput, face and chin, which sweep the perineum and are born by a movement of extension.

Restitution. The twist in the neck of the fetus that resulted from internal rotation is now corrected by a slight untwisting movement. The occiput moves one-eighth of a circle towards the side from which it started (Fig. 27.3A, B).

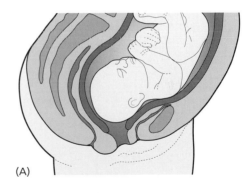
(A)

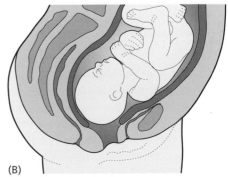
(B)

Fig. 27.2 (A) Internal rotation of the head begins. (B) Upon completion, the occiput lies under the symphysis pubis.

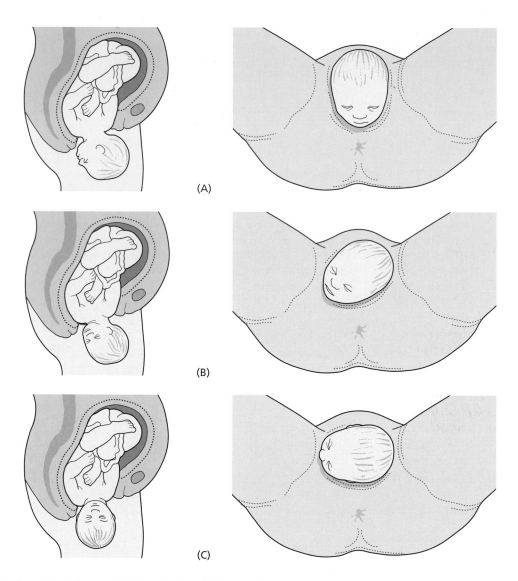

Fig. 27.3 (A) Birth of the head. (B) Restitution. (C) External rotation.

Internal rotation of the shoulders. The shoulders undergo a similar rotation to that of the head to lie in the widest diameter of the pelvic outlet, namely the anteroposterior. The anterior shoulder is the first to reach the levator ani muscle and it therefore rotates anteriorly to lie under the symphysis pubis. This movement can be clearly seen as the head turns at the same time (external rotation of the head) (Fig. 27.3C). It occurs in the same direction as restitution, and the occiput of the fetal head now lies laterally.

Lateral flexion. The shoulders are usually born sequentially. This enables a smaller diameter to distend the vaginal orifice than if both shoulders were born simultaneously. When the mother is in a supported sitting position the anterior shoulder is usually born first, although it has been noted by midwives who commonly use upright or kneeling positions that the posterior shoulder is commonly seen first. In the former case the anterior shoulder slips beneath the subpubic arch and the posterior shoulder passes over the perineum. In the latter the mechanism has been observed to reverse, although there are no formal studies of this phenomenon to date. The remainder of the body is born by lateral flexion as the spine bends sideways through the curved birth canal.

Midwifery care

There are a number of dilemmas of practice relating to midwifery care during the second stage of labour. These are listed in Box 27.2.

Care of the parents

The couple will now realise that the birth of their baby is imminent. They may feel excited and elated but at the same time anxious and frightened by the dramatic change in pace. The midwife's calm approach and information about what is happening can ensure the woman stays in control, and confident of her ability to birth her baby. This is critical at the time of transition when a woman may feel a lack of control over events, which can result in a sensation of panic. Crucially, it is at this point that the mother may request analgesia. This is especially true when a supportive companion is not present. In this situation the relationship of trust the midwife has built up during the earlier stages of labour will help to establish the mother's self-confidence and trust. The midwife may be able to help her over this transient phase with good midwifery support

---

Box 27.2 Dilemmas of practice

- The contrast between the current evidence base and actual practices
- The contrast between knowledge gained from experience (embodied knowledge) and that gained from evidence (authoritative knowledge)
- The problem of using guidelines and clinical risk assessments based on population evidence for individual women/babies
- Balancing maternal choice, institutional demands and midwifery expertise
- Providing optimum care when resources are restricted

---

and without utilising pharmacological analgesia. The decision for or against pain relief at this stage must be made in partnership with the woman. In order to achieve this, it is eminently preferable that the same midwife should support the couple throughout labour. Continuity of carer is one of the key components of a positive birth for both parents and professionals (Hodnett 2001). The mother should be offered every opportunity to ensure that she is supported by birth companion(s) of her choice.

Throughout transition and the second stage of labour the woman and her companion(s) will need frequent explanations of events. The midwife should praise and congratulate the mother on her hard work, recognising that she is probably undertaking the most extreme physical activity she will ever encounter. Birth is an intimate act that often takes place in a public setting. The midwife should work hard to ensure that privacy and dignity are key components of the woman's birth experience. The midwife needs to support the woman with massage, with appropriate nutrition, and with suggestions for changes of position and of scenery, tailored to each woman and her labour. This may encompass techniques such as the use of complementary therapies and optimal fetal positioning if the midwife is competent to undertake them (see Ch. 49). Leg cramp is a common occurrence whichever posture is adopted. It can be relieved by massaging the calf muscle, extending the leg and dorsiflexing the foot.

The midwife should also have regard to the wellbeing of the woman's partner and other companions as far as possible, and recognise that witnessing birth is emotionally taxing. The midwife's attitude to the labour, to the woman and to the partner will have a profound effect on the labour, and is likely to have an effect on the family after the birth (Halldorsdottir & Karlsdottir 1996). It is crucial to respect them, and the meaning that this birth will have for them, both on the day and in the future.

Observations during the second stage of labour

At least five factors determine whether the second stage is continuing optimally, and these must be carefully observed:

Uterine contractions. The strength, length and frequency of contractions should be assessed continuously by observation of maternal responses, and regularly by uterine palpation. They are usually stronger and longer than during the first stage of labour, lasting up to one minute with a longer resting phase between. The posture and position adopted by the mother may influence the contractions.

Descent, rotation and flexion. Initially, descent often occurs slowly, especially in nulliparous women, but it usually accelerates during the active phase. It may occur very rapidly in multigravid women. If descent is progressive, it should not be necessary for the midwife to undertake a vaginal examination. If, however, there is a delay in progress despite regular strong contractions and active maternal pushing, a vaginal examination may be performed with maternal permission. The purpose is to confirm whether or not internal rotation of the head has taken place, to assess the station of the presenting part, and to determine whether a caput succedaneum has formed. If the occiput has rotated anteriorly, the head is well flexed and caput succedaneum is not excessive then it is likely that progress will continue. In the absence of good rotation and flexion, or a weakening of uterine contractions, or both, then a change of position, nutrition and hydration, or use of optimal fetal positioning techniques may be considered. Consultation with a more experienced midwife may provide more suggestions to reorientate the labour. However, if there is evidence that either fetal or maternal condition are compromised, an experienced obstetrician must be consulted.

Fetal condition. If the membranes are ruptured, the liquor amnii is observed to ensure that it is clear. Whereas thin old meconium staining is not always regarded as a sign of fetal compromise, thick fresh meconium is always ominous, and experienced obstetric advice should be sought if this sign appears (Enkin et al 2000, p. 268–269, Ziadeh & Sunna 2000). As the fetus descends, fetal oxygenation may be less efficient owing either to cord or head compression or to reduced perfusion at the placental site. A well-grown healthy fetus will not be compromised by this transitory hypoxia. This will tend to be manifest in early decelerations of the fetal heart, with a swift return to the normal baseline after a contraction. Although early decelerations are always deemed 'suspicious' in the current National Institute of Clinical Effectiveness guidelines (NICE 2001), in practice their occurrence in the active second stage is not usually regarded as pathological in the absence of any other signs of compromise. The midwife should learn to recognise the normal changes in fetal heart rate patterns during the second stage, so that unwarranted interference is avoided. The NICE recommendations for using intermittent auscultation, and for interpreting continuous electronic fetal monitoring, are clearly set out in the clinical practice algorithm bound with the guidelines, and reproduced in Figure 27.4. If the woman is labouring normally, the guideline recommends that a Pinard stethoscope or other handheld system such as a Sonicaid should be used to monitor the fetal heart, and not continuous electronic fetal monitoring. During the second stage this is usually undertaken immediately after a contraction, with some readings being taken through a contraction if the woman can tolerate this.

Suspicious/pathological changes in the fetal heart. Late decelerations, a lack of return to the normal baseline, a rising baseline or diminishing beat-to-beat variation (seen if continuous electronic fetal monitoring is in use) remain signs of concern (NICE 2001). If these are heard for the first time in second stage, they may be due to cord or head compression, which may be helped by a change in position. However, if they persist following such a change then experienced obstetric advice must be sought. If the labour is taking place in a unit that is distant from an obstetric unit, an episiotomy may be considered if the birth is imminent. Midwives who are trained and experienced in ventouse birth may consider expediting the birth at this point. Otherwise, with maternal consent, transfer to an obstetric unit should be arranged.

Maternal condition. The midwife's observation includes an appraisal of the mother's ability to cope emotionally as well as an assessment of her physical well-being. Maternal pulse rate is usually recorded every half hour and blood pressure every hour, provided that these remain within normal limits.

Maternal comfort

As a result of her exertions the woman usually feels very hot and sticky and she will find it soothing to have her face and neck sponged with a cool flannel. Her mouth and lips may become very dry. Sips of iced water are refreshing and a moisturising cream can be

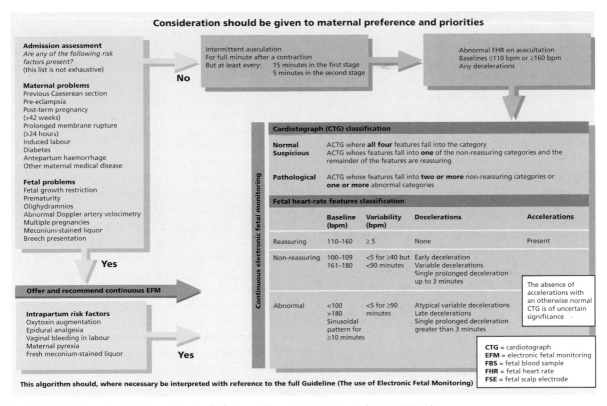

Consideration should be given to maternal preference and priorities

Admission assessment
Are any of the following risk factors present?
(this list is not exhaustive)

Maternal problems
Previous Caeserean section
Pre-eclampsia
Post-term pregnancy
(>42 weeks)
Prolonged membrane rupture
(>24 hours)
Induced labour
Diabetes
Antepartum haemorrhage
Other maternal medical disease

Fetal problems
Fetal growth restriction
Prematurity
Olighydramnios
Abnormal Doppler artery velocimetry
Multiple pregnancies
Meconium-stained liquor
Breech presentation

No

Intermittent auscultation
For full minute after a contraction
But at least every: 15 minutes in the first stage
                        5 minutes in the second stage

Abnormal FHR on auscultation
Baselines ≤110 bpm or ≥160 bpm
Any decelerations

Yes

Offer and recommend continuous EFM

Intrapartum risk factors
Oxytoxin augmentation
Epidural analgesia
Vaginal bleeding in labour
Maternal pyrexia
Fresh meconium-stained liquor

Yes

Continuous electronic fetal monitoring

Cardiotograph (CTG) classification

Normal	ACTG where **all four** features fall into the category
Suspicious	ACTG whoes features fall into **one** of the non-reassuring categories and the remainder of the features are reassuring
Pathological	ACTG whose features fall into **two or more** non-reassuring categpries or **one or more** abnormal categories

Fetal heart-rate features classification

	Baseline (bpm)	Variability (bpm)	Decelerations	Accelerations
Reassuring	110–160	≥ 5	None	Present
Non-reassuring	100–109 161–180	<5 for ≥40 but <90 minutes	Early deceleration Variable decelerations Single prolonged deceleration up to 3 minutes	
Abnormal	<100 >180 Sinusoidal pattern for ≥10 minutes	<5 for ≥90 minutes	Atypical variable decelerations Late decelerations Single prolonged deceleration greater than 3 minutes	

The absence of accelerations with an otherwise normal CTG is of uncertain significance

CTG = cardiotograph
EFM = electronic fetal monitoring
FBS = fetal blood sample
FHR = fetal heart rate
FSE = fetal scalp electrode

This algorithm should, where necessary be interpreted with reference to the full Guideline (The use of Electronic Fetal Monitoring)

Fig. 27.4 Guidelines for fetal monitoring in labour. (From NICE 2001, with permission.)

applied to her lips. Her partner may help with these tasks as a positive contribution to ease her discomfort.

Bladder care

As the fetus descends into the pelvis, the bladder is particularly vulnerable to damage from the pressure of the advancing head. The bladder base may become compressed between the pelvic brim and the fetal head. The risk of trauma is greatly increased if the bladder is distended. The woman should be encouraged to pass urine at the beginning of the second stage unless she has recently done so.

The birth

Preparation

Once the active pushing phase is entered into, the midwife should make preliminary preparations for the birth. There is usually little urgency if the woman is having her first baby, but multigravid women may progress very rapidly.

The room in which the birth is to take place should be warm with a spotlight available so that the perineum can be easily observed if necessary. The woman may wish other family members to witness the birth, especially if it is taking place at home. A clean area should be prepared to receive the baby and waterproof covers provided to protect the bed and floor. Sterile cord clamps, a plastic apron and sterile rubber gloves are placed to hand. These may be in a pack or separate. A uterotonic agent (commonly Syntometrine 1 ml) may be prepared, either in readiness for the active management of the third stage if this is acceptable to the woman, or for use during an emergency. The dose and drug should be checked by a second person, and it must be kept separate from any neonatal drugs such as vitamin K to avoid risk of error. Some units favour the use of oxytocin, 5 or 10 units. Oxytocin avoids the adverse side-effects of ergometrine, but Syntometrine has the advantage of ensuring sustained uterine contraction. A warm cot and clothes should be prepared for the baby. In hospital a heated mattress may be used; at home a warm (but not hot) water bottle can be placed in the cot.

Neonatal resuscitation equipment must be thoroughly checked and readily accessible and should include portable or piped oxygen equipment.

The midwife's skill and judgment are crucial factors in minimising maternal trauma and ensuring an optimal birth for both mother and baby. These qualities are acquired by experience but certain basic principles should be applied whatever the expertise of the midwife. They are:

- observation of progress
- prevention of infection
- emotional and physical comfort of the mother
- anticipation of normal events
- recognition of abnormal developments.

During the birth both mother and fetus are particularly vulnerable to infection. Although there is now evidence that strict antisepsis is unnecessary if the birth is straightforward (Keane & Thornton 1998), meticulous aseptic technique must be observed when preparing sterile equipment such as episiotomy scissors. Surgical gloves should be worn during the birth for the protection of both mother and midwife. In some units, goggles or plain glasses are also advised to minimise the risk of transmission of infection through blood splashes to the eyes. Once she feels the birth is imminent the midwife puts on her apron and gloves and prepares her equipment. This includes the following main items:

- warm swabbing solution, or tap water if this is local practice
- cotton wool and pads
- sterile cord scissors and clamps
- sterile episiotomy scissors.

Birth of the head

Once the birth is imminent, the perineum may be swabbed and a clean pad placed under the woman to absorb any faeces or fluids. If the mother is not in an upright position, it is common practice to place a pad over the rectum on the perineum below the fourchette. Throughout these preparations the midwife observes the progress of the fetus. With each contraction the head descends. As it does so the superficial muscles of the pelvic floor can be seen to stretch, especially the transverse perineal muscles. The head recedes between

contractions, which allows these muscles to thin gradually. The skill of the midwife in ensuring that the active phase is unhurried helps to safeguard the perineum from trauma. She must either watch the advance of the fetal head or control it with light support from her hand, or both. One large study, the HOOP trial, has indicated that, compared with a certain method of guarding the perineum, a hands-off technique is associated with slightly more discomfort at 10 days postnatally (McCandlish et al 1998). The hands-off technique is also associated with a lower risk of episiotomy, but a higher risk of manual removal of placenta. There is some debate about the generalisability of this finding to all settings and positions in labour. However, account should be taken of these findings in working with individual women. Most midwives place their fingers lightly on the advancing head to monitor descent and prevent very rapid crowning and extension, which are believed to result in perineal laceration (Fig. 27.5). However, firm pressure on the head may be associated with vaginal lacerations. Whatever technique the midwife adopts, it should be based on the assumption that it is the woman who is giving birth to her baby, and the midwife is there to add the minimum physical help necessary at any given time.

For her part, once the head has crowned, the mother can achieve control by gently blowing or 'sighing' out each breath in order to minimise active pushing. Birth of the head in this way may take two or three contractions but delicate control may avoid unnecessary maternal trauma.

Once crowned, the head is born by extension as the face appears at the perineum. During the resting phase before the next contraction, the midwife may check that the cord is not around the baby's neck. If it is then the usual practice is to slacken it to form a loop through which the shoulders may pass. If the cord is very tightly wound around the neck, it is common practice to apply two artery forceps approximately 3 cm apart and to sever the cord between the two clamps. Great care must be taken that in this confined space other tissues are not clamped in error. When cutting the cord it is always a wise precaution to hold a swab over the area as it is incised. This will reduce the risk of the attendants being sprayed with blood during the procedure. Once severed, the cord may be unwound from around the neck. There has been controversy over this technique on the basis that, even if

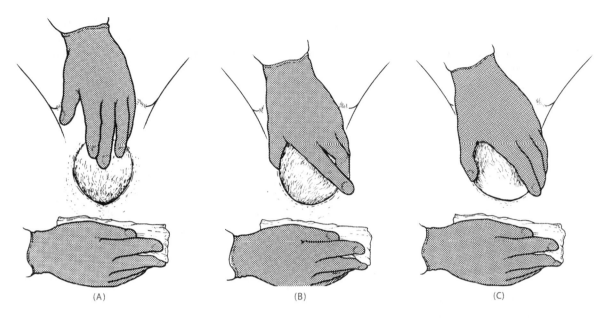

Fig. 27.5 Supporting the head. (A) Preventing rapid extension. (B) Controlling the crowning. (C) Easing the perineum to release the face.

tightly around the neck, the cord is still supplying oxygen. When it is severed there is no oxygen to the baby and it is possible that difficulty with the shoulders later would lead to increased risk of hypoxia. This area remains to be researched.

The mother may now be able to see and touch her baby's head and assist in the birth of the trunk.

Birth of the shoulders

Restitution and external rotation of the head usually occurs, and this maximises the smooth birth of the shoulders and minimises the risk of perineal laceration. However, it is not uncommon for small babies, or for babies of multiparous women, to be born with the shoulders in the transverse position, or even to have a twist in the neck opposite to that expected. Although the hands-on technique in the HOOP trial included perineal support and active delivery of the trunk and shoulders (McCandlish et al 1998), it is not clear which component of this technique was beneficial for women and babies and which, if any, was not. If the position is more upright it is more common for the shoulders to be left to birth spontaneously with the help of gravity. During a water birth, it is important not to touch the emerging fetus to avoid stimulating it to gasp underwater. If there is a problem with the birth in this circumstance, the mother should be asked to stand up out of the water before any manoeuvres are attempted.

If the midwife does physically aid the birth of the shoulders and trunk, she should be absolutely sure that restitution has indeed occurred fully prior to trying to flex the trunk laterally, to avoid the risk of forcing the shoulders out before they are ready. If the midwife does actively assist, one shoulder is released at a time to avoid overstretching the perineum. A hand is placed on each side of the baby's head, over the ears, and gentle downward traction is applied (Fig. 27.6A). This allows the anterior shoulder to slip beneath the symphysis pubis while the posterior shoulder remains in the vagina. If the third stage is to be actively managed, the assistant will give intramuscular Syntometrine 1 ml or oxytocin 5–10 units. When the auxiliary crease is seen, the head and trunk are guided in an upward curve to allow the posterior shoulder to escape over the perineum (Fig. 27.6B). Where the mother is in an upright position, the midwife will usually need only to support the head as it is born. The midwife or mother may now grasp the baby around the chest to aid the birth of the trunk and lift the baby towards the mother's abdomen. This not only allows the mother immediate sighting of her baby and close skin contact, but removes the baby from the gush of liquor which accompanies release of the body. If the

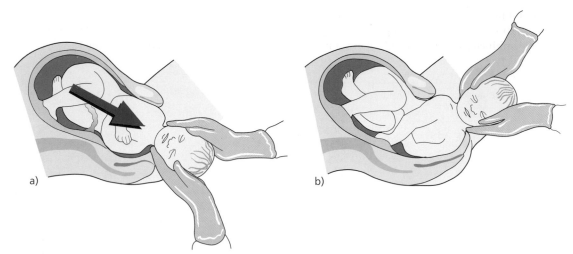

Fig. 27.6 (A) Downward traction releases the anterior shoulder. (B) An upward curve allows the posterior shoulder to escape.

midwife does not actively assist, she should be ready to support the head and trunk as the baby emerges. The time of birth is noted.

The cord is severed between two cord clamps placed close to the umbilicus at whatever time is considered appropriate (see Ch. 28). The cord clamp is applied. The baby is dried and placed in the skin-to-skin position with the mother if she is happy with this (Baby Friendly Initiative 2001). A warm cover is placed over the exposed areas of the baby to prevent cooling. Swabbing of the eyes and aspiration of mucus during and immediately following birth are not considered to be necessary providing the baby's condition is satisfactory. Oral mucus extractors should not be used because of the risks of a mucus that is contaminated with a virus such as the hepatitis virus or HIV entering the operator's mouth.

Episiotomy

As the perineum distends, a decision to undertake an episiotomy may very occasionally be necessary. This is an incision through the perineal tissues that is designed to enlarge the vulval outlet during delivery. As this is a surgical incision it is essential that the mother gives consent prior to the procedure. A detailed discussion should take place during pregnancy so that each woman is aware of the indications for and implications of the intervention. She should be assured that its use is selective and discretional. The

mother's personal wishes for her own care should be clearly documented and respected.

The risks and benefits of episiotomy have been well reviewed (Carroli & Belizan 2001). The rationale for its use depends largely on the need to minimise the risk of severe, spontaneous, maternal trauma and to expedite the birth when there is evidence of fetal compromise. However, during a normal birth the indications for its use are few and the midwife should use her skills to avoid this intervention if at all possible.

The timing of the incision

An episiotomy involves incision of the fourchette, the superficial muscles and skin of the perineum and the posterior vaginal wall. It can therefore successfully speed the birth only when the presenting part is directly applied to these tissues. If the episiotomy is performed too early it will fail to release the presenting part and haemorrhage from cut vessels may ensue. In addition, the levator ani muscles will not have had time to be displaced laterally and may be incised as well. If performed too late there will not be enough time to infiltrate with a local anaesthetic. There is also little reason for superimposing an episiotomy if a tear has already begun.

Types of incision

Mediolateral. This begins at the midpoint of the fourchette and is directed at a 45° angle to the midline towards a point midway between the ischial tuberosity and the anus. This line avoids the danger of damage to both the anal sphincter and Bartholin's gland but it is the more difficult to repair. This is the incision largely used by midwives in the UK.

Median. This is a midline incision that follows the natural line of insertion of the perineal muscles. It is associated with reduced blood loss but a higher incidence of damage to the anal sphincter. It is the easier to repair and results in less pain and dyspareunia. This incision is favoured in the USA.

Procedures

Infiltration of the perineum. The perineum should be adequately anaesthetised prior to the incision. Lidocaine (lignocaine) is commonly used, either 0.5% 10 ml or 1% 5 ml. The advantage of the more concentrated solution is that a smaller volume is needed. It takes 3–4 minutes to have an effect and, if possible, two or three contractions should be allowed to occur between infiltration and incision. The timing is not always easy to calculate but it is better to infiltrate and not perform an episiotomy than to incise the perineum without an effective local anaesthetic.

Method of infiltration. The perineum is cleansed with antiseptic solution. Two fingers are inserted into the vagina along the line of the proposed incision in order to protect the fetal head. The needle is inserted beneath the skin for 4–5 cm following the same line.

The piston of the syringe should be withdrawn prior to injection to check whether the needle is in a blood vessel. If blood is aspirated, the needle should be repositioned and the procedure repeated until no blood is withdrawn. Lidocaine (lignocaine) is continuously injected as the needle is slowly withdrawn. Some practitioners inject the whole amount in one operation. Anaesthesia is, however, more effective if about one-third of the amount is used at first and two further injections are made, one either side of the incision line (Fig. 27.7A). The needle must be redirected just before the tip is withdrawn.

The incision. A straight-bladed, blunt-ended pair of Mayo scissors is usually used. The blades should be sharp to ensure a clean incision. Some practitioners prefer to use a scalpel for this reason. Two fingers are inserted into the vagina as before and the open blades are positioned (Fig. 27.7B). The incision is best made during a contraction when the tissues are stretched so that there is a clear view of the area and bleeding is less likely to be severe. A single, deliberate cut 4–5 cm long is made at the correct angle. Birth of the head should follow immediately and its advance must be controlled in order to avoid extension of the episiotomy. If there is any delay before the head emerges, pressure should be applied to the episiotomy site between contractions in order to minimise bleeding. Postpartum haemorrhage can occur from an episiotomy site unless bleeding points are compressed.

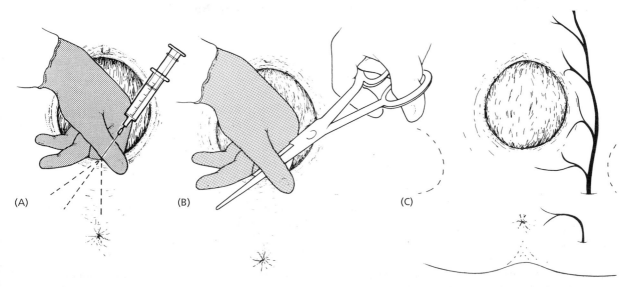

(A)   (B)   (C)

Fig. 27.7 (A) Infiltrating the perineum. (B) Performing an episiotomy. (C) Innervation of the vulval area and perineum.

Perineal repair

Midwives who have had instruction and supervised practice in suturing the perineum and are judged to be proficient may carry out the procedure. Trauma is best repaired as soon as possible after the birth in order to secure haemostasis and before oedema forms. It is also much kinder to the mother to complete this aspect of her care without undue delay and while the tissues are still anaesthetised. Prior to commencement the mother must be made as warm and comfortable as possible. The lithotomy position is usually chosen as it affords a clear view of the area. Other positions may be more appropriate in the home setting. A good, directional light is essential and the operator should be seated comfortably during the procedure.

The trolley, set with the appropriate instruments, antiseptic solution, suture materials and local anaesthetic, should be prepared before the mother's legs are placed in the stirrups. This minimises the time spent in this uncomfortable, undignified position and reduces the risks of complications such as deep vein thrombosis. The midwife scrubs and puts on sterile gown and gloves. The perineum is cleaned with warm antiseptic solution. Blood oozing from the uterus may obscure the field of vision, so a taped vaginal tampon may be inserted into the vault of the vagina. The tape is secured to the towelling drapes by a pair of forceps as a reminder that it must be removed upon completion of the procedure. Both insertion and removal should be recorded. The full extent of the trauma is assessed and explained to the mother. The procedure for repair should also be outlined so that she is aware of what is happening.

Spontaneous trauma may be of the labia anteriorly, the perineum posteriorly, or both. A gentle, thorough examination must be carried out to assess the extent of the trauma accurately and to determine whether an experienced obstetrician should carry out the repair, if it is extensive.

Anterior labial tears. It is debatable whether or not these should be sutured. Much depends upon the control of bleeding as the labia are very vascular. A suture may be necessary to secure haemostasis.

Posterior perineal trauma. Spontaneous tears are usually classified in degrees, which are related to the anatomical structures that have been traumatised. This classification serves only as a guideline because it is often difficult to identify the structures precisely:

- *First degree tear* – this involves the fourchette only.
- *Second degree tear* – this involves the fourchette and the superficial perineal muscles, namely the bulbocavernosus and the transverse perineal muscles and in some cases the pubococcygeus.
- *Third degree tear* – in addition to the above structures there is damage to the anal sphincter.
- *Fourth degree tear* – this classification is sometimes used to describe trauma that extends into the rectal mucosa.

Third and fourth degree tears should be repaired by an experienced obstetrician. A general anaesthetic or effective epidural or spinal anaesthetic is necessary.

Prior to the commencement of repair, infiltration of the wound with local anaesthetic will be required. It is unlikely that any perineal infiltration carried out before delivery will be sufficient to ensure the mother's comfort during the procedure. Lidocaine (lignocaine) 1% is used and time must be allowed for it to take effect before repair begins. If an epidural block is in progress, a 'top up' should be given.

The apex of the vaginal incision is identified and the posterior vaginal wall repaired from the apex downwards (Fig. 27.8). A continuous suture affords better haemostasis (Kettle & Johanson 2001a). The thread should not be pulled too tightly as oedema will develop during the first 24–48 hours. Care must be taken to identify other vaginal lacerations, which should also be repaired. The deeper interrupted sutures are then inserted to repair the perineal muscles. Good approximation of tissue is important. The subsequent strength of the pelvic floor will depend largely upon adequate repair of this layer. Recent studies have indicated that, as long as good approximation is obtained, suturing of the perineal skin is unnecessary and leads to increased maternal discomfort (Gordon et al 1998). If skin closure is carried out, a continuous subcuticular suture (see Fig. 27.8) results in fewer short term problems than interrupted transcutaneous suturing techniques (Kettle & Johanson 2001a).

The suture material recommended is polyglycolic acid (Grant et al 2001, Kettle & Johanson 2001b).

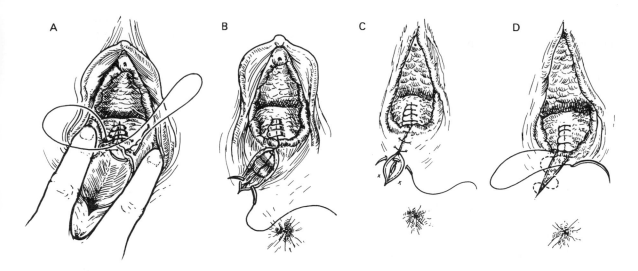

Fig. 27.8 Perineal repair. (A) A continuous suture is used to repair the vaginal wall. (B) Three or four interrupted sutures repair the fascia and muscle of the perineum. (C) Interrupted sutures to the skin. (D) Subcuticular skin suture.

Whatever the choice of material or type of suture, if the skin is sutured then repair should begin at the fourchette so that the vaginal opening is properly aligned. When the wound has been closed, any further vulval lacerations should be repaired. Anterior labial tears occur more frequently when episiotomy has been avoided. This trauma does not appear to cause additional maternal discomfort 10 days after the birth (Sleep et al 1984).

The sutured areas should be inspected in order to confirm haemostasis before the vaginal pack is removed. A vaginal examination is made to ensure that the introitus has not been narrowed. Upon completion a rectal examination is made in order to ensure that no sutures have penetrated the rectal mucosa. Any such sutures must be removed to prevent fistula formation. It is essential to warn the mother before this examination is performed.

The area is cleaned and a sanitary pad positioned over the vulva and perineum. The mother's legs are then gently and simultaneously removed from lithotomy support and she is made comfortable. The nature of the trauma and repair should be explained to her and information given on whether or not sutures will need to be removed.

If the midwife suspects damage to the upper vagina, cervix, anal sphincter or rectal mucosa, a senior obstetrician should be notified as this repair will be outside her province. A general anaesthetic is occasionally necessary if the trauma is extensive.

Records

It is the responsibility of the midwife conducting the birth to complete the labour record. This should include details of any drugs administered, the duration and progress of labour, the reason for performing an episiotomy and perineal repair. This information is recorded on the mother's notes and may be duplicated on her domiciliary record as well as in the birth register. Details of the baby's condition including the Apgar score are also recorded.

The birth notification must be completed within 36 hours of the birth (see Ch. 55).

The development of computerised records has minimised the need for duplication of information and has also reduced the time spent by midwives in completing several sets of documents. All data are subject to the current Data Protection Act (Data Protection Act 1998).

Box 27.3 Examples of areas in need of research

- The areas of controversy, as set out in Box 27.1
- The nature of physiological fetal heart patterns in the normal second stage of labour
- Variation and significance of variation in normal fetal heart tones and rhythms as heard with a Pinard stethoscope
- The mechanisms of labour in upright positions
- The nature of birth in units where no restrictions are imposed as a matter of routine
- The efficacy of midwife observation of maternal behaviours in assessing progress in labour
- The impact of optimal fetal positioning

Box 27.4 Key points relating to the second stage of labour

- The transitional and second stage phases of labour are emotionally intense and physically hard
- The vast majority of labours will progress physiologically
- Maternal behaviour is usually a good indication of progress during this time
- The core midwifery skill is to support the mother in the context of a sound knowledge of the physiology and the mechanisms of this phase of labour
- Support should be unobtrusive
- The woman is the central player
- Clear, comprehensive record keeping is essential
- There are many gaps in the research evidence in this area

Conclusion

The processes of transition and of second stage labour are likely to be very physically and emotionally intense, particularly for the woman, but also for her partner and other birth companions. If maternal behaviour and instinct are respected, in the context of skilled and watchful waiting, the vast majority of labours will progress physiologically. The skill of the midwife is to support the women, guide her when her spirits or the labour are flagging, and to enable her to accomplish her birth safely and in triumph. However, as birth progresses, clear, comprehensive record keeping is essential. Although much practice in this area is not based on formal evidence, new observations about normal birth are beginning to be recorded, and these observations will form the basis for future research (Box 27.3).

Key points relating to the second stage of labour are listed in Box 27.4.

REFERENCES

Albers L L 1999 The duration of labor in healthy women. Journal of Perinatology 19(2):114–119

Aldrich C J, D'Antona D, Spencer J A, Delpy D T, Reynolds E O, Wyatt J S 1995 The effect of maternal pushing on fetal cerebral oxygenation and blood volume during the second stage of labour. British Journal of Obstetrics and Gynaecology 102(6):448–453

Baby Friendly Initiative 2001 Ten steps to successful breastfeeding; step 4. Online. Available: www.babyfriendly.org.uk/matern.htm#top

Benyon C 1990 The normal second stage of labor: a plea for reform in its conduct. In: Kitzinger S, Simkin P 1990 (eds) Episiotomy and the second stage of labor, 2nd edn. Pennypress, Seattle (Originally published in 1957 Journal of Obstetrics and Gynaecology of the British Empire 64:815–820)

Carroli G, Belizan J 2001 Episiotomy for vaginal birth. Cochrane Pregnancy and Childbirth Group Cochrane Database of Systematic Reviews, Issue 3. Update Software, Oxford

Crawford J S 1983 The stages and phases of labour:outworn nomenclature that invites hazard. Lancet July:271–227

Data Protection Act 1998 Online. Available: www.legislation.hmso.gov.uk/acts/acts1998/19980029.htm

Downe S 1996 Concepts of normality in the maternity services: application and consequences. In: Frith L, ed. Ethics and midwifery: issues in contemporary practice. Butterworth Heinemann, Oxford, p 86–103

Downe S 1999 Reducing the risk of adverse outcome for nulliparous women using epidural analgesia in labour: a randomised clinical trial and longitudinal follow-up survey reported in the context of three discourses; the nature of childbirth, the epistemology of research, and the role of participants in clinical trials (PhD thesis). University of Derby

Enkin M, Keirse M J N C, Neilson J et al 2000 A guide to effective care in pregnancy and childbirth, 3rd edn. Oxford University Press, Oxford

Gordon B, Mackrodt C, Fern E, Truesdale A, Ayers S, Grant A 1998 The Ipswich childbirth study: 1. A randomised evaluation of two stage postpartum perineal repair leaving the skin unsutured. British Journal of Obstetrics and Gynaecology 105(4):435–440

Gould D 2000 Normal labour: a concept analysis. Journal of Advanced Nursing 31(2):418–427

Grant A, Gordon B, Mackrodat C, Fern E, Truesdale A, Ayers S 2001 The Ipswich childbirth study: one year follow up of alternative methods used in perineal repair. British Journal of Obstetrics and Gynaecology 108(1):34–40

Gupta J K, Nikodem C 2000 Maternal posture in labour. European Journal of Obstetrics, Gynecology and Reproductive Biology 92(2):273–277

Gupta J K, Nikodem V 2001 Woman's position during second stage of labour. In: The Cochrane Library, Issue 4. Update Software, Oxford

Halldorsdottir S, Karlsdottir S I 1996 Empowerment or discouragement: women's experience of caring and uncaring encounters during childbirth. Health Care for Women International 17(4):361–379

Hobbs L 1998 Assessing cervical dilatation without VEs; watching the purple line. Practising Midwife 1(11):34–35

Hodnett E D 2001 Caregiver support for women during childbirth. In: The Cochrane Library, Issue 4. Update Software, Oxford

Howell C J 2001 Epidural versus non-epidural analgesia for pain relief in labour. Cochrane Pregnancy and Childbirth Group Cochrane Database of Systematic Reviews, Issue 3. Update Software, Oxford

Humphrey M D, Chang A, Wood E C, Morgan S, Hounslow D 1974 A decrease in fetal pH during the second stage of labour when conducted in the dorsal position. Journal of Obstetrics and Gynaecology of the British Commonwealth 81:600–602

Keane H E, Thornton J G 1998 A trial of cetrimide/chlorhexidine or tap water for perineal cleaning. British Journal of Midwifery 6(1):34–37

Kettle C, Johanson R B 2001a. Continuous versus interrupted sutures for perineal repair. Cochrane Pregnancy and Childbirth Group Cochrane Database of Systematic Reviews, Issue 3. Update Software, Oxford

Kettle C, Johanson, R B 2001b Absorbable synthetic versus catgut suture material for perineal repair. Cochrane Pregnancy and Childbirth Group Cochrane Database of Systematic Reviews, Issue 3. Update Software, Oxford

Kurz C S, Schneider H, Hutch R, Hutch A 1982 The influence of maternal position on the fetal transcutaneous oxygen pressure. Journal of Perinatal Medicine 10(suppl 2):74–75

McCandlish R, Bowler U, van Asten H et al 1998 A randomised controlled trial of care of the perineum during second stage of normal labour. British Journal of Obstetrics and Gynaecology 105(12):1262–1272

Minato J F 2000 Is it time to push? Examining rest in second-stage labor. AWHONN Lifelines 4(6):20–23

Montgomery T 1958 Physiologic considerations in labor and the puerperium. American Journal of Obstetrics and Gynecology 76(4):706

NICE (National Institute for Clinical Effectiveness) 2001 The use of electronic fetal monitoring. Online. Available: www.nice.org.uk

Petersen L, Besuner P 1997 Pushing techniques during labor: issues and controversies. Journal of Obstetric, Gynecologic and Neonatal Nursing 26(6):719–726

Roberts J E, Goldstein S A, Gruener J S, Maggio M, Mendez-Bauer C 1987 A descriptive analysis of involuntary bearing-down efforts during the expulsive phase of labour. Journal of Obstetric, Gynecologic and Neonatal Nursing 16(1):48–55

Russell J G B 1969 Moulding of the pelvic outlet. Journal of Obstetrics and Gynaecology 76:817–820

Simkin P, Ancheta R 2000 The labour progress handbook. Blackwell Science, Oxford, p 131

Sleep J, Grant A, Garcia J, Elbourne D, Spencer J, Chalmers 1984 West Berkshire Perineal Management Trial. British Medical Journal 289(6445):587–590

Stewart P, Spiby H 1989 A randomized study of the sitting position for delivery using a newly designed obstetric chair. British Journal of Obstetrics and Gynaecology 96(3):327–333

Sutton J, Scott P 1996 Understanding and teaching optimal fetal positioning, 2nd edn. Birth Concepts, Tauranga, New Zealand

Turner M J, Romney M L, Webb J B, Gordon H 1986 The birthing chair: an obstetric hazard? Journal of Obstetrics and Gynecology 6:232–235

Ziadeh S M, Sunna E 2000 Obstetric and perinatal outcome of pregnancies with term labour and meconium-stained amniotic fluid. Archives of Gynecology and Obstetrics 264(2):84–87

FURTHER READING

Davis E 1992 Heart and hands: a midwife's guide to pregnancy and birth, 2nd edn. Celestial Arts, Berkeley CA

This is a manual of midwifery based on the skills and experiences gained by lay midwives working in America. It offers some unique tips and insights.

Floyd-Davis R, Sargent CF 1997. Childbirth and authoritative knowledge: cross-cultural perspectives. University of California Press, Berkeley CA

A seminal work, which explores how authority is given to certain kinds of knowledge, and how the knowledge and expertise of women and of less dominant cultures is not privileged, even in the area of childbirth, and even in the face of the evidence.

Leap N, Hunter B 1993 The midwife's tale: an oral history from handywoman to professional midwife. Scarlet Press, London

This is an historical account of trained midwives and laywomen practising in the 1950s. The stories of their experiences and responsibilities while attending women in labour are fascinating. The final chapter offers some accounts of labours from the point of view of women themselves.

Simkin P, Ancheta R 2000 The labour progress handbook. Blackwell Science, Oxford

An invaluable practical aid to supporting and facilitating physiological birth.

28 Physiology and Management of the Third Stage of Labour

Sue McDonald

CHAPTER CONTENTS

Postpartum haemorrhage (PPH) is still ranked among the top three major causes of maternal death globally. Although the majority (99%) of deaths reported occur in developing countries, the risk of PPH should not be underestimated for any birth, nor should the potential for the third stage of labour to be the most dangerous stage of labour be underestimated. During this stage the mother's focus and sense of emotional and physical relief often spontaneously shift from the concentrated exertions of the actual birth to that of exploration and familiarisation with her newborn baby. To facilitate a safe and healthy outcome for the mother and her baby, antenatal health as well as the intrapartum preparation, skill, diligence and expertise of the midwife are crucial factors. Research evidence is clearer for some aspects of third stage management than others, so I will attempt to include as broad a discussion as possible.

The chapter aims to:

- describe the normal physiological mechanism of placental separation and descent together with factors that facilitate haemostasis

- consider the types and use of uterotonic drugs in third stage management and the relevance of timing of clamping of the umbilical cord

- describe the risk factors most commonly associated with PPH and discuss the current management strategies for both prophylaxis and treatment of it

- discuss the midwife's care of the mother during and immediately after expulsion of the placenta and membranes.

Physiological processes

These are a continuation of the processes and forces at work during the earlier stages of labour. It is an understanding of these changes that guides the midwife's practice. During the third stage, separation and expulsion of the placenta and membranes occur as the result of an interplay of mechanical and haemostatic factors. The time at which the placenta actually separates from the uterine wall can vary. It may shear off during the final expulsive contractions accompanying the birth of the baby or remain adherent for some considerable time. The third stage usually lasts between 5 and 15 minutes, but any period up to 1 hour may be considered to be within normal limits.

Separation and descent of the placenta

Mechanical factors

The unique characteristic of uterine muscle lies in its power of retraction. During the second stage of labour the uterine cavity progressively empties, enabling the retraction process to accelerate. Thus by the beginning of the third stage the placental site has already begun to diminish in size. As this occurs the placenta itself becomes compressed and the blood in the intervillous spaces is forced back into the spongy layer of the decidua. Retraction of the oblique uterine muscle fibres exerts pressure on the blood vessels so that blood does not drain back into the maternal system. The vessels during this process become tense and congested. With the next contraction the distended veins burst and a small amount of blood seeps in between the thin septa of the spongy layer and the placental surface, stripping it from its attachment (Fig. 28.1). As the surface area for placental attachment reduces, the relatively non-elastic placenta begins to detach from the uterine wall.

Separation usually begins centrally so that a retroplacental clot is formed (Fig. 28.2). This may further aid separation by exerting pressure at the midpoint of placental attachment so that the increased weight helps to strip the adherent lateral borders. This increased weight also helps to peel the membranes off the uterine wall so that the clot thus formed becomes enclosed in a membranous bag as the placenta descends, fetal surface first. This process of separation (first described by Schultze) is associated with more complete shearing of both placenta and membranes and less fluid blood loss (Fig. 28.3A). Alternatively, the placenta may begin to detach unevenly at one of its lateral borders. The blood escapes so that separation is unaided by the formation of a retroplacental clot. The placenta descends, slipping sideways, maternal surface first. This process (first described by Matthews Duncan in the nineteenth century) takes longer and is associated with ragged, incomplete expulsion of the membranes and a higher fluid blood loss (Fig. 28.3B).

Once separation has occurred, the uterus contracts strongly, forcing placenta and membranes to fall into the lower uterine segment (Fig. 28.4) and finally into the vagina.

Haemostasis

The normal volume of blood flow through the placental site is 500–800 ml per minute. At placental separation this has to be arrested within seconds as otherwise serious haemorrhage will occur. The interplay of three factors within the normal physiological processes that control bleeding are critical in minimising blood loss and the serious sequelae of maternal morbidity or mortality, or both, which may result. They are:

1. *Retraction of the oblique uterine muscle fibres in the upper uterine segment through which the tortuous blood vessels intertwine* – the resultant thickening of the muscles exerts pressure on the torn vessels, acting as clamps, so securing a ligature action. This is shown in Figure 28.1. It is the absence of oblique fibres in the lower uterine segment that explains the greatly increased blood loss usually accompanying placental separation in placenta praevia.
2. *The presence of vigorous uterine contraction following separation* – this brings the walls into apposition so that further pressure is exerted on the placental site.
3. *The achievement of haemostasis* – there is evidence to suggest that there is a transitory activation of the coagulation and fibrinolytic systems during, and immediately following, placental separation (Bonnar et al 1970). It is believed that this protective response is especially active at the placental site so that clot formation in the torn vessels is intensified. Following separation, the placental site is rapidly covered by a fibrin mesh utilising 5–10% of the circulating fibrinogen.

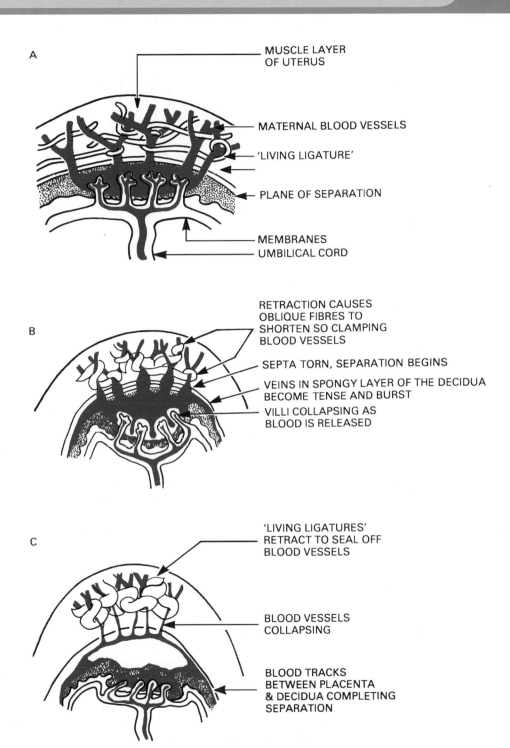

Fig. 28.1 The placental site during separation. (A) Uterus and placenta before separation. (B) Separation begins. (C) Separation is almost complete.

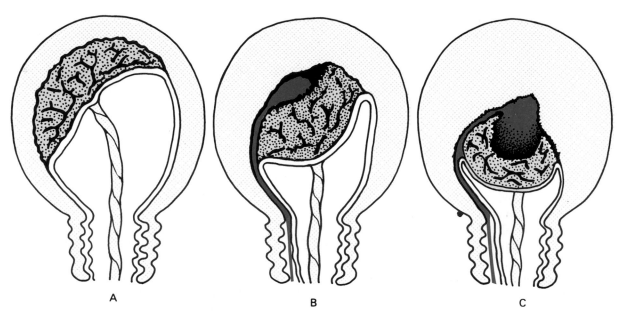

Fig. 28.2 The mechanism of placental separation. (A) Uterine wall is partially retracted, but not sufficiently to cause placental separation. (B) Further contraction and retraction thicken the uterine wall, reduce the placental site and aid placental separation. (C) Complete separation and formation of the retroplacental clot. *Note:* The thin lower segment has collapsed like a concertina following the birth of the baby.

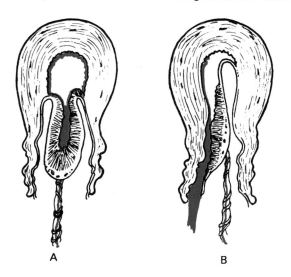

Fig. 28.3 Expulsion of the placenta. (A) Schultze method. (B) Matthews Duncan method.

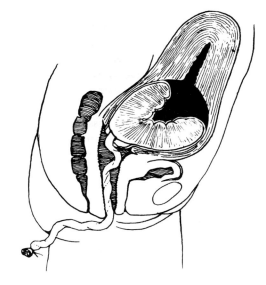

Fig. 28.4 Third stage: placenta in lower uterine segment.

Management of the third stage

The midwife's care of the mother should be based on an understanding of the normal physiological processes at work. Her actions can help to reduce the very real risks of haemorrhage, infection, retained placenta and shock, any of which may increase maternal morbidity and even result in death. A mother's ability to withstand these complications depends, to a large degree, upon her general condition and the avoidance of debilitating, predisposing problems such as anaemia, ketosis, exhaustion and prolonged hypotonic uterine action. Factors that may influence the risk of haemorrhage are discussed in more detail later in this chapter under 'Complications of the third stage of labour'.

Uterotonics or uterotonic agents

These are drugs (e.g. syntometrine, syntocinon, ergometrine and prostaglandins) that stimulate the smooth muscle of the uterus to contract. They may be administered with crowning of the baby's head, at the time of delivery of the anterior shoulder of the baby, at the end of the second stage of labour or following the delivery of the placenta.

Whether women should routinely receive uterotonic drugs, have the umbilical cord clamped or be given assistance with placental delivery has been the subject of a great deal of debate and many research trials. The individual merits of these processes will be discussed in this chapter. What is of primary importance is that the health professional (whether a midwife, GP or obstetrician) providing clinical care and advice should ensure that, in order to facilitate decision making by the woman, adequate time for deliberation and questions should be made available, where possible, during the course of her routine antenatal consultations. Information related to the best available research information on the use of uterotonic drugs during the third stage of labour should be offered in an objective manner, which could perhaps be supported with pamphlets that cover topics such as possible management options for the woman in the setting in which she intends to birth, types of uterotonics, explanation of their different applications, route of administration, timing and method of placental delivery.

Active management. This is a policy whereby *prophylactic* administration of an uterotonic, as a precautionary measure aimed at reduction in the risk for postpartum haemorrhage, is applied regardless of the assessed obstetric risk status of the woman. An active management policy usually includes the routine administration of a uterotonic agent either intravenously, intramuscularly or even orally. This is undertaken in conjunction with clamping of the umbilical cord shortly after birth of the baby and delivery of the placenta by the use of controlled cord traction. In situations where women may also be assessed as being at higher risk for PPH (e.g. multiple birth, grande multiparity), prophylactic infusion of larger doses of uterotonics diluted in intravenous solutions may be administered over several hours following the birth This would also be considered to be part of an active management policy. Active management in the third stage is the policy of third stage labour management most widely practised throughout the developed world.

Expectant or physiological management. In the event of *expectant management*, routine administration of the uterotonic drug is withheld, the umbilical cord is left unclamped until cord pulsation has ceased or the mother requests it to be clamped, or both, and the placenta is expelled by use of gravity and maternal effort. With this approach, *therapeutic* uterotonic administration would be administered either to stop bleeding once it has occurred or to maintain the uterus in a contracted state when there are indications that excessive bleeding is likely to occur.

Emergency use usually indicates an event of uncontrolled haemorrhage. In this situation it is important for the midwife to be aware of whether, what and how much of a uterotonic agent has already been administered.

No matter what an individual midwife's personal practice experience may be or what the best available research evidence recommends, it is still ultimately the woman's decision as to how she would ideally wish her pregnancy and birth plan to be followed. There may be philosophical, religious or cultural beliefs that influence her decision.

However, It is also fair to suggest that the midwife also has rights and responsibilities and, in the very litigious environment in which we may practice, documentation is extremely important, particularly in areas where evidence-based information is relied upon to assess whether due care has been delivered. In the case of third stage management, an example might be: in the circumstance where a woman specifically requests that uterotonic drugs be withheld from routine use in her third stage care, the midwife should clarify the circumstances in which this decision may be reversed. If a uterotonic drug is *not* to be used, the woman's preference for care must be recorded in her notes antenatally. Some would wish the record to be signed by the woman. It would be prudent for the midwife to notify her clinical manager or the attending medical practitioner of such a request if it is contrary to local guidelines.

In practice, one of the following uterotonic drugs is usually used.

Intravenous ergometrine 0.25 mg

This drug acts within 45 seconds; therefore it is particularly useful in securing a rapid contraction where hypotonic uterine action results in haemorrhage. If a doctor is not present in such an emergency, a midwife may give the injection. In an overview of the choice of uterotonics for use in the third stage, Prendiville et al (1988a) found that there was no supportive evidence for the continued routine use of intravenous ergometrine, which is associated with an increased risk of retained placenta. If an intravenous cannula is not already in situ, any difficulty encountered in locating a vein or sudden movement by the woman may result in failed venepuncture or at least a delay in administration.

Combined ergometrine and oxytocin (a commonly used brand is Syntometrine)

A 1 ml ampoule contains 5 international units of oxytocin and 0.5 mg ergometrine and is administered by intramuscular injection. The oxytocin acts within 2½ minutes, and the ergometrine within 6–7 minutes (Fig. 28.5). Their combined action results in a rapid uterine contraction enhanced by a stronger, more sustained contraction lasting several hours. It is usually administered as the anterior shoulder of the baby is delivered, thus stimulating good uterine action at the beginning of the third stage. The use of combined ergometrine/oxytocin or any ergometrine-based drug is associated with side-effects such as elevation of the blood pressure and vomiting (McDonald et al 2002).

Caution. No more than two doses of ergometrine 0.5 mg should be given as it can cause headache, nausea and an increase in blood pressure; it is normally contraindicated where there is a history of hypertensive or cardiac disease.

Oxytocin (a commonly used brand is Syntocinon)

Oxytocin is a synthetic form of the natural oxytocin produced in the *posterior* pituitary, and is safe to use in a wider context than combined ergometrine/oxytocin agents. It can be administered both as an intravenous and as an intramuscular injection. However, an intravenous bolus of oxytocin can cause profound, fatal hypotension, especially in the presence of cardiovascular compromise. The recommendation of the CEMD (Lewis & Drife 2001, p. 21) is that 'when given as an intravenous bolus the drug should be given slowly in a dose of not more than 5 iu'.

Research evidence to date suggests that this is an effective uterotonic choice where routine prophylactic management of the third stage of labour is practised (Choy et al 2002, Khan et al 1995, McDonald et al 1993), more specifically in women who experience a blood loss exceeding 1000 ml (McDonald et al 2002). There still, however, does not appear to be an absolutely decisive guidance for practice with regard to choice of uterotonic. Perhaps it can no longer be discussed in isolation from other issues that surround the management of labour itself, including induction, use of uterotonics in labour, use of epidurals and tolerance of longer second stages.

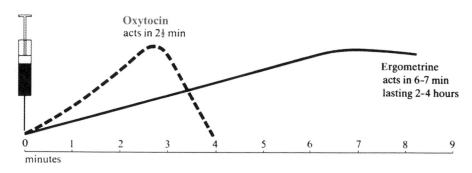

Fig. 28.5 The rapid action of oxytocin in comparison with ergometrine.

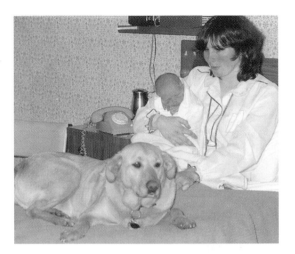

Plate 1 A 26-year-old blind woman with her healthy 7-day-old son and her devoted guide dog. (Reproduced with kind permission from Beischer, Mackay & Colditz 1997.) (See text p. 20.)

The Balance of Good Health

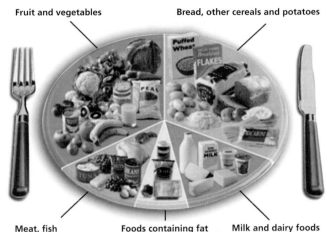

Fruit and vegetables

Bread, other cereals and potatoes

Meat, fish and alternatives

Foods containing fat Foods and drinks containing sugar

Milk and dairy foods

Plate 2 The balance of good health. (Reproduced with kind permission from the Food Standards Agency.) (See text p. 170.)

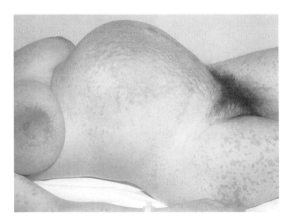

Plate 3 Pemphigoid gestationis (herpes gestationis). The generalised rash appeared at 34 weeks and responded to corticosteroids. This skin disease is rare (1 in 5-10,000 pregnancies), unique to pregnancy and of unknown aetiology. It resolves soon after delivery and may recur in successive pregnancies. Because of the increased risk of intrauterine death, fetal condition must be carefully assessed, and labour induced when the fetus is mature. (Reproduced with kind permission from Beischer, Mackay & Colditz 1997.) (See text p. 311.)

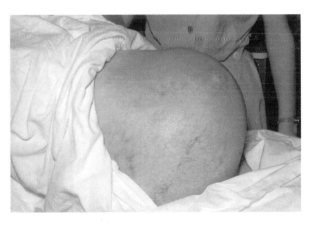

Plate 4 Acute polyhydramnios at 35 weeks' gestation. (Reproduced with kind permission from Beischer, Mackay & Colditz 1997.) (See text p.312.)

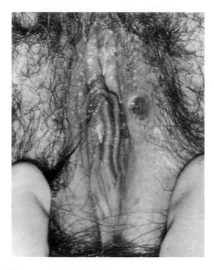

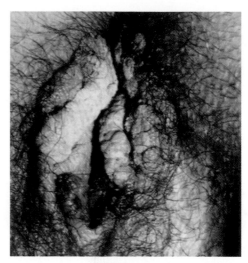

Plate 5 Syphilis: primary chancre on the vulva. (Reproduced with kind permission from the BMJ Publishing Group, from Adler 1998.) (See text p. 379.)

Plate 6 Massive genital warts in pregnancy. (Reproduced with kind permission from the BMJ Publishing Group, from Adler 1998.) (See text p. 381.)

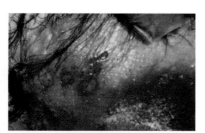

Plate 7 Genital herpes on the vulva. (Reproduced with kind permission from the BMJ Publishing Group, from Adler 1998.) (See text p. 382.)

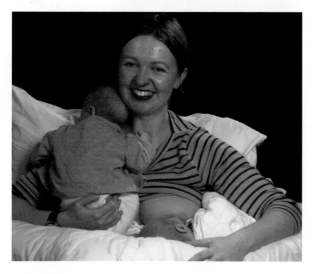

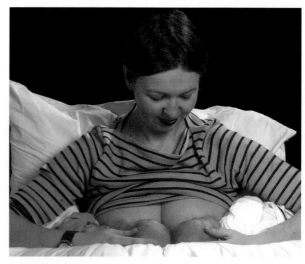

Plate 8 Mother breastfeeding one twin, and winding the other. (See text p. 397.)

Plate 9 Mother breastfeeding both twins simultaneously. (See text p. 397.)

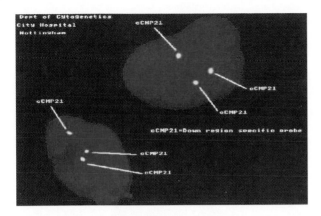

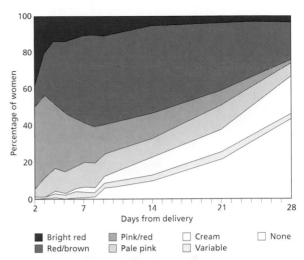

Plate 10 FISH analysis showing Trisomy 21 (Down syndrome). (Reproduced with kind permission from the Department of Cytogenetics, Nottingham City Hospital NHS Trust.) (See text p. 425.)

Plate 11 The colour of vaginal loss reported by women for the first 28 days postpartum. (Reproduced with kind permission from Midwifery 1999 15:80.) (See text p. 631.)

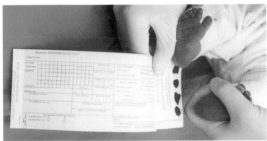

Plate 12 Blood screening. (See text p. 742.)

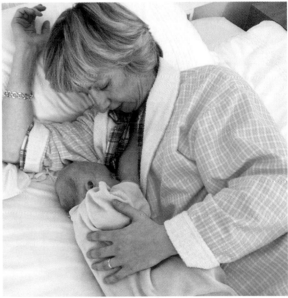

Plate 13 Mother feeding, lying down. (Reproduced with kind permission from the Health Education Board for Scotland.) (See text p. 756.)

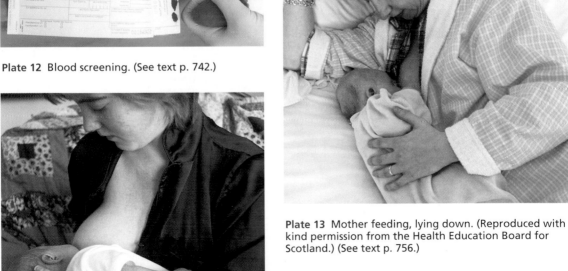

Plate 14 Mother feeding, sitting up. (Reproduced with kind permission from the Health Education Board for Scotland.) (See text p. 756.)

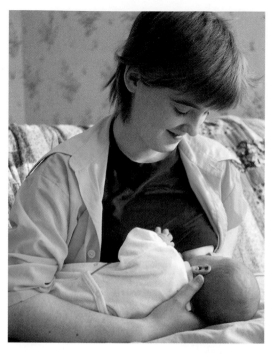

Plate 15 Mother supporting the baby's head with her fingers. (Reproduced with kind permission from the Health Education Board for Scotland.) (See text p. 757.)

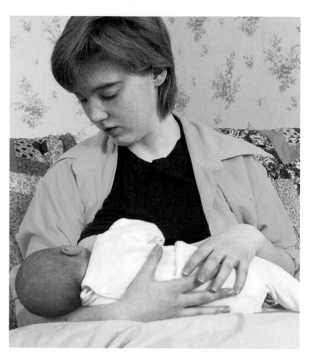

Plate 16 The baby's head is supported by the mother's forearm. (Reproduced with kind permission from the Health Education Board for Scotland.) (See text p. 757.)

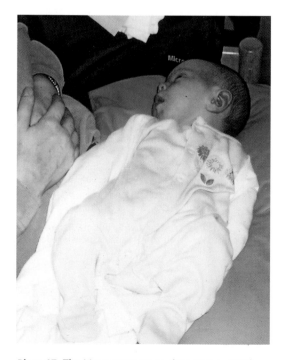

Plate 17 The Vancouver wrap. (See text p. 757.)

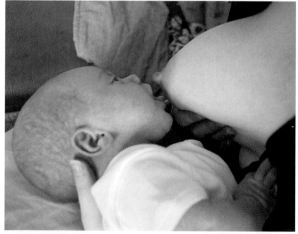

Plate 18 A wide gape. (Reproduced with kind permission from the Health Education Board for Scotland.) (See text p. 757.)

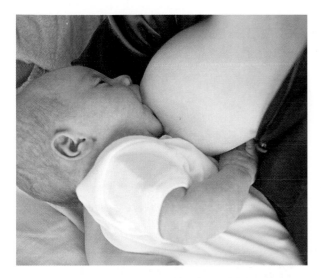

Plate 19 The baby forms a 'teat' from the breast and nipple. (Reproduced with kind permission from the Health Education Board for Scotland.) (See text p. 757.)

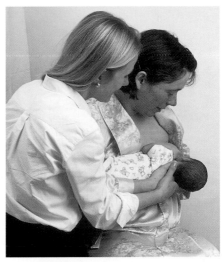

Plate 20 The midwife is kneeling by the mother to help her attach to the baby. (Reproduced with kind permission from Nancy Durrell-McKenna.) (See text p. 758.)

Plate 21 Stool colour comparator. (Reproduced with kind permission from the Midwifery Department, Ninewells Hospital, Dundee, UK.) (See text p. 760.)

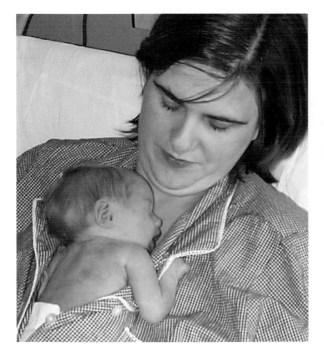

Plate 22 Kangaroo care. (See text p. 792.)

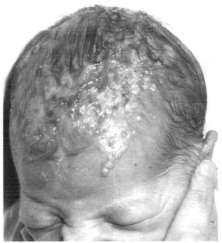

Plate 23 A rash produced by the herpes simplex virus. (See text p. 801.)

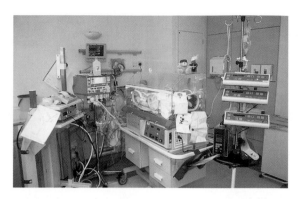

Plate 25 Neonatal intensive care. (See text p. 809, 818.)

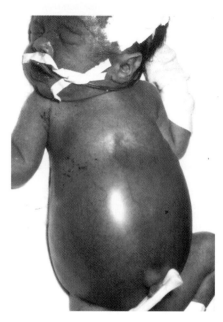

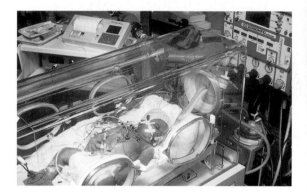

Plate 24 A distended abdomen in necrotising enterocolitis. (See text p. 807.)

Plate 26 A baby receiving intensive care. (See text p. 809, p. 821.)

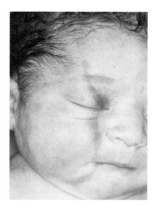

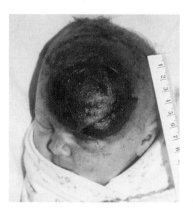

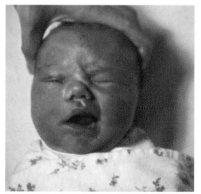

Plate 27 Forceps blade abrasion on cheek. (Reproduced with kind permission from Thomas & Harvey 1997.) (See text p. 826.)

Plate 28 Scalp abrasion suffered during vacuum-assisted birth. Note the chignon. (Reproduced with kind permission from Thomas & Harvey 1997.) (See text p. 826.)

Plate 29 Right-sided facial palsy. Note the eye is open on the paralysed side and the mouth is drawn over to the non-paralysed side. (Reproduced with kind permission from Thomas & Harvey 1997.) (See text p. 827.)

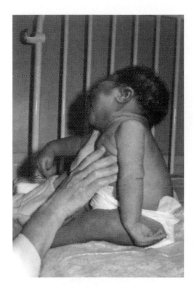

Plate 30 Erb's palsy. (Reproduced with kind permission from Thomas & Harvey 1997.) (See text p. 828, 575.)

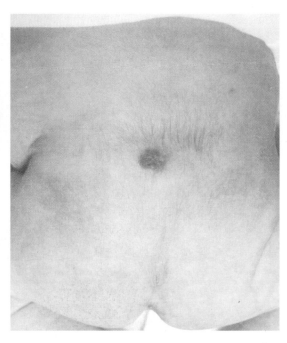

Plate 31 A small meningomyelocele with lower sacral nerve involvement in a 7-day-old baby. (Reproduced with kind permission from Beischer, Mackay & Colditz 1997.) (See text p. 852.)

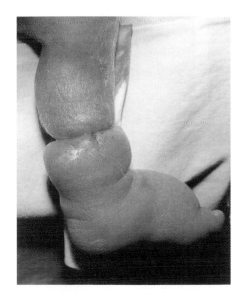

Plate 32 Amniotic band with gross oedema below the deep constriction and transverse fractures at the level of the band. (Reproduced with kind permission from Beischer, Mackay & Colditz 1997.) (See text p. 854.)

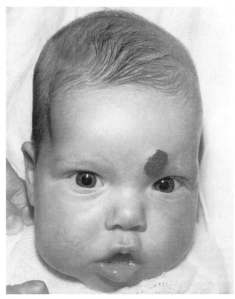

Plate 33 Strawberry naevus (capillary haemangioma) in a female infant aged 12 weeks. Spontaneous regression occurs in more than 90% of cases by the age of 3 years. (Reproduced with kind permission from Beischer, Mackay & Colditz 1997.) (See text p. 856.)

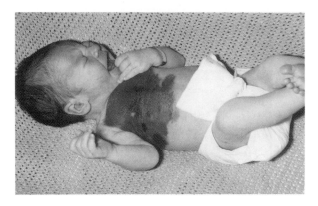

Plate 34 Large, pigmented naevus. (Reproduced with kind permission from Beischer, Mackay & Colditz 1997.) (See text p. 856.)

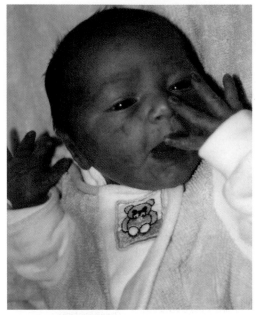

Plate 35 A jaundiced baby. (See text p. 864.)

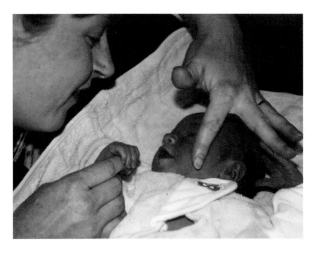

Plate 36 A jaundiced baby and mother. Note the contrast in colour between the jaundiced skin of the baby and the mother's unjaundiced skin. (See text p. 864.)

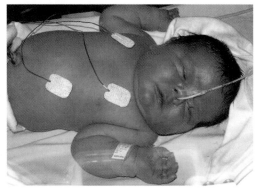

Plate 37 The baby of a diabetic mother, undergoing fibreoptic therapy. (See text p. 876, 877, 893.)

Prostaglandins

The use of prostaglandins for third stage management has up until now been more often associated with the *treatment* of postpartum haemorrhage than with *prophylaxis*. This may be partly due to it being substantially more expensive than the already discussed uterotonics. Prostaglandin agents are also associated with side-effects such as diarrhoea (Chua et al 1995) and cardiovascular complications of increased stroke volume and heart rate (van Selm et al 1995). Prostaglandin administration is most effective when used intramurally (injected directly into the uterine wall) or by intrauterine irrigation (Peyser & Kupfermine 1990). The procedures are time consuming and invasive and the expertise required for undertaking the procedures is unlikely to always be readily available in routine labour management.

More recently, a prostaglandin E_1 analogue (misoprostol), suitable for oral administration and originally prescribed for people suffering from gastric ulcers, has been reported by El-Refaey et al (1997) following use in third stage management. In that study, the authors suggested that misoprostol, which is rapidly absorbed, is not prone to problems of temperature control, does not require the use of sterile syringes and needles and is inexpensive to produce, may be a suitable uterotonic agent for use in the prophylactic management of the third stage of labour. These findings were felt to have an exciting potential, particularly in the developing world, where these issues are very problematic. One of the difficulties with the use of misoprostol has been in elucidating the maximal dosage that can be given without causing unacceptable levels of side-effects such as shivering and raised body temperature. A large randomised controlled multicentre trial involving over 18 000 women throughout 10 countries in both developed and developing countries was undertaken between April 1998 and November 1999. The results of this study were recently published (Gülmezoglu et al 2001). The conclusion of the authors was that 10 i.u. oxytocin (i.v. or i.m.) was more effective than the oral administration of misoprostol in the active management of the third stage of labour in hospital settings where active management is the norm. This is an important finding as it was hoped that, had the drug been effective, it might provide a much-needed approach to third stage

management for developing country settings where approximately 90% of deaths related to PPH occur. In a recent systematic review that included 14 misoprostol and 8 intramuscular prostaglandin trials for prevention of PPH, Gülmezoglu et al (2002) concluded that although neither misoprostol nor injectable prostaglandins could be deemed to be preferable to conventional injectable uterotonics as part of the active management of the third stage of labour, particularly in low risk women, it should not be discounted as a last resort in the management of intractable haemorrhage where other agents were not successful.

Debate will hopefully continue as, although the use of misoprostol may not be an advantage in settings where other uterotonic agents are easily available, there may still be great merit in further exploring its use in areas where maternal deaths related to PPH are all too common and the alternative is no uterotonics at all.

Clamping of the umbilical cord

This may have been carried out during birth of the baby if the cord was tightly around the neck. However, opinions vary as to the most beneficial time for clamping the cord during the third stage of labour (Inch 1985). Early clamping is carried out in the first 1–3 minutes immediately after birth regardless of whether the cord pulsation has ceased. It has been suggested that this practice may have the following effects:

- It may reduce the volume of blood returning to the fetus by as much as 75–125 ml, especially if clamping occurs within the first minute (Montgomery 1960). This may in turn reduce neonatal haemoglobin levels in the short term but, in the only published study to assess longer term outcomes, by 6 weeks after birth the haemoglobin levels in these babies had been restored (Pau-Chen & Tsu-Shan 1960).
- It may prematurely interrupt the respiratory function of the placenta in maintaining O_2 levels and combating acidosis in the early moments of life. This may be of particular importance in the baby who is slow to breathe.
- It may result in lower neonatal bilirubin levels, although the effect on the incidence of clinical jaundice is unclear (Prendiville & Elbourne 1989).

- It may increase the likelihood of fetomaternal transfusion as a larger volume of blood remains in the placenta. Venous pressure is further increased as retraction continues and may be sufficiently high to rupture surface placental vessels, thus facilitating the transfer of fetal cells into the maternal system; this may be a critical factor where the mother's blood group is Rhesus negative (Ladipo 1972) (see also Ch. 46).
- It may result in the truncated umbilical vessels containing a quantity of clotted blood, which provides an ideal medium for bacterial growth. Heavier placental weight has also been associated with early cord clamping (Newton et al 1961).

Proponents of late clamping suggest that no action be taken until cord pulsation ceases or the placenta has been completely delivered, thus allowing the physiological processes to take place without intervention. Postulated advantages of late clamping include:

1. The route to the low resistance placental circulation remains patent, which provides the newborn with a safety valve for any raised systemic blood pressure. This may be critical when the baby is preterm or asphyxiated, as raised pulmonary and central venous pressures may exacerbate the difficulties in initiating respiration and accompanying circulatory adaptation (Dunn 1985).
2. The length of time for the cord to separate postnatally is reduced.
3. There is transfusion of the full quota of placental blood to the newborn. This may constitute as much as 40% of the circulating volume depending on when the cord is clamped and at what level the baby is held prior to clamping (Yao & Lind 1974); it may therefore be important in maintaining haematocrit levels. The neonatal effects associated with increased placental transfusion include higher mean birthweight and higher neonatal haematocrit accompanied by an increase in the incidence of jaundice (Prendiville et al 1988b).

There is very little evidence concerning how much, if any, of a uterotonic agent the baby receives following birth. In five documented cases of accidental administration of an adult dose of Syntometrine to a newborn infant, no long term adverse effects were reported (Whitfield & Salfield 1980).

Another factor that may influence the amount of placental transfusion is the use of an uterotonic agent prior to the completion of labour. This may precipitate a strong uterine contraction with resultant overtransfusion of the baby.

Is the timing of uterotonic administration and cord clamping clinically important in influencing the incidence of PPH?

Background

At the time of birth, the baby is still attached to the mother via the umbilical cord, which is part of the placenta. When the third stage or placental delivery stage is managed actively, an injection of an oxytocic drug is given to the mother at about the same time as the baby's shoulders are born and the umbilical cord is clamped twice. One clamp is placed closer to the baby's navel end. Care should be taken to apply the clamp to the cord end nearer the baby, 3–4 cm clear of the abdominal wall, to avoid pinching the skin or clamping a portion of gut, which, in rare instances, may be in the cord. A greater length of cord is left when umbilical vessels are needed for transfusion, for example in preterm babies and cases of Rhesus haemolytic disease, and the second clamp is placed closer to the placental end of the cord. The cord between the two clamps is then cut. At this time the baby may be placed on the mother's abdomen, put to the breast or be more closely examined on a warmed cot if resuscitation is required. Once the placenta is felt to have separated from the wall of the uterus, downward traction may be applied to the remaining length of umbilical cord to assist delivery of the placenta.

Timing of cord clamping is also supposedly routine, but, in practice it varies greatly. Early cord clamping, which is usually part of active management, is in general regarded as clamping of the umbilical cord within 30 seconds of the birth of the baby. Late cord clamping, a physiological approach, involves clamping of the umbilical cord when cord pulsation has ceased. However, definitions of what constitutes early and late cord clamping vary (Prendiville & Elbourne 1989) and again, in practice, unavoidable factors (e.g. if the cord is around the neck, the number of clinicians in the room, the need for active resuscitation of the infant) can make it difficult to adhere to a particular policy

(McDonald 1996). There is no published evidence that this delay is of consequence in term infants (McDonald 1996, Prendiville & Elbourne 1989, Prendiville et al 1988a).

Investigations have been undertaken into the advantages and disadvantages of maternal–fetal transfusion and the effect of early or late cord clamping in relation to respiratory distress in the preterm infant (Dunn 1966, Inch 1985, Linderkamp 1982). There is a considerable amount of literature published on timing of cord clamping and associated placental transfusion. Debate continues over the effect of the extra 90–100 ml of blood received by the baby when late cord clamping is practised (Rabe & Reynolds 2002).

Although active management leads to reduced risk of PPH, it is important to establish which of the components of this package lead to this reduced risk. Given the difficulties of adhering to an active management policy and the preferences of some women for physiological management, it is important to explore practice behaviours to clarify whether it is necessary to continue to promote the policy as it currently stands.

Recent evidence suggests that the effects of early versus late cord clamping may be different for preterm (Rabe & Reynolds 2002) and term infants. Timing of cord clamping appears to be less of an issue in term infants, probably because the normal physiological process of transfer are completed within the first 1–2 minutes of birth for the majority of these infants

(McDonald 1996). This may suggest that, whereas there is an obvious advantage to the prophylactic administration of a uterotonic drug, future policies may be less prescriptive about the necessity to clamp and cut the cord immediately following the birth.

Delivery of the placenta and membranes

Controlled cord traction (CCT). This manoeuvre is believed to reduce blood loss, shorten the third stage of labour and therefore minimise the time during which the mother is at risk from haemorrhage. It is designed to enhance the normal physiological process. Successful results depend upon understanding the principles of placental separation described at the beginning of this chapter.

If CCT is to be used, there are several checks to be made before proceeding:

- that an uterotonic drug has been administered
- that it has been given time to act
- that the uterus is well contracted
- that countertraction is applied
- that signs of placental separation and descent are present. (At the beginning of the third stage, a strong uterine contraction results in the fundus being palpable below the umbilicus (Fig. 28.6). It feels broad as the placenta is still in the upper

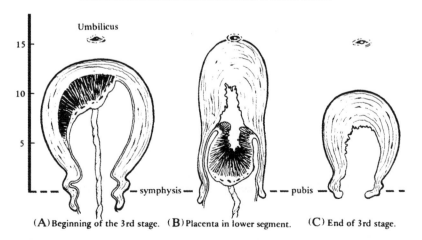

APPROXIMATE FUNDAL HEIGHTS DURING THIRD STAGE

Umbilicus

(A) Beginning of the 3rd stage.   (B) Placenta in lower segment.   (C) End of 3rd stage.

Fig. 28.6 Fundal height relative to the umbilicus and symphysis pubis.

segment. As the placenta separates and falls into the lower uterine segment there is a small fresh blood loss, the cord lengthens, and the fundus becomes rounder, smaller and more mobile as it rises in the abdomen above the level of the placenta.) There is however debate about whether CCT should be applied before or after the signs of placental separation have been noted. Levy & Moore (1985) observed that blood loss was reduced when CCT was delayed until lengthening of the cord and a trickle of fresh blood loss had been observed.

It is important not to manipulate the uterus in any way as this may precipitate incoordinate action. No further step should be taken until a strong contraction is palpable. If tension is applied to the umbilical cord without this contraction, uterine inversion may occur. This is an acute obstetric emergency with life-threatening implications for the mother. The action to be taken in such an event is detailed in Chapter 32.

When CCT is the preferred method of management, the following sequence of actions is usually undertaken.

Once the uterus is found on palpation to be contracted, one hand is placed above the level of the symphysis pubis with the palm facing towards the umbilicus exerting pressure in an upwards direction. This is countertraction. The other hand, firmly grasping the cord, applies traction in a downward and backward direction following the line of the birth canal (Fig. 28.7). Some resistance may be felt but it is important to apply steady tension by pulling the cord firmly and maintaining the pressure. Jerky movements and force should be avoided. The aim is to complete the action as one continuous, smooth, controlled movement. However, it is only possible to exert this tension for 1 or 2 minutes as it may be an uncomfortable procedure for the mother and the midwife's hand will tire.

Downward traction on the cord must be released *before* uterine countertraction is relaxed as sudden withdrawal of countertraction while tension is still being applied to the cord may also facilitate uterine inversion. If the manoeuvre is not immediately successful there should be a pause before the uterine contraction is again checked and a further attempt is made. Should the uterus relax, tension is temporarily released until a good contraction is again palpable.

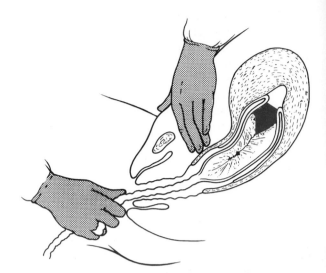

Fig. 28.7 Controlled cord traction.

Once the placenta is visible it may be cupped in the hands to ease pressure on the friable membranes. A gentle upward and downward movement or twisting action will help to coax out the membranes and increase the chances of delivering them intact. Artery forceps may be applied to gradually ease the membranes out of the vagina. This process should not be hurried; great care should be taken to avoid tearing the membranes.

Expectant management. This management policy allows the physiological changes within the uterus that occur at the time of birth to take their natural course with minimal intervention; it normally excludes the administration of uterotonic drugs. The processes of placental separation and expulsion are quite distinct from one another and the signs of separation and descent must be evident before maternal effort can be used to expedite expulsion. If the mother is sitting or squatting at this stage, gravity will aid expulsion.

If good uterine contractions are sustained, maternal effort will usually bring about expulsion. The mother simply pushes as during the second stage of labour. Encouragement is important, as by now she may be exhausted and the contractions will feel weaker and less expulsive than those during the second stage of labour. Providing that fresh blood loss is not excessive, the mother's condition remains stable and her pulse rate normal, there need be no anxiety. This spontaneous process can take from 20 minutes to an hour to complete. It is important that the midwife monitors uterine action by placing a hand lightly on the fundus. She can thus palpate the contraction whilst checking that relaxation does not result in the uterus filling with blood. Vigilance is crucial as it should be remembered that the longer the placenta remains undelivered the greater is the risk of bleeding because the uterus cannot contract down fully whilst the bulk of the placenta is in situ. Dombrowski et al (1995) found that the frequency of haemorrhage increased between 10 and 40 minutes after the birth of the baby. Patience and confidence are required on the part of the midwife to secure a successful conclusion. An uterotonic agent is usually not administered unless uterine tone is poor.

Early attachment of the baby to the breast may enhance these physiological changes by stimulating the reflex release of oxytocin from the posterior lobe of the pituitary gland, which helps to secure good uterine action.

Evidence for active versus expectant management. There is an increasing amount of appropriate, rigorously conducted research evidence available that strongly suggests that the prophylactic administration of an uterotonic significantly reduces the risk of PPH, results in a lower mean blood loss, fewer blood transfusions are required and there is a reduced need for therapeutic uterotonics (Begley 1990, Khan et al 1997, Prendiville et al 1988a, Rogers et al 1998, Thilaganathan et al 1993). It has also been highlighted by the wide range of 'risk status' of women included in several studies that it is in fact very difficult to define a group of women who are not at risk for PPH. Taking all the best available evidence into consideration, a systematic review of the literature recently published (Prendiville et al 2002) recommended that all women who birth in circumstances where this option is available should be encouraged to do so. Although the evidence is strongly in favour of prophylactic administration of a uterotonic, there are still aspects of active vs expectant management that may be worth exploring – for example, uterotonic administration alone versus active management.

Position of the woman

The effect of the position adopted by the woman at the time of placental delivery is still largely unclear. It may vary according to the mother's personal preference, the normality of progress and the experience and confidence of the attendant midwife, and may be influenced by the need for the midwife to monitor closely such factors as uterine contraction and blood loss.

Adoption of a dorsal position allows easy palpation of the uterine fundus. However, blood is more likely to pool in the uterus and vagina, thus disguising the true blood loss. Upright, kneeling and all-fours positions may enhance the effect of gravity and increase intra-abdominal pressure, which may in turn hasten the placental delivery process. Blood loss can be more easily observed as fluids will drain out of the vagina. The squatting position has been reported to increase visible blood loss (Gupta & Nikodem 2002). Whichever position is adopted, the use of aids such as wedges, pillows and physical support from her partner will help to ensure the woman's comfort while completion of the third stage is being accomplished. Some women feel cold and shivery at this time, especially if labour has progressed rapidly. This is usually transient and not abnormal.

Asepsis

The need for asepsis is even greater now than in the preceding stages of labour. Laceration and bruising of the cervix, vagina, perineum and vulva provide a route for the entry of micro organisms. At the placental site, a raw wound provides an ideal medium for infection. Strict attention to the prevention of sepsis is therefore vital.

The abdomen may at this point be draped with a clean towel and a hand placed lightly on the fundus to monitor progress.

Cord blood sampling

This may be required for a variety of conditions:

- when the mother's blood group is Rhesus negative or as a precautionary measure if the mother's Rhesus type is unknown
- when atypical maternal antibodies have been found during an antenatal screening test
- where a haemoglobinopathy is suspected (e.g. sickle cell disease).

The sample should be taken from the fetal surface of the placenta where the blood vessels are congested and easily visible. This must be done before the blood clots, but is a quick procedure if preparation has been made. If the cord has not been clamped prior to placental delivery the fetal vessels will not be congested, but a sample of sufficient volume may still be easily obtained. The appropriate containers should be used for the investigations requested. These may include the baby's blood group, Rhesus type, haemoglobin estimation, serum bilirubin level, Coombs' test or electrophoresis. Maternal blood for Kleihauer testing can be taken upon completion of the third stage.

Completion of the third stage

Once the placenta is delivered, the midwife must first check that the uterus is well contracted and fresh blood loss is minimal. Careful inspection of the perineum and lower vagina is important. A strong light is directed on to the perineum in order to assess trauma accurately prior to instigating repair. This should be carried out as gently as possible as the tissues are often bruised and oedematous. Slight lacerations such as damage to the fourchette may be left unsutured. However, if repair of a more extensive wound such as an episiotomy or a second degree tear is necessary, suturing (see Ch. 27) should be carried out as expediently as possible to prevent unnecessary blood loss and the increased risk of oedema at the site of trauma. Duthie et al (1990) found, in a study of laboratory-measured blood loss compared with delivery room visual estimation, that 17.7% of the primary PPH calculated by laboratory measurement had gone unnoticed on visual estimation in a population of women who were assessed as being at low risk for postpartum haemorrhage.

Blood loss estimation

Moore & Levy (1983) found blood loss over 300 ml to be often underestimated. This is an important factor to be considered when assessing factors. The site of the blood loss does not necessarily alter the impact in terms of potential debility for affected women.

Other blood loss studies have been more specifically related to caesarean section. In his paper on blood loss at caesarean section, Brandt (1966) makes a valid point that haemodynamically women can withstand perhaps a 1000–1500 ml blood loss. However, any further blood loss may not be tolerated so readily.

Women who undergo elective caesarean section will for the most part have been adequately prepared. Women who undergo emergency caesarean section or vaginal birth who are dehydrated or anaemic may not withstand sudden large volumes of blood loss.

In his study of the importance and difficulties of precise estimation of PPH, Brandt (1967) calculated that 20% of women lose more than 500 ml of blood after a vaginal delivery. It was estimated that 3940 ml of circulating blood volume were required to maintain the central venous pressure at 10 cm of water. Most measurement techniques are not sufficiently sensitive to detect a rapid volume change in the immediate setting when decisions need to be made. The study was conducted by collecting all blood-soaked and blood-stained fabric and swabs, collecting spilled blood and clots by wiping the floor and delivery table, and transferring blood and blood clots adherent to the placenta in tubular stockinet to an agitator-model washing machine. After immersion in water the bags were passed several times through the washing machine wringer, ammonium hydroxide was added and the contents of the machine agitated for a further 45 minutes. A sample of the resultant solution was centrifuged and filtered and its oxyhaemoglobin measured in a photoelectric colorimeter. A calculation was then done to ascertain the blood loss. It was concluded that where blood loss had been calculated as less than 500 ml the estimated and measured blood was reasonably accurate. Blood loss over 500 ml was progressively less well estimated. While an amazing effort, calculation of blood loss in this way is highly impractical in the clinical setting where 'best guess' estimations and clinical experience are more likely to be used to determine any immediate need for subsequent treatment of blood loss. It does, however, highlight the tendency to underestimate rather than overestimate blood loss, which may have a bearing on the subsequent well-being of the woman.

Examination of placenta and membranes

This should be performed as soon after delivery as practicable so that, if there is doubt about their completeness, further action may be taken before the woman leaves the birth room or the midwife prepares to leave the home. A thorough inspection must be carried out in order to make sure that no part of the placenta or membranes has been retained. The membranes are the most difficult to examine as they become torn during delivery and may be ragged. Every attempt should be made to piece them together to give an overall picture of completeness. This is easier to see if the placenta is held by the cord, allowing the membranes to hang. The hole through which the infant was delivered can then usually be identified and a hand can be spread out inside the membranes to aid inspection (Fig. 28.8). The placenta should then be laid on a flat surface and both placental surfaces minutely examined in a good light. The amnion should be peeled from the chorion right up to the umbilical cord, which allows the chorion to be fully viewed.

Any clots on the maternal surface need to be removed and kept for measuring. Broken fragments of cotyledon must be carefully replaced before an accurate assessment is possible.

Recent infarctions (areas on the placental surface that indicate deprivation of blood supply) are bright red, old infarctions form grey patches whereas localised calcification can be seen as flattened white plaques feeling gritty to the touch. (None of these is of great significance at this stage, but may provide retrospective evidence of an intrauterine problem.) The lobes of a complete placenta fit neatly together without any gaps, the edges forming a uniform circle. Blood vessels should not radiate beyond the placental edge. If they do this denotes a succenturiate lobe, which has developed separately from the main placenta (see Ch. 10). When such a lobe is visible there is no cause for concern, but if the tissue has been retained the vessels will end abruptly at a hole in the membrane. On the fetal surface the position of insertion of the cord is noted. This is most commonly central but may be lateral (for abnormal insertion, see Ch. 10). In some units the placental weight may be recorded. This will vary according to the time of clamping of the cord. Delayed clamping produces a placenta weighing approximately one-sixth of the infant's birthweight, whereas early clamping results in an additional volume of contained blood, which increases the weight to nearer one-fifth of the birthweight.

If there is any suspicion that the placenta or membranes are incomplete, they must be kept for inspection and a doctor informed immediately. Account

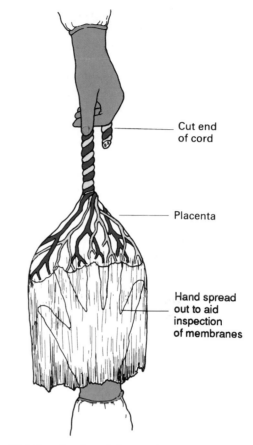

Fig. 28.8 Examination of the membranes.

— Cut end of cord

— Placenta

— Hand spread out to aid inspection of membranes

must be taken of blood that has soaked into linen and swabs as well as measurable fluid loss and clot formation.

Upon completion of the examination, the midwife should return her attention to the mother. The empty uterus should be firmly contracted. If the fundus has risen in the abdomen a blood clot may be present. This should be expelled while the uterus is in a state of contraction by pressing the fundus gently in a downward and backward direction – with due regard to the risk of inversion and acute discomfort to the woman. Force should *never* be used.

Immediate care

It is advisable for mother and infant to remain in the midwife's care for at least an hour after birth, regardless of the birth setting. Much of this time will be spent in clearing up and completion of records but careful observation of mother and infant is very important. If an epidural cannula is in situ it is usually removed and checked at this time.

Most women appreciate being able either to wash or to shower at this stage, which can do much to restore comfort and increase a sense of well-being. Simple comfort measures such as being able to clean the teeth, apply lip balm or cream will be appreciated to alleviate dry mouth and sore lips, especially if inhalational analgesia has been used during labour. The woman should be encouraged to pass urine because a full bladder may impede uterine contraction. She may not actually feel an urge to do so, especially if she has passed urine immediately prior to giving birth or an effective epidural has been in progress, but she should be asked to try. Uterine contraction and blood loss should be checked on several occasions during this first hour. Throughout this same period the midwife should pay regard to the baby's general well-being. She should check the security of the cord clamp and observe general skin colour, respirations and temperature. An infant can quickly chill in the comparative cool following birth, so needs to be thoroughly dried and then wrapped in a clean, dry towel so that body heat is retained. The warmest place for a baby to be placed is in a direct skin-to-skin contact position with the mother or wrapped and cuddled, whichever she prefers. At an early stage a full examination of the baby is made in the presence of the parents (see Ch. 39). Once basic procedures to ensure the woman's and baby's safety and comfort have been completed, there is no evidence to suggest that restriction of food or fluids is necessary, so a meal and fluids may be offered while the midwife completes her tasks and the woman and her support persons enjoy a little privacy with the new family member.

Most women intending to breastfeed will wish to put their babies to the breast during these early moments of contact. This is especially advantageous, as babies are usually very alert at this time and their sucking reflex is particularly strong. There is also evidence to suggest that women who breastfeed soon after delivery successfully breastfeed for a longer period of time (Salariya et al 1979). An additional benefit lies in the reflex release of oxytocin from the posterior lobe of the pituitary gland, which stimulates the uterus to contract. This may result in the mother experiencing a sudden fresh blood loss as the uterus empties and she should be prewarned and reassured that it is a normal response. The desire to feed a newborn baby is a warm, loving and instinctive response. While breastfeeding should be actively encouraged, a formula feed should be available for those who do not wish to breastfeed.

Records

A complete and accurate account of the labour, including the documentation of all drugs and observations, is the midwife's responsibility. This should also include details of examination of the placenta, membranes and cord with attention drawn to any abnormalities. The volume of blood loss is particularly important. This record not only provides information that may be critical in the future care of both mother and infant but is a legal document that may be used as evidence of the care given. Signatures are therefore essential, with co-signatories where necessary. Many mothers now carry their own notes related to pregnancy and details of the birth. The completed records are a vital communication link between the midwife responsible for delivery and other caregivers, particularly those who take over care and provide ongoing community support services once the woman returns home.

It is usually the midwife who completes the birth notification form (see Ch. 55). Timely notification and referral may prevent delay in a woman receiving appropriate assistance should she need it.

Transfer from the birth room

The midwife is responsible for seeing that all observations are made and recorded (as specified above) prior to transfer of mother and baby to the postnatal ward or before the midwife leaves the home following the birth.

The postnatal ward midwife should verify these details prior to transfer of mother and baby. Following a domiciliary birth, the midwife should leave details of a telephone number where she may be contacted should the parents feel any cause for concern.

Complications of the third stage of labour

Postpartum haemorrhage

Postpartum haemorrhage is defined as excessive bleeding from the genital tract at any time following the baby's birth up to 6 weeks after delivery. If it occurs during the third stage of labour or within 24 hours of delivery it is termed *primary postpartum haemorrhage*. If it occurs subsequent to the first 24 hours following birth up until the 6th week postpartum, it is termed *secondary postpartum haemorrhage*.

PPH is one of the most alarming and serious emergencies a midwife may face and is especially terrifying if it occurs immediately following a straightforward birth. It is always a frightening experience for the woman and can undermine her confidence, influence her attitude to future childbearing and delay her recovery. Although the maternal mortality rate (MMR) in developed countries such as the UK has fallen and was 12.2 per 100 000 live births (in the DoH et al 1998 report) the reported MMR for South Africa in 1998 was 150 per 100 000 live births (DoH 1999). A significant number of the deaths recorded were due to PPH. The midwife is often the first and may be the only professional person present when a haemorrhage occurs, so her prompt, competent action will be crucial in controlling blood loss and reducing the risk of maternal morbidity or even death.

Primary postpartum haemorrhage

As described earlier, fluid loss is extremely difficult to measure with any degree of accuracy, especially when the fluid has soaked into dressings and linen. It should also be remembered that measurable solidified clots represent only about half the total fluid loss. With these factors in mind, the best yardstick is that any blood loss, *however small*, that adversely affects the mother's condition constitutes a PPH. Much will therefore depend upon the woman's general well-being. In addition, if the measured loss reaches 500 ml, it must be treated as a PPH, irrespective of maternal condition.

There are several reasons why a PPH may occur, including atonic uterus, retained placenta, trauma and blood coagulation disorder.

Atonic uterus

This is a failure of the myometrium at the placental site to contract and retract and to compress torn blood vessels and control blood loss by a living ligature action (see above). When the placenta is attached, the volume of blood flow at the placental site is approximately 500–800 ml per minute. Upon separation, the efficient contraction and retraction of uterine muscle staunch the flow and prevent a haemorrhage, which would otherwise ensue with horrifying speed. Causes of atonic uterine action resulting in PPH are listed in Box 28.1.

Incomplete placental separation. If the placenta remains fully adherent to the uterine wall it is unlikely to cause bleeding. However, once separation has begun, maternal vessels are torn. If placental tissue remains partially embedded in the spongy decidua, efficient contraction and retraction are interrupted.

Retained cotyledon, placental fragment or membranes. These will similarly impede efficient uterine action.

Box 28.1 Causes of atonic uterine action

- Incomplete separation of the placenta
- Retained cotyledon, placental fragment or membranes
- Precipitate labour
- Prolonged labour resulting in uterine inertia
- Polyhydramnios or multiple pregnancy causing overdistension of uterine muscle
- Placenta praevia
- Placental abruption
- General anaesthesia especially halothane or cyclopropane
- Mismanagement of the third stage of labour
- A full bladder
- Aetiology unknown

Precipitate labour. When the uterus has contracted vigorously and frequently resulting in a duration of labour that is less than 1 hour, then the muscle may have insufficient opportunity to retract.

Prolonged labour. In a labour where the active phase lasts more than 12 hours uterine inertia (sluggishness) may result from muscle exhaustion.

Polyhydramnios or multiple pregnancy. The myometrium becomes excessively stretched and therefore less efficient.

Placenta praevia. The placental site is partly or wholly in the lower segment where the thinner muscle layer contains few oblique fibres: this results in poor control of bleeding.

Placental abruption. Blood may have seeped between the muscle fibres, interfering with effective action. At its most severe this results in a Couvelaire uterus (see Ch. 18).

General anaesthesia. Anaesthetic agents may cause uterine relaxation, in particular the volatile inhalational agents, for example halothane.

Mismanagement of the third stage of labour. It is salutary that this factor remains a frequent cause of PPH. 'Fundus fiddling' or manipulation of the uterus may precipitate arrhythmic contractions so that the placenta only partially separates and retraction is lost.

A full bladder. If the bladder is full, its proximity to the uterus in the abdomen on completion of the second stage may interfere with uterine action. This also constitutes mismanagement.

Aetiology unknown. A precipitating cause may never be discovered.

There are in addition a number of factors that do not directly *cause* a PPH, but do increase the likelihood of excessive bleeding (Box 28.2).

> **Box 28.2** Predisposing factors which might increase the risks of postpartum haemorrhage
>
> - Previous history of postpartum haemorrhage or retained placenta
> - High parity resulting in uterine scar tissue
> - Presence of fibroids
> - Maternal anaemia
> - Ketoacidosis

Previous history of PPH or retained placenta. There is a risk of recurrence in subsequent pregnancies. A detailed obstetric history taken at the first antenatal visit will ensure that arrangements are made for such a mother to give birth in a consultant unit.

High parity. With each successive pregnancy, fibrous tissue replaces muscle fibres in the uterus; this reduces its contractility and the blood vessels become more difficult to compress. Women who have had five or more deliveries are at increased risk.

Fibroids (fibromyomata). These are normally benign tumours consisting of muscle and fibrous tissue, which may impede efficient uterine action.

Anaemia. Women who enter labour with reduced haemoglobin concentration (below 10 g/dl) may succumb more quickly to any subsequent blood loss, however small. Anaemia is associated with debility, which is a more direct cause of uterine atony.

HIV/AIDS. Women who have HIV/AIDS are often in a state of severe immunosuppression; thus lowers the platelet count to such a degree that even a relatively minor blood loss may cause severe morbidity or death.

Ketosis. The influence of ketosis upon uterine action is still unclear. Foulkes & Dumoulin (1983) demonstrated that, in a series of 3500 women, 40% had ketonuria at some time during labour. They reported that if labour progressed well this did not appear to jeopardise either the fetal or maternal condition. However, there was a significant relationship between ketosis and the need for oxytocin augmentation, instrumental delivery and PPH when labour lasted more than 12 hours. Correction of ketosis is therefore advisable and can be facilitated by ensuring women have an adequate intake of fluids and light solid nourishment as tolerated throughout labour. There is no evidence to suggest restriction of food or fluids is necessary during the normal course of labour.

Signs of PPH

These may be obvious such as:

- visible bleeding
- maternal collapse.

However, more subtle signs may present, such as:

- pallor
- rising pulse rate

- falling blood pressure
- altered level of consciousness; the mother may become restless or drowsy
- an enlarged uterus as it fills with blood or blood clot; it feels 'boggy' on palpation (i.e. soft and distended and lacking tone); there may be little or no visible loss of blood.

Prophylaxis

By using the above list, it is possible for the midwife to apply some preventive screening in an attempt to identify women who may be at greater risk and to recognise causative factors. During the antenatal period a thorough and accurate history of previous obstetric experiences will identify risk factors such as previous PPH or precipitate labour. Arrangements can then, after careful explanation and in full consultation with the woman, be made for delivery to take place in a unit where facilities for dealing with emergencies are available. The early detection and treatment of anaemia will help ensure that women enter labour with a haemoglobin level, ideally, in excess of 10 g/dl. The midwife should check that blood tests, if needed, are taken regularly and the results recorded and explained to the woman. If necessary, action can be taken to restore the haemoglobin level before delivery. Women more prone to anaemia should be closely monitored, for example those with multiple pregnancies.

During labour, good management practices during the first and second stages are important to prevent prolonged labour and ketoacidosis. A mother should not enter the second or third stage with a full bladder. Prophylactic administration of a uterotonic agent is recommended for the third stage, by either intramuscular injection or intravenous infusion. Two units of cross-matched blood should be kept available for any woman known to have a placenta praevia.

Treatment of PPH

Whatever the stage of labour or crisis that may occur, the midwife should adhere to the underlying principle of always reassuring the woman and her support persons by continually relaying appropriate information and involving them in decision making.

Three basic principles of care should be applied immediately upon observation of excessive bleeding:

- call for medical aid
- stop the bleeding
  - rub up a contraction
  - give a uterotonic
  - empty the uterus
- resuscitate the mother.

Call for medical aid. This is an important initial step so that help is on the way whatever transpires. If the bleeding is brought under control before the doctor arrives then no action by the doctor will be needed. However, the woman's condition can deteriorate very rapidly, in which case medical assistance will be required urgently. If the mother is at home or in a midwife-led unit, the emergency department of the closest obstetric unit should be contacted and, depending on the policy of the region, an obstetric emergency team summoned or ambulance transfer arranged.

Stop the bleeding. The initial action is always the same, regardless of whether bleeding occurs with the placenta in situ or later.

Rub up a contraction. The fundus is first felt gently with the fingertips to assess its consistency. If it is soft and relaxed, the fundus is massaged with a smooth, circular motion, applying no undue pressure. When a contraction occurs, the hand is held still.

Give a uterotonic to sustain the contraction. In many instances, oxytocin 5 units or 10 units, or combined ergometrine/oxytocin 1 ml, has already been administered and this may be repeated. Alternatively, ergometrine 0.25–0.5 mg may be injected intravenously, which will be effective within 45 seconds. No more than two doses of ergometrine should be given (including any dose of combined ergometrine/oxytocin) as it may cause pulmonary hypertension. Several reports have described the dramatic haemostatic effects of prostaglandins used in cases of uterine atony. A systematic review is currently being undertaken to determine the most effective strategies for treatment of PPH (Mousa & Alfirevic 2002) but, as stated by Thiery in 1986, there is currently no published evidence generated from controlled trials. Nevertheless, its obvious benefits make it worthy of note for use in this dire emergency. The baby may be put to the breast to enhance the physiological secretion of oxytocin from the posterior lobe of the pituitary gland.

Empty the uterus. Once the midwife is satisfied that it is well contracted, she should ensure that the uterus is emptied. If the placenta is still in the uterus, it should be delivered; if it has been expelled, any clots should be expressed by firm but gentle pressure on the fundus.

Resuscitate the mother. An intravenous infusion should be commenced while peripheral veins are easily negotiated. This will provide a route for an oxytocin infusion or fluid replacement. As an emergency measure, the mother's legs may be lifted up in order to allow blood to drain from them into the central circulation. However, the foot of the bed should *not* be raised as this encourages pooling of blood in the uterus, which prevents the uterus contracting.

It is usually expedient to catheterise the bladder in order to minimise trauma should an operative procedure be necessary and to exclude a full bladder as a precipitating cause of further bleeding.

On no account must a woman in a collapsed condition be moved prior to resuscitation and stabilisation.

The flow chart (Fig. 28.9) briefly sets out the possible courses of action that may be taken depending upon whether or not bleeding persists. If the above measures are successful in controlling any further loss, administration of oxytocin, 40 units in 1 litre of intravenous solution (e.g. Hartmann's or saline) infused slowly over 8–12 hours, will ensure continued uterine contraction. This will help to minimise the risk of recurrence. Before the infusion is connected, 10 ml of blood should be withdrawn for haemoglobin estimation and for cross-matching compatible blood. If bleeding continues uncontrolled, the choice of further action will depend largely upon whether the placenta remains undelivered.

Placenta delivered. If the uterus is atonic following delivery of the placenta, light fundal pressure may be used to expel residual clots whilst a contraction is stimulated. If an effective contraction is not maintained, 40 units of Syntocinon in 1 litre of intravenous fluid should be commenced. The placenta and membranes must be re-examined for completeness because retained fragments are often responsible for uterine atony.

Bimanual compression. If bleeding continues, bimanual compression of the uterus may be necessary in order to apply pressure to the placental site. It is desirable for an intravenous infusion to be in progress. The fingers of one hand are inserted into the vagina like a cone; the hand is formed into a fist and placed into the anterior vaginal fornix, the elbow resting on the bed. The other hand is placed behind the uterus abdominally, the fingers pointing towards the cervix. The uterus is brought forwards and compressed between the palm of the hand positioned abdominally and the fist in the vagina (Fig. 28.10). If bleeding persists, a clotting disorder must be excluded before exploration of the vagina and uterus is performed under a general anaesthetic (see also Ch. 54 for aortic compression).

Placenta undelivered. The placenta may be partially or wholly adherent.

Partially adherent. When the uterus is well contracted an attempt should be made to deliver the placenta by applying CCT. If this is unsuccessful a doctor will be required to remove it manually.

Completely adherent. Bleeding does not usually occur if the placenta is completely adherent. However, the longer the placenta remains in situ the greater is the risk of partial separation, which may give rise to profuse haemorrhage.

Retained placenta

This diagnosis is reached when the placenta remains undelivered after a specified period of time (usually ½ to 1 hour following the baby's birth). The conventional treatment is to separate the placenta from the uterine wall digitally, effecting a manual removal. Selinger et al (1986) noted that waiting for 1 hour before resorting to this intervention will almost halve the number of women who will require manual removal with its accompanying risks.

Breaking of the cord. This is not an unusual occurrence during completion of the third stage of labour. Before further action, it is crucial to check that the uterus remains firmly contracted. If the placenta remains adherent, no further action should be taken before a doctor is notified. It is possible that manual removal may be indicated. If the placenta is palpable in the vagina, it is probable that separation has occurred and when the uterus is well contracted then maternal effort may be encouraged (see Expectant management). If there is any doubt, the midwife applies fresh sterile gloves before performing a vaginal examination to ascertain whether this is so. As a last resort, if the woman is unable to push effectively then fundal pressure may be used. A uterotonic must be

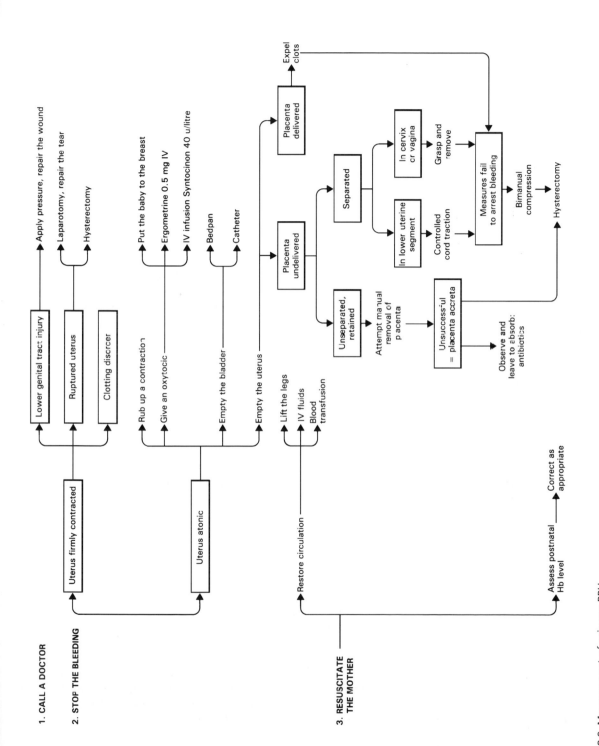

Fig. 28.9 Management of primary PPH.

given prior to this. Great care is exercised to ensure that placental separation has already occurred and the uterus is well contracted. The woman should be relaxed as the midwife exerts downward and backward pressure on the firmly contracted fundus. This method can cause considerable pain and distress to the woman and result in the stretching and bruising of supportive uterine ligaments. If it is performed without good uterine contraction, acute inversion may ensue. This is an extremely dangerous procedure in unskilled hands and is not advocated in everyday practice when alternative, safer methods may be employed.

Manual removal of the placenta. This should be carried out by a doctor. An intravenous infusion must first be sited and an effective anaesthetic in progress. The choice of anaesthesia will depend upon the woman's general condition. If an effective epidural anaesthetic is already in progress, a top-up may be given in order to avoid the hazards of general anaesthesia. A spinal anaesthetic offers an alternative but where time is an urgent factor a general anaesthetic will be initiated. Details of obstetric anaesthesia are given in Chapters 26 and 31.

Management. Manual removal is performed with full aseptic precautions and, unless in a dire emergency situation, should not be undertaken prior to adequate analgesia being ensured for the woman. With the left hand, the umbilical cord is held taut while the right hand is coned and inserted into the vagina and uterus following the direction of the cord. Once the placenta is located the cord is released so that the left hand may be used to support the fundus abdominally, to prevent rupture of the lower uterine segment (Fig. 28.11). The operator will feel for a separated edge of the placenta. The fingers of the right hand are extended and the border of the hand is gently eased between the placenta and the uterine wall, with the palm facing the placenta. The placenta is carefully detached with a sideways slicing movement. When it is completely separated, the left hand rubs up a contraction and expels the right hand with the placenta in its grasp. The placenta should be checked immediately for completeness so that any further exploration of the uterus may be carried out without delay. An uterotonic drug is given upon completion.

In very exceptional circumstances when no doctor is available to be called, a midwife would be expected to carry out a manual removal of placenta. Once she has diagnosed a retained placenta as the cause of PPH the midwife must act swiftly to reduce the risk of onset of

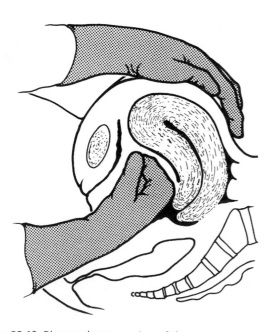

Fig. 28.10 Bimanual compression of the uterus.

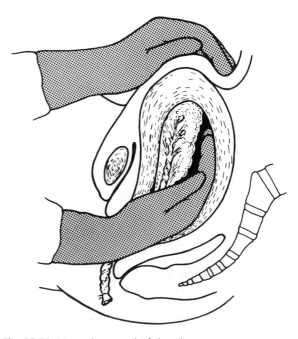

Fig. 28.11 Manual removal of the placenta.

shock and exsanguination. It must be remembered that the risk of inducing shock by performing a manual removal of placenta is greater when no anaesthetic is given. In a developed country the midwife is unlikely to find herself dealing with this situation.

At home. If the placenta is retained following a home confinement, emergency obstetric help must be summoned. Under no circumstances should a woman be transferred to hospital until an intravenous infusion is in progress and her condition stabilised.

It is best if the placenta can be delivered without moving the mother but if this is not possible, or if further treatment is needed, she should be transferred to a consultant unit. The baby should accompany her.

Morbid adherence of placenta. Very rarely, the placenta remains morbidly adherent; this is known as *placenta accreta*. If it is totally adherent, then bleeding is unlikely to occur and it may be left in situ to absorb during the puerperium. If, however, only part of the placenta remains embedded then the risks of fatal haemorrhage are high and an emergency hysterectomy may be unavoidable.

Trauma as a cause of haemorrhage

If bleeding occurs despite a well-contracted uterus, it is almost certainly the consequence of trauma to the uterus, vagina, perineum or labia, or a combination of these. Poeschmann et al (1991) cautioned that episiotomy may contribute up to 30% of total blood loss; in their study the severity of blood loss was linked to the length of time that elapsed between incision of the perineum and the commencement of repair. Predictably, the longer the wait the greater is the blood loss.

In order to identify the source of bleeding, the mother is placed in the lithotomy position under a good directional light. An episiotomy wound or tears to the anterior labia, clitoris and perineum often bleed freely. These external injuries are easily identified and torn vessels may be clamped with artery forceps prior to ligation. Internal trauma to the vagina, cervix or uterus more commonly occurs following instrumental or manipulative delivery. A speculum is inserted to enable the cervix and vagina to be clearly visualised and examined. Tissue or artery forceps may be used to apply pressure prior to suturing under general anaesthesia.

If bleeding persists when the uterus is well contracted and no evidence of trauma can be found, uterine rupture must be suspected. Following a laparotomy this is repaired, but if bleeding remains uncontrolled a hysterectomy may become inevitable.

Blood coagulation disorders

As well as the causes already listed above, PPH may be the result of coagulation failure, which is fully discussed in Chapter 18. The failure of the blood to clot is such an obvious sign that it can be overlooked in the midst of the frantic activity that accompanies torrential bleeding. It can occur following severe pre-eclampsia, antepartum haemorrhage, amniotic fluid embolus, intrauterine death or sepsis. Fresh blood is usually the best treatment as this will contain platelets and the coagulation factors V and VIII. The expert advice of a haematologist will be needed in assessing specific replacement products such as fresh frozen plasma and fibrinogen.

Maternal observation following PPH

Once bleeding is controlled the total volume lost must be estimated as accurately as possible. Large amounts appear less than they are in reality. Maternal pulse and blood pressure are recorded every quarter hour and temperature taken every 4 hours. The uterus should be palpated frequently to ensure that it remains well contracted and lochia lost must be observed. Intravenous fluid replacement should be carefully calculated to avoid circulatory overload. Monitoring the central venous pressure (see Ch. 32) will provide an accurate assessment of the volume required, especially if blood loss has been severe. Fluid intake and urinary output are recorded as indicators of renal function. The output should be accurately measured on an hourly basis by the use of a self-retaining urinary catheter.

The woman will usually remain in the labour ward until her condition is stable. This allows her progress to be closely monitored. All records should be meticulously completed and signed as soon as possible. Continued vigilance will be important for 24–48 hours. As this woman will need a quiet period for recuperation, a single room may be offered and visiting may be restricted to close family members. She will not be suitable for early transfer home.

Secondary postpartum haemorrhage

Secondary PPH is bleeding from the genital tract more than 24 hours after delivery of the placenta; it may occur up to 6 weeks later. However, it is most likely to occur between 10 and 14 days after delivery. Bleeding is usually due to retention of a fragment of the placenta or membranes, or the presence of a large uterine blood clot. Lochial loss is heavier than normal and will consist of a bright red loss that, typically, has recurred during the second week. The lochia may also be offensive if infection is a contributory factor. Subinvolution, pyrexia and tachycardia are usually present. As this is an event that is most likely to occur at home, women should be alerted to the possible signs of secondary PPH prior to discharge from midwifery care.

Management

The following steps should be taken:

- call a doctor
- reassure the woman and her support person(s)
- rub up a contraction by massaging the uterus if it is still palpable
- express any clots
- encourage the mother to empty her bladder
- give an uterotonic drug such as ergometrine maleate by the intravenous or intramuscular route
- keep all pads and linen to assess the volume of blood lost
- if bleeding persists, discuss a range of treatment options with the woman and, if appropriate, prepare the woman for theatre.

If the bleeding occurs at home and the woman has telephoned the midwife, she should be told to lie down flat until the midwife arrives (the front door should be left unlocked if the woman is alone). On arrival, the midwife will assess the amount of blood loss and the woman's condition and attempt to arrest the haemorrhage. If the loss is severe or uncontrolled, she will call the nearest emergency obstetric unit and prepare the mother and baby for transfer to hospital. The doctor, midwife or paramedic who attends will commence an intravenous infusion and ensure that the mother's condition is stable first.

Careful assessment is usually undertaken prior to the uterus being explored under general anaesthetic. The use of ultrasound as a diagnostic tool is invaluable

> **Box 28.3** Key issues in the management of the third stage of labour
>
> - Difficulty of implementing well-documented evidence into practice
>   — prophylactic administration of uteronics have been shown to be of significant benefit in management of the third stage
>   — less clarity of evidence available when talking about choice of uterotonic
>   — how can we accommodate the wishes of women with the responsibilities of the midwife?
> - Possible research
>   — uterotonics alone versus active management
>   — possibilities for use of misoprostol in developing country settings

in minimising the number of mothers who have operative intervention. If retained products of conception cannot be seen on a scan, the mother may be treated conservatively with antibiotic therapy and oral ergometrine. The haemoglobin should be estimated prior to discharge. If it is below 9 g/dl, options for iron replacement should be discussed with the woman. The severity of the anaemia will assist in determining the most appropriate care, which may be dependent on whether the woman is symptomatic (e.g. feeling faint, dizzy, short of breath). Management may vary from increased intake of iron-rich foods, iron supplements or, in extreme cases, blood transfusion. It is also important to discuss the common symptoms that may be experienced as a result of anaemia following PPH, including extreme tiredness and general malaise. Encourage the woman to seek assistance and stress the importance of making an appointment to see her GP to have her general health and haemoglobin levels checked.

Haematoma formation

PPH may also be concealed as the result of progressive haematoma formation. This may be obvious at such sites as the perineum or lower vagina, but it is more difficult to diagnose if it occurs into the broad ligament or vault of the vagina. A large volume of blood may collect insidiously (up to 1 litre). Involution and lochia are usually normal, the main symptom being increasingly severe maternal pain. This is often so acute that the haematoma has to be drained in theatre under a general anaesthetic. Secondary infection is a strong possibility.

Care after a postpartum haemorrhage

Whatever the cause of the haemorrhage, the woman will need the continued support of her midwife until she regains her confidence. Her partner may also be fearful of a recurrence and need much reassurance. If the mother is breastfeeding, lactation may be impaired but this will only be temporary and she should be encouraged to persevere. The midwife is often the first and may be the only professional person present when a haemorrhage occurs, so her prompt, competent action will be crucial in controlling blood loss and reducing the risk of maternal morbidity or even mortality.

Key issues in the management of the third stage of labour are listed in Box 28.3.

REFERENCES

Begley C M 1990 A comparison of 'active' and 'physiological' management of the third stage of labour. Midwifery 6:3–17

Bonnar J, McNicol G P, Douglas A S 1970 Coagulation and fibrinolytic mechanisms during and after normal childbirth. British Medical Journal 25(April):200–203

Brandt II A 1966 Blood loss at caesarean section. Journal of Obstetrics and Gynaecology of the British Commonwealth 73:456–459

Brandt H A 1967 Precise estimation of postpartum haemorrhage: difficulties and importance. British Medical Journal 1:398–400

Choy C M Y, Lau W C, Tam W H, Yuen P M 2002 A randomised controlled trial of intramuscular syntometrine and intravenous oxytocin in the management of the third stage of labour. British Journal of Obstetrics and Gynaecology 109:173–177

Chua S, Shaw S I, Yeoh C L et al 1995 A randomised controlled study of prostaglandin 15 methyl F2 alpha compared with Syntometrine for prophylactic use in the third stage of labour. Journal of Australian and New Zealand Obstetrics and Gynaecology 35(4):413

DoH et al (Department of Health, Welsh Office, Scottish Office Department of Health, Department of Health and Social Services Northern Ireland) 1998 Why mothers die. Report on Confidential Enquiries into Maternal Deaths in the United Kingdom 1994–1996. Stationery Office, London

DoH (Department of Health) 1999 Saving mothers: report on confidential enquiries into maternal deaths in South Africa 1998. Formset Printers Cape (Pty), Pretoria, South Africa

Dombrowski M P, Bottoms S F, Saleb A A A, Hurd W W, Romero R 1995 Third stage of labour: analysis of duration and clinical practice. American Journal of Obstetrics and Gynecology 172:1279–1284

Dunn P M 1985 Management of childbirth in normal women: the third stage and fetal adaptation. In: Perinatal medicine. Proceedings of the IX European Congress on Perinatal Medicine, Dublin, September 1984. MTP Press, Lancaster, ch 7, p 47–54

Dunn P M 1966 The placental venous pressure during and after the third stage of labour following early cord ligation. Journal of Obstetrics and Gynaecology of the British Commonwealth 73:747–756

Duthie S J, Ven D, Yung G L K, Dong Z G, Chan S Y W, Ma H-K 1990 Discrepancy between laboratory determination and visual estimation of blood loss during normal delivery. European Journal of Obstetrics, Gynaecology and Reproductive Biology 38:119–124

El-Refaey H, O'Brien P, Morafa W, Walder J, Rodeck C 1997 Use of oral misoprostol in the prevention of postpartum haemorrhage. British Journal of Obstetrics and Gynaecology 104:336–339

Foulkes J, Dumoulin J G 1983 Ketosis in labour. British Journal of Hospital Medicine 29(6)(June):562–564

Gülmezoglu A M, Villar J, Ngoc T N et al 2001 WHO multicentre randomised trial of misoprostol in the management of the third stage of labour. Lancet 358:689–695

Gülmezoglu A M, Forna F, Villar J, Hofmeyr G J 2002 Prostaglandins for prevention of postpartum haemorrhage (Cochrane review). In: The Cochrane Library, Issue 1. Update Software, Oxford

Gupta J K, Nikodem V C 2002 Position for women during second stage of labour (Cochrane review). In: The Cochrane Library, Issue 1. Update Software, Oxford

Inch S 1985 Management of the third stage of labour – another cascade of intervention. Midwifery 1:114–122

Khan Q K, John I S, Chan T, Wani S, Hughes A O, Stirrat G M 1995 Abu Dhabi third stage trial: oxytocin versus Syntometrine in the active management of the third stage of labour. European Journal of Obstetrics, Gynaecology and Reproductive Biology 58:147–151

Khan G Q, John I S, Wani S, Doherty T, Sibai B M 1997 Abstract 56: 'Controlled cord traction' versus 'minimal intervention' techniques in the delivery of the placenta: a randomised controlled trial. American Journal of Obstetrics and Gynecology 177(4):770–774

Ladipo O A 1972 Management of third stage of labour, with particular reference to reduction of feto-maternal transfusion. British Medical Journal 1:721–723

Levy V, Moore J 1985 The midwife's management of the third stage of labour. Nursing Times 81(5):47–50

Lewis G, Drife J (eds) 2001 Why mothers die 1997–1999. The Confidential Enquiries into Maternal Deaths in the United Kingdom. RCOG Press, London, p 21

Linderkamp O 1982 Placental transfusion: determinants and effects. Clinical Perinatology 9:589–593

McDonald S, Prendiville W J, Elbourne D 2002 Prophylactic syntometrine versus oxytocin for delivery of the placenta (Cochrane review). In: The Cochrane Library, Issue 1. Update Software, Oxford

McDonald S J 1996 Timing of interventions in the third stage of labour. In: McDonald S J. Management in the third stage of labour (Doctoral thesis). Faculty of Medicine, Department of Obstetrics and Gynaecology, University of Western Australia, ch 6, p 60–81

McDonald S J, Prendiville W J, Blair E 1993 Randomised controlled trial of oxytocin alone versus oxytocin and ergometrine in active management of the third stage of labour. British Medical Journal 307:1167–1171

Montgomery T L 1960 The umbilical cord. Clinical Obstetrics and Gynaecology 3:900–910

Moore J, Levy V 1983 Further research into the management of the 3rd stage of labour and the incidence of postpartum haemorrhage. In: Thompson A, Robinson S (eds) Proceedings of the Research and the Midwife Conference, Department of Nursing, University of Manchester, UK

Mousa H A, Alfirevic Z 2002 Treatment for primary postpartum haemorrhage (protocol for a Cochrane Review). In: The Cochrane Library, Issue 1. Update Software, Oxford

Newton M, Mosey L M, Egli G E, Gifford W B, Hull C T 1961 Blood loss during and immediately after delivery. Obstetrics and Gynaecology 17:9–18

Pau-Chen W, Tsu-Shan K 1960 Early clamping of the umbilical cord: a study of its effect on the infant. Chinese Medical Journal 80:351–355

Peyser R M, Kupfermine M J 1990 Management of postpartum haemorrhage by uterine irrigation with prostaglandin. American Journal of Obstetrics and Gynecology 162(3):694–696

Poeschmann R P, Docsburg W H, Eskis T K A B A 1991 Randomised comparison of oxytocin, sulprostone and placebo in the management of the third stage of labour. British Journal of Obstetrics and Gynaecology 98:528–530

Prendiville W, Elbourne D 1989 Care during the third stage of labour. In: Chalmers I, Enkin M, Keirse M J N C (eds) Effective care in pregnancy and childbirth. Oxford University Press, Oxford, p 1145–1169

Prendiville W, Elbourne D, Chalmers I 1988a The effects of routine uterotonic administration in the management of the third stage of labour: an overview of the evidence from controlled trials. British Journal of Obstetrics and Gynaecology 95:3–16

Prendiville W J, Elbourne D R, Chalmers I 1988b The Bristol third stage trial: active versus physiological management of the third stage of labour. British Medical Journal 297:1295–1300

Prendiville W J, Elbourne D, McDonald S 2002 Active versus expectant management of the third stage of labour (Cochrane review). In: The Cochrane Library, Issue 1. Update Software, Oxford

Rabe H, Reynolds G 2002 Delayed cord clamping in preterm infants (protocol for a Cochrane Review). In: The Cochrane Library, Issue 1. Update Software, Oxford

Rogers J, Wood J, McCandlish R, Ayers S, Truesdale A, Elbourne D 1998 Active versus expectant management of third stage of labour: the Hinchingbrooke randomised controlled trial. Lancet 351:693–699

Salariya E, Easton P, Cater J 1979 Early and often for best results. Nursing Mirror 148:15–17

Selinger M, MacKenzie K, Dunlop P, James D 1986 Intraumbilical vein oxytocin in the management of retained placenta. A double blind controlled study. Journal of Obstetrics and Gynaecology 7:115–117

Thiery M 1986 Prostaglandins for the treatment of hypotonic postpartum haemorrhage. Prostaglandin Perspectives 2:10

Thilaganathan B, Cutner A, Latimer J, Beard R 1993 Management of the third stage of labour in women at low risk of postpartum haemorrhage. European Journal of Obstetrics and Gynecology and Reproductive Biology 48:19–22

van Selm M, Kanhai H H H, Keiser M I N C 1995 Preventing the recurrence of atonic postpartum haemorrhage: a double-blind trial. Acta Obstetrica et Gynecologia Scandinavica 74:270–274

Whitfield M F, Salfield S A W 1980 Accidental administration of Syntometrine in adult dosage to the newborn. Archives of Disease in Childhood 55:68–70

Yao A C, Lind J 1974 Placental transfusion. American Journal of Diseases of Children 127:128–141

29 Prolonged Pregnancy and Disorders of Uterine Action

Christine Shiers

CHAPTER CONTENTS

This chapter considers the issues of a pregnancy that continues beyond term, induction of labour and some of the complications that may arise in labour, including abnormal uterine action and obstructed labour.

The chapter aims to:

- discuss the diagnosis and management of a post term pregnancy taking account of current research and practice

- review the indications for induction of labour and the various methods used

- describe how uterine dysfunction may result in a prolonged labour or one that is precipitate

- consider the serious complication of obstructed labour, which may result in the death of mother and baby, or contribute to long term morbidity of both

- highlight the importance of the role of the midwife in the care and management of such situations

- emphasise the involvement of the mother and her partner in the care provided.

Post-term or prolonged pregnancy

Post-term pregnancy is defined as one that exceeds 294 days, from the first day of the last menstrual period (FIGO 1982). Prolonged pregnancy and post-term pregnancy are used synonymously and relate to the duration of the pregnancy, not a maternal condition. *Postmaturity* or postmature are terms that relate to the neonate; they refer to features or condition of the baby and should not be used in relation to the duration of pregnancy.

Incidence

The average incidence of post-term pregnancy is 10% (Bakketeig & Bergsjo 1989) but falls to 1.1% where accurate dating of the pregnancy takes place (Boyd et al 1988). Evidence suggests that the duration of pregnancy varies with parity and race. Primigravid women have a longer mean duration of pregnancy, averaging 288 days. Multigravidae average 283 days, the recurrence risk of post-term birth increasing with parity (Bakketeig & Bergsjo 1989). In multiracial groups in the USA, gestation amongst Afro-Caribbean mothers was measured as being 8.5 days shorter than in similar Caucasian women (Mittendorf et al 1990).

Dating

Statistics quoting the incidence of post-term pregnancy have been influenced by the inaccuracies of dating. Pregnancy cannot be said to be prolonged without accurate dating. Term delivery is one that occurs over a range of 5 weeks from 37 to 42 weeks' gestation. Calculation of the expected date of delivery has been based on Naegele's rule for over a century, giving mothers a single day on which they might be expected to give birth. The accuracy of this is based on gestation being of a standard duration, but does not take account of the variations in length of calendar months. Accuracy also depends on the certainty of the woman's memory of her dates and the length of the menstrual cycle. Additional days need to be added if the cycle exceeds 28 days, and subtracted if it is less than 28. Furthermore, the cycle may be influenced by recent use of the oral contraceptive. A significant number of women are uncertain of, or are unable to recall, the date of their last menstrual period (Hall & Carr Hill 1985).

Estimation of gestational age by clinical assessment can also be flawed. Abdominal examination for fundal height measurements cannot accurately assess gestational age because of the biological variations in size of mother and fetus.

Quickening, or the recognition by the mother of fetal movements, may be felt over a range of weeks, in primigravidae from 18 to 22 weeks and in multigravidae from 16 to 22 weeks, and can help to corroborate the gestation.

An ultrasound scan in early pregnancy can be used to assess duration of pregnancy and fetal age, reducing the numbers of women who are categorised mistakenly as having a prolonged pregnancy. Measurements taken in the first or second trimesters have been found to be accurate to within 5 days, allowing dates to be adjusted (Chua & Arulkumaran 1999). The perinatal mortality associated with prolonged pregnancy has been reduced by allowing pregnancy to be monitored and induction after 41 weeks planned using an accurate dating scan (Crowley 2002).

Risks and clinical implications of post-term pregnancy

Perinatal mortality is lowest at 40 weeks, and increases after 42 weeks, but that risk reduces with the use of modern methods of fetal monitoring. Where the perinatal mortality and morbidity in post-term pregnancy are increased, this may be a result of labour or birth rather than antenatal events (Crowley 1989).

Post-term pregnancy may be associated with the condition defined as postmaturity, but not in all cases. This condition is marked by characteristics including minimal subcutaneous fat, absence of lanugo and vernix and meconium staining. Macrosomia (birth weight of 4000 g or more) also occurs in 10% of prolonged pregnancies, with 1% of newborns weighing 4500 g or more. This influences the outcome of pregnancy, by contributing to cephalopelvic disproportion or shoulder dystocia.

Fetal distress, demonstrated in intrapartum monitoring as decelerations, and meconium aspiration syndrome are likely to complicate the outcome of a post-term pregnancy. Identification of oligohydramnios can reduce risk to the fetus (Divon et al 1995). The production of amniotic fluid reduces at term and, as one of the primary functions of the liquor is to form a protective cushion for the fetus and the umbilical cord, a reduction in fluid volume can result in both cord compression and reduced placental perfusion. The ensuing fetal hypoxia may lead to passage of meconium.

Role of the placenta

Placental ageing was thought to be responsible for fetal and intrapartum complications on the supposition that the demands of the fetus for oxygen and nutrients outstripped the supply and the placenta had come to the end of its functional life. However, the morphological changes attributed to ageing may be a maturation process increasing rather than decreasing the efficiency of the villi. The placenta continues to grow up to and beyond term (Fox 1991). Post-term pregnancy may be complicated by placental insufficiency but the basis of this will have existed from an early stage in pregnancy, rather than have developed as a consequence of prolongation of pregnancy.

Management of post-term pregnancy

The management of post-term pregnancy has taken account of the increased risk to the fetus as pregnancy lengthens. Two forms of care are offered: expectant management with fetal surveillance or elective induction of labour before 42 weeks of gestation. Both aim to diminish the jeopardy to the fetus.

Antenatal surveillance

Biophysical profile. Assessment by a combined ultrasound assessment of fetal breathing, fetal movement, fetal tone, reactivity of the heart rate and amniotic fluid volume is used to predict fetal well-being in a high risk pregnancy. A score of 0–2 is given to each of these variables, a total score of 8–10 indicates the fetus is in good condition. Umbilical artery Doppler velocimetry and fetal growth add additional information (Harman et al 1999). The biophysical profile needs further research as to its effectiveness (Alfirevic & Neilson 2001).

Doppler ultrasound of umbilical artery. This is used to assess fetal and uteroplacental blood flow in pregnancies associated with high risk. Study of the umbilical flow velocity wave forms yields information about vascular resistance within the placenta and perfusion within the fetoplacental circulation. Doppler ultrasound appears to improve fetal outcome in high risk cases (Neilson & Alfirevic 2002).

Cardiotocography (CTG). This is also known as non-stress testing (NST). The fetal heart is monitored and the trace is assessed for the presence of reactivity and whether the baseline rate is within the normal range. The value of CTG in predicting possible compromise is increased if carried out at least twice weekly, and in conjunction with measurement of amniotic fluid volume.

Amniotic fluid measurement. Variation in parameters for defining diminished liquor influence the interpretation and thus the decision to induce labour.

Measurements are taken in several perpendicular planes, to make the diagnosis of oligohydramnios (Harman et al 1999, James 1991).

Elective induction

The active approach to post-term pregnancy, or one approaching the upper limits of term, is for the mother to have labour induced. A statistically significant reduction in perinatal mortality for the normal fetus has been demonstrated where gestation is in excess of 290 days, when this approach is adopted (Crowley 2002).

Hannah et al (1996) published the results of a large multicentre trial comparing induction with antenatal surveillance in post-term pregnancy. Surveillance included twice-weekly CTG and amniotic fluid volume measurements. Those women who were induced were less likely to have a caesarean section than those who were randomised to surveillance. There were no major differences in perinatal mortality or neonatal morbidity between the groups.

It is recognised that the administration of endocervical prostaglandins reduces the incidence of caesarean section. Women in the group for induction were thus managed, whereas women in the surveillance group requiring induction did not have prostaglandin. This may have contributed to the elevated rate of caesarean section in the second group.

Mother's choice

Women should be given information about the options available to them in a manner that allows them to have an informed choice. It is also important that they are aware that management may alter depending on the clinical assessment. Mothers need to know that where there is an alteration in clinical signs such as a reduction in fetal movements or onset of abdominal pain their management may be reviewed. They should be actively involved in the decisions made for their care.

A summary of key points relating to post-term pregnancy is given in Box 29.1.

Induction of labour

Induction of labour is the stimulation of uterine contractions prior to the onset of spontaneous labour. It is an obstetric intervention that should be used when elective birth will be beneficial to mother and baby.

The purpose of induction is to effect the birth of the baby, thereby ending the pregnancy. Successful induction depends on adequate contractions that are effective in bringing about progressive dilatation of the cervix. The procedure is more likely to be successful when the cervix is said to be ripe – that is, it has undergone structural changes to produce softening, dilatation and effacement. The definition of induction of labour includes the stimulation of contractions in the presence of ruptured membranes without labour (NICE 2001, RCOG 2001a).

Parents should be partners in the decision-making process, giving their consent based on full information about the alternatives.

Indications for induction

Induction is indicated when the benefits to the mother or the fetus outweigh those of continuing the pregnancy and it is associated with the following maternal and fetal factors.

Maternal indications

Prolonged or post-term pregnancy. This is the main indication for induction of labour.

Hypertension, including pre-eclampsia. Timing of induction depends on the severity of symptoms, and the possible consequences on maternal and fetal mortality and morbidity (see Ch. 20).

Diabetes. Diabetic women carry an increased risk of pregnancy loss, with a perinatal mortality rate of four or five times greater than the overall population.

Medical problems. Women with concurrent renal, respiratory or cardiac disease may require induction of labour (see Ch. 19).

Placental abruption. Induction may be considered in cases of severe or moderate abruption after the condition of the mother has been stabilised. Caesarean section is more common (see Ch. 18).

Obstetric history, such as previous stillbirth.

Unstable lie. If placenta praevia and pelvic abnormalities have been excluded, induction may be offered. The lie is corrected to longitudinal but as there remains a possibility of cord prolapse, caesarean section may be preferred.

Prelabour rupture of membranes. When rupture occurs at term, spontaneous labour can be anticipated for 86% of mothers within 24 hours and for 90% labour will commence within 72 hours (RCOG 2001a). Delay increases the morbidity to mother and fetus from infection developing (Tan & Hannah 2002). Women should be offered the choice of expectant or active management (NICE 2001). Those known to be group B haemolytic streptococcus positive should be offered immediate oxytocin induction (Hannah et al 1996).

Maternal request. Women may request induction citing social or psychological reasons. Full discussion should take place between the mother, midwife and obstetrician before a decision is made and this should be considered where resources would allow induction; it should be established that the woman's cervix is favourable (NICE 2001).

Fetal indications

Suspected fetal compromise. Evidence of intrauterine growth retardation, diminished fetal movements or abnormal umbilical artery blood flow detected with Doppler ultrasound may provide indication for induction of labour. Where compromise is due to Rhesus isoimmunisation, induction may be indicated so that treatment to arrest haemolysis and rectify its effects can be commenced. In cases of fetal compromise the maturity of the fetus needs to be considered, with any additional risks associated with preterm birth and vaginal delivery reviewed in conjunction with the risk of continuing the pregnancy.

Intrauterine death. Guidance from the Stillbirth and Neonatal Death Society (Kohner, 1995) reminds professionals that parents may not want to be induced swiftly after diagnosis is made. There is, however, a risk of coagulation defects occurring if the pregnancy continues for a long period after fetal death.

Contraindications to induction

These include:

- placenta praevia
- transverse or compound fetal presentation
- cord presentation or cord prolapse
- cephalopelvic disproportion
- severe fetal compromise
- active genital herpes.

If, in these circumstances, delivery is imperative, it should be effected by caesarean section.

Cervical ripening

The cervix is normally 2 centimetres long, firm and closed throughout pregnancy. Its shape is tubular with a rigid structure designed to retain the fetus within the uterus until term. Maturation of the cervix is the result of the physiological processes that soften, efface and dilate the cervix prior to the onset of labour. This can begin as much as 5–6 weeks prior to labour.

Cervical structure

The cervix is composed of dense bundles of collagen fibres, embedded in a protein-based ground substance. These fibres are responsible for the rigidity of the cervix. The cervix also contains elastin fibres, in lesser number. The elastin fibres are thin, running in a line from the internal to the external os. The greatest concentration of elastin fibres is found at the internal os (Leppert 1995). The role of the elastin is to aid expansion in labour and to restore the cervix to prepregnant shape (Calder 1994).

The final component of the cervix is smooth muscle fibres, being 10–15% of cervical tissue. During pregnancy they enlarge and become prominent (Leppert 1995). Traditionally viewed as acting as a sphincter, the quantity of muscle is small. Calder (1994) suggests the muscle protects blood vessels and closes the cervix swiftly on completion of labour.

Structural changes in ripening

Successful induction occurs when the cervix is favourable or so-called 'ripe'. The cervix is then more compliant, offering less soft tissue resistance to the actions of the myometrium and the presenting part. The cervix then dilates as labour becomes established. The muscle, collagen and elastin fibres realign towards term, and water is attracted to the cells of the cervix, softening the tissue. Pressure on the cervix from the presenting part helps the process. With ripening, the ground substance of the cervix changes, cross-linking of fibres occurs and the collagen bundles break down, decreasing in number. There is an increase in the water content of the connective tissue. The process is not dependent on myometrial activity and alters the cervix from a rigid barrier to a pliant structure (Calder & Greer 1992).

Prostaglandins

The spontaneous changes in the cervix can be replicated by the use of prostaglandin compounds, which are available in pharmacological form. They are locally acting chemical compounds derived from fatty acids within cells. Prostaglandins play a significant role in the ripening process and also contribute to the contractibility of the uterus in labour. Although prostaglandins occur throughout the body, specific prostaglandins have been identified as acting on the cervix and the uterus, namely prostaglandin E_2 (PGE_2) and F_2 (PGF_2). In addition to being produced from the cervix, they are known to be produced by the fetal membranes and the decidua and are detectable in liquor in increasing quantities before term. PGF_2 has been the most effective in inducing labour (Kelly et al 2002).

Preinduction prostaglandin can be used to prime or mature the cervix for induction. A low dose prostaglandin is administered to bring about effacement and dilatation but not to stimulate contractions.

Methods of inducing labour

Prostaglandins and induction

In order to decide on method of induction, assessment of the cervix is required. Prior to prescribing the prostaglandin, the Bishop's score is measured (Table 29.1). This is an objective method of assessing

Table 29.1 Modified Bishop's preinduction pelvic scoring system

Inducibility features	0	1	2	3
Dilatation of cervix in cm	0	1–2	3–4	5–6
Consistency of cervix	Firm	Medium	Soft	–
Cervical canal length in cm	> 2	1–2	0.5–1	< 0.5
Position of cervix	Posterior	Mid	Anterior	–
Station of presenting part in cm above or below ischial spine	–3	–2	–1, 0	+1, +2

whether the cervix is favourable for induction of labour. Key elements in the assessment are dilatation, effacement (cervical canal length), position, consistency and station of the presenting part (Bishop 1964). The five different features are considered and each is awarded a score of between 0 and 3. When a total of 6 or over is reached the prognosis for induction is good.

Prostaglandin is most effective when administered by the intravaginal route (Kelly et al 2002). PGE$_2$ preparations are available in gel or slow release tablet form, the latter being recommended for use (NICE 2001). These are inserted close to the cervix within the posterior fornix of the vagina (Fig. 29.1). PGE$_2$ administered locally to the cervix is then absorbed, resulting in changes which can be assessed on vaginal examination, increasing the Bishop's score. Where PGE$_2$ tablets are used the prescribed dose should not exceed 6 mg (MacKenzie & Burns 1997).

Prostaglandin produces frequent, but low intensity, contractions of the uterus. These may not be felt by all women and they wear off after 3–4 hours. Labour will result in 30–50% of cases (Kelly et al 2002). Fetal heart rate and uterine contractions should be monitored continuously for 30–60 minutes thereafter. The mother should remain recumbent or resting for 1 hour.

There is a risk of uterine hyperstimulation and ruptured uterus (CESDI 1998, DoH et al 1998). Systemic side-effects of prostaglandin include pyrexia, diarrhoea and vomiting.

Sweeping or stripping of membranes

Sweeping the membranes can be an effective method of inducing labour where there is an uncomplicated pregnancy. The procedure can be used without admission to hospital, and for some women may be acceptable as an alternative method of inducing labour. During a vaginal examination the clinician inserts a

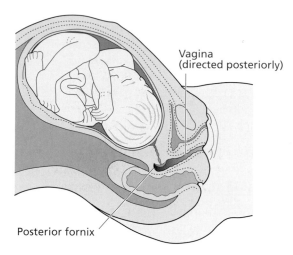

Vagina (directed posteriorly)

Posterior fornix

Fig. 29.1 Insertion of prostaglandins: the posterior fornix of the vagina is used to insert prostaglandins for ripening or induction of labour. The key point is that when undertaking a vaginal examination to assess the cervix midwives should follow the direction of the vagina, which will be directed posteriorly if the woman is semirecumbent. The uterus is anteverted and anteflexed, and the cervix protrudes into the vagina at an angle, creating the posterior fornix. The cervix may appear 'difficult to reach' particularly when unfavourable.

finger through the cervical os, and using a sweeping or circular movement releases the fetal membranes from the lower uterine segment.

Prostaglandins are rapidly produced as the fetal membranes are detached from the decidua. Labour may result as locally produced prostaglandins can be sufficient to stimulate the onset of labour. Prior to undertaking this procedure the woman should be made aware that there may be some discomfort as a result of the examination as some cervical stretching is needed. This provides additional stimulus for prostaglandin release (Boulvain et al 2001).

Amniotomy

Amniotomy is the artificial rupture of the fetal membranes (commonly abbreviated to ARM) resulting in drainage of liquor. It involves the splitting of the amnion and chorion to release the liquor. Informed maternal consent should be given and the reason for the amniotomy clearly stated in the records. An abdominal palpation should precede amniotomy to confirm presentation and degree of engagement of the presenting part. The fetal heart rate should also be noted and these observations recorded in the client records. ARM is carried out during a vaginal examination using an amnihook, a tool with a small hook at one end, or an amnicot, a glove with a small hook on one finger. The membranes over the presenting part are ruptured, the midwife having excluded the presence of low-lying placenta or cord. The colour and quantity of liquor are noted. Presentation, position and station of the fetus are noted again following ARM, and there is further assessment to ensure no cord has prolapsed. On completing the examination, the fetal heart rate should be auscultated. ARM is performed to induce labour when the cervix is favourable or during labour to augment contractions and its use during spontaneous normal (uncomplicated) labour has become common practice. ARM allows the presenting part to descend, improving application to the cervical os. This increased stimulation results in stronger contractions, as levels of prostaglandins rise, causing more pain to the labouring woman but also shortening the duration of labour (Fraser et al 2001). A well-fitting presenting part is essential to prevent cord prolapse.

Amniotomy may be used on its own or in association with oxytocin and may be either low, involving rupture of the forewaters, or, less commonly, high, which requires the hindwaters to be ruptured. The latter uses a curved Drew–Smythe catheter and should be reserved for cases of polyhydramnios with a firm indication for induction (Keirse & Chalmers 1989). Where a high Bishop's score is recorded, a woman may labour spontaneously with ARM alone.

ARM may also be carried out to visualise the colour of the liquor or to attach a fetal scalp electrode for the purposes of continuous electronic monitoring of the fetal heart rate. The use of fetal scalp electrodes has reduced as technology enables abdominal transducers to produce good quality CTG recordings. Only limited information is obtained from visualising liquor, therefore these reasons are not sufficient indications on their own to perform ARM.

Hazards of ARM. These include:

- intrauterine infection, particularly iatrogenic from digital or instrumental contamination
- early decelerations of the fetal heart
- cord prolapse
- bleeding from the following sources: fetal vessels in the membranes (vasa praevia); the friable vessels in the cervix; or a low-lying placental site (placenta praevia).

Systematic review of trials examining the use of amniotomy alone as a means of induction found little research in this area and suggested that further research was needed. Amniotomy alone may be acceptable to women as a means of inducing labour (Bricker & Luckas 2001).

Oxytocin

Oxytocin is a hormone released from the posterior pituitary gland. It acts, at cell level, on smooth muscle and is released in a pulsed manner in response to stimulation. Receptors to oxytocin are found in myometrium and they increase in number towards term and throughout labour (Fuchs et al 1984).

Oxytocin is used in conjunction with amniotomy and may be commenced at the same time as ARM or after a delay of several hours. Systematic review of trials found an increased likelihood of delivery within 12 hours when oxytocin and ARM were used at the same time. Less analgesia was required and the rate of postpartum haemorrhage was reduced.

Administration of oxytocin to induce labour

National recommendations have been made to standardise the administration of oxytocin (RCOG 2001a) and these should form the basis of any local policies and protocols. Oxytocin is used intravenously, diluted in an isotonic solution such as normal saline. Dextrose solutions used over long periods, in conjunction with oxytocin, can alter the electrolyte balance because of the mild antidiuretic effect of the hormone (Singhi et al 1985). The infusion should be controlled through a pump to enable accurate assessment of volume and rate. Dosage should be recorded in milliunits per minute, with the suggested dilution being 30 IU in

Table 29.2 Suggested regimen for intravenous oxytocin in the presence of ruptured membranes

Time in minutes after starting	Dose delivery (milliunits per minute)	
0	1	• Most women should have adequate contractions at 12 milliunits per minute.
30	2	
60	4	
90	8	• Maximum licensed dose is 20 milliunits per minute.
120	12	
150	16	• If regular contractions not established after 5 IU (5 hours on suggested regimen) then induction should be stopped.
180	20	
210	24	
240	28	
270	32	

(From RCOG 2001a, with permission)

500 ml of normal saline. The rate of infusion must be titrated against the assessment of strength and frequency of uterine contractions. The midwife may need to reduce the infusion rate as labour becomes established because the uterus becomes more sensitive to oxytocin as labour progresses. The midwife should aim to administer the lowest dose required to maintain effective, well-spaced uterine contractions, typically occurring every 3 minutes, and lasting 45–50 seconds (Table 29.2).

A summary of key points relating to the induction of labour is given in Box 29.2.

Side-effects of oxytocin

1. Hyperstimulation: oxytocin exposes the mother and fetus to the risk of hyperstimulation of the uterus, which could cause fetal hypoxia and uterine rupture. Hyperstimulation may cause the uterus to contract continuously for several minutes. This is a tonic contraction. The uterus may contract strongly, with the contractions lasting 120 seconds or more, with a frequency greater than 5 contractions in 10 minutes. Relaxation between contractions is inadequate. It may be associated with altered fetal heart rate, in which case the midwife should turn off the infusion, although on occasions decreasing the rate may be adequate. The uterus recovers from the hyperstimulation rapidly as the infusion is discontinued, but in some instances salbutamol may be administered, as an inhalation or infusion, to counteract the effect of the oxytocin. Oxytocin should not be given as a bolus injection during labour because of the risk of hyperstimulation (Alliance Pharmaceuticals 2001).

2. Prolonged use may contribute to uterine atony postpartum.

3. Water retention may occur, and water intoxication when in prolonged use, owing to its antidiuretic effect.

4. Systemic side-effects include direct vascular smooth muscle relaxation leading to transient vasodilatation and hypotension where rapid intravenous bolus doses are given (Alliance Pharmaceuticals 2001).

Responsibilities of the midwife and care of a mother for induction of labour

If the reason for induction allows, planning may include a visit to the delivery suite and special care unit, if appropriate, so the woman is familiar with her surroundings. Communication should be clear between personnel with good liaison between midwifery, obstetric, medical teams and the paediatric services to ensure that support and care are available as needed. Mothers and their birth partners should be given factual and unbiased information about induction of labour. Written information should be available as well as an opportunity to discuss issues relating to induction with both medical and midwifery staff. A record of the mother's and partner's wishes should be made in the maternity notes.

> **Box 29.2** Key points for the induction of labour
>
> - Sweeping of membranes may be effective at initiating labour, and does not require in-hospital assessment.
> - Induction of labour with prostaglandin, in the absence of any additional risk factors, can take place on an antenatal ward.
> - Oxytocin should not be started within 6 hours of the administration of prostaglandins.
> - Prior to any increase in oxytocin, uterine contractions should be assessed by abdominal palpation to ensure the lowest dose is administered to ensure effective uterine action.
> - Continuous fetal monitoring is recommended when oxytocin is used for inducing or augmenting labour.

Care in labour

As with spontaneous labour, all maternal and fetal observations are recorded as contemporaneously as possible on the partogram. A record of discussions and information given during labour should be documented in the mother's notes, with each entry signed, dated and the time of entry noted. The midwife caring for the mother should be aware of her local labour ward protocols and policies for induction of labour.

The midwife is monitoring the well-being of the mother and fetus throughout the process of induction. In addition to assessment of progress in labour, observing for signs of side-effects of oxytocin is essential. For more detailed discussion on care during the first and second stages of labour see Chapters 25 and 27.

Baseline observations. Maternal pulse rate, blood pressure and temperature recorded on the partogram.

Uterine contractions. Uterine contractions can be felt on palpation; their frequency, duration and strength should be recorded on the partogram every 15–30 minutes. It is recommended that continuous tocography be used, in conjunction with monitoring of the fetal heart when oxytocin is in use (RCOG 2001b). The midwife should remain in constant attendance while the rate of oxytocin is increasing, and be able to assess uterine tone both during and after contractions using fingertip palpation.

Fetal well-being. There should be continuous monitoring in conjunction with oxytocin, using an abdominal ultrasound transducer or a fetal scalp electrode. If CTG is not available, the fetal heart rate should be recorded on the partogram every 15 minutes or in accordance with local protocols. The midwife should be vigilant for signs of fetal distress such as a non-reassuring or abnormal trace, or signs of meconium-stained liquor (see Ch. 25).

Assessment of pain. The midwife should note the mother's reaction to pain caused by the contractions. With an oxytocin infusion the build-up in frequency and strength of the contractions may be difficult for the woman to cope with. The midwife should be able to give support and encouragement to the woman to help her cope with the contractions, and appropriate pain relief should be available if it is required. The presence of continuous support has been found to be beneficial to the woman in labour (Hodnett 2001).

Assessment of progress. Before commencing the oxytocin infusion the position of the fetus and relationship of the presenting part to the pelvic brim are assessed by abdominal palpation. A vaginal examination will normally be performed to assess the length, consistency, position and the dilatation of the cervix. Position and station of the presenting part will also be noted and these observations act as a baseline for assessing progress of the labour. Vaginal examinations are usually carried out every 4 hours, but this may vary if progress is slow, or may be dependent on local policies and the woman's choice.

When a woman's labour is induced or augmented with oxytocin and there is a previous history of caesarean section, the midwife should be aware of the risk of uterine rupture associated with excessive use of oxytocin (Leung at al 1993). The rate of oxytocin administration should be closely monitored to ensure uterine activity that is adequate to maintain progress in labour.

Alternative and natural methods of induction

Women seeking to avoid medical or surgical intervention may consider alternative methods of inducing labour. There is little or no research to verify the effectiveness of these methods and mothers should be aware of this.

Box 29.3 Suggestions for further research

Amniotomy (ARM)	• Studies are needed to evaluate the appropriate time interval from amniotomy to additional/further intervention.
	• Women and caregivers' satisfaction need to be explored.
	• Economic analysis of ARM.
Acupuncture	• As the use of complementary medicines increases, the benefits of acupuncture as a means of induction need to be considered. A well-designed RCT is suggested, to test the safety of practice that stretches back centuries.
Castor oil	• Anecdotal evidence has supported the use of this agent for hundreds of years. The efficacy of it as a means of inducing labour has not been rigorously researched

It is known that semen contains high quantities of prostaglandin and one systematic review has been carried out to consider the evidence. Only one clinical trial involving small numbers has been carried out, rendering any conclusions difficult. It is extrapolated that a combination of oxytocin released by the mother during orgasm, prostaglandin released via the semen, and the stimulation of the lower segment of the uterus within intercourse would be helpful to initiate labour (Kavanagh et al 2001).

Similarly insufficient data is available to support the contention that nipple and clitoral stimulation may aid initiation and augmentation of labour. The production of oxytocin as a result of either or both is thought to provide the physiological basis, but the effectiveness of these actions on labour has not been proven.

Anecdotal evidence of the effects of laxatives or foodstuffs exists, with oral histories being passed down through generations of the benefits or otherwise of various methods of inducing labour. Although castor oil has been widely used for many years to initiate labour, despite a poor understanding of its action, there are no methodologically sound studies that support its use (Kelly et al 2001).

The use of acupuncture warrants further investigation as observational data has suggested that acupuncture may stimulate the onset of labour (Smith & Crowther 2001).

Box 29.3 lists suggestions for further research into induction methods.

Prolonged labour

Prolonged labour is associated with the medical model of management of childbirth and for many women, and midwives, the attempts to place time limits on the physiological process of labour is problematic. However, prolonged labour is associated with increasing risks to mother and fetus. The practice of active management and augmentation has been used to reduce the duration of labours, and thus reduce the hazards, but it was reported in the National Sentinel Caesarean Section Audit that failure to progress was a key factor in the UK caesarean section rate, implicated in 20.4% of caesarean sections in England and Wales (Thomas et al 2001, p. 23).

Prolonged labour is most common in primigravidae and may be caused by:

• ineffective uterine contractions
• cephalopelvic disproportion
• an occipitoposterior position (Ch. 30).

Dystocia literally means 'difficult labour' and is associated with slow progress and failure to progress in labour. This can be caused by problems with the contractions:

• not being effective in dilating and effacing the cervix
• being uncoordinated, where the two segments of the uterus fail to work in harmony
• giving inadequate involuntary expulsion.

Other causes of dystocia are abnormalities of presentation and position, of the bony pelvis and of the birth canal, including congenital abnormalities.

The first stage of labour is divided into a latent and an active phase. During the latent phase the uterus contracts regularly, and the mother experiences discomfort and pain. The cervix effaces and dilatation occurs. The duration of the latent phase will vary according to each individual and with parity.

Prolonged latent phase

The latent phase of labour is still poorly understood and its duration difficult to define, therefore a diagnosis of a prolonged latent phase may be arbitrary. A prolonged latent phase of labour can be inaccurately diagnosed when the mother is in false labour. It can also be mistakenly considered to be inefficient uterine activity so that inappropriate intervention occurs.

Prolonged active phase

The active phase is distinguished by an increased rate of dilatation of the cervix, with descent of the presenting part. Slow progress may be defined either as total duration of hours in labour or as failure of the cervix to dilate at a fixed rate per hour. A rate of 1 cm per hour is most commonly used, but vaginal examination is imprecise, with variability between practitioners a possibility (Enkin et al 2000). A prolonged active phase is caused by a combination of factors including the cervix, the uterus, the fetus and the mother's pelvis.

Assessment of the contractions

Clinical assessment by the midwife will give information on the nature of the contractions. Palpation of the fundus during the contraction allows the midwife to assess frequency and duration and gives some indication of the strength. In normal, spontaneous labour this mode of assessment provides adequate information without recourse to further intervention. Using the palm of the hand on the fundus the midwife notes the time the contraction starts, and the duration. The strength of the contractions can be difficult to assess because of the size of the abdomen and the contour of the uterus but can be described in three ways:

- *mild* – the fundus tenses during the contraction but remains easy to indent with fingertip palpation
- *moderate* – the fundus tenses to the extent that it is difficult to indent on palpation
- *strong* – the fundus is hard and rigid to touch.

Assessment by palpation may be subjective, however, so should be used as only part of an overall assessment including the reaction of the mother to the contraction, and her general behaviour.

The use of external tocographic assessment will show the frequency of the contractions and give some indication of their strength and is used as part of electronic fetal monitoring. Assessment of the strength of the contractions can also be made using an internal pressure transducer, although this is rarely used.

Normal uterine action

Normal uterine action is strengthened in labour by the combined effect of increasing levels of prostaglandin and oxytocin receptors. The myometrium contracts and retracts, its efficiency being dependent on fundal dominance and the polarity between the upper uterine segment and the lower segment. The harmony is facilitated by gap junctions in the myometrium. These gaps play a role in allowing electrical impulses to pass between the muscles (Huszar & Naftolin 1984).

The effectiveness of the contractions is further influenced by resistance, especially from the cervix and other soft tissues, the size and position of the fetus and the maternal pelvis.

Inefficient uterine action

Slow progress in labour is often attributed to inefficient uterine contractions. In the absence of effective contractions, descent of the presenting part will be delayed. The practice of restricting food and fluids to mothers in labour may have a detrimental effect on the contractions as muscle needs to have an adequate energy supply to contract effectively (Garfield 1987). The effect of ketones on uterine activity is unclear but some ketosis may be a normal response (Anderson 1998). Mothers who are deemed to be at low risk in labour should be encouraged to continue with a light diet (Grant 1990). Ambulation may promote more effective uterine activity. The upright position of the labouring mother allows the uterus to fall forward, improving the application of the presenting part on to the cervix, and may trigger the neuroendocrine Ferguson reflex. If the mother adopts an upright position, contractions have been found to be less painful although stronger and more efficient than when remaining recumbent (Caldeyro-Barcia 1979a). Stress is also known to affect the contractions, and less tension as a result of mobility enhances the activity (Fenwick & Simkin 1987).

The pelvis offers a rigid canal through which the fetus must manoeuvre. Size of the fetus and size of the pelvis have to permit the mechanism of labour. Where progress is slow, and labour prolonged, consideration of an alternative position may allow the limited opportunity for expansion within the pelvis to be exploited, particularly if there is a malposition of the occiput. Upright positions, or one where the woman adopts a forward-leaning posture, are helpful in encouraging an anterior rotation of the occiput (see Ch. 30). When poor progress of labour is due to hypotonic, inefficient contractions, oxytocin increases the strength and the frequency of the contractions but cephalopelvic disproportion should be excluded before attempts are made to speed up the contractions.

Augmentation of labour

Augmentation of labour refers to intervention to correct slow progress in labour. Correction of ineffective uterine contractions includes amniotomy, administration of oxytocin and amniotomy, or administration of oxytocin in the presence of the previously ruptured membranes. Augmentation is one of the tenets of active management of labour, and as with any intervention its full rationale should be discussed and mother's informed consent documented. At all times the well-being of the mother and her unborn baby are paramount.

Active management of labour

The principles behind active management require that a precise diagnosis of the onset of labour is made, and labour is completed within 12 hours. ARM is carried out routinely, with a dilation rate of 1 cm per hour expected after the cervix is 3 cm dilated. If the labour fails to proceed at the prescribed rate then it is considered prolonged and contractions augmented by the administration of an oxytocin infusion. Progress of labour is plotted on a partogram, having been assessed by vaginal examination. The first assessment occurs within 1 hour of admission, and if labour is diagnosed (i.e. the cervix is 3 cm or more dilated) the membranes will be ruptured. A further examination takes place an hour later, and if the cervix has not dilated sufficiently an intravenous infusion of oxytocin will be commenced.

Assessment of progress relying on vaginal examinations may be subjective, as the nature of the examination itself is unreliable, with no way of accurately measuring dilatation or preventing error on the part of the clinician. Failure to meet the medical rather than physiological expectations of progress in labour may result in labours being described as abnormal. The use of active management in preventing prolonged labour and reducing the caesarean section rate is therefore controversial with high rates of intervention. Forty-five per cent of primigravidae in labour received oxytocin for inefficient uterine action or prolonged labour (O'Driscoll et al 1993). Despite this, it is a model of practice that is used worldwide.

Incoordinate uterine activity

This may be hypertonic and also inefficient. Lacking fundal dominance, the contraction begins and lasts longest in the lower segment. Polarity is reversed. The resting tone of the uterus is raised, the uterus feeling tense on palpation. Pain is intense but out of proportion with the effect of the contraction on the dilatation of the cervix. This pattern of activity is typically found in association with malposition of the occiput and minor degrees of disproportion.

Where co-ordination of the contractions is completely lacking, different areas of the uterus contract independently. This is the so-called 'colicky' uterus. The mother suffers severe generalised pain, as the resting tone of the uterus is raised. Fetal distress may be the result of diminished placental perfusion.

Constriction ring dystocia

This is a localised spasm of a ring of muscle fibres that occurs at the junction of the upper and lower segments of the uterus. It is rare, affecting less than 1 in 1000 labours, and may arise at any stage, although most commonly in the late first or early second stage. It is associated with the use of oxytocin.

Management of prolonged labour

The management of a mother experiencing a prolonged labour will be the responsibility of the obstetric team. Midwives are required to seek medical advice having recognised a deviation from normal, and will normally continue to provide care for the woman, and work with the interprofessional team to ensure a safe outcome (UKCC 1998).

When progress in labour is slow, attempts should be made to determine the cause before deciding on management. Hypotonic uterine activity may be corrected with amniotomy or oxytocin infusion, or both. If, however, there have been strong contractions and slow progress, a decision may be made to carry out a caesarean section. Obvious disproportion or malpresentation are indications for caesarean section.

The midwife should ensure the mother's comfort and offer her and her partner support and information about her management and care. Principles of care for a mother in labour are continued as for normal birth, but with particular attention to the following:

Informed choice and consent to treatment. As with any situation, the couple should be given as much information as is available to ensure that they understand the events and to obtain consent to all aspects of treatment. Accurate records should be made of discussions and details of any management recorded. Where a mother has previously made a birth plan detailing her wishes, the midwife may need to help her through a change of plan in order to attain a successful outcome.

Comfort and analgesia. Adequate analgesia should be offered to the mother. Where labour is prolonged an epidural block may be beneficial and affords complete pain relief in most cases. Attention should be paid to ensuring that the woman is able to adopt the most comfortable position and can avoid immobility, as unrelieved pressure can contribute to the development of pressure injuries. General hygiene is important, especially where the membranes have been ruptured. Prolonged contact with moisture can also give rise to tissue damage and soiled pads and bed linen should be changed as necessary.

Observations. Midwives need to be aware of the total well-being of the woman, including her behaviour. This will entail consideration of how she copes with contractions and whether she is remaining mobile, as well as her ability to engage with companions and caregivers. All relevant observations are noted and should be recorded on the partogram, or written in the client records. Temperature should be taken every 4 hours as infection may develop where there has been prolonged rupture of membranes. Vaginal swabs may be taken and broad spectrum antibiotics commenced when infection is suspected.

Pulse and blood pressure are recorded hourly, or more frequently if the woman's condition requires.

Fluid balance. An accurate record should be kept. A note of urinary output is important and the mother should be offered the opportunity to empty her bladder every 2 hours. A full bladder may affect the uterine action in labour and if she is unable to void then a catheter should be inserted. A reduction in urinary output may be associated with the antidiuretic effect of oxytocin, be linked with pyrexia and dehydration or be a sign of deterioration of the mother's condition, as in pre-eclampsia. A record of output is important where dextrose 5% is the fluid used to administer oxytocin. Fluid overload can occur, which causes hyponatraemia, affecting mother and baby.

Communication. Communication between personnel with liaison between the midwifery, obstetric and paediatric services should be clear to ensure that support and care are available as needed.

Assessment of progress in prolonged labour. Vaginal examination is carried out, usually on a 4-hourly regimen. It should be carried out, if possible, by the same midwife each time as there is a high risk of variability between practitioners. The examination is invasive and intrusive, and a clear rationale for undertaking the assessment should be given to the mother, and recorded in her records.

Progress is noted in terms of increasing dilatation, along with the consistency of the cervix and application of the cervix to the presenting part. Position of the sagittal suture is also noted, as is any caput or moulding of the fetal skull. Moulding is an indication that the fetus is experiencing difficulty in negotiating the pelvis. The degree of moulding should be noted and any increase over successive examinations reported. Caput succedaneum can develop, particularly if labour is prolonged. This can make position and station difficult to assess, as it masks the sutures and fontanelles.

Descent of the presenting part can be demonstrated by correlating findings from an abdominal examination and station of the presenting part on vaginal examination.

The colour of the amniotic fluid needs to be noted and if meconium is present this should be reported (UKCC 1998).

Fetal well-being. It is common practice for the fetal heart to be monitored continuously in a prolonged labour. Intermittent auscultation cannot assess the baseline variability of the fetal heart rate, and it is difficult to hear decelerations during contractions. Late decelerations, occurring after a contraction, may also be missed. The use of oxytocin and epidural analgesia combined with maternal and fetal indications for induction have been cited as reasons for using electronic monitoring (RCOG 2001a). Fetal blood sampling may be used to support a decision to continue with labour or intervene; electronic fetal monitoring combined with fetal blood sampling has been shown to reduce neonatal morbidity (RCOG 2001b, Thacker et al 2001).

The presence of meconium-stained liquor and an abnormal fetal heart tracing is suggestive of fetal hypoxia and, depending on local policy, fetal blood sampling may be carried out. A paediatrician should be present at the birth and precautions taken to prevent aspiration of meconium.

In the event of the mother being in labour at home, it may be necessary to arrange for her to be transferred into hospital. Advice can be sought from local supervisors of midwives and careful records of discussions made.

Prolonged second stage of labour

Provided that there is evidence of descent of the fetus, in the absence of fetal or maternal distress there is no basis for placing a time limit on the duration of the second stage of labour. There is no benefit to the mother or fetus in aggressive pushing to speed up this stage of labour (Caldeyro-Barcia 1979b, Thomson 1993). Adopting an upright position has been found to be advantageous to the mother, although opportunity may be limited by epidural block, infusions or fetal monitors (Gupta & Nikodem 2002).

Causes of delay in the second stage

Ineffective contractions, poor maternal effort, and loss of or absence of a desire to push caused by epidural analgesia may all contribute to a lengthy second stage. A full bladder or a full rectum can also impede progress. A large fetus, malpresentation or malposition may account for delay and an assisted birth may be necessary.

A reduced pelvic outlet, in association with an occipitoposterior position, may result in deep transverse arrest. This occurs where advance of the presenting part is prevented as the occipitofrontal diameter becomes caught at the ischial spines.

Management of a prolonged second stage of labour

A vaginal examination should be carried out to confirm position, attitude and station of the presenting part. The fetal heart should be auscultated after every contraction or electronic monitoring used.

In the presence of inefficient uterine contractions an infusion of oxytocin should be commenced. The usual observations for the use of oxytocin apply.

Where there are related factors such as pre-eclampsia or prematurity, management of the second stage will be assessed constantly.

Where the mother is in labour at home the midwife should arrange for transfer to hospital or seek support via her supervisor of midwives.

Options for birth

Delivery may be expedited where the conditions alter and mother or fetus becomes distressed. The obstetrician will decide on method of delivery. Ventouse or forceps will be utilised where the pelvic outlet is adequate and vaginal birth can be safely carried out. Caesarean section may be necessary where there is evidence of cephalopelvic disproportion.

Cervical dystocia

This occurs rarely and is often acquired as a consequence of scarring of the cervix or a congenital structural abnormality. Despite effective contractions the cervix fails to dilate, although it may efface. Caesarean section is necessary to deliver the baby.

Overefficient uterine activity (precipitate labour)

The contractions are strong and frequent from the onset of labour. Resistance from the soft tissue is low, resulting in rapid completion of the first and second stages. The mother may be distressed by the intensity of the contractions and the unexpected speed of the birth. Soft tissue damage of the cervix or perineum may complicate the birth. The uterus may fail to retract during the third stage, leading to retained placenta or postpartum haemorrhage.

Fetal hypoxia may be detected in labour and rapid moulding can occur. The speed of the birth may result in the baby being born in an inappropriate place, and injury from, for example, hard floors or toilets is a risk.

Precipitate labour tends to recur and the woman may be offered the opportunity to be admitted to hospital in subsequent pregnancies.

Trial of labour

A trial of labour is offered to mothers when, in the presence of a minor degree of cephalopelvic disproportion, there is concern as to the outcome of labour. The outcome of any labour is dependent on:

- the effectiveness of uterine contractions
- the 'give' of the pelvic joints
- flexion of the fetal head
- the degree of moulding of the fetal head.

These factors are unpredictable until labour is established, hence the reason for the trial of labour.

Review of place of birth may be necessary, as care should be offered in a unit that is fully equipped and staffed for operative procedures. The woman will continue her pregnancy until term and may enter labour spontaneously. However, in the presence of other obstetrical indicators, labour may be induced.

Trial of labour will be carried out when the presentation is cephalic and, although the head is likely to be non-engaged, there should be no major disproportion. The position of the fetus and degree of flexion of the head should be noted on abdominal examination and the findings can be correlated with those confirmed by vaginal examination. Progress is recorded on a partograph and any failure to progress is reported. Ambulation and upright positions can be adopted to promote effective uterine contractions, cervical dilatation and flexion of the head. Continuous fetal monitoring is used to assess fetal well-being. If, despite good uterine contractions, cervical dilatation is slow and the head fails to descend, the outlook for vaginal delivery is poor and the decision must be made whether to allow labour to continue.

If at any stage during this labour the mother or fetus are under stress then a caesarean section will be performed. The aim is to ensure a successful outcome of a live mother and child who have sustained minimal trauma.

Obstructed labour

Labour is *obstructed* when there is no advance of the presenting part despite strong uterine contractions. The obstruction usually occurs at the pelvic brim but may occur at the outlet – for example deep transverse arrest in an android pelvis.

Causes of obstructed labour

- *Cephalopelvic disproportion* or *disparity between the size of the mother's pelvis and the fetus that precludes vaginal birth* – this is the most common cause of obstructed labour. The fetus may be large in relation to the pelvis, or the pelvis may be contracted (see Ch. 7).
- *Deep transverse arrest* – this is an outcome of an occipitoposterior position, and can cause obstructed labour (see Ch. 30).
- *Malpresentation* – vaginal birth is impossible in cases of shoulder or brow presentation, or in persistent mentoposterior position (see Ch. 30).
- *Pelvic mass* – fibroids located in the lower segment or on the cervix can prevent descent of the fetal head, causing obstructed labour. Ovarian tumours or rare tumours of the bony pelvis may also prevent the head from entering the pelvis.
- *Fetal abnormalities* – abnormalities such as hydrocephalus resulting in disparity between the size of the fetus and the pelvis may cause obstruction. Conjoined twins, or locked twins, are a rare cause.

Signs of obstructed labour

The presenting part does not enter the pelvic brim despite good contractions. The midwife should exclude reasons such as a full bladder, loaded rectum, or excessive liquor volume as factors contributing to the failure in descent.

As the presenting part is unable to descend, cervical dilatation is affected and dilatation is slow. The cervix is described as hanging loosely like 'an empty sleeve' as the presenting part is not applied to it. The uterine contractions exert pressure on the membranes that are over the cervix, which may result in early rupture or the formation of a large elongated sac of forewaters.

Late signs of obstructed labour

These arise in a badly managed or neglected labour and the diagnosis of obstructed labour should be made before these signs are seen. On examination the mother is dehydrated, ketotic and in constant pain. Clinical signs also include pyrexia and tachycardia. Abdominal palpation is difficult because of maternal distress with the area over the lower segment being particularly tender to the touch. The level of the presenting part may be difficult to assess abdominally but this should be attempted as assessment on vaginal examination is complicated by the presence of caput succedaneum and moulding. Urinary output is poor and haematuria may be present. Evidence of fetal distress may be observed and where the midwife has noted a maternal tachycardia the two rates should be compared. Profound bradycardia or fetal demise may be overlooked as the two rates are misinterpreted.

The uterus becomes moulded round the fetus and it fails to relax properly between contractions. The contractions continue to build in strength and frequency until the uterus is in a continuous state of tonic contraction. The lower segment becomes progressively thinner and longer and the upper segment shorter and thicker. A physiological retraction ring may be seen as an oblique ridge above the symphysis pubis and marks the junction between the upper and lower uterine segment. A visible retraction ring, or Bandl's ring, is similar in appearance to a full bladder. The ridge appears at an oblique angle across the abdomen. Little urine is obtained on catheterisation. Uterine exhaustion, in which contractions cease for a while before recommencing with renewed vigour, may occur in a primigravida.

On examination the vagina feels hot and dry, the presenting part is high and feels wedged and immovable. It may be difficult to assess the station of the presenting part accurately as there is excessive moulding of the fetal skull and a large caput succedaneum present (Fig. 29.2).

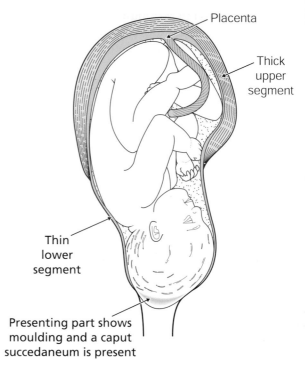

Fig. 29.2 Obstructed labour: the uterus is moulded around the fetus; the thickened upper segment is obvious on abdominal palpation.

Management of obstructed labour

Management includes prevention of obstructed labour in the first instance. Assessment of the risk within the antenatal period begins with noting any history of prolonged labours or difficult births. Antenatal assessment includes abdominal examination, which should alert the midwife to any malpresentation or signs of cephalopelvic disproportion. Appropriate referral can be made prior to the onset of labour and management of the case adjusted to ensure safe delivery. An elective caesarean section may be advocated.

Careful assessment of the progress throughout labour will help detect lack of descent before labour becomes obstructed. Correlation of findings from abdominal examination and vaginal examination helps to confirm descent of the presenting part through the pelvis. This is aided by observation of maternal and fetal condition and assessment of the length, strength and frequency of contractions. If a midwife suspects that labour is obstructed she must seek appropriate medical aid.

An intravenous infusion must be commenced, if not already in progress, to correct dehydration. Blood is taken for cross-matching in case a transfusion is needed. The mother will require treatment with antibiotics to overcome any infection that may be present. An accurate record of observations of maternal and fetal condition, along with any discussions the midwife has with the mother and her family, should be made as contemporaneously as possible.

If obstructed labour is recognised in the first stage of labour, as when the head is extended to brow presentation, delivery should be by caesarean section. In the second stage of labour, failure to progress and descend may be caused by deep transverse arrest. If the obstruction cannot be overcome by rotation and assisted birth, caesarean section should be performed as soon as possible.

If the mother is in labour at home, arrangements should be made to transfer her to the nearest maternity unit with facilities for immediate caesarean section and the staff to care for mother and baby. Both may require specialised care. The midwife should take blood for cross-matching and site an intravenous infusion prior to transfer. Detailed records should be kept as previously stated. The baby is likely to be delivered in a shocked and asphyxiated condition and facilities for resuscitation and expert care should be available. The paediatrician should be present at the birth, and the parents need to be aware that the baby may need special care after birth. If the labour is obstructed and the fetus has died, this will still be the mode of delivery as vaginal birth cannot be achieved. Following the birth of the baby and prior to repair of the uterus and abdomen, the surgeon will check carefully for any indication that the uterus has ruptured.

Complications of obstructed labour

Maternal

Trauma to the bladder may occur as a result of pressure from the fetal head during labour or as a result of trauma during delivery. Vesicovaginal fistula is still a common cause of morbidity in women in developing countries. Prolonged compression of the tissues causes necrosis of the bladder and vaginal walls and results in urinary incontinence. Intrauterine infection may follow prolonged rupture of membranes.

Neglected obstruction will result in rupture of the uterus due to thinning of the lower uterine segment. This in turn results in haemorrhage and possible death for the mother and the fetus (see Ch. 32).

Fetal

Intrauterine asphyxia may result in a fresh stillbirth or, if the baby is born alive, permanent brain damage.

Ascending infection can cause neonatal pneumonia, which may also develop as a consequence of meconium aspiration.

Refusal of treatment

Where a mother and her partner do not consent to the proposed management this does not absolve midwives and doctors of their duty towards the client. The midwife is obliged to continue and provide care and support at a level appropriate to her experience while waiting for assistance. If the mother is at home and refuses to be admitted to hospital, the supervisor of midwives should be informed along with the appropriate obstetrician. Records should be kept of treatment offered and received. The consequences of refusal should be made clear to the family and noted (NMC 2002). The midwife should endeavour to ensure that she maintains the trust of the woman and her family, and that her priorities and accountability are to the woman.

Post-traumatic stress

Untreated distress following a traumatic birth can result in long term psychological problems. Post-traumatic stress disorder results in the client experiencing flashbacks, avoidance to prevent memories and an increased level of anxiety when in similar situations. Opportunities need to be given to the mother and her family to talk through their experience. Labour needs to be explained to help the mother understand and interpret events (Allott 1996). The psychological trauma is caused by pain, a sense of powerlessness and loss of control over events. Lack of information and failure to consent to management add to the sense of disempowerment. The attitude of midwives and obstetricians also contributes to the distress if they are perceived as unsympathetic and uncaring. Debriefing and follow-up support by midwives or trained counsellors has been successful in overcoming stress caused by a traumatic labour or delivery. (See also Ch. 35.)

Mortality

Obstructed labour is a major contributor to maternal mortality figures worldwide, being responsible for the death of approximately 40 000 women each year. It is a major problem in those countries where women may go into labour without the help of trained attendants. As part of the Safe Motherhood Initiative, the WHO has developed and introduced a partograph for use in developing countries. The aim is to increase the detection of women with prolonged or obstructed labour and improve the management of labour. The partograph alerts carers to those women with abnormal progress and enables action to be taken. Maternal and fetal morbidity is thus reduced (WHO 1996).

REFERENCES

Alfirevic Z, Neilson J P 2001 Biophysical profile for fetal assessment in high risk pregnancies (Cochrane review). In: the Cochrane Library, Issue 3. Update Software. Oxford

Alliance Pharmaceuticals 2001 Syntocinon ampoules 5/10 IU/ml. Summary of product characteristics. Alliance Pharmaceuticals, Chippenham, Wilts

Allott H 1996 Picking up the pieces: the post-delivery stress clinic. British Journal of Midwifery 4(10):534–536

Anderson T 1998 Is ketosis in labour pathological? The Practising Midwife 1(9):22–26

Bakketeig L S, Bergsjo P 1989 Post term pregnancy, the magnitude of the problem. In: Chalmers I, Enkin M, Keirse M J N C (eds) Effective care in pregnancy and childbirth. Oxford University Press, Oxford, vol 1, ch 46, p 766

Bishop E M 1964 Pelvic scoring for elective induction. Obstetrics and Gynecology 24(2):266–268

Boulvain M, Stan C, Irion O 2001 Membrane sweeping for induction of labour (Cochrane review). In: The Cochrane Library, Issue 3. Update Software, Oxford

Boyd M E, Usher R H, McLean F H, Kramer M S 1988 Obstetric consequences of postmaturity. American Journal of Obstetrics and Gynecology 158:334–338

Bricker L, Luckas M 2001 Amniotomy alone for induction of labour (Cochrane review). In: The Cochrane Library, Issue 3. Update Software, Oxford

Calder A A 1994 Prostaglandins and biological control of cervical function. Australian and New Zealand Journal of Obstetrics and Gynecology 34(3):347–351

Calder A A, Greer I A 1992 Cervical physiology and induction of labour. In: Bonnar J (ed) Recent advances in obstetrics and gynaecology. Churchill Livingstone, Edinburgh, ch 3, p 33–56

Caldeyro-Barcia R 1979a The influence of maternal position on time of spontaneous rupture of the membranes, progress of labor and fetal head compression. Birth and the Family Journal 6(1):7–15

Caldeyro-Barcia R 1979b The influence of maternal bearing down efforts during the second stage on fetal wellbeing. Birth and the Family Journal 6(1):17–21

CESDI (Confidential Enquiry into Stillbirths and Deaths in Infancy) 1998 5th annual report, 1 January–31 December 1996. Maternal and Child Health Research Consortium, London

Chua S, Arulkumaran S 1999 Prolonged pregnancy. In: James D K, Steer P J, Weiner C P, Gonik B (eds) High risk pregnancy management options, 2nd edn. W B Saunders, Edinburgh, ch 60, pp 1057–1071

Crowley P 1989 Post-term pregnancy: induction or surveillance? In: Chalmers I, Enkin M, Keirse M J N C (eds) Effective care in pregnancy and childbirth. Oxford University Press, Oxford, vol 1, ch 47, p 776–791

Crowley P 2002 Interventions for preventing or improving the outcome of delivery at or beyond term (Cochrane review). In: The Cochrane Library, Issue 1. Update Software, Oxford

Divon M Y, Marko A D, Henderson C E 1995 Longitudinal measurement of amniotic fluid index in postterm pregnancy and its association with pregnancy outcome. American Journal of Obstetrics and Gynecology 136:787–790

DoH (Department of Health), Welsh Office, Scottish Home and Health Department, Department of Health and Social Services, Northern Ireland 1998 Why mothers die. Report on confidential enquiries into maternal deaths in the United Kingdom 1994–1996. Stationery Office, London

Enkin M, Keirse MJNC, Neilson J 2000 A guide to effective care in pregnancy, 3rd edn. Oxford University Press, Oxford, Chapter 31, p 284

Fenwick L, Simkin P 1987 Maternal positioning to prevent or alleviate dystocia in labor. Clinical Obstetrics and Gynecology 30(1):83–89

FIGO 1982 Report of the committee following a workshop in monitoring and reporting perinatal mortality and morbidity. FIGO Standing Committee on Perinatal Mortality. International Federation of Gynaecology and Obstetrics. Chameleon Press, London

Fox H 1991 A contemporary view of the human placenta. Midwifery 7:31–39

Fraser W D, Turcot L, Krauss I, Brisson-Carrol G 2001 Amniotomy for shortening spontaneous labour (Cochrane review). In: The Cochrane Library, Issue 3. Update Software, Oxford

Fuchs A R, Fuchs F, Husslein P, Soloff M S 1984 Oxytocin receptors in pregnant human uterus. American Journal of Obstetrics and Gynecology 150:734–741

Garfield R E 1987 Cellular and molecular bases for dystocia. Clinical Obstetrics and Gynecology 30(1):3–18

Grant J 1990 Nutrition and hydration in labour. In: Alexander J, Levy V, Roch S (eds) Midwifery practice intrapartum care: a research-based approach. Macmillan, Basingstoke, p 66

Gupta J K, Nikodem V C 2002 Position for women during second stage of labour (Cochrane review). In: The Cochrane Library, Issue 1. Update Software, Oxford

Hall M H, Carr Hill R A 1985 The significance of uncertain gestation for obstetric outcome. British Journal of Obstetrics and Gynaecology 92:452–460

Hannah M E, Ohlsson A, Farine D et al 1996 Induction of labor compared with expectant management for prelabor rupture of membranes at term. New England Journal of Medicine 334(6):1005–1010

Harman C R, Menticoglou S M, Manning F A 1999 Assessing fetal health. In: James D K, Steer P J, Weiner C P, Gonik B (eds) High risk pregnancy management options, 2nd edn. W B Saunders, Edinburgh, ch 17, p 249–289

Hodnett E D 2001 Caregiver support for women during childbirth (Cochrane review). In: The Cochrane Library, Issue 3. Update Software, Oxford

Huszar G, Naftolin F 1984 The myometrium and uterine cervix in normal and pre-term labor. New England Journal of Medicine 311(9):571–581

James D 1991 Limitation of fetal biophysical assessment. Contemporary Reviews in Obstetrics and Gynaecology 3:69–74

Kavanagh J, Kelly A J, Thomas J 2001 Sexual intercourse for cervical ripening and induction of labour (Cochrane review). In: The Cochrane Library, Issue 3. Update Software, Oxford

Keirse M J N C, Chalmers I 1989 Methods for inducing labour. In: Chalmers I, Enkin M, Keirse M J N C (eds) Effective care in pregnancy and childbirth. Oxford University Press, Oxford, vol 2, ch 62, p 1058, 1063

Kelly A J, Kavanagh J, Thomas J 2001 Castor oil, bath and/or enema for cervical priming and induction of labour (Cochrane review). In: The Cochrane Library, Issue 3. Update Software, Oxford

Kelly A J, Kavanagh J, Thomas J 2002 Vaginal prostaglandin (PGE$_2$ and PGF$_{2a}$) for induction of labour at term (Cochrane review). In: The Cochrane Library, Issue 1. Update Software, Oxford

Kohner N 1995 Pregnancy loss and the death of a baby. Guidelines for professionals. SANDS, London, p 19–20

Leppert P C 1995 Anatomy and physiology of cervical ripening. Clinical Obstetrics and Gynecology 38(2):267–279

Leung A S, Farmer R M, Leung E K, Medearis A L, Paul R H 1993 Risk factors associated with uterine rupture during trial of labor after cesarean delivery: a case–control study. American Journal of Obstetrics and Gynecology 168:1358–1363

MacKenzie I Z, Burns E 1997 Randomised trial of one versus two doses of prostaglandin E$_2$ for induction of labour: 1 Clinical outcome. British Journal of Obstetrics and Gynaecology 104:1062–1067

Mittendorf R, Williams M A, Berkley C S, Cotter P F 1990 The length of uncomplicated human gestation. Obstetrics and Gynecology 75(6):929–932

Neilson J P, Alfirevic Z 2002 Doppler ultrasound for fetal assessment in high risk pregnancies (Cochrane review). In: The Cochrane Library, Issue 1. Update Software, Oxford

NICE (National Institute for Clinical Excellence) 2001 Induction of labour inherited clinical guideline D. NICE, London

NMC (Nursing and Midwifery Council) 2002 Code of professional conduct. NMC, London

O'Driscoll K, Meagher D, Boylan P 1993 Active management of labour. The Dublin experience, 3rd edn. Mosby, London

RCOG (Royal College of Obstetricians and Gynaecologists) 2001a Induction of labour. Evidence based clinical guideline 9. RCOG Press, London

RCOG (Royal College of Obstetricians and Gynaecologists) 2001b Electronic fetal monitoring. Evidence based clinical guideline 8. RCOG Press, London

Singhi S, Chookang E, Hall J, Kalghatgi S 1985 Iatrogenic neonatal and maternal hyponatraemia following oxytocin and aqueous glucose infusion during labour. British Journal of Obstetrics and Gynaecology 92:356–363

Smith C A, Crowther C A 2001 Acupuncture for induction of labour (Cochrane review). In: The Cochrane Library, Issue 3. Update Software, Oxford

Tan B P, Hannah M E 2002 Oxytocin for prelabour rupture of membranes at or near term (Cochrane review). In: The Cochrane Library, Issue 1. Update Software, Oxford

Thacker S B, Stroup D, Chang M 2001 Continuous electronic heart rate monitoring for fetal assessment during labor (Cochrane review). In: The Cochrane Library, Issue 3. Update Software, Oxford

Thomas J, Paranjothy S, Royal College of Obstetricians and Gynaecologists Clinical Effectiveness Support Unit 2001 National sentinel caesarean section audit report. RCOG Press, London, p 23

Thomson A M 1993 Pushing techniques in the second stage of labour. Journal of Advanced Nursing 18:171–177

UKCC (United Kingdom Central Council for Nursing, Midwifery and Health Visiting) 1998 Midwives rules and code of practice. UKCC, London

WHO (World Health Organisation) 1996 Safe motherhood care in normal birth: a practical guide. Report of a technical working group. Family and Reproductive Health Unit, WHO, Geneva

30 Malpositions of the Occiput and Malpresentations

Terri Coates

Malpositions and malpresentations of the fetus present the midwife with a challenge of recognition and diagnosis both in the antenatal period and during labour.

The chapter aims to:

- outline the causes of these positions and presentations
- discuss the midwife's diagnosis and management
- describe the possible outcomes.

Occipitoposterior positions

Occipitoposterior positions are the most common type of malposition of the occiput and occur in approximately 10% of labours. A persistent occipitoposterior position results from a failure of internal rotation prior to delivery. This occurs in 5% of deliveries (Pearl et al 1993).

The vertex is presenting, but the occiput lies in the posterior rather than the anterior part of the pelvis. As a consequence, the fetal head is deflexed and larger diameters of the fetal skull present (Fig. 30.1).

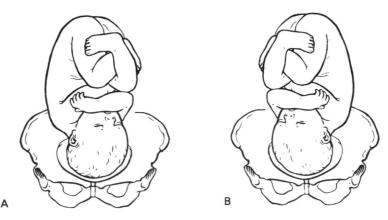

Fig. 30.1 (A) Right occipitoposterior position. (B) Left occipitoposterior position.

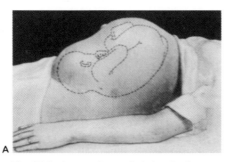
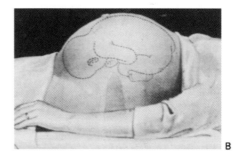

Fig. 30.2 Comparison of abdominal contour in (A) posterior and (B) anterior positions of the occiput.

Causes

The direct cause is often unknown, but it may be associated with an abnormally shaped pelvis. In an android pelvis the forepelvis is narrow and the occiput tends to occupy the roomier hindpelvis. The oval shape of the anthropoid pelvis, with its narrow transverse diameter, favours a direct occipitoposterior position.

Antenatal diagnosis

Abdominal examination

On inspection. There is a saucer-shaped depression at or just below the umbilicus. This depression is created by the 'dip' between the head and the lower limbs of the fetus. The outline created by the high, unengaged head can look like a full bladder (Fig. 30.2).

On palpation. Whilst the breech is easily palpated at the fundus the back is difficult to palpate as it is well out to the maternal side, sometimes almost adjacent to the maternal spine. Limbs can be felt on both sides of the midline.

The head is usually high, a posterior position being the most common cause of non-engagement in a primigravida at term. This is because the large presenting diameter, the occipitofrontal (11.5 cm), is unlikely to enter the pelvic brim until labour begins and flexion occurs. The occiput and sinciput are on the same level (Figs 30.3 and 30.4). Flexion allows the engagement of the suboccipitofrontal diameter (10 cm).

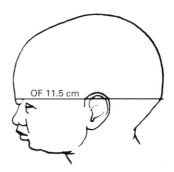

Fig. 30.3 Engaging diameter of a deflexed head: occipitofrontal (OF) 11.5 cm.

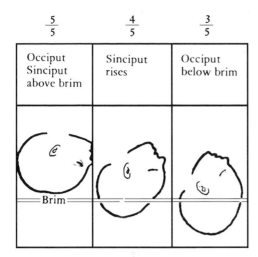

Fig. 30.4 Flexion with descent of the head.

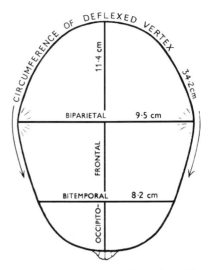

Fig. 30.5 Presenting dimensions of a deflexed head.

The cause of the deflexion is a straightening of the fetal spine against the lumbar curve of the maternal spine. This makes the fetus straighten its neck and adopt a more erect attitude.

On auscultation. The fetal back is not well flexed so the chest is thrust forward, therefore the fetal heart can be heard in the midline. However, the heart may be heard more easily at the flank on the same side as the back.

Antenatal preparation

There is anecdotal evidence to suggest that active changes of maternal posture may help to achieve an optimal fetal position before labour (El Halta 1995, 1998, Sutton 1996). It may be possible that the mother adopting a knee–chest position several times a day may achieve rotation of the fetus to an anterior position. However, this possibility needs to be researched as there is insufficient evidence to evaluate the effectiveness of maternal posture on the presenting part (Hofmeyr & Kulier 2002).

Diagnosis during labour

The woman may complain of continuous and severe backache worsening with contractions. However, the absence of backache does not necessarily indicate an anteriorly positioned fetus (Biancuzzo 1993).

The large and irregularly shaped presenting circumference (Fig. 30.5) does not fit well on to the cervix.

Therefore the membranes tend to rupture spontaneously at an early stage of labour and the contractions may be inco-ordinate. Descent of the head can be slow even with good contractions. The woman may have a strong desire to push early in labour because the occiput is pressing on the rectum.

Vaginal examination

The findings (Fig. 30.6) will depend upon the degree of flexion of the head; locating the anterior fontanelle in the anterior part of the pelvis is diagnostic but this may be difficult if caput succedaneum is present. The direction of the sagittal suture and location of the posterior fontanelle will help to confirm the diagnosis.

Care in labour

Labour with a fetus in an occipitoposterior position can be long and painful. The deflexed head does not fit well on to the cervix and therefore does not produce optimal stimulation for uterine contractions.

First stage of labour

The woman may experience severe and unremitting backache, which is tiring and can be very demoralising especially if the progress of labour is slow. Continuous support from the midwife will help the mother and her partner to cope with the labour (Thornton & Lilford 1994) (see Chs 24 and 26). The midwife can help to provide physical support such as massage and

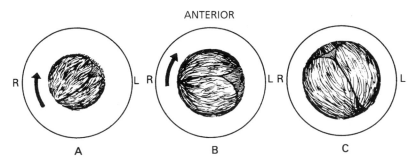

Fig. 30.6 Vaginal touch pictures in a right occipitoposterior position. (A) Anterior fontanelle felt to left and anteriorly. Sagittal suture in the right oblique diameter of the pelvis. (B) Anterior fontanelle felt to left and laterally. Sagittal suture in the transverse diameter of the pelvis. (C) Following increased flexion the posterior fontanelle is felt to the right and anteriorly. Sagittal suture in the left oblique diameter of the pelvis. The position is now right occipitoanterior.

other comfort measures and suggest changes of posture and position. The all-fours position may relieve some discomfort; anecdotal evidence suggests that this position may also aid rotation of the fetal head.

A study using ultrasound to confirm fetal position and presentation has shown that most (68%) persistent occipitoposterior positions develop through a malrotation during labour from an occipitoanterior position; only 32% of persistent cases were occipitoposterior at the start of labour (Gardberg et al 1998). In the same study, 87.5% of occipitoposterior positions that presented at the start of labour rotated to an anterior position for delivery.

Labour may be prolonged and the midwife should do all she can to prevent the mother from becoming dehydrated or ketotic (see Ch. 24).

Incoordinate uterine action or ineffective contractions may need correction with an oxytocin infusion (see Ch. 29).

The woman may experience a strong urge to push long before her cervix has become fully dilated. This is because of the pressure of the occiput on the rectum. However, if the woman pushes at this time, the cervix may become oedematous and this would delay the onset of the second stage of labour. The urge to push may be eased by a change in position and the use of breathing techniques or Entonox to enhance relaxation. The woman's partner and the midwife can assist throughout labour with massage, physical support and suggestions for alternative methods of pain relief (see Ch. 26). The mother may choose a range of pain control methods throughout her labour depending on the level and intensity of pain that she is experiencing at that time.

Second stage of labour

Full dilatation of the cervix may need to be confirmed by a vaginal examination because moulding and formation of a caput succedaneum may bring the vertex into view while an anterior lip of cervix remains. If the head is not visible at the onset of the second stage, then the midwife could encourage the woman to remain upright (see Ch. 27). This position may shorten the length of the second stage and may reduce the need for operative delivery. In some cases where contractions are weak and ineffective an oxytocin infusion may be commenced to stimulate adequate contractions and achieve advance of the presenting part. As with any labour, the maternal and fetal conditions are closely observed throughout the second stage. The length of the second stage of labour is increased when the occiput is posterior, and there is an increased likelihood of operative delivery (Gimovsky & Hennigan 1995, Pearl et al 1993).

Mechanism of right occipitoposterior position (long rotation) (Figs 30.7–30.10)

- The lie is longitudinal.
- The attitude of the head is deflexed.
- The presentation is vertex.
- The position is right occipitoposterior.
- The denominator is the occiput.

- The presenting part is the middle or anterior area of the left parietal bone.
- The occipitofrontal diameter, 11.5 cm, lies in the right oblique diameter of the pelvic brim. The occiput points to the right sacroiliac joint and the sinciput to the left iliopectineal eminence.

Flexion. Descent takes place with increasing flexion. The occiput becomes the leading part.

Internal rotation of the head. The occiput reaches the pelvic floor first and rotates forwards 3/8 of a circle along the right side of the pelvis to lie under the symphysis pubis. The shoulders follow, turning 2/8 of a circle from the left to the right oblique diameter.

Crowning. The occiput escapes under the symphysis pubis and the head is crowned.

Extension. The sinciput, face and chin sweep the perineum and the head is born by a movement of extension.

Restitution. In restitution the occiput turns 1/8 of a circle to the right and the head realigns itself with the shoulders.

Internal rotation of the shoulders. The shoulders enter the pelvis in the right oblique diameter; the anterior shoulder reaches the pelvic floor first and rotates forwards 1/8 of a circle to lie under the symphysis pubis.

External rotation of the head. At the same time the occiput turns a further 1/8 of a circle to the right.

Lateral flexion. The anterior shoulder escapes under the symphysis pubis, the posterior shoulder sweeps the perineum and the body is born by a movement of lateral flexion.

Possible course and outcomes of labour

As with all labours, complicated or otherwise, the mother should be kept informed of her progress and proposed interventions so that she can make informed choices and give informed consent, ensuring the optimum outcome for herself and her baby.

Long internal rotation

This is the commonest outcome, with good uterine contractions producing flexion and descent of the head so that the occiput rotates forward 3/8 of a circle as described above.

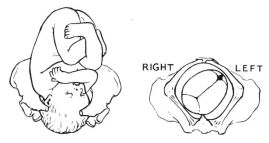

Fig. 30.7 Head descending with increased flexion. Sagittal suture in right oblique diameter of the pelvis.

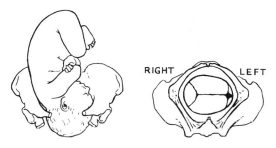

Fig. 30.8 Occiput and shoulders have rotated 1/8 of a circle forwards. Sagittal suture in transverse diameter of the pelvis.

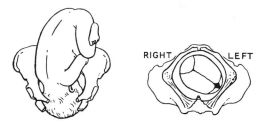

Fig. 30.9 Occiput and shoulders have rotated 2/8 of a circle forwards. Sagittal suture in the left oblique diameter of the pelvis. The position is right occipitoanterior.

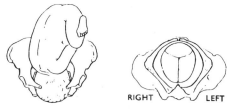

Fig. 30.10 Occiput has rotated 3/8 of a circle forwards. Note the twist in the neck. Sagittal suture in the anteroposterior diameter of the pelvis.

Figs 30.7–30.10 Mechanism of labour in right occipitoposterior position.

Short internal rotation – persistent occipitoposterior position (Figs 30.11 and 30.12)

The term 'persistent occipitoposterior position' indicates that the occiput fails to rotate forwards. Instead the sinciput reaches the pelvic floor first and rotates forwards. The occiput goes into the hollow of the sacrum. The baby is born facing the pubic bone (face to pubis).

Cause.

Failure of flexion. The head descends without increased flexion and the sinciput becomes the leading part. It reaches the pelvic floor first and rotates forwards to lie under the symphysis pubis.

Diagnosis.

In the first stage of labour. Signs are those of any posterior position of the occiput, namely a deflexed head and a fetal heart heard in the flank or in the midline. Descent is slow.

In the second stage of labour. Delay is common. On vaginal examination the anterior fontanelle is felt behind the symphysis pubis, but a large caput succedaneum may mask this. If the pinna of the ear is felt pointing towards the mother's sacrum, this indicates a posterior position.

The long occipitofrontal diameter causes considerable dilatation of the anus and gaping of the vagina while the fetal head is barely visible, and the broad biparietal diameter distends the perineum and may cause excessive bulging. As the head advances, the anterior fontanelle can be felt just behind the symphysis pubis; the baby is born facing the pubis. Characteristic upward moulding is present with the

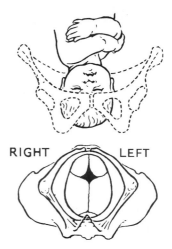

Fig. 30.12 Persistent occipitoposterior position after short rotation: position direct occipitoposterior.

caput succedaneum on the anterior part of the parietal bone (Fig. 30.13).

The birth (Figs 30.14–30.17). The sinciput will first emerge from under the symphysis pubis as far as the root of the nose and the midwife maintains flexion by restraining it from escaping further than the glabella, allowing the occiput to sweep the perineum and be born. She then extends the head by grasping it and bringing the face down from under the symphysis pubis. Owing to the larger presenting diameters, perineal trauma is common and the midwife should watch for signs of rupture in the centre of the perineum ('button-hole' tear). An episiotomy may be required.

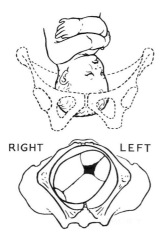

Fig. 30.11 Persistent occipitoposterior position before rotation of the occiput: position right occipitoposterior.

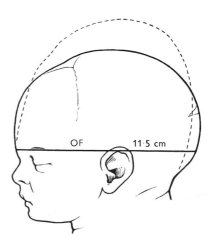

Fig. 30.13 Upward moulding (dotted line) following persistent occipitoposterior position. OF = occipitofrontal.

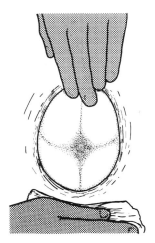

Fig. 30.14 Allowing the sinciput to escape as far as the glabella.

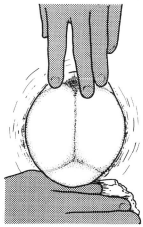

Fig. 30.15 The occiput sweeps the perineum, sinciput held back to maintain flexion.

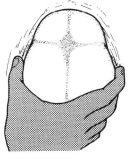

Fig. 30.16 Grasping the head to bring the face down from under the symphysis pubis.

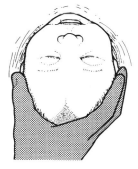

Fig. 30.17 Extension of the head.

Figs 30.14–30.17 Delivery of head in a persistent occipitoposterior position.

Undiagnosed face to pubis. If the signs are not recognised at an earlier stage, the midwife may first be aware that the occiput is posterior when she sees the hairless forehead escaping beneath the pubic arch. She may have been misguidedly extending the head and should therefore now flex it towards the symphysis pubis.

Deep transverse arrest

The head descends with some increase in flexion. The occiput reaches the pelvic floor and begins to rotate forwards. Flexion is not maintained and the occipitofrontal diameter becomes caught at the narrow bispinous diameter of the outlet. Arrest may be due to weak contractions, a straight sacrum or a narrowed outlet.

Diagnosis. The sagittal suture is found in the transverse diameter of the pelvis and both fontanelles are palpable. Neither sinciput nor occiput leads. The head is deep in the pelvic cavity at the level of the ischial spines although the caput may be lower still. There is no advance.

Management. The mother must be kept informed of progress and participate in decisions. Pushing at this time may not resolve the problem; the midwife and the woman's partner can help by encouraging SOS breathing (see Ch. 15). A change of position may help to overcome the urge to bear down.

If an operative delivery is required for the safe delivery of a healthy baby then the mother's informed consent is required. The procedure would be undertaken under local, regional or more rarely general anaesthesia (see Ch. 31). The considerations are the choice of the mother and the condition of the mother and fetus.

Vacuum extraction has been associated with lower incidence of trauma to both the mother and the infant (Pearl et al 1993) (see Ch. 31). The doctor may choose to use forceps to rotate the head to an occipitoanterior position before delivery. Whichever procedure is undertaken, the mother should first be given adequate analgesia or anaesthesia.

Conversion to face or brow presentation

When the head is deflexed at the onset of labour, extension occasionally occurs instead of flexion. If extension is complete then a face presentation results, but if incomplete the head is arrested at the brim, the brow presenting. This is a rare complication of posterior positions, and is more commonly found in multiparous women (see also below).

Complications

Apart from prolonged labour with its attendant risks to mother and fetus (see Ch. 29) and the increased likelihood of instrumental delivery, the following complications may occur.

Obstructed labour (see Ch. 32)

This may occur when the head is deflexed or partially extended and becomes impacted in the pelvis.

Maternal trauma

Forceps delivery may result in perineal bruising and trauma. Delivery of a fetus in the persistent occipitoposterior position, particularly if previously undiagnosed, may cause a third degree tear (Pearl et al 1993).

Neonatal trauma

Neonatal trauma occurring following delivery from an occipitoposterior position has been associated with forceps or ventouse delivery. The outcome for a neonate delivered from an occipitoposterior position is comparable to that expected for an infant delivered from an occipitoanterior position (Gimovsky & Hennigan 1995, Pearl et al 1993).

Cord prolapse (see Ch. 32)

A high head predisposes to early spontaneous rupture of the membranes, which, together with an ill-fitting presenting part, may result in cord prolapse.

Cerebral haemorrhage (see Ch. 44)

The unfavourable upward moulding of the fetal skull, found in an occipitoposterior position, can cause intracranial haemorrhage, as a result of the falx cerebri being pulled away from the tentorium cerebelli. The larger presenting diameters also predispose to a greater degree of compression. Cerebral haemorrhage may also result from chronic hypoxia, which may accompany prolonged labour.

Face presentation

When the attitude of the head is one of complete extension, the occiput of the fetus will be in contact with its spine and the face will present. The incidence is about 1 : 500 or less (Bhal et al 1998) and the majority develop during labour from vertex presentations with the occiput posterior; this is termed *secondary face presentation*. Less commonly the face presents before labour; this is termed *primary face presentation*. There are six positions in a face presentation (Figs 30.18–30.23); the denominator is the mentum and the presenting diameters are the submentobregmatic (9.5 cm) and the bitemporal (8.2 cm).

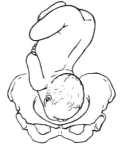

Fig. 30.18 Right mentoposterior.

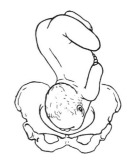

Fig. 30.19 Left mentoposterior.

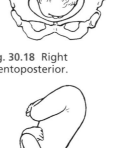

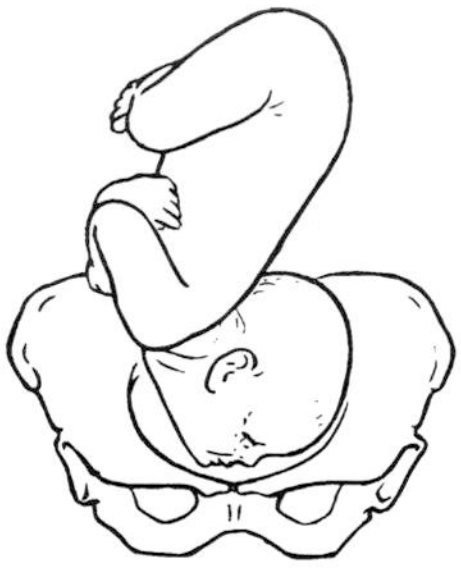

Fig. 30.20 Right mentolateral.

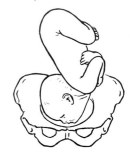

Fig. 30.21 Left mentolateral.

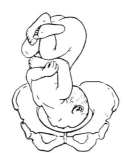

Fig. 30.22 Right mentoanterior.

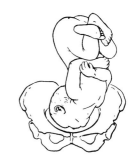

Fig. 30.23 Left mentoanterior.

Fig. 30.18–30.23 Six positions of face presentation.

Causes

Anterior obliquity of the uterus. The uterus of a multiparous woman with slack abdominal muscles and a pendulous abdomen will lean forward and alter the direction of the uterine axis. This causes the fetal buttocks to lean forwards and the force of the contractions to be directed in a line towards the chin rather than the occiput, resulting in extension of the head.

Contracted pelvis. In the flat pelvis, the head enters in the transverse diameter of the brim and the parietal eminences may be held up in the obstetrical conjugate; the head becomes extended and a face presentation develops. Alternatively, if the head is in the posterior position, vertex presenting, and remains deflexed, the parietal eminences may be caught in the sacrocotyloid dimension, the occiput does not descend, the head becomes extended and face presentation results. This is more likely in the presence of an android pelvis, in which the sacrocotyloid dimension is reduced.

Polyhydramnios. If the vertex is presenting and the membranes rupture spontaneously, the resulting rush of fluid may cause the head to extend as it sinks into the lower uterine segment.

Congenital abnormality. Anencephaly can be a fetal cause of a face presentation. In a cephalic presentation, because the vertex is absent the face is thrust forward and presents. More rarely, a tumour of the fetal neck may cause extension of the head.

Antenatal diagnosis

Antenatal diagnosis is rare since face presentation develops during labour in the majority of cases. A cephalic presentation in a known anencephalic fetus may be presumed to be a face presentation.

Intrapartum diagnosis

On abdominal palpation

Face presentation may not be detected, especially if the mentum is anterior. The occiput feels prominent, with a groove between head and back, but it may be mistaken for the sinciput. The limbs may be palpated on the side opposite to the occiput and the fetal heart is best heard through the fetal chest on the same side as the limbs. In a mentoposterior position the fetal heart is difficult to hear because the fetal chest is in contact with the maternal spine (Fig. 30.24).

On vaginal examination

The presenting part is high, soft and irregular. When the cervix is sufficiently dilated, the orbital ridges, eyes, nose and mouth may be felt. Confusion between the mouth and anus could arise, however. The mouth may be open, and the hard gums are diagnostic. The fetus may suck the examining finger. As labour progresses

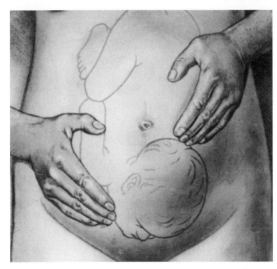

Fig. 30.24 Abdominal palpation of the head in a face presentation. Position right mentoposterior.

the face becomes oedematous, making it more difficult to distinguish from a breech presentation. To determine position the mentum must be located; if it is posterior, the midwife should decide whether it is lower than the sinciput; if so, it will rotate forwards if it can advance. In a left mentoanterior position, the orbital ridges will be in the left oblique diameter of the pelvis (Fig. 30.25). Care must be taken not to injure or infect the eyes with the examining finger.

Mechanism of a left mentoanterior position

- The lie is longitudinal.
- The attitude is one of extension of head and back.
- The presentation is face (Fig. 30.26).
- The position is left mentoanterior.
- The denominator is the mentum.
- The presenting part is the left malar bone.

Extension. Descent takes place with increasing extension. The mentum becomes the leading part.

Internal rotation of the head. This occurs when the chin reaches the pelvic floor and rotates forwards 1/8 of a circle. The chin escapes under the symphysis pubis (Fig. 30.27A).

Flexion. This takes place and the sinciput, vertex and occiput sweep the perineum; the head is born (Fig. 30.27B).

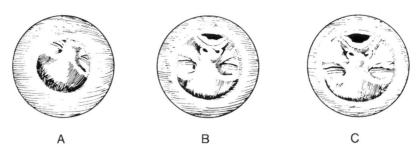

Fig. 30.25 Vaginal touch pictures of left mentoanterior position: (A) The mentum is felt to left and anteriorly. Orbital ridges in left oblique diameter of the pelvis. (B) Following increased extension of the head, the mouth can be felt. (C) The face has rotated 1/8 of a circle forwards. Orbital ridges in transverse diameter of the pelvis. Position direct mentoanterior.

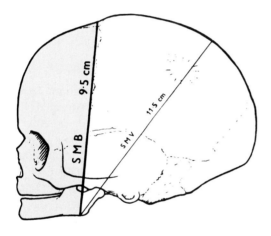

Fig. 30.26 Diameters involved in delivery of face presentation. Engaging diameter, submentobregmatic (SMB) 9.5 cm. The submentovertical (SMV) diameter, 11.5 cm, sweeps the perineum.

Restitution. This occurs when the chin turns 1/8 of a circle to the woman's left.

Internal rotation of the shoulders. The shoulders enter the pelvis in the left oblique diameter and the anterior shoulder reaches the pelvic floor first and rotates forwards 1/8 of a circle along the right side of the pelvis.

External rotation of the head. This occurs simultaneously. The chin moves a further 1/8 of a circle to the left.

Lateral flexion. The anterior shoulder escapes under the symphysis pubis, the posterior shoulder sweeps the perineum and the body is born by a movement of lateral flexion.

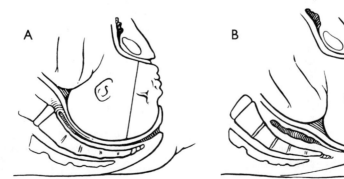

Fig. 30.27 Birth of head in mentoanterior position: (A) The chin escapes under symphysis pubis. Submentobregmatic diameter at outlet. (B) The head is born by a movement of flexion.

Possible course and outcomes of labour

The mother should be kept informed of her progress and any proposed intervention throughout labour.

Prolonged labour

Labour is often prolonged because the face is an ill-fitting presenting part and does not therefore stimulate effective uterine contractions. In addition the facial bones do not mould and, in order to enable the mentum to reach the pelvic floor and rotate forwards, the shoulders must enter the pelvic cavity at the same time as the head. The fetal axis pressure is directed to the chin and the head is extended almost at right angles to the spine, increasing the diameters to be accommodated in the pelvis.

Mentoanterior positions

With good uterine contractions, descent and rotation of the head occur (see above) and labour progresses to a spontaneous delivery.

Mentoposterior positions

If the head is completely extended, so that the mentum reaches the pelvic floor first, and the contractions are effective, the mentum will rotate forwards and the position becomes anterior.

Persistent mentoposterior position

In this case the head is incompletely extended and the sinciput reaches the pelvic floor first and rotates forwards 1/8 of a circle, which brings the chin into the hollow of the sacrum (Fig. 30.28). There is no further mechanism. The face becomes impacted because, in order to descend further, both head and chest would have to be accommodated in the pelvis. Whatever emerges anteriorly from the vagina must pivot around the subpubic arch; if the chin is posterior this is impossible because the head can extend no further.

Reversal of face presentation

A face presentation in a persistent mentoposterior position may, in some cases, be manipulated to an occipitoanterior position using bimanual pressure (Gimovsky & Hennigan 1995, Neuman et al 1994). This method was developed to reduce the likelihood of an operative delivery for those women who refused caesarean section. Using a ritodrine bolus to relax the

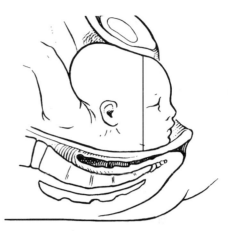

Fig. 30.28 Persistent mentoposterior position.

uterus, the fetal head is disengaged using upward transvaginal pressure. The fetal head is then flexed with bimanual pressure under ultrasound guidance to achieve an occipitoanterior position.

Management of labour

First stage

When she diagnoses a face presentation, the midwife should inform the doctor of this deviation from the normal. Routine observations of maternal and fetal conditions are made as in a normal labour (see Ch. 25). A fetal scalp electrode must not be applied, and care should be taken not to infect or injure the eyes during vaginal examinations.

Immediately following rupture of the membranes, a vaginal examination should be performed to exclude cord prolapse; such an occurrence is more likely because the face is an ill-fitting presenting part. Descent of the head should be observed abdominally, and a vaginal examination performed every 2–4 hours to assess cervical dilatation and descent of the head.

In mentoposterior positions the midwife should note whether the mentum is lower than the sinciput, since rotation and descent depend on this. If the head remains high in spite of good contractions, caesarean section is likely. The woman may be prescribed oral ranitidine, 150 mg every 6 hours throughout labour, if it is considered that an anaesthetic may be necessary.

Birth of the head (Fig. 30.29)

When the face appears at the vulva, extension must be maintained by holding back the sinciput and permitting

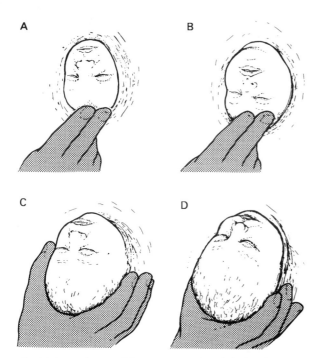

Fig. 30.29 Delivery of face presentation: (A) The sinciput is held back to increase extension until the chin is born. (B) The chin is born. (C) Flexing the head to bring the occiput over the perineum. (D) Flexion is completed; the head is born.

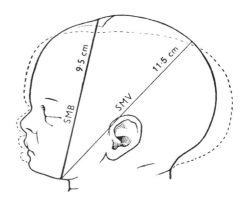

Fig. 30.30 Moulding in a face presentation (dotted line). SMB = submentobregmatic; SMV = submentovertical.

the mentum to escape under the symphysis pubis before the occiput is allowed to sweep the perineum. In this way the submentovertical diameter (11.5 cm) instead of the mentovertical diameter (13.5 cm) distends the vaginal orifice. Because the perineum is also distended by the biparietal diameter (9.5 cm), an elective episiotomy may be performed to avoid extensive perineal lacerations.

If the head does not descend in the second stage, the doctor should be informed. In a mentoanterior position it may be possible for the obstetrician to deliver the baby with forceps; when rotation is incomplete, or the position remains mentoposterior, a rotational forceps delivery may be feasible. If the head has become impacted, or there is any suspicion of disproportion, a caesarean section will be necessary.

Complications

Obstructed labour (see Ch. 32)

Because the face, unlike the vertex, does not mould, a minor degree of pelvic contraction may result in obstructed labour. In a persistent mentoposterior position the face becomes impacted and caesarean section is necessary.

Cord prolapse (see Ch. 32)

A prolapsed cord is more common when the membranes rupture because the face is an ill-fitting presenting part. The midwife should always perform a vaginal examination when the membranes rupture in order to detect such an occurrence.

Facial bruising

The baby's face is always bruised and swollen at birth with oedematous eyelids and lips. The head is elongated (Fig. 30.30) and the baby will initially lie with head extended. The midwife should warn the parents in advance of the baby's 'battered' appearance, reassuring them that this is only temporary; the oedema will disappear within 1 or 2 days, and the bruising will usually resolve within a week.

Cerebral haemorrhage

The lack of moulding of the facial bones can lead to intracranial haemorrhage caused by excessive compression of the fetal skull or by rearward compression, in the typical moulding of the fetal skull found in this presentation (see Fig. 30.30).

Maternal trauma

Extensive perineal lacerations may occur at delivery owing to the large submentovertical and biparietal diameters distending the vagina and perineum. There is an increased incidence of operative delivery, either forceps delivery or caesarean section, both of which increase maternal morbidity.

Brow presentation

In the *brow presentation* the fetal head is partially extended with the frontal bone, which is bounded by the anterior fontanelle and the orbital ridges, lying at the pelvic brim (Fig. 30.31). The presenting diameter of 13.5 cm is the mentovertical (Fig. 30.32), which exceeds all diameters in an average-sized pelvis. This presentation is rare, with an incidence of approximately 1 in 1000 deliveries (Bhal et al 1998).

Causes

These are the same as for a secondary face presentation (see above); during the process of extension from a vertex presentation to a face presentation, the brow will present temporarily and in a few cases this will persist.

Diagnosis

Brow presentation is not usually detected before the onset of labour.

On abdominal palpation

The head is high, appears unduly large and does not descend into the pelvis despite good uterine contractions.

On vaginal examination

The presenting part is high and may be difficult to reach. The anterior fontanelle may be felt on one side

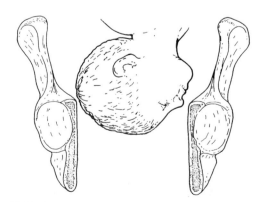

Fig. 30.31 Brow presentation.

of the pelvis and the orbital ridges, and possibly the root of the nose, at the other (Fig. 30.33). A large caput succedaneum may mask these landmarks if the woman has been in labour for some hours.

Management

The doctor must be informed immediately this presentation is suspected. This is because vaginal delivery is extremely rare and obstructed labour usually results. It is possible that a woman with a large pelvis and a small baby may deliver vaginally. When the brow reaches the pelvic floor the maxilla rotates forwards

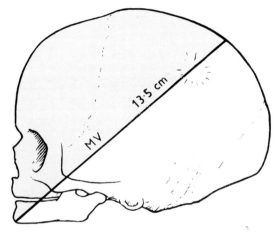

Fig. 30.32 Brow presentation. The mentovertical (MV) diameter, 13.5 cm, lies at the pelvic brim.

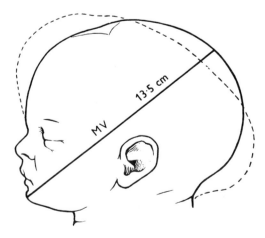

Fig. 30.33 Moulding in a brow presentation (dotted line). MV = mentovertical.

and the head is born by a mechanism somewhat similar to that of a persistent occipitoposterior position. However, the midwife should never expect such a favourable outcome. The mother should be warned about the possible course of labour and that a vaginal delivery is unlikely.

If there is no evidence of fetal compromise, the doctor may allow labour to continue for a short while in case further extension of the head converts the brow presentation to a face presentation. Occasionally spontaneous flexion may occur, resulting in a vertex presentation. If the head fails to descend and the brow presentation persists, a caesarean section is performed, with maternal consent.

Complications

These are the same as in a face presentation, except that obstructed labour requiring caesarean section is the probable rather than a possible outcome.

Breech presentation

Here the fetus lies longitudinally with the buttocks in the lower pole of the uterus. The presenting diameter is the bitrochanteric (10 cm) and the denominator the sacrum. This presentation occurs in approximately 3% of pregnancies at term. In mid-trimester the frequency is much higher because the greater proportion of amniotic fluid facilitates free movement of the fetus (Gimovsky & Hennigan 1995).

Types of breech presentation and position

There are six positions for a breech presentation, illustrated in Figures 30.34–30.39.

Breech with extended legs (frank breech) (Fig. 30.40)

The breech presents with the hips flexed and legs extended on the abdomen. Seventy per cent of breech presentations are of this type and it is particularly common in primigravidae whose good uterine muscle tone inhibits flexion of the legs and free turning of the fetus.

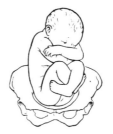

Fig. 30.34 Right sacroposterior.

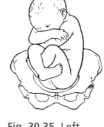

Fig. 30.35 Left sacroposterior.

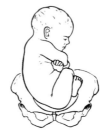

Fig. 30.36 Right sacrolateral.

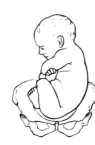

Fig. 30.37 Left sacrolateral.

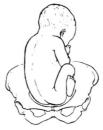

Fig. 30.38 Right sacroanterior.

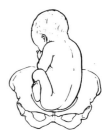

Fig. 30.39 Left sacroanterior.

Figs 30.34–30.39 Six positions in breech presentation.

Complete breech (Fig. 30.41)

The fetal attitude is one of complete flexion, with hips and knees both flexed and the feet tucked in beside the buttocks.

Footling breech (Fig. 30.42)

This is rare. One or both feet present because neither hips nor knees are fully flexed. The feet are lower than the buttocks, which distinguishes it from the complete breech.

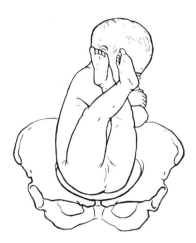

Fig. 30.40 Frank breech.

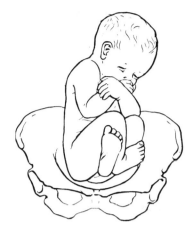

Fig. 30.41 Complete breech.

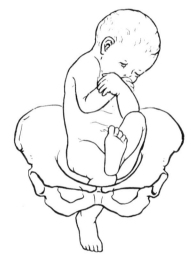

Fig. 30.42 Footling presentation.

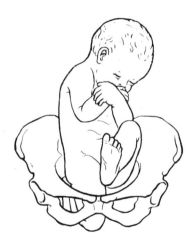

Fig. 30.43 Knee presentation.

Figs 30.40–30.43 Types of breech presentation.

Knee presentation (Fig. 30.43)

This is very rare. One or both hips are extended, with the knees flexed.

Causes

Often no cause is identified, but the following circumstances favour breech presentation.

Extended legs. Spontaneous cephalic version may be inhibited if the fetus lies with the legs extended, 'splinting' the back.

Preterm labour. As breech presentation is relatively common before 34 weeks' gestation, it follows that breech presentation is more common in preterm labours.

Multiple pregnancy. Multiple pregnancy limits the space available for each fetus to turn, which may result in one or more fetuses presenting by the breech.

Polyhydramnios. Distension of the uterine cavity by excessive amounts of amniotic fluid may cause the fetus to present by the breech.

Hydrocephaly. The increased size of the fetal head is more readily accommodated in the fundus.

Uterine abnormalities. Distortion of the uterine cavity by a septum or a fibroid may result in a breech presentation.

Placenta praevia. Some authorities believe that this may be a cause of breech presentation but there is some disagreement on this.

Antenatal diagnosis

Abdominal examination

Palpation. In primigravidae, diagnosis is more difficult because of their firm abdominal muscles. On palpation the lie is longitudinal with a soft presentation, which is more easily felt using Pawlik's grip (see Fig. 16.4, p. 264) The head can usually be felt in the fundus as a round hard mass, which may be made to move independently of the back by ballotting it with one or both hands. If the legs are extended, the feet may prevent such nodding. When the breech is anterior and the fetus well flexed, it may be difficult to locate the head but use of the combined grip in which the upper and lower poles are grasped simultaneously may aid diagnosis. The woman may complain of discomfort under her ribs, especially at night, owing to pressure of the head on the diaphragm.

Auscultation. When the breech has not passed through the pelvic brim the fetal heart is heard most clearly above the umbilicus. When the legs are extended the breech descends into the pelvis easily. The fetal heart is then heard at a lower level.

Ultrasound examination

This may be used to demonstrate a breech presentation.

X-ray examination

Although largely superseded by ultrasound, X-ray has the added advantage of allowing pelvimetry to be performed at the same time.

Diagnosis during labour

A previously unsuspected breech presentation may not be diagnosed until the woman is in established labour. If the legs are extended, the breech may feel like a head abdominally, and also on vaginal examination if the cervix is less than 3 cm dilated and the breech is high.

Abdominal examination

Breech presentation may be diagnosed on admission in labour.

Vaginal examination

The breech feels soft and irregular with no sutures palpable, although occasionally the sacrum may be mistaken for a hard head and the buttocks mistaken for caput succedaneum. The anus may be felt and fresh meconium on the examining finger is usually diagnostic. If the legs are extended (Fig. 30.44) the external genitalia are very evident but it must be remembered that these become oedematous. An oedematous vulva may be mistaken for a scrotum.

If a foot is felt (Fig. 30.45), the midwife should differentiate it from the hand. Toes are all the same length, they are shorter than fingers and the big toe cannot be opposed to other toes. The foot is at right angles to the leg, and the heel has no equivalent in the hand.

Presentation may be confirmed by ultrasound scan or X-ray.

Antenatal management

If the midwife suspects or detects a breech presentation at 36 weeks' gestation or later, she should refer the woman to a doctor. The presentation may be confirmed by ultrasound scan or occasionally by abdominal X-ray. There are differing opinions amongst obstetricians as to the management of breech presentation during pregnancy and a decision on management is usually deferred until near term.

External cephalic version

External cephalic version (ECV) is the use of external manipulation on the mother's abdomen to convert a breech to a cephalic presentation. The Royal College of

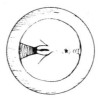

Fig. 30.44 No feet felt; the legs are extended.

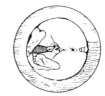

Fig. 30.45 Feet felt; complete breech presentation.

Figs 30.44 & 30.45 Vaginal touch pictures of left sacrolateral position.

Obstetricians and Gynaecologists (RCOG 1993) recommend that ECV should be offered at term by a practitioner skilled and experienced in the procedure and should be undertaken only in a unit where there are facilities for emergency delivery (CESDI 2000). The success of the procedure depends not only upon the skill and experience of the operator, but also upon the position and engagement of the fetus, liquor volume and maternal parity (Hofmeyr 2002).

It has been demonstrated that ECV can reduce the number of babies presenting by the breech at term by two-thirds, and therefore reduce the caesarean section rate for breech presentations (Hofmeyr 2002).

Turning the fetus from a breech to a cephalic presentation before 37 weeks' gestation does not reduce the incidence of breech birth or rate of caesarean section as it is likely to turn itself back spontaneously (Zhang et al 1993). The reasons for attempting ECV and the procedure itself should be explained to the woman so that she can give her informed consent to have ECV performed.

Method. An ultrasound scan is performed to localise the placenta and to confirm the position and presentation of the fetus.

If the procedure is to be performed under tocolysis then a cannula will be sited to allow venous access. A 30 minute CTG is performed to establish that the fetus is not compromised at the start of the procedure and maternal blood pressure and pulse are recorded.

The woman is asked to empty her bladder. The midwife then assists the woman into a comfortable supine position. The foot of the bed may be elevated to help free the breech from the pelvic brim. The abdomen is usually dusted with talcum powder to prevent pinching of the mother's skin during the procedure. Whilst ECV may be uncomfortable for the mother it should not be painful. The breech is displaced from the pelvic brim towards an iliac fossa. Simultaneous force is then used as with one hand on each pole the operator makes the fetus perform a forward somersault (Figs 30.46–30.48). If this is not successful then a backward somersault can be attempted. If the fetus does not turn easily, then the procedure is abandoned but may be tried again a few days later.

The fetal heart should be auscultated after the procedure, or a CTG performed.

If the woman is Rhesus negative an injection of anti-D immunoglobulin is given as prophylaxis against iso-immunisation caused by any placental separation. If the version is performed immediately prior to the onset of labour, this can be delayed until after delivery when the blood group of the baby is known. In this case if anti-D is needed, it must be given within 72 hours of the version.

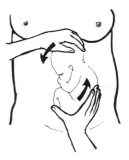

Fig. 30.46 The right hand lifts the breech out of the pelvis. The left hand makes the head follow the nose. Flexion of head and back is maintained throughout.

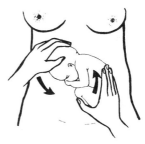

Fig. 30.47 Flexion is continued. The left hand brings the head downwards. The right hand pushes the breech upwards.

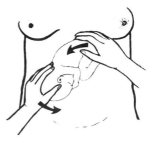

Fig. 30.48 Pressure is exerted on head and breech simultaneously until the head is lying at the pelvic brim.

Figs 30.46–30.48 External cephalic version.

Complications

Knotting of the umbilical cord. This should be suspected if bradycardia occurs and persists. The fetus is immediately turned back to a breech presentation. The woman is admitted for observation and, if necessary, caesarean section.

Separation of the placenta. The midwife should ask the woman to report pain or vaginal bleeding during and after the procedure.

Rupture of the membranes. If this occurs the cord may prolapse because neither the head nor the breech is engaged.

Relative contraindications. The presence of a uterine scar was previously thought to be an absolute contraindication to performing an ECV. Recent evidence, however, suggests that it is a safe and effective procedure used selectively in those women who have previously had a caesarean section (Flamm et al 1991, Shalev et al 1993).

Contraindications. These include:

- *pre-eclampsia or hypertension* – because of the increased risk of placental abruption
- *multiple pregnancy*
- *oligohydramnios* – because too much force has to be applied directly to the fetus and the version is likely to be unsuccessful
- *ruptured membranes*
- *a hydrocephalic fetus* – if a vaginal delivery is contemplated in preference to a caesarean section, the second stage is managed more easily when the fetus presents by the breech
- any condition that would require delivery by caesarean section.

Persistent breech presentation

When external version has been unsuccessful or has not been attempted, then at 37 weeks' gestation a discussion of the available options should take place between the mother and an experienced practitioner (CESDI 2000) and a decision made as to whether to perform an elective caesarean section or to attempt a vaginal delivery. The discussion and the plan formulated should be recorded. A planned caesarean section at term reduces the perinatal and neonatal mortality and morbidity but there is an increased risk of maternal morbidity (Hofmeyr & Hannah 2002). 'An increased effort should be made to diagnose presentation at 37 weeks for all women planning to deliver outside an obstetric unit' (CESDI 2000, p. 37).

Assessment for vaginal delivery. Any doubt as to the capacity of the pelvis to accommodate the fetal head must be resolved before the buttocks are delivered and the head attempts to enter the pelvic brim. At this point the fetus begins to be deprived of oxygen and a last minute decision to perform caesarean section may be too late.

Fetal size. This, especially in relation to maternal size, can be assessed on abdominal palpation but is more accurately judged in association with an ultrasound examination.

Pelvic capacity. This can be judged on vaginal assessment (see Ch. 16), but it is usual to perform a lateral pelvimetry. This will show the shape of the sacrum and give accurate measurements of the anteroposterior diameters of the pelvic brim, cavity and outlet. No studies have confirmed the value of this procedure in selecting women who are likely to succeed in achieving a vaginal delivery of a breech or in improving perinatal outcome (Hannah 1994). In a multigravida, information about the type of delivery and the size of previous babies when compared with the size of the present fetus can be helpful.

Mechanism of left sacroanterior position

- The lie is longitudinal.
- The attitude is one of complete flexion.
- The presentation is breech.
- The position is left sacroanterior.
- The denominator is the sacrum.
- The presenting part is the anterior (left) buttock.
- The bitrochanteric diameter, 10 cm, enters the pelvis in the left oblique diameter of the brim.
- The sacrum points to the left iliopectineal eminence.

Compaction. Descent takes place with increasing compaction, owing to increased flexion of the limbs.

Internal rotation of the buttocks. The anterior buttock reaches the pelvic floor first and rotates forwards 1/8 of a circle along the right side of the pelvis to lie underneath the symphysis pubis. The bitrochanteric diameter is now in the anteroposterior diameter of the outlet.

Lateral flexion of the body. The anterior buttock escapes under the symphysis pubis, the posterior buttock sweeps the perineum and the buttocks are born by a movement of lateral flexion.

Restitution of the buttocks. The anterior buttock turns slightly to the mother's right side.

Internal rotation of the shoulders. The shoulders enter the pelvis in the same oblique diameter as the buttocks, the left oblique. The anterior shoulder rotates forwards 1/8 of a circle along the right side of the pelvis and escapes under the symphysis pubis; the posterior shoulder sweeps the perineum and the shoulders are born.

Internal rotation of the head. The head enters the pelvis with the sagittal suture in the transverse diameter of the brim. The occiput rotates forwards along the left side and the suboccipital region (the nape of the neck) impinges on the undersurface of the symphysis pubis.

External rotation of the body. At the same time the body turns so that the back is uppermost.

Birth of the head. The chin, face and sinciput sweep the perineum and the head is born in a flexed attitude.

Management of labour

Vaginal delivery should be presented to the woman as the norm for breech delivery (MIDIRS 1997), provided there are no complications, and it should be made clear that there is a risk of delivery by caesarean section.

In a retrospective study of breech births (Hofmeyr 1989) the outcome for breech presentation diagnosed in labour has been shown to be as good, in all respects, as that for those who were selected as suitable for a vaginal birth; if vaginal delivery is selected with a breech presentation there is approximately a 50% chance of a successful vaginal delivery. Careful assessment should be made at the start of labour and anticipated labour management should be reviewed and a 'consultant obstetrician informed of a breech presentation in labour' (CESDI 2000, p. 37).

First stage

Basic care during this stage is the same as in normal labour (see Chs 24, 25). Although the breech with extended legs fits the cervix quite well, the complete breech is a less well-fitting presenting part and the membranes tend to rupture early. For this reason there is an increased risk of cord prolapse, and a vaginal examination is performed to exclude this as soon as the membranes rupture. If they do not rupture spontaneously at an early stage, it is considered safer to leave them intact until labour is well established and the breech is at the level of the ischial spines. Meconium-stained liquor is sometimes found owing to compression of the fetal abdomen and is not always a sign of fetal compromise.

Analgesia. (See Ch. 26 for analgesia and Ch. 25 for support in labour.) An epidural block may be offered to a woman with a breech presentation as it inhibits the urge to push prematurely. However, there is no evidence to suggest that this is indicated. Epidural analgesia has been associated with prolongation of the second stage of labour and has not been associated with any unique advantages for a woman delivering a breech at term (Chadha et al 1992).

Second stage

Full dilatation of the cervix should always be confirmed by vaginal examination before the woman commences active pushing. This is because in a footling presentation a foot may appear at the vulva when the cervix is only partially dilated; or when the legs are extended, particularly if the fetus is small, the breech may slip through an incompletely dilated cervix. In either case, the head may be trapped by the cervix when the fetus is partially delivered.

If the delivery is taking place in hospital it is usual to inform the obstetrician of the onset of the second stage; a paediatrician should be present for delivery and it is usual to inform the anaesthetist also in case a general anaesthetic is required. Active pushing is not commenced until the buttocks are distending the vulva. Failure of the breech to descend on to the perineum in the second stage despite good contractions may indicate a need for caesarean section.

Types of delivery

Spontaneous breech delivery. The delivery occurs with little assistance from the attendant.

Assisted breech delivery. The buttocks are born spontaneously, but some assistance is necessary for delivery of extended legs or arms and the head.

Breech extraction. This is a manipulative delivery carried out by an obstetrician and is performed to hasten delivery in an emergency situation such as fetal compromise.

Management of delivery

The midwife should discuss this with the woman beforehand so that she understands the need for the attendance of the doctors. The delivery is explained in order to help her to appreciate the importance of not pushing until full dilatation of the cervix has been confirmed.

When the buttocks are distending the perineum, the woman is placed in the lithotomy position (unless an upright position is chosen – see below) and the vulva is swabbed and draped with sterile towels. The bladder must be empty and it is usually catheterised at this stage. If epidural analgesia is not being used, the perineum is infiltrated with up to 10 ml of 0.5% plain lidocaine (lignocaine) prior to an episiotomy being performed. (Pudendal block is sometimes used by a doctor.)

The woman is encouraged to push with the contractions and the buttocks are delivered spontaneously. If the legs are flexed, the feet disengage at the vulva and the baby is born as far as the umbilicus. A loop of cord is gently pulled down to avoid traction on the umbilicus. Spasm of the cord vessels can be caused by manipulating the cord or by stretching it. If the cord is being nipped behind the pubic bone it should be moved to one side. The midwife should feel for the elbows, which are usually on the chest. If so, the arms will escape with the next contraction. If the arms are not felt, they are extended.

Delivery of the shoulders. The uterine contractions and the weight of the body will bring the shoulders down on to the pelvic floor where they will rotate into the anteroposterior diameter of the outlet.

It is helpful to wrap a small towel around the baby's hips, which preserves warmth and improves the grip on the slippery skin. The midwife now grasps the baby by the iliac crests with her thumbs held parallel over his sacrum and tilts the baby towards the maternal sacrum in order to free the anterior shoulder.

When the anterior shoulder has escaped, the buttocks are lifted towards the mother's abdomen to enable the posterior shoulder and arm to pass over the perineum (Fig. 30.49). As the shoulders are born the head enters the pelvic brim and descends through the pelvis with the sagittal suture in the transverse diameter. The back must remain lateral until this has happened but will afterwards be turned uppermost. If the back is turned upwards too soon, the anteroposterior diameter of the head will enter the anteroposterior diameter of the brim and may become extended. The shoulders may then become impacted at the outlet and the extended head may cause difficulty.

Delivery of the head. When the back has been turned the infant is allowed to hang from the vulva without support. The baby's weight brings the head on to the pelvic floor on which the occiput rotates forwards. The sagittal suture is now in the anteroposterior diameter of the outlet. If rotation of the head fails to take place, two fingers should be placed on the malar bones and the head rotated. The baby can be allowed to hang for 1 or 2 minutes. Gradually the neck elongates, the hair-line appears and the suboccipital region can be felt. Controlled delivery of the head is vital to avoid any sudden change in intracranial pressure and subsequent cerebral haemorrhage. There are three methods used.

Forceps delivery. Most breech deliveries are performed by an obstetrician, who will apply forceps to the after-coming head to achieve a controlled delivery.

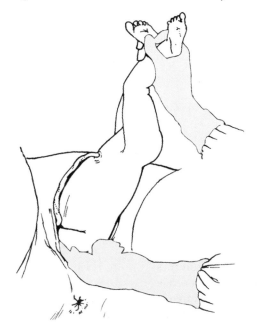

Fig. 30.49 Delivery of the posterior shoulder in a breech presentation.

Burns Marshall method. The midwife or doctor stands facing away from the mother and, with the left hand, grasps the baby's ankles from behind with forefinger between the two (Fig. 30.50A). The baby is kept on the stretch with sufficient traction to prevent the neck from bending backwards and being fractured. The sub-occipital region, and not the neck, should pivot under the apex of the pubic arch or the spinal cord may be crushed. The feet are taken up through an arc of 180° until the mouth and nose are free at the vulva. The right hand may guard the perineum in order to prevent sudden escape of the head. An assistant may now clear the airway and the baby will breathe. The mother should be asked to take deliberate, regular breaths which allow the vault of the skull to escape gradually, taking 2 or 3 minutes (Fig. 30.50B).

Mauriceau–Smellie–Veit manoeuvre (jaw flexion and shoulder traction; Fig. 30.51). This is mainly used when there is delay in descent of the head because of extension. Excessive shoulder traction may cause Erb's palsy.

The baby is laid astride the right arm with the palm supporting the chest. Two fingers are inserted well back into the mouth to pull the jaw downwards and flex the head. (If they can be accommodated, two fingers may be placed on the malar bones with the middle finger in the mouth.) Two fingers of the left hand are hooked over the shoulders with the middle finger pushing up the occiput to aid flexion. Traction is applied to draw the head out of the vagina and, when the suboccipital region appears, the body is lifted to assist the head to pivot around the symphysis pubis. The speed of delivery of the head must be controlled so that it does not emerge suddenly like a cork popping out of a bottle. Once the face is free, the airways may be cleared and the vault is delivered slowly.

Alternative positions. When the woman has chosen to deliver in an alternative position, it is the upright or supported squat that is the most suitable. The delivery techniques described above will be adapted accordingly and the midwife will observe and encourage the spontaneous mechanism of delivery.

Use of uterotonics for third stage. These are withheld until the head is delivered.

Delivery of extended legs. The frank breech descends more rapidly during the first stage of labour. The cervix dilates more quickly and there is a risk of the cord becoming compressed between the legs and the body.

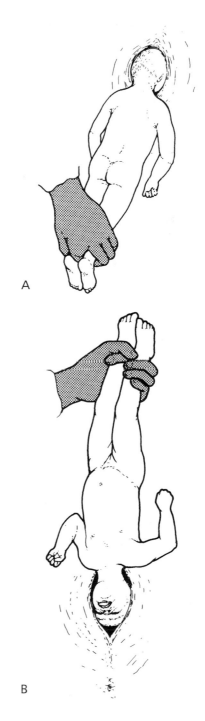

A

B

Fig. 30.50 Burns Marshall method of delivering the after-coming head of a breech presentation: (A) The baby is grasped by the feet and held on the stretch. (B) The mouth and nose are free. The vault of the head is delivered slowly.

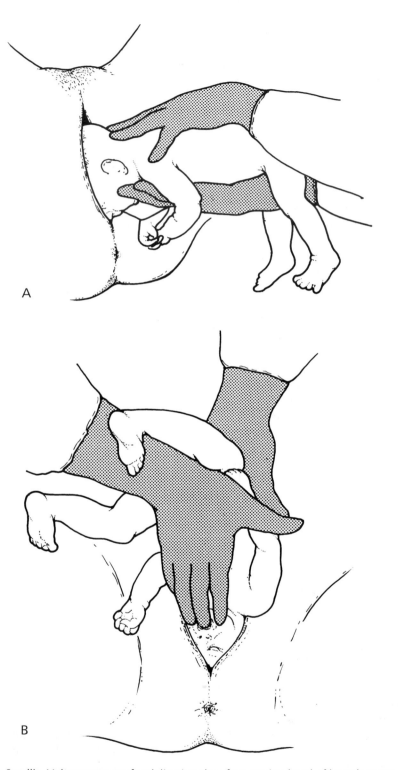

Fig. 30.51 Mauriceau–Smellie–Veit manoeuvre for delivering the after-coming head of breech presentation (see text): (A) The hands are in position before the body is lifted. (B) Extraction of the head.

Cord prolapse is less likely than in other breech presentations because the frank breech is a better-fitting presenting part. Delay may occur at the outlet because the legs splint the body and impede lateral flexion of the spine.

The baby can be born with legs extended but assistance is usually required. When the popliteal fossae appear at the vulva, two fingers are placed along the length of one thigh with the fingertips in the fossa. The leg is swept to the side of the abdomen (abducting the hip) and the knee is flexed by the pressure on its under surface. As this movement is continued the lower part of the leg will emerge from the vagina (Fig. 30.52). This process should be repeated in order to deliver the second leg. The knee is a hinge joint, which bends in one direction only. If the knee is pulled forwards from the abdomen, severe injury to the joint can result.

Delivery of extended arms. Extended arms are diagnosed when the elbows are not felt on the chest after the umbilicus is born. Prompt action must be taken to avoid delay and consequent hypoxia. This may be dealt with by using the Løvset manoeuvre (Figs 30.53 and 30.54). This is a combination of rotation and downward traction that may be employed to deliver the arms whatever position they are in. The direction of rotation must always bring the back uppermost and the arms are delivered from under the pubic arch.

When the umbilicus is born and the shoulders are in the anteroposterior diameter, the baby is grasped by the iliac crests with the thumbs over the sacrum. Downward traction is applied until the axilla is visible.

Maintaining downward traction throughout, the body is rotated through half a circle, 180°, starting by turning the back uppermost. The friction of the posterior arm against the pubic bone as the shoulder becomes anterior sweeps the arm in front of the face. The movement allows the shoulders to enter the pelvis in the transverse diameter.

The arm which is now anterior is delivered. The first two fingers of the hand that is on the same side as the baby's back are used to splint the humerus and draw it down over the chest as the elbow is flexed.

The body is now rotated back in the opposite direction and the second arm delivered in a similar fashion.

Delay in delivery of the head.

Extended head. If, when the body has been allowed to hang, the neck and hair-line are not visible, it is probable that the head is extended. This may be dealt

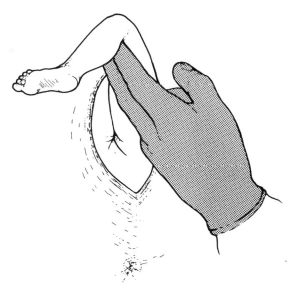

Fig. 30.52 Assisting delivery of extended leg by pressure on popliteal fossa.

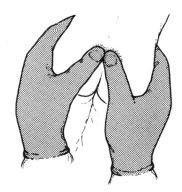

Fig. 30.53 Correct grasp for Løvset manoeuvre.

with by the use of forceps or the Mauriceau–Smellie–Veit manoeuvre. If the head is trapped in an incompletely dilated cervix, an air channel can be created to enable the baby to breathe pending intervention. This is done by inserting two fingers or a Sim's speculum in front of the baby's face and holding the vaginal wall away from the nose. Moisture is mopped away and the airways are cleared. Attempts to release the head from the cervix result in high fetal morbidity and mortality. The McRoberts manoeuvre has been suggested as a method to facilitate the release of the fetal head (Shushan & Younis 1992). The McRoberts manoeuvre requires the woman to lie flat on her back and bring her knees up to her abdomen with hips abducted. This manoeuvre, more commonly used to relieve shoulder dystocia, is described in detail in Chapter 32.

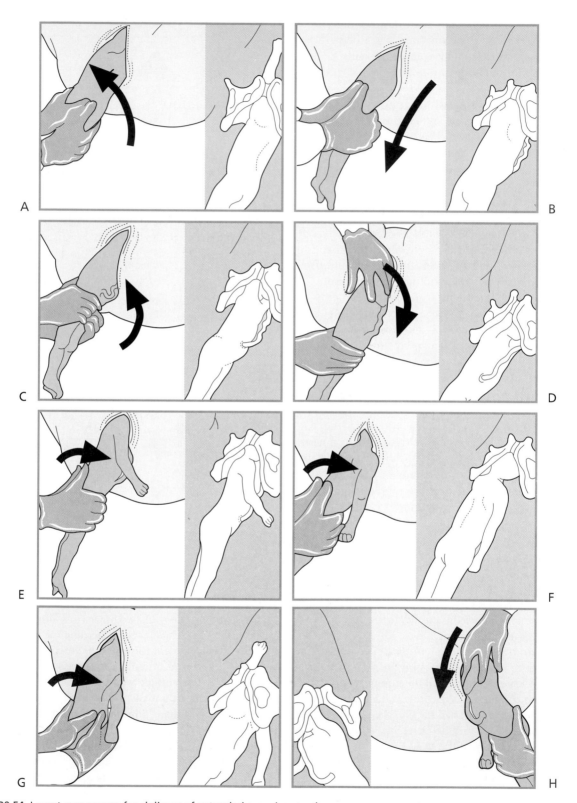

A

B

C

D

E

F

G

H

Fig. 30.54 Løvset manoeuvre for delivery of extended arms (see text).

Posterior rotation of the occiput. This malrotation of the head is rare and is usually the result of mismanagement, for the back should be turned upwards after the shoulders are born.

To deliver the head with the occiput posterior, the chin and face are permitted to escape under the symphysis pubis as far as the root of the nose and the baby is then lifted up towards the mother's abdomen to allow the occiput to sweep the perineum.

Complications

Apart from those difficulties already mentioned, other complications can arise, most of which affect the fetus. Many of these can be avoided by allowing only an experienced operator, or a closely supervised learner, to deliver the baby.

Impacted breech

Labour becomes obstructed when the fetus is disproportionately large for the size of the maternal pelvis.

Cord prolapse (see Ch. 32)

This is more common in a flexed or footling breech, as these have ill-fitting presenting parts.

Birth injury

Superficial tissue damage. The midwife must warn the mother and her partner of the bruising that may be expected following delivery. Oedema and bruising of the baby's genitalia may be caused by pressure on the cervix. In a footling breech a prolapsed foot that lies in the vagina or at the vulva for a long time may become very oedematous and discoloured.

If the delivery is performed correctly the following are less likely to occur:

Fractures of humerus, clavicle or femur or dislocation of shoulder or hip. These can be caused during delivery of extended arms or legs.

Erb's palsy. This can be caused when the brachial plexus is damaged. The brachial plexus can be damaged at delivery by twisting the baby's neck (see Plate 30).

Trauma to internal organs. There may be especially a ruptured liver or spleen, which is produced by grasping the abdomen.

Damage to the adrenals. This can be caused by grasping the baby's abdomen, leading to shock caused by adrenaline release.

Spinal cord damage or fracture of the spine. This can be caused by bending the body backwards over the symphysis pubis while delivering the head.

Intracranial haemorrhage. This may be caused by rapid delivery of the head, which has had no opportunity to mould. *Hypoxia* may also cause intracranial haemorrhage.

Fetal hypoxia

This may be due to cord prolapse or cord compression or to premature separation of the placenta.

Premature separation of the placenta

Considerable retraction of the uterus takes place while the head is still in the vagina and the placenta begins to separate. Excessive delay in delivery of the head may cause severe hypoxia in the fetus.

Maternal trauma

The maternal complications of a breech delivery are the same as found in other operative vaginal deliveries (see Ch. 32).

Shoulder presentation

When the fetus lies with its long axis across the long axis of the uterus (*transverse lie*) the shoulder is most likely to present. Occasionally the lie is oblique but this does not persist as the uterine contractions during labour make it longitudinal or transverse.

Shoulder presentation occurs in approximately 1 : 300 pregnancies near term. Only 17% of these cases remain as a transverse lie at the onset of labour; the majority are multigravidae (Gimovsky & Hennigan 1995). The head lies on one side of the abdomen, with the breech at a slightly higher level on the other. The fetal back may be anterior or posterior (Figs 30.55 and 30.56).

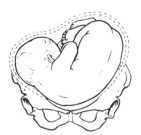 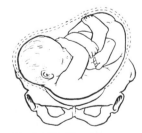

Fig. 30.55 Shoulder presentation, dorsoanterior.

Fig. 30.56 Shoulder presentation, dorsoposterior.

Causes

Maternal

Before term, transverse or oblique lie may be transitory, related to maternal position or displacement of the presenting part by an overextended bladder prior to ultrasound examination (Hofmeyr 1989). Other causes are described below.

Lax abdominal and uterine muscles. This is the most common cause and is found in multigravidae, particularly those of high parity.

Uterine abnormality. A bicornuate or subseptate uterus may result in a transverse lie – as, more rarely, may a cervical or low uterine fibroid.

Contracted pelvis. Rarely, this may prevent the head from entering the pelvic brim.

Fetal

Preterm pregnancy. The amount of amniotic fluid in relation to the fetus is greater, allowing the fetus more mobility than at term.

Multiple pregnancy. There is a possibility of poly-hydramnios but the presence of more than one fetus reduces the room for manoeuvre when amounts of liquor are normal. It is the second twin that more commonly adopts this lie after delivery of the first fetus.

Polyhydramnios. The distended uterus is globular and the fetus can move freely in the excessive liquor.

Macerated fetus. Lack of muscle tone causes the fetus to slump down into the lower pole of the uterus.

Placenta praevia. This may prevent the head from entering the pelvic brim.

Antenatal diagnosis

On abdominal palpation. The uterus appears broad and the fundal height is less than expected for the period of gestation. On pelvic and fundal palpation, neither head nor breech is felt. The mobile head is found on one side of the abdomen and the breech at a slightly higher level on the other.

Ultrasound. An ultrasound scan may be used to confirm the lie and presentation.

Intrapartum diagnosis

On abdominal palpation. The findings are as above but when the membranes have ruptured the irregular outline of the uterus is more marked. If the uterus is contracting strongly and becomes moulded around the fetus, palpation is very difficult. The pelvis is no longer empty, the shoulder being wedged into it.

On vaginal examination. *This should not be performed without first excluding placenta praevia.* In early labour the presenting part may not be felt. The membranes usually rupture early because of the ill-fitting presenting part, with a high risk of cord prolapse.

If the labour has been in progress for some time the shoulder may be felt as a soft irregular mass. It is sometimes possible to palpate the ribs, their characteristic grid-iron pattern being diagnostic (Fig. 30.57). When the shoulder enters the pelvic brim an arm may prolapse; this should be differentiated from a leg. The hand is not at right angles to the arm, the fingers are longer than toes and of unequal length and the thumb can be opposed. No os calcis can be felt and the palm is shorter than the sole. If the arm is flexed, an elbow feels sharper than a knee.

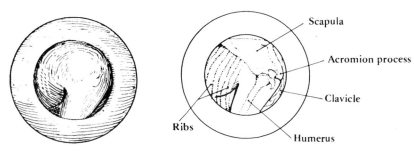

Fig. 30.57 Vaginal touch picture of shoulder presentation.

Possible outcome

There is no mechanism for delivery of a shoulder presentation. If this persists in labour, delivery must be by caesarean section to avoid obstructed labour and subsequent uterine rupture (see Ch. 32).

Whenever the midwife detects a transverse lie she must obtain medical assistance.

Management

Antenatal

A cause must be sought before deciding on a course of management. Ultrasound examination can detect placenta praevia or uterine abnormalities, whilst X-ray pelvimetry will demonstrate a contracted pelvis (see Ch. 7). Any of these causes requires elective caesarean section. Once they have been excluded, ECV (see p. 566) may be attempted. If this fails, or if the lie is again transverse at the next antenatal visit, the woman is admitted to hospital while further investigations into the cause are made. She frequently remains there until delivery because of the risk of cord prolapse if the membranes rupture.

Intrapartum

If a transverse lie is detected in early labour while the membranes are still intact, the doctor may attempt an ECV followed, if this is successful, by a controlled rupture of the membranes. (This may be considered before labour in some cases (Hofmeyr 2002).) If the membranes have already ruptured spontaneously, a vaginal examination must be performed immediately to detect possible cord prolapse.

Immediate caesarean section must be performed:

- if the cord prolapses
- when the membranes are already ruptured
- when ECV is unsuccessful
- when labour has already been in progress for some hours.

Complications

Prolapsed cord (see Ch. 32)

This may occur when the membranes rupture.

Prolapsed arm

This may occur when the membranes have ruptured and the shoulder has become impacted. Delivery should be by immediate caesarean section.

Neglected shoulder presentation

The shoulder becomes impacted, having been forced down and wedged into the pelvic brim. The membranes have ruptured spontaneously and if the arm has prolapsed it becomes blue and oedematous. The uterus goes into a state of tonic contraction, the overstretched lower segment is tender to touch and the fetal heartbeat may be absent. All the maternal signs of obstructed labour are present (see Ch. 29) and the outcome, if not treated in time, is a ruptured uterus and a stillbirth.

With adequate supervision both antenatally and during labour this should never occur.

Treatment. An immediate caesarean section is performed under general anaesthetic regardless of whether the fetus is alive or dead, as attempts at manipulative procedures or destructive operations can be dangerous for the mother and may result in uterine rupture.

Unstable lie

The lie is defined as *unstable* when after 36 weeks' gestation, instead of remaining longitudinal, it varies from one examination to another between longitudinal and oblique or transverse.

Causes

Any condition in late pregnancy that increases the mobility of the fetus or prevents the head from entering the pelvic brim may cause this.

Maternal

These include:

- lax uterine muscles in multigravidae
- contracted pelvis.

Fetal

These include:

- polyhydramnios
- placenta praevia.

Management

Antenatal

It may be advisable for the woman to be admitted to hospital to avoid unsupervised onset of labour with a transverse lie. An alternative is for the woman to admit herself to the labour ward as soon as labour commences. The risk associated with the possibility of rupture of membranes and cord prolapse should be emphasised if the mother chooses to remain at home.

Ultrasonography is used to rule out placenta praevia. Attempts will be made to correct the abnormal presentation by ECV. If unsuccessful, caesarean section is considered.

Intrapartum

Many obstetricians induce labour after 38 weeks' gestation, having first ensured that the lie is longitudinal; the induction may be performed by commencing an intravenous infusion of oxytocin to stimulate contractions. A controlled rupture of the membranes is performed so that the head enters the pelvis.

The midwife should ensure that the woman has an empty rectum and bladder before the procedure, as a loaded rectum or full bladder can prevent the presenting part from entering the pelvis. She should palpate the abdomen at frequent intervals to ensure that the lie remains longitudinal and to assess the descent of the head. Labour is regarded as a trial (see Ch. 29).

Complications

If labour commences with the lie other than longitudinal, the complications are the same as for a transverse lie.

Compound presentation

When a hand, or occasionally a foot, lies alongside the head, the presentation is said to be *compound*. This tends to occur with a small fetus or roomy pelvis and seldom is difficulty encountered except in cases where it is associated with a flat pelvis. On rare occasions the head, hand and foot are felt in the vagina – a serious situation that may occur with a dead fetus.

If diagnosed during the first stage of labour, medical aid must be sought. If, during the second stage, the midwife sees a hand presenting alongside the vertex, she could try to hold the hand back.

REFERENCES

Bhal P S, Davies N J, Chung T 1998 A population study of face and brow presentation. Journal of Obstetrics and Gynaecology 18(3):231–235

Biancuzzo M 1993 How to recognise and rotate an occiput posterior fetus. American Journal of Nursing 93(3):38–41

CESDI (Confidential enquiry into stillbirths and deaths in infancy) 2000 7th annual report. Maternal and Child Health Research Consortium, London

Chadha Y C, Mahmood T A, Dick M J 1992 Breech delivery and epidural analgesia. British Journal of Obstetrics and Gynaecology 99(2):96–100

El Halta V 1995 Posterior labour: a pain in the back. Midwifery Today 36:19–21

El Halta 1998 Preventing prolonged labour. Midwifery Today 46:22–27

Flamm B L, Fried M, Lonky N M, Giles W A 1991 External cephalic version after previous cesarean section. American Journal of Obstetrics and Gynecology 165(2):370–372

Gardberg M, Laakkonen E, Salevaara M 1998 Intrapartum sonography and persistent occiput posterior position: a study of 408 deliveries. Obstetrics and Gynecology 91(5):1, 746–749

Gimovsky M, Hennigan C 1995 Abnormal fetal presentations. Current Opinion in Obstetrics and Gynecology 7(6):482–485

Hannah W J 1994 The Canadian consensus on breech management at term. Society of Obstetricians and Gynaecologists of Canada policy statement. Journal of the Society of Obstetricians and Gynaecologists of Canada 16(6):1839–1848

Hofmeyr G J 1989 Breech presentation and abnormal lie in late pregnancy. In: Chalmers I, Enkin M W, Keirse M J N C (eds) Effective care in pregnancy and childbirth. Oxford University Press, Oxford, p 653–665

Hofmeyr G J 2002 External cephalic version at term. In: Neilson J P, Crowther C A, Hodnett E D, Hofmeyr G J, Keirse M J N C (eds) Pregnancy and childbirth module of the Cochrane Database of Systematic Reviews (updated 05 December 1996). In: The Cochrane Library, Issue 1. Update Software, Oxford

Hofmeyr G J, Hannah M E 2002 Planned caesarean section for term breech delivery (Cochrane review). In: The Cochrane Library, Issue 1. Update Software, Oxford

Hofmeyr G J, Kulier R 2002 Hands/knees posture in pregnancy in late pregnancy or labour for fetal malposition (lateral or posterior) (Cochrane review) In: The Cochrane Library, Issue 1. Update Software, Oxford

MIDIRS 1997 Informed choice for professionals. Number 9 breech presentation – options for care. MIDIRS and The NHS Centre for Reviews and Dissemination, Bristol

Neuman M, Beller U, Lavie O 1994 Intrapartum bimanual tocolytic-assisted reversal of face presentation: preliminary report. Obstetrics and Gynecology 84(10):146–148

Pearl M L, Roberts J M, Laros R K, Hurd W W 1993 Vaginal delivery from the persistent occiput posterior position. Influence on maternal and neonatal morbidity. Journal of Reproductive Medicine 38(12):955–961

RCOG (Royal College of Obstetricians and Gynaecologists) 1993 Effective procedures in obstetrics suitable for audit. Medical Audit Unit, RCOG, Manchester, p 2

Shalev E, Battino S, Giladi Y 1993 External cephalic version at term using tocolysis. Acta Obstetrica et Gynecologica Scandinavica 72(6):455–457

Shushan A, Younis J S 1992 McRoberts manoeuvre for the management of the aftercoming head in breech deliveries. Gynecology and Obstetric Investigations 34(3):188–189

Sutton J 1996 Birth: medical emergency or engineering miracle? A midwifery approach to keeping birth normal. MIDIRS Digest 6(2):170–173

Thornton J G, Lilford R J 1994 Active management of labour: current knowledge and research issues. British Medical Journal 309(6951):366–369

Zhang J, Bowes W A, Fortney J A 1993 Efficacy of external cephalic version: a review. Obstetrics and Gynecology 82(2):306–312

FURTHER READING

Ben-Arie A, Kogan S, Schachter M 1995 The impact of external cephalic version on the rate of vaginal and cesarean breech deliveries: a 3-year cumulative experience. European Journal of Obstetrics and Gynecology and Reproductive Biology 63(2):125–129

This paper remains relevant to current practice, an interesting European perspective on the experience of ECV and breech deliveries.

Bhal P S, Davies N J, Chung T 1998 A population study of face and brow presentation. Journal of Obstetrics and Gynaecology 18(3):231–235

Brow and face presentations are rare and there are few papers written on the subject, this is an interesting and useful paper for both the student and qualified midwives.

CESDI (Confidential enquiry into stillbirths and deaths in infancy) 2000 7th annual report. Maternal and Child Health Research Consortium, London

The 7th CESDI report focuses on breech presentation at the onset of labour. Recommendations for management of breech presentation and training of staff should be read in full.

Chapman K 2000 Aetiology and management of the secondary brow. Journal of Obstetrics and Gynaecology 20:(1)39–44

Six cases of vaginal delivery from a brow presentation over a career of 39 years are recorded in this article. Most midwives will never see a brow presentation deliver vaginally, this is a fascinating record from a long career.

Gardberg M, Tuppurainen M 1994 Anterior placental location predisposes for occiput posterior presentation near term. Acta Obstetrica et Gynecologica Scandinavica 73(2):151–152

In a series of 325 ultrasound examinations the authors demonstrated an association between an anteriorly situated placenta and OP position after 36 weeks of pregnancy.

Gardberg M, Laakkonen E, Salevaara M 1998 Intrapartum sonography and persistant occiput posterior position: a study of 408 deliveries. Obstetrics and Gynecology 91(5):1, 746–749

This study showed that in most cases occipitoposterior position develops through a malrotation and only one-third through absence of rotation from an initially occiput posterior position.

31 Operative Deliveries

Adela Hamilton

CHAPTER CONTENTS

The aim of this chapter is to examine alternative methods of delivery that are used when the mother is unable to give birth without medical or surgical assistance. The role of the midwife will be explored and the importance of providing complete and comprehensive information to the woman will be emphasised.

This chapter aims to:

- identify the midwifery care in relation to preparation for caesarean, forceps and ventouse birth

- describe the role of the midwife in relation to prevention of complications following assisted birth and also in relation to informed consent

- consider the various techniques used for caesarean, forceps and ventouse birth, and the skills required by the midwife to improve the experience of assisted childbirth, for the mother and her partner

- discuss the changing role of the midwife in relation to medical intervention, considering such innovations as the midwife ventouse practitioner.

Caesarean section

Caesarean section is described as being an operative procedure, that is carried out under anaesthesia whereby the fetus, placenta and membranes are delivered through an incision in the abdominal wall and the uterus. This is usually carried out after viability has been reached (i.e. 24 weeks of gestation onwards).

The operative procedure

There are two layers of pelvic peritoneum and the non-gravid uterus is a pelvic organ closely covered by a layer of pelvic peritoneum. As pregnancy advances, the uterus grows up into the abdomen and this peritoneum rises up with the uterus and comes into contact with the abdominal peritoneum. Each of these layers must be incised and repaired. The abdominal peritoneum is situated below the abdominal muscle layer. The anatomical layers are:

- skin
- fat
- rectus sheath
- muscle (rectus abdominis)
- abdominal peritoneum
- pelvic peritoneum
- uterine muscle.

The operation most commonly carried out is the lower uterine segment caesarean section (LUSCS). A pfannensteil or bikini line incision is usually performed. The lower segment incision is in the less muscular and active part of the uterus and heals better. The main reason for preferring the lower uterine segment technique is the reduced incidence of dehiscence of the uterine scar in subsequent pregnancy (Al-Azzawi 1990). A classical or vertical incision of the uterus may be the only choice in such situations as implantation of the placenta on the lower anterior uterine wall, in the presence of dense adhesions from previous surgery, or in the case of a large fetus with the shoulder impacted in the maternal pelvis. The risk and disadvantage of this is that the uterine incision is more likely to rupture during a subsequent birth.

The abdomen is opened and the loose fold of the peritoneum over the anterior aspect of the lower uterine segment and above the bladder is incised. The operator continues to incise this further, to visualise the fundus of the bladder, which is then pushed down and away from the surgeon. The uterus is incised transversely. The surgeon directs the fetal head out while the assistant applies fundal pressure to help the delivery of the baby. Oxytocics may be given by the anaesthetist after delivery of the baby and clamping of the cord. When the baby and placenta have been delivered the uterus is sutured. This is usually done in two layers. The peritoneum may then be closed over the uterine wound to exclude it from the peritoneal cavity. The rectus sheath is closed, then the layer of fat and finally the skin is sutured with the surgeon's choice of material; commonly vicryl, a braided polyglactin preparation, is used for this.

Preparation

The usual preoperative preparation is observed – that is, an anaesthetic chart/preoperative assessment, weight, and observations of blood pressure, pulse and temperature – which serve as a baseline. Gowning and removal of make-up and jewellery (or taping of rings) will be carried out. The woman is visited by the anaesthetist preoperatively, and assessed.

Results of any blood tests that have been requested are obtained and a full blood count is carried out. Blood is grouped and saved. In the case of pre-eclampsia, urea and electrolyte levels will be examined and clotting factors acquired. The woman will have fasted and have taken the prescribed antacid therapy. Attitudes and practices vary regarding pubic shaving.

The woman may prefer to be catheterised in the theatre under epidural or general anaesthetic, but it may be more private to do this in her room, before entering the operating theatre where others are present.

Positioning of the woman

As the woman will need to lie flat it is essential that a wedge or cushion is used, or the table is tilted, to direct the weight of the gravid uterus away from the inferior vena cava. Supine hypotensive syndrome is thus avoided.

Aortocaval compression is caused by the weight of the gravid uterus partially occluding the inferior vena cava. Venous return is then reduced, followed by a fall in cardiac output. The effect can be a compromise of placental perfusion and a fall in blood pressure, which is often referred to as *supine hypotension syndrome*. This sequence of events is not only associated with general anaesthesia but may occur at any time in late pregnancy or during labour. It will always occur if the woman lies supine in late pregnancy. Most women do not find it comfortable to lie flat but the midwife must take steps to ensure that the woman in labour does not do so. If emergency caesarean section is being performed because of fetal compromise, aortocaval occlusion will increase this and cause further fetal hypoxia.

Caesarean section – some statistics

Internationally, the caesarean section rate is on the increase, with the exception of Norway and Sweden (Chaffer & Royle 2000). It is also well known that the northern European countries have not only the lowest caesarean section rates, but also the lowest perinatal mortality rates (Currie 1987).

The World Health Organization recommends that a caesarean section rate of 10–15% should not be exceeded and a survey of UK consultants advise a 12% rate (Francome et al 1993). Dimond (1999) states that caesarean section rates rose from 4.8% in 1970 to 15.6% in 1995. The results of the National Sentinel Caesarean Section Audit (RCOG 2001) show that caesarean section rates in 2000 were highest in Wales, at 24.2% in 2000 and in Northern Ireland, at 23.9% in 2000–1. Fear of litigation is thought to be a major contributing factor, but in Canada, where litigation is not widespread, the rates are still rising.

The drive to lower caesarean section rates is economic, but other vital perspectives must be appraised. Chaffer & Royle (2000) state that, by reducing the caesarean section rate by 5%, two to seven maternal deaths could be prevented annually in Britain. The fifth report of the Confidential Enquiries into Maternal Deaths in the UK (Lewis & Drife 2001) states that there have been significant decreases in deaths from pulmonary embolism and sepsis following caesarean section. This is said to be due to implementation of guidelines proposed by former reports. It is also stated that, although the benefits of prophylactic antibiotics for emergency caesarean sections are clearly evidenced, such a policy is still not universally employed.

Reasons for the increase in caesarean section rates

There are many reasons for the increase in caesarean section rates. These may be attributed to both technological and social changes. The expectation is perhaps that every pregnancy should have a healthy outcome (Silverton 1993), perhaps the more so because many women work full time and are choosing to delay and restrict the number of pregnancies they have (Callwood & Thomas 2000). Fear of litigation may be a reason for early recourse to caesarean birth.

Women's request for caesarean section

Some writers insist that the reasons behind the 'demand' for caesarean section are complex and involved (Robinson 1999). Accounts of women who have had difficult experiences of childbirth describe knowing something was wrong, and believing they were not listened to. They then go on to request caesarean section for a subsequent birth. According to Robinson (1999) these demands stem from previous bad experiences, expressed even as 'nightmare' by some women. There is much evidence to support the fact that very few women actually request caesarean section in the absence of medical indications (Chaffer & Royle 2000, Robinson 1999, Weaver et al 2001).

Maternal age and caesarean section

Opinions on this vary and remain equivocal. Women over the age of 34 are more likely to have a caesarean section (Chaffer & Royle 2000, Marwick & Lynn 2001, Weaver et al 2001). There is interest in this subject as a growing proportion of childbearing women are delaying pregnancy (Bell et al 2001).

There is literature to show that more research is required on obstetrical practices and complications that occur in older women who have had caesarean section, to understand the relationship between these two. It is true that interventions are a consequence of complications (Bell et al 2001), but complications may also result from intervention. The variation in rates of caesarean section between obstetricians and how maternal age affects these requires more consideration.

Other reports show that caesarean section rates rise from teenage years onwards (Marwick & Lynn 2001). These writers state that as findings were particularly uniform, and this from very diverse countries, clinical practice and societal pressures were unlikely to be the cause of the increase in intervention with the increase in maternal age. One author states that 'concern about complications might be as much of a problem as the complications themselves' (Weaver et al 2001, p. 285). The midwife should understand the fears of the childbearing woman, and provide information and support appropriately to disperse these.

Shearer (1993) states that the four major indicators provided for caesarean section in the United States were previous caesarean section (35%), failure to progress

(30%), breech presentation (10%) and fetal distress (8%). This supports the Scottish initiative to lower the rate of caesarean section carried out for previous caesarean and for breech presentation (McIlwaine et al 1994–5). Both these indications are not included in the 'definite' category; therefore they can be worked on and lowered, whereas an indication such as fetal compromise is an absolute indicator for caesarean section, and cannot be changed.

Psychological support and the role of the midwife

The Changing Childbirth report (DoH 1993) clearly states that women are to be involved in the decision-making process concerning their maternity care. Choice is an important element in this sequence. One writer makes recommendations following a study on the rise of caesarean section rates, in the attempt to decipher the various reasons why there is such a variation in practice (Chaffer & Royle 2000). Five of the 11 propositions for practice relate to information giving, involvement of the woman in the decision-making process and the provision of consistent advice.

Women expect to be actively involved in their care and the midwife must ensure that recent, valid and relevant information is provided in a straightforward manner for women. This will help women to decide what is best for them, in their circumstances. An informed, confident and competent practitioner will relieve the stress of the situation and help the woman make a decision, supporting her in the midst of her misgivings. The midwife has a pivotal role in giving women clear and unbiased information concerning the choices available (McAleese 2000).

One-to-one care from a support person during labour can influence caesarean section rates (Walker & Golois 2001). It is important that midwives recognise that this is a positive tactic and should value their role and skills. A continual, supportive presence in labour is widely reported as being of considerable benefit. Churchill (1997) states that a friend or partner is appreciated because they are able to act as a mediator on behalf of the woman. They are also able to describe the occurrences and happenings during the operation.

Clarifying the indications for caesarean section

In an effort to try to clarify the precise motive behind women's request for caesarean section, the National Caesarean Section Audit (RCOG 2001) formulated the following objectives:

- to determine the frequency of caesarean sections in all maternity units in England and Wales
- to determine the factors associated with variations in the rates of caesarean section including maternal request
- to assist in the development of new standards.

The aim of the study was to ascertain the contribution of maternal requests to caesarean section rates and also to interpret the variation of caesarean section rates. There is evidence to support the notion that caesarean section is being used too liberally (Dimond 1999). Many authors state that the number of women who request caesarean section purely for convenience is low (Page 1999, Weaver et al 2001). The same writers observe that, although women are not aware of the morbidity for mother and the baby, they are generally well informed as to the incapacitating consequences of major surgery.

Not all caesarean sections that are non-elective are of an emergency nature. A caesarean section, for example carried out after a few hours of labour when the CTG shows that there may be a degree of fetal compromise present, may be carried out urgently. This will not be an emergency in the strict sense of the word.

Elective caesarean section

This indicates that the decision to carry out the procedure has been taken during the pregnancy, therefore before labour has commenced. If the indication for caesarean section has been a non-recurring one, for example placenta praevia, vaginal delivery after caesarean may be attempted. Repeat caesarean section may be indicated in, for example, cephalopelvic disproportion, or on a uterus that has been scarred twice.

Within the umbrella of 'elective' caesarean there could be merit in reclassification. For example, there are those operations that are truly 'elective' in that they are booked around term at a time convenient for mother and surgeon. The other category includes 'scheduled' caesarean sections when it becomes clear that early delivery is required, but there is no immediate compromise to mother or fetus.

Definite indications. These include:

- cephalopelvic disproportion
- major degree of placenta praevia
- high order multiple pregnancy.

Possible indications. These include:

- breech presentation
- moderate to severe pre-eclampsia
- a medical condition that warrants the exclusion of maternal effort
- diabetes mellitus
- intrauterine growth restriction
- antepartum haemorrhage
- certain fetal abnormalities (e.g. hydrocephalus).

There is much literature to substantiate the thought that there is no overall consensus among obstetricians concerning the indications for caesarean section (Chaffer & Royle 2000). Hence there is a need for reflective, careful and vigilant practice on the part of the midwife. The information given and the decision concerning the care to be administered must be done in discussion with the woman. The clarity of the discussion and the detail of the midwife's observations, together with all aspects of the history, will contribute to the enhancement of the care of the woman. The midwife also has an important role in multidisciplinary team discussions to review decisions taken regarding medical or surgical interventions.

Emergency caesarean section

This is carried out when adverse conditions develop during pregnancy or labour. Standards have been suggested for the maximum time that should elapse from the decision to deliver to the actual time the baby is born. However, this is less straightforward as in some cases there is a real 'emergency' and everything needs to be in place for immediate delivery of the baby if it is to survive (e.g. cord prolapse with fetal compromise). Then there are other situations where delivery is 'urgent' but more time can be taken to prepare for the operation and proposed actions can be discussed with the parents in a more relaxed manner. The following are examples of urgent/emergency reasons for caesarean birth:

- antepartum haemorrhage
- cord prolapse
- uterine rupture (dramatic/scar dehiscence)
- cephalopelvic disproportion diagnosed in labour
- fulminating pre-eclampsia
- eclampsia
- failure to progress in the first or second stage of labour and fetal compromise if delivery is not imminent.

Vaginal delivery following caesarean section

Ziadeh & Sunna (1995) state that widespread adoption of a policy whereby 80% of women with prior caesarean section have a trial of labour could potentially eliminate up to a third of caesarean sections. Reports state less than a 1% frequency of uterine rupture and no maternal deaths from this cause (Taffel et al 1992, Ziadeh & Sunna 1995). Walmsley & Hobbs (1994) state that uterine rupture is indeed very rare, and the risk of dehiscence very low.

Often, it is the inflexible nature of the management of vaginal birth following caesarean section that disempowers women, hindering them from making a valid choice. According to Walmsley & Hobbs (1994), vaginal birth after a previous caesarean section is a safe option. The fact that women who have had previous caesarean section and who go into labour spontaneously have a greater chance of delivering normally (Coltart et al 1990, Walmsley & Hobbs 1994) is evidenced by the literature. Women should then be given every opportunity to start labour spontaneously as induction of labour after a previous caesarean section leads to increased risk of scar rupture or dehiscence (Lydon-Rochelle et al 2001).

Trial of labour

A trial of labour is carried out whenever there is doubt about the outcome of the labour because of a previous caesarean section. Criteria include:

- after adequate supervision, it is established that the presenting part is capable of flexing adequately to pass through the brim of the pelvis
- all the facilities for assisted birth are readily available
- progress of the labour is sufficient, observed both in the descent of the presenting part and by the dilatation of the cervix
- time limits as to the duration of the trial are set.

Some of the literature shows that pain at the site of the scar does not reliably indicate rupture and that caesarean section carried out for this reason often found intact scars (Goer 1995). Coltart et al (1990) claim that women admitted in active labour have higher vaginal birth rates following caesarean section than those admitted in early labour. Birthweight in previous pregnancies should not exert undue influence on management procedures (Peterson & Saunders 1991). Peterson & Saunders (1991) suggest that units allowing longer labours had higher vaginal birth rates following caesarean section, and Walmsley & Hobbs (1994) state that placing time limits on the duration of these labours is neither helpful nor reassuring for the woman. Concerning elective caesarean section after two caesarean sections, Roberts (1991) maintains that there is no conclusive proof of an increased risk of scar dehiscence during labour after two caesarean sections. He goes on to say that there is no scientific evidence to substantiate the notion that such hazard exists, but equally absence of proof is not proof of absence.

As there seem to be very divided practices and judgements relating to the management of trial of labour following caesarean section, it is even more important that the midwife has critically appraised the literature. This will enable her to provide appropriate and timely care and advice for the woman she is responsible for, based on the relevant and valid evidence.

General anaesthesia

Despite the increasing use of regional anaesthesia, general anaesthesia is sometimes required. Regional anaesthesia is incompatible with any maternal coagulation disorder. General anaesthesia can be more rapidly administered, and is of value when speed is important, such as when the fetus is in serious jeopardy (Enkin et al 2000). According to Holdcroft et al (1995) about a third of women choose general rather than regional anaesthesia. Women are preoxygenated prior to induction of anaesthesia; that is, they are given oxygen-rich gas mixtures to breathe for several minutes. A muscle relaxant (suxamethonium) is given to allow safe orotracheal intubation; a cuffed tube and cricoid pressure are essential to prevent aspiration of stomach contents. Induction agents include thiopental and propofol. Maternal unconsciousness ensues within

seconds. There are minimal side-effects and relatively little negative fetal consequences at the time of birth provided meticulous practices are in place. Regional anaesthesia, however, normally remains the safer option for caesarean birth. Anaesthesia is sustained by inhalational anaesthetic means using Fluothane or Ethrane.

Twenty-five 'anaesthetic incidents' were reported in 1998 (CESDI 2000). These fell into three categories, involving:

- serious complications related to giving anaesthetic
- delays with personnel
- delays in the provision of anaesthesia once the anaesthetist was available.

When the midwife recognises an abnormality she must report it to the appropriate person, giving adequate details, as it is obvious that efficiency and clarity will prevent major incidents from occurring. Speed is essential and the midwife can assist by making sure that optimal care is given and by being an advocate for the mother.

Mendelson's syndrome

This condition was described by Mendelson in 1946 (Stables 1999). It is caused if acid gastric contents are inhaled and result in a chemical pneumonitis. This regurgitation may occur during the induction of a general anaesthetic and go unheeded. The acidic gastric contents then damage the alveoli, impairing gaseous exchange. It may become impossible to oxygenate the woman and death may result. The predisposing factors are: the pressure from the gravid uterus when the woman is lying down, the effect of the progesterone relaxing smooth muscle, and the cardiac sphincter of the stomach possibly being relaxed by the effect of the anaesthetic. Analgesics such as pethidine cause significant delay in gastric emptying, thereby exacerbating the above (Mander 1998).

One writer summarises the results of research as showing that aspiration is an extremely rare event and is almost always associated with substandard anaesthetic practice (Goer 1995). This is confirmed in the seventh CESDI report (CESDI 2000), which featured complications of anaesthesia as one of the main themes for investigation. Goer (1995) goes on to say that it is actually the management of labour and surgical interventions that increases the likelihood of vomiting and aspiration. Various studies substantiate this statement (Broach & Newton 1988, Elkington 1991).

Prevention of Mendelson's syndrome.

Antacid therapy. Although there are now relatively few cases where general anaesthesia is used for caesarean section, the prevention of Mendelson's syndrome is essential. Prophylactic treatment is given to all women in whom a caesarean is planned or anticipated. A usual regimen is for women having an elective operation to be given two doses of oral ranitidine 150 mg approximately 8 hours apart, plus 30 ml sodium citrate immediately before transfer to theatre. Women in labour who are thought to have a high risk of caesarean section should have ranitidine 150 mg every 8 hours. These drugs inhibit the secretion of hydrochloric acid in the stomach.

Cricoid pressure. This is the most important measure in preventing pulmonary aspiration (Enkin et al 2000). The oesophagus is occluded by the use of cricoid pressure. Cricoid pressure is a technique whereby the pressure exerted on the one whole ring of tracheal cartilage, the cricoid cartilage, thus occludes the oesophagus and prevents reflux. Cricoid pressure is maintained by an assistant until the tracheal tube is positioned by the anaesthetist, and the seal of the cuff is verified for its essential. The correct use of this manoeuvre is essential in preventing major incidents from occurring (Fig. 31.1).

Difficult or failed intubation

This condition is more likely to occur in pregnant women and particularly with those who have pregnancy-induced hypertension. Laryngeal oedema arises more frequently in these women, therefore anticipation of the disorder is key to its management. If laryngeal oedema is anticipated, a very experienced and well-briefed anaesthetist should carry out the intubation. A well-lubricated stylet or bougee may be used to aid endotracheal intubation. Management of failed intubation is: continued cricoid pressure (but not at the expense of oxygenation) and ventilation by face mask until the effects of suxamethonium and thiopental have worn off (and the woman has regained consciousness and her cough reflex).

Complications

It is suggested that, with the increase in caesarean section rates, there is likely to be a subsequent rise in maternal mortality (Chaffer & Royle 2000, Dimond 1999, Hillan 1995, Lilford 1990). There is documentation that maintains this may be as much as five times greater in women who have had caesarean section (Silverton 1993). Morbidity reports reveal that only 9.5% of a sample of women delivered by caesarean section (*n* = 619) had no reported morbidity in the postnatal period (Magill-Cuerdin 1996). The evidence suggests that there is also a wide variation in reported

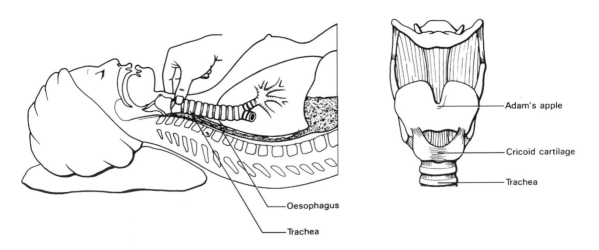

Fig. 31.1 Cricoid pressure, showing occlusion of the oesophagus by pressure applied to the cricoid cartilage.

morbidity (Hillan 1995) and scanty research on this. Although surgical and anaesthetic techniques have improved, women are still more liable to suffer from complications and to have increased morbidity following caesarean section (Stables 1999).

Infection. Maternal morbidity following caesarean section has not been studied methodically, but the problem of postoperative infection is considerable (Enkin at al 2000). In one study that considered wound infection (Chaffer & Royle 2000), this was confirmed as being as high as 34%. In the same study, the wound infection rate was even greater, when data covering the first 6 weeks following caesarean section were included. There is now persuasive evidence to indicate that antibiotic prophylaxis markedly reduces the risk of serious postoperative infection such as pelvic abscess, septic shock and septic pelvic vein thrombophlebitis. There is similar evidence to support the fact that women are also safeguarded against endometritis. Protection against wound infection is less sure, but remains considerable (Enkin et al 2000).

Infection is associated with previous rupture of membranes and other factors such as obesity. The prophylactic use of antibiotics was recommended in the 1998 CEMD report (DoH et al 1998) and there is clear evidence showing its benefits, from controlled trials. This report recommends that guidelines for the use of antibiotics should be implemented and audited in each maternity unit. One writer states that one way of reducing the infection morbidity is to reduce the number of unnecessary caesarean sections (Enkin et al 2000). There is a much greater incidence of infection following emergency caesarean section (Enkin et al 2000, Hillan 1995). The length of stay in hospital prior to operation also influences this incidence. Enkin et al (2000) also state that delaying shaving of the operation site until immediately before operating, ensuring sterilisation of all swabs and instruments and a general good sterile and surgical technique would all contribute to a reduction in infection postoperatively.

Urinary tract infection. This was the most consistent of the infectious morbidity described by Hillan's (1995) comprehensive and informative investigation into postoperative morbidity following caesarean section. Urinary tract infection was present in 10.9% of women who had elective and 10.3% of women who had emergency caesarean section. Wound infection rose from 4.1 to 8.3%, intrauterine infection from 1.4 to 6% and chest infection from 0.9 to 5.3% respectively in elective and emergency caesarean section. Hence the need for attentive and careful observation and care by the midwife of women who have had caesarean section in an emergency.

Thromboembolic disorders. These remain the leading direct cause of maternal death, accounting for 35 of the total 106 direct maternal deaths (Lewis & Drife 2001). Although there was a marked reduction in deaths after caesarean section, further improvements are necessary. Pregnancy carries with it an increased risk of thrombosis and all women on bedrest, and all women undergoing caesarean section, should be assessed for thromboembolic prophylaxis (Lewis & Drife 2001, pp. 72–73).

Postoperative care

Immediate care

Observations. The blood pressure and pulse should be recorded every quarter hour in the immediate recovery period. The temperature should be recorded every 2 hours. The wound must be inspected every half hour to detect any blood loss. The lochia should also be inspected and drainage should be small initially. Following general anaesthesia the woman is nursed in the left lateral or 'recovery' position until she is fully conscious, since the risks of airway obstruction or regurgitation and silent aspiration of stomach contents are still present.

Analgesia. This is prescribed and is given as required. If the mother intends to breastfeed, the baby should be put to the breast as soon as possible. This can usually be achieved with minimal disturbance to the mother. Postoperative analgesia may be given in a variety of ways:

- an epidural opioid
- rectal analgesia, such as diclofenac (this is contraindicated if there is continuing bleeding, poor urine output, a history of sensitivity to NSAIDs, or peptic ulcer)
- intramuscular analgesia (though this is never given in conjunction with epidural opioids because of the risk of cumulative effects)
- oral drugs (e.g. dihydrocodeine, paracetamol).

Antiemetics (e.g. cyclizine; prochlorperazine) are usually prescribed by the anaesthetist.

Care following regional block. Following epidural or spinal anaesthesia the woman may sit up as soon as she wishes, provided her blood pressure is not low. All observations are recorded as described above. Fluids are introduced gradually followed by a light diet. The intravenous infusion remains in progress for about 12 hours. Care must be taken to avoid any damage to the legs, which will gradually regain sensation and movement.

As it is possible that an opiate administered via the epidural route may cause some respiratory depression, the woman's respiratory rate must be recorded. This means of pain relief offers the advantage of excellent analgesia without motor block and also seems to give a feeling of well-being. Women are usually able to become mobile very quickly, which reduces the risk of deep venous thrombosis. It is also more conducive to the woman's psychological health.

Ideally the baby should remain with his mother and they should be transferred to the postnatal ward together as soon as possible.

Care in the postnatal ward

When mother and baby are transferred to the postnatal ward, the blood pressure, temperature and pulse are usually checked every 4 hours. The intravenous infusion will continue, and the urinary catheter may remain in the bladder until the woman is able to get up to the toilet. The wound and lochia must initially be observed at least hourly. The baby should remain with his mother, and the midwife should offer extra help to ensure that the mother has adequate rest. The mother is encouraged to move her legs and to perform leg and breathing exercises. The physiotherapist will usually teach these and may give chest physiotherapy. Prophylactic low dose heparin and TED antiembolism stockings are often prescribed. The woman is helped to get out of bed as soon as possible following caesarean section, and is encouraged to become fully mobile.

Urinary output must be monitored carefully both before and after removal of the urinary catheter; women may have some difficulty with micturition initially and the bladder may be incompletely emptied. Any haematuria must be reported to the doctor.

Women who have had a general anaesthetic for caesarean section may feel very tired and drowsy for some hours. A woman may complain of a feeling of detachment and unreality and may feel that she does not relate well to the baby. The woman who is concerned

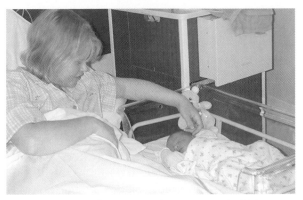

Fig. 31.2 Baby in clip-on cot, adjacent to and within easy reach of mother when in bed.

should be reassured and be given the opportunity to talk freely.

Appropriate analgesia must be given as frequently as necessary (see above).

The mother must be encouraged to rest as much as possible and tactful advice may need to be given to her visitors. If the mother becomes too tired, help is needed with care for the baby. This should preferably take place at the mother's bedside and should include support with breastfeeding. The new clip-on cots, which may be attached to the mother's bed, can facilitate the handling of baby for the mother (Fig. 31.2).

Some women may have a lingering feeling of failure or disappointment at having had a caesarean section and may value the opportunity to talk this over with the midwife.

Research and the incidence of caesarean section

Low caesarean section rates are associated with low levels of intervention and high levels of psychological support (Henderson 1996). It is difficult to decipher whether caesarean section rates have been affected by interventions such as proactive management of labour – that is, artificial rupture of membranes and use of oxytocin – or whether other factors have influenced these. As the protocol of O'Driscoll et al (1993) requires a continuous and supportive presence during labour, this may also have influenced the outcome of the labour and birth; this trial shows an impressive 5% caesarean section rate in Dublin. Other researchers have attempted to interpret these results. Beart et al

(1992) found no significant difference in the outcomes of labours in those who had been actively managed and those in the control group. Lopez-Zeno et al (1992) did find a significant difference in caesarean section rates between women who were actively managed and those who were not; the actively managed group had much lower caesarean section rates.

There are many other motives and factors that greatly affect the outcome of labour, the giving of food in labour being one. Haire & Elsberry (1991) recount that a caesarean rate of 11% in the Bronx rose to 38% when women were fasted in labour. Another reseacher relates that even the procedure of monitoring the unit's caesarean section rates had the effect of reducing these by 4% (Urquhart et al 1987).

It has been demonstrated that by a systematic and reflective approach, and a certain amount of will, caesarean section rates *can* be lowered. One American teaching hospital launched a course of action to reduce caesarean section rates (Myers & Gleicher 1988), which included the following criteria:

- second opinion for all non-emergency caesarean sections
- trial of labour for all women with previous caesarean section
- diagnosis of dystocia after 2 hours of non-progress with adequate contractions
- diagnosis of fetal distress to be corroborated with fetal gas analysis
- vaginal delivery of breech (except for true hyperextension)
- peer review process.

Primary caesarean section rates in this study dropped from 17 to 7.5%. Apgar scores and neonatal mortality were unaffected.

Corresponding findings were described by Sanchez-Ramos et al (1990) where a similarly impressive drop in caesarean section rates was witnessed, from 27.5% and 19.5% (total and primary rates of caesarean section) to 10.5% and 7.5% respectively. Comparable guidelines were used in both of these studies. Ziadeh & Sunna (1995) examined the increase of caesarean section rates in Jordan. By introducing guidelines that managed dystocia, previous caesarean section delivery, fetal distress and breech presentation in a similar fashion to the researchers above (Myers & Gleicher 1988, Sanchez-Ramos et al 1990), the same objective was achieved in Jordan. There are many instances where caesarean section rates have fallen well below the 10–15% rate recommended by WHO. Single figures are commonplace: O'Driscoll et al 1993 (6%), De Muylder & Thiery 1990 (8%), Wright et al 1991 (4.4%). All these writers agree that caesarean section rates can be reduced and accompanied by low perinatal mortality.

Birth by forceps

Forceps are most commonly employed to expedite delivery of the fetal head or to protect the fetus or the mother, or both, from trauma and exhaustion. They are also used to assist the delivery of the after-coming head of the breech or to draw the head of the baby up and out of the pelvis at caesarean section birth.

Stephenson (1992) reports that assisted vaginal delivery may be carried out as frequently as 15% in Australia and Canada. Johanson & Menon (1997) state that, in general, maternal outcomes would be improved by lowering instrumental birth rates.

Characteristics of obstetric forceps

Obstetric forceps are composed of two separate blades, a right and a left, and are identified on these as such. The forceps are inserted separately on each side of the head. The forceps are locked together by either an English or a Smellie lock. Rotational forceps have a sliding lock. The blades are spoon shaped (cephalic curve) to accommodate the form of the baby's head and are fenestrated to minimise trauma to the baby's head. In most modern obstetric forceps, the blade is attached to the handle at an angle that corresponds to the pelvic curve. When the blades are correctly positioned the handles will be neatly aligned in the hands of the doctor who applies them.

Classification of obstetric forceps

Forceps operations fall into two categories: low and mid cavity. *Low cavity forceps* are used when the head has reached the pelvic floor and is visible at the vulva. *Mid cavity forceps* are used when the head is engaged and the leading part is below the level of the ischial spines. High cavity forceps are now considered unsafe and a caesarean section will be carried out.

Types of obstetric forceps

Forceps are often described as non-rotational or rotational (Fig. 31.3). Adequate analgesia is required prior to their application to the fetal head.

Wrigley's forceps. These are designed for use when the head is on the perineum. This is a short and light type of forceps, with both pelvic and cephalic curves and an English lock. They are also used for the aftercoming head of a breech delivery, or at caesarean section.

Neville-Barnes or Simpson's forceps. These are generally used for a low or mid cavity forceps delivery when the sagittal suture is in the anteroposterior diameter of the cavity/outlet of the pelvis. They have cephalic and pelvic curves and the handles are longer and heavier than those of the Wrigley's. Anderson's and Haig-Ferguson's forceps are also similar in shape and size.

Keilland's forceps. These were originally designed to deliver the fetal head at or above the pelvic brim. They are generally used for the rotation and extraction of the head that is arrested in the deep transverse or in the occipitoposterior position. The blades have little pelvic curve and are for traction. The shallow curve allows safe rotation of the forceps in the vagina. Downward traction encourages rotation of the head. The claw lock allows sliding and corrects asynclitism of the fetal head. These should be used only by an obstetrician skilled in their application and use.

Indications for the use of obstetric forceps

The three main indications for the use of forceps are delay in the second stage of labour, fetal compromise and maternal distress.

Delay in the second stage of labour may be due to:

- insufficient contractions (but this is better corrected by oxytocin infusion)
- epidural analgesia
- malrotation of the head
- maternal fatigue.

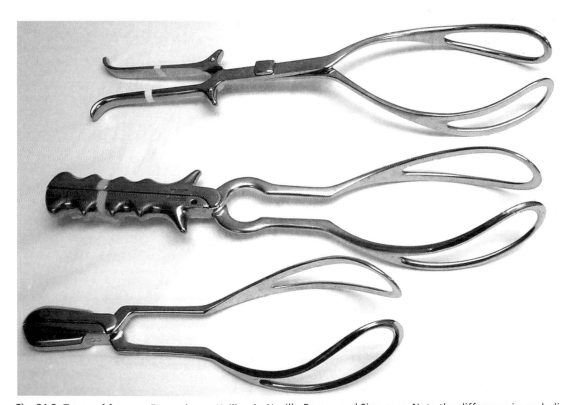

Fig. 31.3 Types of forceps. From above: Keillands, Neville-Barnes and Simpsons. Note the difference in cephalic curve. The rotational forceps (Keillands) have a long shaft and little pelvic curve.

Fetal compromise may be due to:

- prematurity
- hypoxia
- intrauterine growth restriction
- a maternal obstetric or medical condition (e.g. pre-eclampsia).

Maternal distress may be caused by:

- hypertension
- cardiac condition
- maternal exhaustion or long labour.

Prerequisites for forceps delivery

Care of the bladder. To prevent harm or injury, the bladder must be kept empty.

Analgesia. This is generally by epidural or pudendal block plus perineal infiltration of local anaesthetic.

Information giving and consent. The couple must be kept informed of the course of events, and must be involved in the decision-making process.

Paediatric presence. The paediatrician may not be required at birth, but should be kept informed of circumstances.

Neonatal resuscitation equipment. This must be checked and prepared in case it becomes necessary. (See also Technique.)

A useful **FORCEPS** pneumonic is:

Full dilatation of the cervix
0 fifths of the head palpable abdominally
Room in pelvis and Ruptured membranes
Cephalic presentation
Empty bladder
Position recognized
Suitable pain relief.

Procedure

Pudendal block

This is the infiltration of the area around the pudendal nerve by local anaesthetic. The transvaginal route is used to locate the ischial spine, as the pudendal nerve emerges from vertebrae S2–S4 and crosses this. A particular needle that possesses a ring or guard is employed, called a pudendal block needle. About 10 ml of local anaesthetic, usually 1% lidocaine (lignocaine), are injected into the region just below the ischial spine (Fig. 31.4). Both motor and sensory nerves are affected as both lie in this region. The pudendal nerve supplies the levator ani muscle, also the deep and superficial perineal muscles (Al-Azzawi 1990). It may be used to provide analgesia for the lower vagina and perineum, and is therefore used for forceps and ventouse deliveries. The advantage of this technique is that it does not harm the baby.

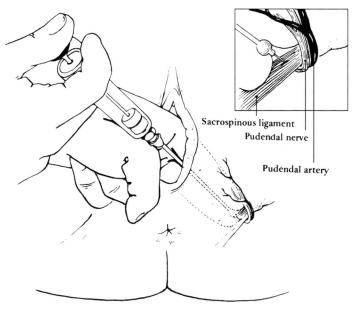

Sacrospinous ligament
Pudendal nerve

Pudendal artery

Fig. 31.4 Locating the pudendal nerve per vaginam.

Perineal infiltration

A local anaesthetic is used to infiltrate the perineum prior to episiotomy or suturing (see Ch. 27).

Technique (Figs 31.5–31.8)

After careful vaginal examination by the obstetrician, the presentation and position are identified. There

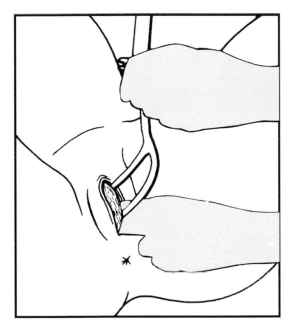

Fig. 31.5 Left blade being inserted. The fingers of the right hand guard the vaginal tissue.

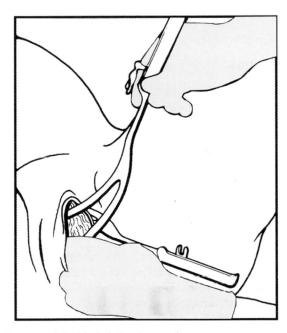

Fig. 31.6 Right blade being inserted.

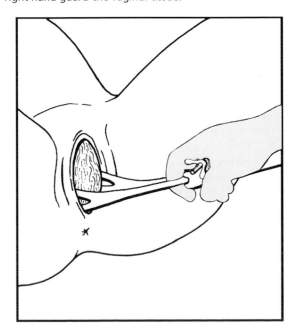

Fig. 31.7 Traction of the head is downwards until this point; when the head is low, the direction of pull is outward, towards the operator.

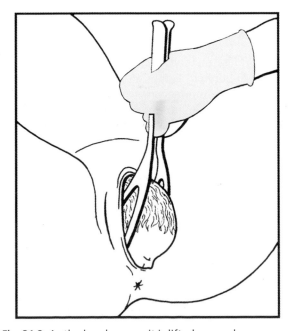

Fig. 31.8 As the head crowns it is lifted upwards.

Figs 31.5–31.8 Technique for forceps delivery.

must be no apparent obstruction. The membranes must be ruptured and full dilatation of the cervix must be confirmed. The head must be engaged and there should be no cephalopelvic disproportion. Episiotomy is not routinely carried out.

Complications

Maternal. These include:

- trauma or soft tissue damage, which may occur to the perineum, vagina, or cervix
- haemorrhage from the above
- dysuria or urinary retention, which may result from bruising or oedema to the urethra
- painful perineum
- postnatal morbidity, which is higher in any birth intervention.

Neonatal (see Ch. 44). These include:

- marks on the baby's face, which can be caused by the pressure of the forceps, but resolve quite rapidly
- excessive bruising from the forceps
- facial palsy, which may result from pressure from a blade compressing a facial nerve, and is usually temporary.

Birth by the ventouse method

The ventouse method is used more commonly than forceps in northern Europe and in Africa. The vacuum extractor is an instrument that applies traction. It can be used as an alternative to forceps. The cup cleaves to the baby's scalp by suction and is used to assist maternal effort.

The use of the ventouse

The ventouse may be used when there is a delay in labour, when the cervix is not quite fully dilated (Miller & Hanretty 1997). As with forceps, the ventouse should be applied when the head is engaged and there is no cephalopelvic disproportion. It may be useful in the case of a second twin, when the head remains relatively high. It may be safer and simpler to use the ventouse in this event than forceps.

Application of the cup

There remains some controversy as to the application of the vacuum in ventouse extraction (Lim et al 1997). It is important that the midwife has an understanding of this principle as it is frequently the midwife who is called upon to manage the vacuum. The stepwise or conventional method recommends a gradual or stepwise increase in the vacuum, in an effort to achieve a closely applied cup to the presenting part. A few studies have compared the stepwise method with the one-step technique (Lim et al 1997, Svenningssen 1987). These have not observed any difference in the number of detachments, which is the main factor to consider. This is because the number of detachments lengthens the duration of the procedure and neonatal asphyxia is related to the time of traction and to the number of compression forces (Moolgaoker et al 1979). It is strongly recommended that an experienced obstetrician or midwife carry out this responsibility.

Soft and rigid vacuum extractor cups

The metal cups used are the Bird variety (Johanson & Menon 1997) and have a central traction chain and a vacuum conduit. These come in 4, 5 and 6 cm diameters. The preferred new silicone rubber cup is shaped to the contour of the baby's head. This allows the cup to be placed further back on the baby's head to increase flexion, reduce the diameter of the head and facilitate delivery (Fig. 31.9).

The advantage of the new malleable silicone cup is that it effects much less of a 'chignon' on the baby's scalp (Miller & Hanretty 1997). Soft cups have a poorer success rate than the metal, but are less likely to be associated with scalp trauma (Chenoy & Johanson 1992). They are also more favoured by both women and midwives (Johanson & Menon 1997). Most of the research shows that the two main outcomes, the occurrence of trauma and the likelihood of vaginal delivery, have been well investigated. However, many studies have not considered other important maternal consequences such as the pain experienced, satisfaction or the mother's anxiety about the baby (Johanson & Menon 1997). One writer states that there is an absence of mature assessment in relation to the research on vacuum. This is due to the continual development of new cups, and after introduction a certain

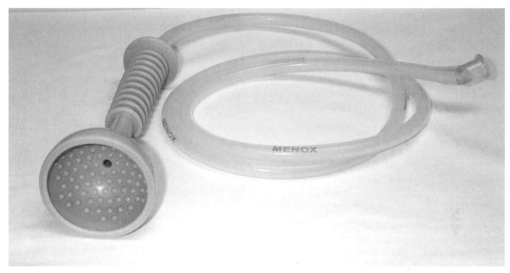

Fig. 31.9 The soft cup ventouse.

time lapse is necessary before it is possible to judge which is preferable and more efficient (Drife 1996). The evidence is also rather inconclusive as to whether vacuum or forceps should be chosen. Drife (1996) maintains that there are other important issues that require consideration, such as the reasons for the increase in assisted birth, or whether caesarean section is a more preferable option. A significant factor is the carrying out of instrumental manoeuvres by registrars (52%) and by senior house officers (45%); the choice of instrument should therefore be dependent upon the experience of the accoucheur. There is also a reasonable argument to support the notion that women should be involved in the choice.

Procedure

The woman is usually in the lithotomy position and the same precautions are observed as for a forceps birth. Local anaesthesia may be used or inhalational analgesia may be sufficient. Pudendal nerve block may be employed or epidural, if already in situ, may be topped up. Episiotomy is not routinely carried out.

The procedure is explained and consent obtained; then adequate analgesia is assured and the bladder is emptied. The fetal heart rate is recorded regularly. The cup of the ventouse is placed as near as possible to, or on, the flexing point of the fetal head. The vacuum in the cup is increased gradually so as to achieve a close application of this to the fetal head. Usually a vacuum of 0.8 kg/cm^2 is reached, by an increase of 0.2 kg/cm^2 in stages, or an increase from 0.2 to 0.8 kg/cm^2 is achieved directly. When the vacuum is achieved, traction is applied with a contraction, with maternal effort, in an attempt to involve and include the woman in the birth experience. This traction is done in a downwards and backwards direction, then in forwards and upwards, thus following the natural curve of the pelvis, the curve of Carus. The vacuum is released and the cup then removed at the crowning of the fetal head, as it will no longer regress. The mother can then push the baby for the final part of the birth, thus involving her in this and giving the mother the opportunity to participate. This will result in a more satisfactory experience for the mother and the family.

Precautions in use. These include the following:

- Care should be taken to ensure that no vaginal skin is trapped in the edges of the cup.
- Prolonged or excessive traction should not be used.

Complications

As the vacuum actually works by raising an artificial caput, it is not logical to then say that caput is a complication of this intervention, as the aim is to form a chignon. However, prolonged traction will increase the likelihood of scalp abrasions, cephalhaematoma or subaponeurotic bleeding (Miller & Hanretty 1997).

Failure of the ventouse may arise in as much as 20% of cases (Drife 1996). This is more likely in the presence of excessive caput, and in the hands of less experienced obstetricians. The role of the midwife is to improve the overall efficiency of the manoeuvre, and to support the mother and her partner.

The midwife ventouse practitioner

Some midwives feel that women will be better served by the midwife ventouse practitioner and embrace such innovations, whereas others see it as exceeding the limits of normal midwifery practice (Charles 1999). The fact is that, with the advancement of midwife-led care and the increased demand for less interference in the birth process and also the development of consultant midwives and other resource key persons, midwifery care is changing and developing. There was a similar reaction when midwives commenced suturing, and yet women have been well served by midwives carrying out this activity. The response of women has been positive, with continuity of care being confirmed as the main advantage (Mulholland 1997).

One advantage of the midwife ventouse practitioner role is that women are not traumatised by a change of carer as the midwife is able to provide the panoply of care required by the woman, and this at a very crucial and critical moment. Midwife ventouse practitioners must be well educated and trained before carrying out this procedure. There is more likelihood of the indication being maternal fatigue than for any other reason. Midwives in developing countries and in a few birth centres in the UK are already familiar with this technique.

Symphysiotomy

This is an incision of the fibrocartilage partly through the symphysis pubis and is performed in labour to enlarge the transverse diameter of the pelvis. It is rarely carried out in the UK, but is carried out in countries where the risk of caesarean section is particularly high for the management of cephalopelvic disproportion. A urinary catheter is inserted into the bladder to empty it and to displace the urethra laterally whilst the symphysis is being divided. The fibrocartilage is incised over the centre of the symphysis pubis. A vacuum extractor or forceps may be used to facilitate delivery. Following the operation a bandage is applied around the pelvis to provide support. The catheter may remain in situ for a few days as oedema is likely.

REFERENCES

Al-Azzawi F 1990 A colour atlas of childbirth and obstetric techniques. Wolfe, London

Beart G, Garel M, Milka-Cabane N 1992 Evaluation of different policies of the management of labour for primiparous women. Journal of Gynaecology, Obstetrics and Biology of Reproduction (11):43–56

Bell J S, Campbell D M, Graham W J, Penney G C, Ryan M, Hall M H 2001 Do obstetric complications explain high caesarean section among women over 30? British Medical Journal (322):894–895

Broach J, Newton N 1988 Food and beverages in labour. Part ii. The effects of oral intake during labour. Birth 15(2):89–92

Callwood A, Thomas J 2000 The National Sentinel Caesarean Section Audit. Practising Midwife 3(6):34–35

CESDI (Confidential Enquiry into Stillbirths and Deaths in Infancy) 2000 7th annual report, 1 January–31 December 1998. Maternal and Child Health Research Consortium, London, p 1–113

Chaffer D, Royle L 2000 The use of audit to explain the rise in caesarean section. British Journal of Midwifery 8(11):677–684

Charles C 1999 How it feels to be a midwife practitioner. British Journal of Midwifery 7(6):380–382

Chenoy R, Johanson R 1992 A randomised prospective study comparing delivery with metal and silicone rubber vacuum extraction caps. British Journal of Obstetrics and Gynaecology (99):360–364

Churchill H 1997 Caesarean birth experience, practice and history. Books for Midwives Press, Hale, Cheshire

Coltart T, Davies J, Katesmark M 1990 Outcome of second pregnancy after a previous caesarean section. British Journal of Obstetrics and Gynaecology (97):1140–1143

Currie E 1987 Parliamentary written answer. House of Commons report (Hansard) 24 July, 120 col 713 (no. 26 part ii)

De Muylder X, Thiery M 1990 The cesarean delivery rate can be safely reduced in a developing country. Obstetrics and Gynaecology 75(3 Pt 1):360–364

Dimond B 1999 Is there a legal right to choose a caesarean? British Journal of Midwifery 7(8):515–518

DoH (Department of Health) 1993 Changing childbirth part 1: report of the Expert Maternity Group. HMSO, London

DoH (Department of Health), Welsh Office, Scottish Office Department of Health, Department of Health and Social Services Northern Ireland 1998 Why mothers die. Report on Confidential Enquiries into Maternal Deaths in the United Kingdom, 1994–1996. Stationery Office, London

Drife J 1996 Choice and instrumental delivery. British Journal of Obstetrics and Gynaecology (103):608–611

Elkington K W 1991 At the water's edge: where obstetrics and anaesthesia meet. Obstetrics and Gynecology 77(2):304–308

Enkin M, Keirse M, Neilson J et al 2000 A guide to effective care in pregnancy and childbirth, 3rd edn. Oxford University Press, Oxford

Francome C, Savage W, Churchill H, Lewison H 1993 Caesarean section birth in Britain. Middlesex University Press, Middlesex

Goer H 1995 Obstetrical myths versus research realities. A guide to the medical literature. Bergin & Garvey, London

Haire D B, Elsberry C C 1991 Maternity care and outcomes in a high risk service: the North Bronx Hospital experience. Birth 18(1):33–37

Henderson J 1996 Active management of labour and caesarean section rates. British Journal of Midwifery 4(3):132–149

Hillan E M 1995 Postoperative morbidity following caesarean delivery. Journal of Advanced Nursing (22):1035–1042

Holdcroft A, Parshall A M, Knowles M G et al 1995 Factors associated with mothers selecting general anaesthesia for lower segment caesarean section. Journal of Psychosomatic Obstetrics and Gynaecology 16(3):167–170

Johanson R B, Menon V J 1997 Vacuum extraction versus forceps delivery. In: Neilson J P, Crother C A, Hodnett E D, Hofmeyr G J, Keirse M J (eds) Pregnancy and childbirth module of the Cochrane Database of Systematic Reviews, The Cochrane Library. Update Software, Oxford

Kitzinger S 2000 Who would choose to have a caesarean? British Journal of Midwifery 9(5):284–285

Lewis G, Drife J (eds) (2001) Why mothers die 1997–1999. The fifth report of the confidential enquiries into maternal deaths in the United Kingdom. RCOG Press, London

Lilford R 1990 Maternal mortality and caesarean section. British Journal of Obstetrics and Gynaecology 97:883–892

Lim F T H, Holm J P, Schuitemaker N W E, Jansen F H M, Hermans J 1997 Stepwise compared with rapid application of vacuum in ventouse extraction procedures. British Journal of Obstetrics and Gynaecology 104:33–36

Lopez-Zeno J A et al 1992 A controlled trial of a program for the active management of labour. New England Journal of Medicine 326(17):450–454

Lydon-Rochelle M, Holt V L, Easterling T R, Martin D P 2001 Risk of uterine rupture during labor among women with a prior cesarian delivery. New England Journal of Medicine 345(1):3–8

McAleese S 2000 Caesarean section for maternal choice? Midwifery Matters 84:1–7

McIlwaine G, Boulton-Jones C, Cole S, Wilkinson C 1994–1995 Caesarean section in Scotland: a national audit

Magill-Cuerden J 1996 Intervention in a natural process. Modern Midwife, May: 4

Mander R 1998 Pain in childbearing and its control. Blackwell Science, London

Marwick J C, Lynn R 2001 High caesarean rates among women over 30. British Medical Journal 323:284

Miller A W F, Hanretty K P 1997 Obstetrics illustrated, 5th edn. Churchill Livingstone, London

Moolgaoker A S, Ahamed S O S, Payne P R 1979 A comparison of different methods of instrumental delivery based on electronic measurements of compression and traction. Obstetrics and Gynecology 81:689–694

Mulholland L 1997 Midwife ventouse practitioners. British Journal of Midwifery 5(5): 255

Myers S A, Gleicher N 1988 A successful program to lower cesarean section rates. New England Journal of Medicine 319(23):1511–1516

O'Driscoll K, Meagher D, Boylan P 1993 Active management of labour, 3rd edn. Mosby, London

Page L 1999 Caesarean birth: the kindest cut? British Journal of Midwifery 7(5):296

Peterson C M, Saunders N J 1991 Mode of delivery after one caesarean section: audit of current practice in a health region. British Medical Journal 303(6806):818–821

RCOG (Royal College of Obstetricians and Gynaecologists) 1994 Clinical Audit Unit information leaflet. RCOG, London

RCOG (Royal College of Obstetricians and Gynaecologists) 2001 Clinical Effectiveness Support Unit. The National Sentinel Caesarean Section audit report. RCOG, London

Roberts L J 1991 Elective section after two sections – Where's the evidence. British Journal of Obstetrics and Gynaecology 98(12):1199–1202

Robinson J 1999 The demand for caesareans: fact or fiction? British Journal of Midwifery 7(5):306

Sanchez-Ramos L et al 1990 Reducing cesarean sections in a teaching hospital. American Journal of Obstetrics and Gynaecology 163(3):1081–1088

Shearer E 1993 Caesarean section: medical benefits and costs. Social Science in Medicine 37(10):1223–1231

Silverton L 1993 The art and science of midwifery. Prentice Hall, London

Stables D 1999 Physiology in childbearing with anatomy and related biosciences. Baillière Tindall, London

Stephenson P A 1992 International differences in the use of obstetrical inventions. WHO, Copenhagen 112

Stratham H, Weaver J, Richards M 2001 Why choose caesarean section? Lancet 357:635

Svenningssen L 1987 Birth and progression and traction forces developed under vacuum traction after slow or rapid application of suction. European Journal of Obstetrics, Gynecology and Reproductive Biology 26:105–112

Taffel S M, Placek P J, Kosary C L 1992 US Cesarean section rates 1990: an update. Birth 19(1):21–22

Urquhart D R, Grieve R M K, Geals M F 1987 The rising caesarean section rate: a year's audit to assess the trend. Health Bulletin 45(6):316–328

Walker R, Golois E 2001 Why choose caesarean section? Lancet 357:636–637

Walmsley K, Hobbs L 1994 Vaginal birth after lower segment caesarean section. Modern Midwife, April: 20–21

Weaver J, Stratham H, Richards M 2001 High rates may be due to perceived potential for complications. British Medical Journal 323:284–285

Wright E A, Kapu M M, Onwuhafua H I 1991 Perinatal mortality and caesarean section in University Teaching Hospital, Nigeria. International Journal of Gynaecology and Obstetrics 35:299–304

Ziadeh S M, Sunna E I 1995 Decreased cesarean birth rates and improved perinatal outcome: a seven year study. Birth 22(3):144–147

FURTHER READING

Churchill H 1997 Caesarean birth experience, practice and history. Books for Midwives Press, Hale

This presents a comprehensive overview of caesarean birth, containing an historical account, from preindustrial times to the present. Developments in operative technique and indications for, and effects of, caesarean section are discussed in depth. Women's experience of this type of birth are considered.

Francome C, Savage W, Churchill H, Lewison H 1993 Caesarean birth in Britain. Middlesex University Press, London

A book for health professionals and parents, this presents an international and an historical narration of issues such as causes of, coping with, and policies of British consultants in relation to, caesarean section. Vaginal birth after caesarean section is reviewed.

32 Midwifery and Obstetric Emergencies

Christine Shiers and Terri Coates (Section on 'Shoulder dystocia')

CHAPTER CONTENTS

The immediate management of the emergencies discussed in this chapter is dependent on the prompt action of the midwife. The speed of this action while calling for medical aid will often help to determine the outcome for the mother or the baby. Recognition of the problem and the instigation of emergency measures allow time for help to arrive.

The chapter aims to:

- describe emergency situations including vasa praevia, cord prolapse and shoulder dystocia, with discussion on possible causes and action to be taken

- consider the rare conditions of uterine rupture and acute inversion, neither of which need occur with good management

- discuss amniotic fluid embolism, which remains an unpredictable catastrophe in which prompt action is needed to preserve the mother's life

- recommend strongly the practising of procedures for basic resuscitation on a regular basis

- provide information on shock, focusing on the conditions of hypovolaemic shock and septic shock, both of which may be seen in midwifery practice.

The midwife should remain alert to the possibility that the emergency, as in the case of sudden collapse, may not be directly associated with the mother's pregnancy. Basic life-support measures are included in this chapter.

Vasa praevia

The term *vasa praevia* is used when a fetal blood vessel lies over the os, in front of the presenting part. This occurs when fetal vessels from a velamentous insertion of the cord cross the area of the internal os to the placenta. The fetus is in jeopardy, owing to the risk of rupture of the vessels, which could lead to exsanguination.

Vasa praevia may sometimes be palpated on vaginal examination when the membranes are still intact. It may also be visualised on ultrasound. If it is suspected a speculum examination should be made.

Ruptured vasa praevia

When the membranes rupture in a case of vasa praevia, a fetal vessel may also rupture. This leads to exsanguination of the fetus unless birth occurs within minutes.

Diagnosis

Slight fresh vaginal bleeding, particularly if it commences at the same time as rupture of the membranes, may be due to ruptured vasa praevia. Fetal distress disproportionate to blood loss may be suggestive of vasa praevia.

Management

The midwife should call for assistance, requesting urgent medical aid. The fetal heart rate should be monitored. If the mother is in the first stage of labour and the fetus is still alive, an emergency caesarean section is carried out. If in the second stage of labour, delivery should be expedited and a vaginal birth may be achieved. Caesarean section may be carried out but mode of delivery will be dependent on parity and fetal condition.

A paediatrician should be present at delivery and, if the baby is alive, haemoglobin estimation will be necessary after resuscitation. The baby will require a blood transfusion but there is a high mortality associated with this emergency.

Presentation and prolapse of the umbilical cord (Box 32.1)

Predisposing factors

These are the same for both presentation and prolapse of the cord. Any situation where the presenting part is neither well applied to the lower uterine segment nor well down in the pelvis may make it possible for a loop of cord to slip down in front of the presenting part. Such situations include:

- high or ill-fitting presenting part
- high parity
- prematurity
- malpresentation
- multiple pregnancy
- polyhydramnios (Mesleh et al 1993, Murphy & MacKenzie 1995).

High head. If the membranes rupture spontaneously when the fetal head is high, a loop of cord may be able to pass between the uterine wall and the fetus, resulting in its lying in front of the presenting part. As the presenting part descends the cord becomes occluded.

Multiparity. The presenting part may not be engaged when the membranes rupture and malpresentation is more common.

Prematurity. The size of the fetus in relation to the pelvis and the uterus allows the cord to prolapse. Babies of very low birthweight (less than 1500 g) are particularly vulnerable (Mesleh et al 1993).

Malpresentation (see Ch. 30). Cord prolapse is associated with breech presentation, especially complete or footling breech. This relates to the ill-fitting nature of the presenting parts and also the proximity of the umbilicus to the buttocks. In this situation the degree of compression may be less than with a cephalic presentation, but there is still a danger of asphyxia.

Box 32.1 Definitions

Cord presentation

This occurs when the umbilical cord lies in front of the presenting part, with the fetal membranes still intact.

Cord prolapse

The cord lies in front of the presenting part and the fetal membranes are ruptured (see Fig. 32.1).

Occult cord prolapse

This is said to occur when the cord lies alongside, but not in front of, the presenting part.

Shoulder and compound presentation and transverse lie carry a high risk of prolapse of the cord, occurring with spontaneous rupture of the membranes.

Face and brow presentations are less common causes of cord prolapse.

Multiple pregnancy. Malpresentation, particularly of the second twin, is more common in multiple pregnancy.

Polyhydramnios. The cord is liable to be swept down in a gush of liquor if the membranes rupture spontaneously. Controlled release of liquor during artificial rupture of the membranes is sometimes performed to try to prevent this.

Murphy & MacKenzie (1995) found in 55 cases out of a total 132 that none of the above factors could be attributed as the reason for cord prolapse.

Cord presentation

This is diagnosed on vaginal examination when the cord is felt behind intact membranes. It is, however, rarely detected but may be associated with aberrations in fetal heart monitoring such as decelerations, which occur if the cord becomes compressed.

Management

Under no circumstances should the membranes be ruptured. The midwife should discontinue the vaginal examination, in order to reduce the risk of rupturing the membranes. Help should be summoned, including medical aid. If continuous electronic fetal monitoring is available, a recording may be commenced to assess fetal well-being. The mother should be helped into a position that will reduce the likelihood of cord compression. In the absence of continuous fetal monitoring the fetal heart should be auscultated as continuously as possible, particularly during contractions.

Caesarean section is the most likely outcome.

Cord prolapse (Fig. 32.1)

Diagnosis

The diagnosis of cord prolapse is made when the cord is felt below or beside the presenting part on vaginal examination. A loop of cord may be visible at the vulva. The cord is more commonly felt in the vagina or, in cases where the presenting part is very high, it may be felt in the cervical os.

Whenever there are factors present that predispose to cord prolapse, a vaginal examination should be performed immediately on spontaneous rupture of membranes.

An abnormal heart rate, particularly bradycardia, may indicate cord prolapse. Suspected cord prolapse may be the result of a suspicious CTG. Variable decelerations and prolonged decelerations of the fetal heart are associated with cord compression, which may be caused by cord prolapse.

Immediate action

Where the diagnosis of cord prolapse is made, the midwife should call for urgent assistance. The midwife should explain her findings to the mother and her birth partner(s) and the emergency measures that will be needed.

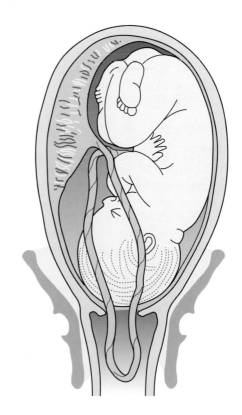

Fig. 32.1 Cord prolapse: cord prolapse with ruptured membranes.

If an oxytocin infusion is in progress this should be stopped. The midwife carries out a vaginal examination and assesses the degree of cervical dilatation. She identifies the presenting part and station. The time should also be noted. If the cord can be felt pulsating, it should be handled as little as possible. Spasm of the cord may occur through handling or be due to reduction in temperature. If the cord lies outside the vagina, then it should be gently replaced to try to maintain temperature. An assistant should be asked to auscultate the fetal heart and a record of the fetal heart rate is made.

Pressure on the cord must be relieved. In order to do this the midwife keeps her fingers in the vagina and, especially during a contraction, holds the presenting part off the umbilical cord. The mother is helped to change position so that her pelvis and buttocks are raised. The knee–chest position causes the fetus to gravitate towards the diaphragm, relieving the compression on the cord (Fig. 32.2). Alternatively the mother can be helped to lie on her left side, with a wedge or pillow elevating her hips (exaggerated Sims' position) (Fig. 32.3). The foot of the bed may be raised. These measures need to be maintained until the delivery of the baby, either vaginally or by caesarean section.

Management

The risks to the fetus are hypoxia and death as a result of cord compression. The risks are greatest with prematurity and low birthweight (Murphy & MacKenzie 1995). Delivery must be expedited with the greatest possible speed to reduce the mortality and morbidity associated with this condition. Caesarean section is the treatment of choice in those instances where the fetus is still alive and delivery is not imminent, or vaginal birth cannot be indicated.

In the second stage of labour the mother may be able to push and the midwife may perform an episiotomy to expedite the birth. This may be possible with a multiparous mother. Where the presentation is cephalic, assisted birth may be achieved through ventouse or forceps.

If cord prolapse occurs in the community and the fetus is thought to still be alive, emergency transfer to hospital is essential. The midwife should carry out the same procedures to relieve the compression on the cord, with the mother adopting a left lateral position, as above, with buttocks elevated. Consultant unit staff should be informed and be prepared to perform an emergency caesarean section on arrival.

Shoulder dystocia

Definition

The term 'shoulder dystocia' is used in this chapter to describe failure of the shoulders to traverse the pelvis spontaneously after delivery of the head (Smeltzer 1986). However, a universally accepted definition of shoulder dystocia has yet to be produced (Roberts 1994).

The anterior shoulder becomes trapped behind or on the symphysis pubis, whilst the posterior shoulder may be in the hollow of the sacrum or high above the sacral promontory (Fig. 32.4). This is, therefore, a bony dystocia, and traction at this point will further impact the anterior shoulder, impeding attempts at delivery.

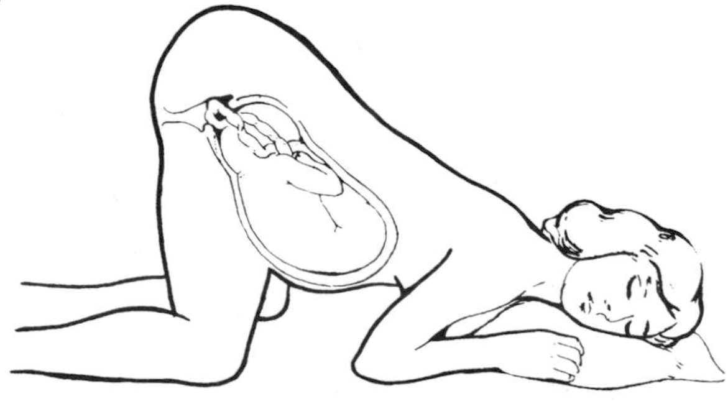

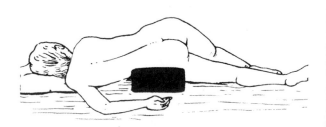

Fig. 32.2 Knee–chest position. Pressure on the umbilical cord is relieved as the fetus gravitates towards the fundus.

Fig. 32.3 Exaggerated Sims' position. Pillows or wedges are used to elevate the woman's buttocks to relieve pressure on the umbilical cord.

Incidence

Shoulder dystocia is not a common emergency: the incidence is reported as varying between 0.37% and 1.1% (Bahar 1996).

Risk factors

Although it would be useful to identify those women at risk from a delivery complicated by shoulder dystocia, most risk factors can give only a high index of suspicion (Al-Najashi et al 1989). Antenatally these risk factors include post-term pregnancy, high parity, maternal age over 35 and maternal obesity (weight over 90 kg at delivery).

Fetal macrosomia (birthweight over 4000 g) has been associated with an increased risk of shoulder dystocia, the incidence increasing as birthweight increases (Acker et al 1985, Delpapa & Mueller-Heubach 1991, Hall 1996). However, ultrasound scanning for prediction of macrosomia to prevent shoulder dystocia has a poor record of success (Combs et al 1993, Hall 1996). If a large baby is suspected then this fact must be communicated clearly to the team caring for the woman in labour (CESDI 1999, p. 47).

Maternal diabetes and gestational diabetes have been identified as important risk factors (Bahar 1996, Benedetti & Gabbe 1978, Gross et al 1987, Spellacy et al 1985). In diabetic women a previous delivery complicated by shoulder dystocia increases the risk of recurrence to 9.8%; this compares with a risk of recurrence of 0.58% in the general population (Smith et al 1994).

In labour, risk factors that have been consistently linked with shoulder dystocia include oxytocin augmentation, prolonged labour, prolonged second stage of labour and operative deliveries (Acker et al 1986, Al-Najashi et al 1989, Bahar 1996, Benedetti & Gabbe 1978, Keller et al 1991). For a clinically suspected large baby the delivery team must be alert for the possibility of shoulder dystocia (CESDI 1999).

Warning signs and diagnosis

The delivery may have been uncomplicated initially (Morris 1955), but the head may have advanced slowly and the chin may have had difficulty in sweeping over the perineum. Once the head is delivered it may look as if it is trying to return into the vagina, which is caused by reverse traction.

Shoulder dystocia is diagnosed when manoeuvres normally used by the midwife fail to accomplish delivery (Resnik 1980).

Management

Upon diagnosing shoulder dystocia the midwife must summon help immediately. An obstetrician, an anaesthetist and a person proficient in neonatal resuscitation should be called.

Shoulder dystocia is a frightening experience for the mother, for her partner and for the midwife. The midwife should keep calm and try to explain as much as possible to the mother to ensure her full cooperation for the manoeuvres that may be needed to complete the delivery.

The purpose of all these manoeuvres is to disimpact the shoulders and accomplish delivery. The principle of using the most simple manoeuvres first should be applied.

The midwife will need to make an accurate and detailed record of the type of manoeuvre(s) used and the time taken, the amount of force used and the outcome of each manoeuvre attempted.

Non-invasive procedures

Change in maternal position. Any change in the maternal position may be useful to help release the fetal shoulders. However, certain manoeuvres have

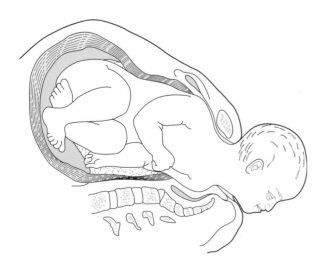

Fig. 32.4 Shoulder dystocia.

proved useful and are described below. It is anticipated that following the use of one or more of these manoeuvres the midwife should be able to proceed with the delivery.

The McRoberts manoeuvre. This manoeuvre involves helping the woman to lie flat and to bring her knees up to her chest as far as possible (Fig. 32.5).

This manoeuvre will rotate the angle of the symphysis pubis superiorly and use the weight of the mother's legs to create gentle pressure on her abdomen, releasing the impaction of the anterior shoulder (Gonik et al 1983, 1989). It is the manoeuvre associated with the lowest level of morbidity and requires the least force to accomplish delivery (Bahar 1996, Gross et al 1987, Nocon et al 1993).

Suprapubic pressure. Pressure should be exerted on the side of the fetal back and towards the fetal chest. This manoeuvre may help to adduct the shoulders and push the anterior shoulder away from the symphysis pubis (Fig. 32.6).

Manipulative procedures

Where non-invasive procedures have not been successful, direct manipulation of the fetus must now be attempted.

Positioning of the mother. The McRoberts position as detailed above can be used, or the mother could be placed in the lithotomy position with her buttocks well over the end of the bed so that there is no restriction on the sacrum. If neither the McRoberts nor lithotomy positions are appropriate, then the all-fours position may prove useful. Any of the following

manoeuvres can be undertaken with the mother in one of these positions.

Episiotomy. It must be remembered that the problem facing the midwife is an obstruction at the pelvic inlet and is a bony dystocia, not an obstruction caused by soft tissue. Although episiotomy will not help to release the shoulders per se, the midwife should nevertheless perform one (see Ch. 27) to gain access to the fetus without tearing the perineum and vaginal walls.

Rubin's manoeuvre. This manoeuvre (Rubin 1964) requires the midwife to identify the posterior shoulder on vaginal examination, then to push the posterior shoulder in the direction of the fetal chest, thus rotating the anterior shoulder away from the symphysis pubis. By adducting the shoulders this manoeuvre reduces the 12 cm bisacromial diameter (Fig. 32.7).

Woods' manoeuvre. Woods' (1943) manoeuvre requires the midwife to insert her hand into the vagina and identify the fetal chest. Then, by exerting pressure on to the posterior fetal shoulder, rotation is achieved. Although this manoeuvre does abduct the shoulders it will rotate the shoulders into a more favourable diameter and enable the midwife to complete the delivery (Fig. 32.8).

Delivery of the posterior arm. To deliver the posterior arm the midwife has to insert her hand into the vagina making use of the space created by the hollow of the sacrum (Fig. 32.9A, B). Then two fingers splint the humerus of the posterior arm (Fig. 32.9C), flex the elbow, and sweep the forearm over the chest to deliver the hand (Fig. 32.9D) (O'Leary 1992). If the rest of the delivery is not then accomplished, the second arm can

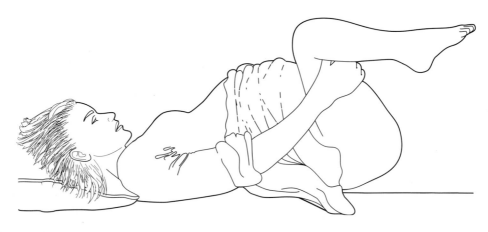

Fig. 32.5 The McRoberts manoeuvre position.

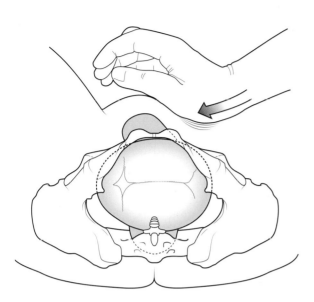

Fig. 32.6 Correct application of suprapubic pressure for shoulder dystocia. (After Pauerstein C 1987 with permission.)

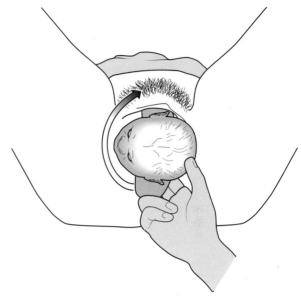

Fig. 32.7 The Rubin manoeuvre.

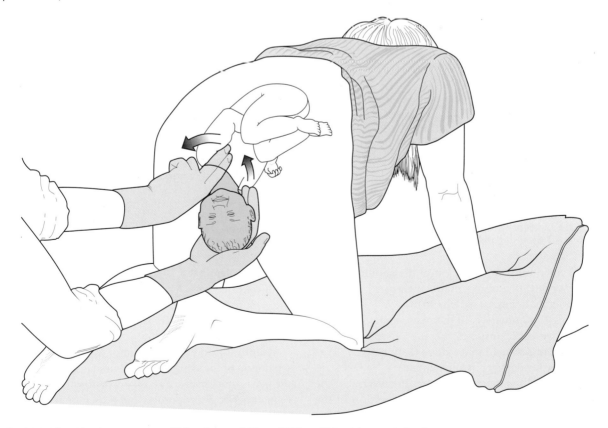

Fig. 32.8 The Woods manoeuvre. (After Sweet & Tiran 1996, p. 664, with permission.)

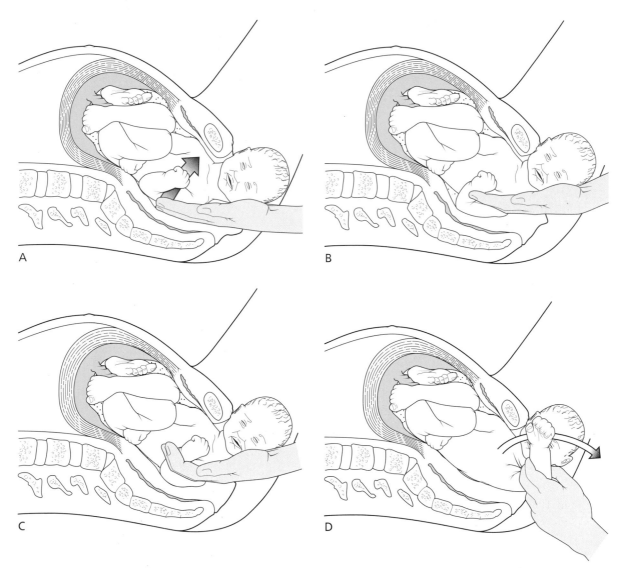

Fig. 32.9 Delivery of the posterior arm: (A) Location of the posterior arm. (B) Directing the arm into the hollow of the sacrum. (C) Grasping and splinting the wrist and forearm. (D) Sweeping the arm over the chest and delivering the hand.

be delivered following rotation of the shoulder using either Woods' or Rubin's manoeuvre or by reversing the Løvset manoeuvre (see Ch. 30).

Zavanelli manoeuvre. If the manoeuvres described above have been unsuccessful, the obstetrician may consider the Zavanelli manoeuvre (Sandberg 1985) as a last hope for delivery of a live infant.

The Zavanelli manoeuvre requires the reversal of the mechanisms of delivery so far and reinsertion of the fetal head into the vagina. Delivery is then completed by caesarean section.

Method. The head is returned to its pre-restitution position (Fig. 32.10A). Pressure is then exerted on to the occiput and the head is returned to the vagina (Fig. 32.10B). Prompt delivery by caesarean section is then required.

Symphysiotomy. Symphysiotomy is the surgical separation of the symphysis pubis and is used to enlarge the pelvis for delivery. It is usually performed in cases of cephalopelvic disproportion and is used more routinely in Third World countries. There are a few recorded cases where symphysiotomy has been used successfully to

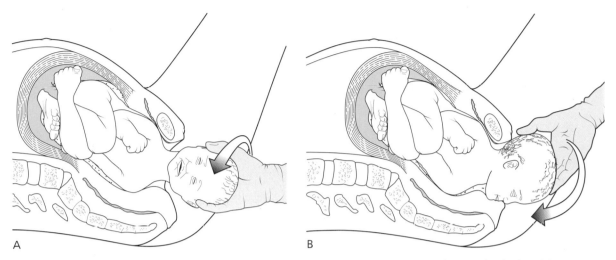

Fig. 32.10 The Zavanelli manoeuvre: (A) Head being returned to direct anteroposterior (pre-restitution) position. (B) Head being returned to the vagina. (After Sandberg 1985, with permission.)

relieve shoulder dystocia (Reid & Osuagwu 1999), but the procedure has usually been associated with a high level of maternal morbidity. The rarity of reported cases makes it difficult to assess the technique for the relief of shoulder dystocia.

Outcomes following shoulder dystocia

Maternal

Approximately two-thirds will have a blood loss of more than 1000 ml from injury associated with the delivery (Benedetti & Gabbe 1978). Maternal death from uterine rupture has been reported following the use of fundal pressure (Seigworth 1966) and from haemorrhage during and following the delivery (O'Leary 1992).

Fetal

Neonatal asphyxia may occur following shoulder dystocia in 5.7–9.7% of cases and the attending paediatrician must be experienced in neonatal resuscitation (Acker et al 1985, Brook & Weindling 1995, CESDI 1999, Modaniou et al 1980, Naef & Morrison 1994).

Brachial plexus injury with damage to cervical nerve roots 5 and 6 may result in an Erb's palsy (see also Ch. 44). This is commonly associated with shoulder dystocia when the head and neck have been twisted (Ubachs et al 1995).

Neonatal morbidity may be as high as 42% following shoulder dystocia. Fetal damage may occur even with excellent management using appropriate obstetric manoeuvres (Naet & Morrison 1994). Shoulder dystocia remains a cause of intrapartum fetal death (CESDI 1999).

Rupture of the uterus

Rupture of the uterus is one of the most serious complications in midwifery and obstetrics. It is often fatal for the fetus and may also be responsible for the death of the mother. With effective antenatal and intrapartum care this complication should be avoided; however, it remains a significant problem worldwide.

Rupture of the uterus is defined as being complete or incomplete:

- *complete rupture* – involves a tear in the wall of the uterus with or without expulsion of the fetus
- *incomplete rupture* – involves tearing of the uterine wall but not the perimetrium.

Life of both mother and fetus may be endangered in either situation.

Dehiscence of an existing uterine scar may also occur. This involves rupture of the uterine wall but the fetal membranes remain intact. The fetus is retained within the uterus and not expelled into the peritoneal cavity (Cunningham et al 1997).

Causes

Spontaneous rupture of the uterus can be precipitated in the following circumstances:

- high parity
- injudicious use of oxytocin, particularly where the mother is of high parity
- use of prostaglandins to induce labour, in the presence of an existing scar (Lydon-Rochelle et al 2001, Vause & Macintosh 1999)
- obstructed labour: the uterus ruptures owing to excessive thinning of the lower segment
- neglected labour, where there is previous history of caesarean section
- extension of severe cervical laceration upwards into the lower uterine segment – this may be the result of trauma during an assisted birth (DoH et al 1996)
- trauma, as a result of a blast injury or an accident (Awwad et al 1993)
- perforation of the non-pregnant uterus, resulting in rupture of the uterus in a subsequent pregnancy; perforation and rupture occur in the upper segment (Howe 1993)
- antenatal rupture of the uterus, where there has been a history of previous classical caesarean section.

Cases of spontaneous rupture of an unscarred uterus in primigravid mothers are also reported in the literature (Guirgis & Kettle 1989, Roberts & Trew 1991), but are rare.

Signs of intrapartum rupture of the uterus

Complete rupture of a previously non-scarred uterus may be accompanied by sudden collapse of the mother, who complains of severe abdominal pain. The maternal pulse rate increases; simultaneously, alterations of the fetal heart may occur, including the presence of variable decelerations (Flannelly et al 1993, Phelan 1990). Heart sounds may be lost (Rachagan et al 1991). There may be evidence of fresh vaginal bleeding. The uterine contractions may stop and the contour of the abdomen alters. The fetus becomes palpable in the abdomen as the presenting part regresses. The degree and speed of the mother's

collapse and shock depend on the extent of the rupture and the blood loss (Box 32.2).

Incomplete rupture of the uterus

Incomplete rupture may have an insidious onset or be silent, and found only after delivery or during a caesarean section. This type is more commonly associated with previous caesarean section. Blood loss associated with dehiscence, or incomplete rupture, can be scanty, as the rupture occurs along the fibrous scar tissue (O'Connor & Gaughan 1993).

Incomplete rupture may also be manifest as a cause of postpartum haemorrhage following vaginal birth. Whenever shock during the third stage of labour is more severe than the type of delivery or blood loss warrants, or the mother fails to respond to treatment given, the possibility of incomplete rupture should be considered.

Management

An immediate caesarean section is performed, in the hope of delivering a live baby. Following the delivery of the fetus and placenta, the extent of the rupture can be assessed. Choice between the options to perform a hysterectomy or to repair the rupture depends on the extent of the trauma and the mother's condition. Further clinical assessment will include evaluation of the need for blood replacement and management of any shock.

The mother will be unprepared for the events that have occurred and therefore may be totally opposed to hysterectomy. Reports of successful pregnancy following repair of uterine rupture are available (O'Connor & Gaughan 1993).

Box 32.2 Signs of rupture of uterus

- Maternal tachycardia
- Scar pain and tenderness (where previous caesarean section)
- Abnormalities of the fetal heart rate and pattern
- Poor progress in labour
- Vaginal bleeding

Rupture of the uterus following previous caesarean section

The risk of uterine rupture is increased for those women who have a uterine scar. The fifth annual report of the Confidential Enquiry into Stillbirths and Deaths in Infancy (CESDI 1998) found 42 intrapartum fetal deaths that were the result of uterine rupture. It estimated that uterine rupture occurs in 1 in 140 to 1 in 300 labours where mothers present with an existing uterine scar. Additional studies cite figures of between 0.3 and 0.7% of labours following a previous caesarean section (Miller et al 1994, Vause & Macintosh 1999). It is evident that both mothers and babies are at risk, and that mortality and morbidity from uterine rupture can be reduced if appropriate care is given. Rupture can be in the form of total rupture or dehiscence. Rates of rupture are lowest following a lower segment caesarean section, which is the commonest type of incision.

The Confidential Enquiries into Maternal Deaths in the UK for the triennium 1997–1999 record one death due to ruptured uterus where there is a history of previous caesarean section (Lewis & Drife 2001). Uterine rupture associated with the use of prostaglandin was reported in the previous report of the Confidential Enquiry into Maternal Deaths in the UK (DoH 1998). The use of prostaglandins for induction in the presence of a uterine scar is contraindicated (British National Formulary 2001). Induction with oxytocin is also associated with increased risk of rupture where a previous caesarean section has been carried out.

Amniotic fluid embolism/ anaphylactoid syndrome of pregnancy

This rare but potentially catastrophic condition occurs when amniotic fluid enters the maternal circulation via the uterus or placental site. The presence of amniotic fluid in the maternal circulation triggers an anaphylactoid response and the term 'embolus' is a misnomer (Clark et al 1995).

The body responds in two phases. The initial phase is one of pulmonary vasospasm causing hypoxia, hypotension, pulmonary oedema and cardiovascular collapse. The second phase sees the development of left ventricular failure, with haemorrhage and coagulation disorder and further uncontrollable haemorrhage. Mortality and morbidity are high (Clark 1990).

Predisposing factors

Amniotic fluid embolism can occur at any gestation. It is mostly associated with labour and its immediate aftermath but cases in early pregnancy and postpartum have been documented. There is no evidence to suggest that parity places mothers at any increased risk nor can the condition be attributed to the use of oxytocics (Clark 1990, Clark et al 1995, Morgan 1979).

The risk of amniotic fluid infusion is associated with the exposure of the maternal circulation to even small quantities of amniotic fluid. Transfer of amniotic fluid from the uterus to the maternal circulation can be insidious, and associated with a tear in the membranes. Chance entry of amniotic fluid into the circulation under pressure may occur, although the hypertonic uterine activity seen in some cases may be a consequence of uterine hypoxia that occurs in the first phase rather than as a precursor to the condition. Uterine hypertonus occurs in response to the cardiovascular collapse and protects against liquor transferring into the maternal circulation, rather than being responsible for pumping liquor across (Clark et al 1995) (Box 32.3).

The barrier between the maternal circulation and the amniotic sac may be breached in the presence of a placental abruption, when the placental bed is disrupted. Procedures such as insertion of an intrauterine catheter and ARM are also associated with this. Amniotic fluid embolism can occur during a caesarean section and is not prevented by performing a caesarean section. It may also occur in association with a perforated or ruptured uterus. Trauma may occur during an intrauterine manipulation, such as internal podalic version. The opportunity for amniotic fluid to enter the mother's circulation may also occur during termination of pregnancy.

It is a condition that is difficult to predict and equally difficult to prevent. Amniotic fluid embolism is associated with a high maternal mortality rate. Eight women died in the years 1997–1999, the diagnosis having been confirmed by postmortem. Based on the UK Confidential Enquiry Reports, age has been seen to be a consistent risk factor, with women over the age of 30 being found to be at risk (Lewis & Drife 2001).

Box 32.3 Process of amniotic fluid embolism/anaphylactoid syndrome of pregnancy

Amniotic fluid enters maternal circulation

↓

Pathophysiology	Possible clinical signs
Phase 1	
Pulmonary vasospasm	Fetal compromise
Hypoxia	Shock
Hypotension	Uterine hypertonus
Cardiovascular collapse	Tachycardia
	Cyanosis
	Breathlessness
	Tachypnoea
	Anxiety
	Shivering
	Sweating
	Convulsions
	Cardiac arrest
Phase 2	
Left ventricular failure	Bleeding
Pulmonary oedema	Thrombolysis (bleeding from intravenous sites)
Haemorrhage	Cardiovascular
Coagulation disorder	collapse

Clinical signs and symptoms

There is sudden onset of maternal respiratory distress. The woman becomes severely dyspnoeic and cyanosed. There is maternal hypotension and uterine hypertonus. The latter will induce fetal compromise and is in response to uterine hypoxia. Cardiopulmonary arrest follows quickly. Only minutes may elapse before arrest. There is evidence that many mothers present with convulsions immediately preceding the collapse (Clark 1990).

Blood coagulopathy develops following the initial collapse, if the mother survives. Where cases have been confirmed, mortality within 1 hour from onset is 50% (Chatelain & Quirk 1990).

Emergency action

Any one of the above symptoms is indicative of an acute emergency. As the mother is likely to be in a state of collapse, resuscitation needs to be commenced at once. An emergency team should be called, since the midwife responsible for the care of the mother requires immediate help. If collapse occurs in a community setting, basic life support should be commenced prior to the arrival of emergency services.

Despite improvements in intensive care the outcome of this condition is poor. Specific management for the condition is life support, and high levels of oxygen are required. Mothers who survive are likely to have suffered a degree of neurological impairment (Clark et al 1995).

Complications of amniotic fluid embolism

Disseminated intravascular coagulation (DIC) is likely to occur within 30 minutes of the initial collapse. In some cases the mother bleeds heavily prior to developing amniotic fluid embolism, which contributes to the severity of her condition. It has also been reported that the amniotic fluid has the ability to suppress the myometrium, resulting in uterine atony. This further compounds the haemorrhage (Courtney 1970).

Acute renal failure is a complication of the excessive blood loss and the prolonged hypovolaemic hypotension. The mother will require continuous assessment of urinary output, using an indwelling catheter. Accurate records of fluid intake and urinary output and urinalysis should be maintained by the midwife. A urinary output of less than 30 ml per hour should be reported, as should the presence of proteinuria. Transfer to an intensive therapy unit for specialised nursing care is indicated. Midwifery care and advice should be continued for the family.

Effect of amniotic fluid embolism on the fetus

Perinatal mortality and morbidity are high where amniotic fluid embolism occurs before the birth of the baby. Delay in the time from initial maternal collapse to delivery needs to be minimal if fetal compromise or death is to be avoided. However, maternal resuscitation may, at that time, be a priority.

Box 32.4 is a summary of the key points relating to amniotic fluid embolism.

Box 32.4 Summary of key points for amniotic fluid embolism

- Amniotic fluid embolism is a major cause of maternal death worldwide.
- Its common name is a misnomer: there is no embolism.
- Is now understood to be an anaphylactoid response to amniotic fluid entering the maternal circulation.
- Universal features are maternal shock and fetal distress, followed by dysnoea and cardiovascular collapse.
- It can be a response to *any* amniotic fluid, not merely the response to large quantities.
- It can occur at any time, but labour and its immediate aftermath are most common.
- It should be suspected in cases of sudden collapse or uncontrollable bleeding.

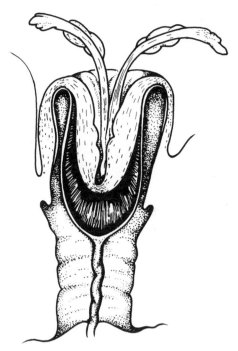

Fig. 32.11 Second degree inversion of the uterus.

Acute inversion of the uterus

This is a rare but potentially life-threatening complication of the third stage of labour. It occurs in approximately 1 in 2500 births (Brar et al 1989).

In the most serious cases the inner surface of the fundus appears at the vaginal outlet, as in *total inversion*. In less severe cases the fundus is dimpled, which is known as a *partial inversion*.

A midwife's awareness of the precipitating factors enables her to take preventive measures to avoid this emergency.

Classification of inversion

Inversion can be classified according to severity as follows:

- *First degree* – the fundus reaches the internal os
- *Second degree* – the body or corpus of the uterus is inverted to the internal os (Fig. 32.11)
- *Third degree* – the uterus, cervix and vagina are inverted and are visible.

It is also classified according to timing of the event:

- *acute inversion* – occurs within the first 24 hours
- *subacute inversion* – occurs after the first 24 hours, and within 4 weeks

- *chronic inversion* – occurs after 4 weeks and is rare (Brar et al 1989).

It is the first of these, acute inversion, that the remainder of this section considers.

Causes

Causes of acute inversion are associated with uterine atony and cervical dilatation, and include:

- mismanagement in the third stage of labour, involving excessive cord traction to manage the delivery of the placenta actively
- combining fundal pressure and cord traction to deliver the placenta
- use of fundal pressure while the uterus is atonic, to deliver the placenta
- pathologically adherent placenta (Kitchin et al 1975)
- spontaneous occurrence, of unknown cause
- primiparity (Brar et al 1989, Platt & Druzin 1981)
- fetal macrosomia (Brar et al 1989)
- short umbilical cord (Kitchin et al 1975)
- sudden emptying of a distended uterus.

Careful management of the third stage of labour is needed to prevent inversion. In active management of the third stage, palpation of the fundus is essential to confirm that contraction has taken place, prior to controlled cord traction.

Warning signs and diagnosis

The major sign of acute inversion is haemorrhage, which occurs in 94% of documented cases. The blood loss is within a range of 800–1800 ml (Platt & Druzin 1981, Watson et al 1980).

Shock and sudden onset of pain are seen in 40% of affected mothers. The pain is thought to be caused by the stretching of the peritoneal nerves and the ovaries being pulled as the fundus inverts. Bleeding may or may not be present, depending on the degree of placental adherence to the uterine wall. The cause of the symptoms may not be readily apparent.

The fundus will not be palpable on abdominal examination and diagnosis may be missed if inversion is incomplete and therefore the fundus not visible at the introitus. A mass may be felt on vaginal examination.

Management

Immediate action

A swift response is needed to reduce the risks to the mother.

1. Help is summoned, including appropriate medical support.
2. The midwife in attendance should immediately attempt to replace the uterus. This may be achieved by pushing the fundus with the palm of the hand, along the direction of the vagina, towards the posterior fornix. The uterus is then lifted towards the umbilicus and returned to position with a steady pressure (Johnson's manoeuvre). This, if successful, will reduce the risk to the mother.
3. An intravenous cannula should be inserted and fluids commenced. Blood should be taken for cross-matching prior to starting the infusion.
4. If the placenta is still attached, it should be left in situ as attempts to remove it at this stage may result in uncontrollable haemorrhage.
5. Once the uterus is repositioned, the operator should keep the hand in situ until a firm contraction is palpated. Oxytocics should be given to maintain the contraction (Cunningham et al 1997).

Medical management

If manual replacement fails, then medical or surgical intervention is required. The use of the hydrostatic method of replacement involves the instillation of warm saline infused through a giving set into the vagina. The pressure of the fluid builds up as several litres are run into the vagina and restores the uterus to the normal position, while the operator seals off the introitus by one hand inserted into the vagina.

If the inversion cannot be manually replaced, it may be due to the development of a cervical constriction ring. Drugs can be utilised to relax the constriction and facilitate the return of the uterus to its normal position.

Throughout the events the mother and her partner should be kept informed of what is happening. Assessment of vital signs, including level of consciousness, is of utmost importance.

Basic life-support measures

Standards of basic life support have been agreed for health professionals and lay people throughout Europe. Basic life support refers to the maintenance of an airway and support for breathing, without any specialist equipment other than possibly a pharyngeal airway. Before starting any resuscitation, assessment of any risk to the carer and the patient is needed. The space available, size of patient* and her condition may place those undertaking resuscitation in danger of injury. Slide sheets should be available to move patients. The position of the patient may result in the midwife being unable to undertake chest compression or ventilation effectively and cause personal injury as a result of twisting, or straining back muscles (Resuscitation Council UK 2001).

The basic principles are:

A – airway
B – breathing
C – circulation.

1. The level of consciousness is established by shaking the woman's shoulders and enquiring whether she can hear.
2. Assistance is called for by ringing the emergency bell or asking the partner to call for help and then return to the midwife who must remain with the woman.

---

* 'Patient' rather than 'mother' or 'woman' is used, as the reference is to any collapsed person who requires resuscitation.

3. The woman is laid flat, removing pillows. A pregnant woman should be further positioned with a left lateral tilt to prevent aortocaval compression. This can be achieved by the use of pillows or a wedge under the right side.

4. The head is tilted back and the chin lifted upwards to improve the patency of the airway (Fig. 32.12).

5. The airway is cleared of any mucus or vomit. Any well-fitting dentures are left in place.

6. The chest is observed for signs of respiratory effort. The midwife listens for breathing sounds and feels for breath being exhaled from the mouth and nose. An oropharyngeal airway of the correct size is inserted if available.

7. If no breathing is detected, the midwife will pinch the nose closed, take a deep breath in and exhale into the woman's mouth, so that her chest can be seen to rise. The air is then allowed to escape and the chest should be observed to fall. She repeats this to achieve two effective breaths. If after five attempts the woman remains unresponsive the signs of circulation should be assessed.

8. The midwife should quickly check for a carotid pulse. If there is no pulse, external chest compression is needed. The xiphisternum is located. The hands are placed palm downwards one on top of the other with the fingers interlinked. The heel of the lower hand is positioned on the lower two-thirds of the sternum. With arms straight, the midwife leans on to the sternum, depressing it 4–5 cm, and releases it slowly at the same rate as compression. The action should be repeated 100 times a minute. The midwife may need to kneel over the woman or find something to stand on to ensure that she is suitably positioned to carry out resuscitation (Fig. 32.13). The surface under the woman must be firm for the manoeuvre to succeed.

9. Chest compression and rescue breathing should be continued until help arrives and until those experienced in resuscitation are able to take over. A rate of 15 chest compression to 2 breaths is carried on if only one person is present; if two people are available the rate is 15 compressions to 2 breaths (Resuscitation Council UK 2000).

These measures are summarised in Box 32.5.

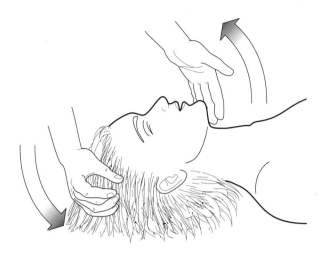

Fig. 32.12 The airway is opened by tilting the head backwards and lifting the chin upwards.

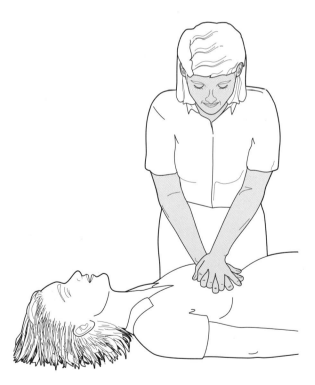

Fig. 32.13 Chest compression. The midwife leans well over the patient, with arms straight. Hands are one on top of the other with fingers interlinked. The heel of the hand is used to compress the chest.

Box 32.5 Summary of basic life-support guidelines

1. Shake and shout
2. Call for help
3. Check breathing
4. Check pulse
5. Cardiac arrest – precordial thump to chest
6. Check pulse
7. Use 2 breaths to 15 compressions
8. Continue until help arrives

Shock

Shock is a complex syndrome involving a reduction in blood flow to the tissues with resulting dysfunction of organs and cells. It entails progressive collapse of the circulatory system and, if left untreated, can result in death. Shock can be acute but prompt treatment results in recovery, with little detrimental effect on the mother. However, inadequate treatment or failure to initiate effective treatment can result in a chronic condition ending in multisystem organ failure, which may be fatal.

Shock can be classified as follows:

- *hypovolaemic* – the result of a reduction in intravascular volume
- *cardiogenic* – impaired ability of the heart to pump blood
- *distributive* – an abnormality in the vascular system that produces a maldistribution of the circulatory system; this includes septic and anaphylactic shock (Rice 1991).

This section deals with the principles of hypovolaemic shock and septic shock, either of which may develop as a consequence of events of childbearing.

Hypovolaemic shock

This is caused by any loss of circulating fluid volume that is not compensated for, as in haemorrhage, but may also occur when there is severe vomiting. The main causes and management of both these conditions are dealt with elsewhere.

The body reacts to the loss of circulating fluid in stages as follows:

Initial stage. The reduction in fluid or blood decreases the venous return to the heart. The ventricles of the heart are inadequately filled, causing a reduction in stroke volume and cardiac output. As cardiac output and venous return fall, the blood pressure is reduced. The drop in blood pressure decreases the supply of oxygen to the tissues and cell function is affected.

Compensatory stage. The drop in cardiac output produces a response from the sympathetic nervous system through the activation of receptors in the aorta and carotid arteries. Blood is redistributed to the vital organs. Vessels in the gastrointestinal tract, kidneys, skin and lungs constrict. This response is seen by the skin becoming pale and cool. Peristalsis slows, urinary output is reduced and exchange of gas in the lungs is impaired as blood flow diminishes. The heart rate increases in an attempt to improve cardiac output and blood pressure. The pupils of the eyes dilate. The sweat glands are stimulated and the skin becomes moist and clammy. Adrenaline (epinephrine) is released from the adrenal medulla and aldosterone from the adrenal cortex. Antidiuretic hormone (ADH) is secreted from the posterior lobe of the pituitary. Their combined effect is to cause vasoconstriction, an increased cardiac output and a decrease in urinary output. Venous return to the heart will increase but, unless the fluid loss is replaced, will not be sustained.

Progressive stage. This stage leads to multisystem failure. Compensatory mechanisms begin to fail, with vital organs lacking adequate perfusion. Volume depletion causes a further fall in blood pressure and cardiac output. The coronary arteries suffer lack of supply. Peripheral circulation is poor, with weak or absent pulses.

Final, irreversible stage of shock. Multisystem failure and cell destruction are irreparable. Death ensues.

Effect of shock on organs and systems

The human body is able to compensate for loss of up to 10% of fluid volume, principally by vasoconstriction. When that loss reaches 20–25%, however, the compensatory mechanisms begin to decline and fail. In pregnancy the plasma volume increases, as does the red cell mass. The increase is not proportionate, but allows a healthy pregnant woman to sustain significant blood loss at birth as the plasma volume is reduced with little disturbance to normal haemodynamics. In a woman who has not had a healthy increase in plasma volume, or has sustained an antepartum haemorrhage, a much lower blood loss is required to have a pathological effect on the body and its systems. Individual organs are affected as follows:

Brain. The level of consciousness deteriorates as cerebral blood flow is compromised. The mother will become increasingly unresponsive. She may not respond to verbal stimuli and there is a gradual reduction in the response elicited from painful stimulation.

Lungs. Gas exchange is impaired as the physiological dead space increases within the lungs. Levels of carbon dioxide rise and arterial oxygen levels fall. Ischaemia within the lungs alters the production of surfactant and, as a result of this, the alveoli collapse. Oedema in the lungs, due to increased permeability, exacerbates the existing problem of diffusion of oxygen. Atelectasis, oedema and reduced compliance impair ventilation and gaseous exchange, leading ultimately to respiratory failure. This is known as *adult respiratory distress syndrome* (ARDS).

Kidneys. The renal tubules become ischaemic, owing to the reduction in blood supply. As the kidneys fail, urine output falls to less than 20 ml per hour. The body does not excrete waste products such as urea and creatinine, so levels of these in the blood rise.

Gastrointestinal tract. The gut becomes ischaemic and its ability to function as a barrier against infection wanes. Gram negative bacteria are able to enter the circulation.

Liver. Drug and hormone metabolism ceases, as does the conjugation of bilirubin. Unconjugated bilirubin builds up and jaundice develops. Protection from infection is further reduced as the liver fails to act as a filter. Metabolism of waste products does not occur, so there is a build-up of lactic acid and ammonia in the blood. Death of hepatic cells releases liver enzymes into the circulation.

Management

Urgent resuscitation is needed to prevent the mother's condition deteriorating and causing irreversible damage. The priorities are to:

1. *Call for help* – Shock is a progressive condition and delay in correcting hypovolaemia can lead ultimately to maternal death.

2. *Maintain the airway* – if the mother is severely collapsed she should be turned on to her side and 40% oxygen administered at a rate of 4–6 litres per minute. If she is unconscious an airway should be inserted.

3. *Replace fluids* – two wide-bore intravenous cannulae should be inserted to enable fluids and drugs to be administered swiftly. Blood should be taken for crossmatching prior to commencing intravenous fluids. A crystalloid solution such as Hartmann's or Ringer's lactate is given until the woman's condition has improved. A systematic review of the evidence found that colloids were not associated with any difference in survival and were more expensive than crystalloids (Alderson et al 2001). Crystalloids are, however, associated with loss of fluid to the tissues, and therefore to maintain the intravascular volume colloids are recommended after 2 litres of crystalloid have been infused. No more than 1000–1500 ml of colloid such as Gelofusine or Haemocell should be given in a 24 hour period. Packed red cells and fresh frozen plasma are infused when the condition of the woman is stable and these are available.

4. *Warmth* – it is important to keep the woman warm, but not overwarmed or warmed too quickly as this will cause peripheral vasodilatation and result in hypotension.

5. *Arrest haemorrhage* – the source of the bleeding needs to be identified and stopped. Any underlying condition needs to be managed appropriately.

Assessment of clinical condition

Once the mother's immediate condition is stable, the midwife should assess her condition constantly. An interprofessional team approach to management should be adopted to ensure that the correct level of expertise is available. A clear protocol for the management of shock should be used, with the midwife fully aware of key personnel required.

Hypovolaemic shock in pregnancy will reduce placental perfusion and oxygenation to the fetus. This will result in fetal distress and possibly death. Where maternal shock is caused by antepartum factors, the midwife should determine whether the fetal heart is present, but as swift and aggressive treatment may be required to save the mother's life this should be the first priority.

Clinical observations for the mother in shock

1. Assessment of level of consciousness should be undertaken in association with the Glasgow coma

score. This is a reliable, objective tool for measuring coma, using eye opening, motor response and verbal response. A total of 15 points can be achieved, and one of less than 12 is cause for concern. Any signs of restlessness or confusion should be noted (Mallett & Dougherty 2000).

2. Respiratory rate, depth and pattern – pulse oximetry and blood gases will be taken to assess respiratory status. Humidified oxygen will be used if oxygen therapy is to be maintained for some time

3. Monitoring of blood pressure should be continuous, or at least every 30 minutes, with note taken of any drop in blood pressure.

4. Cardiac rhythm will be monitored continuously.

5. Urine output is measured hourly, using an indwelling catheter.

6. Skin colour, core and peripheral temperature are assessed hourly.

7. Haemodynamic measures of pressure in the right atrium (central venous pressure) are taken to monitor infusion rate and quantities. The fluid balance is maintained accurately (see below).

8. The mother is observed for the occurrence of further bleeding, including oozing from a wound or puncture sites.

9. Haemoglobin and haematocrit are measured to assess the degree of blood loss.

10. The mother is likely to be nursed flat in the acute stages of shock. Clinical assessment will also include review of pressure areas, with positional changes made as necessary to prevent deterioration. A lateral tilt should be maintained to prevent aortacaval compression if a gravid uterus is likely to compress the major vessels.

Detailed observation charts should be accurately maintained. The extent of the mother's illness may require her transfer to a critical care unit.

Box 32.6 is a summary of key points relating to hypovolaemic shock.

Central venous pressure

In the presence of acute peripheral circulatory failure, which accompanies severe shock, the monitoring of central venous pressure (CVP) aids assessment of blood loss and indicates the fluid replacement required. In such a situation it is extremely dangerous to base an intravenous regimen on guesswork.

> **Box 32.6** Key points for hypovolaemic shock
>
> - Call for help
> - Gain venous access and insert two wide-bore cannulae
> - Immediate rapid infusion of fluid is needed to correct loss
> - Identify the source of bleeding and control temporarily if necessary
> - Assess for coagulopathy and correct
> - Manage the underlying condition

Hyper- or hypovolaemia, cardiac and renal failure may result. CVP is the pressure in the right atrium or superior vena cava. It is an indicator of the volume of blood returning to the heart and reflects the competence of the heart as a pump and the peripheral vascular resistance.

The normal pressure varies between 5 and 10 cm H_2O. In shock the pressure will be persistently low (i.e. below 5 cm) and may even register a negative reading, indicating hypovolaemia. The correct volume of replacement fluids may then be assessed with greater accuracy.

Method of measuring CVP

A catheter is inserted into a major vein such as the subclavian or external jugular vein and advanced into the right atrium. The catheter is then connected to a manometer and an intravenous infusion using a three-way tap.

To take a manometer reading, the mother should be lying flat and the base of the manometer should be calibrated to measure 0 cm of water when aligned with the level of the right atrium (Fig. 32.14). This point is level with a midaxillary line for most people. The three-way tap is opened and filled with intravenous fluid. The fluid will fall and rise with respiratory effort and should be allowed to stabilise before a reading is taken. The highest level the fluid reaches is used for the CVP measurement. Once the reading is completed the tap is returned to the infusion position.

A baseline observation is taken when the CVP catheter is inserted and the position in which the mother was lying is noted. Minor changes in position should be noted, as they may alter the CVP reading.

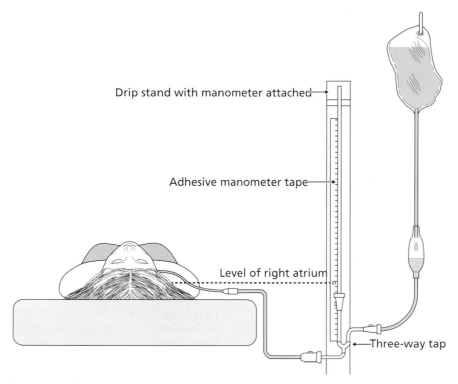

Drip stand with manometer attached

Adhesive manometer tape

Level of right atrium

Three-way tap

Fig. 32.14 Monitoring central venous pressure.

Principles of care of CVP lines

1. *Prevention of infection* – insertion of the catheter requires strict asepsis. The site should be inspected regularly for signs of infection and precautions taken to protect against inadvertent contamination during clinical procedures.

2. *Maintaining a closed system* – the mother will bleed profusely if the catheter becomes disconnected, or incur a possible air embolus. Connections in particular should be checked (Mallett & Dougherty 2000).

3. *Maintaining patency of the catheter by preventing clot formation* – positive pressure of the infusion should be maintained.

Additional complications include pneumothorax, hydrothorax, trauma to lung or veins and cardiac arrhythmias during and due to insertion.

Septic shock

This is a distributive form of shock, where an overwhelming infection develops. The commonest form of sepsis in childbearing in the UK is reported to be that caused by beta haemolytic *Streptococcus pyrogenes* (lancefield Group A) (Lewis & Drife 2001). This is a Gram positive organism, responding to intravenous antibiotics, specifically those that are penicillin based. In the general population, infections from Gram negative organisms such as *Escherichia coli*, *Proteus* or *Pseudomonas pyocyaneus* are predominant, which are common pathogens in the female genital tract.

The placental site is the main point of entry for an infection associated with pregnancy and childbirth. This may occur following prolonged rupture of fetal membranes, obstetric trauma, septic abortion or in the presence of retained placental tissue. Endotoxins present in the organisms release components that trigger the body's immune response culminating in multiple organ failure.

The Confidential Enquiries into Maternal Deaths in the UK (Lewis & Drife 2001) reports that 14 mothers died as a result of genital tract sepsis, and infection was the principal cause of death for 10 women admitted to intensive care for treatment. Sepsis is also a common development in those admitted to intensive care for other reasons.

Clinical signs

The mother may present with a sudden onset of tachycardia, pyrexia, rigors and tachypnoea. The mother may also exhibit a change in her mental state. Signs of shock, including hypotension, develop in septic shock as the condition takes hold.

Haemorrhage may be present. This could be a direct result of events due to childbearing, but it occurs in septic shock because of DIC.

The body responds to septic shock in the following way. The primary responses to the infection are alterations in the peripheral circulation. Cells damaged by the infecting organism release histamine and enzymes that contribute to vasodilatation and increased permeability of the capillaries. Mediators are also produced that have the opposite action and cause vasoconstriction. The overall response, however, is one of vasodilatation, which reduces the systemic vascular resistance. Cardiac output remains elevated.

Vasodilatation and continued hypotension lead to kidney damage, with reduced glomerular filtration, acute tubular necrosis and oliguria. ARDS occurs in many cases; DIC is also a feature of septic shock.

Multisystem organ failure will result as an effect of the continued hypotension and myocardial depression. Failure of the liver, brain and respiratory systems follows, and death ensues.

Management

This is based on preventing further deterioration by restoring circulatory volume and eradication of the infection. Replacement of fluid volume will restore perfusion of the vital organs. Satisfactory oxygenation is also needed.

Measures are needed to identify the source of infection and to protect against reinfection by maintaining high standards of care in clinical procedures. A full infection screening should be carried out including a high vaginal swab, midstream specimen of urine and blood cultures. Infusion sites and indwelling catheters should be checked for signs of contamination and changed as appropriate. Rigorous treatment with intravenous antibiotics, after blood cultures have been taken, is necessary to halt the illness.

Retained products of conception can be detected on ultrasound, and these can then be removed.

In situations where the mother requires to be transferred for critical or intensive care, relatives should be kept informed of progress. The midwife may be the person with whom the relatives have formed a relationship and therefore is relied on to give information.

Conclusion

The emergency situations included in this chapter are rare, but the actions of the midwife are fundamental to the well-being of mother, baby and also the partner. Awareness of local emergency procedures and knowledge of correct use of any supportive equipment are essential. Midwives in all practice settings should maintain skills that enable them to act in an emergency. The use of multiprofessional workshops to rehearse simulated situations can ensure that all members of the care team know exactly what is required when needed. Midwives should also engage in reviews of practice to ensure that policies and protocols are regularly reviewed to incorporate best practice and current evidence.

REFERENCES

Acker D B, Sachs B P, Friedman E A 1985 Risk factors for shoulder dystocia. Obstetrics and Gynecology 66(6):762–768

Acker D B, Sachs B P, Friedman E A 1986 Risk factors for shoulder dystocia in the average weight infant. Obstetrics and Gynecology 67(5):614–618

Alderson P, Schierhout G, Roberts I, Bunn F 2001 Colloids versus crystalloids for fluid resuscitation in critically ill patients (Cochrane review). In: The Cochrane Library, Issue 3. Update Software, Oxford

Al-Najashi S, Al-Suleiman S A, El-Yahia A, Raman M S, Raman J 1989 Shoulder dystocia – a clinical study of 56 cases. Australian and New Zealand Journal of Obstetrics and Gynaecology 29:129–131

Awwad J T, Azar G B, Aswad N K, Suidan F J, Karam K S 1993 Uterine rupture in pregnancy caused by blast injury with fetal survival. Journal of Obstetrics and Gynaecology 13(6):448

Bahar A M 1996 Risk factors and fetal outcome in cases of shoulder dystocia compared with normal deliveries of a similar birthweight. British Journal of Obstetrics and Gynaecology 103:868–872

Benedetti T J, Gabbe S G 1978 Shoulder dystocia: a complication of fetal macrosomia and prolonged second stage of labour with mid pelvic delivery. Obstetrics and Gynecology 52(5):526–529

Brar H S, Greenspoon J S, Platt L D, Paul R H 1989 Acute puerperal uterine inversion. New approaches to management. Journal of Reproductive Medicine 34(2):173–177

British National Formulary 2001 Number 40, March 2001. British Medical Association and The Royal Pharmaceutical Society of Great Britain, London

Brook L A, Weindling A M 1995 The paediatric. Clinical focus: shoulder dystocia. Clinical Risk 1(2):55–60

Chatelain S M, Quirk J G 1990 Amniotic and thromboembolism. Clinical Obstetrics and Gynecology 33(3):473–481

Clark S L 1990 New concepts of amniotic fluid embolism: a review. Obstetrical and Gynecological Survey 45(6):360–368

Clark S L, Hankins G D V, Dudley D A, Dildy G A, Porter T F 1995 Amniotic fluid embolism: an analysis of the national registry. American Journal of Obstetrics and Gynecology 172(4 part 1):1158–1169

Combs C A, Singh N B, Khoury J C 1993 Elective induction versus spontaneous labour after sonographic diagnosis of fetal macrosomia. Obstetrics and Gynecology 81(4):492–496

CESDI (Confidential Enquiry into Stillbirths and Deaths in Infancy) 1998 5th annual report. London, Maternal and Child Health Research Consortium, ch 7, p 63–72

CESDI (Confidential enquires into stillbirths and deaths in infancy) 1999 6th annual report. Maternal and Child Health Research Consortium London

Courtney L D 1970 Coagulation failure in pregnancy. British Medical Journal 1:691

Cunningham F G, MacDonald P C, Gant N F, Leveno K J, Gilstrap L C 1997 Williams obstetrics, 20th edn. Prentice Hall, London, ch 32, p 773

Delpapa E, Mueller-Heubach E 1991 Pregnancy outcome following ultrasound diagnosis of macrosomia. Obstetrics and Gynecology 78(1):340–343

DoH (Department of Health), Welsh Office, Scottish Home and Health Department, Department of Health and Social Services, Northern Ireland 1996 Report on confidential enquiries into maternal deaths in the United Kingdom 1991–1993. HMSO, London

DoH (Department of Health), Welsh Office, Scottish Home and Health Department, Department of Health and Social Services, Northern Ireland 1998 Why mothers die. Report on confidential enquiries into maternal deaths in the United Kingdom 1994–1996. Stationary Office, London

Flannelly G M, Turner M J, Rassmussen M J, Stronge J M 1993 Rupture of the uterus in Dublin: an update. Journal of Obstetrics and Gynaecology 13:440–443

Gonik B, Allen Stringer C, Held B 1983 An alternate maneuver for management of shoulder dystocia. American Journal of Obstetrics and Gynecology 145:882–883

Gonik B, Allen R, Sorab J 1989 Objective evaluation of the shoulder dystocia phenomenon: effect of maternal pelvic orientation on force reduction. Obstetrics and Gynecology 74(1):44–48

Gross S J, Shime J, Forrine D 1987 Shoulder dystocia: predictors and outcome. A five year review. American Journal of Obstetrics and Gynecology 56(2):334–336

Guirgis R R, Kettle M J 1989 Uterine rupture in a primigravid patient. Journal of Obstetrics and Gynaecology 9(3):214–215

Hall M 1996 Guessing the weight of the baby. British Journal of Obstetrics and Gynaecology 103:734–736

Howe R S 1993 Third trimester uterine rupture following hysteroscopic uterine perforation. Obstetrics and Gynecology 81(5, part 2):827–829

Keller J D, Lopez J A, Dooley S L, Socol M L 1991 Shoulder dystocia and birth trauma in gestational diabetes: a five year experience. American Journal of Obstetrics and Gynecology 165:928–930

Kitchin J D, Thiagarajah H, May H V, Thornton W N 1975 Puerperal inversion of the uterus. American Journal of Obstetrics and Gynecology 123(1):51–58

Lewis G, Drife J (eds) 2001 Why mothers die 1997–1999. Report of the Confidential Enquiries into Maternal Deaths in the UK 1997–1999. RCOG Press, London

Lydon-Rochelle M, Holt V L, Easterling T R, Martin D P 2001 Risk of uterine rupture among women with a prior cesarean delivery. New England Journal of Medicine 345(1):3–8

Mallett J, Dougherty L (eds) 2000 The Royal Marsden NHS Trust manual of clinical nursing procedures, 5th edn. Blackwell Science, Oxford

Mesleh R, Sultan M, Sabagh T, Algwiser A 1993 Umbilical cord prolapse. Journal of Obstetrics and Gynaecology 13(1):24–28

Miller D A, Diaz F G, Paul R H 1994 Vaginal birth after cesarean: a ten year experience. Obstetrics and Gynecology 84:255–258

Modanlou H D, Dorchester W L, Thorosian A, Freeman R K 1980 Macrosomia – maternal fetal and neonatal implications. Obstetrics and Gynecology 55(4):420–424

Morgan M 1979 Amniotic fluid embolism. Anaesthesia 34:20–32

Morris W I C 1955 Shoulder dystocia. Journal of Obstetrics and Gynaecology of the British Empire 62:302–306

Murphy D J, MacKenzie I Z 1995 The mortality and morbidity associated with umbilical cord prolapse. British Journal of Obstetrics and Gynaecology 102:826–830

Naef R W, Morrison J C 1994 Guidelines for management of shoulder dystocia. Journal of Perinatology 15(6):435–441

Nocon J J, McKenzie D K, Thomas L J, Hansell R S 1993 Shoulder dystocia: an analysis of risk and obstetric maneuvers. American Journal of Obstetrics and Gynecology 168(6):1732–1739

O'Connor R A, Gaughan B 1993 Rupture of the gravid uterus and its management. Journal of Obstetrics and Gynaecology 13:29–33

O'Leary J A 1992 Shoulder dystocia and birth injury: prevention and treatment. McGraw-Hill, New York

Pauerstein C (ed) 1987 Clinical obstetrics. Churchill Livingstone, New York

Phelan J P 1990 Uterine rupture. Clinical Obstetrics and Gynecology 33(3):432–437

Platt L D, Druzin M L 1981 Acute puerperal inversion of the uterus. American Journal of Obstetrics and Gynecology 141(2):187–190

Rachagan S P, Raman S, Balasundram G, Balakrishnan S 1991 Rupture of the uterus – a 21 year review. Australian and New Zealand Journal of Obstetrics and Gynaecology 31(1):37–40

Reid P C, Osuagwu F I 1999 Symphysiotomy in shoulder dystocia. Journal of Obstetrics and Gynaecology 19(6):664–666

Resnik R 1980 Management of shoulder girdle dystocia. Clinical Obstetrics and Gynecology 23(2):559–564

Resuscitation Council UK 2000 Resuscitation guidelines. Resuscitation Council UK, London

Resuscitation Council UK 2001 Guidance for safer handling during resuscitation in hospitals. Resuscitation Council UK, London

Rice V 1991 Shock, a clinical syndrome: an update part 1. An overview of shock. Critical Care Nurse 11(4):20–27

Roberts L 1994 Shoulder dystocia. In: Studd J (ed) Progress in obstetrics and gynaecology. Churchill Livingstone, Edinburgh, vol 11, ch 12, p 201–216

Roberts L, Trew G 1991 Uterine rupture in a primigravida. Journal of Obstetrics and Gynaecology 11(4):261–262

Rubin A 1964 Management of shoulder dystocia. Journal of the American Medical Association 189:835

Sandberg E C 1985 The Zavanelli maneuver: a potentially revolutionary method for the resolution of shoulder dystocia. American Journal of Obstetrics and Gynecology 152:479–487

Seigworth G R 1966 Shoulder dystocia: review of five years experience. Obstetrics and Gynecology 25(6):764–767

Smeltzer J S 1986 Prevention and management of shoulder dystocia. Clinical Obstetrics and Gynecology 29(2):299–308

Smith R B, Lane C, Pearson J F 1994 Shoulder dystocia: what happens at the next delivery? British Journal of Obstetrics and Gynaecology 101:713–715

Spellacy W N, Miller S, Winegar A, Peterson P Q 1985 Macrosomia maternal characteristics and infant complications. Obstetrics and Gynecology 66(2):158–161

Sweet B R, Tiran D 1996 Mayes' midwifery. Baillière Tindall, London

Ubachs J M H, Slooff A C J, Peeters L L H 1995 Obstetric antecedents of surgically treated obstetric brachial plexus injuries. British Journal of Obstetrics and Gynaecology 102:813–817

Vause S, Macintosh M 1999 Use of prostaglandins to induce labour in women with a caesarean scar. British Medical Journal 318:1056–1058

Watson P, Besch N, Bowes W A 1980 Management of acute and subacute puerperal inversion of the uterus. Obstetrics and Gynecology 55(1):12–16

Woods C E 1943 A principle of physics as applied to shoulder delivery. American Journal of Obstetrics and Gynecology 45:796–805

FURTHER READING

Allott H 1994 A grief shared. British Medical Journal 6308:602

A chilling contemporary account of a delivery complicated by shoulder dystocia.

Brook L A, Weindling A M 1995 The paediatric. Clinical focus: shoulder dystocia. Clinical Risk 1(2):55–60

Shoulder dystocia from the paediatrician's perspective; useful descriptions of possible sequelae.

CESDI (Confidential enquires into stillbirths and deaths in infancy) 1999 6th annual report. Maternal and Child Health Research Consortium, London

This edition covers the recommendations from the working group on shoulder dystocia.

Coates T 1995 Shoulder dystocia. In: Alexander J, Levy V, Roch S (eds) Aspects of midwifery practice. Macmillan, Basingstoke, ch 4, p 69–94

Gives a broad overview of the clinical problem from a midwifery perspective.

Hofmeyr G J, Mohlala B K F 2001 Hypovolaemic shock best practice in research. Clinical Obstetrics and Gynaecology 15(4):645–662

This article presents best practice for the management of hypovolaemic shock in childbearing. It revisits the pathophysiology of the condition and examines some of the evidence that informs current practice.

Jevon P, Raby M 2001 Resuscitation in pregnancy. A practical approach. Books for Midwives, Hale, Cheshire

The authors of this book are a resuscitation officer and midwife respectively and they have provided a concise guide that addresses the key issues of resuscitation. The topics covered include those required for effective practice, as well as ethical and professional issues.

Johnstone F D, Myerscough P R 1998 Shoulder dystocia. British Journal of Obstetrics and Gynaecology 105.811–815

Gives clinically useful overview of shoulder dystocia from an obstetric perspective.

Lewis G, Drife J (eds) 2001 Why mothers die. Report on confidential enquiries into maternal deaths in the United Kingdom 1997–1999. RCOG Press, London

Published triennially; every midwife should read and take account of the issues reported. This report covers the UK as a whole and critically reviews all reported cases of maternal death. Clinical practice may alter according to the principles of care recommended within this and subsequent documents.

O'Leary J A 1992 Shoulder dystocia and birth injury: prevention and treatment. McGraw-Hill, New York

The only book on the subject. Currently out of print but available in many medical libraries. A comprehensive overview to 1992.

RCM (Royal College of Midwives) 2000 Clinical risk management. Paper 2. Shoulder dystocia. RCM Midwives Journal 3(11):348–351

Looks at shoulder dystocia from a risk management perspective with the authority of the RCM.

Reid P C, Osuagwu F I 1999 Symphysiotomy in shoulder dystocia. Journal of Obstetrics and Gynaecology 19(6):664–666

Symphysiotomy is rarely used for shoulder dystocia in the West; where it is used, it is usually associated with maternal morbidity. This is a useful article giving a balanced overview.

Resuscitation Council UK 2000 Resuscitation for the citizen, 6th edn. Resuscitation Council UK, London

This publication provides straightforward information and guidance on resuscitation and emergency life support. It is uncomplicated and as such can be used for professionals and lay people alike. The web site http://www.resus.org.uk contains a range of publications that can be downloaded.

5

Section 5
The Puerperium

SECTION CONTENTS

33

Physiology and Care in the Puerperium

Sally Marchant

This chapter concentrates on the normal processes
that lead to the physical recovery of the newly
delivered woman in the days and weeks following
the birth event. Midwives have historically been
responsible for providing the majority of care for
women at this time (CMB 1983). Current care
involves midwives, health visitors, general
practitioners and others within the primary health
care network working together on behalf of the
new mother, baby and family members (HEA 1999).
The role and responsibility of the midwife to the
mother and new baby for the first 28 days after the
birth will be discussed in relation to the
management of care with regard to the expectation
of normal recovery and restitution of health and
well-being. (Where there are deviations from these
normal processes, the role and responsibility of the
midwife with regard to detection and referral
related to pathology and potential morbidity for
the mother is discussed in Ch. 34.)

The chapter aims to:

- explore the role of the midwife in the assessment
  of women's postpartum health and psychosocial
  needs

- review the current evidence for the normal
  parameters of women's health after childbirth

- discuss the current challenges to the provision of
  postpartum care in the light of women's
  experiences.

Defining the puerperium and the postnatal period

Following the birth of the baby and expulsion of the
placenta, the mother enters a period of physical and
psychological recuperation (Ball 1994, Hytten 1995).

From a medical and physiological viewpoint this period, called the *puerperium*, starts immediately after delivery of the placenta and membranes and continues for 6 weeks. The exact rationale for the 6 week, or 42 day, period is unclear but appears to relate to a range of cultural customs and traditions in addition to the physiological processes that occur over this time. The relationship between these factors has historically been the topic of some debate (Hytten 1995). The overall expectation is that by 6 weeks after the birth all the systems in the woman's body will have recovered from the effects of pregnancy and returned to their non-pregnant state (Beischer & Mackay 1986, Cunningham et al 1993). However, recent research into the morbidity experienced by women in the weeks after childbirth suggests that some women continue to experience problems related to childbirth that extend well beyond the 6 week period defined as the puerperium (Alexander et al 1997, Ball 1994, Glazener et al 1995, MacArthur et al 1991, Rome 1975).

Midwives and the management of postpartum care

The first 4 weeks after the birth is referred to as the *postnatal* or *postpartum period*; this is defined as 'not less than ten and not more than 28 days after the end of labour during which the continued attendance of a midwife on the mother and baby is requisite' (UKCC 1998a, p. 9). Over this time the activity of the midwife is one of care and support and monitoring of the health of the new mother and her baby (UKCC 1998a, p. 26).

Statutory framework and regulation for the practice of midwifery

Over the past century the rules and codes of practice for midwives have changed in terms of the amount of detail they contain about specific aspects of care and the role and responsibility of the midwife (Garcia & Marchant 1996). For the majority of women, postnatal care was a continuation of their care by the midwife who was familiar to them antenatally and in labour. The woman's home was the central point for normal births, with the majority of care being undertaken by domiciliary midwives and the local GP. Over the past 50 years, changes have occurred in obstetric care.

Active management of labour is associated with more women giving birth in the hospital environment, and increased rates for instrumental and operative births has initially led to longer periods in hospital postnatally (Donnison 1988).

The effect of these changes meant that the hospitalised postpartum woman was then in an environment related more to sickness than to the normal physiological processes. It is likely that this affected the framework of hospital postnatal care, in which the undertaking of routine observations was considered pivotal to the essence of 'good' and viewed therefore as effective care (Garcia & Marchant 1996). When considering the current practice of transfer home soon after the birth, it is of interest that there was initially resistance and concern to the suggestion that there should be shorter hospital stays after the birth (Theobald 1959) and arguably this debate continues (McCourt & Percival 2000, RCM 2000, Singh & Newburn 2000). It is only within the last decade or so that postpartum care has been reviewed with regard to its content, purpose or effectiveness (Garcia and Marchant 1993, Marchant & Garcia 1993, Marsh & Sargent 1991, Twaddle et al 1993); as a result there are now moves to review and make changes to the traditional pattern of postpartum care (Bick et al 2002, Lewis 1987, Walsh 1997).

The provision of postnatal care

In the UK, it is usual for a midwife to 'attend' a postpartum woman on a daily basis for the first 4–5 days regardless of whether the mother is in hospital or at home. During the course of this contact, current midwifery practice has been to undertake a regular physical examination to assess the new mother's recovery from the birth (Garcia et al 1994, Marsh & Sargent 1991, Murphy-Black 1989). From an international perspective this practice is unusual; it is only comparatively recently that postpartum home visits, and postpartum support programmes, have been initiated in America and Canada (Evans 1995, Gupton 1995). In Europe there appear to be different patterns of postpartum care depending on the health care framework for that country (Mackay 1993). In The Netherlands it is usual for the majority of postnatal care to be undertaken in the home by a maternity aide who has access to a midwife if needed (van Teijlingen 1990). Recent studies have reviewed the use of support workers in the community in the UK and this continues to be an area for ongoing review (Morrell et al 2000).

What is postnatal care?

When the extraordinary changes in physiology that occur throughout pregnancy are considered, it should come as no surprise that the period of physiological adjustment and recovery following the end of pregnancy is both complex and closely related to the overall health status of the individual. The intricate relationships between physiological, psychological and sociological factors are encompassed in the remit of postnatal care (Ball 1994, MaGuire 2000, Wiggins 2000). The management of postpartum care for women in the developed world presents with very different health needs from those in countries with sparse resources (WHO 1999). Thus the picture of public health can be seen to have a direct relationship on the role and responsibility of the midwife to postpartum women and their newborn infants. Where resources are scarce it is even more important to be able to offer the care appropriate to that woman as an individual rather than to adhere to a care pattern predominantly based on routine tasks or procedures (WHO 1999).

Postnatal care in the UK

Brief historical background

The background to the current postpartum observations routinely undertaken by midwives is unclear. It is likely that key observations that were associated with signs of potential morbidity became part of the routine procedures undertaken by those employed to care for the lying-in woman. In the 1920s the work of the midwife was to undertake a range of housekeeping tasks in addition to monitoring the health of the new mother and her baby (Donnison 1988, Garcia & Marchant 1996). With the introduction of the National Health Service in 1947, social changes influenced the duties of the midwife and focused care on assessment of health needs rather than domestic duties. As the health service developed and new statutory regulations emerged there were moves to alter the statutory framework away from a task-orientated approach. This has led to postpartum care in the UK facing challenges from women, midwives and other health care professionals to identify ways in which it

can re-establish its place of value as a means towards improving the health of women and their babies (Audit Commission 1997, RCM 2000, Singh & Newburn 2000). The effect of such criticism has resulted in a small number of research studies that have attempted to explore the needs of postpartum women and the advantages and disadvantages where the framework for care is based around a series of routine tasks (Abbott, unpublished MSc dissertation, 1994, Cluett et al 1995, 1997, Marchant et al 1999).

What are we doing and why?

It is common for midwifery textbooks on this topic to describe the activities of the midwife with regard to physical examination of the mother and the baby (Ball 1993, Silverton 1993, Sweet & Tiran 1997). However, there is now a move towards viewing care for postpartum women as a partnership where the woman is encouraged to explore how she is feeling physically and emotionally and seeks the advice and support of the midwife where she needs it (MaGuire 2000, Proctor 1999, RCM 2000). It is nevertheless important that all postpartum women still have access to, and appropriately receive, postpartum midwifery care. To facilitate this, midwives may need to assess a woman's capability with regard to self-knowledge and communication skills. Midwives will need to have the appropriate knowledge and skills to determine when to be proactive with regard to undertaking specific observations where these might be required. Therefore the midwife must be able to identify signs of morbidity that require further investigation and discuss the future management of these with the woman. Such a model of care can be challenging to practitioners who lack confidence in their autonomy and decision-making skills, or feel a lack of support in a community setting (McCourt & Percival 2000). In addition, greater numbers of women now experience birth in the form of a caesarean section. Whether this was planned or undertaken as an emergency procedure, these woman will require a different approach to their postpartum care, especially with regard to information and support.

The purpose of any textbook is to provide reference points for factual information and to suggest a plan of direction for clinical management. Where possible, such information should be clearly underpinned by research evidence for its effectiveness. In the area of postpartum physiology, information included in the past in standard textbooks has been inconsistent and lacking in what is now considered to be authoritative evidence based on valid and reliable research (Hytten 1995, Marchant et al 1999). This chapter aims to assist the practitioner to explore the environment surrounding the woman as a new mother. Within this context, any decisions made by the midwife in relation to reassurance of normality or referral for actual or potential morbidity must centre on the circumstances of the individual woman.

Midwifery postpartum visits

Culture and respect

The majority of postpartum care in the UK now occurs in the community setting of the woman or a relative's home. Expectations of women about the nature and purpose of the visits by the midwife may vary according to their cultural backgrounds, from one of welcoming enthusiasm to views that reflect negativity and suspicion (McCourt & Percival 2000). Although the 10 day period following the birth is recognised as a period within which statutory visits are made, it is important for midwives to have insight into how women might view the timing of these visits. For example, some faiths hold important ceremonies for the baby soon after the birth. This might involve many family members gathering in the home and the visit from the midwife in the middle of these celebrations might not be convenient (McCourt & Percival 2000, Schott & Henley 1996). The concept of postpartum care is one that aims to assist the mother and her baby towards attaining an optimum health status. Where the visit from the midwife can be seen as supportive and useful to the mother and her family, this purpose is more likely to be achieved. The social changes that have occurred over the past 20 years will have an effect on how different members of society view the need for care for new mothers, both from health professionals and from family members. In the light of the effects of such changes, it is a challenge to midwives in the twenty-first century to become involved by being advocates for women and their babies. This goes beyond the midwife's role of physical assessments of women's health to public debate about the use of national resources and support for women and their

families at this time. Although the timing of midwifery postpartum care has traditionally been a period of not less than 10 and for up to 28 days, this timing is now being questioned (Bick et al 2002).

Physiological observations

Regardless of whether the birth is at home or in a hospital setting, the midwife is primarily concerned with the observation of the health of the postpartum mother and the new baby. As such, it has been common practice to have an overall framework upon which to base the assessment of the mother's state of health. It is also common for the observations contained within the examination to link with pre-stated categories in the postnatal midwifery records. This formalised approach to the postpartum review might be an appropriate tool to use if there is concern about a woman who is feeling unwell and there is a need for a comprehensive picture of the woman's state of health (see Ch. 34). Where this is not the case such an approach might be less useful from the viewpoint of the healthy postpartum woman (Gready et al 1997, McCourt & Percival 2000, MaGuire 2000). Of more concern is that, by taking the time to complete a 'top to toe' examination as a thorough review of the woman's health, the midwife might ignore or give less attention to what the mother really wants to talk about (Garcia et al 1998).

The skill of the midwife's care is to achieve a balance when deciding which observations are appropriate so that she does not fail to detect potential aspects of morbidity. The next part of this chapter identifies areas of physiology that are likely either to cause women the most anxiety or to have the greatest outcome with regard to morbidity. These descriptions relate to observations undertaken for women who have had vaginal births and uncomplicated pregnancies. It is assumed that, where women have pre-existing medical or obstetric problems, individualised care will have been defined to assist in the management of their postpartum care. Taking the premise that pregnancy and childbirth are predominantly normal events from which the body will recuperate, where there is prolonged or unexpected pain, or the woman feels unwell or reports signs that are different from her previous experience, these will lead the midwife to further enquiry as appropriate.

The uterus and vaginal fluid loss

It should be recalled that the structure of the uterus is largely composed of muscle, blood vessels and connective tissue and its location in the non-pregnant state is deep in the pelvis. This structure allows for substantial enlargement in pregnancy when the uterus can be palpated abdominally as the fetus develops (Cunningham et al 1993, Hytten 1995). The activity of the uterus during normal labour involves the uterine muscles of the upper uterine segment systematically contracting and retracting, resulting in gradual shortening as labour progresses (Cunningham et al 1993) (see Ch. 24).

After the birth, oxytocin is secreted from the posterior pituitary gland to act upon the uterine muscle and assist separation of the placenta (see Ch. 28). Following expulsion of the placenta, the uterine cavity collapses inwards; the now opposed walls of the uterus compress the newly exposed placental site and effectively seal the exposed ends of the major blood vessels (Cunningham et al 1993, Hytten 1995, Williams 1931). The muscle layers of the myometrium are said to simulate the action of ligatures that compress the large sinuses of the blood vessels exposed by placental separation (Cunningham et al 1993, Hytten 1995). These occlude the exposed ends of the large blood vessels and contribute further to reducing blood loss. In addition, vasoconstriction in the overall blood supply to the uterus results in the tissues being denied their previous blood supply; de-oxygenation and a state of ischaemia arise. Through the process of autolysis, autodigestion of the ischaemic muscle fibres by proteolytic enzymes occurs resulting in an overall reduction in their size (Cunningham et al 1993, Hytten 1995). There is phagocytic action of polymorphs and macrophages in the blood and lymphatic systems upon the waste products of autolysis, which are then excreted via the renal system in the urine. Coagulation takes place through platelet aggregation and the release of thromboplastin and fibrin (Cunningham et al 1993, Hytten 1995).

Renewal of the uterine lining and renewal of the placental site involve different physiological processes. What remains of the inner surface of the uterine lining apart from the placental site, regenerates rapidly to produce a covering of epithelium. Partial coverage is said to have occurred within 7–10 days after the birth; total coverage is complete by the 21st day (Cunningham et al 1993, Williams 1931).

Once the placenta is expelled the circulating levels of oestrogen, progesterone, human chorionic gonadotrophin and human placental lactogen are reduced. This leads to further physiological changes in muscle and connective tissues as well as having a major influence on the secretion of prolactin from the anterior pituitary gland.

Once empty, although the uterus retains its muscular structure, it can be likened to an empty sac. It is therefore important to remember that the uterus, although at this point markedly reduced in size, still retains the potential to be a much larger cavity. This underpins the requirement to undertake immediate and then regular observations of fundal height and the degree of uterine contraction in the first few hours after the birth. Abdominal palpation of the uterus is usually performed soon after placental expulsion to ensure that the physiological processes described above are, in fact, beginning to take place. On abdominal palpation, the fundus of the uterus should be located centrally, its position being at the same level or slightly below the umbilicus, and should be in a state of contraction, feeling firm under the palpating hand. The woman may experience some uterine or abdominal discomfort especially where uterotonic drugs have been administered to augment the physiological process (Anderson et al 1998).

Traditionally textbooks have described precise measurements for the size of the uterus at various points in this process. The sources related to these measurements are poorly described and the inconsistencies in these descriptions in the various textbooks cast doubt on the validity of the information overall (Marchant et al 1999). It is arguable that these anatomical measurements are of little use to the practitioner in the day-to-day practice setting. The *process of involution*, however, is essential background knowledge for midwives monitoring the physiological process of the return of the uterus to its non-pregnant state. Current research would suggest that the information required by both midwives and women is that a well-contracted uterus will gradually reduce in size until it is no longer palpable above the symphysis pubis (Cluett et al 1995, 1997, Marchant et al 2000). The rate at which this occurs and the duration of time taken have been demonstrated to be highly individual (Cluett et al 1997) rather than occurring specifically at a daily rate.

Overall the uterus should not be tender during this process and, although women may be experiencing afterpains (see below), the presence of these should be defined separately from any uterine tenderness. The observations obtained by the midwife about the state of involution of the uterus should be placed into context alongside the colour, amount and duration of the woman's vaginal fluid loss and her general state of health at that time.

Assessment of postpartum uterine involution

Palpation of the uterus is a midwifery skill that is used throughout pregnancy, labour and postpartum but the skill required to palpate the same organ at different stages in childbirth differs in subtle ways (Marchant et al 1999). Acquiring this clinical skill requires observing expert practitioners and then undertaking the procedure under their guidance to achieve personal competence. There are several aspects to the abdominal palpation of the postpartum uterus that contribute to the observation as a whole. The first is to identify the position in the abdomen of the height and location of the fundus (the upper parameter of the uterus). Assessment should then be made of the condition of the uterus with regard to uterine muscle contraction and finally whether palpation of the uterus causes the woman any pain. When all these dimensions are combined, this provides an overall assessment of the state of the uterus and the progress of uterine involution can be described. Findings from such an assessment should clearly record the position of the uterus in relation to the umbilicus or the symphysis pubis, the state of uterine contraction and the presence of any pain during palpation. A suggested approach to how this is undertaken in clinical practice can be found in Box 33.1.

Record keeping, appropriate use

Clear and accurate records of any observation that has been undertaken are essential tools to competent practice (UKCC 1998a, b). They provide a reference point of information for those providing subsequent care and the contemporaneous nature of the written report is of sufficient importance that it is viewed as a legal document in the case of any forthcoming litigation. This is a particular challenge when changes to the

---

Box 33.1 Suggested approach to undertaking postpartum assessment of uterine involution

- Discuss the need for uterine assessment with the woman and obtain her agreement to proceed. She should have emptied her bladder in the previous half an hour.

- Ensure privacy and an environment where the woman can lay down on her back with her head supported. Locate a covering to put over her legs and abdomen.

- The midwife should have clean, warm hands and should help the woman to expose her abdomen; the assessment should not be done through clothing.

- The midwife faces the woman and, placing the lower edge of her hand at the umbilical area, gently palpates inwards towards the spine until the uterine fundus is located.

- The fundus is palpated to assess its location and the degree of uterine contraction. Any pain or tenderness should be noted.

- Once the midwife has completed the assessment she should help the woman to dress and to sit up.

- The midwife should then ask the woman about the colour and amount of her vaginal loss and whether she has passed any clots or is concerned about the loss in any way.

- Following the assessment, the woman should be informed about what has been found and any further action that is required, and then a record of the assessment is made by the midwife in the midwifery notes.

---

practice of assessment of involution are discussed as this has been held to be pivotal to the examination of postpartum women for so many years. Although the usefulness of uterine assessment is not in doubt where this contributes to the confirmation of abnormality, it is questionable whether this assessment when it is carried out routinely (regardless of clinical indication) contributes to the prediction of potential problems associated with involution (Marchant et al 2000). Recording of the findings from assessment of uterine involution has been found to be inconsistent between midwives and examples have demonstrated many varied forms of abbreviation and hieroglyphics (Marchant et al 2000). When undertaken in accordance with the UKCC guidance, the record of the assessment should be written contemporaneously, clearly and be devoid of abbreviation and ambiguity (UKCC 1998a, b).

Postpartum vaginal blood loss (whatever happened to lochia?)

Blood products constitute the major part of the vaginal loss immediately after the birth of the baby and expulsion of the placenta. As involution progresses the vaginal loss reflects this and changes from a predominantly fresh blood loss to one that contains stale blood products, lanugo, vernix and other debris from the unwanted products of the conception. This loss varies from woman to woman, being a lighter or darker colour, but for any woman the shade and density tends to be consistent.

'Lochia' is a Latin word traditionally used to describe the vaginal loss following the birth (Cunningham et al 1993). Medical and midwifery textbooks have described three phases of lochia and have given the duration over which these phases persist. Recent research has explored the relevance of these descriptions for women and raised questions about the use of these descriptions in clinical practice. One study identified that not all women were even aware that they would have a vaginal blood loss after the birth (Marchant et al 1999), but of more importance was the wide variation experienced by women in colour, amount and duration of vaginal loss in the first 12 weeks' postpartum (Marchant et al 1999, Oppenheimer et al 1986). This suggests that, overall, descriptions of normality ascribed to the traditional descriptions of lochia are outdated and unhelpful to women and midwives in accurately describing a clinical observation. Women also appreciate the use of language that is familiar to them and therefore it is recommended that the description of vaginal loss as 'lochia' should be abandoned and replaced with postpartum 'vaginal blood' or 'fluid' loss (Marchant et al 1999, 2000, Oppenheimer et al 1986).

Plate 11 illustrates the colour of vaginal blood loss reported by women in the first 28 days' postpartum.

Assessment of vaginal blood loss

The majority of women are well aware of the variability of their own vaginal loss from their menstruation experiences or from previous pregnancies. Most women can clearly identify colour and consistency if asked and, more importantly, will be able to describe key changes from what has happened previously. Therefore it is of more use to the midwife to ask focused questions about the current vaginal loss: whether this is more or less, lighter or darker than previously and whether the mother has any concerns about it herself. When asking these questions, women should be asked an open question first: 'can you tell me the colour/amount of your vaginal loss today?' rather than asking whether the vaginal loss is brown or red, etc. (Marchant et al 1999, 2000). It is of particular importance to record any clots passed and when these occurred. Clots can be associated with future episodes of excessive or prolonged bleeding postpartum; this is described further in Chapter 34.

Assessment that attempts to quantify the amount of loss or the size of clot is problematic. For example, how large is 'large', how heavy is 'heavy'? The use of descriptions that are common to both woman and midwife can improve accuracy in these assessments. Examples are asking the woman to describe the size of the spread of the vaginal loss on a sanitary pad, the frequency of changing the pad because of the saturation level, or comparison of the size of clots to familiar items such as a 50 pence coin or a plum. To use these approaches will substantially improve the detail obtained by the observer and add valuable clinical information if this is required at a later date (Marchant et al 1999, 2000).

The following areas are concerned with the overall physiology of the human body. It is important that women are encouraged to discuss with the midwife any problems that concern them or impede their recovery to health, regardless of whether these have origins in the pregnancy or are additional to it. Of most importance is the underlying knowledge that women are recovering from fundamental changes to the major systems that support life as well as adapting to major psychological changes. Although this recovery is in turn a part of the normal physiological process, as with pregnancy, there are occasions when deviations from the normal occur. It is in this area that the skills of the midwife of listening and focused observations are at their most significant.

Perineal pain

Regardless of whether the birth resulted in actual perineal trauma, women are likely to feel bruised around the vaginal and perineal tissues for the first few days after the birth. Women who have undergone any degree of actual perineal injury will experience pain for several days until healing takes place (McCandlish et al 1998, Sleep 1995, Wylie 2002). It has been said that the effects of perineal trauma significantly blight the first experiences of motherhood for many women because of the degree of pain experienced and the effects of this on the activities of daily living (McCandlish et al 1998, Sleep 1995). Long term psychological and physiological trauma is also evident.

Whose perineum is it?

As with palpation of the uterus, the perineum is not easily viewed by the woman herself and so midwifery care should involve observing the progress of healing from any trauma (WHO 1999). However, the woman will be well aware of how it feels with regard to degrees of pain and discomfort, or the absence of these. Appropriate care immediately after the birth or suturing can help to reduce oedema and bruising (Bick et al 2002, Sleep 1995). When the midwife is undertaking the postpartum review it is recommended that, particularly in the first few days after the birth, all women are asked about discomfort in the perineal area regardless of whether there is a record of actual perineal trauma. Advice from the midwife may be welcomed and clear information and reassurance are helpful where women have poor understanding of what happened and are anxious about urinary, bowel or sexual function in the future.

Where women appear to have no discomfort or anxieties about their perineum, it is not essential for the midwife to examine this area. The basic principles of morbidity or infection (Beischer & Mackay 1986) indicate that it is unusual for morbidity to occur without inflammation and pain; therefore, although the area might be causing discomfort from the original trauma, where this is unchanged or absent a pathological condition should not be developing. There may be occasions, however, where the midwife might consider that the woman is declining this observation because she is embarrassed or anxious. In such cases, the midwife should use her skills of communication to explore whether there is a clinical need for this observation to be undertaken and, if so, to advise the woman accordingly. For the majority of women, the perineal wound gradually becomes less painful and healing should occur by 7–10 days after the birth. (Chapter 34 reviews the morbidity associated with perineal trauma where this is not the case.)

Advice on what might help perineal pain

This is an area of high commercial interest and, with regard to practice, it is important that midwives attempt to seek out the current information available so that they can give advice based on the best available evidence. Advice might also be sought by women from a variety of people and the effectiveness of such advice may therefore be questionable. In a review of treatments for perineal pain in 1995, Sleep identified a number of studies aimed at providing evidence of effectiveness in this area. Treatments included the use of salt or Savlon in bathwater, pulsed electromagnetic energy, infra-red heat and ultrasound. None of these trials produced evidence that was persuasive about overall benefit in the area of reducing pain or improving healing (Sleep 1995). Further enquiry is still needed within the overall aim of giving relief without destabilising the most suitable environment for healing. However, women may still find soaking in a bath of great comfort to them regardless of any additive, and relief may be derived from the use of a bidet or cool water poured over the area that is tender. Appropriate information and advice are important components in pain management and should take into account women's individual experiences of their pain and their preferences for its relief.

There is increasing interest and research being undertaken into the use of complementary therapeutic preparations. Essential oils such as lavender and tea tree have been found to be beneficial when used as bath additives or topical compresses (Duke & Cornwall 1994, Harrison 1995, Steen & Cooper 1998). Homeopathic remedies such as Arnica, Calendula and Bellis perennis can be applied topically or taken orally. Midwives need to practise within their code of practice (UKCC 1998a) with regard to the use of complementary therapies and information about specific substances should be obtained from, or women referred to, appropriately trained complementary therapists (see Ch. 49).

Vital signs and general health

The following information is based on the premise that the midwife is exploring the health of the postpartum women from a viewpoint of confirming normality. 'Common sense' is an important part of midwifery care and in this instance an overall assessment of the woman's physical appearance will add considerably to the management of what will be undertaken prior to continuing any further investigation for either the woman or her baby.

Observations of pulse, temperature, respiration and blood pressure

Making a note of the pulse rate is probably one of the least invasive and most cost effective observations a midwife can undertake. If undertaken when seated alongside or at the same level as the woman, it can create positive feelings of care whilst also obtaining valuable clinical information. While observing the pulse rate, particularly if this is done for a full minute, the midwife can also observe a number of related signs of well-being: the respiratory rate, the overall body temperature, any untoward body odour, skin condition and the woman's overall colour and complexion, as well as just listening to what the woman is saying.

It is not necessary to undertake observations of temperature routinely for women who appear to be physically well and who do not complain of any symptoms that could be associated with an infection. However, where the woman complains of feeling unwell with flu-like symptoms, or there are signs of possible infection or information that might be associated with a potential environment for infection, the midwife should undertake and record the temperature. This will enhance the amount of clinical information available where further decisions about potential morbidity may need to be made.

Blood pressure. Following the birth of the baby a baseline recording of the woman's blood pressure will be made. In the absence of any previous history of morbidity associated with hypertension, it is usual for the blood pressure to return to a normal range within 24 hours after the birth. Routinely undertaking observations of blood pressure without a clinical reason is therefore not required.

Circulation

The body has to reabsorb a quantity of excess fluid following the birth (Hytten 1995). For the majority of women this results in passing large quantities of urine, particularly in the first day, as diuresis is increased (Cunningham et al 1993, Hytten 1995). Women may also experience oedema of their ankles and feet and this swelling may be greater than that experienced in pregnancy. These are variations of normal physiological processes and should resolve within the puerperal time scale as the woman's activity levels also increase. Advice should be related to taking reasonable exercise, avoiding long periods of standing, and elevating the feet and legs when sitting where possible. Swollen ankles should be bilateral and not accompanied by pain; the midwife should note particularly if this is present in one calf only as it could indicate pathology associated with a deep vein thrombosis.

Skin and nutrition

Women who have suffered from urticaria of pregnancy or cholestasis of the liver should experience relief once the pregnancy is over. The pace of life once the baby is born might lead to women having a reduced fluid intake or eating a different diet than they had formerly. This in turn might affect their skin and overall physiological state. Women should be encouraged to maintain a balanced fluid intake and a diet that has a greater proportion of fresh food in it (HEA 1999). This will improve gastrointestinal activity and the absorption of iron and minerals, and reduce the potential for constipation and feelings of fatigue.

Urine and bowel function

Labour has associations with loss of personal privacy and dignity and, for some women, discussions about bladder and bowel functions may be too personal and embarrassing for them despite or possibly because they have undergone a degree of loss of privacy in labour. Women may subsequently find it difficult to give information about possible problems in these areas. Midwives need to consider that women might either think that problems are 'to be expected' (because they have just had a baby) or that they are unique to them. Women may be unable to tell the midwife about it in case it is either worse than they had dreamed or too trivial to worry someone about. These primarily psychological and sociological barriers can result in women suffering from serious and debilitating urinary or bowel problems for years after the birth (MacArthur et al 1991, WHO 1998). Taking again the aspect of the range for normal function after childbirth, women need reassurance that, in the first few days after the birth, minor disorders of urinary and bowel function are common. These may be associated with retention or incontinence of urine or constipation, or both. The skill of midwifery care is to try to explore the possible cause of this and decide whether it will resolve spontaneously or requires further investigation.

Expectations of health

Following 9 months of 'renting out' your uterus and large parts of your body in the interests of another human being (or two or more!), it is reasonable for women to look forward to regaining their body for themselves once the baby is born (Gready et al 1997, MaGuire 2000). However, this is not the immediate outcome for many women and, once again, individual women will have their own expectations about the nature and speed at which they would like this recovery to occur. The role of the midwife at this point is to assist the woman to identify actual symptoms of disorder from the gradual process of reorder and advise what action the woman can do for herself in the way of progressive recovery. Advice for new parents in the matter of recovery from the birth is sparse and often superficial; also women may feel they should know what to do (HEA 1999, Marchant et al 2001, Proctor 1999). Offering women an opportunity to talk about a range of peripheral issues that might be worrying them could be of more benefit that day than a range of routine clinical observations.

Exercise and healthy activity versus rest, relaxation and sleep

Within the current national policy for health promotion there is an emphasis on increasing the understanding in the general population about the value of different forms of exercise and health. It is difficult to imagine that a woman with a new baby will not undertake quite a substantial amount of exercise once she has recovered from the birth event, but women vary considerably in their perception of exercise. One woman will be wanting to get back to her weight lifting whilst another may be having a struggle just going up and down stairs more often than previously. Exploring each person's level of activity will encourage advice in relation to appropriate exercise and, by association, nutritional intake and rest or relaxation and sleep. Undertaking regular pelvic floor exercises is of benefit to women's long term health (Enkin et al 1995). It is becoming increasingly common for obstetric physiotherapists to provide women with advice leaflets while they are in the postnatal ward. Midwives need to support the work of the obstetric physiotherapist by reminding and encouraging women to do the exercises advised.

Afterpains

It has been traditional to associate afterpains with multiparity and breastfeeding. However, women experience afterpains regardless of whether they have had previous pregnancies and when they are not breastfeeding (Mander 1998, Marchant et al 1999). The description of afterpains in parent education books suggests that they are mildly uncomfortable and more an issue of inconvenience. Women themselves, however, have described the pain as equal to the severity of moderate labour pains (Marchant et al 1999). Management of afterpains is by an appropriate analgesic, where possible taken prior to breastfeeding as it is the production of the oxytocin in relation to the letdown response that initiates the contraction in the uterus and causes pain. It is helpful to explain the cause of afterpains to women and that they might experience a heavier loss at this time, even to the extent of passing clots. Pain in the uterus that is constant or present on abdominal palpation is unlikely to be associated with afterpains and further enquiry should be made about this. Women might also confuse afterpains with flatus pain, especially after an operative birth or where they are constipated. Relief of the cause is likely to relieve the symptoms.

Future health, future fertility

It is not uncommon in a hospital setting for the first visitor to women who have given birth during the night to be the family planning advisor. This provokes some interesting responses from the women, suggesting that this is not a high priority for them at that time. Advice on managing fertility is within the sphere of practice of the midwife and it is an important aspect of postpartum care (see Ch. 36). Midwives need to be aware of a range of different needs with regard to women's sexuality and should be able to offer sensitive and appropriate advice on contraception where this is needed.

Weighing up the 'evidence'

The midwife should have gained a considerable amount of information during her contact with the mother and baby. The wide range for normality and the individuality within this can make it difficult for the midwife to decide whether an observation is related to morbidity. It is more likely to be the relationship between several observations that may cause concern and, where these appear to be more related to abnormality than normality, the midwife has a responsibility to make appropriate referral to a medical practitioner or other health care professional. The role of the midwife in the care of women and their babies is regulated under the Midwives rules with additional guidance being available within the code of practice (UKCC 1998a). The ethical framework that encompasses the philosophy of the work of any health care professional should act as additional guidance for the practitioner about individual management where circumstances are outside expected normal parameters (NMC 2002).

Care and the philosophy of dependence to independence

It has been the presumption in this chapter that women will welcome or even actively seek the help and advice of the midwife once the baby has been born. Within this is also the assumption that she will have the capability to do this. What about women who do not seek this or who actively reject advice or contact with health care professionals? There may be various reasons why some women do not seem to be so welcoming of the care offered as others. As noted previously, women from different cultural backgrounds may have traditions that conflict with the current management of postpartum care. Not being able

to speak or understand English may also inhibit the woman from seeking advice, or may appear to the midwife as being withdrawn and uncommunicative (Schott & Henley 1996). Aspects of domestic disharmony may also lead the woman to decline visits from an outsider. The midwife may have an important role with regard to referral and support for these women, where the worst outcome has been identified within the statistics for maternal death (Lewis & Drife 2001).

Although a visit to the home might have been planned, there will also be times when women are not at home when the midwife visits. It is important to keep in mind individual circumstances and whether these might have any bearing on a failed visit. For example, people with disabilities such as hearing loss or poor mobility might not hear a doorbell. It is important to make arrangements for contact to be made by alternative means (using a visual alarm or telephone to alert women of the visit beforehand, for example). A very loud television set can prevent the people inside from hearing a doorbell and, simplest of all, although the doorbell has been rung it is not working and no one is aware that the midwife is standing on the doorstep. Such events may lead to misunderstandings and a breakdown of communication between women and the caregivers.

Some women who have had previous children may not consider that the midwife or health visitor has much to offer them once they have returned home (Murphy-Black 1989). Where this appears to be the case, the midwife needs to recognise that the situation is one where the mother perceives that she has different priorities from those of the health care services. The midwife can ensure that the woman has access to sufficient information (in a format that she can utilise) to feel able to make contact with any of the services if she or the baby requires it in the future (Gready et al 1997, McCourt & Percival 2000). Where there are concerns about the safety or protection of the newborn infant, the supervisor of midwives should be informed and advice sought from the local social services (child protection team).

It is important that those undertaking postpartum care, whether in an active or passive format, are appropriately educated and supported so that they can meet the diverse health needs of the mother and baby over the postnatal period. In addition, there is a need for midwives to work in collaboration with other health and social care professionals during this time. The social environment has a marked impact on the overall health outcomes for both mother and baby and the acknowledgement of this has drawn midwifery care into the overall public health arena and long term outcomes for health initiatives (or lack of them) at this time.

REFERENCES

Alexander J, Garcia J, Marchant S 1997 The BliPP study – final report for the South and West Research and Development Committee. IHCS, Bournemouth University

Anderson B, Torvin Anderson L, Sørensen T 1998 Methylergometrine during the early puerperium; a prospective randomised double blind study. Acta Obstetricia et Gynecologica Scandinavica 77:54–57

Audit Commission for Local Authorities and the National Health Service in England and Wales 1997 First class delivery, improving maternity services in England and Wales (national report). Audit Commission Publications, Abingdon

Ball J 1993 Physiology, psychology and management of the puerperium. In: Bennett V R, Brown L K (eds) Myles textbook for midwives, 12th edn. Churchill Livingstone, Edinburgh, ch 12, p 234–250

Ball J 1994 Reactions to motherhood, 2nd edn. Books for Midwives Press, Hale, Cheshire

Beischer N, Mackay E 1986 Obstetrics and the newborn. The normal puerperium, anatomy and physiology, 2nd British edn. Baillière Tindall, London, ch 55, p 519–523

Bick D, MacArthur C, Knowles H et al 2002 Postnatal care: evidence and guidelines for management. Churchill Livingstone, Edinburgh

Cluett E R, Alexander J, Pickering R M 1995 Is measuring postnatal symphysis–fundal distance worthwhile? Midwifery 11(4):174–183

Cluett E R, Alexander J, Pickering R M 1997 What is the normal pattern of uterine involution? An investigation of postpartum involution measured by the distance between the symphysis pubis and the uterine fundus using a tape measure. Midwifery 13:9–16

CMB (Central Midwives Board) 1983 The role of the midwife. Spottiswood Ballantyne, London

Cunningham F G, MacDonald P C, Gant N F, Leveno K J, Gilstrap L C (eds) 1993 Williams obstetrics, 19th edn. Prentice Hall International, Appleton & Lange UK, London, ch 13, p 245–256, ch 27, p 615–625

Donnison J 1988 Midwives and medical men. Historical Publications, London, chs 1, 10

Duke A, Cornwall S 1994 The role of lavender oil in relieving perineal discomfort following childbirth: a blind randomised controlled trial. Journal of Advanced Nursing 19(1):89–96

Enkin M, Keirse M J N C, Renfrew M, Neilson J 1995 A guide to effective care in pregnancy and childbirth, 2nd edn. Oxford University Press, Oxford

Evans C 1995 Postpartum home care in the United States. Journal of Obstetrics, Gynecology and Neonatal Nursing 24(2):180–187

Garcia J, Marchant S 1993 Back to normal? Postpartum health and illness. In: Research and the Midwife Conference Proceedings, University of Manchester, Manchester, p 2–9

Garcia J, Marchant S 1996 The potential of postnatal care. In: Kroll D (ed) Issues in midwifery care for the future. Baillière Tindall, London, p 58–74

Garcia J, Renfrew M, Marchant S 1994 Postnatal home visiting by midwives. Midwifery 10(1):40–43

Garcia J, Redshaw M, Fitzsimmons B et al 1998 First class delivery, a national survey of women's views of maternity care. Audit Commission Publications, Abingdon

Glazener C, Abdalla M, Stroud P, Naji S, Templeton A, Russell I 1995 Postnatal maternal morbidity: extent, causes, prevention and treatment. British Journal of Obstetrics and Gynaecology 102(4):282–287

Gready M, Buggins E, Newburn et al 1997 Hearing it like it is: understanding the views of users. British Journal of Midwifery 5(8):496–500

Gupton A 1995 The Canadian perspective on postpartum care. Journal of Obstetrics and Gynecologic and Neonatal Nursing (February):173–179

Harrison J 1995 The use of complementary medicine in postnatal care. British Journal of Midwifery 3(1):31–34

HEA (Health Education Authority) 1999 The pregnancy book. HEA, London

Hytten F 1995 The clinical physiology of the puerperium. Farrand Press, London, ch 7, p 121–145, ch 8, p 146–162

Lewis G, Drife J (eds) 2001 Why mothers die: 1997–1999. The Fifth Confidential Enquiries into Maternal Death in the United Kingdom. RCOG Press, London

Lewis P 1987 The discharge of mothers by midwives. Midwives Chronicle and Nursing Notes (January):16–18

MacArthur C, Lewis M, Knox G 1991 Health after childbirth: an investigation of long term health problems beginning after childbirth in 11701 women. HMSO, London

McCandlish R, Bowler U, van Asten H et al 1998 A randomised controlled trial of care of the perineum during the second stage of normal labour. British Journal of Obstetrics and Gynaecology 105(12):1262–1272

McCourt C, Percival P 2000 Social support in childbirth. In: Page L (ed) The new midwifery: science and sensitivity in practice. Churchill Livingstone, Edinburgh, p 245–268

MacKay S 1993 Models of midwifery care: Denmark, Sweden and The Netherlands. Journal of Nurse Midwifery 38(2):114–120

MaGuire M 2000 The transition to parenthood. In: Life after birth: reflections on postnatal care, report of a multi-disciplinary seminar, 3 July 2000. RCM, Cardiff

Mander R 1998 Postnatal pain. In: Pain in childbearing and its control. Blackwell Science, Oxford, p 165–194

Marchant S, Garcia J 1993 The NPEU postnatal care project. Proceedings of the International Confederation of Midwives, 23rd international congress, Vancouver, May 9–14, p 343–344

Marchant S, Alexander J, Garcia J, Ashurst H, Alderdice F, Keene J 1999 Blood loss in the postnatal period – the BLiPP study. A survey of women's experiences of vaginal loss from twenty four hours to three months after childbirth. Midwifery 15:72–81

Marchant S, Alexander J, Garcia J 2000 How does it feel to you? Uterine palpation and lochial loss as guides to postnatal recovery 2 – the Blipp study (blood loss in the postnatal period). Practising Midwife 3(7):31–33

Marchant S, Alexander J, Garcia J 2001. One small drop in the ocean: blood loss in the postnatal period: the development and pilot testing of information leaflets for women about vaginal loss after childbirth (Blipp2). MIDIRS Midwifery Digest 11 (suppl 1):S9–S13

Marsh J, Sargent E 1991 Factors affecting the duration of postnatal visits. Midwifery 7:177–182

Morrell C J, Spiby H, Stewart P, Walters S, Morgan S 2000 Costs and benefits of community postnatal support workers: randomised controlled trial. British Medical Journal 321:593–598

Murphy-Black T 1989 Postnatal care at home: a descriptive study of mother's needs and the maternity services. University of Edinburgh

NMC (Nursing and Midwifery Council) 2002 Code of professional conduct. NMC, London

Oppenheimer L W, Sherrif E, Goodman D S, Shah D, James C 1986 The duration of lochia. British Journal of Obstetrics and Gynaecology 93:754–757

Proctor S 1999 Women's reactions to their experience of maternity care. British Journal of Midwifery 7(8):492–498

RCM (Royal College of Midwives) 2000 Life after birth: reflections on postnatal care, report of a multi-disciplinary seminar, 3rd July 2000. RCM, Cardiff

Rome R 1975 Secondary postpartum haemorrhage. Journal of Obstetrics and Gynaecology 82:289–292

Schott J, Henley A 1996 Culture. In: Schott J, Henley A Religion and childbearing in a multi-racial society. Butterworth Heinemann, Oxford, p 172–185

Silverton L 1993 Postnatal care. In: The art and science of midwifery. Prentice Hall, New York, ch 28

Singh D, Newburn M 2000 Women's experiences of postnatal care. National Childbirth Trust, London

Sleep J 1995 Postnatal perineal care revisited. In: Alexander J, Levy V, Roche C (eds) Aspects of midwifery practice: a research based approach. MacMillan, Chatham, Kent, p 132–153

Steen M, Cooper K 1998 Cold therapy and perineal wounds: too cool or not too cool? British Journal of Midwifery 6(9):572–579

Sweet B, Tiran D 1997 Mayes midwifery, a textbook for midwives, 12th edn. Baillière Tindall, London, part 9, p 474–475

Theobald G 1959 Home on the second day: the Bradford experiment. British Medical Journal Dec 19:1364–1376

Twaddle S, Liao X, Fyvie H 1993 An evaluation of postnatal care individualised to the needs of the woman. Midwifery 9:154–160

UKCC (United Kingdom Central Council for Nursing, Midwifery and Health Visiting) 1998a Midwives rules and code of practice. UKCC, London, p 9, 26

UKCC (United Kingdom Central Council for Nursing, Midwifery and Health Visiting) 1998b Guidelines for records and record keeping. UKCC, London

van Teijlingen E R 1990 The profession of maternity home care assistant and its significance for the Dutch midwifery profession. International Journal of Nursing Studies 27(4):355–366

Walsh D 1997 Hospital postnatal care: the end is nigh. British Journal of Midwifery 5(9):516–518

WHO (World Health Organisation) 1998 Postpartum care of the mother and newborn. Report of a technical working group. WHO, Geneva

WHO (World Health Organisation) 1999 Postpartum care of the mother and newborn: a practical guide. Birth 26(4):255–258

Wiggins M 2000 Psychosocial needs after childbirth. In: Life after birth: reflections on postnatal care, report of a multi-disciplinary seminar, 3rd July 2000. RCM, Cardiff

Williams J W 1931 Regeneration of uterine mucosa after delivery, with especial reference to the placental site. American Journal of Obstetrics and Gynecology 22:664–696

Wylie L 2002 Postnatal pain. Practising Midwife 5(1):13–15

FURTHER READING

Bick D, MacArthur C, Knowles H et al 2002 Postnatal care: evidence and guidelines for management. Churchill Livingstone, Edinburgh

This publication draws on the tools used in a recent trial of selective home visits by midwives. The pattern of midwifery visits continued throughout the 28 day statutory postnatal period and care was based upon the use of a series of checklists to systematically identify physical and psychological health problems. These initial checklists were then formulated into guidelines based on current evidence and contributions from a panel of experts.

Singh D, Newburn M 2000 Women's experiences of postnatal care. National Childbirth Trust, London

This is a report of a survey undertaken by the NCT to review the experiences of women after the birth of their baby and the extent to which their care (from a variety of sources) met their needs within the first 30 days after giving birth in either 1999 or 2000. The study group comprised of 960 women who completed questionnaires after the survey was advertised in the NCT journal in March 2000. As such they are a self-selected group and this raises concerns about bias; however, where women communicate in this way this enables caregivers to have access to their views and as such can be valuable even though these views may not be generalisable.

WHO (World Health Organisation) 1998 Postpartum care of the mother and newborn. Report of a technical working group. WHO, Geneva

This report, from one of the WHO technical working groups, attempts to gather together key aspects of care that are recommended for adoption worldwide as overall minimum standards to reduce morbidity for the postpartum woman and her newborn child. Of interest is the number of issues for women and their infants that are not necessarily related to wealth but to cultural environments and the role of education in the reduction of morbidity.

34 Physical Problems and Complications in the Puerperium

Sally Marchant

CHAPTER CONTENTS

This chapter reviews the care of women who either entered the postpartum period having experienced obstetric or medical complications, including those who did not undergo a vaginal birth, or whose postpartum recovery, regardless of the mode of delivery, did not follow a normal pattern. It includes the care for women with obvious risks for increased postpartum physical morbidity; the effects of morbidity related to psychological trauma are covered in Chapter 35.

The chapter aims to:

- discuss the role of midwifery care in the detection and management of postpartum morbidity
- review best practice in the management of problems associated with trauma and pathology arising from pregnancy and childbirth
- review the role of the midwife where postpartum health is complicated by an instrumental or operative birth.

The need for women-centred and women-led postpartum care

A women-centred approach to care in the postpartum period should assist physical and psychological recovery by being focused on the needs of women as individuals rather than fitting women into a routine care package (MaGuire 2000). The context of postpartum care within the woman's social and ethnic environment should take into account women's individual perceptions and experiences surrounding the pregnancy and the birth event. The midwife needs to be familiar with this background and be aware of the possible implications when assessing whether or not the woman's progress is following the expected post-partum pattern (DoH 1993, Garcia et al 1998).

The effects of obstetric or medical complications will be described within the context of the ongoing review by the midwife of the woman's health over the postnatal period. The role of the midwife in these cases is first to identify whether a potentially pathological condition exists and if so, to refer the woman for appropriate investigations and care (UKCC 1998). Where the birth involves obstetric or medical complications, a woman's postpartum care is likely to differ from those women whose pregnancy and labour is considered straightforward with regard to such factors. However, it must also be considered that some women have a perception of the whole birth experience as traumatic, although to the obstetric or midwifery staff no untoward events occurred (Singh & Newburn 2000).

Maternal mortality and morbidity after the birth

Death of a mother following childbirth causes devastation to family members and all those involved in her care; the course of history has been changed on a number of occasions because of such untimely death (Donnison 1988). Historically an unacceptably high proportion of women who had undergone a normal or straightforward birth then died shortly afterwards from puerperal sepsis (Loudon 1986). Where the birth was complicated by life-threatening haemorrhage this was often untreatable and also resulted in a fatal outcome (Loudon 1987). The activities of supposed caregivers such as 'the monthly nurse' led to concerns about the use of untrained women and the relationship of their practices to the increasing and unacceptable mortality and morbidity after childbirth (Donnison 1988, Loudon 1987). As knowledge increased about the dangers of cross-infection and the impact of the woman's social circumstances on the incidence of ill health (Donnison 1988), the high rates of mortality after childbirth became to be seen as avoidable rather than inevitable outcomes of pregnancy. Medical influences on the education and training for the registration of midwives included competence in a range of procedures that aimed to reduce the risk of disease as well as to identify signs of potential pathological conditions in the postpartum woman (Calder 1912, Longridge 1906). Such thinking was key to the campaign for the statutory registration of midwives early in the twentieth century (Cowell & Wainwright 1981).

The discovery of penicillin, the development of antibiotic treatment and the introduction of the blood transfusion service also dramatically changed the picture of puerperal mortality (Loudon 1987). Maternal death after childbirth where there has been no preceding antenatal complication is now a rare occurrence in the United Kingdom. In the most recent review of maternal deaths associated with pregnancy and childbirth over the period 1997–1999, 106 direct maternal deaths were identified giving a maternal mortality rate of 5.0 per 100 000 maternities (Lewis & Drife 2001). Thrombosis or thromboembolism remains a major cause of death but, despite the apparent advances in medication and practice, women still die postpartum as a result of haemorrhage or from sepsis associated with genital tract infection. The value of this information is to raise awareness of the degree to which care can contribute to the prevention as well as the detection and management of potentially fatal outcomes (Lewis & Drife 2001).

Within recent years, the extent of maternal ill health after childbirth has been more clearly described. This morbidity is remarkable in the extensive nature of the problems and the duration of time over which such problems continue to be experienced by women (Bick & MacArthur 1995, Brown & Lumley 1998, Glazener et al 1995, MacArthur et al 1991). As described in the previous chapter, where women have entered pregnancy in a state of health and have subsequently undergone a normal pregnancy and labour the midwife has a duty to undertake midwifery care over the first 28 days postpartum. The activities of the midwife are to support the new mother and her family unit by monitoring her recovery after the birth and to offer her appropriate information and advice (UKCC 1998). This role remains in keeping with current government health promotion principles that aim to improve the health status of the population overall and within which a healthy mother and her newborn baby are integral parts (DOH 1999a, b).

Immediate untoward events for the mother following the birth of the baby

Immediate (primary) postpartum haemorrhage (PPH) is the most immediate and potentially life-threatening event occurring at the point of or within 24 hours of delivery of the placenta and membranes and presents as a sudden, and excessive vaginal blood loss. Secondary, or delayed PPH is where there is excessive or prolonged vaginal loss from 24 hours after delivery and for up to 6 weeks' postpartum (Cunningham et al 1993). Unlike primary PPH, which includes a defined volume of blood loss (500 ml or more) as part of its definition (Prenderville et al 1988), there is no specified volume of blood for a secondary PPH.

Regardless of the timing of any haemorrhage, it is most frequently the placental site that is the source. Alternatively, a cervical or deep vaginal wall tear or trauma to the perineum might be the cause in women who have recently given birth. Retained placental fragments or other products of conception are likely to inhibit the process of involution, or reopen the placental wound. The diagnosis is likely to be determined more by the woman's condition and pattern of events (Dewhurst 1966) and is also often complicated by the presence of infection (see Ch. 28).

Maternal collapse within 24 hours of the birth without overt bleeding

Where no signs of haemorrhage are apparent other causes need to be considered; these will include, for example, inversion of the uterus or an amniotic fluid embolism (see Ch. 32). Other rare complications can present where the woman suffers collapse that suggests total or partial paralysis. This might occur following a cerebral vascular accident arising as a result of uncontrolled hypertension or a thrombosis. A woman may also suffer a fit shortly after the birth where there have been no previous signs of a rising blood pressure, pre-eclampsia or a previous history of epilepsy. Management of all these conditions requires ensuring the woman is in a safe environment until appropriate treatment can be administered, and meanwhile maintaining the woman's airway, basic circulatory support as needed and providing oxygen. It is important to remember that, regardless of the apparent state of collapse, the woman may still be able to hear and so verbally reassuring the woman (and her partner or relatives if present) is an important aspect of the immediate care.

Postpartum complications and identifying deviations from the normal

Following the birth of their baby, women recount feelings that are, at one level, elation that they have experienced the birth and survived and, at another, the reality of pain or discomfort from a number of unwelcome changes as their bodies recover from pregnancy and labour (Gready et al 1997). Chapter 33 reviewed how midwifery care can encompass an holistic approach to help women prioritise their concerns and needs at this time. However, women may experience symptoms that might be early signs of pathological events. These might be presented by the woman as 'minor' concerns, or not actually be in a form that is recognised as abnormal by the woman herself. Where the postpartum visit is undertaken as a form of review of the woman's physical and psychological health, led by the woman's needs, the midwife is likely to obtain a random collection of information that lacks a specific structure. Women will probably give information about events or symptoms that are the most worrying or most painful to her at that time. At this point the midwife needs to 'play detective' to establish whether there are any other signs of possible morbidity and determine whether these might indicate the need for referral. Figure 34.1 suggests a model for linking together key observations that suggest potential risk of, or actual, morbidity.

The central point, as with any personal contact, is the midwife's initial review of the woman's appearance and psychological state. This is underpinned by a review of the woman's vital signs where any general state of illness is evident. It is suggested that a pragmatic approach be taken with regard to evidence of pyrexia as a mildly raised temperature may be related to normal physiological hormonal responses, for

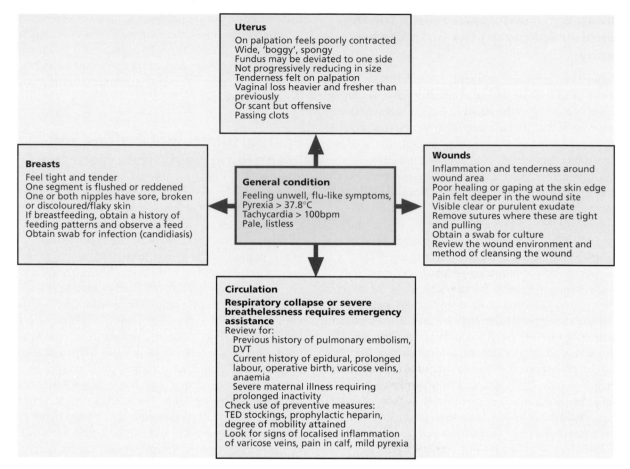

Uterus
On palpation feels poorly contracted
Wide, 'boggy', spongy
Fundus may be deviated to one side
Not progressively reducing in size
Tenderness felt on palpation
Vaginal loss heavier and fresher than previously
Or scant but offensive
Passing clots

Breasts
Feel tight and tender
One segment is flushed or reddened
One or both nipples have sore, broken or discoloured/flaky skin
If breastfeeding, obtain a history of feeding patterns and observe a feed
Obtain swab for infection (candidiasis)

General condition
Feeling unwell, flu-like symptoms,
Pyrexia > 37.8°C
Tachycardia > 100bpm
Pale, listless

Wounds
Inflammation and tenderness around wound area
Poor healing or gaping at the skin edge
Pain felt deeper in the wound site
Visible clear or purulent exudate
Remove sutures where these are tight and pulling
Obtain a swab for culture
Review the wound environment and method of cleansing the wound

Circulation
Respiratory collapse or severe breathelessness requires emergency assistance
Review for:
  Previous history of pulmonary embolism, DVT
  Current history of epidural, prolonged labour, operative birth, varicose veins, anaemia
  Severe maternal illness requiring prolonged inactivity
Check use of preventive measures:
TED stockings, prophylactic heparin, degree of mobility attained
Look for signs of localised inflammation of varicose veins, pain in calf, mild pyrexia

Fig. 34.1 Diagrammatic demonstration of the relationship between deviation from normal physiology and potential morbidity.

example the increasing production of breastmilk. The accumulation of a number of clinical signs will assist the midwife in making decisions about the presence or potential for morbidity. Where there is a rise in temperature above 37.8° centigrade it is usual for this to be considered a deviation from normal and of clinical significance.

The pulse rate is also a significant observation when accumulating clinical evidence. Although there may be no evidence of vaginal haemorrhage for example, a weak and rapid pulse rate in conjunction with a woman who is in a state of collapse with signs of shock and a low blood pressure may indicate the formation of a haematoma, where there is an excessive leakage of blood from damaged blood vessels into the surrounding tissues. A rapid pulse rate in an otherwise well woman might suggest that she is anaemic but could also indicate increased thyroid or other dysfunctional hormonal activity.

The midwife needs to be alert to any possible relationship between the observations overall and their potential cause with regard to common illnesses – for example, that the woman has a common cold, and that the morbidity is associated with or affected by having recently given birth. Where the midwife is in conversation with the woman as part of the postpartum review, if she receives information that suggests the woman has signs deviating from what is expected to be normal, it is important that a range of clinical observations are undertaken to refute or confirm this.

The uterus and vaginal loss following vaginal birth

Normal uterine involution should follow a progressive pattern that demonstrates reduction in uterine size in the days following the birth until the uterus is no longer palpable abdominally. It is expected that the midwife will undertake assessment of uterine involution at intervals throughout the period of midwifery care. It is recommended that this should always be undertaken where the woman is feeling generally unwell, has abdominal pain, a vaginal loss that is markedly brighter red or heavier than previously, is passing clots or reports her vaginal loss to be offensive (Marchant, unpublished PhD thesis, 1999). The progress of involution of the uterus is individual and largely unaffected by parity, birthweight or method of feeding (Cluett et al 1997, Montgomery & Alexander 1994).

Where the palpation of the uterus identifies that it is deviated to one side, this might be as a result of a full bladder. Where the midwife has ensured that the woman had emptied her bladder prior to the palpation, the presence of urinary retention must be considered. Catheterisation of the bladder in these circumstances is indicated for two reasons: to remove any obstacle that is preventing the process of involution taking place and to provide relief to the bladder itself. If the deviation is not as a result of a full bladder, further investigations need to be undertaken to determine the cause.

Morbidity might be suspected where the uterus fails to follow the expected progressive reduction in size, feels wide or 'boggy' on palpation and is less well contracted than expected. This might be described as subinvolution of the uterus, which can indicate postpartum infection, or the presence of retained products of the placenta or membranes, or both (Dewhurst 1966, Howie 1995, Khong & Khong 1993).

Treatment is by antibiotics, oxytocic drugs that act on the uterine muscle, hormonal preparations or evacuation of the uterus (ERPC), usually under a general anaesthetic (RCOG 1994). Guidelines have been compiled that identify key pointers to assist the midwife in making decisions about a condition that is indicative of potential morbidity and the need for further medical review (Bick et al 2002).

Vulnerability to infection, potential causes and prevention

Infection is the invasion of tissues by pathogenic microorganisms; the degree to which this results in ill health relates to their virulence and number. Vulnerability is increased where conditions exist that enable the organism to thrive and reproduce and where there is access to and from entry points in the body. Organisms are transferred between sources and a potential host by hands, air currents and fomites (i.e. agents such as bed linen). Hosts are more vulnerable where they are in a condition of susceptibility because of poor immunity or a pre-existing resistance to the invading organism. The body responds to the invading organisms by forming antibodies, which in turn produce inflammation initiating other physiological changes such as pain and an increase in body temperature.

Acquisition of an infective organism can be *endogenous*, where the organisms are already present in or on the body (e.g. *Streptococcus faecalis* (Lancefield group B), *Clostridium welchii* (both present in the vagina) or *Escherichia coli* (present in the bowel)) or organisms in a dormant state are reactivated (notably tuberculosis bacteria). Other routes are *exogenous*, where the organisms are transferred from other people (or animal) body surfaces or the environment. Other transfer mechanisms include *droplets* – inhalations of respiratory pathogens on liquid particles (e.g. beta-haemolytic streptococcus and *Chlamydia trachomatis*), *cross-infection* and *nosocomial* (hospital acquired) transfer from an infected person or place to an uninfected one (e.g. *Staphylococcus aureus*).

The bacteria responsible for the majority of puerperal infection arise from the streptococcal or staphylococcal species. The *Streptococcus* bacterium has a chain-like formation and may be haemolytic or non-haemolytic, and aerobic or anaerobic; the most common species associated with puerperal sepsis is the beta-haemolytic *S. pyogenes* (Lancefield group A). The *Staphylococcus* bacterium has a grape-like structure, of which the most important species is *S. aureus* or *pyogenes*. Staphylococci are the most frequent cause of wound infections; where these bacteria are coagulase positive they form clots on the plasma which can lead to more widely spread systemic morbidity. There is additional concern about their resistance to antibiotics and subsequent management to control spread of the infection. Regardless of the location of care, postpartum women and health care professionals should be aware of how infection can be acquired and should pay particular attention to effective hand-washing techniques and the use of gloves where there is direct contact with wounds or areas in the body where bacteria of potential morbidity are prevalent.

The uterus and vaginal loss following operative delivery

The most common approach to the uterus in a lower segment caesarean section (C/S) is via an incision in the skin at or just above the symphysis pubis. Although this leaves the upper abdomen free from any wound, the operation will have involved cutting of the major abdominal muscles and damage to other soft tissues. Palpation of the abdomen is therefore likely to be very painful for the woman in the first few days after the operation. The woman who has undergone a C/S will have a very different level of physical activity from the woman who has had a vaginal birth. It may be some hours after the operation until the woman sits up or moves about at all. Blood and debris will have been slowly released from the uterus during this time and, when the woman begins to move, this will be expelled though the vagina and may appear as a substantial fresh-looking red loss. Following this initial loss, it is usual for the amount of vaginal loss to lessen and for further fresh loss to be minimal. All this can be observed without actually palpating the uterus. For women who have undergone an operative delivery, once 3 or 4 days have elapsed then abdominal palpation to assess uterine involution (as described in Ch. 33) can be undertaken by the midwife where this appears to be clinically appropriate. By this time the uterus or area around the uterus should not be painful on palpation.

Where clinically indicated, for example where the vaginal bleeding is heavier than expected (as described above), the uterine fundus can be gently palpated. If the uterus is not well contracted then medical intervention is needed. Uterine stimulants (uterotonics) are usually prescribed in the form of an intravenous infusion of oxytocin or an intravenous or intramuscular injection of ergometrine (see Ch. 28). If the bleeding continues where such treatment has been commenced, further investigations required might be to obtain blood for clotting factors, or the woman might need to return to theatre for further exploration of the uterine cavity.

Wound problems

Perineal problems

Where women have undergone perineal trauma that has required suturing, the most immediate problem that occurs soon after the birth is that the woman complains of severe perineal pain. This might be as a result of the analgesia no longer being effective, of increased oedema in the surrounding tissues or, more seriously, of haematoma formation. Haematoma usually develops deep in the perineal fascia tissues and may not be easily visible to the observer if the perineal tissues are already oedematous and discoloured. The blood contained within such a haematoma can exceed 1000 ml and may significantly affect the overall state of the woman, who can present with signs of acute shock. Treatment is by evacuation of the haematoma and resuturing of the perineal wound, usually under a general anaesthetic.

Perineal pain that is severe and is not caused by a haematoma might arise as a result of oedema, causing the stitches to feel excessively tight. Local application of cold packs can bring relief as they reduce the immediate oedema. The use of oral analgesia as well as complementary medicines such as arnica and witch hazel are said to have a beneficial effect, although the effectiveness of such therapies has to date not been confirmed by research findings (Bick et al 2002).

Pain in the perineal area that occurs at a later stage, or reoccurs, might be associated with an infection. The skin edges are likely to have a moist, puffy and dull appearance; there may also be an offensive odour and evidence of pus in the wound. A swab should be obtained for microorganism culture and referral made to a GP. Antibiotics might be commenced immediately when there is specific information about any infective agent. Where the perineal tissues appear to be infected, it is important to discuss with the woman about cleaning the area and making an attempt to reduce constant moisture and heat. Women might be advised about using cotton underwear, avoiding tights and trousers and frequently changing sanitary pads. They should also be advised to avoid using perfumed bath additives or talcum powder.

If the perineal area fails to heal, or continues to cause pain once the initial healing process should have occurred, resuturing or refashioning might be advised. Women need information about the time scale by which healing should have occurred. They may also need to be encouraged to discuss this with their GP, and may need to be given other support where the vaginal or perineal tissues still cause discomfort within the course of daily activities. Women should be pain free and have been able to resume sexual intercourse without pain by 6 weeks after the birth, although some discomfort might still be present depending on the degree of trauma experienced. Recent discussion and research related to sexual health after childbirth identifies that health care professionals and women alike may encounter difficulties discussing sexual health issues. Although high levels of sexual morbidity after childbirth have been identified, the approach to discussion and management of this area appears to be problematic (Barrett et al 2000). In giving health advice and support, health care professionals are advised to identify an appropriate time, not to make assumptions with regard to sexual activity after childbirth and to be conversant with support agencies relevant to a range of cultural and sexual diversities and associated needs (Barrett et al 2000, Glazener 1997, RCM 2000).

Caesarean section wounds

It is now common practice for women undergoing an operative birth to have prophylactic antibiotics at the time of the surgery (Smaill & Hofmeyr 2000). This has been demonstrated to reduce significantly the incidence of subsequent wound infection and endometritis. In addition it is now usual for the wound dressing to be removed after the first 24 hours as this also aids healing and reduces infection. Advice needs to be offered to the woman about care of their wound and adequate drying when taking a bath or shower, or for more obese women where abdominal skin folds are present and are likely to create an environment that is constantly warm and moist. For these women, a dry dressing over the suture line might be appropriate.

A wound that is hot, tender and inflamed and is accompanied by a pyrexia is highly suggestive of an infection. Where this is observed, a swab should be obtained for microorganism culture and medical advice should be sought. Haematoma and abscesses can also form underneath the wound and women may identify increased pain around the wound where these are present. Rarely a wound may need to be probed to reduce the pressure and allow infected material to drain, reducing the likelihood of the formation of an abscess. With the hospital stay now being much shorter than previously, these problems increasingly occur after the woman has left hospital and wound care may need to be undertaken by the primary health care team alongside normal midwifery care.

Circulation

Pulmonary embolism remains the major cause of maternal deaths in the UK; the most recent Confidential Enquiry into Maternal Deaths report continues to identify the need for midwives and general practitioners to be more alert to the possibility of thromboembolism in puerperal women with chest or leg symptoms (Girling 2000, Lewis & Drife 2001). Women who have a *previous* history of pulmonary embolism, a deep vein thrombosis or who have varicose veins have a higher risk of postpartum problems. Postpartum care of women who have pre-existing or pregnancy-related medical complications relies on prophylactic precautions and should be undertaken for women who undergo surgery and have these pre-existing factors. Thromboembolitic D (TED) stockings should be provided during, or as soon as possible after, the birth and prophylactic heparin prescribed until women attain normal mobility. All women who undergo an epidural anaesthetic, are anaemic, or have a prolonged labour or an operative birth are slightly more at risk of developing complications linked to blood clots. Women with pre-existing problems are at higher risk because of their overall health status and environment of care postpartum. For example, women who undergo a C/S as a result of maternal illness are more likely to spend longer in bed, thereby reducing their mobility and increasing their risk of morbidity.

Clinical signs that women might report include the following (from the most common to the most serious). The signs of circulatory problems related to varicose veins are usually localised inflammation or tenderness around the varicose vein, sometimes accompanied by a mild pyrexia. This is superficial thrombophlebitis, which is usually resolved by applying support to the affected area and administering anti-inflammatory drugs, where these are not in conflict with other medication being taken or with breast feeding. Unilateral oedema of an ankle or calf accompanied by stiffness or pain and a positive Homan's sign might indicate a deep vein thrombosis that has the potential to cause a pulmonary embolism. Urgent medical referral must be made to confirm the diagnosis and commence anticoagulant or other appropriate therapy. The most serious outcome is the development of a pulmonary embolism. The first sign might be the sudden onset of breathlessness, which may not be associated with any obvious clinical sign of a blood clot. Women with this condition are likely to become seriously ill and could suffer a respiratory collapse with very little prior warning.

Some degree of oedema of the lower legs and ankles and feet can be viewed as being within normal limits where it is not accompanied by calf pain (especially unilaterally), pyrexia or a raised blood pressure.

Hypertension

Women who have had previous episodes of hypertension in pregnancy may continue to demonstrate this postpartum. There is still a risk that women who have clinical signs of pregnancy-induced hypertension can develop eclampsia in the hours and days following the birth although this is a relatively rare outcome in the normal population (Atterbury et al 1998). Some degree of monitoring of the blood pressure should be continued for women who suffered hypertension antenatally, and postpartum management should proceed on an individual basis. For these women the medical advice should determine optimal systolic and diastolic levels, with instructions for treatment with antihypertensive drugs if the blood pressure exceeds these levels. Occasionally women can develop postnatal pre-eclampsia without having antenatal problems associated with this. Therefore, if a postpartum woman presents with signs associated with pre-eclampsia, the midwife should be alert to this possibility and undertake observations of the blood pressure and urine and obtain medical advice.

For women with essential hypertension, the management of their overall medical condition will be reviewed postpartum by their usual caregivers. Undertaking clinical observation of blood pressure for a period after the birth is advisable so that information is available upon which to base the management of this for the woman in the future.

Headache

As with backache, this is a common ailment in the general population; concern in relation to postpartum morbidity should therefore centre around the history of the severity, duration and frequency of the headaches, the medication being taken to alleviate them and how effective this is. In taking the history, if an epidural anaesthetic was administered for the birth (or at any time postpartum), medical advice should be sought and the anaesthetist who sited the epidural might need to be contacted. Headaches from a dural tap typically arise once the woman has become mobile after the birth and they are at their most severe when standing, lessening when the woman lies down. They are often accompanied by neck stiffness, vomiting and visual disturbances. These headaches are very debilitating and are best managed by stopping the leakage of cerebral spinal fluid by the insertion of 10–20 ml of blood into the epidural space; this should resolve the clinical symptoms. Where women have returned home after the birth, they would need to return to the hospital to have this procedure.

Headaches might also be precursors of psychological distress and it is important that other issues related to the birth event are explored, taking the time and opportunity to do this in a sensitive manner. Factors that might be overlooked include dehydration, sleep loss and a greater than usual stressful environment. Screening, investigations and management of psychological factors are discussed in Chapter 35. However, the midwife should take time to discuss the woman's feelings and offer advice or reassurance about these where possible and act as an important source of support to the new mother at this time.

Backache

Many women experience pain or discomfort from backache in pregnancy as a result of separation or diastasis of the abdominal muscles (rectus abdominis diastasis, or RAD). RAD occurs where the collagen fibres of the abdominal muscles stretch under the effects of the hormones progesterone and relaxin, which increase the extensibility of the connective tissues (see Ch. 15). As the weight of the growing fetus increases this adds stress to the spine and causing backache (Russell et al 1996). It might be sufficient to give advice on skeletal support to attain a good posture when feeding and lifting, to suggest a feasible personal exercise plan and how to achieve this as well as to discuss a range of relaxation techniques (Richardson & Jull 1995). Where backache is causing pain that affects the woman's activities of daily living, referral can be made to local physiotherapy services; usually this is via the woman's GP, although direct referral by the woman can be made in some areas. Where the symphysis pubis has been affected in pregnancy this should resolve in the weeks after the baby is born, with relief from no longer having to carry the weight of the fetus and gradual resolution of the problem as the non-pregnant hormonal levels return.

Urinary problems

With the changes to the management of labour over the past 30 years, it appears to be less common nowadays for women who have experienced an uncomplicated labour to experience acute retention of urine following the birth. However, it is still important to monitor urinary function and to ask women about this and the sensations associated with normal bladder control. For some women a short period of poor bladder control may be present for a few days after the birth, but this should resolve within a week at the most. Women with perineal trauma may have difficulty in deciding whether they have normal urinary control; as noted earlier, retention of urine might be detected by the midwife as a result of abdominal palpation of the uterus. Abdominal tenderness in association with other urinary symptoms, for example a poor output, dysuria or offensive urine and a pyrexia or general flu-like symptoms, might indicate a urinary tract infection. Very rarely urinary incontinence might be a result of a urethral fistula following complications from the labour or birth.

Where women have undergone an epidural or spinal anaesthetic, this can have an effect on the neurological sensors that control urine release and flow. This might cause acute retention in some women and be identified within hours of the birth where, as a result of the physiological diuresis, large volumes of urine are produced. In other cases, women may appear to be voiding urine without difficulty but not emptying the bladder each time. They may pass small amounts of urine and be unaware that more urine has remained in the bladder (Lee et al 1999). The main complication of any form of urine retention is that the uterus might be prevented from effective contraction, which leads to increased vaginal blood loss. There is also increased potential for the woman to contract a urine infection with possible kidney involvement and potential long term effects on bladder function.

It is not uncommon for some women to have a small degree of leakage of urine or retention within the first 2 or 3 days while the tissues recover from the birth, but this should resolve with the practice of postnatal exercise and healing of any localised trauma. Women might feel embarrassed about having urinary problems and midwives may need to consider appropriate ways of encouraging women to talk about any problems so that they can advise women about their future management. Referral to a physiotherapist might be an appropriate first step as pelvic floor exercises and bladder training have been found to improve the outcome significantly in women with long term urinary incontinence (Glazener et al 2001). Specific enquiry about these issues should be made when women attend for their 6 week postnatal examination; further investigations should be made for women who are encountering these problems.

Bowels and constipation

It is the relationship of the regularity of bowel movements to the woman's previous experience that is likely to assist the midwife in determining whether or not there is a problem. The occurrence of haemorrhoids and constipation is not uncommon during pregnancy and is a result of the influence of progesterone on smooth muscle. Additional factors are following an altered diet, a degree of dehydration during labour and concern about further pain from any perineal trauma. A diet that includes soft fibre, increased fluids and the use of prophylactic laxatives that are non-irritant to the bowel can be prescribed to alleviate constipation, the most common of these being lactulose. Women need advice that any disruption to their normal bowel pattern should resolve within days of the birth, taking into consideration the recovery required by the presence of perineal trauma. They should also be reassured about the effect of a bowel movement on the area that has been sutured as many women may be unnecessarily anxious about the possibility of tearing their perineal stitches. Where women have prolonged difficulty with constipation, anal fissures can result (Corby et al 1997). These are painful and difficult to resolve and therefore advice about bowel management is important in avoiding this situation. Women who have haemorrhoids should also be given advice on following a diet high in fibre and fluids, preferably water and the use of appropriate laxatives to soften the stools as well as topical applications to reduce the oedema and pain.

It is also of concern where women might experience loss of bowel control and whether this is faecal incontinence. It is important to determine the nature of the incontinence and distinguish it from an episode of diarrhoea. It might be helpful to ask whether the woman has taken any laxatives in the previous 24 hours and explore what food was eaten. Where the problems do not seem to be associated with other factors the woman should first be advised to see her GP. Faecal incontinence is not always associated with a third degree tear and its prevalence is unclear, with recent reports suggesting that it is more common than was previously thought (MacArthur et al 1997). The role of the midwife is to facilitate women to talk about these problems by being proactive in asking women about any problems with bowel control. Where women identify any change to their prepregnant bowel pattern by the end of the puerperal period, they should be advised to have this reviewed further whether it is constipation or loss of bowel control.

Anaemia

The impact of the events of the labour and birth may leave many women looking pale and tired for a day or so afterwards. Where it is evident that a larger than normal blood loss has occurred, it can be valuable to obtain an overall blood profile within which the red blood cell volume and haemoglobin can be assessed so as to provide appropriate treatment to reduce the effects of anaemia (Paterson et al 1994). The degree to which the haemoglobin level has fallen should determine the appropriate management. Where the haemoglobin level is less than 9.0 g/dl a blood transfusion might be appropriate, otherwise oral iron and appropriate dietary advice are advocated where women decline a blood transfusion or where the level is less

than 11.0 g/dl. However, where the woman has returned home soon after the birth, the postpartum woman's haemoglobin values might not have been undertaken where there was no history of anaemia prior to labour and the blood loss at delivery was not assessed as excessive. If there is no clinical information to hand, the midwife needs to rely on the women's clinical symptoms; if these include lethargy, tachycardia and breathlessness as well as a clinical picture of pale mucous membranes, it would be prudent to arrange for the blood profile to be reviewed. Some researchers have questioned blood loss estimation after childbirth and the timing of blood tests taken to assess the physiological impact of this (Paterson et al 1994). Therefore the postnatal day when the haemoglobin test was taken might have a clinically significant bearing on the subsequent management.

Breast problems

Regardless of whether women are breastfeeding, they may experience tightening and enlargement of their breasts towards the 3rd or 4th day as hormonal influences encourage the breasts to produce milk. For women who are breastfeeding (see Ch. 40) the general advice is to feed the baby and avoid excessive handling of the breasts. Simple analgesics may be required to reduce discomfort. For women who are not breast feeding the advice is to ensure that the breasts are well supported but that this is not too constrictive and, again, that taking regular analgesia for 24 to 48 hours should reduce the discomfort. Heat and cold applied to the breasts via a shower or a soaking in the bath may temporarily relieve acute discomfort. From the midwife's point of view, it is important to gauge whether the duration of the engorgement is excessive and whether there are any other signs of a possible infection. Apart from the overall heaviness of the engorged breast there should not be overt tenderness or inflammation. Other signs, such as whether the woman is pyrexial or has flu-like symptoms, should assist the midwife to decide whether or not the mastitis is due to an infective organism. If infective mastitis is suspected then urgent referral should be made to a GP for antibiotics. If a woman is breastfeeding it is important that this continues, or that the breastmilk is still expressed (see Ch. 40).

Practical skills for postpartum midwifery care after an operative birth

In the immediate period after an operative birth, the attendant will be closely monitoring recovery from the anaesthetic used for the caesarean section. If the operation was performed under a general anaesthetic, the attendant will observe for signs of cognitive recovery and reorientation as well as taking the usual recording of temperature, pulse, respiration rate and blood pressure. Women who have undergone a spinal anaesthetic will also require monitoring of the level of sensation of their lower body and limbs. Regular observation of vaginal loss, leakage on to wound dressings and fluid loss in any 'redivac' drain system should also be undertaken.

Once the woman has fully recovered from the operation she is transferred to a ward environment and intensive observations are no longer required. Midwifery care for these women with regard to assessment of the woman's physical and psychological needs involves the overall framework described in Chapter 33, but there are a few variations. Appropriate care is to assess the needs of the individual woman and to formalise this within a stated pattern of care so that she and caregivers have similar and agreed expectations (RCM 2000). Women who have undergone an operative delivery need time to recover from a major physical shock to the systems of the body, for optimal conditions to allow tissue repair to take place as well as psychological adjustment to the events of the birth.

In addition to the observations undertaken to monitor the woman's state of health, women who have undergone an operative birth will require assistance with a number of activities they would otherwise have done themselves. This might mean that, for a short period of time, they are very dependent on the hospital staff for the majority of their needs. In the hospital environment, they will need help to maintain their personal hygiene, to get out of bed and to start to care for their baby. The rate at which each woman will be able to regain control over these areas of activity is *highly individual*. It is strongly suggested that caregivers should not expect all women to have reached a certain level of recovery in line with their 'postnatal day'. Using such a framework to assess the degree to which a woman is recovering from a major operation leads to a tendency to become judgmental. Opinions are then voiced about how well or otherwise women appear to be achieving these goals from the viewpoint of the hospital routine, rather than an appreciation of their individual circumstances and progress. Women may view undergoing a caesarean section or any complication in the birth in different ways depending on their social and cultural background.

It is now common for women to have a much shorter period in hospital after the birth; some women might return home 72 hours after a major operation with very minimal support. Practical advice about the management of their recovery and use of resources at home is also within the remit of midwifery postpartum care. For example; the midwife might suggest that the woman identifies what she will need for herself and the baby and gather this together in one place at the start of the day to reduce the need to go upstairs too often. Alongside this, women can be encouraged to go out with their baby when someone is available to help with all the baby transportation equipment; this will encourage venous return and cardiac output at a level that is beneficial rather than exhausting.

One aspect of current care that can be misunderstood is the need for mobility after surgery. Although women may be supplied with thromboembolitic stockings prior to the operation and be prescribed an anticoagulant regimen such as heparin, women need to be encouraged to mobilise as soon as practical after the operation to reduce the risk of circulatory problems. Although women need an explanation that mobility is of benefit soon after the birth, it is also an important part of care to recognise when the woman has reached her limit of activity and may need to rest. This is particularly important where women who have undergone an operative birth are in hospital settings alongside women who have given birth vaginally. Regular use of appropriate analgesia should be made available to women where this is required.

Psychological deviation from normal

Psychological distress and psychiatric illness in relation to childbirth are covered in depth in Chapter 35. However, it is relevant to reflect here on the possible importance of the relationship that develops between the woman and the midwife during these postpartum visits. Clearly such relationships are of greater depth where there has been antenatal contact or a degree of continuity postpartum, or both, and women have commented positively where such continuity has been achieved (Singh & Newburn 2000). This prior knowledge can mean that the midwife might detect or be concerned about a change in the woman's behaviour that has not been noticed by her family. At the outset of any contact made with the postpartum mother, the skilled midwife will make effective use of verbal and non-verbal communication skills to establish a relationship that will enable a situation of mutual trust and respect to develop. Any initial concerns of the mother or the family should be explored by the midwife making use of open questions and listening skills during the visit in the home or the contact time in the hospital setting. Behavioural changes may be very subtle, but, however small, they might be of importance in the woman's overall psychological state; it is the balance between the woman's physical condition and her psychological state that might influence an eventual decision to refer for expert advice. An appropriate example of this relates to the issue of sleep and tiredness described below.

Although the woman and her partner are likely to have an expectation of reduced sleep once the baby is born, the actual experience of this can have very varied effects on individual women. The cause of the lack of sleep or tiredness is what is important – is it being *unable to get to sleep* as a result of anxiety about the future and what is, as yet, unknown? This might include fears about the possibility of a cot death, or a lack of confidence in coping as a mother, or financial or relationship worries. The *opportunity to sleep* might be reduced because the feeding is not yet established or the baby is not in a settled environment and so the mother is constantly disturbed when she tries to sleep. In addition, other people may not be allowing the mother to sleep when the baby does not need her

attention. Unravelling these issues can help the midwife and the women to determine what is the underlying cause and whether management of this could improve the situation. As a result of this enquiry, women who come into the category where anxiety prevents them from sleeping when the opportunity arises may benefit from interagency support. The midwife is an important member of the primary health care team and should operate within an interagency context; therefore she should have access to a range of services with regard to information about ongoing child care and services related to mental health (see Ch. 35).

Talking after childbirth

The essence of the contact between the woman and the midwife after the birth event is to strive to maintain a framework of support and advice that existed antenatally. Within the current provision of care it is not always possible to achieve the continuity of carer postnatally and some women will have postnatal home visits from several different midwives possibly previously unknown to them.

Once the birth is over and the woman has returned to her home environment, there may be aspects of the birth that she does not understand or that even distress her to think about. Where appropriate, a midwife undertaking postnatal care in the woman's home might be able to help the woman review and reflect on the birth by talking about it and identifying her concerns and anxieties. Where necessary, the midwife can facilitate referral to the key people involved in order that the woman can discuss the birth or see the notes kept of the birth and clarify any outstanding issues (Allen 1999, Charles & Curtis 1994). Other forms of support, for instance specific counselling for those with traumatic emotional experiences, might also be appropriate (see Ch. 35).

REFERENCES

Allen H 1999 Debriefing for postnatal women: does it help? Professional Care of Mother and Child 9(3):77–79

Atterbury J L, Groome L, Hoff C et al 1998 Clinical presentation of women re-admitted with postpartum severe pre-eclampsia or eclampsia. Journal of Obstetrics, Gynecology and Neonatal Nursing 27(2):134–141

Barrett G, Pendry E, Peacock J et al 2000 Women's sexual health after childbirth. British Journal of Obstetrics and Gynaecology 107(2):186–195

Bick D, MacArthur C 1995 The extent, severity and effect of health problems after childbirth. British Journal of Midwifery 3:27–31

Bick D, MacArthur C, Knowles H et al 2002 Postnatal care: evidence and guidelines for management. Churchill Livingstone, Edinburgh

Brown S, Lumley J 1998 Maternal health after childbirth: results of an Australian population based study. British Journal of Obstetrics and Gynaecology 105:156–161

Calder A B 1912 Lectures on midwifery, 2nd edn. Baillière Tindall, London, p 121–131, 174–177

Charles J, Curtis L 1994 Birth afterthoughts: a listening and information service. British Journal of Midwifery 2(7):331–334

Cluett E R, Alexander J, Pickering R M 1997 What is the normal pattern of uterine involution? An investigation of postpartum involution measured by the distance between the symphysis pubis and the uterine fundus using a tape measure. Midwifery 13(1):9–16

Corby H, Donnelly V S, O'Herlihy C et al 1997 Anal canal pressures are low in women with postpartum anal fissure. British Journal of Surgery 84(1):86–88

Cowell B, Wainwright D 1981 Behind the blue door: the history of the Royal College of Midwives. Baillière Tindall, London

Cunningham F G, MacDonald P C, Gant N F, Leveno K J, Gilstrap L C (eds) 1993 Williams obstetrics, 19th edn. Prentice Hall International, Appleton & Lange UK, London, ch 13 p 245–256, ch 27 p 615–625

Dewhurst C J 1966 Secondary postpartum haemorrhage. Journal of Obstetrics and Gynaecology of the British Commonwealth 73:53–58

DoH (Department of Health) 1993 Changing childbirth, the report of the Expert Maternity Group. HMSO, London

DoH (Department of Health) 1999a Making a difference. Stationery Office, London

DoH (Department of Health) 1999b Saving lives: our healthier nation. Stationery Office, London

Donnison J 1988 Midwives and medical men. Historical Publications, London, chs 1, 10

Garcia J, Redshaw M, Fitzsimmons B et al 1998 First class delivery, a national survey of women's views of maternity care. Audit Commission, Abingdon

Girling J 2000 Physical adaptations to pregnancy. In: Page L (ed) The new midwifery: science and sensitivity in practice. Churchill Livingstone, Edinburgh, ch 15, 319–339

Glazener C, Abdalla M, Stroud P, Naji S, Templeton A, Russell I 1995 Postnatal maternal morbidity: extent, causes, prevention and treatment. British Journal of Obstetrics and Gynaecology 102(4):282–287

Glazener C 1997 Sexual function after childbirth: women's experiences, persistent morbidity and lack of professional recognition. British Journal of Obstetrics and Gynaecology 104:330–335

Glazener C, Herbison G P, Wilson C D et al 2001 Conservative management of persistent postnatal urinary and faecal incontinence: a randomised controlled trial. British Medical Journal 323:593–598

Gready M, Buggins E, Newburn M et al 1997 Hearing it like it is: understanding the views of users. British Journal of Midwifery 5(8):496–500

Howie P W 1995 The puerperium and its complications. In: Whitfield C (ed) Dewhurst's textbook of obstetrics and gynaecology, 5th edn. Blackwell Science, Oxford, ch 29, p 421–437

Khong T Y, Khong T K 1993 Delayed postpartum haemorrhage: a morphologic study of causes and their relation to other pregnancy disorders. Obstetrics and Gynecology 82(1):17–22

Lee S N S, Lee C P, Tang O S F et al 1999 Postpartum urinary retention. International Journal of Gynaecology and Obstetrics 66:287–288

Lewis G, Drife J (eds) 2001 Why mothers die 1997–1999: The fifth report of the Confidential Enquiries into Maternal Deaths in the United Kingdom. RCOG Press, London

Longridge C N 1906 The puerperium or management of the lying-in woman and newborn infant. Adlard, London, ch 5, p 95–111

Loudon I 1986 Obstetric care, social class, and maternal mortality. British Medical Journal 293:606–608

Loudon I 1987 Puerperal fever, the streptococcus, and the sulphonamides, 1911–1945. British Medical Journal 295:485–490

MacArthur C, Bick D E, Keighley M 1997 Faecal incontinence after childbirth. British Journal of Obstetrics and Gynaecology 104:46–50

MacArthur C, Lewis M, Knox G 1991 Health after childbirth: an investigation of long term health problems beginning after childbirth in 11 701 women. HMSO, London

MaGuire M 2000 The transition to parenthood. In: Life after birth: reflections on postnatal care, report of a multi-disciplinary seminar, 3rd July. Royal College of Midwives, London

Montgomery E, Alexander J 1994 Assessing postnatal uterine involution: a review and a challenge. Midwifery 10(2):73–86

Paterson J, Davis J, Gregory M et al 1994 A study on the effects of low haemoglobin on postnatal women. Midwifery 16:77–86

Prenderville W, Elbourne D, Chalmers I 1988 The effects of routine oxytocic administration in the management of the third stage of labour: an overview of the evidence from controlled trials. British Journal of Obstetrics and Gynaecology 95:3–16

RCM (Royal College of Midwives) 2000 Midwifery practice in the postnatal period: recommendations for practice. Davies Communications, London

RCOG (Royal College of Obstetricians and Gynaecologists) 1994 Bleeding after childbirth. RCOG Press, London

Richardson C A, Jull G A 1995 Muscle control – pain control. What exercises would you prescribe? Manual Therapy 1:2–10

Russell R, Dundas R, Reynolds F 1996 Long term backache after childbirth: prospective search for causative factors. British Medical Journal 321:1384–1388

Singh D, Newburn M (eds) 2000 Access to maternity information and support: the experiences and needs of women before and after giving birth. National Childbirth Trust, London

Smaill F, Hofmeyr G J 2000 Antibiotic prophylaxis for caesarean section (Cochrane review). The Cochrane Library, Issue 3. Update Software, Oxford

UKCC (United Kingdom Central Council for Nursing, Midwifery and Health Visiting) 1998 Midwives rules and code of practice. UKCC, London

35

The Psychology and Psychopathology of Pregnancy and Childbirth

Maureen D. Raynor   Margaret R. Oates

Pregnancy and childbirth are normal life events, yet women are exposed to a significant amount of stress. Ball (1994) chronicles many causes of unhappiness in some women's lives as being related to poor socioeconomic status, poverty, lack of social support and domestic violence. Many mothers may also experience unnecessary distress and anxiety simply because they did not anticipate or did not know about the normal psychological upheavals, emotional changes and adjustment that are integral to the childbearing process.

Midwives, therefore, have a pivotal role to play in assisting women and their partners to prepare for the physical, social, emotional and psychological demands of pregnancy, labour, the puerperium and, perhaps more importantly, parenthood (RCM 1999). To achieve this, midwives must consider the impact of antecedent factors alongside the array of emotional responses pregnant women may encounter. An underpinning knowledge and understanding of the psychology of pregnancy and childbirth is therefore essential. This must be distinct from the psychopathology that may affect some women during the childbearing continuum.

The chapter aims to:

- differentiate between normal and psychopathological changes in childbearing

- consider the psychological issues in midwifery practice, and motherhood as a transitional phase

- examine the contribution of pregnancy and childbirth to the development of mental illness

- illustrate the interface between theory and practice via the use of case scenarios and the identification of key points for best practice

- assess the safety of psychotropic medication in the context of breastfeeding.

Importance of psychological issues in midwifery practice

Evidence suggests that pregnancy, labour and the post-natal period are times of tremendous stress, anxiety, emotional turmoil and readjustment (Ball 1994, Bick & MacArthur 1995, Nieland & Roger 1997). Careful consideration must be given, therefore, to the exploration and identification of risk factors during the antenatal period. This is one way of ensuring that early and robust interventions are effected in the face of the undue emotional turbulence that some women may encounter (DoH 1998). Research by Clement (1995) suggests that antenatal 'listening interventions' may be a useful strategy for preventing psychological morbidity. This is based on the premise that midwives are skilled in recognising reasonable emotional distress as a response to adversity and pregnancy-related events.

Predicting risk is an important facet of antenatal care because elevated levels of stress during pregnancy not only affect the woman's emotional and psychological health, but have physiological implications for the physical well-being of the fetus (Teixeira et al 1999). The deleterious effects for both mother and fetus of raised levels of the stress hormone, cortisol, during pregnancy have been reported (Evans et al 2001, Teixeira et al 1999). Although these studies have raised the profile of antenatal stress factors as a possible precursor to mental illness, they have provided very little insight as to how antenatal stress may be alleviated. Equally worryingly, Murray et al (1999) reported that poor mental health might have a long-lasting impact on the quality of life both for the mother and for her child's cognitive development.

The ramifications of poor mental health are addressed in a number of social policies, not least being the National Services Framework for mental health (DoH 1999). This report has identified a key issue for the government of raising the public health role of health care professionals such as midwives, in promoting the mental health of women. The national strategy in conjunction with recommendations from the Royal College of Psychiatrists (RCOP 2000) seeks to improve access to perinatal mental health services, strengthen interprofessional and interagency collaboration and generally widen the role of health care professionals, especially those in primary care. Indeed, primary care facilities should be valued as not all women who are mentally ill or at risk of psychological morbidity need to be referred to the perinatal mental health service. Midwives are therefore required to work in partnership with women and families, as well as across professional boundaries.

Research has shown that the increased stress during pregnancy is both essential and normal for the psychological adjustment of pregnant women (Ball 1994). Johnstone (1994) surmises that the 'worry work' that women encounter assists in their psychological adaptation to the emotional changes of pregnancy. Stress in manageable doses is a normal phenomenon of our everyday lives; it acts as a great motivator, for example in preparing for an interview. Conversely, elevated levels of stress hormones and unnecessary anxiety will stretch our coping reserves, and could prove crippling. During periods of stress, supportive and holistic care from midwives will not only assist in promoting emotional well-being of women, but will also help to ameliorate threatened psychological morbidity in the postnatal period (Clement 1995, Hodnett 2000, Wesseley, Rose & Bisson 2000).

In an increasingly litigious society, the Audit Commission (1997) stated that poor communication is the single most common factor that is associated with women's dissatisfaction with their care. Being provided with adequate information will serve to diminish women's anxiety levels and the possibility of emotional distress (Newton & Raynor 2000).

The social construction of motherhood

The transition to motherhood cannot be fully understood without first examining the contested meanings and ideology of motherhood. The social context of birth has changed over time. Most births now occur within the confines of the hospital setting, and many mothers embark upon a journey for which they are ill prepared. Childbirth by television and other popular media is now the dominant image. Consequently, there are many assumptions about mothering and motherhood that may prove damaging (Phoenix & Wollett 1991). Following birth, a woman may need time to readjust, to become herself again and to feel her separateness from the baby before she can reach out her arms to it (Price 1988). The feelings that mothers have for their babies are nothing but complex and contradictory. At the positive end of the spectrum is a mother who is overwhelmed with love for her baby, one who feels completely euphoric and satisfied with her birth experience. However, at the negative end of the spectrum is the mother who feels traumatised by her experience of pregnancy and childbirth, as depicted in Case scenario 35.1. This case illustrates how care can be disempowering and, not surprisingly, women so affected may find the whole magnitude of motherhood particularly distressing.

Competing images of motherhood compound many women's lives (Nicholson 1998). Newborn babies are supposed to bring nothing but utter joy and fulfilment. Motherhood, it is thought, ensures that a woman has fulfilled her biological destiny, confirms a woman's femininity and raises her status in society, but without financial gain (Symonds & Hunt 1996). It therefore seems rather curious that women should indeed experience displeasure, harbour feelings of unhappiness and feel dismayed or even disappointed in their role as new mothers (Price 1988). Many women may feel afraid to speak out about their feelings in case they are judged a 'bad' mother. Therefore painful emotions may be internalised, magnifying difficulties with coping and sleeping. This leads many women to suffer in silence; distress may then manifest as mothers rage against their impossible situation. Nicholson (1998) contends that health care professionals have defined women's postnatal experience through proposing that well-adjusted, 'normal' and therefore 'good' mothers are those who are happy and fulfilled, but those who are unfulfilled, anxious or distressed are 'ill' and may be perceived as 'bad' mothers.

Clearly the ideology of motherhood is an assumption and a paradox, which is based on a flawed mythology (Riley 1995). Not surprisingly, the dichotomies inherent in the experience of motherhood often lead to feelings of isolation, inadequacy and confusion. However, the social construction of motherhood in part assists in our understanding of the complexities inherent in the definitions, meanings and historical context of the term.

The transition to motherhood

Pregnancy and childbirth is often a journey into the unknown. Ball (1994) describes the transition to motherhood as a life crisis, an emotional watershed, a period of heightened sensitivity when the woman will be extremely vulnerable. Many women find coping

> **Case scenario 35.1**
>
> Beth and James are in their late thirties; the couple are self-employed managing their own soft furnishing company. Both are delighted that Beth is finally pregnant after two failed attempts at IVF. At 12 weeks' gestation Beth had a chorionic villi biopsy to exclude Down's syndrome and was very worried that she would miscarry. The pregnancy continued to term without any complications, and labour commenced at 41 weeks' gestation. Beth's birth plan reflected that she wanted to breast feed and would like to initiate skin-to-skin contact as early as possible. She also indicated her wishes to have a natural and active birth and use of the birthing pool when labour was established. Upon hospitalisation, Beth was assessed by the midwife and informed that she was in very early labour and would be better off being transferred to the mixed ante/postnatal ward to await events, as the labour suite was very busy. It was close to midnight, therefore James was advised to go home to have a 'good night's rest'. This was despite Beth's protestations that she wanted James to stay to massage her back and provide moral support. James reluctantly left his tearful wife only to return some 4 hours later after being notified that Beth had been transferred back to the labour suite for pain relief. On his return, James was concerned to see that Beth was having an epidural sited. Beth said she was encouraged by the midwife to have this means of analgesia as she felt she was not coping. According to the dictates of the unit's protocol, labour was determined to be progressing slowly and Syntocinon was commenced. Ten hours later, Beth was taken to theatre for an emergency caesarean section for 'failure to progress'.

with the physiological adaptation to pregnancy, the plethora of antenatal screening tests, issues around choice, control and communication emotionally draining. As illustrated in Case scenario 35.1, labour also poses its own challenges in relation to the birth environment, coping strategies, birth companion, pain management, intervention, technology and the actual process of birth. Postnatally, parents may find coping with the demands of a new baby – infant feeding, the financial constraints and adjusting to the changes in their roles and relationships – a particularly testing time emotionally. For new mothers, this will involve diverse emotional responses ranging from joy and elation to sadness or a profound lowering of their mood, to utter exhaustion (Bick & MacArthur 1995).

Exhaustion, pain and discomfort commonly result once the elation that follows the safe arrival of the baby wears off. Disturbed sleep is inevitable with a new baby. Mothers who are trying to establish breast-feeding, older women, women who have had an operative delivery or those who have had a long and difficult birth may feel wretched and constantly weary for months following the birth (Bick & MacArthur 1995, Bick et al 2002). Soreness and pain being experienced from perineal trauma will affect libido, so too will feelings of exhaustion, despair and unhappiness that may be associated with the round-the-clock demands of caring for a new baby.

Women may be left feeling bereft and quite miserable after giving birth (DoH 1998). Therefore, postnatal care from midwives should be a continuation of the care given during pregnancy. Its contribution plays a significant factor in the positive adjustment to motherhood, as it assists in the acquisition of confident and well-informed parenting skills (Ball 1994, RCM 1999). The work by Bick et al (2002) has provided much-needed evidence regarding the psychosocial benefits of midwifery care well beyond the end of the traditionally defined postnatal period of 28 days, as identified by the UKCC (1998). The transition to motherhood is a testing time, bringing about changes in the usual order of things. It raises heightened vulnerabilities and weaknesses, feelings of insecurity, fear and anxiety and it is a period of loss as well as gain – including loss of expectations, of identity, of self-confidence and in terms of changes in relationships (Johnstone 1994). Some women may grieve for the loss of their former lifestyle, career or status (Symonds & Hunt 1996). Barclay & Lloyd (1996) identified that the losses involved in the whole process of parenthood are often not accounted for, or could be completely overlooked, by mothers and health professionals; they concluded that (p. 138):

> in Western cultures the misery of motherhood is carelessly labelled depression when it may be a response to a decline in life satisfaction and the experience of unexpected loss

Distress or depression?

Pregnancy and childbirth will bring episodes of repeated contact between the woman, midwives and other health professionals. Such contacts afford a wealth of opportunity to explore feelings, experience and emotions, and for midwives to provide clear explanations to women about the differences between distress – a normal reaction to major life events – and depression – an abnormal reaction to life crises. But are midwives adequately prepared to be able to assess the significance of the information they receive? Can they, for example, recognise when it is appropriate to refer the woman to a specialist perinatal mental health service, when it is appropriate to refer her to a social worker and when to alert the primary care services?

Barclay & Lloyd (1996) illuminate how the medical model, which still influences midwifery care, is used to describe women's moods and is therefore limited, serving only to pathologise or medicalise normal emotional changes. A pathological approach for understanding normal psychological events, such as transitional crises, denies the heterogeneity of women and is therefore limited. It trivialises non-pathological distress that may occur during times of transitional crisis, or it takes this distress seriously only if it is given a medical label or diagnosis. Nicholson (1998) explains that this perspective is confining and fails to validate women's feelings. Midwives who are educated and trained with such rigidity cannot meet the holistic needs of women in an informed and responsive way. Such a one-dimensional approach may fail to harmonise the depth of women's feelings (Barclay & Lloyd 1996).

Furthermore the dangers of labelling, misdiagnosis and misuse of terminology can do inexplicable damage from the viewpoint of a woman's mental health (Nicholson 1998). Once wrongly labelled as depressed, everything the woman does will be carefully scrutinised and interpreted within the stated confines of the label. The primary cause of the woman's distress will be ignored and only the clinical symptoms addressed (Barclay & Lloyd 1996, Nicholson 1998).

Relevant psychological perspective

There are many psychological theories relating to developmental crises such as adapting to change, the coping process and the resolution of stress, anxiety and internal conflict, but only the work of Erikson (1980) will be examined here.

Erikson (1980) framework

Psychological paradigms such as the psychoanalytical approach of Erikson (1980, 1995) are useful in developing an understanding of the changes, adjustments and general transitional phases involved when an individual encounters and has to deal with conflicts arising from major life events, for example motherhood. Eight stages of development during the life span are identified; these are commonly referred to as 'developmental or maturational crises' – that is, dilemmas or periods of difficulty rather than disasters or catastrophes (Johnstone 1994). The stages of Erikson's model may involve:

- transitions or turning points
- stress from having to resolve dilemmas.

To ensure psychological well-being, effective coping mechanisms and secure emotional adjustment, each stage will need to be satisfactorily resolved or negotiated by the person in order to effectively move on to the next step.

Stage 1: basic trust versus mistrust (birth–1 year). This stage relates to the ability of the child to establish safe, secure and trustful relationships with mother, father or significant others.

Stage 2: autonomy versus shame and doubt (1–3 years). The crisis within this developmental phase is between establishing a sense of self-control, self-worth or self-esteem, as well as confidence and independence, versus shame and self-doubt.

Stage 3: initiative versus guilt (3–6 years). This developmental phase is concerned with encouragement of the child to exercise freedom and initiative, whilst developing knowledge about social rules and norms.

Stage 4: industry versus inferiority (7–11 years). This phase addresses the influence of peer group versus parental pressure and expectations.

Stage 5: identity versus role confusion (12–18 years). This developmental phase is peppered with role confusion and indecisiveness. The adolescent might be in a state of flux in pursuit of a sense of identity, which may be social, educational, occupational or sexual. In the context of teenage mothers, this stage is very important for midwives.

Stage 6: intimacy versus isolation (young adulthood). This phase of the developmental crisis enables midwives to consider the importance of a well-integrated identity emerging from stage 5 of Erikson's (1980) framework.

Stage 7: generativity versus stagnation (middle adulthood). This penultimate stage is concerned with reproduction, childrearing, advancement of the species and doing good. Erikson (1980) defines this phase as the interest in guiding and establishing the next generation, which is of particular relevance to midwifery practice.

Stage 8: integrity versus despair (late adulthood). This final phase of the developmental crises relates to negotiating all the previous stages successfully, and accepting the limitations of life.

The work of Erikson (1980, 1995) though limited at times, serves to inform midwives that pregnancy and childbirth are punctuated by developmental crises. When such periods of increased emotionality are not resolved positively, psychological disturbances may ensue (Ball 1994, Johnstone 1994). During pregnancy, labour and the puerperium the importance of pre-existing or antecedent factors and their influence on a woman's emotional state should therefore account for her personality, past experiences, sociocultural influences, quality of psychosocial support, major life events and the responses of others. These pre-existing events will determine the way in which the woman will react to change. Conflicts around self-esteem, body image, femininity and adulthood might therefore be intensified during pregnancy. So too could a woman's unresolved feelings around previous birth events, such as birth trauma, grief around the death of a baby or previous experience of congenital abnormality. Careful assessment by the midwife during the antenatal period, noting past history and how this may affect the present, is a good way of identifying vulnerable groups of women.

The importance of psychosocial support during pregnancy has emerged in a number of studies (Hodnett 2000, Oakley et al 1996). Such evidence suggests that a woman's perception of events is extremely important to her emotional well-being. For example, if the woman perceives that she has psychosocial

> **Case scenario 35.2**
>
> Lisa is an 18-year-old single mother of three young children. She had twin boys when she was 16 and a girl 18 months ago. At 12 weeks' gestation, Lisa attends the antenatal 'booking' clinic as she is pregnant with her fourth child. She is tearful and says she can't cope, and reveals that her mother has recently been diagnosed with breast cancer.

support it will buffer the effects of the life changes she is currently experiencing. Furthermore, the systematic review on psychosocial support by Hodnett (2000) highlighted the benefits of this intervention in improving outcomes for both mother and baby. Case scenario 35.2 illustrates that vulnerable groups of women will need to be identified in order for that extra support to be mobilised.

Normal emotional changes during pregnancy, labour and the puerperium

These are many and varied as many decisions have to be made, hence it is perfectly normal for women to have periods of self-doubt and crises of confidence (Ball 1994). The reality for many women will encompass fluctuations between positive and negative emotions (Riley 1995), and according to Johnstone (1994) may include the following:

First trimester:

- pleasure, excitement, elation
- dismay, disappointment
- ambivalence
- emotional lability (e.g. episodes of weepiness exacerbated by physiological events such as nausea, vomiting and tiredness)
- increased femininity.

Second trimester:

- a feeling of well-being especially as physiological effects of tiredness, nausea and vomiting start to abate
- a sense of increased attachment to the fetus; the impact of ultrasound scanning generating images

for the prospective parents may intensify the experience
- stress and anxiety about antenatal screening and diagnostic tests
- increased demand for knowledge and information as preparations are now on the way for the birth
- feelings of the need for increasing detachment from work commitments.

Third trimester:

- loss of or increased libido
- altered body image
- psychological effects from physiological discomforts such as backache and heartburn
- anxiety about labour (e.g. pain)
- anxiety about fetal abnormality, which may disturb sleep or cause nightmares
- increased vulnerability to major life events such as financial status, moving house, or lack of a supportive partner.

Antenatal depression

According to findings of the Avon longitudinal cohort study of depressed mood during pregnancy and after childbirth, antenatal depression is emerging as an important entity, and not just a forerunner to postpartum depression (Evans et al 2001). However, previous research about antenatal psychopathology has tended to focus on just that (O'Hara et al 1990). Midwives must therefore be knowledgeable and confident in their skills to differentiate between distress and depression. It is crucial to recognise that the majority of cases of emotional distress in the first trimester of pregnancy are normal, and do not pose a risk to a woman's mental health following birth. However, the midwife should be alert to the importance of social support. Nevertheless an Australian study conducted to determine the level of a woman's social support at antenatal 'booking' interview concluded that measurement of social support is rather 'ad hoc and non-quantifiable' (Webster et al 2000). The researchers suggested that an assessment tool (e.g. the Edinburgh postnatal depression scale) provides a simple and meaningful strategy for measuring antenatal depression.

Box 35.1 lists key points for practice relating to antenatal emotional changes.

> **Box 35.1** Key points for practice
>
> - Prevalence of mental illness at conception is the same as the general population.
> - Antenatal depression will improve over the course of the pregnancy.
> - Prevalence of antenatal depression has not been accurately determined.
> - Incidence of mild morbidity in the first trimester increases, but then decreases in the second and third trimesters.
> - An elevated anxiety state is often a reaction to events and is therefore understandable, but the woman will need careful assessment and support.

Emotional changes during labour

For many women, labour will be greeted with varied emotional responses ranging from:

- great excitement and anticipation to utter dread
- fear of the unknown
- fear of technology, intervention and hospitalisation
- tension, fear and anxiety about pain and the ability to exercise control during labour
- concerns about the well-being of the baby and ability of the partner to cope
- fear of death – hospitals may be construed as places of illness, death and dying; the magnitude of such feelings may intensify if the woman experiences complications such as major postpartum haemorrhage, shoulder dystocia or even an emergency caesarean section
- the process of birth thrusts a lot of private data into the realms of the public, so there could be a fear of lack of privacy or utter embarrassment.

Evidence from Green et al's (1998) prospective study of women's expectations and experiences of childbirth suggests that having choice in pregnancy and childbirth, and a sense of being in control, leads to a more satisfying birth experience. The main issues for practice emerging from this research are:

- Women's perception of labour and childbirth are crucial to their emotional adjustment.

- Interventions per se do not equate to postnatal psychological sequelae, provided that the woman feels that the right decision was made.
- Adequate information decreases the likelihood of psychological morbidity.
- Being involved in the discussion of what happened is not enough for women, but having some say in the outcome may be viewed more positively.
- Being unable to be assertive in the face of health care professionals is more likely to result in lowering of women's mood.
- Emergency caesarean section is linked with more negative feelings about the baby.
- A woman's view of her baby is linked with her prior sense of control.
- There is a slight increase in the incidence of antenatal anxiety and depression compared with postnatal depression.

During labour, midwives must consider the factors that induce stress, and these should be prevented, or at least minimised, as the woman's long term emotional health may be severely compromised by an adverse birth experience.

The puerperium

The puerperium is hailed as the 'fourth trimester' (Johnstone 1994), and by definition it is the period from birth to 6–8 weeks postpartum, when the woman is readjusting physiologically and psychosocially to motherhood. Emotional responses may be just as intense and powerful for experienced as well as for new mothers. The major psychological changes are therefore emotional, and the woman's mood appears to be a barometer, reflecting the baby's needs of feeding, sleeping and crying patterns. New mothers tend to be easily upset and oversensitive. A sense of proportion is easily lost, as women may feel overwhelmed and agitated by minor mishaps. The woman might start to regain a sense of proportion and 'normality' between 6 and 12 weeks. Perhaps the most important factor in regaining any semblance of normality is the mother's ability to sleep throughout the night. This seems to happen at the time that the baby also starts to develop a predictable pattern, settle into a routine and become more responsive. Nevertheless, feelings of sheer exhaustion may persist for women who are breastfeeding or if solids are not yet introduced for babies who are artificially fed. Thus a woman's sexual urges, emotional stability and intellectual acuity may take months, if not a year or more, to return and for the woman to feel whole again. Normal emotional changes in the puerperium are therefore eclectic and complex and may encompass the following (Ball 1994, Barclay & Lloyd 1996, Bick & MacArthur 1995, Bick et al 2002, Johnstone 1994):

- contradictory and conflicting feelings ranging from satisfaction, joy and elation to exhaustion, helplessness, discontentment and disappointment as the early weeks seem to be dominated by the novelty and unpredictability of this stranger
- relief – 'thank goodness that's over' – may be chorused by many women immediately following birth; sometimes the woman conveys a cool detachment from events, especially if labour was protracted, complicated and difficult
- some may experience closeness to partner or baby; equally the woman may feel disinterested in the baby, though some who intend to breastfeed will want to initiate skin-to-skin contact and feed straight away
- disinterest or being very attentive towards the baby
- fear of the unknown and sudden realisation of overwhelming responsibility
- exhaustion and increased emotionality
- pain (e.g. perineal, in nipples)
- increased vulnerability, indecisiveness (e.g. in feeding); loss of libido, disturbed sleep and anxiety.

Postnatal 'blues'

Due to the influence of the medical model of care this normal and transient phase, experienced by 50–80% of women depending on parity (Cox & Holden 1994), is erroneously categorised as a form of mental illness. Perhaps because it has been identified as an antecedent to postnatal depression (Cooper & Murray 1997, Gregoire 1995). The mean onset typically occurs between 3 and 4 days postpartum, but may last up to a week or more, though rarely persisting longer than a few days. The features of this state are mild and transitory and may include a state whereby women usually experience labile emotions (e.g. tearfulness, euphoria and laughter). The actual aetiology is unclear but hormonal influences (e.g. changes in oestrogen, progesterone and prolactin levels) seem to be implicated as the period of increased emotionality appears to coincide with the production of milk in the breasts (Cooper & Murray 1997, Gregoire 1995). Although self-limiting, occurrence of the postnatal 'blues' illuminates the need for psychosocial support.

Emotional distress associated with traumatic birth events

Over recent years the label 'post-traumatic stress disorder' (PTSD) has emerged in midwifery practice (Crompton 1996a, b, Lyons 1998). What is intended to be one of the happiest days in a woman's life can quickly turn into anguish and distress. Effects of intense pain, use of technological interventions, insensitive and disrespectful care may prove very distressing and frightening (see Case scenario 35.1 p. 655). Many women will eventually overcome the pain, fear and crippling anxiety of labour and childbirth. However, for others, the traumatic events surrounding their birth experience will remain ingrained in their psyche, and may blight their lives and affect the relationship with their partner and baby (Lyons 1998). However, the concept of PTSD in maternity care is fraught with difficulties. Not only does it evoke images of negligence and suboptimal care, but PTSD is most commonly associated with individuals who have suffered the onslaught of war (Crompton 1996a). Nevertheless PTSD following childbirth may result in nightmares and 'flashbacks', which could be very distressing and frightening when women are again confronted with real images of labour. Unlike postnatal depression, which seems to have its roots in the biophysical and psychosocial domains, obstetric distress after childbirth appears to be directly linked to the stress, fear and trauma of birth, yet its prevalence is unrecognised (Lyons 1998). Charles & Curtis (1996) recommend brief psychological interventions, which they refer to as 'debriefing', for managing immediate symptomatology related to obstetric distress. However, there is no reliable evidence that psychological 'debriefing' is a useful intervention in reducing psychological morbidity (Bick et al 2002, Wesseley, Rose and Bisson 2000).

Key points for practice relating to emotional distress linked to giving birth are listed in Box 35.2.

The psychopathology of pregnancy and childbirth

There is a steep rise in the prevalence of psychotic illness and, to a lesser extent, mild to moderate 'postnatal

- Each woman should be treated as an individual; some may find the normal emotional changes quite distressing, and others will find them less so and be more realistic in their expectations.

- Women who experience nightmares should be reassured that, in many instances, bad dreams can be expressions of fear and anxiety.

- Women do not freely express their fears but a supportive midwife who the woman knows and trusts may encourage and persuade the woman to be open and honest.

- Midwives should possess good communication skills and be able to listen and attend to women's concerns in order to meet their emotional needs.

- Psychological morbidity in 'normal' pregnancies may be missed because:
  — it is not given enough recognition
  — it is thought to be self-limiting
  — it is not identified, especially where there are difficulties realising continuity of care
  — it is attributable to the 'normal' emotionality of pregnancy.

Table 35.1 Prevalence of psychopathology (Oates 1998)

10–15%	Postnatal depressive illness (depending on the diagnostic tool and criteria used)
3–5%	Moderate to severe depressive illness
2%	Referred to psychiatrist
2/1000	Admitted puerperal psychosis
4/1000	Admitted all conditions

Mild to moderate postnatal depression

Over 10–15% of mothers will suffer from a mild to moderate postnatal depressive illness for the first time (Cox et al 1993), and there is now widespread acknowledgement that PND is an important public health problem. Considerable evidence now highlights the fact that it can become chronic, damages the relationship between the woman and her partner, and has adverse effects on the emotional and cognitive development of the child (Murray et al 1999). Although PND is widely accepted by the lay public, and it is distinctive from serious forms of depressive illness in terms of its onset, clinical features and management, it is not included in the international classification and definition of ICD10 depression criteria (National Screening Committee 2001). A substantial evidence base suggests the 1 year incidence of PND is no higher than that of depression in age-matched non-postpartum women (O'Hara et al 1990). However, the incidence of PND in the first 3 months postpartum is higher and more severe (Cox et al 1993). No matter whether or not the incidence of PND increases, the presence of distressing depression in a critical time in women's lives when they expect to be happy is of heightened importance, not least because of its implications for child development. The recent report on Confidential Enquiries into Maternal Deaths in the United Kingdom 1997–1999 (Lewis & Drife 2001) identified that the term 'postnatal depression' should be used only to describe a mild to moderate non-psychotic depressive state, with its onset associated with pregnancy and childbirth. It should *not* be used as a generic term for all forms of mental health disturbances following childbirth.

Postnatal depression has a later onset than the postnatal 'blues'. Beck (1996) undertook a meta-analysis to identify the risk factors associated with mild to

depression' ('PND') associated with having children (Table 35.1). For women with pre-existing mental health problems, childbirth increases the risk of recurrence. For those with chronic illness such as schizophrenia, pregnancy and childbirth pose an even greater concern about their risk of relapse and their ability to care for the baby (Oates 1995a, b). Although the risk of a serious depressive illness increases significantly postpartum, difficulties may also emerge during pregnancy. The range of severity and types of mental health problems are very varied, but in this chapter mild to moderate PND, severe depressive illnesses and puerperal psychosis will be discussed. However, it should be realised that these illnesses form part of a continuum.

moderate postnatal depression (Box 35.3). The majority of women with identified risk factors will not subsequently suffer from postnatal depression. The non-specificity of these risk factors means that they are widely found in the population, but are helpful for targeting vulnerable groups of women who may need special resources. However, their predictive power is weak and limited as an antenatal index for predicting women at risk of developing postnatal depression (Cooper & Murray 1997, Forman et al 2000, Oates 1995b).

Recognition and aetiology

Evidence from an epidemiological study links causative factors of a psychosocial nature to postnatal depression, for instance stressful life events such as the presence of relationship conflict, absence of a supportive partner, higher levels of obstetric stressors and unemployment (Appleby et al 1994, O'Hara et al 1991). Postnatal depressive illnesses may take different forms. But generally, in the mildest forms, it could be an exaggeration of the various emotional changes during the puerperium, and may not be easily distinguishable from the emotional upheavals being experienced during the transition to motherhood. Postnatal depression may occur in the first month postpartum, at a time when midwives are often withdrawing care, and may last up to a year (Brockington 1996). However, in its more severe forms it may be clearly distinguishable from the norm.

Early signs of postnatal depression may include anxiety and worries about the baby. Feelings of inability to cope and feeling overwhelmed by the demands of motherhood and having a new baby may lead to sleep disturbance. Commonly there are feelings of sadness, inadequacy, worthlessness, loss of appetite, low self-esteem, a persistently lowered mood and loss of enjoyment and spontaneity. These associated features are not hard to detect but may be missed by health care professionals. There is the added problem that postnatal depression is still a taboo subject in some social circles, which silences many women. Women may feel guilty, isolated and a failure at a time when they should feel victorious and contented to embrace the powerful role of motherhood. Some women and their partners may not be fully informed about the signs and symptoms of postnatal depression. This is further compounded where the woman is having repeated contact with health professionals, who may fail

> **Box 35.3** Risk factors for mild to moderate postnatal depression based on Beck (1996) meta-analysis
>
> - Antenatal depression
> - History of previous postnatal depression
> - Quality of psychosocial support
> - Stressful life events
> - Stress related to child care
> - Postnatal `blues'
> - Quality of relationship with partner
> - Antenatal anxiety

to recognise the signs of postnatal depression. Furthermore, a woman may disguise her true emotional state from those around her, which only serves to complicate things further.

With thought and innovation the antenatal 'booking' visit and selective postnatal visits could be modified to include screening for psychological morbidity (Clement 1995, Webster et al 2000). The midwifery-led postnatal care trial (IMPaCT study), a randomised controlled trial conducted in Birmingham by Bick et al (2002), suggests benefits in reviewing the organisation of traditional postnatal care. The study involved selective postnatal visits of women up to 10–12 weeks postpartum. This new way of working fits with the public health agenda, as this extended visiting pattern provided a window of opportunity to identify the majority of cases of psychological morbidity.

Value of using a screening tool

The Edinburgh postnatal depression scale (EPDS) was developed by Cox et al (1987) for research in the postnatal period, because other tools were not suitable for use. Its use as a valid screening tool in risk identification in clinical practice has been well documented (Bick et al 2002, Cooper & Murray 1997). Nationally, many health visitors administer the EPDS postpartum at 6 weeks, allowing time for the mother to reflect on feelings and how well she is adjusting to and coping with motherhood. The EPDS is a simple 10-item self-completion questionnaire that takes only minutes to complete. Scores for each item range from 0 to 3, according to the woman's mood and responses. Cox et al (1987) suggest an aggregated cut-off score of 12/13 as being a predictive risk. The validity of the EPDS has been tested on a large community sample (Murray & Carothers 1990), with encouraging results. An 11/12 cut-off threshold has been highlighted as having a specificity of 92.5%, a predictive value of 35.1% and a sensitivity of 88% (Cooper & Murray 1997). Nevertheless concerns have been raised about the misuse and limitations of the EPDS with respect to primary carers (Elliott 1994, Leverton & Elliott 2000). These authors remind us that it should add to clinical judgement, not replace it. Inadequate preparation of midwives in predicting risk, as few have mental health education and training, may result in the danger of a significant number of false positive situations developing – that is, women who have high scores but are not depressed may swamp already stretched mental health services. The value and limitations of the EPDS are summarised in Box 35.4.

Because obtaining an EPDS result for a woman is a very complex exercise with many steps along the way, involving many variables, a recent report by the National Screening Committee (2001) concluded that more work needs to be done in relation to the EPDS. It stressed that this is especially important to determine its validity in routine primary care, and that the widespread implementation of screening for PND with the EPDS throughout the UK is indeed a matter of concern.

Care and management and the role of the midwife

Given that many cases of mild to moderate PND go undetected, the condition is usually self-limiting, and many mothers will recover by about 6 months postpartum. However, 30% of women will remain ill at 1 year and over 10% at 2 years postpartum (Oates 2000), with consequences for the cognitive development of the infant (Cooper & Murray 1997, Murray et al 1999). Midwives should be vigilant when observing the mother–baby relationship to assess how the mother interacts with her child, taking into account cultural influences. Any untoward problems with infant feeding, sleeping and general temperament should alert the midwife to the need for psychosocial support. The partner should also be involved in these interactions to help address and alleviate any simmering tensions that may exist within the couple's relationship.

Despite evidence of the efficacy of antidepressants in the treatment of PND, as in depressive illness at other times, a study by Appleby et al (1997) suggests another possibility. Psychological interventions such as non-directive counselling have also been shown to be effective. This means that many women can be cared for in their own communities via the primary care team. However, this option is dependent on early detection and the possession of appropriate referral and consultation with the mental health team; where

---

Box 35.4 Value and limitations of the Edinburgh postnatal depression scale

Value

- Useful screening tool
- Acceptable to women
- Takes minutes to complete and score
- Results can be discussed immediately leading to early identification of problems.
- A score of 12+ indicates the likelihood of depression
- Provides women with tangible 'permission' to talk, be listened to and have feelings validated.

Limitations

- May lead to misdiagnosis, i.e. false positives and medicalisation of low moods and situational distress
- Depression about depression
- Only *predictive*, not *diagnostic*
- Is not a magic wand
- Does not replace and should not replace clinical judgement
- Does not give women opportunity to describe symptoms fully.

this service is non-existent, referral to out of area services must be considered. Collaboration with voluntary support agencies (e.g. postnatal support groups) is also valuable.

Motherhood and mental illness

Severe depressive illness

The risk of women being referred to a psychiatrist in the year following pregnancy and childbirth is five times greater than at other times in their lives (Oates 1994). This incidence of referred mental illness is much greater than for men and women in the general population (Oates 2000, O'Hara et al 1990). Approximately 3–5% of mothers will be affected by the more severe form of depressive illness (Oates 2000). While health care professionals might be forgiven for experiencing problems in recognising mild to moderate postnatal depression, the identification of severe depressive illness should not be too taxing. It develops in the early postpartum period, and women who are severely depressed may look mentally anguished and ill.

Recognition and aetiology

The actual aetiology is unclear; however, the most powerful predictor appears to be a previous history of depressive illness either postpartum or at other times (O'Hara & Swain 1996). It is generally thought that neuroendocrine factors play a part; particularly precipitous is the part played by oestradiol (Wieck et al 1991). The onset is insiduous and often starts slowly in the first 2–3 weeks postpartum. It usually commences when midwifery care and general social support from partner, family and friends may be significantly curtailed. Again the 6 week postnatal examination is a useful watershed in detecting the condition. If not, two-thirds will present later, between 10 and 12 weeks postdelivery (Brockington 1996, Oates 1995a); the main characteristics are:

- 'biological syndrome' of sleep disturbance, of waking early in the morning; the woman will feel most depressed and her symptoms will be worst at the start of the day
- impaired concentration, disturbed thought processes, indecisiveness and an inability to cope with everyday life

- emotional detachment and profound lowering of mood
- loss of ability to feel pleasure (anhedonia)
- feelings of guilt, incompetence and of being a 'bad' mother
- in approximately one-third of women, distressing intrusive obsessional thoughts and ruminations
- commonly extreme anxiety and even panic attacks
- impaired appetite and weight loss
- in a small number, a depressive psychosis and morbid, delusional thoughts and hallucinations.

Variations

Phobic anxiety, panic disorders and obsessive compulsive disorders (OCD) might be a variation on the theme (Case scenario 35.3). For example, anxiety might be the dominating feature leading to feelings of apprehension, palpitations, tension headaches and dizziness. An acute attack of anxiety associated with intense fear of losing control, hyperventilating or overbreathing is called a panic attack. These feelings could be triggered when the woman is out shopping or travelling on public transport leading to agoraphobia, and resulting in the woman not wanting to leave her home. Hence the habit of avoidance soon sets in.

OCD may present with unpleasant, intrusive and distressing thoughts. The thoughts often relate to obscenities, dirt or disease, which are incongruent with the woman's true nature. Thoughts may also include harm coming to the baby or a member of the family, excessive cleanliness, disproportionate anxiety about the baby and obsession with personal health and hygiene.

Puerperal psychosis

Puerperal psychosis has been known since antiquity; consistent evidence over 100 years notes that it affects approximately 2–3 per 1000 births (Kendell et al 1987), leading to a psychiatric admission. Although the least common of the postpartum syndromes, puerperal psychosis is regarded as the most severe and dramatic of the psychiatric disturbances to occur in the postpartum period.

Recognition and aetiology

Symptoms are florid, presenting dramatically and very early and tending to change rapidly, altering from day

Case scenario 35.3

Mary Flower is a 42-year-old psychiatric nurse, married for 16 years to Bob, a telecommunications engineer. She has neither a family history of mental illness nor a previous personal history. However, she had always been anxious with marked obsessional (perfectionist) personality traits, and had not coped well in the past with changes. She had a long history of infertility investigations and had conceived her two children with IVF. Following the birth of her first child, she found it difficult to adjust to her new lifestyle, suffering from self-doubt, mild anxiety attack and depression, which spontaneously resolved following her return to work at 6 months postpartum. Four years later, following the birth of her second child, she became severely depressed and at 6 weeks postpartum developed psychomotor slowing, impaired concentration and efficiency. She had early morning wakening, with her mood and coping abilities being worst in the morning (*diurnal variation of mood*). She was very anxious and had panic attacks triggered by intrusive thoughts of some terrible harm coming to her baby. She had overvalued ideas of guilt and incompetence, and actively concealed her state from her midwife (who continued to visit because Mary was experiencing problems with breastfeeding), health visitor and GP. A good friend insisted that she seek help. Within 2 weeks of starting tricyclic antidepressants, dosulepin (dothiepin) 150 mg, Mary began to recover and was quite well by 3 months postpartum. She reduced and discontinued her antidepressants 6 months later and remained well.

Features may include:

- restlessness and agitation
- confusion and perplexity
- suspicion and fear
- insomnia
- episodes of mania, making the woman hyperactive (e.g. talking rapidly and incessantly, and being very overactive and elated)
- neglect of basic needs (e.g. nutrition and hydration)
- hallucinations and morbid delusional thoughts involving the woman and her baby
- major behavioural disturbance
- profound depressive mood.

Puerperal psychosis appears to be much less related to stress factors (Cooper & Murray 1997) and more related to biochemical changes. However, the evidence about its biophysical origins, though plausible, remains equivocal (Gregoire 1995, Harris et al 1994). Most mothers with puerperal psychosis will be experiencing mental illness for the first time. The strong association between family history of a manic depressive disorder (mother or father) and puerperal psychosis suggests a genetic link (Oates 2000).

Care and management and the role of the midwife

Great care must be taken to ensure effective communication and to avoid the ambiguous label of 'postnatal depression', which serves only to underestimate the profound nature of the illness and may subsequently lead to missed opportunities and suboptimal care. Documentation of any past history of psychiatric disturbances should clearly spell out the precise onset, duration, diagnosis and treatment regimen (Lewis & Drife 2001). In the case of psychosis, where delusional thoughts and hallucinations are implicated, the woman must be referred urgently to the mental health team, as it is likely that she will need admission. This should be to a specialist mother and baby unit, with an out-of-area referral if necessary.

Perinatal mental health services make an important contribution to the management of this condition (Oates 1998). Ideally, care and management should be based primarily on preventative measures and begin preconception, or at least during the antenatal

to day during the acute phase of the illness. These typically include changes of mood state, irrational behaviour and disturbed agitation, fear and perplexity as the woman quickly loses touch with reality. The onset is very sudden, commonly occurring within the 1st postnatal week and rarely before the 3rd postpartum day, with the majority presenting before the 16th postnatal day (Kendell et al 1987).

period, for women with a past history and known risk factors. Tremendous cooperation and interprofessional collaboration are required during the acute phase of the illness. Safety should be at the forefront of care; hospitalisation of mother and baby should never occur on a general psychiatric ward (Lewis & Drife 2001). In a specialist mother and baby unit, skilled staff will be able to undertake an assessment of the mother's ability to care for her baby and her needs to continue this care back in the community.

Hospitalisation also serves to provide the distressed and ill mother with an understanding and a therapeutic environment in which she can develop an effective relationship with her infant and the skills necessary to be an able mother. However, sensitive care is vital, as it may be difficult for the woman or her partner and family to accept the symptoms and diagnosis of a psychotic illness.

Antipsychotic (neuroleptic) medication is often an essential initial part of treatment. Such medication will not only sedate, but will also reduce the perplexity, distress and fear, and within 48 hours should make some impact on hallucinations and delusions (Oates 1995a, 2000). Manic features are often managed effectively with medication such as lithium carbonate; however, this is contraindicated if the woman is breastfeeding. Although is widely believed that electroconvulsive therapy (ECT) is the treatment of choice, modern management has resulted in much lower usage than in the past. However, it remains useful in states where there is a threat of suicide. Antidepressants could take up to 2 weeks to have any therapeutic effect so may not be appropriate for first line management, but are useful to maintain recovery after ECT treatment has been terminated (Oates 1998). Risk of relapse is high, therefore medication will need to be continued for 6 months, by which time the majority of women would have recovered. But if this happens on more than one occasion the psychiatrist may consider using lithium carbonate or other mood stabilisers to stabilise the woman's mood for 6 months to 1 year postpartum, and up to 2 years prophylactically if the woman presents with a non-postpartum manic depressive disorder.

Suicide

Suicide is substantially less common in pregnant and postpartum women (DoH 1998). Despite this the findings of the recent Confidential Enquiries into Maternal Deaths (Lewis & Drife 2001) found that suicide is now the leading cause of maternal mortality in the UK. Appleby et al (1994) reveal that suicide and infanticide are rare events, but nevertheless the majority of postpartum maternal suicides were the sequelae of puerperal psychosis and severe depressive illness. Furthermore, there is little evidence to implicate severe postpartum mental illness as a major contributor to non-accidental injury in children. The most consistent findings are linked to parental youth, previous abusive relationships and, in men, a previous criminal record for violence (Lewis & Drife 2001). Unequivocally, the most important factors in the reduction of risk to both mother and baby from mental illness are prompt detection, appropriate referral, early intervention and effective and vigorous management (Lewis & Drife 2001).

Prognosis

Research by Cooper & Murray (1995) suggests that not only does postpartum psychopathology respond well to psychological interventions, but they generally have a good prognosis. Although there is a risk of mental illness with subsequent pregnancies, the good news is that women do recover to carry on with their lives. Women will recover from puerperal psychosis, but those who have a personal history of psychosis, whether or not related to childbirth, have between a 1:2 and 1:3 risk of having the disorder after the birth of any other children (Wieck et al 1991). Furthermore the risk of recurrence of a severe mental illness is at its greatest in the first 30 days postpartum (Lewis & Drife 2001). The risk is estimated to be highest if the woman has another child within 2 years of recovery.

Psychotropic medication during pregnancy and implications for breastfeeding

Given that there has been a paucity of systematic research on the efficacy and risks of pharmacological intervention in the management of postnatal depression, balancing risk to the fetus against the risk of not treating the mother is a challenge (Cooper & Murray 1997). Women should be actively supported to breast feed their baby, if this is their wish. Apart from all the well-established reasons for doing so, it may protect the infant from the consequences of maternal post-partum mental health problems. This may be the only positive contribution the woman feels she can make as a mother in the midst of all the emotional chaos and confusion. Management should therefore always be case specific and based on a risk–benefit analysis.

General principles

- Whenever possible, conception and birth should be medication free, but approximately half of all pregnancies are unplanned.
- Most new episodes of mental illness in pregnancy are early and improve as pregnancy progresses with appropriate psychosocial interventions. Therefore, the initiation of psychotropic medication should be infrequent.
- Liaison between the midwife, GP, obstetrician, psychiatrist, community psychiatric nurse, health visitor and, where necessary, social worker is of great importance.
- If medication is known to cross the placenta it is likely to be present in breastmilk.

- No medication is of proven safety.
- However, those with significant increases in risk of teratogenesis are still low risk (1–2% of exposed pregnancies). Nevertheless they may contribute to fetal demise, intrauterine growth restriction, organ dysgenesis and adverse effects on the neonate such as withdrawal.
- Babies more than 12 weeks old are at low risk of exposure to antidepressants in breastmilk.
- breastmilk levels will reflect the serum levels of the medication. Therefore women should be advised to avoid feeding at times of peak plasma level, and preferably should time their medication after a feed and before the baby's longest sleep.
- The baby should be monitored for any deleterious effects, particularly weight gain and drowsiness.

Psychotropic medication and their implications for breastfeeding are summarised in Table 35.2.

Conclusion

A summary of key recommendations for best practice is given in Box 35.5.

Table 35.2 Psychotropic medication and breastfeeding

Category/name of medication	Considered safe	Considered unsafe
1. Tricyclic antidepressants, e.g. dosulepin (dothiepin)	✓	✗
2. Selective serotonin reuptake inhibitors (SSRIs), e.g. fluvoxamine, fluoxetine, paroxetine and Sertraline	✗	Controversial Not in last trimester
3. Monoamine oxidase inhibitors (MAOIs), e.g. phenelzine, isocarboxazid and, the most hazardous, tranylcypromine	✗	✓
4. Lithium carbonate	✗	✓
5. Neuroleptics, e.g. chlorpromazine, trifluoperazine and fluphenazine: —moderate oral dosage —high dosage, e.g. intramuscular injection	 ✓ ✗	 ✗ ✓
6. New 'atypical' antipsychotics, e.g. olanzapine, risperidone	No data	No data
7. Benzodiazepines, e.g. lorazepam and flurazepam	✗	✓
7. Alcohol and marijuana	✗	✓

Box 35.5 Summary of key recommendations for best practice

- *Prevention*:
  - Realistic preparation of couples to aim for achievable birth expectations and to deal ably with the demands and challenges of parenthood.
  - Value interagency networking to afford more responsive helplines and points of contact for parents in crisis.
  - Development of evidence base of effective mental health promotion strategies.
  - The risk of recurrence of a severe mental illness is at its greatest in the first 30 days postpartum.
  - Antenatally, screen for risk factors that may culminate in antenatal or postnatal depression, personal or family history of mental illness, history of substance (drug or alcohol) abuse, domestic violence and self-harm and suicidal traits (Lewis & Drife 2001).
  - Be vigilant with record keeping to ensure good communication and continuity of care. Good liaison between interprofessional team.
  - Avoid misdiagnosis, prevent errors and missed opportunities in care by employing the correct terminology. The umbrella term of 'PND' to describe all types of postpartum mental health problems must cease. In accordance with the 2001 CEMD report (Lewis & Drife 2001), the acronym 'PND' must be used only when referring to mild to moderate severity of non-psychotic depressive illness that has an onset following childbirth.
- *Standards and targets*:
  - Set national targets for perinatal mental health services.
  - Develop clear care pathways for women with a history of mental health problems, substance abuse, and those in abusive relationships.
  - Set targets to establish the incidence of antenatal depression and reduce the prevalence of postnatal depression; one way of achieving this is to standardise the criteria used for screening.
- *Services*:
  - Improve access to perinatal mental health services.
  - Increase consultants specialising in perinatal mental health problems.
  - Increase specialist facilities to avoid risk of mother and baby being admitted to a general psychiatric ward.
  - Formulate strategy groups reflective of all key members of the multiprofessional team to review services for the childbearing woman with perinatal mental health problems.
  - Interprofessional and interagency collaboration, especially within the primary and secondary care sectors.
- *Research, education and training*:
  - Evaluation of perinatal mental health services.
  - Interprofessional or interagency education programmes to aid learning and to improve and understand lines of communication or delineate professional boundaries.
  - To distinguish between psychology and pathology in order to avoid or reduce inappropriate referrals.

REFERENCES

Appleby L, Gregoire A, Platz C, Martin P, Kumar R 1994 Screening women for high risk of postnatal depression. Journal of Psychosomatic Research 38:539–545

Appleby L, Warner R, Whitton A, Faragher B 1997 A controlled study of fluoxetine and cognitive-behavioural counselling in the treatment of postnatal depression. British Medical Journal 314:932–936

Audit Commission 1997 First class delivery: improving maternity services in England and Wales. Audit Commission, London

Ball J A 1994 Reactions to motherhood: the role of postnatal care, 2nd edn. Books for Midwives Press, Hale, Cheshire

Barclay L, Lloyd B 1996 The misery of motherhood: alternative approaches to distress. Midwifery 12(3):136–138

Beck C 1996 Meta-analysis of predictors of postnatal depression. Nursing Research 45(5):297–302

Bick D, MacArthur C, Knowles H, Winter H 2002 Postnatal care: evidence and guidelines for management. Churchill Livingstone, Edinburgh

Bick D E, MacArthur C 1995 The extent, severity and effect on health problems after childbirth. British Journal of Midwifery 3:27–31

Brockington I 1996 Maternal mental health. Oxford University Press, Oxford

Charles J, Curtis L 1996 Birth after thoughts: a listening information service. British Journal of Midwifery 2(7):331–334

Clement C 1995 Listening visits in pregnancy: a strategy for preventing postnatal depression? Midwifery 11(2):75–80

Cooper P J, Murray L 1995 The course and recurrence of postnatal depression. British Journal of Psychiatry 166:191–195

Cooper P J, Murray L 1997 Effects of postnatal depression on infant development. Archives of Disease in Childhood 77:97–101

Cox J L, Holden J (eds) 1994 Perinatal psychiatry: use and misuse of the Edinburgh postnatal depression scale. Gaskell, London

Cox J L, Holden J M, Sagovsky R 1987 Detection of postnatal depression: development of the Edinburgh postnatal depression scale. British Journal of Psychiatry 150:782–786

Cox J L, Murray D, Chapman G 1993 A controlled study of the onset, duration and prevalence of postnatal depression. British Journal of Psychiatry 163:27–31

Crompton J 1996a Post-traumatic stress disorder and childbirth. British Journal of Midwifery 4(6):290–294

Crompton J 1996b Post-traumatic stress disorder and childbirth: 2. British Journal of Midwifery 4(7):354–356, 373

DoH (Department of Health) 1993 Report of the expert maternity group: changing childbirth: parts 1 and 2. HMSO, London

DoH (Department of Health) 1998 Why mothers die: Report of the confidential enquiries into maternal deaths in the United Kingdom 1994–1996. HMSO, London

DoH (Department of Health) 1999 National service framework for mental health: modern standards and service models. DoH, London

Elliot S 1994 Uses and misuses of Edinburgh postnatal depression score in primary care: a comparison of models developed in health visiting. In: Cox J L, Holden J M (eds) Perinatal psychiatry: use and misuse of the Edinburgh postnatal depression scale. Gaskill, London, ch 14, p 221–228

Erikson E 1980 Identity and the life cycle: a re-issue. Norton, New York

Erikson E 1995 Childhood and society, 3rd edn. Norton, New York

Evans J, Heron J, Francomb H, Oke S, Golding J 2001 Cohort study of depressed mood during pregnancy and childbirth. British Medical Journal 323:257–260

Forman D N, Videbech P, Hedegraad M, Salvig J D, Secher N J 2000 Postnatal depression: identification of women at risk. British Journal of Obstetrics and Gynaecology 107:1210–1217

Green J M, Coupland V A, Kitzinger J V 1998 Great expectations: a prospective study of women's expectations and experiences of childbirth. Books for Midwives, Hale, Cheshire

Gregoire A 1995 Hormones and postnatal depression. British Journal of Midwifery 3(2):99–104

Harris B, Lovett L, Newcombe R G 1994 Maternity blues and major endocrine changes: Cardiff puerperal mood and hormone study 2. British Medical Journal 308:949–953

Hodnett E D 2000 Support during pregnancy for women at increased risk. Cochrane Database of Pregnancy and Childbirth Module of Systematic Reviews, Issue 2. Update Software, Oxford

Johnstone M 1994 The emotional effects of childbirth: a distance learning course for midwives, health visitors and others who care for women aound the time of birth. London: Marće Society

Kendell R E, Chalmers L, Platz C 1987 The epidemiology of puerperal psychoses. British Journal of Psychiatry 150:662–673

Leverton T J, Elliott S A 2000 Is the EPDS a magic wand? 1. A comparison of the Edinburgh postnatal depression scale and health visitor report as predictors of diagnosis on the present state examination. Journal of Reproductive and Infant Psychology 18(4):280–296

Lewis G, Drife J (eds) 2001 Why mothers die 1997–1999: The fifth report of the Confidential Enquiries into Maternal Deaths in the United Kingdom. RCOG, London

Lyons S 1998 Post-traumatic stress disorder following childbirth: causes, prevention and treatment. In: Clement S (ed) Psychological perspectives on pregnancy and childbirth. Churchill Livingstone, London, ch 7, p 123–143

Murray L, Carothers A D 1990 The validation of the Edinburgh postnatal depression scale on a community sample. British Journal of Psychiatry 157:288–290

Murray L, Sinclair D, Cooper P, Ducournau P, Turner P 1999 The socioemotional development of 5 year olds with postnatally depressed mothers. Journal of Child Psychology and Psychiatry 40:1259–1271

National Screening Committee 2001 Screening for postnatal depression. Online. Available: http://www.nelh.nhs.uk/screening/adult_pps/postnatal_depression.html

Newton C, Raynor M D 2000 Routine intrapartum care. In: Kean L H, Baker P N, Edelstone D I (eds) Best practice in labor ward management, 1st edn. W B Saunders, Edinburgh, ch 2, p 19–40

Nicholson P 1998 Postnatal depression: psychology, science and the transition to motherhood. Routledge, London

Nieland M N S, Roger D 1997 Symptoms in postpartum and non-postpartum samples: implications for postnatal depression. Journal of Reproduction and Infant Psychology 15(1):31–42

Oakley A, Hickey D, Rajan L, Rigby A 1996 Social support in pregnancy – does it have long term effects? Journal of Reproduction and Infant Psychology 14:7–22

Oates M R 1994 Postnatal mental illness: organisation and function of services. In: Cox J, Holden J (eds) Perinatal psychiatry: use and misuse of the Edinburgh Postnatal Depression Scale. Gaskell, London, p 8–33

Oates M R 1995a Psychiatric disorder and childbirth. Current Obstetrics and Gynaecology 5:64–69

Oates M R 1995b Risk and childbirth in psychiatry. Advances in Psychiatric Treatment 1:146–153

Oates M R 1998 Psychiatric disorders in childbirth. In: Symonds E M, Symonds I M (eds) Essential obstetric and gynaecology, 3rd edn. Churchill Livingstone, New York, ch 17, p 169–179

Oates M R 2000 Psychiatric disorders in pregnancy and the puerperium. In: Campbell S, Lees C (eds) Obstetrics by ten teachers, 17th edn. Arnold, London, ch 21, p 319–330

O'Hara M W, Zekosi E M, Phillips L H, Wright E J 1990 Controlled prospective study of postpartum mood disorders: comparison of childbearing and non-childbearing women. Journal of Abnormal Psychology 99:3–15

O'Hara M W, Schlechte J A, Lewis D A, Varner M W 1991 A controlled prospective study of postpartum mood disorders: psychological, environmental and hormonal variables. Journal of Abnormal Psychology 100:63–73

O'Hara M W, Swain A M 1996 Rates and risk of postpartum psychosis: a meta-analysis. Psychiatry 8:37–54

Phoenix A, Woollett A 1991 Motherhood: meanings, practices and ideologies. Sage, London

Price J 1988 Motherhood what it does to your mind. Pandora, London

RCM (Royal College of Midwives) 1999 The transition to parenthood: an open learning resource for midwives. RCM, London

RCOP (Royal College of Psychiatrists) 2000 Report on recommendations for the provision of mental health services for childbearing women 2000. RCOP, London

Riley D 1995 Perinatal mental health: a resource book for health professionals. Radcliffe, Oxford

Symonds A, Hunt SC 1996 The midwife and society: perspective, policies and practice. Macmillan, London

Teixeira J M A, Fisk N M, Glover V 1999 Association between anxiety in pregnancy and increased uterine artery resistance index: cohort based study. British Medical Journal 318:153–157

UKCC (United Kingdom Central Council for Nursing, Midwifery and Health Visiting) 1998 Midwives rules and code of practice. UKCC, London

Webster J, Linnane J W J, Dibley L M, Hinson J K, Starrenburg S E, Roberts J A 2000 Measuring social support during pregnancy: can it be simple and meaningful? Birth 27(2):97–103

Wessely S, Rose S, Bisson J 2000 Brief psychological interventions ('debriefing') for treating immediate trauma related symptoms and prevention of post traumatic stress disorder. The Cochrane Library of Systematic Reviews, Issue 3. Update Software, Oxford

Wieck A, Kumar R, Hirst A D, Marks M N, Campbell I, Checkley S A 1991 Increased sensitivity of dopamine receptors and recurrence of affective psychosis after childbirth. British Medical Journal 303:613–616

FURTHER READING

Clement S (ed) 1998 Psychological perspectives on pregnancy and childbirth. Churchill Livingstone, London

A useful text for understanding the psychological issues arising from pregnancy and childbirth.

Enkin M, Keirse M J N C, Neilson J et al 2000 A guide to effective care in pregnancy and childbirth, 3rd edn. OUP, Oxford

Chapter 3 'support for pregnancy' and Chapter 28 'social and professional support in childbirth' are useful for strengthening understanding of these key psychosocial issues.

Irion O, Boulvain M, Straccia A T, Bonnet J 2000 Emotional, physical and sexual violence against women before or during pregnancy. British Journal of Obstetrics and Gynaecology 107:1306–1308

Provides some evidence around the vexed issue of women in abusive relationships and the implications for their psychological well-being.

Shaw F 1997 Out of me: the story of a postnatal breakdown. Viking, London

This is a powerful, reflective and personal narrative of the author's experience of severe postnatal depressive illness.

USEFUL ADDRESSES

Association for Post Natal Illness 145 Dawes Road Fulham London SW6 7BE Tel: 0207 386 0868 Website: http://www.pni.org/

CRY-SIS (support for mothers with crying babies) BM CRY-SIS London SW1 3XX Tel: 0207 2400953

Home-Start UK 9 (voluntary domestic support) 2 Salisbury Road Leicester LE1 7QR Tel: 0116 233 9955

(MAMA) Meet-A-Mum Association 14 Willis Road Croydon Surrey CR0 2XX Tel: 0208 665 0357

MIND (National Association of Mental Illness) 22 Harley Street London W1N 2ED Tel: 0207 6370741 Website: http://www.mind.org.uk/mindpdfs/ understanding_postnatal_depression.pdf

Useful websites:
Most offer factsheets, information about postnatal depressive illnesses, guidance for partners, links for support groups and a discussion forum as well as contact with other sufferers online:

Access to government reports such as the national services framework for mental health: http://www.doh.gov.uk

An introduction to postpartum illness http://www.chss.iup.edu/postpartum

Babyworld (provides general information for new parents) http://www.babyworld.co.uk/information/ newparents/post_natal_depression.htm

BBC PND Page http://www.bbc.co.uk/education/health/parenting/ yoblues.shtml

36 Family Planning

Jennifer Lennox   Yvonne S. Watson

Contraception is an important factor in many women's lives, with needs varying according to the particular stage of the life continuum, and should also be viewed in the wider context of sexual and reproductive health. It has been argued that control of their own fertility is the largest single factor affecting the independence of women (Roberts 1981).

The capacity to enjoy and control sexual and reproductive behaviour is a key element of sexual health (WHO 1992), yet this is not the experience of many women. Unintended pregnancies can have long-lasting effects on the quality of life of parents and children, and prevention could save the NHS over £2.5bn a year (DoH 2001).

In the UK, the Government's white paper 'Health of the Nation' (DoH 1992) heralded the rising number of unintended pregnancies, highlighting the need to improve access to family planning services for all women, particularly the young (Kishen & Presho 1996). The strategy 'Making a Difference' (DoH 1999a) identified the need for midwives to recognise their transferable, and often underutilised, skills by applying them to the wider care of women in areas such as fertility advice.

The chapter aims to:

- consider the role of the midwife in family planning and related issues

- review contraceptive methods

- explore the provision of family planning services.

The role of the midwife in family planning and related issues

The role of the midwife in family planning is acknowledged by the WHO, International Confederation of

Midwives, International Confederation of Gynaecologists and Obstetricians and the EC Midwives Directives (UKCC 1998). The midwife must be able to facilitate client knowledge and choice by providing 'sound family planning information and advice' (UKCC 1998).

The issues surrounding contraceptive use can promote needs that women are unable to express; midwives are in a key position to use and create opportunities that may enable women to express their needs. Opportunistic discussion around sexual health issues may influence not only the woman, her partner and children but also her friends, and this in turn could perhaps help them make choices that are pertinent to their sexual health.

Barrett et al (2000) suggest health professionals assume that women will resume intercourse after delivery and consequently discuss contraception, however at 6 weeks' postpartum as many as 60% of women will not have resumed intercourse. Contraception is only one aspect of an overall sexual health strategy and the midwife could use this opportunity to promote issues such as breast awareness, cervical screening and safer sex. Difficulties may arise if the midwife is uncomfortable when discussing sexual issues, especially if she does not know the woman well, or if her knowledge is out of date.

Issues such as loss of libido, adjustment to motherhood, breastfeeding, perineal discomfort, vaginal dryness and body image can all influence the choice and compliance of a particular method. The midwife's knowledge of the woman will enable her to appreciate implicit influences such as religion, culture, relationships, lifestyle, age, motivation and socioeconomic status, which also affect the mother's choice. She should be familiar with the family planning services available in the area in which she practises and be aware of the system of referral to practitioners with specialist training.

Guillebaud (1999) suggests that the ideal contraceptive would be 100% effective, perfectly safe, and painlessly reversible. There would be no interruption of spontaneity, mess, unpleasant odour or taste. It would be easy to use, cheap, not reliant on the user's memory and independent of the medical profession. The method would also need to be culturally acceptable to its users. One of the most pertinent considerations today is protection against sexually transmitted infections.

Currently this contraceptive does not exist, but if the midwife has an up-to-date knowledge of available contraceptive methods and postpartum considerations she may be able to facilitate the most suitable choice for the woman and her partner.

For most contraceptive methods discussed in the following section, the failure rate is given per 100 woman years (HWY) of use. This is the number who would become pregnant if 100 women used the method for 1 year. This rate does not reflect the fact that fertility decreases with age and may be suppressed during lactation; and that the success of a method is partially dependent on motivation, experience in using the method and the teaching received. It is also noteworthy that unprotected intercourse in women results in 80–90 pregnancies per HWY, and not 100.

Bounds (1994) suggests it is important to relate failure rates to a specific period of time, such as in the 'first year of use', since with most methods the risk of failure decreases with time. When discussing failure rates with women, it may be more relevant to give individualised advice, which takes into account such factors as age, lactation, frequency of intercourse and the importance of avoiding pregnancy.

Contraceptive methods

Hormonal methods

Combined oral contraceptive pill

The combined oral contraceptive pill (COC or 'the pill') contains synthetic steroid hormones oestrogen and progestogen in varying amounts depending on which preparation is prescribed. The most commonly used pills in the UK are monophasic pills, which contain a constant dose of steroids throughout the packet. 'Everyday' pills contain 28 pills in the packet, 21 of which are active monophasic pills whilst the seven remaining pills contain no hormones and are thus inactive.

Also available are biphasic and triphasic pills, in which the dose of steroids administered varies in two or three phases throughout the packet to mimic the natural fluctuations of the hormones during the menstrual cycle. These pills are less commonly used in Britain.

The pill is a popular method of contraception chosen by 25% of British women. Usage varies with age and marital status. In their study of sexual lifestyle, Wellings et al (1994) found it is most popular with women under 24 years of age and with those who are single or cohabiting, rather than married.

Mode of action. Oestrogen and progestogen suppress FSH and LH production causing the ovaries to go into a resting state; ovarian follicles do not mature and ovulation does not normally take place. Progestogen also causes cervical mucus to thicken, making penetration by spermatozoa difficult. The pill also renders the endometrium unreceptive to implantation by the blastocyst. These actions provide additional contraception in the event of breakthrough ovulation occurring. Progestogens in the combined oral contraceptive pill are of two types, described as second and third generation. Third generation progestogens were reported to be associated with an increased risk of venous thromboembolism. A meta-analysis by Kemmeren et al (2001) supported this view. The DoH (1999b) advised that third generation progestogens can be offered provided that the woman accepts this slightly increased risk.

Failure rate. Provided that the pill is taken correctly and consistently, is absorbed normally and interaction with other medication does not affect its metabolism, its reliability is almost 100% (Guillebaud 1999).

Important considerations. The pill is a reliable contraceptive that is independent of intercourse and has many advantages, and some drawbacks, to its use.

The main advantages of the combined oral contraceptive pill include:

- *regular, lighter, less painful periods* – as the normal menstrual cycle is inhibited and the usual proliferation of the endometrium does not occur
- *possible reduction in premenstrual symptoms* – again because the menstrual cycle is inhibited
- *protection against pelvic inflammatory disease (PID)* – because of the thickened cervical mucus
- *decreased incidence of ectopic pregnancy* – as ovulation is inhibited.

Other advantages include protection against ovarian and endometrial cancers (Thorogood & Villard-Mackintosh 1993), and prevention of ovarian cysts and fibroids (Szarewski & Guillebaud 2000).

Over recent years the steroid dosage of all oral contraceptives has been greatly reduced or modified in order to minimise the disadvantages of the pill.

However, many of the metabolic effects of the pill result in potential drawbacks, for example:

- *Venous or arterial thrombosis* – as clotting factors and platelet function are modified (Thorogood & Villard-Mackintosh 1993). The risk of venous thrombosis is greatest in women with a BMI over 30, those with a family history of venous thrombosis and those who are immobile.
- *Hypertension* – the pill causes a slight rise in blood pressure in most users, but some women may develop a greater degree of hypertension, which could increase the potential for haemorrhagic stroke (Guillebaud 1999). In their guidelines for clinical practice, the Faculty of Family Planning and Reproductive Health Care (FFPRHC 2000) suggest the relevant risk of haemorrhagic stroke in current users of the COC with hypertension may be 10 times that of non-hypertensive COC users and suggest that if the blood pressure is repeatedly over 160/95 the woman should change to a progestogen-only method.

Following reanalysis of worldwide epidemiological data, women currently using the pill are considered to be at a slightly increased risk of developing breast cancer (Collaborative Group on Hormonal Factors in Breast Cancer 1996). This risk declines in the first 10 years after discontinuing the pill. Studies show a small increase in relevant risk of cervical cancer, which is associated with long duration of use (Beral et al 1999). However, understanding of the influence of the COC is complicated by the effects of confounding factors such as STIs, non-use of barrier methods and number of sexual partners. Cigarette smoking is known to potentiate most of the risks associated with pill use such as ischaemic and haemorrhagic stroke and myocardial infarction (Dunn et al 1999).

Pill use may also lead to other side-effects such as breast tenderness, nausea, weight increase, depression and loss of libido. These effects often diminish with continued use, or may improve with a change of pill. Contraindications to pill use include:

- pregnancy
- history of arterial or venous thrombosis, or predisposing factors such as immobility
- hypertension
- focal or crescendo migraines

- current liver disease
- undiagnosed abnormal vaginal bleeding
- hydatidiform mole (until serum HCG is no longer detectable)
- smoking, if the woman is over 35 years old
- BMI over 30.

This is not an exhaustive list and, as the pill is not suitable for everyone, women wishing to consider using this form of contraception should have a full history recorded and be fully informed and counselled regarding possible side-effects. Women should be warned to stop taking the pill and seek urgent medical advice if any of the following occur:

- sudden, severe chest pain
- sudden breathlessness
- severe, unilateral calf pain
- severe abdominal pain
- unusual, severe, prolonged headache (BMA & RPS 1996).

Using the pill. When initially commencing the pill, the very first pill is usually taken on the first day of the menstrual period (for postpartum use, see later). If a 21 day pill has been prescribed, the contraceptive effect is immediate, provided that the remainder of pills in the packet are taken correctly. If the pill is initially commenced on any day other than the first day of the period, additional contraception (such as a condom) should be used in conjunction with the pill for the first 7 days. One pill is taken every day for 21 days, then no pills for the next 7 days. Vaginal bleeding usually occurs within the 7 day break before the next packet of pills is commenced. The woman should be informed that this is the result of hormone withdrawal and is not a true menstrual period.

When commencing the everyday pill the inactive pills are taken first and thus the contraceptive effect is not immediate. It is important to advise the use of additional contraceptive measures, such as condoms, for the duration of the inactive pills. Thereafter one pill is taken daily, care being taken to take the pills in the correct order. Vaginal bleeding will usually occur when the inactive pills are taken, which are usually denoted by a different coloured section on the pill packet.

It is important to emphasise taking the pill at an easily remembered time each day. If a pill is forgotten, the

woman will then have some idea of when the previous pill was taken and how late she is in taking the next pill. If the woman is less than 12 hours late taking a pill, she can take the pill immediately and continue the pack as normal. If the pill is forgotten by more than 12 hours, the advice given in Figure 36.1 should be followed.

It is commonly thought that pills missed at the beginning or the end of the packet do not matter, this is a mistake. If these pills are forgotten, the pill-free interval is lengthened and ovulation may be more likely to occur (Guillebaud 1999). If a woman is concerned about a missed or late pill, she can contact the local family planning clinic or GP for reassurance or advice, as emergency contraception may be indicated (see later).

Other factors that may render the pill less effective include interaction with other medication, vomiting within 3 hours of taking a pill, and severe diarrhoea. Medications that may hinder the effectiveness of the pill include broad spectrum antibiotics (such as ampicillin), liver-enzyme-inducing drugs such as rifampicin, some anticonvulsants and some herbal remedies, for example St Johns wort.

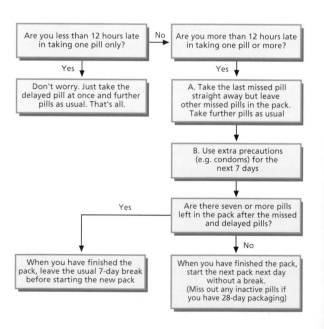

Fig. 36.1 Advice regarding missed combined 21 day oral contraceptive pills over 12 hours late. (After Guillebaud 1998, with permission.)

After absorption, synthetic oestrogen and progestogen are transported to the liver via the hepatic portal vein. Liver-enzyme-inducing drugs reduce the efficacy of the pill by increasing the metabolism, and subsequent elimination, of oestrogen and progestogen in the bile. Newer antiepileptics are not enzyme inducers (Guillebaud 1999). Some antibiotics may affect the normal action of certain gut flora that enable the breakdown products of oestrogen to be reconverted into a reabsorbable form. If this action is impaired by antibiotics the reactivated oestrogen is disposed of with progestogen, therefore reducing the amount available in the body for contraception.

The advice in cases of vomiting within 3 hours of taking the pill is similar to that in Figure 36.1. Additional contraception is recommended during the illness and for 7 days afterwards. Similar advice is given for diarrhoea, although Guillebaud (1999) suggests that to affect the action of the COC the diarrhoea must be very severe.

It is important that women are made aware of possible drug interactions and inform their medical practitioner that the pill is being taken whenever other medications are prescribed.

Preconception considerations. As the pill disrupts vitamin and mineral metabolism, some authorities advise stopping the pill 2–3 months before attempting to conceive; however, Guillebaud (1995) suggests that there is no objective evidence to support this, although it would not do any harm. As the pill causes folic acid levels to fall, it is worthwhile ensuring that any woman planning conception is aware of the recommendation to take folic acid supplements (see Ch. 12). Any woman who does conceive whilst taking the pill may be reassured that studies appear to conclude that the incidence of birth defects following periconception exposure to the pill is no greater than to be expected among any group of women expecting a planned baby (Guillebaud 1999).

For conceptions occurring after the pill has been discontinued, there is no evidence of increased risk of miscarriage, ectopic pregnancy or stillbirth, or of any adverse effects on the fetus (Guillebaud 1999).

Postpartum considerations. The combined oral contraceptive pill reduces milk supply, particularly if lactation is not well established, and is therefore not recommended for use in the early months in lactating women (Tankeyoon et al 1988). If the mother is bottle

feeding, the pill may be commenced 21 days postpartum. This allows the high oestrogen levels of pregnancy to fall before introducing the pill (Guillebaud 1999), thus reducing the risk of thromboembolism, but allowing the contraceptive effect to be initiated before ovulation resumes.

Women who have experienced pregnancy-induced hypertension may use the combined oral contraceptive pill once their blood pressure has returned to normal levels (Speroff & Darney 2001). Women who experienced severe pregnancy-induced hypertension with persistent biochemical abnormalities are at greater risk of thrombosis and, if no alternative method is acceptable, should delay starting the pill until at least 8 weeks postpartum (Guillebaud 1999).

The pill can be commenced immediately following spontaneous abortion or therapeutic termination of pregnancy. Due to the risk of thromboembolism, the pill should be stopped 4 weeks before major surgery and a progestogen-only method used; if this is not possible then thromboprophylaxis and compression hosiery are advised (BMA & RPS 2001). Women who have minor surgery do not need to discontinue the pill.

Further postpartum considerations for discussion with the mother may include whether remembering to take the pill will fit into her current lifestyle and if she can easily access a clinic or surgery. Research evidence for optimum follow-up intervals is lacking (FFPRHC 2000), but blood pressure recordings must be reviewed. Common practice is at about 10 to 12 weeks after the initial visit and then at 6-monthly intervals. If this proves difficult for the woman, she may be referred to a domiciliary family planning service, if available, or her health visitor.

Once they experience motherhood with its attendant responsibilities, some women have an increased awareness of their own mortality. Given the rare but potentially catastrophic side-effects of the pill, the midwife may need to assist the mother to explore these aspects in greater depth.

Progestogen-only methods

Progestogen-only methods of contraception were introduced partly to avoid the side-effects of oestrogen in the combined pill, as discussed above. They also offer increased choice for women and their partners. For contraceptive purposes, progestogen can be administered in several formats. Currently available in the UK are progestogen-only pills (POP), two kinds of intramuscular injection, depot medroxyprogesterone acetate (DMPA or 'Depo-provera') and norethisterone enanthate (NET-EN or 'Noristerat'), and subdermal implants (such as Implanon). Also available are progestogen-releasing intrauterine systems (IUS), which combine the contraceptive effects of progestogen and an IUCD (see later). The dose of progestogen administered varies with each method, as shown in Figure 36.2.

Mode of action. The POP exerts its contraceptive effects at different levels. Originally the main action was thought to be thickening of cervical mucus, making it impenetrable to spermatozoa, and modification of endometrium, thus preventing implantation; it also has a variable effect on the uterine tubes (Guillebaud 1991). Subsequently it has been shown that only 40% of women using the POP have normal ovulation. As progestogens have many actions within the body, Fraser (1995) suggests that the importance of each contraceptive action is likely to depend on the type of progestogen and the dose. The contraceptive action of the POP does not rely on prevention of ovulation, although there is some suppression of FSH and LH release. However, it is thought that follicular development and ovulation are effectively suppressed in some other progestogen-only methods, such as the injection, because of the higher dose of progestogen (Fraser 1995).

Important considerations. Each individual progestogen-only method has pros and cons to its specific use; these will be considered following the discussion of each method.

General advantages to progestogen-only use include:

- fewer metabolic side-effects than oestrogen and progestogen combined; therefore these methods may be useful in cases where the combined pill is contraindicated
- can be used during lactation (see below)
- probable reduction in premenstrual symptoms (Guillebaud 1999)
- protection against PID.

Other advantages include possible protection against endometrial and ovarian cancers (Fraser 1995).

Drawbacks to use include the following:

- *Menstrual disturbances*, encompassing erratic, sometimes prolonged, bleeding, oligomenorrhoea or amenorrhoea – Fraser (1995) comments that little is known about the mechanism causing such disturbances, which most women experience to some degree. Newton (1993) suggests that menstrual disruption is the most common reason for discontinuation of progestogen-only methods. This illustrates the need for careful explanation to potential users.

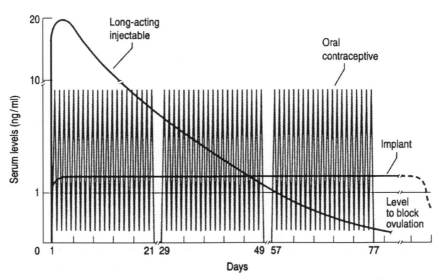

Fig. 36.2 The different blood serum levels of progestogen resulting from progestogen-only methods of contraception. (From Szarewski 1991, with permission.)

- *Functional ovarian cysts* – an increased prevalence of these has been demonstrated in women using progestogen-only methods (Newton 1993). McCann & Potter (1994) suggest these may settle with continuation of use and will resolve if the POP is discontinued.

Contraindications to use include:

- pregnancy
- undiagnosed abnormal vaginal bleeding
- severe arterial disease
- hydatidiform mole (until serum HCG is no longer detectable).

The rate of ectopic pregnancy is no higher than in women using no contraception; however, the POP prevents uterine pregnancy more effectively than tubal pregnancy (McCann & Potter 1994). This is not a problem with other progestogen-only methods as they usually inhibit ovulation.

Antibiotics do not adversely affect progestogen-only methods, but women should be advised to consult the doctor regarding possible interactions if any other medications (especially enzyme inducers such as rifampicin) are prescribed.

General considerations.

Preconception considerations. McCann & Potter (1994) conclude there is no evidence of teratogenic effect of the POP at normal doses.

Postpartum considerations. The use of progestogen-only methods for contraception in the puerperium has been associated with an increased incidence of vaginal bleeding. As the dose of progestogen differs for each method, current recommendations of postnatal starting times vary.

Generally progestogen has either no effect, or a slightly enhancing effect, on the volume of breast milk (Foxwell & Howie 1995). Therefore these methods are usually recommended for breastfeeding mothers who cannot, or do not wish to, use non-hormonal methods. However, transmission of the steroid to the infant via breast milk may concern some mothers. Studies by the WHO (1994) have demonstrated that such transmission and absorption by the neonate are minimal and do not affect the short term growth and development of infants. Nevertheless, some authors (Diaz & Croxatto 1993, Pardue 1994) comment that the long term potential effects have not been fully evaluated.

For this reason several authorities (IPPF 1990, WHO 1994) advocate that progestogen-only methods, particularly the higher dose varieties, are not commenced until 6 weeks postpartum. This delay avoids early, unnecessary exposure of the infant to the hormone. Because of this concern, the mother may choose the POP, rather than other progestogen-only methods, as it provides a lower dose of steroid.

Progestogen-only methods can be used immediately following spontaneous or therapeutic termination.

Using the POP. The POP is taken every day; there are no pill-free days and thus tablets are taken throughout periods. If the first tablet is taken on the first day of menstruation the contraceptive effect is immediate. If the POP is started on any other day of the cycle then additional contraception, for example a condom, should be used for the first 7 days.

If a pill is forgotten, the woman has only 3 hours in which to remember to take it. This is because the effect on cervical mucus is at its maximum between 4 and 22 hours after the tablet has been taken. For this reason, it is also recommended that the daily tablet is taken about 4 hours before the usual time of intercourse and at the same time each day. If the woman is over 3 hours late in taking a tablet, she should continue taking her pills and use additional contraception for the next 7 days. Similarly, following vomiting or severe diarrhoea, additional contraception should be used until 7 days after the illness ceases. Women concerned about missed or late pills should be advised to contact their family planning clinic or GP, as emergency contraception may be indicated (see later). Antibiotics do not affect the action of the POP.

Failure rate. The effectiveness of the POP is dependent upon meticulous compliance. Vessey et al (1985) found that the failure rate of this method is clearly related to age, with failure rates ranging from 3 per HWY in a population aged 25–29 to only 0.3 per HWY in women aged 40 years or over. For women under 25 the failure rate is approximately 4 per HWY, suggesting this method is less appropriate for younger women.

Specific considerations. As success of this method depends on very precise compliance, it may not be suitable for those with a poor memory or hectic lifestyle.

Preconception considerations. As above.

Postpartum considerations. Early postnatal use of the POP is associated with breakthrough bleeding (BMA & RPS 1996). The Family Planning Association (FPA

2000a) recommends that women begin this method 21 days after delivery (although some authorities, such as the International Planned Parenthood Federation (IPPF 1990) suggest waiting until 4–6 weeks).

Progestogen injections

This is a commonly used reversible form of contraception and is the method of choice for many women, not simply those for whom other methods are contraindicated. Over 6 million women use this method worldwide and in some countries it is the most commonly used reversible method (Newton 1993). In England in 1998 to 1999 figures show that 6% of women attending community family planning clinics used injectables. A similar pattern was seen in other parts of the UK (FPA 2000b). Injections act in a similar way to the POP but in addition always inhibit ovulation.

The two contraceptive progestogen injections currently available in the UK are DMPA (Depo-provera) and NET-EN (Noristerat). Both methods are given by deep intramuscular injection. DMPA is the most commonly used injectable and is given in a 150 mg dose at 12 week intervals, although the interval may be less for some women. This high dose of progestogen inhibits ovulation and is formulated to be released slowly into the circulation.

NET-EN is used as a short term contraceptive method – for example when the partner has undergone vasectomy until the procedure is confirmed as effective, and is given in a 200 mg dose at 8 week intervals. It is used more commonly in developing countries.

Failure rate. Both methods are very effective, the failure rate of DMPA being below 0.5 per HWY for DMPA (Guillebaud 1999). The failure rate for NET-EN is slightly higher, although still below 1 per HWY (Fraser 1995).

Using injectable progestogens. The initial injection is given within the first 5 days of the menstrual period. If given on day 1 the contraceptive effect is immediate; however, if given at any other time then additional contraception should be used for the next 7 days (FPA 2000b). (For postpartum use see below.)

Specific considerations. Progestogen injections are highly effective methods of contraception and do not rely on the woman remembering to take a daily tablet, only to attend regularly for injections. This method is irreversible for the term of action, therefore any side-effects may also be present until the injection wears off. These may include breast discomfort, nausea, vomiting and depression or mood swings. The major side-effect is often menstrual irregularities, although amenorrhoea becomes prominent with long term DMPA use (Fraser 1995). Other disadvantages to use include weight gain and a possible link with loss of bone density, which is yet to be resolved (Fraser 1995). The results of a prospective study are awaited.

Preconception considerations. Return of fertility is slow once the injection is stopped, especially with DMPA. The median delay to conception following the presumed end of contraceptive effect is 5–7 months (IPPF 1988). Therefore injectable progestogen is not recommended as contraception for women who plan to conceive soon after its use.

Postpartum considerations. Early postpartum use of DMPA increases the possibility of heavy, prolonged bleeding (BMA & RPS 1966) and currently in the UK the recommended timing for the first dose is 5–6 weeks following delivery. An alternative form of contraception may be required in the interim and for 7 days after the injection. Guillebaud (1999) suggests that, if a woman is not breastfeeding, DMPA can be given prior to day 21 thus preventing the earliest ovulation; however, the woman must be warned about the increased risk of bleeding.

Subdermal implants

Implants have been used internationally for several years but the first licensed use in the UK was in 1993.

Using implants. Implants (Fig. 36.3) are capsules containing progestogen that are inserted under local anaesthetic into the inner aspect of the non-dominant upper arm. The steroid is released at a constant rate and this steady circulating blood level ensures high contraceptive efficacy by producing a cervical mucus blockade, which prevents sperm penetration. Progestogen may also affect the maturation of the endometrium (Cullins 1992). 'Implanon' is a single contraceptive rod measuring 40 mm by 2 mm and containing 68 mg of etonogestrel, which is released at 30–40 µg per day inhibiting ovulation. Implanon has been available in Britain since 1999.

The implant should be inserted during the first 5 days of the menstrual cycle and no additional contraceptive cover will be required. It remains in place and is effective for 3 years but can be removed at any time if the woman wishes.

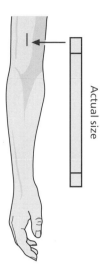

Actual size

Fig. 36.3 Subdermal implant.

Norplant, the previously used implant in the UK, comprises five rods and does not inhibit ovulation. It is effective for 5 years and is still available in other parts of the world.

Failure rate. To date there have been no reported pregnancies with the single rod implant (Croxatto & Makarainen 1998). Norplant has a cumulative failure rate of 1 per 100 users after 5 years.

Specific considerations. Irregular bleeding is the most common problem in women using this method. Some women become amenorrhoeic (Affandi 1998). Headache, nausea and weight gain have also been reported as disadvantages. Insertion and removal require a minor surgical procedure, with accompanying risks of bleeding and infection. These aspects should be discussed prior to the woman making her decision.

Preconception considerations. The action of the implant is quickly reversible and ovulation can return within 30 days of removal (Davies et al 1993), making it suitable for women wishing to 'space' pregnancies.

Postpartum considerations. The implant can be inserted from day 21 to day 28 post delivery or after second trimester termination without any extra contraceptive precautions. The implant is not routinely recommended for women who are breastfeeding.

Future developments

Alternative delivery systems reducing the need for daily pill taking are being explored. Vaginal rings using combined oestrogen and progestogen, and progestogen alone, are being developed; research into the use of transdermal patches for the delivery of oestrogen and progestogen is ongoing. POPs inhibiting ovulation, thus allowing a 12 hour, rather than 3 hour window, are available in parts of Europe and a new combined hormonal monthly injectable is available in America. Effective methods for men are still problematic; however longer-acting testosterone injections with implanted progestogens may be available in a few years (Szarewski & Guillebaud 2000).

Intrauterine contraceptive device (IUCD)

As the name suggests, this device is inserted into the uterus, as illustrated in Figure 36.4. All standard IUCDs currently available in the UK contain copper, which increases contraceptive efficacy. About 4% of women in the UK use an IUCD (Durex Report 2001), whereas according to Guillebaud (1999) this number is rising and 110 million women use it worldwide, of which 50 million are in China.

Mode of action. The IUCD creates an inflammatory response, with the increased number of leucocytes destroying spermatozoa and ova. Gamete viability is further impaired by alteration of uterine and tubal fluids (Drife 1995). Copper affects endometrial enzymes, glycogen metabolism and oestrogen uptake, thus rendering the endometrium hostile to implantation.

Failure rate. The failure rate is less than 0.2–2 HWY (Guillebaud 1999).

Using the IUCD. A copper IUCD can be inserted up to 5 days following the earliest estimated date of ovulation – that is, day 19 in a 28 day cycle (Mansour 2000). Some practitioners prefer to insert a routine IUCD from day 4 to day 14 (Guillebaud 1999). The woman may experience some discomfort during the procedure, which should be performed using aseptic techniques.

Depending upon the type of IUCD used, it may be left in place from 3 to 10 years and longer in some instances; for example, if a woman aged 40 years or over has an IUCD fitted, it may remain in place until

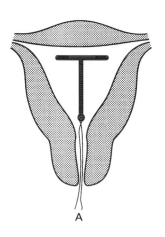
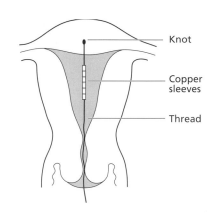
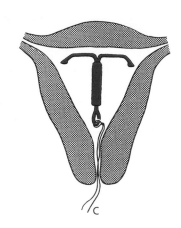

Fig. 36.4 Intrauterine contraceptive devices. After insertion through the cervix, the framed devices assume the shape shown; the threads attached to it protrude into the vagina. (A) Copper-carrying device. (B) Frameless copper device. (C) Levonorgestrel-releasing system.

1 year after the menopause, if this occurs after the age of 50. Once in situ the device requires little action on behalf of the user and does not interfere with intercourse. Women are usually taught to feel the threads as reassurance that it remains in place, and they are usually reviewed annually. Side-effects may include menorrhagia and, as with implants, the woman will need to consult with a doctor before discontinuing use.

The suggestion that IUCDs promote PID has been refuted, although there is evidence to suggest that pre-existing asymptomatic, cervical STI may be introduced at the time of insertion. Selective screening for chlamydia and other STIs prior to insertion may decrease pelvic infections and permit contact tracing (Mansour 2000). IUCDs are associated with a decreased risk of ectopic pregnancies because of their effectiveness. However, the ratio of ectopic to intrauterine pregnancies is greater among women using IUCDs as, in general, it prevents more intrauterine pregnancies than ectopic pregnancies (Ross & Frankenburg 1993). Thus a woman who has the device inserted should be advised to seek early medical advice should she suspect that she is pregnant.

If uterine pregnancy occurs, there is an increased risk of spontaneous abortion; therefore gentle removal of the device is preferred to prevent miscarriage, infection and premature labour. If removal is not possible it is reassuring to know there is no evidence of teratogenicity (Szarewski & Guillebaud 2000).

A newer frameless device (see Fig. 36.4B), comprising six copper sleeves threaded onto a suture, is embedded into the fundal myometrium of the uterus. This is associated with lower expulsion rates, less pain and less blood loss (Wildermeersch et al 1999).

Progestogen-releasing intrauterine systems (IUS)

These were developed to overcome some of the problems associated with conventional IUCDs and vaginal bleeding. The device in current use consists of a small plastic 'T'-shaped frame carrying a Silastic sleeve containing levonorgestrel (see Fig. 36.4C). It is inserted into the uterus and the steroid hormone is released gradually. Both the steroid and the IUCD acting as a carrier have contraceptive properties, as discussed above. The system is usually initially fitted within the first 7 days of the menstrual period; the contraceptive effect is then immediate. It is licensed for 5 years of use.

Failure rate. Failure rates of less than 0.2–2 per HWY have been reported (Guillebaud 1999).

Specific considerations. Irregular vaginal bleeding is common initially, then gradually ceases. The menstrual bleeding is lighter than with copper IUCDs, with possible amenorrhoea.

Postpartum considerations. The copper IUCD has no effect on lactation (Drife 1995). It is recommended that copper devices can be inserted 6 weeks after delivery. Following miscarriage or termination, immediate insertion is practised, and 6 to 8 weeks after caesarean section (Guillebaud 1999).

The IUS should be inserted about 6–8 weeks post-partum to prevent prolonged bleeding. Following termination of pregnancy or miscarriage, it can be inserted immediately. A new frameless device suitable for postpartum and post-termination use will be marketed soon and another containing progestogen is under discussion (Mansour 2000).

Barrier methods

Barrier methods prevent spermatozoa coming into contact with the ovum. They comprise male and female condoms, caps and diaphragms, which are usually used with spermicides.

General advantages include the easy availability of condoms and the fact that using barrier methods (once a diaphragm has been fitted) is independent of professional intervention and they are used only when required. As condoms afford some (although not absolute) protection against sexually transmissible infections, including HIV, the concurrent use of condoms with another method such as the pill is becoming more popular and is known as the 'double Dutch method'. Barrier methods also confer some protection against cervical cancer (Mindel & Estcourt 2000). The main disadvantage, of possible interruption to intercourse, may constitute a drawback for some couples.

General consideration for use. It is good practice to ensure that anyone choosing a barrier method is made aware of emergency contraception (see below), and how to access it if required.

Condom (or sheath)

Condom use has increased in recent years in response to publicity given to HIV infection. In their study of sexual attitudes in the UK, Wellings et al (1994) found that over 25% of women and 36.9% of men had used a condom in the previous year. Condom use is more prevalent in younger age groups (Durex Report 2001).

Many varieties of condom are available, including latex, hypoallergenic and polyurethane. Polyurethane is less sensitive to heat and humidity and is not affected by oil-based lubricants (FPA 2000c). Condoms are available free from family planning clinics, but not on prescription, and can be purchased from outlets such as pharmacies, supermarkets and vending machines.

Using a condom. The condom is rolled on to the erect penis and must be applied before any genital contact occurs as some semen may escape prior to ejaculation. About 1 cm of air-free space must be left at the tip to accommodate the ejaculate, otherwise the condom may burst (some designs incorporate a teat end for this purpose). Care should be taken when handling the condom to prevent tearing. The condom must be held in place during withdrawal of the still erect penis so that it does not slip off. The condom should be used only once and disposed of responsibly.

Some sheaths are impregnated with spermicides (see below), which increases their efficacy. This lubrication may be helpful in cases of vaginal dryness, which is not uncommon postnatally. Water-based lubricants should be used, as oil-based lubricants will damage rubber but not polyurethane.

Failure rate. This is dependent on the age and experience of the user and failure rates vary widely between 1 and 10 per HWYs.

Important considerations. Only condoms with a CE mark should be used. The condom should not be used after the expiry date and should be stored away from extremes of heat, light and damp.

Female condom

This consists of a polyurethane sheath that is inserted into the vagina. The closed inner end is anchored in place by a polyurethane ring, whilst the open outer edge lies flat against the vulva (Fig. 36.5). This is not currently available on prescription, but is available free of charge from family planning clinics and may be purchased from chemists. Some studies (Bounds et al 1992, Ford & Mathie 1993) have questioned its acceptability to users; however, the method is another contraceptive option.

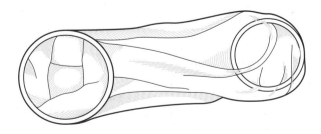

Fig. 36.5 Female condom: 'Femidom'.

Failure rate. There have been few studies on efficacy but findings suggest it is comparable to other barrier methods (Young 2000).

Diaphragm

This is a thin rubber dome with a circumference of metal to help maintain its shape. It is available in a range of types and sizes and the woman is individually fitted. About 1% of women in Britain use this method (Durex Report 2001).

Using the diaphragm. When in place, the rim of the diaphragm should lie closely against the vaginal walls and rest between the posterior fornix and the symphysis pubis (Fig. 36.6). Before insertion, spermicide should be applied. After insertion, the woman must check that her cervix is covered. In order to preserve spontaneity during intercourse, the diaphragm can be inserted every evening as a matter of routine. This should be done after bathing, if applicable, rather than before.

If intercourse occurs more than 3 hours after insertion then additional spermicide is required. The diaphragm must be left in place for at least 6 hours after the last intercourse. On removal, the diaphragm should be washed with a mild soap, dried and inspected for any damage. A new diaphragm should be fitted annually and following any alteration in weight by more than 3 kilograms.

Failure rate. This depends on age and experience of use. If used according to instructions, they are between 92 and 96% effective (FPA 2000d).

Important considerations. In order to feel confident in using this method, the woman must feel comfortable touching her genitalia and have the physical ability to do this. If she is unable to do this, her partner could position the diaphragm. The woman will also need privacy and access to water to clean the diaphragm.

Cystitis may occur owing to pressure on the urethra and bladder base from the rim of the diaphragm. This may be remedied by a change in size or type of diaphragm.

Postpartum considerations. After delivery, the woman should not rely on her previous diaphragm. The size should be assessed 5–6 weeks postpartum when the vagina and pelvic floor muscles will have regained some of their tone, and any repairs will have

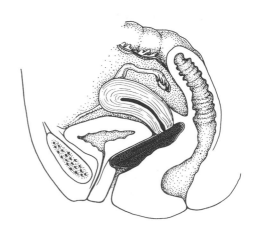

Fig. 36.6 The diaphragm in place.

healed. Size should also be checked following spontaneous or therapeutic termination of pregnancy.

Cervical and vault caps. These cover only the cervix, adhering to it by suction. Their use is similar to that of the diaphragm. Two new disposable caps made from silicone can now be bought from pharmacies. Currently there is little data on efficacy, however, a multicentre trial is in progress.

Spermicidal creams, jellies, aerosols, films, vaginal tablets and pessaries

These preparations kill spermatozoa, but as they are not able to penetrate the cervical mucus and are thus probably only active in the vagina, they are not recommended for use on their own (Gebbie 1995). They must be applied immediately before, or in the case of pessaries 10 minutes before, intercourse. Allergies can occur and the couple may need to experiment to find the most suitable preparation. Some spermicides are available free from family planning clinics and on prescription, or they may be bought from pharmacies.

Nonoxynol-9 (N-9) is the reagent of choice. Although there is evidence of inactivation of STIs including HIV in vitro, Jeffries & Aitken (2000) suggest there is no conclusive evidence that any spermicide will prevent infection in vivo. Concern has been expressed about possible teratogenicity if spermicides are used around the time of conception, but most studies are reassuring (Guillebaud 1999).

Failure rate. Spermicides are not as effective when used alone.

A new vaginal sponge impregnated with spermicide is now available over the counter.

Fertility awareness methods (FAM)

The term *fertility awareness methods* includes all family planning methods based on the identification of the fertile time (WHO 1988). The effectiveness of these methods depends on two factors – accurately identifying the fertile time and modifying sexual behaviour. To avoid pregnancy, couples can either abstain from intercourse (*natural family planning*, or NFP) or use a barrier method consistently during the fertile time. These methods are attractive to those who, for any reason, cannot or do not wish to use hormonal (or mechanical) methods.

As NFP involves abstaining from intercourse during the fertile time, the commitment and cooperation of both partners is essential. The communication between a couple, which is necessary to use these methods effectively, may enhance the quality of their relationship. Women may also feel empowered by a deeper knowledge of their own bodies.

Successful use of FAM to avoid pregnancy depends on adequate teaching by qualified FAM teachers. Such instruction may be beyond the scope of many midwives; however, they should be able to provide basic information on these methods to promote informed family planning choices and refer to local service providers (Knight a Pyper 1999).

Physiological signs of fertility include the following indicators:

Cervical secretions (Billings or ovulation method)

The woman needs to learn to identify the characteristic changes that occur in the cervical secretions (mucus) throughout the menstrual cycle. Following menstruation she will experience dryness at the vaginal entrance. As oestrogen levels rise, the fluid and nutrient content of the secretions increases to facilitate sperm motility. At first a sticky white, creamy or opaque secretion is noticed. As ovulation approaches, the secretions become wetter, more transparent and slippery with the appearance of raw egg white and capable of considerable stretching between finger and thumb (known as 'Spinnbarkeit'). The last day of the transparent slippery secretions is known as the peak day. This day coincides closely with ovulation (Depares et al 1986). Following ovulation, progesterone causes the secretions to thicken forming a plug blocking the cervical canal, acting as a barrier to sperm. The woman will experience a sensation of stickiness or dryness until the next menstruation.

The cervical secretions are observed throughout the day. The fertile time starts when secretions are first noticed and ends on the fourth morning after the peak day. If the secretions are used as a single indicator of fertility, the presence of seminal fluid can make observation difficult; therefore during the preovulatory relatively infertile dry days, it is recommended that intercourse takes place only on alternate dry evenings. Intercourse should be avoided during menstruation as this can mask the first appearance of cervical secretions. Changes in secretions will be also affected by spermicide, vaginal infections and some medications.

Postpartum considerations. In the first 6 months postpartum, the majority of women who are fully breastfeeding will be able to rely on the lactational amenorrhoea (LAM) method (see p. 687) for up to 6 months. Woman who wish to continue using their fertility awareness knowledge should start observing cervical secretions for at least 2 weeks before the LAM criteria will no longer apply in order to establish their basic infertile pattern. Once the basic infertile pattern is established, intercourse may take place on alternate evenings. Abstinence should follow any change in the basic infertile pattern for 4 days from the last day of change.

Basal body (waking) temperature

The woman is taught to take her temperature immediately on waking each day (if she has had to get up during the night, she must have been resting in bed for at least 3 hours). After ovulation, progesterone produced by the corpus luteum causes the temperature to rise by about 0.2°C and to remain at the higher level until the next menstruation. Hence the postovulatory infertile phase of the menstrual cycle is said to begin on the 3rd day after the temperature shift has been observed (WHO 1988). However, factors such as illness, stress, alcohol consumption or a late night may affect the temperature and therefore great care should be taken when interpreting charts.

Postpartum considerations. Day-to-day variation is greater at this time, producing a swinging pattern. It is a sign of infertility, and to be expected during breast-feeding. Recording the temperature has its advantages, but many women prefer to rely on cervical secretions alone or combine this with cervical changes.

Cervical palpation

Changes in the cervix throughout the menstrual cycle can be detected by daily palpation by the woman or her partner. After menstruation, the cervix is low, easy to reach, feels firm and dry and the os is closed. As ovulation approaches the cervix shortens, softens and dilates slightly under the influence of oestrogen.

Postpartum considerations. The hormonal changes of pregnancy take around 12 weeks to settle. The cervix will not revert completely to its prepregnant state – the os will always be slightly dilated even in its infertile state.

Calendar calculation

The calendar calculation is a personalised calculation based on the length of a woman's previous 6–12 menstrual cycles. The shortest cycle (S) and longest cycle (L) are used to identify the likely fertile time. If (S) or (L) changes, she recalculates her fertile time. The first fertile day is calculated by subtracting 20 days from (S) and the last fertile day is calculated by subtracting 10 days from (L). Cycle length is constantly reassessed and appropriate calculations made. Although present research (Kambric & Lamprecht 1996) indicates that the calendar method is not sufficiently reliable to be recommended as a single indicator, the information gained by recording cycle lengths is useful when combining indicators.

Postpartum considerations. Personalized calendar calculations must be recalculated following resumption of normal fertile cycles postnatally.

Combining the indicators of fertility (symptothermal method)

This method combines temperature charting with observation of cervical secretions, calendar calculation (shortest cycle data) and optional cervical palpation to identify the fertile time.

When combining indicators, a couple avoid intercourse from the first sign of any cervical secretions (or first fertile day by calculation, or first change in the cervix – whichever occurs earlier) until the 3rd day of elevated temperature, provided all high temperatures

occur after the peak day. Use of more than one indicator increases the accurate identification of the fertile time, and generally reduces the length of abstinence.

Failure rate of FAM. This is hotly debated. Reports range from 2 to 20 per HWY and are dependent upon crucial factors such as which indicator or indicators are used, motivation (spacing or limiting children), quality of teaching and the use of abstinence or barrier methods during the fertile time (Pyper & Knight 2001). The most recent prospective study using a combination of indicators reported an overall failure of 2.6 (Freundi 1999).

Fertility-monitoring devices

Persona is a personal hormone-monitoring system comprising an electronic monitor and urine test sticks. The test sticks determine the levels of an oestrogen metabolite and LH. The woman checks the monitor daily and a red or green light indicate the fertile or infertile times. Persona is not available on prescription.

Failure rate. The system has a 6% failure rate when used according to instructions (Bonnar et al 1999).

Postpartum considerations. The monitor is not recommended for use during lactation. Following delivery or after cessation of breastfeeding, the manufacturer recommends that a woman should wait until she has had at least two normal menstruations with cycle length 23–35 days before using the monitor with the beginning of the third period.

The contraceptive effect of breastfeeding

Before modern forms of contraception, lactation, with its inhibitory action on ovulation, was a major factor in ensuring adequate intervals between births (IPPF 1997).

Mode of action. Full understanding of the process is still incomplete but it is thought that the action of the infant suckling at the nipple causes neural inputs to the hypothalamus, resulting in the inhibition of gonadotrophin release (especially LH) from the anterior pituitary gland, leading to suppression of ovarian activity (Short 1993). The role of high levels of prolactin is unclear (Diaz & Croxatto 1993).

The delay in return of postpartum fertility in lactating mothers varies greatly as it depends on patterns of breastfeeding, which are influenced by local culture, custom and socioeconomic status. The time taken for return of ovulation is directly related to suckling frequency, intensity and duration, the maintenance of night-time feeding and the introduction of supplementary food.

Lactational amenorrhoea method (LAM)

Lactation can be considered as a method of family planning when used according to the Bellagio Consensus statement (Kennedy et al 1989). This concludes that there is a 98% protection against pregnancy during the first 6 months following delivery if the mother is still amenorrhoeic and fully or nearly fully breastfeeding her infant (Fig. 36.7). Pardue (1994) suggests that even mothers who work outside

the home can be considered to be 'nearly fully breast-feeding' provided they stimulate the nipples by expressing breast milk several times a day. The LAM is not recommended for use after 6 months postpartum because of the increased likelihood of ovulation. A recent WHO multicentre study (WHO 1999) reported that in the first 6 months after childbirth the cumulative pregnancy rate ranged from 0.9% to 1.2% during full breastfeeding. This provides further evidence to support previous research that LAM offers at least 98% protection against pregnancy during this period. The FPA recommends that much more recognition should be given to LAM, provided the guidelines are strictly adhered to (Belfield 1999). In spite of these recent findings, health professionals still lack confidence in discussing this method postnatally with breastfeeding women.

Coitus interruptus (withdrawal)

This involves withdrawal of the penis from the vagina prior to ejaculation and when referring to it many euphemisms are used for example 'being careful'. It necessitates tremendous self-control and both partners may find this interruption of intercourse frustrating. The practice is widely used, however, especially among young couples; Wellings et al (1994) found it more commonplace than diaphragm use. The failure rate may be as high as 25 per HWY, although it is more effective than no contraception at all.

Male and female sterilisation

This is the contraceptive choice of approximately 23% of couples in the UK (FPA 2000f). Although, technically, sterilisation procedures may be reversible, they should be viewed as permanent. Couples need thorough and careful counselling to ensure that they have considered all eventualities, including possible changes in family circumstances, and accept the permanence of the procedures. Although consent of a spouse is not required, joint counselling of both partners is desirable. The operation is available for both sexes under the NHS, but waiting lists may be long. With the commonly used techniques, neither male nor female sterilisation results in any hormonal changes. Diminished libido may result for psychological reasons, but some couples find the freedom from fear of pregnancy very liberating.

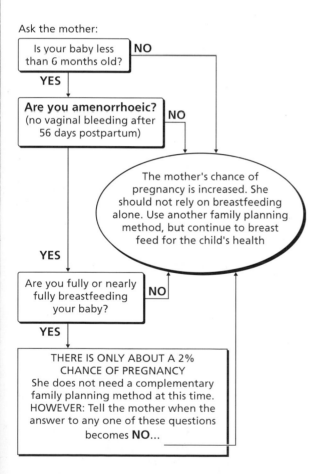

Fig. 36.7 Lactational amenorrhoea method of contraception. (Courtesy Institute for Reproductive Health, Georgetown University Medical Center, under cooperative agreement with the US Agency for International Development, Washington, DC.)

Female sterilisation

The uterine tube is occluded using division and ligation, application of clips or rings, diathermy or laser treatment. Modern methods aim at minimal tissue destruction and the isthmus is chosen (it is of static diameter here) as it increases the chance of successful reversal. The operation, performed under either local or general anaesthetic, may be carried out via laparotomy, mini-laparotomy or laparoscopy. New advances may include non-surgical methods of occluding the tubes using a hysteroscope, which does not leave a scar (Szarewski & Guillebaud 2000).

Failure rate. This is about 1 in 200, depending on the method used (FPA 2000e).

Important considerations. The effect is immediate, although the woman may be advised to use contraception until her next menstrual period in case ovulation had already occurred prior to the operation. For this reason, some women are asked to abstain from sexual intercourse for 7 days prior to the procedure.

In the case of failure, there may be an increased chance of ectopic pregnancy (Glasier 1995) and women should be advised to seek medical help urgently if they suspect pregnancy following sterilisation.

Postpartum considerations. Hepburn (1995) suggests that immediate postpartum female sterilisation may be associated with increased risk of thromboembolism and regret. This highlights the need for thorough counselling prior to the procedure. Guillebaud (1999) suggests that laparoscopic sterilisation after 12 weeks may be more appropriate.

Male sterilisation (vasectomy)

This procedure, which is usually performed under local anaesthetic, involves occlusion of the vas deferens by division and ligation, diathermy or application of clips. A 'no-scalpel' technique may be used, using a small puncture instead of a skin incision.

Failure rate. The FPA (2000e) comments that in about 1 in 2000 cases fails within a few months and that, very rarely, late recanalisation can occur.

Important considerations. The effect is not immediate as it takes some time for spermatozoa to be cleared from the distal part of the vas. Therefore an additional means of contraception must be used until two samples of ejaculate have been shown to be clear of sperm. This may take several months.

Emergency or postcoital contraception (PCC)

PCC is reserved for use when contraception was not used, used incorrectly or failed (as in a condom mishap). Two methods are commonly used.

The copper intrauterine device is the most effective method, with a failure rate of less than 1%. If it is inserted within 5 days of the unprotected intercourse or earliest estimated date of ovulation, implantation of a fertilised ovum can be avoided. If appropriate, it could also be left in place for future contraception.

Alternatively, a progestogen-only method comprising two pills, each containing 750 μg of the progestogen levonorgestrel, can be used. The first is taken within 72 hours of unprotected intercourse and the second 12 hours later. The method works by delaying ovulation or preventing implantation of a fertilised ovum, depending on the stage of the menstrual cycle.

A large randomised controlled trial (WHO 1998) compared the progestogen-only method with the previously used combined oestrogen and progestogen method. Results showed the progestogen method as more effective, with less side-effects.

Nausea is less of a problem with the progestogen-only method, but an additional tablet should be taken if the woman vomits within 3 hours of taking either dose. The next period may begin earlier or later than expected and the need to use contraception until the next period should be stressed. The woman should be advised to have a pregnancy test if her period is more than 7 days late.

Failure rate. The WHO (1998) trial demonstrated a failure rate of 1% if used within 48 hours of unprotected intercourse and 3% when use was delayed to 72 hours.

Important considerations. There are very few contraindications to the progestogen-only method, other than pregnancy and certain pre-existing medical conditions. Hormonal PCC may be contraindicated if there has been more than one episode of unprotected intercourse during the cycle, as the earlier intercourse may already have resulted in a pregnancy.

Postpartum considerations: Breastfeeding mothers can use both methods.

Hormonal PCC can be used as frequently as needed, however it is not recommended as regular contraception. The method is available from family planning clinics, GPs and some accident and emergency departments. Since 2001, postcoital contraception has been available as an 'over the counter medicine' from pharmacies.

Future developments. Mifepristone (RU 486) is an antiprogestogen and studies have shown it to act effectively as an emergency contraceptive (WHO 1999).

Family planning services

History

Modern family planning provision owes much to workers such as Marie Stopes, who opened the first clinic in 1921. Initially, family planning services were provided by independent agencies, such as the FPA. These services were handed over to the NHS only following the 1973 NHS Reorganisation Act, with family planning supplies and advice available free of charge irrespective of marital status and age. General practitioners began providing family planning services within the NHS from 1975.

Services today

Health authorities or trusts run family planning clinics in most areas, often in premises away from hospital sites, providing ease of access for the client. Many clinics operate a self-referral system and partners are welcome. Staff normally have a specialist interest in family planning and related issues, usually having completed postbasic educational courses in this field.

Clinics may also provide a wide range of services including psychosexual and genetic counselling and well-woman sessions. In the UK, addresses of family planning clinics are available from health centres, community health councils, telephone directories or from the FPA and its web site. Lists of GPs are kept in libraries, advice centres and are available from family health service authorities. GPs who provide contraceptive advice have the letter 'C' after their names. Clients may choose a GP other than their own to consult for contraceptive services if they wish.

In recent years there has been concern regarding family planning clinic closures (FPA 1995g) although the provision of family planning services by both clinics and GPs is seen as necessary and complementary. Clients may choose to attend a family planning clinic for its relative anonymity and specialism of staff, whereas others may consult their GP for reasons of familiarity (Fleissing 1992). Combining contraception and genito-urinary medicine (GUM) services in one clinic has advantages for certain clients

and this type of provision is available in some areas.

Some health authorities provide domiciliary family planning services that can be used by clients who, for a variety of reasons such as physical disability, learning or language difficulties or cultural considerations, are unable to access conventional services. However, this service makes up less than 1% of contacts (FPA 2000g). In 1998 to 1999 attendance at NHS family planning clinics (GPs and community clinics) reached almost 6 million (FPA 2000g).

Private services and some run by charitable organisations, such as Brook, also exist. Additionally, the majority of health authorities now provide clinics and projects specifically for young people and the report of the Social Exclusion Unit (DoH 1999c) had as one of its specific targets the need to halve the rate of conceptions in under-eighteens by 2010. In England, Wales and Northern Ireland, following the House of Lords' decision in the Gillick case (*Gillick* v. *West Norfolk and Wisbech Area Health Authority* 1985) it is legal to give contraceptive advice to young people under 16 years, providing parental involvement is encouraged and the client understands the nature and consequences of treatment. The practitioner should also be of the opinion that, if contraception were withheld, sexual intercourse would still be likely to take place and the young person's physical and mental health could be compromised. There is no specific government guidance in Scotland. Under-sixteens may consent to medical treatment if the doctor feels they are capable of understanding its nature and consequences (FPA 1997).

Whoever a woman chooses to consult regarding contraceptive advice, she must be assured of confidentiality.

Box 36.1 lists some contentious issues in the area of family planning.

Box 36.1 Midwives and family planning: contentious issues

- Do midwives have sufficient knowledge or use appropriate opportunities to discuss fertility control?
- In the light of the proposals contained within 'Making a Difference' (DoH 1999a), how can midwives expand their role to include women's sexual health?
- Are midwives adequately prepared and confident in discussing sexual issues with their clients?

ACKNOWLEDGEMENTS

The authors wish to acknowledge the work of Jocelyn Franey. This chapter is largely based on her work in the previous edition.

The authors would like to thank Jane Knight, Director of Fertility UK, Cathleen Anderson, NFP Teacher Marriage Care, Newcastle and Dr Cecilia Piper, NHS Primary Care Career Scientist, University of Oxford.

REFERENCES

Affandi B 1998 An integrated analysis of vaginal bleeding patterns in clinical trials of Implanon. Contraception 58: 99s–107s

Barrett G, Pendry E, Peacock J, Victor C, Thakar R, Manyonda I 2000 Women's sexual health after childbirth. British Journal of Obstetrics and Gynaecology 107(2):186–195

Belfield T 1999 Contraception handbook, 3rd edn. FPA, London

Beral V, Kay C, Hannaford P, Darby S, Reeves G 1999 Mortality associated with oral contraceptive use: 25 year follow up of a cohort of 46 000 women from the RCGP's oral contraception study. British Medical Journal 318:96–100

BMA & RPS (British Medical Association & Royal Pharmaceutical Society of Great Britain) 1996 British National Formulary No 32. BMA & The Pharmaceutical Press, London and Oxon

BMA & RPS (British Medical Association & Royal Pharmaceutical Society of Great Britain) 2001 British National Formulary No 41. BMJ Books & The Pharmaceutical Press, London and Oxon.

Bonnar J, Flynn A, Freundi G, Kirkman P, Royston P, Snowden R 1999 Personal hormone monitoring for contraception. British Journal of Family Planning 24:128–134

Bounds W 1994 Contraceptive efficacy of the diaphragm and cervical caps used in conjunction with spermicides – a fresh look at the evidence. British Journal of Family Planning 20:84–87

Bounds W, Guillebaud J, Newman G 1992 Female condom (Femidom). A clinical study of its use-effectiveness and patient acceptability. British Journal of Family Planning 18:36–41

Collaborative Group on Hormonal Factors in Breast Cancer 1996 Breast cancer and hormonal contraceptives: collaborative reanalysis of individual data on 53 297 women with breast cancer and 100 239 women without breast cancer from 54 epidemiological studies. Lancet 347:1713–1727

Croxatto H, Makarainen L 1998 The pharmacodynamics and efficacy of Implanon. An overview of data. Contraception 58:91S–97S

Cullins V 1992 Injectable and implantable contraceptives. Current Opinion in Obstetrics and Gynaecology 44:536–543

Davies G, Feng L, Newton J 1993 Release characteristics, ovarian activity and menstrual bleeding pattern with a single contraceptive implant releasing 3-ketodesogestrel. Contraception 47:251–261

Depares J, Ryder R, Walker S, Scanlon M 1986 Ovarian ultrasonography highlights precision of symptoms of ovulation as markers of ovulation; British Medical Journal 292:1562

Diaz S, Croxatto H 1993 Contraception in lactating women. Current Opinion in Obstetrics and Gynaecology 5(6): 815–822

DoH (Department of Health) 1992 Health of the nation. Cm 1986. HMSO, London

DoH (Department of Health) 1999a Making a difference: strengthening the nursing, midwifery and health visiting contribution to health and healthcare. HMSO, London

DoH (Department of Health) 1999b Medicines Commission advice on third generation oral contraceptives and risk of venous thromoembolism. Online Available: http://www.mca.gov.uk/ourwork/monitorsafequalmed/safetymessages/cocepinet.htm (accessed 12/7/01)

DoH (Department of Health) 1999c Teenage pregnancy. Report by the Social Exclusion Unit. Stationery Office, London

DoH (Department of Health) 2001 The national strategy for sexual health and HIV. DoH, London

Drife J 1995 Intrauterine contraceptive devices. In: Louden N, Glasier A, Gebbie A (eds) Handbook of family planning and reproductive health care, 4th edn. Churchill Livingstone, Edinburgh, p. 124

Dunn N, Thorogood M, Faragher B et al 1999 Oral contraceptives and myocardial infarction: results of the MICA case control study. British Medical Journal 318:1579–1584

Durex Report 2001 Survey into sexual attitudes and behaviour in Britain. SSL International, England

FFPRHC (Faculty of Family Planning and Reproductive Health Care) 2000 First prescription of combined oral contraception: recommendations for clinical practice. British Journal of Family Planning 26(1):27–38

Fleissing A 1992 Family planning services – use and preference of recent mothers. British Journal of Family Planning 17:110–114

Ford N, Mathie E 1993 The acceptability and experience of the female condom, Femidom, among family planning clinic attenders. British Journal of Family Planning 19:187–192

Foxwell M, Howie P 1995 Natural regulation of fertility. In: Louden N, Glasier A, Gebbie A (eds) Handbook of family planning and reproductive health care, 3rd edn. Churchill Livingstone, Edinburgh, p. 200

FPA (Family Planning Association) 1997 Factsheet 12: young people, confidentiality and the law. FPA, London

FPA (Family Planning Association) 2000a Your guide to the progestogen-only pill. FPA, London

FPA (Family Planning Association) 2000b Your guide to injections and implants. FPA, London

FPA (Family Planning Association) 2000c Your guide to male and female condoms. FPA, London

FPA (Family Planning Association) 2000d Your guide to diaphragms and caps. FPA, London

FPA (Family Planning Association) 2000e Your guide to male and female sterilisation. FPA London

FPA (Family Planning Association) 2000f Factsheet 5: contraception: patterns of use. FPA, London

FPA (Family Planning Association) 2000g Factsheet 2: use of family planning services. FPA, London

Fraser I 1995 Progesterone-only contraception. In: Louden N, Glasier A, Gebbie A (eds) Handbook of family planning and reproductive health care, 3rd edn. Churchill Livingstone, Edinburgh, p 116

Freundi G 1999 European multi-centre study of natural family planning (1989–1995). Advances in Contraception 15:69–83

Gebbie A 1995 Barrier methods. In: Louden N, Glasier A, Gebbie A (eds) Handbook of family planning and reproductive health care, 4th edn. Churchill Livingstone, Edinburgh, p 172

Gillick v West Norfolk and Wisbech Area Health Authority 1986 1 AC 112

Glaser A 1995 Emergency postcoital contraception. In: Louden N, Glasier A, Gebbie A (eds) Handbook of family planning and reproductive health, 3rd edn. Churchill Livingstone, Edinburgh, p 211

Guillebaud J 1991 The pill. Oxford University Press, Oxford

Guillebaud J 1995 Combined hormonal contraception. In: Louden N, Glasier A, Gebbie A (eds) Handbook of family planning and reproductive health care, 4th edn. Churchill Livingstone, Edinburgh, p 42

Guillebaud J 1998 Contraception today, 3rd edn. Martin Dunitz, London

Guillebaud J 1999 Contraception: your questions answered, 3rd edn. Churchill Livingstone, Edinburgh

Hepburn M 1995 Factors influencing contraceptive choice. In: Louden N, Glasier A, Gebbie A (eds) Handbook of family planning and reproductive health care, 4th edn. Churchill Livingstone, Edinburgh, p 33

IPPF (International Planned Parenthood Federation) 1988 Family planning handbook for doctors. IPPF, London

IPPF (International Planned Parenthood Federation) 1990 New IPPF statement on breastfeeding, fertility and postpartum contraception. IPPF Medical Bulletin 24(2):2–4

IPPF (International Planned Parenthood Federation) 1997 Family planning handbook for health professionals. IPPF Medical Publications, London

Jeffries D, Aitken R 2000 Spermicides and virucides. In: Mindel A (ed) Condoms. BMJ Books, London, p 85

Kambric R T, Lamprecht V 1996 Calendar rhythm efficacy: a review. Advances in Contraception 12:123–128

Kemmeren J, Algra A, Grobbee D 2001 Third generation oral contraceptives and risk of venous thrombosis: a meta-analysis. British Medical Journal 323:131–139

Kennedy K, Rivera R, McNeilly A et al 1989 Consensus statement on the use of breast-feeding as a family planning method. Contraception 39:477–496

Kishen M, Presho M 1996 Emergency contraception – a prescription for change. British Journal of Family Planning 22:25–27

Knight J, Pyper C 1999 Integrating fertility awareness into family planning consultations. FPA Contraceptive Education Bulletin Spring: 5

McCann M, Potter L 1994 Progestin only contraception: a comprehensive review. Contraception 50 (6 Suppl 1): S3–S195

Mansour D 2000 Intrauterine contraceptive devices and systems. Postgraduate Centre Series, Excerpta Medica Medical Communications BV, Amsterdam

Mindel A, Estcourt C 2000 Condoms for the prevention of sexually transmitted infections. In: Mindel A (ed) Condoms. BMJ Books, London, p 91

Newton J 1993 Long acting methods of contraception. British Medical Bulletin 49(1):40–61

NHS Reorganisation Act 1973. HMSO, London

Pardue N 1994 On the LAM. Mothering 72:76–81

Pyper C M M, Knight J 2001 Fertility awareness methods of family planning: The physiological background, methodology and effectiveness of fertility awareness methods. Journal of Family Planning and Reproductive Health Care 27(2):103–110

Roberts H (ed) 1981 Women, health and reproduction. Routledge, London

Ross J, Frankenburg E 1993 Findings from two decades of family planning research. Population Council, New York.

Short R 1993 Lactational infertility in family planning. Annals of Medicine 25(2):175–180

Speroff L, Darney P 2001 A clinical guide for contraception, 3rd edn. Lippincott, Philadelphia

Szarewski A 1991 Hormonal contraception. Macdonald Optima, London

Szarewski A, Guillebaud J 2000 Contraception: a users guide, 3rd edn. Oxford University Press, Oxford

Tankeyoon M, Dusitin N, Chalapati S et al 1988 Effects of hormonal contraceptives on breast milk composition and infant growth. Studies in Family Planning 19(6):361–369

Thorogood M, Villard-Mackintosh L 1993 Combined oral contraceptives: risks and benefits. British Medical Bulletin 49(1):124–139

UKCC (United Kingdom Central Council for Nursing, Midwifery and Health Visiting) 1998 The midwives rules and code of practice. UKCC, London

Vessey M, Lawless M, Yeates D, McPherson K 1985 Progestogen-only oral contraception. Findings in a large prospective study with special reference to effectiveness. British Journal of Family Planning 10:117–121

Wellings K, Field J, Johnson A, Wadsworth J 1994 Sexual behaviour in Britain. Penguin Books, London

WHO (World Health Organization) 1988 Natural family planning. WHO, Geneva

WHO (World Health Organization) 1992 Reproductive health: a key to a brighter future. WHO, Geneva

WHO (World Health Organization) 1994 Progestogen-only contraceptives during lactation: I. Infant growth. Contraception 50 (July):35–52

WHO (World Health Organisation) 1998 Task force on postovulatory methods of fertility regulation. Randomised controlled trial of levonorgestrel versus the yuzpe regimen of combined oral contraceptives for emergency contraception. Lancet 332:428–433

WHO (World Health Organization) 1999 Task force on postovulatory methods of fertility regulation. Comparison of three single doses mifepristone as emergency contraception: a randomised trial. Lancet 353:697–702

WHO (World Health Organization) 1999 Multinational study of breast-feeding and lactational amenorrhoea method. 111 Pregnancy during breastfeeding. Fertility and Sterility 72(3):431–440

Wildemeersch D, Batar I, Webb A et al 1999 Gynefix. The frameless intrauterine contraceptive implant – an update for interval, emergency and postabortal contraception. British Journal of Family Planning 24:149–159

Young A, 2000 The female condom. In: Mindel A (ed) Condoms. BMJ Books, London, p 195

FURTHER READING

Andrews G 2001 (ed) Women's Sexual Health, Baillière Tindall, London

This book covers a wide range of women's health issues and will act as a valuable reference book for midwives.

Mindel A 2000 (ed) Condoms. BMJ Books, London

This is an in-depth readable guide to an often neglected area as health professionals can presume clients know about condoms. There are many studies, which make it an objective valuable source of information.

Szarewski A, Guillebaud J 2000 Contraception: a users guide, 3rd edn. Oxford University Press, Oxford

A comprehensive text written in an easy style with clear description of methods. Useful information for clinicians, which can be applied in discussion with clients.

Guillebaud J 1999 Contraception – your questions answered, 3rd edn. Churchill Livingstone, London.

A book for the clinician discussing in some depth the most frequently asked questions on contraception. The reader requires a working knowledge of contraceptive methods.

USEFUL ADDRESSES

Brook Advisory Centres www.brook.org.uk

FPA (including Contraceptive Education Service) www.fpa.org.uk

International Planned Parenthood Federation www.ippf.org

Fertility UK (NFP, fertility awareness and infertility) www.fertilityuk.org

The Association to Aid the Sexual and Personal Relationships of People with a Disability (SPOD) 286 Camden Road London N7 0BJ

37 Bereavement and Loss in Maternity Care

Rosemary Mander

This chapter introduces the reader to the issues which those working in the maternity area are likely to have to face in the event of bereavement or loss. It is hoped that it will help the reader to be better able to cope with the situation and, thus, be able to care for those who are more directly involved and affected. Throughout the chapter the assumption is made that care in situations of loss is more likely to be effective if it is based on research or, where possible, evidence.

The chapter aims to:

- consider the meaning of bereavement and loss and their significance in maternity care

- discuss the forms of loss that may be encountered

- draw on the available research and evidence to review the care of those who are likely to be affected by the loss.

Introduction

In Western society by the beginning of the twenty-first century, bereavement has become inextricably linked with loss through death. In this chapter, to make these concepts more relevant to the midwife, I am broadening the focus to include other sources of grief that may impinge on care of the childbearing woman. In widening out the topic, I reflect the original meaning of 'bereavement', which carries connotations of plundering, robbing, snatching or otherwise removing traumatically and without consent. This meaning may appear to conflict with the other part of my title – 'loss' – which is also widely used in this context. Such inconsistency is fallacious because, although the baby may be 'taken' in any of a variety of ways, the unspoken hopes and expectations invested in that child remain irretrievably lost.

In many ways loss in childbearing is unique. This uniqueness may be due to the awful contrast between the sorrow of death and the mystical joy of a new life emerging from a woman. Additionally, there is the cruel paradox of simultaneous birth and death; we tend to assume that these events are ordinarily separated by a lifetime and the experience becomes incomprehensible when they become unified (Bourne 1968). Although any perinatal loss is unique, the uniqueness of both the individual's experience and the phenomenon itself must be contrasted with the frequency with which a woman may encounter 'lesser' losses during childbearing. Such lesser losses may include the woman's loss of her previous independence, her loss of her special relationship with her fetus at birth, or her loss of her expectations for a perfect baby when she comes to recognise that her actual baby is all too real (Raphael-Leff 1991).

In this chapter I focus mainly on the reactions of the woman and the care that the midwife provides for her. The midwife is in the privileged position of being able to be with the woman when she first faces such losses. It is the responsibility of the midwife to draw on her theoretical knowledge, which, as in any area of her care, should be based as far as possible on the best research evidence. Such knowledge is utilised in the skilled care of the woman to assist her adjustment to these greater and lesser losses.

Grief and loss

Grief, like death and other fundamentally important matters, is a fact of life. It is something that human beings invariably meet in one form or another at a relatively early age. In spite of its universality, a woman in a developed country who experiences loss in childbearing is likely to be young enough not to have previously encountered grief due to death. This is another reason for the uniqueness of loss in childbearing.

Attachment

A limited understanding of mother–baby attachment, sometimes known as 'bonding', for a long time prevented midwives and others from recognising the significance of perinatal loss. This situation resulted in care being based largely on assumptions that later were proved by research to be incorrect. The strength of the relationship that develops during pregnancy between the woman and her fetus emerged in a small research project involving bereaved mothers (Kennell et al 1970). This relationship is facilitated by the woman feeling fetal movements and by her experience of pregnancy, as well as by investigations that may be undertaken, such as ultrasound scans. Katz Rothman (1988) showed the damaging effect that such investigations may have on attachment. Ordinarily the process of attachment continues well beyond the birth. The development of attachment during pregnancy does mean, however, that should the relationship not continue it has to be ended or completed in the same way as any parting. Thus, the existence and the reality of the relationship between the mother and the baby during pregnancy must be recognised before the loss is accepted. These processes are crucial to the initiation of healthy grieving.

Grief

It is through grieving that we are able to adjust to the more serious as well as the lesser losses that confront us throughout life (Marris 1986). Healthy grief means that we are able to move forward, although not necessarily directly, from our initial feelings of distraught hopelessness. We eventually achieve some degree of resolution, which permits our usual functioning for a large part of life; we may even find that in the process we have grown by learning something about ourselves and the resources available to us.

Although grief may be viewed as a state of apathetic passivity, it is better regarded as a time during which the bereaved person actively strives to complete the emotional tasks facing her; to describe this active striving, the term 'grief work' has been coined (Éngel 1961).

The stages of grief through which the person is likely to have to work have been described in a number of ways, but Kübler-Róss's (1970) account is well known and may be useful. These stages (Box 37.1) are not necessarily negotiated in a consistent sequential order, but there will be individual variation and often the person moves back and forth through them before eventually achieving some degree of resolution.

The initial response to learning of a loss comprises a defence mechanism, which serves to protect from the full impact of the news or realisation. This reaction may

> **Box 37.1** Stages of grief
>
> **Shock and denial**
>
> **Increasing awareness**
>
> - Emotions
>   - —sorrow
>   - —guilt
>   - —anger
> - Searching
> - Bargaining
>
> **Realisation**
>
> - Depression
> - Apathy
> - Bodily changes
>
> **Resolution**
>
> - Equanimity
> - Anniversary reactions

comprise shock or denial, which helps by insulating the bereaved person from the unthinkable reality. This initial response allows the woman a 'breathing space' in which she is able to marshal her emotional resources, which will facilitate coping with the eventual realisation.

Denial soon ceases to be effective, and awareness of the reality of the loss gradually dawns. Awareness brings with it powerful emotional reactions, together with their physical manifestations. Feelings of sorrow may be apparent but other, less acceptable, emotions may simultaneously overwhelm the bereaved person; such emotions may include guilt and dissatisfaction, as well as compulsive searching and, still more worryingly, feelings of anger. Realisation dawns in waves as the bereaved person tries out various coping strategies to 'bargain' with herself to delay accepting reality.

When such fruitless strategies are exhausted, the despair of full realisation of the loss materialises, bringing with it apathy and poor concentration as well as some bodily changes. At this point in her grief, the bereaved person may show the anxiety and physical symptoms of a true depression.

After the loss has eventually been accepted, it is integrated into the person's life. As mentioned already, this process is not straightforward and may involve slow progress and many setbacks. Such uncertain progress has been described in terms of 'oscillation and hesitation' (Stroebe & Stroebe 1987). Although the person is never likely to 'get over' her loss, she will probably eventually be able to integrate it into her experience of life. This ultimate degree of 'resolution' is recognisable in the bereaved person's ability to contemplate realistically and with equanimity the strengths, and the weaknesses, of her lost relationship.

Significance

Healthy grieving matters because of its contribution to the resumption of some degree of balance or homeostasis in the life of the bereaved person. Grief is crucial in helping people to recover from the wounding effects that the greater and the lesser losses of life inflict. The hazards of being unable to grieve healthily have long been recognised in emotional terms, but more recently research has revealed the association between perinatal loss and the woman's physical ill health (Ney et al 1994). This research suggests the woman's need for support, regardless of the nature of the loss or the extent to which it is recognised, or her grief sanctioned, by society.

Culture

I have described a general picture of healthy grieving, and mentioned the likelihood of individual variation, which has been shown to be common to people of many ethnic backgrounds (Cowles 1996). It is now necessary to emphasise that the overt manifestations of grief, and the mourning rituals that accompany it, vary even more. These variations are influenced by a number of factors. In her book, Cecil (1996) shows us the massive differences between ethnic groups in their attitudes towards loss in childbearing. In my own research I found that a midwife may encounter difficulty in accepting the different attitudes to loss in women belonging to cultures other than her own, possibly illustrating the fundamental nature of these attitudes (Mander 1994). The extent to which midwives are able to work through such feelings, to permit them to support fully women whose attitudes are different, is uncertain.

Closely bound up with culture, and certainly influencing mourning, is the religious persuasion of the grieving person. These aspects, however, may be difficult to dissociate from the influence of social class and the prevalent societal attitudes.

Despite the huge variations in the manifestation of grief, the underlying purpose of mourning is universal. It serves to establish support for those most closely affected by strengthening the links between those who remain. In perinatal loss it is the midwife who initially provides this support; the role of the midwife is to be with the woman at the time when she is beginning to realise the extent of her loss. The midwife aims to prevent any interference with the mother's healthy initiation of her grieving.

Forms of loss

As I have mentioned already, the terms 'loss' and 'bereavement' may be applied to a wide range of experiences, which vary hugely in their severity and effects. We must be careful, however, to avoid making assumptions about the meaning of a childbearing loss to a particular woman. It is difficult, if not impossible, for anybody else to understand the significance of a pregnancy or a baby to another person. This is because childbearing carries with it a vast range of profoundly deep feelings, which include unspoken hopes and expectations based on personal as well as cultural values. We need to accept that grief, like pain, 'is what the person experiencing it says it is' (McCaffery 1979).

I mention here some of the situations in which we may expect to encounter grief. I emphasise, however, that this list is not exclusive. There may well be situations of childbearing grief that are not included here and, conversely, some of the situations mentioned here may not invariably engender grief.

Perinatal loss

When loss in childbearing is mentioned, loss in the perinatal period comes quickly to mind. This includes babies who are stillborn (that is, in the UK, who show no sign of life after complete expulsion from the mother after 24 weeks' gestation) and babies who die in the first week of life (sometimes referred to as 'early neonatal death').

Attempts have been made to compare the severity of grief following loss at different stages, perhaps to demonstrate that certain women deserve more sympathy or care. A study investigating this point, however, showed no significant differences in the grief response between mothers losing a baby by miscarriage, stillbirth or neonatal death (Peppers & Knapp 1980). This study serves to emphasise the crucial role of the developing mother–baby relationship – the understanding of which has facilitated great improvements in care of the mother.

Stillbirth

The long term recovery of the mother from stillbirth was the subject of a retrospective study undertaken in Sweden. Rådestad and colleagues (1996a) compared the recovery of 380 women who had given birth to a stillborn baby with 379 women who had borne a healthy child. Judging from the 84% response rate, the mothers were comfortable to participate in this study. These researchers found that the bereaved mother made a better recovery if she was able to decide how long to keep her baby with her after the birth and if she was able to keep tokens or mementoes of her baby's birth. The mother who was less likely to make a good recovery was the one in whom there was some delay between her realisation of fetal demise and the birth of her baby. Clearly, these findings have important implications for the midwifery and obstetric care of the mother (see The mother, p. 701). Additionally, they emphasise that stillbirth may be 'known', when the mother realises in advance of the birth that her baby has died. This situation has been termed in the past 'intrauterine death' or 'IUD'. Alternatively, the loss may be unexpected. While avoiding any comparison of the two mothers' grief, it is understandable that the mother who knows that she is to give birth to a dead baby carries a particular emotional burden. This burden, compounded by maceration causing deterioration in the baby's appearance, may impede her healthy grieving.

Early neonatal death

Grieving the loss of a baby who has lived independently, albeit briefly, may be facilitated by three factors. The first is that the mother is likely to have been able to see and hold her real live baby, thus giving her a genuine memory of her experience. Secondly there is the legal requirement that a baby who dies neonatally must have both her or his birth and death registered, providing written evidence of the baby having lived. The third factor relates to the investment of the staff in their care of this dying baby, which Littlewood (1992) suggests increases the likelihood of their providing effective support for the parents.

Accidental loss in early pregnancy: miscarriage

Early pregnancy loss may be due to one of a number of pathological processes, such as ectopic pregnancy or spontaneous abortion. The word 'abortion' is avoided in this context, because it carries with it connotations of deliberate interference, which may be unacceptable to a grieving mother. The term 'miscarriage' is preferable to include all of these accidental forms of loss. The grief of miscarriage has been ignored in the past, largely owing to the frequency with which it happens. This has been estimated as up to 31% of pregnancies in USA (Bansen & Stevens 1992), though the figure may be higher in the UK (Oakley et al 1990).

Understanding of the woman's experience of miscarriage was sought through a qualitative research project (Bansen & Stevens 1992). Among the 10 mothers whom they interviewed 2–5 months after the miscarriage, these researchers identified profound grief, which was associated with anger that their bodies had allowed them to miscarry, and anxiety about their future childbearing. Far from being an insignificant event, these mothers were so ill during the miscarriage that they became fearful that they might die. Although each mother found reassurance in the conception of the pregnancy that was lost, each experienced reduced confidence in her own fertility. As may happen in other forms of childbearing loss, each mother found difficulty in locating suitable support and encountered comments that belittled her loss and denigrated its significance.

It may be necessary to seek the cause of a woman's miscarriage, especially if this happens repeatedly. Miscarriage has been found to be significantly correlated with stressful life events (O'Hare & Creed 1995). Unfortunately the research was unable to identify whether stressful events are actually the cause of the miscarriage. It may be that both the woman's stressful life event and her miscarriage are caused by some other factor, such as her environment or lifestyle.

The former lack of recognition of miscarriage is now being addressed, and women are encouraged to create their own rituals to assist their grieving. Speakman (1996) discusses the helpful nature of a religious service, of suitable photographs or of communicating sorrow through writing a poem or a letter.

Infertility

The grief associated with involuntary infertility is less focused than that experienced when grieving for a particular person and it has been termed 'genetic death' (Crawshaw 1995). In this situation the couple grieve for the hopes and expectations that are integral to the conception of a baby. The realisation of their infertility, and the grief it brings, is aggravated by the widespread assumption that conception is easy. This is sufficiently prevalent for the emphasis, in society in general and in health care in particular, to be on the prevention of conception. The complex investigations and prolonged treatment associated with infertility result in grief that has been compared with a 'rollercoaster' of hope and despair.

As with any grief, the woman and the man in the infertile relationship are likely to grieve differently, engendering tensions. Being told the diagnosis or cause of their infertility may resolve some of their uncertainty about their predicament, but it also raises other difficulties. These may include the problems associated with one partner being 'labelled' as infertile and, hence, being blamed as the cause of the couple's difficulty. A complex spiral of blame and recrimination may escalate to damage further what may already be a vulnerable relationship.

Obviously, counselling an infertile couple must differ markedly from counselling those who are bereaved through death. Because of the nature of our society, infertility counselling tends to focus on the woman (Crawshaw 1995). Bearing in mind the limited success of assisted reproduction techniques, the infertility counsellor has a duty to encourage the couple to contemplate their continuation of investigations or treatment. They may need to consider other options open to them in the creation of their family.

Relinquishment for adoption

Although it has long been widely accepted that relinquishment is followed by grief (Sorosky et al 1984) the view still persists among some health care personnel that, because of relinquishment's voluntary nature, grief is unlikely (Mander 1995). Each mother in my study was quite clear that her relinquishment was in no way a voluntary action and that she was presented with no alternative but to give up her baby for adoption. These mothers really were 'bereaved' in the original meaning of the word (see Introduction, p. 693).

The grief of relinquishment differs from the grief of death in certain crucial ways, however. First, following relinquishment the grief is likely to be delayed. This is partly because of the woman's lifestyle at the time and partly because of the secrecy imposed on the woman who does not mother her baby in the conventional way. Secondly, the grief of relinquishment is unable to be resolved in the short or medium term. This is because, ordinarily, the acceptance of the loss is fundamental to the resolution of grief. Following relinquishment, such acceptance is impossible because of the likelihood that the one who was relinquished will seek to make contact with her mother when she is legally assisted to do so. The possibility of being reunited with the relinquished one was fundamentally important to the mothers who spoke with me. The words of 'Rosa' reflect what many mothers said: 'I'd be delighted if she would turn up on the doorstep'.

Termination of pregnancy (TOP)

Grief associated with elective termination of an uncomplicated pregnancy is problematic and it may be for this reason that it tends not to be included in the research-based literature on grief (Bewley 1993). The experience of grief following TOP for fetal abnormality and of guilt following TOP do, however, tend to be recognised and accepted. In view of the frequency with which TOP happens and the grief likely to be engendered, this deserves more attention.

TOP for fetal abnormality (TFA)

The package of investigations available to the pregnant woman that has become known as 'prenatal diagnosis' may ultimately lead to the decision to undergo TFA. Although it may be assumed that the mother's reaction is solely one of relief at avoiding giving birth to a baby with a disability, Iles (1989) suggests several reasons why this mother may experience conflicting emotions, which may impede her grieving:

- the pregnancy is likely to have been wanted
- the TFA is a serious event in both physiological and social terms

- the reason for TFA may arouse guilty feelings
- the recurrence risk may constitute a future threat
- the woman's biological clock will be ticking away
- her failure to achieve a 'normal' outcome may engender guilt.

Interventions have been introduced to facilitate the grieving of the mother who has undergone TFA. These may involve the creation of memories, as are attempted in other forms of childbearing loss (see The baby, p. 699), and counselling. A study of the effectiveness of psychotherapeutic counselling in such mothers with no other risk factors was undertaken in the form of a randomised controlled trial (Lilford et al 1994). This study suggested that bereavement counselling does not make a difference in terms of the difficulty or duration of grieving and, additionally, the researchers concluded that mothers who attend for counselling would probably have resolved their grief more satisfactorily than the other group anyway.

TOP for other reasons

The non-recognition of grief associated with TOP may be partly because the mother who decides to have her pregnancy ended may be regarded as 'undeserving' of the luxury of grief. Additionally, this may be aggravated by her being held responsible or blamed for her situation (Hey 1996). Research on the psychological sequelae of TOP has focused largely on the guilt of having decided to end the pregnancy, as opposed to grief reactions; it may be that this focus is associated with the acrimonious abortion debate in some countries. Thus, the 'post-abortion blues' have been identified, presenting as grief, regret and tearfulness, and have been linked by Raphael-Leff (1991) with feelings of 'feminine inadequacy'. This researcher suggests that these reactions may be prevented by counselling before as well as after the TOP.

On the basis of the limited material on grief following TOP, it is necessary to question the extent to which grief is still a luxury in which people may allow themselves to wallow, or whether it is a painful way of coming to terms with a traumatic experience.

The baby with a disability

For a variety of reasons a baby may still be born with a disability, which may or may not be expected. Disabilities vary hugely in their severity and in their implications for the future of the baby. It may be that a mother will have to adjust to the possibility of her baby not surviving, but many conditions will be compatible with the continuation of life.

The mother's reaction to the birth of a baby with a disability will involve some elements of grief. This is particularly true if the condition was unexpected, as the mother must grieve for her expected baby before beginning her relationship with her real baby. The mother may be shocked to find herself thinking that her baby might be better off not surviving (Lewis & Bourne 1989). Although the mother may be reassured that she is not unique in experiencing such thoughts, she may nevertheless find it difficult to complete her grieving.

In the case of a baby born with an unexpected disability, the problem of breaking the news emerges. There are no easy answers to how this can be done with the minimum of trauma, but clear, effective and honest communication is crucial (Crowther 1995).

The 'inside baby'

It may be hard to understand that, even in uncomplicated, healthy childbearing, grief may feature. This is because, in spite of obstetric technology, the mother is unable to see her baby before the birth; inevitably the real baby will differ from the one with whom she developed a relationship during pregnancy. These differences are likely to be minor, such as hair colour or crying behaviour. Lewis (1979) coined the term 'inside baby' to denote the one she came to love during pregnancy and who was perfect. The 'outside baby' is the real one, for whom she will care and who may have some imperfections, such as having the wrong hair colour. Clearly the mother may have a few moments of regret, during which she grieves the loss of her fantasy baby, while at the same time beginning her relationship with her real baby.

The mother's birth experience

A further form of loss, over which the mother may need to grieve, is her loss of the birth experience that she was anticipating. If she was hoping for a quite uncomplicated birth, even some of the more common interventions may leave her with a sense of failure (Niven 1992, p. 167). Thus, as with the woman grieving the loss of her 'inside baby', even though all may appear to be satisfactory this disappointed mother will have some grief work to complete.

Care

In considering the care that midwives provide in the event of loss, there are difficulties in deciding where to begin. Thus, I have organised this section by focusing first on those who are involved or affected and then on other crucial issues. From this material will emerge the principles on which our care in this situation is based. While I recognise the artificiality of distinguishing care for individuals in this complex situation, this approach may help us to consider the different needs among people affected by a single event.

The baby

It is particularly hard to separate the care of the baby from the care of those who are grieving, because much of our care comprises the creation of memories of the baby, which will facilitate the grieving (Box 37.2).

Box 37.2 Creating memories

Midwifery activities
- Information giving
- Arranging for/taking photographs*
- Cutting a lock of hair*
- Taking a footprint*
- Giving a cot card and/or nameband

Parental activities
- Naming baby
- Seeing baby
- Holding baby
- Caring for baby
  —bathing
  —dressing
- Taking photographs

Other activities
- Writing in a book of remembrance
- Service/funeral/burial/cremation
- Tree planting
- Writing a letter and/or poem

* Parents' informed consent will be needed.

We may think of the care of the baby beginning before the birth by considering the presence of the cot in the labour room (Mander 1994). Although the presence of the cot may cause the staff some discomfort, it reminds all concerned of the reality of the baby. If possible, that is if the baby's demise is known, the midwife discusses with the parents prior to the birth the contact which will be made with the baby. This contact may take any of a number of forms, beginning with just a sight of the wrapped baby. Contact with the baby resolves some of the confusion surrounding the birth, and mothers who do choose to make some contact do not regret their decision (Kellner & Lake 1993).

The midwife faces the quandary of whether, and how much, she will encourage the mother to make contact with her baby, drawing on her knowledge of its beneficial effect on grief (Mander 1995). This quandary is difficult, but midwives tend to be overcautious in encouraging the mother to make contact with her baby. This was an important finding from a study of 380 mothers who had experienced perinatal loss (Rådestad et al 1996b). These researchers found that one-third of the mothers would have appreciated more encouragement to make contact with their babies.

The mother may choose to have considerable contact with her baby, perhaps keeping the baby with her for some time. During this time the mother may wish to have her baby baptised which, as well as its religious significance, emphasises the reality of the baby. This simple act, which may be undertaken by the midwife, additionally presents an opportunity to name the baby. The mother may also during this time take advantage of other opportunities to create memories of her experience; these include doing some of the things a mother ordinarily does for a baby, such as bathing and dressing him or her. Whether or not the mother chooses to make contact with her baby immediately, it is usual to collect certain mementoes at the time of the birth, such as a lock of hair, a footprint or photographs. If the mother chooses to make no contact at the birth she may later avail herself of these mementoes. Taking photographs of a suitable quality may present a challenge to the midwife who is not skilled in using a camera, giving rise to dissatisfaction (Rådestad et al 1996b). Figure 37.1 shows the sensitive way in which a photograph may be used to help create memories of the birth.

In the hope of preventing a future loss, the parents may be advised that the baby should have a postmortem examination. This raises many difficult issues for parents, who may consider that their baby has suffered enough already. In the UK, the guidelines about information given to the parents prior to seeking their consent for the postmortem has recently been redrafted. These new guidelines aim to prevent certain abuses, such as the retention of body parts, which have previously caused anguish to some bereaved parents (Dimond 2001, DoH 2000).

The funeral serves a multiplicity of purposes, including a demonstration of general support as well as establishing the reality of the loss. A young woman with no experience of death may have difficulty imagining how such a ritual could possibly be beneficial. She may be helped, though, by being reminded how cemetery and crematorium staff are becoming more sensitive to the need to provide a suitable ceremony and a suitable environment in which the child may subsequently be remembered (Kohner 1995). In some situations, such as early miscarriage, a funeral might not be considered appropriate. The mother may find that an impromptu service is helpful near the time of her loss or, later, she may create her own memorial by writing a letter to her lost baby or by planting a tree (Speakman 1996).

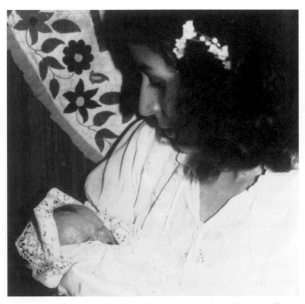

Fig. 37.1 Photograph showing a grieving mother cradling her baby, who has been named Baby Shane.

The mother

Much of the midwife's care of the grieving mother comprises helping her to make some sense of the incomprehensible experience that has happened to her. As mentioned already, the mother may need help to recognise that she has given birth, even though she no longer has that baby. Integral to this is assisting her realisation that she is a mother, which may be achieved through midwifery care.

The mother may start to make sense of her loss by talking about it. Although this sounds simple enough, 'opening up' may present the mother with a number of challenges. For example, she may have little experience of and be uncomfortable talking about such profound feelings. Further, she may have difficulty finding a suitable and willing listener at the precise time when she feels ready. The problem of her finding a listener was identified in a research project showing that senior hospital staff appear too busy, and other staff insufficiently experienced, for her to unburden herself (Lovell et al 1986). Family members who might be expected to listen have been shown to have their own difficulties in coping, making them less receptive to the mother's needs (Rajan 1994).

In a situation involving loss, any of us may feel that our control over our lives is slipping away. Such feelings of losing control may be exacerbated when the loss involves a physiological process such as childbearing, which many people seem to achieve successfully and relatively effortlessly. Midwives should be able to help the mother to retain some degree of, or at least some sense of, control. They can do this is by giving her accurate information about the choices open to her and on which she is able to base her decision making.

The reality of the grieving mother's control over her care was the subject of Gohlish's research (1985). She interviewed 15 mothers of stillborn babies and asked them to identify the 'nursing' behaviours that they considered most helpful. This study showed the importance to the grieving mother of assuming control over her environment. The difficulty mentioned already that the mother experiences in identifying a suitable listener may be more generally associated with the support that she is able to locate. Women's support at this time was the subject of a systematic review, which found that there is no evidence to indicate the effectiveness of psychological support at this time (Chambers & Chan 2001). A randomised controlled trial by Forrest et al (1982) investigated the effects of support following perinatal loss. The experimental group, comprising 25 bereaved mothers, received ideal supported midwifery care together with counselling; the control group comprised another 25 bereaved mothers who received the standard care. Unlike Lilford and colleagues' more psychotherapeutically oriented study (1994), Forrest found that the well-supported and counselled group recovered from their grief more quickly than did the control group. It is unfortunate that both of these studies found difficulty in retaining contact with the grieving mothers.

The mother may find helpful support in any of a number of people, who may provide such support on a more or less formal basis (Forrest et al 1982). Although we may assume that identifying support is easy, research by Rådestad et al (1996b) has shown that, like finding a suitable listener, locating support may be problematic for the mother. These researchers found that for just over one-quarter of bereaved mothers the support lasted for less than 1 month; while for just over another quarter of them the support was non-existent.

Of particular significance to midwives is the contribution of the lay support and self-help groups. My research showed that midwives are happy to recommend that a mother may find a support group, such as the Stillbirth and Neonatal Death Society (SANDS), helpful (Mander 1994). Unfortunately, little is known about their effectiveness or about the experiences of those who attend.

The family

Although it is the mother who is clearly most intimately involved with, and likely to be most affected by, a perinatal loss, to a greater or lesser extent those close to her will share her grief. In this context, as well as conventional family members, I would include a range of non-blood and non-marital relationships.

The father

The effect of the loss on the father may in the past have been underestimated (Murphy & Hunt 1997). This may be partly because men tend to show their grief differently from women and partly because they are socialised into providing support for their womenfolk, possibly at the cost of their own emotional well-being. Additionally, men are less likely to avail themselves of the therapeutic effects of crying and communicating their sorrow in words. Men's coping mechanisms may also involve resorting to other less healthy grieving strategies, which may include an early return to work and the use of potentially harmful substances such as nicotine or alcohol.

Possibly in association with their different patterns of grieving (Samuelsson et al 2001), the parental relationship is likely to change following perinatal loss. Whether the couple find that their relationship is strengthened or otherwise is unpredictable.

Other family members

Perhaps because they are less closely involved, the grandparents may be disproportionately adversely affected by the loss. This may be due to their inability to protect their children (the bereaved parents) from their painful loss. Inevitably and additionally they will experience their own sense of loss at the threat to the continuity of their family and what it means to them.

The effects of perinatal loss on a sibling may be problematic because of uncertainty about the young child's understanding of the event (Mahan & Calica 1997). This difficulty is compounded by the parents' limited ability to articulate their pain in a suitable form. The parents may seek to solve these problems by 'protecting' their other child(ren) from the truth. They little know that such protection may create a pattern of unhealthy grieving, which leaves the family with a legacy of dysfunctional relationships (Dyregrov 1991).

Although my own research found that midwives tend to assume that the family are the best people to support a grieving mother (Mander 1994, 1996), it has also been found that family responses may not invariably be healthy or helpful (Kissane & Bloch 1994).

The formal carers

The difficulty that staff face in caring for a grieving mother has been linked with their own personal reactions to the loss of a baby (Bourne 1968). This may be part of the reason for the longstanding neglect of such mothers in particular and this topic in general. Furthermore, the loss of a baby may represent all too clearly the failure of the health care system, and those who work in it, to provide the mother with a successful outcome to her pregnancy. The fear of failure in turn engenders a cycle of avoidance, which continues the neglect of the mother.

Even though, as mentioned already, this vicious cycle has been interrupted to the extent that the care of the mother has been changed, it is necessary to question whether the care of staff has kept pace (Askey & Moss 2001). The emotional costs of providing care are now being recognised. Phillips (1996) describes how the devaluation of the emotional component of care is associated with increasing use of the medical model. This devaluation may contribute to the increasing recognition of the phenomenon sometimes known as 'burnout'. The remedy has been identified in a midwifery setting to comprise support in the form of development of 'team spirit' (Foster 1996). The need for extra support is particularly important for less experienced staff when they are providing care for families who are grieving (Mander 2000). The education of staff for their counselling role is another solution, which is enhanced by the availability of a supervisor for the counsellors. The role of the midwife manager in creating a suitably supportive environment for staff working in stressful situations should not be underestimated. The midwife may also be able to locate support in other personnel alongside whom she works, such as the hospital minister or chaplain. Additionally, there are a number of helpful agencies which may be located within or outwith the health care system (Stoter 1997).

The extent of the involvement of staff in the mother's grief raises some difficult questions. First there is the helpfulness or otherwise of the midwife sharing the tears of the bereaved mother. Although some midwives may be prepared to cry alongside the mother, others feel that such behaviour is 'unprofessional' and would not be comfortable shedding even a few tears. The midwives in my research told me that, on the whole, crying was not a problem, but that any loss of control that impeded their ability to provide care needed to be avoided at all costs (Mander 1994). A further difficult decision relates to whether the staff should attend the funeral for the baby. Some of the midwives I interviewed had found this helpful and they had not been uncomfortable being present. It is easy to imagine circumstances, however, in which this might not apply.

Other aspects of care

Not least because of the possibility of their impeding the initiation of grieving, other aspects of care assume greater importance.

Documentation

Record keeping is always a fundamentally important part of the midwife's role, but in this context it becomes even more significant. This is because of the importance of communication in ensuring consistent care, which will facilitate the mother's grieving. Although far from ideal, it may be difficult to avoid this care being provided by a number of personnel. Thus, it is crucial that each midwife should be able to learn from the mother's records about decisions and actions already taken. Horsfall (2001) lists the large number of personnel who are likely to be involved in this mother's care, emphasising the need for good communication.

A checklist may be helpful to ensure good continuity but we are warned that such devices may impede individualised care at the time of this most uniquely individual of experiences (Leon 1992).

The cremation or burial

The documents required for the 'disposal' of the baby differ according to whether the baby was born before or after 24 weeks' gestation (the current legal limit of viability in the UK), according to whether the baby was born alive or not and according to the part of the UK in which the baby was born. If the baby was pre-viable, there is no legal requirement for the baby to be buried or cremated. It is, however, essential to ensure that the baby's remains are removed according to the mother's wishes. If she decides not to participate in the removal of the baby's remains, they should still be removed sensitively (SODoH 1996). A book of remembrance, housed in the maternity unit, is likely to be available to parents to record their names, their baby's details and some thoughts about the baby.

For a baby born after 24 weeks, burial or cremation may be organised by the hospital, with the parents' permission, or by the parents. The municipal cemetery is likely to have a special plot for babies to be buried individually. This may include the provision of a small tree or rose bush, and a religious or other service may be available. There is also the possibility that the parents may erect a headstone (Mortonhall, Edinburgh City Council, personal communication, 2001).

The statutory documentation is specific to each of the countries of the UK (McDonald 1996). Details of the registration requirements in each of the four countries of the UK are provided in the websites listed in the Useful addresses (p. 705).

The mother's choices

At the time of the loss of her baby, as well as her grief work, the mother has certain choices. In terms of how the baby's remains should be disposed of, the mother should decide whether she would prefer to arrange this privately or leave it to the hospital. The mother also needs to decide the extent to which she would like to be involved in organising the funeral service, or the blessing or the memorial ceremony (Kohner 1995). In some hospitals, services of remembrance are arranged on a regular basis, and bereaved parents are able to choose whether to attend. As mentioned above, the mother needs appropriate information in order to make decisions about the funeral and the postmortem.

The death of a mother

A form of loss that fortunately happens even less frequently than the death of a baby is when the mother dies; this is usually known as maternal death. In the UK the rate of maternal death is approximately 1 in 8771 births (Lewis & Drife 2001). This means that in a moderately large maternity unit a mother is likely to die about once every 3 years.

Although the obstetric and epidemiological aspects of maternal death have been well addressed, the personal aspects seem to have been avoided. The family's loss has been addressed anecdotally (Cooke, unpublished work, 1990, Dunn 1987). There appears to be, however, no systematic research on the family's experience of loss, or on the life of the motherless baby. However, the experience of the midwife providing care at this time is beginning to be addressed (Mander 2001).

Conclusion

I have shown in this chapter that the midwife's care of the mother grieving a loss in childbearing requires research-based knowledge. Although undertaking such research is not easy for any who are involved, it is only by obtaining and using such knowledge that we are able to give this mother and family care of the highest standard. In this way, the midwife facilitates healthy grieving in the mother, having avoided any impediments that may interfere with or complicate her grief and prevent its resolution. In this most human of situations, we must remember that 'being nice' is not enough; we need to ensure that our care is based on the strongest evidence available if the woman is eventually to come to terms with her loss.

REFERENCES

Askey K, Moss L 2001 Termination for fetal defects: the effect on midwifery staff. British Journal of Midwifery 9(1):17–24

Bansen S, Stevens H 1992 Women's experience of miscarriage in early pregnancy. Journal of Nurse Midwifery 37(2):84–90

Bewley C 1993 The midwife's role in pregnancy termination. Nursing Standard 8(12):25–28

Bourne S 1968 The psychological effects of stillbirth on women and their doctors. Journal of the Royal College of General Practitioners 16:103–112

Cecil R 1996 The anthropology of pregnancy loss: comparative studies in miscarriage, stillbirth and neonatal death. Berg, Oxford

Chambers H M, Chan F Y 2001 Support for women/families after perinatal death. The Cochrane Database of Systematic Reviews, Issue 1. Update Software, Oxford

Cowles K 1996 Cultural perspectives of grief: an expanded concept analysis. Journal of Advanced Nursing 23(2):287–294

Crawshaw M 1995 Offering woman-centred counselling in reproductive medicine. In: Jennings S (ed) Infertility counselling. Blackwell Science, Oxford, pp 38–65

Crowther M 1995 Communication following a stillbirth or neonatal death: room for improvement. British Journal of Obstetrics and Gynaecology 102(12):952–956

Dimond B 2001 Alder Hey and the retention and storage of body parts. British Journal of Midwifery 9:3 173–176

DoH (Department of Health) 2000 Organ retention interim guidance on postmortem examination. DoH, London. Available online at: http://www.doh.gov.uk/pm2.htm

Dunn S E 1987 Suddenly, at home … Midwives Chronicle 100(1192):132–134

Dyregrov A 1991 Grief in children: a handbook for adults. Kingsley, London

Engel G C 1961 Is grief a disease? A challenge for medical research. Psychosomatic Medicine 23:18–22

Forrest G, Standish E, Baum J 1982 Support after perinatal death: a study of support and counselling after perinatal bereavement. British Medical Journal 285:1475–1479

Foster A 1996 Perinatal bereavement: support for families and midwives. Midwives 109(1303): 218–219

Gohlish M 1985 Stillbirth. Midwife Health Visitor and Community Nurse 21(1):16

Hey V 1996 A feminist exploration. In: Hey V, Itzin C, Saunders L, Speakman A (eds) Hidden loss: miscarriage and ectopic pregnancy, 2nd edn. The Women's Press, London, pp 125–149

Horsfall A 2001 Bereavement: tissues, tea and sympathy are not enough. Royal College of Midwives Journal 4(2):54–57

Iles S 1989 The loss of early pregnancy. In: Oates M R (ed) Psychological aspects of obstetrics and gynaecology. Baillière Tindall, London, ch 5, pp 769–790

Katz Rothman B 1988 The tentative pregnancy: prenatal diagnosis and the future of motherhood. Pandora, London

Kellner K, Lake M 1993 Grief counselling. In: Knuppel R A, Drukker J E (eds) High risk pregnancy. W B Saunders, Philadelphia, ch 34, pp 717–732

Kennell J, Slyter H, Klaus M 1970 The mourning response of parents to the death of newborn infant. New England Journal of Medicine 283(7):344–349

Kissane D, Bloch S 1994 Family grief. British Journal of Psychiatry 164:728–740

Kohner N 1995 Pregnancy loss and the death of a baby: guidelines for professionals. SANDS, London

Kübler-Ross E 1970 On death and dying. Tavistock Publications, London

Leon I G 1992 Choreographing loss on the obstetric unit. American Journal of Orthopsychiatry 62: 7–8

Lewis E 1979 Mourning by the family after a stillbirth or neonatal death. Archives of Disease in Childhood 54:303–306

Lewis E, Bourne S 1989 Perinatal death. In: Oates M (ed) Psychological aspects of obstetrics and gynaecology. Baillière Tindall, London, pp 935–954

Lewis G, Drife J 2001 Why mothers die 1997–1999. The fifth report of the Confidential Enquiry into Maternal Deaths in the United Kingdom. NICE/SeHD/DoHSSPS, London

Lilford R, Stratton P, Godsil S, Prasad A 1994 A randomised trial of routine versus selective counselling in perinatal bereavement from congenital disease. British Journal of Obstetrics and Gynaecology 101(4):291–296

Littlewood J 1992 Aspects of grief: bereavement in adult life. Tavistock/Routledge, London

Lovell H, Bokoula C, Misra S, Speight N 1986 Mothers' reactions to perinatal death. Nursing Times 82(46):40–42

McCaffery M 1979 Nursing management of the patient with pain. Lippincott, Philadelphia

McDonald M 1996 Loss in pregnancy: guidelines for midwives. Baillière Tindall, London

Mahan C K, Calica J 1997 Perinatal loss: considerations in social work practice. Social Work in Health Care 24(3/4):141–152

Mander R 1994 Loss and bereavement in childbearing. Blackwell Scientific, Oxford

Mander R 1995 The care of the mother grieving a baby relinquished for adoption. Avebury, Aldershot

Mander R 1996 The grieving mother: care in the community? Modern Midwife 6(8):10–13

Mander R 2000 Perinatal grief: understanding the bereaved and their carers. In: Alexander J, Levy V, Roth C (eds) Midwifery practice: core topics 3. ch 3, pp 29–50. Macmillan, London

Mander R 2001 The midwife's ultimate paradox: a UK-based study of the death of a mother: Midwifery 17(4):248–259

Marris P 1986 Loss and change. Routledge, London

Murphy F A, Hunt S C 1997 Family issues. Early pregnancy loss: men have feelings too. British Journal of Midwifery, 5(2):87–90

Ney P, Tak F, Wickett A, Beaman-Dodd C 1994 The effects of pregnancy loss on women's health. Social Science and Medicine 38(9):1193–1200

Niven K 1992 Psychological care for families: before, during and after birth. Butterworth Heinemann, Oxford, p 167

O'Hare T, Creed F 1995 Life events and miscarriage. British Journal of Psychiatry 167(6):799–805

Oakley A, McPherson A, Roberts H 1990 Miscarriage. Penguin, London

Peppers L, Knapp R 1980 Maternal reactions to involuntary fetal/infant death. Psychiatry 43:55–59

Phillips S 1996 Labouring the emotions: expanding the remit of nursing work? Journal of Advanced Nursing 24(1):139–143

Rådestad I, Steineck G, Nordin C, Sjogren B 1996a Psychological complications after stillbirth. British Medical Journal 312(7045):1505–1508

Rådestad I, Nordin C, Steineck G, Sjogren B 1996b Stillbirth is no longer managed as a non-event: a nationwide study in Sweden. Birth 23(4):209–216

Rajan L 1994 Social isolation and support in pregnancy loss. Health Visitor 67(3):97–101

Raphael-Leff J 1991 Psychological processes of childbearing. Chapman & Hall, New York

Samuelsson M, Rådestad I, Segesten K 2001 A waste of life: fathers' experience of losing a child before birth. Birth 28(2):124–130

SODoH (Scottish Office Department of Health) 1996 The management of early pregnancy loss. National Medical Advisory Committee, Edinburgh

Sorosky A D, Baran A, Pannor R 1984 The adoption triangle. Anchor, New York

Speakman M A 1996 Letting go and holding on. In: Hey V, Itzin C, Saunders L, Speakman M A (eds) Hidden loss: miscarriage and ectopic pregnancy, 2nd edn. The Women's Press, London

Stoter D J 1997 Staff support in health care. Blackwell Science, Oxford

Stroebe W, Stroebe M S 1987 Bereavement and health: the psychological and physical consequences of partner loss. Cambridge University Press, Cambridge

FURTHER READING

Jones A 1996 Psychotherapy following childbirth. British Journal of Midwifery 4(5): 239–243

An in-depth exploration of relevant psychoanalytical issues.

Moulder C 1998 Understanding pregnancy loss: perspectives and issues in care. Macmillan, London

A wide-ranging account of a qualitative research project.

Schott J, Henley A 1996 Childbearing losses. British Journal of Midwifery 4(10): 522–526

The implications of cultural and religious variations in the context of childbearing loss.

USEFUL ADDRESSES

Registration and other statutory documentation of a stillborn baby

England & Wales:
http://www.statistics.gov.uk/nsbase/registration/registering_still_birth.asp

Scotland: http://www.gro-scotland.gov.uk/grosweb/grosweb.nsf/pages/groreg

Northern Ireland:
http://www.belfastcity.gov.uk/bdm/howto3.htm

Support groups

The Miscarriage Association
http://www.the-ma.org.uk/

SANDS (Stillbirth and Neonatal Death Society)
http://www.uk-sands.org/contact.html

6

Section 6
The Newborn Baby

SECTION CONTENTS

38 The Baby at Birth

Philomena Farrell   Norma Sittlington

A newborn baby's survival is dependent on his ability to adapt to an extrauterine environment. This involves adaptations in cardiopulmonary circulation and other physiological adjustments to replace placental function and maintain homeostasis. It is also the commencement of the early parent–baby relationship.

The chapter aims to:

- describe the physiological changes taking place at birth

- discuss the care of the baby during and immediately after birth

- consider the early responses of both parents and baby, identifying steps that can be taken to promote good parent–baby relationships.

- identify factors to be considered when the baby fails to establish respiration at birth and describe the principles of neonatal resuscitation.

Introduction

The transition from intrauterine to extrauterine life is a dramatic one and demands considerable and effective physiological alterations by the baby in order to ensure survival. The fetus leaves the uterine environment, which has been completely life sustaining for oxygenation, nutrition, excretion and thermoregulation. The aquatic amniotic sac has permitted movement but freedom to extend the limbs has been limited towards the end of pregnancy as the size of the fetus has increased in relation to the capacity of the uterus. Though the fetus is sensitive to sound, the dim uterine environment has dulled the impact of the noise of the outside world.

Subjected to intermittent diminution of the oxygen supply during uterine contractions, compression followed by decompression of the head and chest, and extension of the limbs, hips and spine during birth, the baby emerges from the mother to encounter light, noises, cool air, gravity and tactile stimuli for the first time. Simultaneously the baby has to make major adjustments in the respiratory and circulatory systems as well as controlling body temperature. These initial adaptations are crucial to the baby's subsequent wellbeing and should be understood and facilitated by the midwife at the time of birth.

Respiratory and cardiovascular changes are interdependent and concurrent.

Adaptation to extrauterine life

Onset of respiration

At birth a baby is transposed from the warm contentment of the uterine environment to the outside world where the role of independent existence is assumed. The baby must be able to make this sharp transition swiftly, and in order to achieve this a series of adaptive functions have been developed to accommodate the dramatic change from the intrauterine to extrauterine environment.

Pulmonary adaptation

Until the time of birth, the fetus depends upon maternal blood gas exchange via the maternal lung and the placenta. Following the sudden removal of the placenta after delivery, very rapid adaptation takes place to ensure continued survival. Prior to birth, the fetus makes breathing movements and the lungs will have matured both biochemically and anatomically to produce surfactant and have adequate numbers of alveoli for gas exchange. Before birth, the fetal lung is full of fluid, which is excreted by the lung itself. During birth, this fluid leaves the alveoli either by being squeezed up the airway and out of the mouth and nose, or by moving across the alveolar walls into the pulmonary lymphatic vessels and into the thoracic duct or to the lung capillaries.

The stimuli of respiration include mild hypercapnia, hypoxia and acidosis, which result from normal labour, due partially to the intermittent cessation of maternal–placental perfusion with contractions. The rhythm of respiration changes from episodic shallow fetal respiration to regular deeper breathing as a result of a combination of chemical and neural stimuli, notably a fall in pH and P_aO_2 and a rise in P_aCO_2. Other stimuli include cold, light, noise, touch and pain. Considerable negative intrathoracic pressure of up to 9.8 kPa (100 cm water) is exerted as the first breath is taken. The pressure exerted to effect inhalation diminishes with each breath taken until only 5 cm water pressure is required to inflate the lungs. This effect is caused by surfactant, which lines the alveoli, lowering the surface tension thus permitting residual air to remain in the alveoli between breaths. Surfactant is a complex of lipoproteins and proteins produced by the alveolar type 2 cells in the lungs, and is primarily concerned with the reduction in surface tension at the alveolar surface, thus reducing the work of breathing (Halliday et al 1998).

Cardiovascular adaptation

Prior to birth the fetus relies solely on the placenta for all gas exchanges and excretion of metabolic waste. Separated from the placenta at birth, the baby's circulatory system must make major adjustments in order to divert deoxygenated blood to the lungs for reoxygenation. This involves several mechanisms, which are influenced by the clamping of the umbilical cord and also by the lowered resistance in the pulmonary vascular bed.

During fetal life (see Ch. 11) only approximately 10% of the cardiac output is circulated to the lungs through the pulmonary artery. With the expansion of the lungs and lowered pulmonary vascular resistance, virtually all of the cardiac output is sent to the lungs. Oxygenated blood returning to the heart from the lungs increases the pressure within the left atrium. At almost the same time, pressure in the right atrium is lowered because blood ceases to flow through the cord. As a result, a functional closure of the foramen ovale is achieved. During the first days of life this closure is reversible; reopening may occur if pulmonary vascular resistance is high, for example when crying, resulting in transient cyanotic episodes in the baby (Perry 1995). The septa usually fuse within the 1st year of life, forming the interatrial septum, though in some individuals perfect anatomical closure may never be achieved.

The ductus arteriosus, which is nearly as wide as the aorta, provides a diversionary route to bypass the lungs of the fetus. Contraction of its muscular walls occurs almost immediately after birth. This is thought to occur because of sensitivity of the muscle of the ductus arteriosus to increased oxygen tension and reduction in circulating prostaglandin (Heyman 1989). As a result of altered pressure gradients between the aorta and pulmonary artery, a temporary reverse left-to-right shunt through the ductus may persist for a few hours, although there is usually functional closure of the ductus within 8–10 hours of birth. Intermittent patency has been demonstrated in most healthy infants in the first 3 days of life (Lim et al 1992), but complete closure takes several months. Persistence or reopening of the ductus, with associated cyanosis or cyanotic attacks, may occur if pulmonary vascular resistance is high or hypoxia is present. This is a common problem in preterm infants with respiratory distress syndrome (see Ch. 43). Persistence of the foramen ovale or ductus arteriosus, or both, may be lifesaving in some forms of congenital heart abnormality (see Ch. 45).

The remaining temporary structures of the fetal circulation – the umbilical vein, ductus venosus and hypogastric arteries – close functionally within a few minutes after birth and constriction of the cord. Anatomical closure by fibrous tissue occurs within 2–3 months, resulting in the formation of the ligamentum teres, ligamentum venosum and the obliterated hypogastric arteries. The proximal portions of the hypogastric arteries persist as the superior vesical arteries.

Thermal adaptation

The baby enters a much cooler atmosphere at delivery, with a birthing room temperature of 21°C contrasting sharply with an intrauterine temperature of 37.7°C. This causes rapid cooling of the baby as amniotic fluid evaporates from the skin. Each millilitre that evaporates removes 560 calories of heat (Rutter 1992). The baby's large *surface area : body mass* ratio potentiates heat loss, especially from the head, which comprises 25% of body mass. The subcutaneous fat layer is thin and provides poor insulation, allowing rapid transfer of core heat to the skin, then to the environment, and it also effects blood cooling. In addition to heat loss by *evaporation*, further heat will be lost by *conduction* when the baby is in contact with cold surfaces, by *radiation* to cold objects in the environment, and by *convection* caused by currents of cool air passing over the surface of the body (Fig. 38.1) (Brueggemeyer 1993, Greer 1988, Rutter 1992, Thomas 1994).

The heat-regulating centre in the baby's brain has the capacity to promote heat production in response to stimuli received from thermoreceptors. However, this is dependent on increased metabolic activity, compromising the baby's ability to control body temperature especially in adverse environmental conditions. The

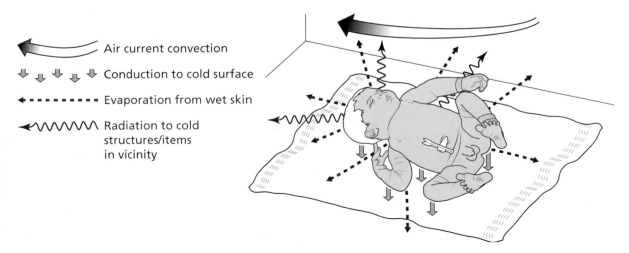

Air current convection

Conduction to cold surface

Evaporation from wet skin

Radiation to cold structures/items in vicinity

Fig. 38.1 Modes of heat loss in the neonate.

baby has a limited ability to shiver and is unable to increase muscle activity voluntarily in order to generate heat. This means that the baby must depend on his ability to produce heat by metabolism.

The neonate is endowed with brown adipose tissue, which assists in the rapid mobilisation of heat resources (namely free fatty acids and glycerol) in times of cold stress. This mechanism is called *nonshivering thermogenesis* (Dawkins & Hull 1964). Babies derive most of their heat production from the metabolism of brown fat. The term 'brown fat' refers to the reddish-brown colouring of the fat, which is caused by the high degree of vascularisation of the tissue. Brown fat is stored in pockets throughout the baby's body. The majority of brown fat is located around the neck, along the line of the spinal column between the scapulae, across the clavicle line and down the sternum (Fig. 38.2). It also surrounds the major thoracic vessels and pads the kidneys (Holdcroft 1980). The term baby has sufficient brown fat to meet minimum heat needs for 2–4 days after birth, but cold stress results in increased oxygen consumption as the baby strives to maintain sufficient heat for survival. Brown fat uses up to three times as much oxygen as other tissue (Wong 1995), with the undesired effect of diverting oxygen and glucose from vital centres such as the brain and cardiac muscle. In addition, cold stress causes vasoconstriction, thus reducing pulmonary perfusion, and respiratory acidosis develops as the pH and PaO_2 of the blood decrease and the $PaCO_2$ increases leading to respiratory distress, exhibited by tachypnoea (Box 38.1), and grunting respirations (see Ch. 43). This, together with the reduction in pulmonary perfusion, may result in the reopening or maintenance of the right-to-left shunt across the ductus arteriosus. Anaerobic glycolysis (i.e. the metabolism of glucose in the absence of oxygen) results in the production of acid compounding the situation by adding a metabolic acidosis. Protraction of cold stress should therefore be avoided. The peripheral vasoconstrictor mechanisms of the baby are unable to prevent the fall in core body temperature, which occurs within the first few hours after birth. It is important, therefore, for the midwife to ensure that she employs measures to minimise heat loss at birth (Dahm & James 1972, Rutter 1992).

Immediate care of the baby at birth

Prevention of heat loss

With the midwife's knowledge of the baby's transitional requirements it is her responsibility to ensure appropriate preparations are made for the birth of the baby. Whether the baby is born at home or in hospital, it is important that the midwife endeavours to provide an ambient temperature in the range 21–25°C. It is accepted that in some remote parts of the world and

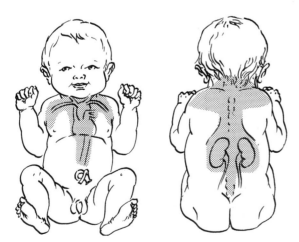

Fig. 38.2 Sites of brown fat. (From Brendan Ellis, medical illustrator, Royal Group of Hospitals, Belfast, with permission.)

Box 38.1 Transient tachypnoea of the newborn

This condition is characterised by rapid respirations of up to 120 per minute; it is especially common after a caesarian section. The baby may be cyanosed but maintains normal blood gases apart from PaO_2. Little or no recession of the rib cage is evident and there is minimal, if any, grunt on expiration. The respiratory rate may remain elevated for up to 5 days. Treatment consists of oxygen therapy to maintain adequate oxygenation. It is essential that other causes of respiratory distress are excluded, especially infective causes (which mimic this condition) and respiratory distress syndrome (see also Ch. 43).

in emergency situations this may not be possible. However, within controlled circumstances, provision of an optimal thermal environment is paramount in facilitating a successful transition to extrauterine life. Switching off fans prior to delivery helps to minimise heat loss by convection, and closing curtains reduces the radiant heat loss to windows (Karlsson 1996). The baby's temperature can drop by as much as 3–4.5°C within the first minute (Dahm & James 1972, Greer 1988, Sinclair 1992, Thomas 1994). Drying the baby at birth helps to minimise heat loss by evaporation and it is important to ensure that the wet towel is then removed and the baby wrapped in a dry prewarmed towel. Skin-to-skin contact with the mother, for example obtaining permission to place the baby on her abdomen at the time of birth, may assist the baby to conserve heat although transfer of heat from the mother to the baby is minimal. However, considerable heat loss continues by convection, conduction and radiation, particularly from exposed areas of the baby's skin (Karlsson 1996). This can be minimised by covering the baby with an insulating blanket, swaddling or putting on loose clothing. Covering the baby's head is of particular importance, and fabric-insulated hats are significantly more effective than stockinette hats in preventing heat loss (Greer 1988). (**NB** electric heating pads in cots must be used with care to avoid burning or overheating the baby.)

Prevention of heat loss after birth remains important throughout, and after, the initiation and establishment of respirations.

Clearing the airway

As the baby's head is born, excess mucus may be wiped gently from the mouth. However, care must be taken to avoid touching the nares as such action may stimulate reflex inhalation of debris in the trachea. Although fetal pulmonary fluid is present in the mouth, most babies will achieve a clear airway unaided. If necessary, the airway can be cleared with the aid of a soft suction catheter attached to low pressure (10 cm water) mechanical suction. It is important to aspirate the oropharynx prior to the nasopharynx so that, if the baby gasps as his nasal passages are aspirated, mucus or other material is not drawn down into the respiratory tract. Excess suction can result in vagal stimulation, with laryngospasm and bradycardia.

The time of birth and sex of the baby are noted and recorded once the baby has been completely expelled from his mother.

Cutting the cord

The umbilical cord is the lifeline of the fetus and of the baby in the first few minutes after birth. Separation of the baby from the placenta is achieved by dividing the umbilical cord between two clamps, which should be applied approximately 8–10 cm from the umbilicus. Application of a gauze swab over the cord while cutting it with scissors will prevent blood spraying the delivery field. The cord should not be cut until it has been clamped securely. Failure to comply with this procedure may result in excessive blood loss from the baby. In some delivery suites it is now common practice for the father of the baby to assist the midwife and cut the umbilical cord. Care of the umbilical cord and stump in the immediate period varies according to social, cultural and geographic factors. The optimal time for umbilical cord clamping after birth remains unknown. Research continues into cord clamping (Mercer et al 2000).

Some centres advocate delay in cutting until respirations are established and cord pulsation has ceased, thus ensuring that the infant receives a placental transfusion of some 70 ml of blood (Nelle et al 1993). This view is countered by those who maintain that the placental transfusion so acquired may predispose to neonatal jaundice (see Ch. 46). What is agreed is that a term baby at birth can be drawn up on to the mother's abdomen, but raised no higher, and a preterm baby should be kept at the level of the placenta. This is because if a preterm baby is held above the placenta then blood can drain from the baby to the placenta, resulting in anaemia, and if held below can cause the baby to receive a blood transfusion.

Identification

It is the practice in many units to apply namebands to the baby before the cord is cut. Within the baby's own home, unless a twin delivery, identification does not present a problem. However, when babies are born in hospital it is essential that they are readily identifiable from one another. Various methods of indicating identity can be employed, for example namebands or identity tags. In the UK two namebands are applied, each of which should indicate *legibly* in indelible pen the family name, sex of the baby, date and time of birth. In some centres the namebands are number coded with the baby's case records; in others the number coding corresponds with that of the mother. The amount of information written on the namebands may vary slightly according to local policy. The mother or father, or both, should verify that the information on the bands or tags is correct prior to these being attached to the baby. The midwife should ensure that the namebands are fastened securely and are neither too tight, impeding circulation or likely to excoriate the skin, nor too loose, risking loss of the means of identification. Namebands or tags should remain on the baby until discharged from hospital. The midwives must advise the mother to inform a member of the midwifery or nursing staff if the nameband or tag becomes detached or is removed for any reason.

By the end of 2002, England and Wales, Scotland and Northern Ireland hope to issue each baby from birth with a national unique reference number for receipt of health and social care. Each area will have its own range within the numbering system and will issue their own guidance.

Assessment of the baby's condition

As soon as the baby has been born the midwife can proceed with drying the skin, which will help minimise heat loss. In the vast majority of cases, babies are well and can be handed directly to their parents. Whether a home or hospital birth, the midwife at 1 minute and 5 minutes after the birth will make an assessment of the baby's general condition using the Apgar score (Apgar 1953) (Table 38.1). The assessment at 1 minute is important for the further management of resuscitation. However, it has been shown that an assessment at 5 minutes is more reliable as a predictor of the risk of death during the first 28 days of life, and of the child's neurological state and risk of major disability at the age of 1 year. The higher the score the better the outcome for the baby. The Apgar score must be fully documented in the baby's records.

A mnemonic for the Apgar score is:

A   Appearance (i.e. colour)
P   Pulse (i.e. heart rate)
G   Grimace (i.e. response to stimuli)
A   Active (i.e. tone)
R   Respirations.

Continued early care

Prior to leaving the mother's home, or transferring the baby to the ward, the midwife undertakes a detailed examination of the baby checking for obvious abnormalities such as spina bifida, imperforate anus, cleft lip or palate, abrasions, fractures or haemorrhage due to trauma. The initial cord clamp is replaced with another method of securing haemostasis by applying a disposable plastic clamp (or rubber band or three cord ligatures) approximately 2–3 cm from the umbilicus and cutting off the redundant cord. The baby's temperature is now recorded. The midwife should ensure that the environmental temperature remains warm, between 21–25°C as previously discussed. Early transfer of the baby to a postnatal ward has been advocated as a means of minimising heat loss. The baby should be transferred with the mother, in her arms, to avoid heat loss and to promote mother–baby attachment.

Table 38.1 The Apgar score. The score is assessed at 1 minute and 5 minutes after birth. Medical aid should be sought if the score is less than 7. 'Apgar minus colour' score omits the fifth sign. Medical aid should be sought if the score is less than 6

Sign	Score		
	0	1	2
Heart rate	Absent	Less than 100 b.p.m.	More than 100 b.p.m.
Respiratory effort	Absent	Slow, irregular	Good or crying
Muscle tone	Limp	Some flexion of limbs	Active
Reflex response to stimulus	None	Minimal grimace	Cough or sneeze
Colour	Blue, pale	Body pink, extremities blue	Completely pink

Instillation of eyedrops as prophylaxis against gono-coccal infection is not practised in the UK. In other parts of the world drops or antibiotic ointment may be instilled (Wong 1995). It is suggested that, to be effective, such treatments should be administered within one hour of birth (Tyson 1992). Localised reactions to silver nitrate drops have been shown to impair eye-to-eye contact with the mother and it has been noted that this may interfere with early mother–baby relationships (de Château 1987).

The first bath and other non-urgent procedures may be deferred in order to minimise thermal stress. (Further care is discussed in Ch. 39.) All babies should remain with their mother during the first few hours of life, providing both mother and baby are in good condition that is, as this is the time when parent–baby interactions are initiated and the reality of parenthood begins.

Early parent–baby relationships

The safe delivery of a healthy baby engenders considerable emotion in most parents and indeed in attendants at the birth. The efforts of the preceding hours are temporarily forgotten as the mother sees her baby for the first time. Characteristically her first query relates to the sex of the baby speedily followed by an anxious enquiry about the baby's state of health – 'is he all right?' Reassured on these points, a mother progresses to an examination of her baby, which follows a fairly predictable pattern unless the condition of either the mother or the baby is impaired by the process of labour or by narcotic drugs. Fathers too are involved in this early exploration of the newborn baby. The response of both parents is influenced not only by their prenatal understanding and previous experiences with babies but also by the appearance, behaviour and responses of their baby, who takes an active part in the proceedings (Salariya 1990, White & Woollet 1987, Williams 1995). Cultural background may also play a part in parental behaviours at this time (Callister 1995).

The first hour after birth is a time of particular sensitivity for the mother. Close contact with her baby during this time facilitates the attachment process (Klaus & Kennell 1989). This sensitive period of interaction between mother and baby should promote ideal later development of the baby.

Regardless of age, parity or marital status, mothers are likely to display a similar behavioural pattern when touching their babies for the first time. This sequence of touching behaviour is enhanced if the baby is naked. The mother begins her examination of her baby by exploring the extremities and head with her fingertips. Thereafter, she caresses her baby's body with her entire hand before gathering her baby in her arms often in the *en face* position where eye-to-eye contact can be established. She talks to her baby with great emotion, looking for positive reinforcement from her partner and other birth attendants (Klaus et al 1975).

Her emotions at this time may be mixed. She may display great excitement and happiness – laughing, talking or even crying with joy, or she may feel too tired to react positively towards her baby. Factors which may predispose to this latter reaction include prolonged labour, instrumental delivery, baby of the 'wrong' sex or congenital abnormality. Lack of support from partner or parents may influence the behaviour of an unmarried mother and, for some mothers, high parity may dampen their response. Childhood deprivation can inhibit some women from reacting in the anticipated manner.

For some mothers, the sight of an unwashed, wet and sometimes bloody infant is profoundly distasteful and they are not appreciative of skin-to-skin contact with a baby in this condition. A good midwife will ascertain the mother's attitude during pregnancy or early labour. This will allow her to modify her delivery technique and immediate care of the baby to meet the mother's wishes and so assist the mother to feel comfortable at her first meeting with her baby. Some, though not all, mothers are keen to encourage their babies to suckle at birth. This practice should be facilitated and encouraged by the midwife as it has been shown that early skin-to-skin contact and breastfeeding are significantly associated with exclusive breastfeeding at discharge and also promote good mother–baby relationships and stimulate lactation (Catlaneo & Buzzetti 2001) (see Ch. 40).

Many fathers are surprised at their profound emotional response to the birth of their baby. Sometimes a man's reactions are stronger than those of his wife or partner, who may be rather tired initially. The father feels a sense of deep satisfaction and self-esteem, and is elated and keen to touch and hold his baby and his partner and share his excitement (Barclay & Lupton 1999, Bedford & Johnson 1988, Wildman 1995). Intimacy shared between the father and mother at this time is extended to include the baby within an exclusive family group, often oblivious to their surroundings. The baby at birth is alert and wakeful, reactive to surroundings. His rounded, soft features provide an appealing image to which other human beings react protectively. The reaction of parents is increased by their emotional ties with their baby.

Having accomplished the immediate physiological adaptations of respiration and circulation, the baby displays interest in sound, light and nutrition, responding to the mother's voice by moving limbs in synchrony. The response to touch is illustrated in the grasp reflex and in suckling of the breast if offered – or the fist. Newborn babies appear to focus on their mother's face at a distance of 20 cm and respond to movement of bright shiny objects, such as their mother's eyes, by tracking them visually. These responsive behaviours evoke reinforcing responses from parents, thus promoting the interactions essential for survival, which is dependent on good parenting. A slightly darkened delivery room encourages babies to open their eyes widely and look around them, whereas bright lights cause frowning. The midwife's understanding of these responses allows her to create optimal conditions for interaction to occur.

Promotion of parent–baby interaction

The term 'bonding' has been used to describe the establishment of parent–baby relationships in the early neonatal period. The implication of the desirability to feel instant love for one's child can lead to feelings of guilt in some parents who do not identify a strong emotional tie with their baby at birth. It is important to recognise that, as individuals, parents develop a loving relationship with their child at their own pace, some taking longer than others – days, weeks or months. Parents should feel able to express their disappointments as well as their joys without fear of being thought a 'bad' parent (Barclay & Lupton 1999, Herbert & Sluckin 1985, Parkinson & Harvey 1987, Sluckin et al 1984).

A good rapport between the parents and the midwife should enable the development of their love for

their baby to progress happily and at its own speed. However, the midwife must be alert to report and document marked negative reactions from either or both parents, as this may be an early sign of future parenting difficulties. Adverse behaviours of note include hostile verbal or non-verbal attitude, lack of supportive interaction between the parents, disinclination to touch or hold their baby, disparaging remarks about the baby or marked disappointment about the sex of the baby.

Involvement of the father in the birth of the baby's body, clamping of the cord and early bathing have been introduced in some centres to help to promote father–baby relationships. The midwife can do much to promote the beginnings of loving relationships by encouraging both parents to handle and examine their baby, by her positive comments about the baby and by examining the baby beside the parents.

Privacy to talk, touch and be alone together with their baby is important for parents and opportunities to do so should be provided whether their baby is born at home or in hospital. The midwife should be sensitive to this often-unexpressed need and leave the family together for some time before progressing with further care of the baby.

The opportunity for this initial intimate family moment is dependent on the baby's condition being satisfactory. A baby whose Apgar score is below 7 requires some form of resuscitation, which may necessitate speedy removal to a special resuscitation area. It is essential that parents receive a reassuring explanation and adequate information about the need for this separation, which can be totally unexpected and therefore very frightening.

Vitamin K

Depending on local policy vitamin K, intramuscular or orally may be given as prophylaxis against bleeding disorders (see Ch. 44). Vitamin K is fat soluble; it can only be absorbed from the intestine in the presence of bile salts. The body's capacity to store vitamin K is very low and the half-life of the vitamin-K-dependent coagulation factors is short (Zipursky 1999). However, since Golding et al (1990, 1992) reported an increased risk of developing childhood cancer after parenteral vitamin K prophylaxis, this has been a cause for concern.

After this report several studies were carried out:

1. oral vitamin K versus placebo or nothing (Motohara et al 1985, Sharma et al 1995, Ulusahin et al 1996)
2. single dose oral versus intramuscular vitamin K (Bakhshi et al 1996, Cornelissen et al 1992, Sharma et al 1995, Ulusahin et al 1996)
3. three oral doses versus intramuscular vitamin K (Greer et al 1998).

A review of these studies concluded that a single dose (1.0 mg) of intramuscular vitamin K after birth is effective in the prevention of classic haemorragic disease of the newborn (Puckett & Offringa 2000). Either intramuscular or oral (1.0 mg) vitamin K prophylaxis improves biochemical indices of coagulation status at 1–7 days. Neither intramuscular nor oral vitamin K has been tested in randomised trials with respect to effect in late haemorrhagic disease of the newborn (HDN). Oral vitamin K, either single or multiple doses, has not been tested in randomised trials for its effect on either classic or late HDN. When three doses of oral vitamin K are compared with a single dose of intramuscular vitamin K the plasma vitamin K levels are higher in the oral group at 2 weeks and 2 months, but again there is no evidence of a difference in coagulation studies. Midwives must be aware of and follow their local hospital policy regarding consent and administration of vitamin K.

Failure to establish respiration at birth

Although the majority of babies gasp and establish respirations within 60 seconds of birth, some do not. Failure to initiate and sustain respiration at birth necessitates prompt and effective intervention. The midwife must therefore be aware of the predisposing factors and causes of respiratory depression and be proficient in the resuscitative measures, which can be employed in the absence of medical aid.

Intrauterine hypoxia

Oxygenation of the fetus is dependent on oxygenation of the mother, adequate perfusion of the placental site, placental function, fetoplacental circulation and

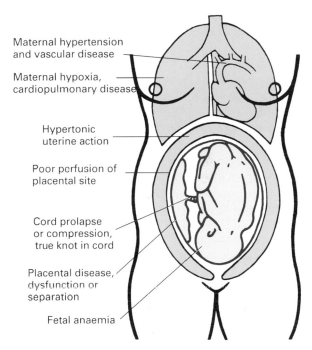

Fig. 38.3 Factors predisposing to intrauterine hypoxia.

adequate fetal haemoglobin. Absence or impairment of any of these factors will result in a reduction of oxygen supply to the fetus (Fig. 38.3).

Oxygenation of the mother may be impaired as a result of cardiac or respiratory disease, an eclamptic fit or during induction of general anaesthesia if difficulties arise during intubation. Perfusion of the placental site is dependent on satisfactory blood supply. This may be reduced in the presence of maternal hypertension or if hypotension occurs in response to haemorrhage, shock or aortocaval occlusion. Hypertonic uterine action, when uterine resting tone is elevated, will impede the blood supply to the placental site. This is sometimes due to hyperstimulation of the uterus by oxytocin and necessitates discontinuation of the oxytocic agent to allow the uterus to relax, thus restoring circulation to the placental bed. The umbilical cord transports oxygenated blood to the fetus. If prolapsed or compressed, fetal oxygenation will be reduced. The transport of oxygen within the fetus necessitates the availability of adequate haemoglobin, which may be reduced if Rhesus incompatibility is present. Abnormal fetal cardiac function may also diminish the supply of oxygen to the fetal brain.

The fetus responds to hypoxia by accelerating the heart rate in an effort to maintain supplies of oxygen to the brain. If hypoxia persists, glucose depletion will stimulate anaerobic glycolysis resulting in a metabolic acidosis. Cerebral vessels will dilate and some brain swelling may occur. Peripheral circulation will be reduced. As the fetus becomes acidotic and cardiac glycogen reserves are depleted, bradycardia develops, the anal sphincter relaxes and the fetus may pass meconium into the liquor. Gasping breathing movements triggered by hypoxia may result in the aspiration of meconium-stained liquor into the lungs, which presents an additional problem after birth.

Auscultation of the fetal heart, use of cardiotocography and observation of meconium staining of the liquor draining from the vagina should alert the midwife to fetal compromise (see Ch. 25). Subsequent fetal blood sampling may confirm a compromised fetus by revealing acidosis. However, Apgar scores do not always correlate with these findings (Jacobs & Phibbs 1989, Silverman et al 1985).

The length of time during which the fetus or neonate is subjected to hypoxia determines the outcome. It is considered that the human neonate responds to hypoxia in a similar manner to other young mammals (Roberton 1992). This involves an initial response of gasping respirations followed by a period of apnoea lasting $1\frac{1}{2}$ minutes – *primary apnoea* – which, if not resolved by intervention techniques, is followed by a further episode of gasping respirations, which accelerate while diminishing in depth until, approximately 8 minutes after birth, respirations cease completely – *terminal apnoea*. The essential difference between primary and terminal apnoea is the baby's circulatory status. During primary apnoea, the circulation and heart rate are maintained and such babies respond quickly to simple resuscitation measures. In secondary apnoea the circulation is impaired, the heart rate is slow and the baby looks shocked (Table 38.2).

Respiratory depression

Obstruction of the baby's airway by mucus, blood, liquor or meconium is one of the most common reasons for a baby failing to establish respirations. Depression of the respiratory centre may be due to:

- the effects of drugs administered to the mother, for example narcotic drugs, or diazepam
- cerebral hypoxia during labour or traumatic delivery
- immaturity of the baby, which causes mechanical dysfunction because of underdeveloped lungs, lack of surfactant and a soft pliable thoracic cage
- intranatal pneumonia, which can inhibit successful establishment of respirations and should be considered, especially if the membranes have been ruptured for some time
- severe anaemia, caused by fetomaternal haemorrhage or Rhesus incompatibility, which diminishes the oxygen-carrying capacity of the blood
- respiratory function that may be compromised by major congenital abnormalities, particularly by abnormalities of the central nervous system or within the respiratory tract
- a congenital abnormality such as choanal or tracheal atresia (choanal atresia should be suspected when a baby is pink when crying but becomes cyanosed at rest).

Table 38.2 Degrees of respiratory depression

Mildly depressed	Severely depressed
Heart rate not severely depressed (60–80 b.p.m.)	Slow feeble heart rate (less than 40 b.p.m.)
Short delay in onset of respiration	No attempt to breathe
Good muscle tone	Poor muscle tone
Responsive to stimuli	Limp, unresponsive to stimuli
Deeply cyanosed	Pale, grey
Apgar score 5–7	*Apgar score less than 5*
No significant deprivation of oxygen during labour (Primary apnoea)	Oxygen lack has been prolonged before or after delivery, circulatory failure is present, baby is shocked (Secondary apnoea)

Failure to establish respirations compounds hypoxia as previously described. It is necessary therefore for midwives to be able and prepared to undertake specific resuscitative measures for any infant who has difficulty establishing respirations at birth.

Resuscitation of the newborn

Though the need for resuscitation can be anticipated in some situations, in many instances a baby is born in poor condition without forewarning. It is essential that resuscitation equipment (Box 38.2) is always available and in working order and that personnel in attendance at the birth of a baby are familiar with the equipment, resuscitation techniques and local policies regarding the provision of medical aid.

In some units resuscitation of babies is undertaken in a specific area, whereas in others each birthing room is equipped to deal with this emergency. Whenever problems are anticipated, such as preterm delivery, instrumental or breech delivery or fetal compromise, it is desirable that a paediatrician, neonatal nurse or midwife experienced in resuscitation techniques is present at the delivery. (In some centres an anaesthetist may be the person responsible for neonatal resuscitation.) At home the midwife is the responsible person.

Aims of resuscitation. These are to:

- establish and maintain a clear airway, by ventilation and oxygenation
- ensure effective circulation
- correct acidosis
- prevent hypothermia, hypoglycaemia and haemorrhage.

As soon as the baby is born, the clock timer should be started. The Apgar score is assessed in the normal manner at 1 minute. In the absence of any respiratory effort, resuscitation measures are commenced. The baby's upper airways should be cleared by gentle suction of the oro- and nasopharynx and the presence of a heartbeat verified. The baby is dried quickly and transferred to a well-lit resuscitaire and placed on a flat, firm surface at a comfortable working height and under a radiant heat source to prevent hypothermia. The baby's shoulders may be elevated on a small towel, which causes slight extension of the head and

---

Box 38.2 Resuscitation equipment

- Resuscitaire with overhead radiant heater (switched on) and light, piped oxygen, manometer, suction and clock timer
- Two straight-bladed infant laryngoscopes, spare batteries and bulbs size 0 and 1
- Neonatal endotracheal tubes 2.0, 2.5, 3.0, and 3.5 mm and connectors
- Neonatal airways sizes 0,00,000
- Suction catheters sizes 6, 8 and 10 FG
- Neonatal bag and mask and face masks of assorted sizes (clear, soft masks)
- Magills forceps
- Endotracheal tube introducer
- Syringes 1 ml, 2 ml, 5 ml and 20 ml and assorted needles
- Drugs
    - Naloxone hydrochloride 1 ml ampoules 400 mcg/ml (adult Narcan)
    - adrenaline (epinephrine) 1:10 000 and 1:1000
    - human albumin solution 4.5%
    - THAM (tris-hydroxymethyl-amino-methane) 7%
    - sodium bicarbonate 4.2%
    - dextrose 10%
    - vitamin K_1 1 mg ampoules
    - normal saline 0.9%
- Stethoscope
- Cord clamps
- Warmed dry towels
- Adhesive tape for tube fixation

---

straightens the trachea (Fig. 38.4). Hyperextension may cause airway obstruction owing to the short neck of the neonate and large, ill-supported tongue.

Stimulation

Rough handling of the baby merely serves to increase shock and is unnecessary. Gentle stimulation by drying the baby and clearing the airway may initiate

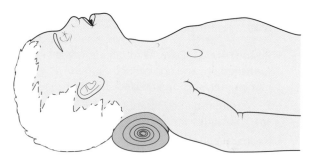

Fig. 38.4 Small towel under the neck.

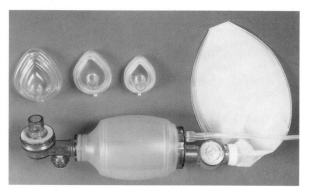

Fig. 38.5 Face-mask sizes, self-inflating bag and face mask. (From Medical Photography Department, Royal Group of Hospitals, Belfast, with permission.)

breathing, but there are a number of different methods that can be used, for example a single finger flick to the sole of the foot, or gentle back rubbing; this will give an indication as to whether tactile stimulation is likely to be effective. Under no circumstances should the method used cause significant pain or bruising. A number of unsafe methods of stimulation have been used including back slapping and sternal pressure, which could physically damage the baby. Directing a low flow (2–4 L/min) of oxygen over the baby's face may be all that is needed to stimulate a gasp reflex (Drew et al 2000).

Warmth

Hypothermia exacerbates hypoxia as essential oxygen and glucose are diverted from the vital centres in order to create heat for survival. Wet towels should be removed and the baby's body and head should be covered with a prewarmed blanket leaving only the chest exposed. **NB** It is hazardous to use a silver swaddler under a radiant heater because this could cause burning.

Clearing the airway

Most babies require no airway clearance at birth; however, if there is obvious respiratory difficulty a suction catheter may be used size 10 FG (8 FG in preterm babies). It is recommended that the catheter tip should be inserted not further than 5 cm and that each suction attempt should last not longer than 5 seconds (Royal College of Paediatrics and Child Health 1997). Even with a soft catheter it is still possible to traumatise the delicate mucosa, especially in the premature baby. If meconium is present in the airway, suction

under direct vision should be performed by passing a laryngoscope and visualising the larynx (Roberton 1992). Care should be taken to avoid touching the vocal cords as this may induce laryngospasm, apnoea and bradycardia. Thick meconium may need to be aspirated out of the trachea through an endotracheal tube.

Ventilation and oxygenation

If the baby fails to respond to these simple measures, assisted ventilation is necessary. This can be achieved in a variety of ways. Face-mask ventilation is the most commonly used method of inflating the baby's lungs. It is effective and relatively safe in experienced hands. Choose an appropriately sized mask (usually 00 or 0/1) (Fig. 38.5) and position it on the face so that it covers the nose and mouth and ensures a good seal. Use a 500 ml bag (Fig. 38.5) as a smaller 250 ml bag does not permit sustained inflation. Care should be taken not to apply pressure on the soft tissue under the jaw as this may obstruct the airway. To aerate the lungs deliver five sustained inflations using oxygen or air, or a combination of both, with a pressure of 30 cmH_2O applied for 2–3 seconds and repeated five times, then continue to ventilate at a rate of 40 respirations per minute (Drew et al 2000, Vyas et al 1981). Insertion of a neonatal airway helps to prevent obstruction by the baby's tongue. Note that overextension of the baby's head causes airway obstruction. A longer inspiration phase improves oxygenation. Higher inflation pressures may be required to produce chest movement (Milner 1991). Bag and mask technique therefore

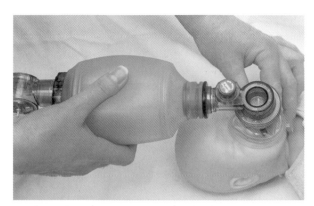

Fig. 38.6 Bagging demonstration. (From Medical Photography Department, Royal Group of Hospitals, Belfast, with permission.)

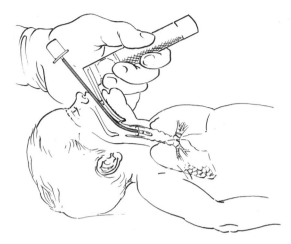

Fig. 38.7 Endotracheal intubation. (From Brendan Ellis, medical illustrator, Royal Group of Hospitals, Belfast, with permission.)

requires a skilled operator to achieve success (Fig. 38.6). Used correctly this method can avoid the need for endotracheal intubation (Palme-Kilander 1992).

Endotracheal intubation. If the baby fails to respond to intermittent positive pressure ventilation (IPPV) by bag and mask, or if bradycardia is present, an endotracheal tube should be passed without delay. Intubating a baby requires special skill that, once acquired, must be practised to be retained. The midwife can learn this skill by practice on models.

Technique for intubation

Ensure that all the equipment listed in Box 38.2 is available and in working order. Position the baby on a flat surface, preferably a resuscitaire, and extend the neck into the 'neutral position'. A rolled-up towel placed under the shoulders will help maintain proper alignment. The blade of the laryngoscope is introduced over the baby's tongue into the pharynx until the epiglottis is seen. Elevation of the epiglottis by the tip of the laryngoscope reveals the vocal cords. Any mucus, blood or meconium obstructing the trachea should be cleared by careful suction prior to passing the endotracheal tube a distance of 1.5–2 cm into the trachea (Fig. 38.7). (Pressure on the cricoid cartilage may facilitate visualisation of the larynx.) Intubation may be easier if a tracheal introducer made of plastic-covered soft metal wire is used. This will increase the stiffness and curvature of the tube. After the laryngoscope is removed, oxygen is administered by IPPV to the endotracheal tube via the Ambu bag. A maximum of 30 cm water pressure should be applied, as there is

risk of rupture of alveoli or tension pneumothorax if higher pressure is applied. The rise and fall of the chest wall should indicate whether the tube is in the trachea. This can be confirmed by auscultation of the chest. Distension of the stomach indicates oesophageal intubation necessitating resiting of the tube.

Mouth-to-face/nose resuscitation

In the absence of specialised equipment, assisted ventilation can be achieved by mouth-to-face resuscitation. With the baby's head in the 'sniffing' position the operator places her mouth over the baby's mouth and nose and, using only the air in her buccal cavity, breathes gently into the baby's airway at a rate of 20 breaths per minute, allowing the infant to exhale between breaths. It may be easier with larger babies to use mouth-to-nose resuscitation (Tonkin et al 1995).

External cardiac massage

Chest compressions should be performed if the heart rate is less than 60, or between 60 and 100 and falling despite adequate ventilation. The most effective way of achieving this is by encircling the baby's chest with the fingers on the spine and thumbs on the lower midsternum (Fig. 38.8) (David 1988, Graves 1988, Milner 1991, Roberton 1992). The chest is depressed at a rate of 100–120 times per minute, at a ratio of

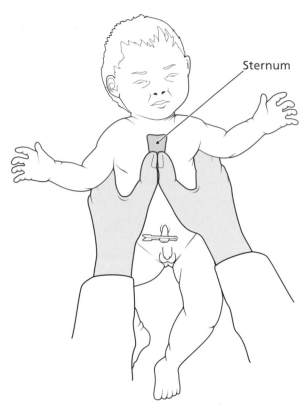

Sternum

Fig. 38.8 External cardiac massage.

three compressions to one ventilation, and at a depth of a third of the baby's chest. (Excessive pressure over the lower end of the sternum may cause rib, lung or liver damage.)

Use of drugs

If the baby's response is slow or he remains hypotonic after ventilation is achieved, consideration will be given to the use of drugs. In specialist obstetric units, pulse oximetry (see Ch. 39) may be employed to monitor hypoxia (Letko 1996) and blood obtained through the umbilical artery or vein to ascertain biochemical status (Harris et al 1996). Results will enable appropriate administration of resuscitation drugs, as discussed below.

Naloxone hydrochloride. This is not an emergency drug per se and should be used with caution and only in specific circumstances. It is a powerful antiopioid drug used to reverse the effects of maternal narcotic drugs given in the preceding 3 hours. Ventilation

should be established prior to its use. *It must not be given to apnoeic babies.* A dose of up to 100 micrograms per kilogram body weight may be administered intramuscularly for prolonged action (Drew et al 2000). As opioid action may persist for some hours the midwife must be alert for signs of relapse when a repeat dose may be required. *NB It should not be administered to babies of narcotic-addicted mothers as this may precipitate acute withdrawal* (Gibbs et al 1989). Policies relating to dosage and route of administration may vary in different hospitals.

Sodium bicarbonate. This is not recommended for brief periods of cardiopulmonary resuscitation. Once tissues are oxygenated by lung inflation with 100% oxygen and cardiac compression, the acidosis will self-correct unless asphyxia is very severe. If the heart rate is less than 60 despite effective ventilation, chest compression and two intravenous doses of adrenaline (epinephrine), then sodium bicarbonate 4.2% solution (0.5 mmol/ml), can be administered using 2–4 ml/kg (1–2 mmol/kg) by slow intravenous injection at a rate of 1 ml/min in order to avoid rapid elevation of serum osmolality with the attendant risk of intracranial haemorrhage (Drew et al 2000, Howell 1987). *It should not be given prior to ventilation being established.* THAM 7% (tris-hydroxymethyl-aminomethane), 0.5 mmol/kg may be used in preference to sodium bicarbonate (Roberton 1992).

Adrenaline (epinephrine). This is indicated if the heart rate is less than 60 despite 1 minute of effective ventilation and chest compression. An initial dose of 0.1–0.3 ml/kg of 1:10 000 solution (10–30 mcg/kg) can be given intravenously; this can be repeated after 3 minutes for a further two doses. The Royal College of Paediatrics and Child Health (1997) recommends a higher dose of 100 mcg/kg i.v. if there is no response to the boluses. It is reasonable to try giving one dose via the endotracheal tube of adrenaline (epinephrine) 0.1 ml/kg of 1:1000 as this sometimes has an immediate effect (Halliday et al 1998).

Human albumin 4.5%. This is infrequently needed in practice. If pulmonary haemorrhage or sign of shock persists despite adequate resuscitation then 4.5% human albumin 10–20 ml/kg as a volume expander should be administered as quickly as possible. Despite the ongoing controversy over the use of human albumin solution, there is currently insufficient evidence on which to base the choice between crystalloid and colloid for resuscitation. The use of human albumin solution in neonates is widespread and based on clinical experience (Drew et al 2000).

Hypoglycaemia is not usually a problem unless resuscitation has been prolonged. A solution of dextrose 10% 3 ml/kg may be given intravenously to correct a blood sugar of less than 2.5 mmol/L.

Observations and aftercare

Throughout the resuscitation procedure the baby's response should be monitored and recorded. An accurate written record detailing the resuscitation events is essential, not only because it forms an integral part of the medical and midwifery management of the baby, but also because it can help to protect the practitioner if defence of her actions is required. The endotracheal tube may be left in place for a few minutes after the baby starts to breathe spontaneously. Suction may be applied through the endotracheal tube as it is removed. There are some babies who at birth may be somewhat distressed but improve with good resuscitation, so that they require observations for a while before a decision is made whether to admit to a postnatal ward or the neonatal unit. The delivery suite is an ideal place for this form of transitional care to take place. A baby whose Apgar score was less than 6 at 5 minutes, or who was slow to respond to resuscitation, or who requires continued ventilatory assistance, should be transferred to the neonatal unit for a period of observation in order to monitor behaviour and detect early signs of hypoxic ischaemic encephalopathy (HIE) (see Ch. 44).

Explanation about the resuscitation and the need for transfer to hospital (if born at home) or to the neonatal unit must be given to the parents and, provided that the baby's condition permits, the mother should have the opportunity to see and hold her baby prior to separation. This assists the attachment process previously described. Babies who respond quickly to resuscitation can be reunited with their parents, remaining in the delivery room until the usual transfer time to the postnatal ward where their care continues as normal.

The principles of resuscitation of the newborn are applicable wherever and whenever apnoea occurs. The midwife must be able to implement emergency care whilst awaiting medical assistance (Box 38.3).

It can be seen that the midwife's role at the time of delivery is one both of privilege and of immense responsibility. Her wish to meet the psychological needs of the parents and the baby must be tempered with the need to accommodate the baby's necessary adaptations at the time of birth and to institute emergency care when required. Continued care of the newborn takes the history of the baby's condition at delivery into account and is discussed in Chapter 39.

Box 38.3 Resuscitation action plan

A	Anticipation	assessment (Apgar)	airway – clear debris
B	Breathing	bag + mask	endotracheal tube
C	Circulation	cardiac massage	caring-warmth, comfort
D	Doctor	drugs	documentation
E	Explanation	Family	
F	Follow-up care	Environment	

Key points of resuscitation

1. Anticipate problems
2. Check resuscitation equipment
3. Start clock
4. Suctioning
5. Keep warm
6. Apgar score
7. Oxygen
8. Bag and mask ventilation
9. Endotracheal ventilation
10. Cardiac massage
11. Drugs
12. Other problems

REFERENCES

Apgar V 1953 A proposal for a new method of evaluation of the newborn infant. Current Research in Anaesthesiology and Analgesics 40:340

Bakhshi S, Deorari A K, Roy S et al 1996 Prevention of subclinical vitamin K deficiency based on PIVKA-11 levels: oral versus intramuscular route. Indian Pediatrics 33:10040–10043

Barclay L, Lupton D 1999 The experiences of new fatherhood: a socio-cultural analysis. Journal of Advanced Nursing April 29(4):1013–1020

Bedford V, Johnson N 1988 The role of the father. Midwifery 4:190–195

Brueggemeyer A 1993 Neonatal thermoregulation. In: Kenner C, Brueggemeyer A, Gunderson L P (eds) Comprehensive neonatal nursing: a physiologic perspective. W B Saunders, Philadelphia

Callister L C 1995 Cultural meanings of childbirth. Journal of Obstetric, Gynecologic, and Neonatal Nursing 24(4):327–331

Catlaneo A, Buzzetti P 2001 effects on rates of breastfeeding in training for the baby friendly hospital initiative. British Medical Journal 323:1358–1362

Cornelissen E A M, Kolee L A A, De Abreu R A et al 1992 Effects of oral and intramuscular vitamin K prophylaxis on vitamin K1, PIVKA-11, and clotting factors in breast fed infants. Archives of Disease in Childhood 67:1250–1254

Dahm L S, James L S 1972 Newborn temperature and calculated heat loss in the delivery room. Pediatrics 49(4):504–513

David R 1988 Closed chest cardiac massage in the newborn infant. Pediatrics 81(4):552–554

Dawkins M, Hull D 1964 Brown adipose tissue in the response of newborn rabbits too cold. Journal of Physiology 172:215–238

de Château P 1987 Promotion of mother–infant relationship during delivery. In: Harvey D (ed) Parent–infant relationships. Wiley series on perinatal practice. John Wiley, Chichester, vol 4

Drew D, Jevon P, Ravy M 2000 Resuscitation of the newborn: a practical approach. Butterworth-Heinemann, Oxford

Gibbs J, Newson T, Williams J, Davidson D C 1989 Naloxone hazards in infants of opioid abusers. Lancet 2(8655):159–160

Golding J, Paterson M, Kinlen L J 1990 Factors associated with childhood cancer in a national cohort study. British Journal of Cancer 62:304–308

Golding J, Greenwood R, Birmingham K, Mott M 1992 Childhood cancer, intramuscular vitamin K and pethidine given during labour. British Medical Journal 305:341–346

Graves B 1988 Challenges of neonatal resuscitation for nurse-midwives. Journal of Nurse-Midwifery 33(5):217–224

Greer F R, Marshall S P, Severson R R et al 1998 A new mixed micellar preparation for oral vitamin K prophylaxis: randomised controlled comparison with an intramuscular formulation in breast fed infants. Archives of Disease in Childhood 79:300–305

Greer P S 1988 Head coverings for newborns under radiant warmers. Journal of Obstetric, Gynecologic, and Neonatal Nursing 17:265–271

Halliday H L, McClure B G, Reid M 1998 Handbook of neonatal intensive care, 4th edn. W B Saunders, London

Harris M, Beckley S L, Garibaldi J M, Keith R D F, Greene K R 1996 Umbilical cord blood analysis at the time of delivery. Midwifery 12(3):146–150

Herbert M, Sluckin A 1985 A realistic look at mother–infant bonding. In: Chiswick M (ed) Recent advances in perinatal medicine 2. Churchill Livingstone, Edinburgh

Heyman M 1989 Arachidonic acid derivatives in the perinatal period. In: Barness L, De Vivo D, Morrow G, Oski F, Rudolph A (eds) Advances in pediatrics 36. Year Book Medical, Chicago, p 151–176

Holdcroft A 1980 Body temperature control in anesthesia, surgery and intensive care. Baillière Tindall, London

Howell J 1987 Sodium bicarbonate in the perinatal setting – revisited. Clinics in Perinatology 14(4):807–816

Jacobs M, Phibbs R 1989 Prevention, recognition and treatment of perinatal asphyxia. Clinics in Perinatology 16(4):785–807

Karlsson H 1996 Skin to skin care: heat balance. Archives of Disease in Childhood 75(2):F130–F132

Klaus M H, Kennell J H 1989 Parent infant bonding, 3rd edn. C V Mosby, St Louis

Klaus M H, Trause M A, Kennell J H 1975 Does human maternal behaviour after delivery show a characteristic pattern? In: CIBA Foundation Symposium 33, parent–infant interaction. Associated Scientific, Amsterdam

Letko M D 1996 Understanding the Apgar score. Journal of Obstetric, Gynecologic, and Neonatal Nursing 25(4):299–303

Lim M K, Hanretty K, Houston A B, Lilley S, Murtagh E P 1992 Intermittent ductal patency in healthy newborn infants: demonstration by colour Doppler flow mapping. Archives of Disease in Childhood 67(10):1217–1218T

Mercer J S, Nelson C C, Skovgaard R L 2000 Umbilical cord clamping: beliefs and practices of American nurse-midwives. Journal of Midwifery and Women's Health 45(1):58–65

Milner A D 1991 Resuscitation of the newborn. Archives of Disease in Childhood 66(1):66–69

Motohara K, Endo F, Matsuda I Effect of vitamin K administration in acarboxy prothrombin (PIVKA-11) levels in newborns. Lancet 1985 2:242–244

Nelle M, Zilow E P, Kraus M 1993 The effect of Leboyer delivery on blood viscosity and other hemorheologic parameters in term neonates. American Journal of Obstetrics and Gynecology 169(1):189–193

Palme-Kilander C 1992 Methods of resuscitation in low-Apgar-score newborn infants – a national survey. Acta Paediatrica 81:739–744

Parkinson C E, Harvey D 1987 Child development and the maternal–infant relationship. In: Harvey D (ed) Parent–infant relationships. Wiley series on perinatal practice. John Wiley, Chichester, vol 4

Perry S E 1995 The newborn. In: Bobak I M, Lowdermilk D L, Jensen M D (eds) Maternity nursing, 4th edn. CV Mosby, St Louis

Puckett R M, Offringa M 2000 The Dutch Cochrane Centre, The Netherlands

Roberton N R C 1992 Resuscitation of the newborn. In: Roberton N R C (ed) Textbook of neonatology. Churchill Livingstone, Edinburgh.

Royal College of Paediatrics and Child Health 1997 Resuscitation of babies at birth. BMJ Publishing, London

Rutter N 1992 Temperature control and its disorders. In: Roberton N R C (ed) Textbook of neonatology. Churchill Livingstone, Edinburgh

Salariya E 1990 Parental–infant attachment. In: Alexander J, Levy V, Roch S (eds) Postnatal care – a research based approach. Macmillan, Basingstoke

Salariya E, Easton P, Cater J 1979 Early and often for best results. Nursing Mirror 148(22):15–17

Sharma R K, Marwaha N, Kumar P, Narang A 1995 Effect of oral water soluble vitamin K on PIVKA-11 levels in newborns. Indian Pediatrics 32:863–867

Silverman F, Suidan J, Wasserman J, Antoine C, Young B 1985 The Apgar score: is it enough? Obstetrics and Gynaecology 66:331–336

Sinclair J C 1992 Management of the thermal environment. In: Sinclair J C, Bracken M B (eds) Effective care of the newborn infant. Oxford University Press, Oxford

Sluckin W, Sluckin A, Herbert M 1984 On mother-to-infant bonding. Midwife, Health Visitor and Community Nurse 20(11):404–407

Thomas K 1994 Thermoregulation in neonates. Neonatal Network 13(2):15–22

Tonkin S L, Davis S L, Gunn T R 1995 Nasal route for infant resuscitation by mothers. Lancet 345(8961):1353–1354

Tyson J E 1992 Immediate care of the newborn infant. In: Sinclair J E, Bracken M B (eds) Effective care of the newborn infant. Oxford University Press, Oxford

Ulusahin N, Arsan S, Ertogan F 1996 Effects of oral and intramuscular vitamin K prophylaxis on PIVKA-11 assay parameters in breastfed infants in Turkey. Turkish Journal of Pediatrics 38:295–300

Vyas H, Milner A D, Hopkin I E 1981 Physiologic responses to prolonged slow rise inflation in the resuscitation of the asphyxiated newborn infant. Journal of Paediatrics 99:635–639

White D G, Woollet E A 1987 The father's role in the neonatal period. In: Harvey D (ed) Parent–infant relationships. Wiley series on perinatal practice. John Wiley, Chichester, vol 4

Wildman J 1995 Is this finally it? New Generation 14(2):5

Williams R P 1995 Family dynamics after childbirth. In: Bobak I M, Lowdermilk D L, Jensen M D (eds) Maternity nursing, 4th edn. CV Mosby, St Louis

Wong D L (ed) 1995 Whaley and Wong's nursing care of infants and children, 5th edn. CV Mosby, St Louis

Zipursky A 1999 Prevention of vitamin K deficiency bleeding in newborns. British Journal of Haematology 19 104:430–437

FURTHER READING

Beachy P, Deacon J 1993 The core curriculum for neonatal intensive care nursing. W B Saunders, Philadelphia

This book is written for nurses caring for high risk babies. As well as providing information regarding the physiological problems of the sick newborn, it also deals with problems concerning the family, legal and ethical issues.

Bracken M, Sinclair J 1992 Effective care of the newborn infant. Oxford University Press, Oxford

This informative textbook covers all aspects of neonatal conditions with contributions from many neonatal specialists. It should be used as a reference to complement conditions discussed in the chapter.

Drew D, Jevon P, Raby M 2000 Resuscitation of the newborn, a practical approach. Butterworth-Heinemann, Oxford

This book gives very practical knowledge regarding resuscitation; it is a clear well-researched book, with learning objectives clearly defined for each chapter.

Halliday H L, McClure B G, Reid M 1998 Handbook of neonatal intensive care, 4th edn. W B Saunders, London

This is an up-to-date handbook on neonatal care with recommendations of care derived from evidence-based medicine. It gives step-by-step management guidelines for both common and uncommon disorders of the newborn, based on current knowledge and clinical experience.

Kenner C, Wright Lott J, Flandermeyer A 1998 Comprehensive neonatal nursing: a physiologic perspective, 2nd edn. W B Saunders, Philadelphia

This book provides a comprehensive approach to neonatal care, and is an essential text for those caring for newborn babies and their families.

Rennie J M, Roberton N R C (eds) 1999 Textbook of neonatology, 3rd edn. Churchill Livingstone, Edinburgh

This is a valuable book for resource material; as well as covering all the conditions that effect the baby it covers topics such as litigation and how the law relates to the baby. It also looks at ethical and moral questions raised because of modern intensive care.

39 The Normal Baby

Philomena Farrell Norma Sittlington

CHAPTER CONTENTS

The normal neonate continues to adapt to extrauterine life in the first weeks after delivery, remaining vulnerable to airway obstruction, hypothermia, hypoglycaemia and infection. This necessitates the provision of an environment that is optimal for physiological needs. The provision of this environment, normally by the mother, is sustained by the developing mother–baby relationship. Extrauterine life presents a challenge to the newborn baby. The most important changes, those in the heart and lungs, take place at birth (see Ch. 38); however, continued adaptations are necessary in the first weeks of life as the baby assumes independence from the maternal and placental nurturing which was enjoyed before birth. The baby remains dependent on the mother or other caregiver for nutrition and protection, but is responsible for maintaining metabolism and homeostasis among other functions essential for survival.

The chapter aims to:

- describe the external features of the normal newborn baby

- discuss the functioning of the different body systems in relation to their stage of maturity and the changes taking place at birth

- describe the behaviour of the baby during the first weeks of life

- detail the systematic examination of the baby at birth and the subsequent daily examinations

- discuss the care of the baby and the measures employed to ensure security and safety and promotion of normal growth and development

- highlight the role of the midwife in promoting confidence and competence in the parents and encouraging interaction between them and their baby.

General characteristics

Appearance

A normal term baby weighs approximately 3.5 kg, when fully extended measures 50 cm from the crown of the head to the heels, has on average an occipito-frontal head circumference of 34–35 cm. Most babies are plump and have a prominent abdomen. They lie in an attitude of flexion, with arms extended their fingers reach upper thigh level.

Vernix caseosa is a white sticky substance, present on the baby's skin at birth. The amount of vernix is variable. It is thought to have a protective function in utero and after birth dries up and flakes off within a few hours.

The skin

One of the largest organs in the body, the skin has an important role in temperature regulation and provides protection from acquired infection. It can also give the carer a guide to the overall well-being of the baby. The midwife must be knowledgeable about the normal parameters of neonatal skin, which differs somewhat from adult skin (Michie 1996).

The skin of a newborn baby is thin, delicate, and easily traumatised by friction, pressure or substances with a different pH. This renders the skin prone to blistering, excoriation and infection. Although sterile at birth, the skin is colonised by microorganisms within 24 hours. The skin of babies born at term has a pH of 6.4, which reduces to 4.9 over 3–4 days (Irving 2001). The low pH of the skin surface (pH < 5) creates an 'acid mantle', which protects against infection.

The umbilical cord's position on the anterior abdominal wall predisposes to its contamination from excreta. The stump is rapidly colonised and necroses and separates by a process of dry gangrene, usually within the first 10 days of life.

Downy hair, called lanugo, covers the skin and is plentiful over the shoulders, upper arms and thighs. The general colour of the skin depends on the baby's ethnic origin, ranging from pink and white to olive or dark brown. Peripheral cyanosis is common and is usually of no significance. Pigmentation of nipples and genitalia is deeper in babies with darker skins and a linea nigra may be present. Another feature of racial origin is the Mongolian blue spot, which presents as a diffuse bluish-black area usually over the sacral region. Dark-skinned babies become more pigmented in the first weeks of life though the palms of the hands and soles of the feet remain paler than the rest of the body.

A mature baby has many skin creases on the palms of the hands and soles of the feet. The nails are fully formed and adherent to the tips of the fingers, sometimes extending beyond the fingertips. The hair is soft and silky: some babies have virtually no hair, whereas others have a significant amount of straight or curly hair. The eyebrows and eyelashes present a similar variation. The cartilage of the ears is well formed.

Sebaceous glands, though present in the skin, are relatively inactive. Distended glands, milia, may be present over the nose and cheeks. Sweat glands are present but inactive in the first days of life. The vasoconstrictor mechanism is inefficient because the vascular plexuses are underdeveloped. The baby's poor melanin production renders a vulnerability to sunburn.

Sensitivity to touch and pressure, heat and cold, and pain are mediated through the skin.

Physiology

Respiratory system

At birth the respiratory system is developmentally incomplete, growth of new alveoli continuing for several years. The lumen of the peripheral airways is narrow, which predisposes to atelectasis. Respiratory secretions are more plentiful than in an adult and the mucous membranes are delicate and sensitive to trauma, the area below the vocal cords being particularly prone to oedema (see also Ch. 38).

The normal baby has a respiratory rate of 30–60 breaths per minute, and breathing is diaphragmatic, chest and abdomen rising and falling synchronously. The breathing pattern is erratic. Respirations are shallow and irregular, being interspersed with brief 10–15 second periods of apnoea (Perry 1995). This is known as *periodic breathing*. Apart from the initial profound respiratory efforts at birth, no nasal flaring, sternal or subcostal recession or grunting is present. The pattern of respiration alters during sleeping and waking states. Babies are obligatory nose breathers and do not convert automatically to mouth breathing when nasal obstruction occurs. Respiratory difficulties can occur because of neurological, metabolic, circulatory or thermoregulatory dysfunction as well as infection, airway obstruction or abnormalities of the respiratory tract itself.

Babies have a lusty cry, which evokes an immediate response from carers. The cry is normally loud and of medium pitch unless neurological damage, infection or hypothermia is present, when it may be high pitched or weak. Transient cyanosis may arise in the first few days when the baby is crying and altered pressure gradients recreate right-to-left shunts within the heart and great vessels. This is of no clinical significance (see Ch. 38).

Cardiovascular system and blood

The changes in the baby's heart at birth have been described in Chapter 38. The heart rate is rapid, 120–160 beats per minute, and fluctuates in accordance with the baby's respiratory function and activity or sleep state. Peripheral circulation is sluggish. This results in mild cyanosis of hands, feet and circumoral areas and in generalised mottling when the skin is exposed. Blood pressure fluctuates according to activity and ranges from 50–55/25–30 mmHg to 80/50 mmHg in the first 10 days of life (Roberton 1996). It is considered that, even at rest, the baby's heart probably functions at full capacity, rendering the baby vulnerable to additional stress (Blackburn & Loper 1992).

The total circulating blood volume at birth is 80 millilitres per kilogram bodyweight. However, this may be raised if there is delay in clamping the umbilical cord at birth. The haemoglobin level is high (13–20 g/dl), of which 50–85% is fetal haemoglobin (Blackburn & Loper 1992). Conversion from fetal to adult haemoglobin, which commenced in utero, is completed in the first 1–2 years of life. Haemoglobin, red cell count ($5–7 \times 10^{12}$/L) and haematocrit (55%) levels decrease gradually during the first 2–3 months of life, during which time erythropoiesis is suppressed. The white cell count is high initially (18.0×10^{9}/L) but decreases rapidly (Perry 1995, Roberton 1992).

Breakdown of excess red blood cells in the liver and spleen predisposes to jaundice in the first week. Because colonisation of the intestine by the bacteria, which synthesise vitamin K, is delayed until feeding is established, vitamin-K-dependent clotting factors II (prothrombin), VII, IX and X are low. This inhibits blood clotting during the first week. Platelet levels equal those of the adult, but there is a reduced capacity for adhesion and aggregation (Blackburn & Loper 1992).

Temperature regulation

Thermal control in the neonate remains poor for some time. Initial thermal adaptation and modes of heat loss and gain have been described in Chapter 38. Owing to the immaturity of the hypothalamus, temperature regulation is inefficient and the baby remains vulnerable to hypothermia particularly when exposed to cold or draughts, when wet, when unable to move about freely, or when deprived of nutrition. Cold babies are unable to shiver; therefore they attempt to maintain body heat by adopting a flexed fetal posture, increasing their respiratory rate and activity. These activities increase calorie consumption and may result in hypoglycaemia, which in turn will compound the effects of hypothermia, as do hypoxia, acidosis and hyperbilirubinaemia (see Chs 32 and 46).

The baby's normal core temperature is 36–37°C. A healthy, clothed, term baby will maintain this body temperature satisfactorily provided the environmental temperature is sustained between 18 and 21°C, nutrition is adequate and movements are not restricted by tight swaddling. However, like adults, babies are individuals with differing metabolic rates. This makes finite statements of thermoneutral range difficult (Hull et al 1996a,b). Hyperthermia can occur when the baby is exposed to a radiant heat source. Sweating may occur, especially over the forehead, although the neonate's ability to sweat is limited. An unstable temperature may indicate infection.

Renal system

Though the kidneys are functional in fetal life, their workload is minimal until after birth. They are functionally immature. The glomerular filtration rate is low and tubular reabsorption capabilities are limited. The baby is not able to concentrate or dilute urine very well in response to variations in fluid intake, nor compensate for high or low levels of solutes in the blood. This results in a narrow margin between homeostasis and fluid imbalance (see Ch. 47). The ability to excrete drugs is also limited and the baby's renal function is vulnerable to physiological stress (Blackburn & Loper 1992, Perry 1995, Roberton 1992). The first urine is passed at birth or within the first 24 hours and there-after with increasing frequency as fluid intake rises. The urine is dilute, straw coloured and odourless. Cloudiness caused by mucus and urates may be present initially until fluid intake increases. Urates may cause pink staining, which is insignificant. As the neonatal pelvis is small, the bladder becomes palpable abdominally when full.

Gastrointestinal system

The gastrointestinal tract of the neonate is structurally complete though functionally immature in comparison with that of the adult (Blackburn & Loper 1992, Perry 1995, Roberton 1992). The mucous membrane of the mouth is pink and moist. The teeth are buried in the gums and ptyalin secretion is low. Small epithelial pearls are sometimes present at the junction of the hard and soft palates. Sucking pads in the cheeks give them a full appearance. Sucking and swallowing reflexes are coordinated.

The stomach has a small capacity (15–30 ml), which increases rapidly in the first weeks of life. The cardiac sphincter is weak, predisposing to regurgitation or posseting. Gastric acidity, equal to that of the adult within a few hours after delivery, diminishes rapidly within the first few days and by the 10th day the baby is virtually achlorhydric, which increases the risk of infection. Gastric emptying time is normally 2–3 hours.

In relation to the size of the baby the intestine is long, containing large numbers of secretory glands and a large surface area for the absorption of nutrients. Enzymes are present though there is a deficiency of amylase and lipase, which diminishes the baby's ability to digest compound carbohydrates and fat. When food enters the stomach a gastrocolic reflex results in the opening of the ileocaecal valve. The contents of the ileum pass into the large intestine and rapid peristalsis means that feeding is often accompanied by reflex emptying of the bowel.

The gut is sterile at birth but is colonised within a few hours. Bowel sounds are present within 1 hour of birth. Meconium, present in the large intestine from 16 weeks' gestation, is passed within the first 24 hours of life and is totally excreted within 48–72 hours. This first stool is blackish-green in colour, is tenacious and contains bile, fatty acids, mucus and epithelial cells.

From the 3rd to 5th day the stools undergo a transitional stage and are brownish-yellow in colour. Once feeding is established, yellow faeces are passed. The consistency and frequency of stools reflect the type of feeding. breastmilk results in loose, bright yellow and inoffensive acid stools. The baby may pass 8 to 10 stools a day, or pass stools as infrequently as every 2 or 3 days. The stools of the bottle-fed baby are paler in colour, semiformed, less acidic and have a slightly sharp smell (Roberton 1992).

Physiological immaturity of the liver results in low production of glucuronyl transferase for the conjugation of bilirubin. This, together with a high level of red cell breakdown, and stimulation of hepatic blood flow may result in a transient jaundice, which is manifest on the 3rd to 5th days (see also Ch. 46). Glycogen stores are rapidly depleted, so early feeding is required to maintain normal blood glucose levels (2.6–4.4 mmol/L). Feeding stimulates liver function and colonisation of the gut, which assists in the formation of vitamin K.

Infant-feeding practices are designed to meet the physiological needs and capabilities of the baby and are discussed in Chapter 40.

Immunological adaptations

Neonates demonstrate a marked susceptibility to infections, particularly those gaining entry through the mucosa of the respiratory and gastrointestinal systems. Localisation of infection is poor, 'minor' infections having the potential to become generalised very easily.

The baby has some immunoglobulins at birth but the sheltered intrauterine existence limits the need for learned immune responses to specific antigens (Blackburn & Loper 1992, Crockett 1995, Perry 1995, Stern 1992). There are three main immunoglobulins, IgG, IgA and IgM, and of these only IgG is small enough to cross the placental barrier. It affords immunity to specific viral infections. At birth the baby's levels of IgG are equal to or slightly higher than those of the mother. This provides passive immunity during the first few months of life. IgM and IgA do not cross the placental barrier but can be manufactured by the fetus. Levels of IgM at term are 20% those of the adult, taking 2 years to attain adult levels (elevation of IgM levels at birth is suggestive of intrauterine infection). This relatively low level of IgM is thought to render the baby more susceptible to enteric infections. IgA levels are very low and increase slowly, although secretory salivary levels attain adult values within 2 months. IgA protects against infection of the respiratory tract, gastrointestinal tract and eyes. breastmilk, and especially colostrum, provides the baby with passive immunity in the form of *Lactobacillus bifidus*, lactoferrin, lysozyme and secretory IgA among others (see Ch. 40).

The thymus gland, where lymphocytes are produced, is relatively large at birth and continues to grow until 8 years of age.

Reproductive system: genitalia and breasts

In boys the testes are descended into the scrotum, which has plentiful rugae; the urethral meatus opens at the tip of the penis and the prepuce is adherent to the glans. In girls born at term the labia majora normally cover the labia minora; the hymen and clitoris may appear disproportionately large. Spermatogenesis in boys does not occur until puberty, but the total complement of primordial follicles containing primitive ova is present in the ovaries of girls at birth. In both sexes withdrawal of maternal oestrogens results in breast engorgement, sometimes accompanied by secretion of 'milk' by the 4th or 5th day. Baby girls may develop pseudomenstruation for the same reason. Both boys and girls have a nodule of breast tissue around the nipple. Midwives should have the knowledge to reassure and explain the physiological nature of these events to the parents.

Skeletomuscular system

The muscles are complete, subsequent growth occurring by hypertrophy rather than by hyperplasia. The long bones are incompletely ossified to facilitate growth at the epiphyses. The bones of the vault of the skull also reveal lack of ossification. This is essential for growth of the brain and facilitating moulding during labour. Moulding is resolved within a few days of birth. The posterior fontanelle closes at 6–8 weeks. The anterior fontanelle remains open until 18 months of age, making assessment of hydration and intracranial pressure possible by palpation of fontanelle tension.

Psychology and perception

The newborn baby is alert and aware of his surroundings when he is awake. Far from being impassive he reacts to stimuli and begins at a very early age to amass information about his environment (Brazelton 1984).

Special senses

Vision

Though immature, the structures necessary for vision are present and functional at birth. Babies are sensitive to bright lights, which cause them to frown or blink. They demonstrate a preference for bold black and white patterns and the shape of the human face, focusing at a distance of approximately 15–20 cm. This gives babies the ability to establish eye contact with their mother while being nursed and so enhance the bonding process. They can track a moving object briefly within the first 5 days, and by 2 weeks of age can differentiate their mother's face from that of a stranger. Interest in colour, variety and complexity of patterns develops within the first 2 months of life (Blackburn & Loper 1992, Perry 1995, Roberton 1992). The shape of the baby's eyes may reflect racial origin; for instance the epicanthic folds of Oriental babies alter the appearance of the orbital region. No tears are present in the eyes of the newborn, therefore they become infected easily.

Hearing

Newborn babies' eyes turn towards sound. On hearing a high-pitched sound they first blink or startle and then become agitated, and are comforted by low-pitched sounds. They prefer the sound of the human voice to other sounds and within a few weeks the patterns of adult speech are mimicked by reactive movements. Newborn babies can discriminate between voices, giving preference to their mother's (DeCasper & Fifer 1987). This, too, promotes mother–baby interaction.

Smell and taste

Babies prefer the smell of milk to that of other substances and show a preference for human milk. Within a few days babies can differentiate the smell of their mother's milk from that of another woman (MacFarlane

1975). They prefer the smell of an unwashed breast to that of a washed one (Righard 1995). They turn away from unpleasant smells and show preference for sweet taste as is demonstrated by vigorous and sustained sucking and a speedy grimacing response to bitter, salty or sour substances (Blackburn & Loper 1992).

Touch

Babies are acutely sensitive to touch, enjoying skin-to-skin contact, immersion in water, stroking, cuddling and rocking movements (Blackburn & Loper 1992, Perry 1995). A puff of air on the face induces an inspiration or gasp reflex. The grasp reflexes enhance relationship with the mother. Facial coding of pain in babies is expressed by brow bulging, eyelid squeezing, nasolabial furrowing and open lipped crying (Grunau & Craig 1987, Rushforth & Levene 1994).

Sleeping and waking

Following the initiation of respiration at birth, the baby remains alert and reactive for a period of approximately 1 hour, and then relaxes and sleeps. The length of this first sleep varies from a few minutes to several hours and is followed by a second period of reactivity, during which mucus accumulation in the oropharynx may occur, causing choking or gagging (Perry 1995). Subsequent sleeping and waking rhythms show marked variations and the baby takes some time to settle into an individual pattern. Initially, waking periods are related to hunger, but within a few weeks the waking periods last longer and meet the need for social interaction.

Sleep states

Two sleep states are identifiable:

• In *deep sleep*, the baby's eyes are closed, respirations are regular, no eye movements are present and response to stimuli is delayed and quickly suppressed. Jerky movements may occur at intervals.
• In *light sleep*, rapid eye movements are observable through the closed eyelids. Respirations are irregular and sucking movements occur intermittently. Response to stimuli occurs more readily and may result in an alteration of sleep state. Random movements are noted.

Wakeful states

A wider range of awake states is observed, ranging from drowsiness to crying:

• In the *drowsy state*, the baby's eyes may be open or closed with some fluttering of the eyelids. Smiling may occur. Limb movements are variable, generally smooth, but are interspersed by startle responses. Alteration in state occurs more readily following stimulation.
• In the *quiet alert state*, though motor activity is minimal, the baby is alert to visual and auditory stimuli.
• In the *active alert state*, the baby is generally active and reactive to the surrounding environment.
• In the *active crying state*, the baby cries vigorously and may be difficult to console. Muscular activity is considerable. The amount of time that the baby spends in each state varies tremendously and influences the response to stimuli, whether visual, auditory or tactile (Brazelton 1984).

Crying

The crying repertoire of babies distinguishes different needs and is the way in which they communicate discomfort and summon assistance. With experience it is possible to differentiate the cry and identify the need, which may be hunger, thirst, pain, general discomfort (e.g. wanting a change of position or feeling too cold or too hot), boredom, loneliness or a desire for physical and social contact. Maternal anxiety and difficulties related to baby crying can be allayed by information and advice from the midwife. The mother needs to learn how to comfort her baby. Rapid rocking induces sleep, swaddling and an upright position appear to be soothing (Downey & Bidder 1990).

Growth and development

Babies because of their physiological limitations are dependent on their mothers (or other caregiver) for continued survival, growth and development. These will progress satisfactorily only if the baby is physiologically and neurologically normal, is in a safe environment, nutritional needs are met, and psychological development is promoted by appropriate stimulation and loving care. Abnormality of the baby's body systems, inadequate nutrition or emotional deprivation will compromise the baby's ability to grow and develop to full potential (Fry 1994). The relatively immature organ functions and the vulnerability to infection and hypothermia demand that care must be designed to meet needs and capabilities.

Normality of the baby is assessed by a variety of means. This assessment begins at birth.

Examination at birth

All newborn babies should have a quick overall examination performed in the delivery suite as soon as possible after birth to ascertain that, externally at least, the baby is normal, and to assess adaptation to normal extrauterine life. If any defects are identified, medical assistance should be sought. Examination of the baby should, whenever possible, be performed beside the parents. The midwife should talk to them as she proceeds, explaining her findings. Prior to examining the baby the midwife should wash her hands to prevent the spread of infection. Her hands should be warm to prevent chilling of the baby. During the examination the baby should be naked in a warm, draught-free environment. There should be sufficient light to allow the midwife to see the baby clearly. The examination is performed in an orderly manner from the crown to heel. Overall symmetry should be verified and skin blemishes or abrasions noted.

Colour and respirations

Babies are obligatory nose breathers; patency can be assessed by watching the baby breathe in a quiet state. If one nostril is blocked, occlusion of the other results in cyanosis with unsuccessful attempts to breathe through the mouth. Bilateral nasal obstruction is of major significance if due to bilateral choanal atresia, which is a major medical emergency. Observe the colour of the baby's skin and mucous membranes. In the normal baby, the lips and mucous membranes are pink and well perfused.

Face, head and neck

After a general observation of the face, the midwife should inspect the eyes and mouth of the baby. Each eye should be visualised to confirm that it is present and that the lens is clear. The eyes open spontaneously if the baby is held in an upright position. Any slight oedema or bruising is noted but may be insignificant. The normal space between the eyes is up to 3 cm.

The mouth. The mouth can be opened easily by pressing against the angle of the jaw. This allows visual inspection of the tongue, gums and palate. The palate should be high arched, intact and the uvula central. Epithelial pearls (*Epstein's pearls*) may be observed. They occur as a cluster of several white spots in the mouth at the junction of the soft and hard palate in the midline. Less commonly they occur in the alveolar margin or on the prepuce. They are of no significance, but occasionally are mistaken for infection, and they disappear spontaneously. The midwife uses her little finger to feel the palate for any submucous cleft. A normal baby will respond by sucking the finger. Precocious teeth may protrude through the central part of the lower gum. (Though usually covered by epithelial tissue, such teeth may have erupted and be loose, requiring extraction in the early neonatal period to prevent their inhalation.) A tight frenulum will give the appearance of tongue-tie: no treatment is necessary for this.

The ears. These are inspected, noting their position. The upper notch of the pinna should be level with the canthus of the eye. Patency of the external auditory meatus is verified. Accessory auricles, small tags of tissue, are sometimes noted lying in front of the ear. Ear abnormalities can be associated with chromosomal anomalies and syndromes, and should be reported to a paediatrician.

The head and neck bones. By palpating the vault of the skull the midwife can determine the degree of moulding by the amount of overriding of the bones at the sutures and fontanelles. The bones should feel hard in a term baby. A wide anterior fontanelle and splayed sutures may indicate hydrocephalus or immaturity. The shape of the baby's head as a result of moulding gives an indication of the presentation in utero (Fig. 39.1). An oedematous swelling, caput succedaneum, may be noted overlying the part that was presenting. This is a result of pressure from the cervical os and will disappear spontaneously within 24 hours. Parents can be reassured that moulding usually resolves within a few days after birth.

The short thick neck of the baby must be examined to exclude the presence of swellings and to ensure that rotation and flexion of the head are possible.

Chest and abdomen

Observation of respiratory movement should reveal that chest and abdominal movements are synchronous.

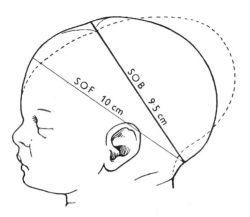

Fig. 39.1 Type of moulding in a vertex presentation (SOB = suboccipitobregmatic; SOF = suboccipitofrontal).

The respirations may still be irregular at this stage. The space between the nipples should be noted, widely spaced nipples being associated with chromosomal abnormality.

The shape of the abdomen should be rounded. The midwife notes any variation, including a scaphoid (boat-shaped) abdomen (which may indicate a malnourished fetus or diaphragmatic hernia) or any protrusions, particularly at the base of the umbilical cord.

The artery forceps securing the umbilical cord should be replaced by a plastic disposable clamp, or elastic bands (according to hospital policy) applied approximately 2 cm from the umbilicus. Excess cord is discarded.

Haemostasis of the umbilical cord is vital. A blood loss of 30 ml from a baby is equivalent to almost half a litre of blood from an adult. Prophylactic vitamin K 1 mg can be given orally or intramuscularly to promote prothrombin formation (Jørgensen et al 1991, Shearer 1995). Midwives must be aware of their local hospital policy (see Ch. 38).

Normally three cord vessels are present. Absence of one of the arteries is occasionally associated with renal anomalies and must be reported to the paediatrician.

Genitalia and anus

The genitalia should be examined carefully. If the sex is uncertain, the paediatrician will initiate investigations. Depending on local policy, the baby's temperature may be taken rectally to detect any excessive cooling and to confirm patency of the anus. This method is less commonly used today. The preferred methods are via the axilla (under the arm), tympanic (ear), or in the groin. The normal baby's skin temperature should range from 36.6 to 37°C.

Limbs and digits

In addition to noting length and movement of the limbs, it is essential that the digits are counted and separated to ensure that webbing is not present. The hands should be opened fully as any accessory digits may be concealed in the clenched fist. The feet are examined for any deformity such as talipes equinovarus, as well as looking for extra digits. The axillae, elbows, groins and popliteal spaces should also be examined for abnormalities. Normal flexion and rotation of the wrist and ankle joints should be confirmed.

Spine

With the baby lying prone the midwife should inspect and palpate the baby's back. Any swellings, dimples or hairy patches may signify an occult spinal defect. (All abnormalities must be reported to a paediatrician.)

Measurements

The baby's head circumference, length and weight are measured to provide parameters against which future growth can be monitored. The head circumference is measured, encircling it at the occipital protuberance and the supraorbital ridges with a measuring tape. Moulding may reduce this measurement and for this reason this estimate is sometimes delayed until the 3rd day when the head shape has resumed its normal contours.

Accurate measurement of the baby's crown–heel length is extremely difficult; this can only be measured accurately using calibrated equipment. In circumstances where this is not available only an approximation of length can be achieved. The midwife should comply with local policy and procedures in this regard. When using calibrated equipment it is essential that the baby's legs are fully extended and that the head and feet are in full contact with the measuring device (Fig. 39.2). This requires assistance from a second person (which may be the mother). The practice of suspending the baby upside down for measuring purposes is outmoded and hazardous for the reasons stated in Ch. 38. It is advisable to record the method by which the baby was measured in order that the validity of this basic parameter can be taken into

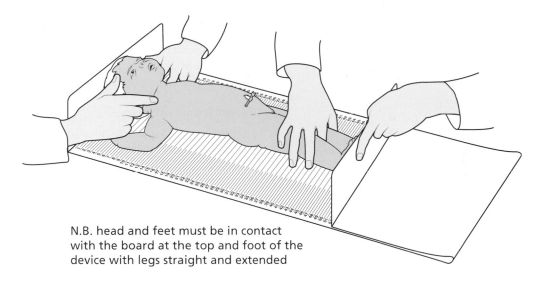

N.B. head and feet must be in contact
with the board at the top and foot of the
device with legs straight and extended

Fig. 39.2 Calibrated equipment length measurement.

account if future assessments reveal a discrepancy. It is suggested that serial length measurements monitoring growth should be made by the same individual to improve reliability (Doull et al 1995).

When the baby is weighed and the identity bands are verified as correct, they are then attached one to the arm and one on the leg, though this may vary according to local hospital policy. The baby is then dressed and wrapped in warm blankets.

Documentation

The midwife records her findings in the case notes, and any abnormalities are brought to the attention of the paediatrician, or GP if a home birth, and receiving midwife in the postnatal ward. Midwives must adhere to the Guidelines for records and record keeping (UKCC 1998).

Observation and general care

Identification and security procedures

In hospital, the midwife receiving the baby from the delivery suite staff should verify that the baby's name, sex, date and time of birth on the two namebands match the information in the case notes and are entered on to the cot card. The namebands should remain on the baby until discharge from hospital. It is recommended that the presence of two legible, matching,

correct namebands is verified daily, on transfer to other wards and on discharge from hospital. If the information becomes illegible, or a nameband is lost, new nameband(s) should be prepared, verified with the mother *and replaced in her presence*. The replacement of the namebands should be documented in the case notes. In the event of a baby being found without any namebands the midwife must notify the unit manager and comply with local policy and procedures for their replacement. No mother should ever be in any doubt about her baby's identity (Laurent 1992).

Abduction of babies from hospitals has led to the development of security tagging and other monitoring devices being employed in recent years (Day 1995). It is advisable that the mother accompanies her baby at all times and she should be able to identify members of staff who are involved in her baby's care. Staff must be alert to the movement of babies and mothers in their care.

Rest

Following the necessary administrative procedures, the baby should be warmly dressed and placed in a pre-heated cot beside the mother to allow him to rest until feeding time. During these first few hours after birth, the midwife should observe the baby frequently for any colour changes, patency of airway and haemorrhage from the umbilical cord. Temperature should also be monitored to ensure that it is maintained within the normal range. The mother's wishes regarding feeding should be determined early on so that the midwife can plan the baby's nutritional needs (see Ch. 40). Promotion of parent–baby relationships is integral to all aspects of care.

Neonatal care

In caring for the normal baby it is the midwife's duty to ensure that the baby is made comfortable, fed and that facilities are available for the parents to help them with the attachment process. It is also important to ensure that the baby is protected from:

- airway obstruction
- hypothermia
- infection
- injury and accident.

Prevention of airway obstruction

Choking can occur during feeding if coordination is poor, and also following vomiting or regurgitation of mucus or feed. According to guidelines it is important for a baby to sleep in the supine position (on his back) or side with the feet at the foot of the cot (Fig. 39.3) (Foundation for the Study of Infant Deaths 1996, Lerner 1993). Suction apparatus should be readily available so that aspiration of the baby's airway can be effected quickly.

Prevention of hypothermia

Overexposure of the baby should be avoided to prevent heat loss. Where possible the room temperature should be maintained at 18–21°C. In hospital, and where higher ambient temperatures are able to be maintained, the baby should be dressed in a cotton gown or baby grow and covered by two cellular blankets. An additional blanket underneath the bottom sheet will provide extra warmth for babies who are having difficulty in maintaining a stable body temperature. At home, or in cold environments, extra blankets may be required. Bath water should be warm (36°C) and wet clothing should be changed as soon as possible. It is essential also to avoid overheating (Bacon 1991, Rutter 1992, Thomas 1994). Advice regarding clothing and bedding can only be a guide as babies have marked individual variations in their metabolic rates (Hull et al 1996a). Parents should be advised to take account of environmental temperature when dressing their baby. Swaddling should be loose enough to permit movement of arms and legs, allowing adjustment to posture in response to the need for a change in temperature (Hull et al 1996b).

Prevention of infection

The baby's skin is a barrier to infection provided its integrity and pH balance are maintained. Babies should be provided with their own equipment. Adequate linen supplies are essential. This is especially important in hospital. The number of people handling the baby should be restricted. Members of staff who are liable to be a source of infection should not handle babies, and friends and relatives who have colds or sore throats (especially children) should not visit. Hand washing before and after handling babies is essential. Cross-infection can be a particular problem in hospitals. For this reason rooming-in and explicit instructions to parents regarding the importance of hand washing are recommended. The wearing of gowns when handling babies is not necessary.

Skin care. Promotion of skin integrity is enhanced by avoiding friction against hard fabrics or soiled or wet clothing, and by minimising the length of time the skin is in contact with irritants such as gastric contents, urine and stool. Cleansing of the skin should be carried out gently to prevent damage to the epidermis. Soaps, creams, isopropyl alcohol and other skin care preparations should be used with caution to prevent

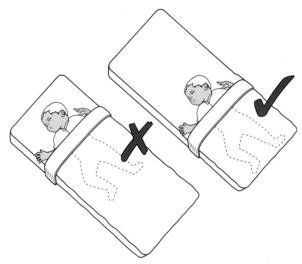

Fig. 39.3 'Feet-to-foot' sleeping position.

irritation and disturbance of the skin pH and absorption of topical agents. Baby soaps and other baby-washing solutions are usually pH adjusted. Grapeseed oil and aqueous cream have also been recommended for baby care. In some centres hexachlorophane-based soap or liquid preparations (maximum concentration 3%) are used for cleansing the baby's skin (excluding the face). It is important to remember that these preparations should be rinsed off the skin, as the risk of absorption of hexachlorophane has to be considered. The use of biological powders, fabric softeners and starch should be avoided when laundering babies' clothing (Michie 1996).

The timing of the first bath is not critical, although it has been suggested that removal of blood and liquor reduces the risk of transmission of HIV and other organisms to staff (Penny-MacGillivray 1996). Bathing should be deferred until the baby's temperature is above 36.5°C. The temperature of the bath water should be 36°C. The hair is washed and dried carefully at the first bath but need not be washed daily. If the baby has been regurgitating mucus, a thin layer of petroleum jelly may be applied to the cheek to prevent soreness. Petroleum jelly applied to the buttocks will prevent meconium adhering to the skin and causing excoriation.

Daily bathing is not essential but the mother should be given sufficient opportunities to bath her baby in order to increase her confidence. 'Topping and tailing' (cleansing the baby's face, skin flexures and napkin area only) may be carried out once or twice a day. It should be noted that greater heat loss may be incurred during this procedure than when the baby is bathed (Perry 1995).

The baby's eyes do not need to be cleansed unless a discharge is present. Attention should be paid to the washing and drying of skin flexures to prevent excoriation. The buttocks must be washed and dried carefully at every napkin change. Sore buttocks may occur if the stools are loose, if there is protracted delay in changing a soiled napkin or if the skin is traumatised by over-enthusiastic rubbing. Regular use of a barrier cream is recommended by some people (Jethwa 1994) but may interfere with the 'one-way' membrane in disposable nappies.

Cleanliness of the umbilical cord is essential. Hand washing is required before and after handling the cord. No specific cord treatment is required, although a wide variety of preparations have been used to promote early separation. However, it should be noted that topical applications could interfere with the normal process of colonisation and delay separation. Cleansing with tap water and keeping the cord dry have been shown to promote separation (Barclay et al 1994, Mugford et al 1986, Rush 1990, Salariya & Kowbus 1988, Verber & Pagan 1993). It is advisable to ensure that the cord is not enclosed within the baby's napkin where contamination by urine or faeces may occur. The cord clamp is removed on the third day provided the cord is dry and necrosed.

Circumcision. Although not commonly practised in the UK, in other parts of the world neonatal circumcision may be undertaken whilst the baby is in hospital. There is little evidence to support this practice as beneficial; rather it is a traditional cultural custom (Gonik & Barrett 1995). It is recommended that appropriate anaesthesia, dorsal penile nerve block is used for this procedure and that postoperative analgesia is also prescribed (Rabinowitz & Hulbert 1995). After care involves the use of a non-adherent dressing, observing for haemorrhage and keeping the area clean and dry.

Vaccination and immunisation. BCG vaccination may be given during the early neonatal period in some areas where early protection is desirable. Vaccination against hepatitis B and poliomyelitis may also be given in some parts of the world (Roberton 1992).

Prevention of injury and accident

Sensible precautions should be observed by all staff in their own practice and explained to the parents. A baby should not be left unattended unless in a cot as vigorous activity may result in the baby falling off a bed or table. A baby should be moved from place to place in a cot rather than in the arms and the bassinet of the cot should be flat, not elevated, to prevent accidents if uneven floors are encountered. If a larger crib is used, the cot sides should be up and secured. The cot design should comply with safety standards. Babies do not require a pillow until the age of 2 years and mothers should be advised that placing a pillow behind the baby's head is unsafe. Similarly, polythene bags or sheeting should not be used near a baby and waterproof mattress covers must be tight fitting and enclose the mattress completely to prevent suffocation of the baby by a loose cover.

The temperature of bath water should be tested prior to immersing the baby to avoid scalding or chilling. The temperature of a bottle feed should also be tested before it is offered to the baby.

If safety pins are used to secure the napkin they should be inserted into the cloth from side to side (not vertically) and with one hand protecting the baby's abdomen to avoid penetration of the skin or genitalia. The baby with long or ragged nails may cause facial scratches. Mittens worn to prevent this should be made from cotton material with French seams to prevent loose threads entwining the fingers and occluding the circulation.

Advice should also be given to mothers about safety in the home. This should address such issues as bed sharing, use of cat-nets, fireguards, cooker guards, stair gates, pram brakes and car seats. 'Smoking', 'Back to sleep' and 'Feet-to-foot' advice should be reinforced (Foundation for the Study of Infant Deaths 1996).

Daily examination

Each day, the baby should be examined by a midwife, to evaluate progress and identify problems as they arise. The examination is similar to that undertaken at birth but is now concerned with monitoring daily changes in the baby and detecting any signs of infection.

A newborn baby usually sleeps for most of the time between feeds but should be alert and responsive when awake. Erratic sleep patterns may prove disconcerting to new parents and they should be reassured by the midwife that this can be normal if the baby looks healthy, is alert and is feeding well. Undue lethargy or irritability may indicate cerebral damage or sepsis.

The skin is a barometer of the baby's hydration and general well-being. The midwife's knowledge of its normal parameters and minor variations assists in the interpretation of her findings.

The examination begins by noting the baby's posture, colour and respirations. Any cyanosis should be reported to the paediatrician immediately. Jaundice may be noted from the 3rd day and is abnormal if it arises earlier, deepens or persists beyond the 7th day. If a baby remains jaundiced on discharge from hospital the midwife must instruct the parent to report to their GP if the baby's stools become pale or if the urine becomes dark, which may be suggestive of bilary atresia (see Ch. 46).

Palpation of the head permits assessment of the anterior fontanelle (which should be level), resolution of the caput succedaneum and moulding, and allows identification of any new swellings, for example cephalhaematoma (see Ch. 44).

The baby's eyes and mouth are inspected for signs of infection. Sticky eyes are cleaned with sterile water after obtaining a swab for culture and sensitivity testing. The mouth should be clean and moist. Adherent white plaques indicate oral thrush infection. Sucking blisters on the baby's lips may be observed, especially after feeding. These do not require any treatment.

It is important for the midwife to note responses to handling and noise as she undresses the baby. She can use this time to inspect the identity bands, and have a discussion with the mother about feeding or any other concerns that the latter may have.

The skin, especially in flexures and between the digits, is inspected for rashes, septic spots, excoriation or abrasions. Skin rashes such as erythema toxicum, a red blotchy rash, are of little significance. Sometimes a harlequin colour change may be noted; this is a very rare but dramatic colour change, with vivid midline demarcation of colour. The baby is red on one side of the trunk and pale on the other side. This is caused by vasomotor instability and is of little importance. However, its appearance is startling and can alarm the mother.

The fingertips and toes are examined for ragged nails and paronychia. Septic spots must be differentiated from milia, which do not require treatment. Even a few septic spots must be taken seriously. The paediatrician may prescribe topical applications or systemic antibiotics and consider possible isolation of the baby.

The umbilical cord base is inspected for redness and the mother is reminded about care. In some areas the baby's temperature is recorded with a low-recording thermometer. This may be taken in the axilla, ear, in the groin or rectally. If the rectal route is used it is essential that the baby's legs and the thermometer are held firmly to prevent sudden movement, which could cause the thermometer to break and perforate the rectum. The midwife should ensure that the bulb of the thermometer is inserted no further than 2.5 cm into the rectum. Concern regarding the risk of injury has led to an increased use of alternative methods of measuring babies' temperatures. This concern must be balanced against the need for an accurate estimate of core temperature when babies are ill (Morley 1992). Midwives should comply with local policy in regard to rectal temperature taking.

The phase of stools are observed in relation to the baby's age and the type of milk ingested. Non-passage of stools or vomiting helps to identify abnormalities of the gastrointestinal tract, inborn errors of metabolism and infection. Constipation may be alleviated by offering the baby water between feeds. Loose, watery stools may signify sugar intolerance or infection and may cause sore buttocks. Sore buttocks may be treated by exposure to the air, but care must be taken to avoid chilling the baby. The frequency of passing urine and stools in the preceding 24 hours should be noted.

During feeds the midwife should observe the baby's eagerness or reluctance to feed and the coordination of sucking and swallowing reflexes, as well as noting the frequency with which the baby demands feeds. During feeding, babies clench their fists, tuck them under the chin and wriggle their toes while grasping their mother's fingers. Eye contact also occurs, which enhances communication between mother and baby. Sucking is interspersed with rest periods. Abnormal feeding behaviour may signify cerebral damage, congenital abnormality or illness. Breast engorgement and pseudomenstruation require no treatment but explanation to the mother is essential. No attempt should be made to express engorged breasts.

If the baby is to be weighed, this is done before dressing, and the result compared with his birthweight. A common regimen is weighing every 3rd day. Weight loss is normal in the first few days but more than 10% bodyweight loss is abnormal and requires investigation. Most babies regain their birthweight in 7–10 days, thereafter gaining weight at a rate of 150–200 g per week.

All findings at the daily examination are entered in the baby's records and abnormalities reported. Parents can be introduced to the concept of daily examination and gradually assume this responsibility as their confidence increases. This helps to enhance parent–baby interaction.

Examination by the paediatrician (or competent other)

All newborn babies should be examined by one of the following: paediatrician, obstetrician, general practitioner, advanced neonatal nurse practitioner or midwife with appropriate training, within the first 24 hours of life. Moss et al (1991) assert that a second examination is of little value, apart from a repeat examination of the hips. The mother should be present for the examination. Some of the examination duplicates what has been described above and so only the medical aspects are considered here. In some areas the midwife incorporates, and is accountable for, these additional elements of examination following appropriate in-service education (MacKeith 1995, Michaelides 1995, Rose 1994). A general appraisal of the baby's colour, overall appearance, muscular activity and response to handling is made throughout the examination.

Head assessment

To start this assessment the occipital frontal circumference (OFC) is measured using a non-stretchable tape measure. The average OFC in a term baby is 31–38 cm. Next check the size and tension of the anterior fontanelle are checked and suture lines palpated noting cranial moulding, caput succedaneum and cephalhaematoma. Any abnormality detected should be reported to a senior paediatrician and documented in the baby's case notes. Parents should be reassured that moulding, caput and cephalhaematoma usually resolve within a few weeks after birth.

Examination of the face should begin with observing the relationships between all the facial components: eyes, ears, nose and mouth, remembering that unusual facial characteristics may be familial (Boyer Johnson 1996). A general inspection of the eyes for conjunctivitis, cataracts, aniridia and coloboma is carried out before using an ophthalmoscope. The ophthalmoscope is held in the right hand, with the viewing aperture as close as possible to the right eye, and using the right index finger to turn the lens selector dial to the appropriate lens for proper focus (Honeyfield 1996). While positioning the baby's head with the free hand, the illuminating light is aligned along the baby's visual plane (Honeyfield 1996), observing for the red reflex and pupil reaction. Parents will need reassurance about common eye trauma such as bruising or oedema of the eyelids and haemorrhage seen around the iris (Boyer Johnson 1996). These can occur after a normal vaginal delivery and usually resolve within 1–2 weeks. The ears should be assessed for size, shape and placement; abnormal formation or placement can be associated with chromosomal anomalies and syndromes. The nose should be symmetric and placed vertically in the midline. Its size and shape may be familial (Boyer Johnson 1996).

To examine the mouth a gloved finger should be inserted into the baby's mouth with the fingerpad up, to ensure continuity of the hard and soft palates and to assess suck and gag reflexes. Small white clusters of Epstein's pearls may be seen at the junction of the hard and soft palate and on the gums (Boyer Johnson 1996); these should not be mistaken for the white plaque of oral thrush.

Cardio/respiratory assessment

This assessment requires great skills in the techniques of inspection, palpation and auscultation. After inspection of the baby's colour, the next step is to auscultate the heart sounds. It is necessary to have a paediatric stethoscope with a double-headed chest piece; both sides are necessary to listen to the heart. The stethoscope should be placed firmly on bare skin, to assess the heart rate and evaluate cardiac rhythm and regularity (Honeyfield 1996). The practitioner carefully listens to the rhythm of the heart to determine whether there is any irregularity, a note is made of patterns and frequencies of the irregularity, which help identify the type of arrhythmia (Fraser Askin 1996). Murmurs are described as additional heart sounds and must be discussed and reported to a senior paediatrician.

To assess the chest and lungs, the shape of the chest is noted, and the rate and regularity of the respirations. Normal respirations are 40–60 per minute and relaxed, symmetrical diaphragmatic respirations are normal. Breath sounds can now be assessed using a stethoscope; sounds are louder and coarser in the baby than in the adult. Breath sounds should be assessed for pitch, intensity and duration. The practitioner begins at the top of the chest and moves the stethoscope systematically from side to side. Breath sounds in the lower lobes can be assessed adequately only through the baby's back (Fraser Askin 1996). Any irregularities detected must be reported to the paediatrician.

Abdomen

This assessment requires inspection, palpation, and auscultation. The practitioner palpates the abdomen with warm hands and observes for pain responses, starting at the groin by placing the index finger just above the groin parallel to the right costal margin and, with a gentle compressing motion, gradually moving the finger upward until the liver edge is felt. The normal liver is smooth and firm with a sharp and well-defined edge, and is felt 1–2 cm below the right costal margin (Keels Conner 1996). The spleen is normally not palpable unless infection is present. Next the kidneys and bladder are examined. The bladder when full is easily palpated 1–4 cm above the symphysis pubis, and can be associated with abnormalities if frequently or continuously distended. The kidneys are sometimes difficult to palpate; the left kidney is more easily palpated than the right, unless the descending colon is filled with meconium. The kidney is palpated using a deep smooth firm pressure by placing one hand under the baby's flank and pressing downward with the other (Keels Conner 1996). Next the practitioner auscultates for bowel sounds; using a stethoscope to listen to all four abdominal quadrants, breath sounds are usually heard in the upper abdominal region. Bowel sounds are absent immediately after birth. With crying and sucking, the abdomen begins to fill with air, and bowel sounds become audible within the first 15 minutes after birth. The sounds have a metallic, tinkling quality and are usually heard every 15–20 seconds (Keels Conner 1996).

Neurological system

The baby's reflex responses are elicited in order to establish normality of the neurological system. These are tested while the baby is in a quiet alert state. Absent or weak responses may indicate immaturity, cerebral damage or abnormality.

In comparison with the other body systems, the nervous system is remarkably immature both anatomically and physiologically at birth. This results in predominantly brain stem and spinal reflex activity with minimal control by the cerebral cortex in the early months, though social interaction occurs early. After birth, brain growth is rapid, requiring constant and adequate supplies of oxygen and glucose. The immaturity of the brain renders it particularly vulnerable to hypoxia, biochemical imbalance, infection and haemorrhage. Temperature instability and uncoordinated muscle movement reflect the incomplete state of brain development and incomplete myelination of nerves.

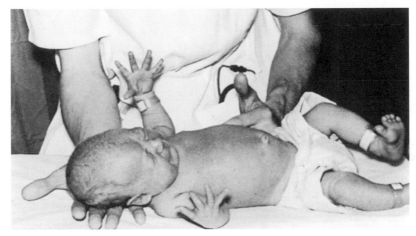

Fig. 39.4 Moro reflex.

The baby is equipped with a wide range of reflex activities, the presence of which at varying ages provides an indication of the normality and integrity of the neurological and skeletomuscular systems (Gandy 1992, Roberton 1992).

Moro reflex. This reflex occurs in response to a sudden stimulus. The baby is held supine, with the trunk and head supported from below. When the head and shoulders are suddenly allowed to fall back, the baby responds by abduction and extension of arms with fingers fanned, and sometimes accompanied by a tremor. The arms then flex and embrace the chest. A similar response may be seen in the legs which, following extension, flex on to the abdomen (Fig. 39.4). The Moro reflex is often accompanied by a cry and may be demonstrated unintentionally when briskly placing a baby in the supine position. Babies do not seem to like this reflex, so it should not be elicited as a routine procedure. The reflex is symmetrical and is present for the first 8 weeks of life. The most common cause of an asymmetric Moro response is a fracture of the humerus or clavical, or a brachial plexus palsy. Absence of the Moro reflex may indicate brain damage or immaturity. Persistence of the reflex beyond the age of 6 months is suggestive of mental retardation (Thomas & Harvey 1992).

Rooting reflex. In response to stroking of the cheek or side of the mouth the baby will turn towards the source of stimulus and open the mouth ready to suckle.

Sucking and swallowing reflexes. These are well developed in the normal baby and are coordinated with breathing. This is essential for safe feeding and adequate nutrition.

Gag, cough and sneeze reflexes. These protect the baby from airway obstruction.

Blinking and corneal reflexes. These protect the eyes from trauma.

Grasp reflexes. A palmar grasp is elicited by placing a finger or pencil in the palm of the baby's hand. The finger or pencil is grasped firmly. A similar response can be demonstrated by stroking the base of the toes (plantar grasp).

Walking and stepping reflexes. When supported upright with his feet touching a flat surface, the baby simulates walking. If held with the tibia in contact with the edge of a table the baby will step up on to the table (limb placement reflex).

Asymmetrical tonic neck reflex. In the supine position the limbs on the side of the body to which the head is turned extend, while those on the opposite side flex. Muscle tone is reflected in the baby's response to passive movements.

Traction response. When pulled upright by the wrists to a sitting position the head will lag initially (Fig. 39.5) then right itself momentarily before falling forward on to the chest.

Ventral suspension. When held prone, and suspended over the examiner's arm, the baby momentarily holds the head level with the body and flexes the limbs (Fig. 39.6).

These reflexes and responses are self-defence mechanisms, which are designed to attract the mother to her baby and so promote the mother–child attachment.

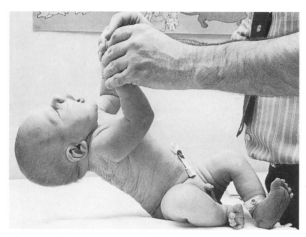

Fig. 39.5 Traction response. (From Gandy 1992, with permission.)

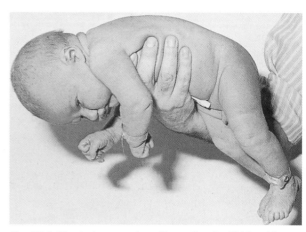

Fig. 39.6 Ventral suspension. (From Gandy, 1992, with permission.)

Examination of hips

It is essential that all babies undergo specific examination to detect developmental dysplasia of the hips (Aronsson et al 1994, Beverley & Nathan 1995). In some centres the midwife performs this; in others the paediatrician is the person responsible. Care must be taken in order to avoid producing an iatrogenically unstable hip (Beverley & Nathan 1995). The examination should not be undertaken by inexperienced staff. To examine the hips the examiner must place the baby on a firm flat surface at waist height.

Ortolani's test (Fig. 39.7). The baby's legs are grasped with the flexed knees in the palms of the examiner's hands and the femur splinted between the index and middle fingers and the thumb. Both hips are examined simultaneously. The baby's thighs are flexed on to the abdomen and rotated and abducted through an angle of 70–90° towards the examining surface. *No force should be exerted.* If the hip is dislocated a 'clunk' will be felt as the head of the femur slips into the acetabulum during adduction and the dislocation is reduced.

Barlow's test (Fig. 39.7). With the baby's legs flexed (as above), the head of the femur is held between the examiner's thumb and index finger while the other hand steadies the pelvis. Following the initial movement of flexion and rotation, as the hip is abducted to 70° *gentle* pressure is exerted in a backward and lateral direction. A 'clunk' will be felt as the head of the femur dislocates out of the acetabulum.

In some centres a modified Ortolani/Barlow procedure is followed. This incorporates the essential elements of both of the above manoeuvres (Hall et al 1994). Early referral to a paediatrician is essential if effective treatment for a dislocated, or dislocatable, hip is to be achieved (see Ch. 41).

Blood tests

Certain inborn errors of metabolism and endocrine disorders are detected by means of a blood test, for example the Guthrie test. Blood, obtained from a heel prick made with a stilette on the lateral aspect of the heel to avoid nerves and blood vessels, is dripped on to circles on an absorbent card on to which full details of the baby's identity are entered (see Plate 12). For detection of phenylketonuria, hypothyroidism and cystic fibrosis the baby must have had at least 4–6 days of milk feeding, and if for any reason the baby or mother is receiving antibiotics, this information should be recorded on the card. Some centres also test routinely for galactosaemia (see Ch. 47.)

Child health surveillance

Following discharge from the care of the midwife into that of the health visitor, the screening of the baby is continued on a regular basis at the child health clinic (see Ch. 46). The specific screening procedures described in this section are complemented by the daily care and observations by the midwife during the first 10–28 days of life, and possibly up to the end of the puerperium. The new public health policy in particular advocates the continuing role of the midwife beyond 28 days and suggests that midwives further

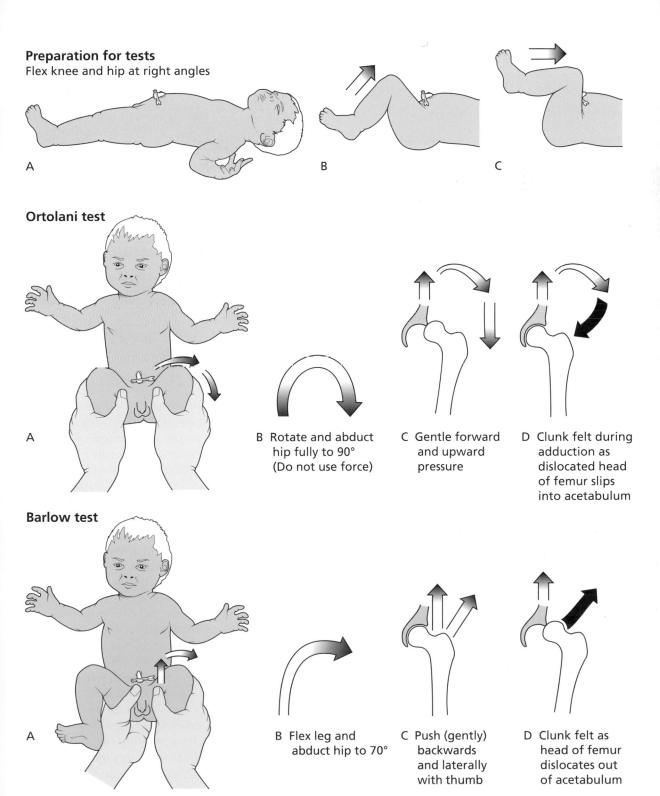

Preparation for tests
Flex knee and hip at right angles

A

B

C

Ortolani test

A

B Rotate and abduct hip fully to 90° (Do not use force)

C Gentle forward and upward pressure

D Clunk felt during adduction as dislocated head of femur slips into acetabulum

Barlow test

A

B Flex leg and abduct hip to 70°

C Push (gently) backwards and laterally with thumb

D Clunk felt as head of femur dislocates out of acetabulum

Fig. 39.7 Examination of the hips. Ortolani's and Barlow's test.

build and expand on their roles around public health (DoH 1999, RCM 2000).

Promoting family relationships

Parent–infant attachment

Positive responses from the baby to his parents reinforce parental attachment and stimulate further interaction. Knowledge of the reflexes, general abilities and sleep and awake states of babies enables the midwife to teach the parents how to take advantage of the occasions when their baby is likely to be most responsive. The resulting interactions continue the process of attachment initiated at delivery (see Ch. 38). To help the mother in her new role it is important to use the baby's name and to speak positively about his appearance and activities.

Parents develop their relationship with their babies in individual ways and at their own pace. Some mothers feel somewhat distant from their baby at first; others experience an overwhelming protective urge and intense absorption with their baby (Jowitt 1996). It is important not to overemphasise 'bonding' as this may create non-productive guilt feelings in parents who do not experience instant love for their child and result in negative attitudes towards the baby (Barclay & Lupton 1999, Billings 1995, Rutter 1995).

It is suggested that the parents' relationship with one another is enhanced when the father is encouraged to be involved in discussions, choices and decisions about baby care and to share the responsibility for care. The resultant maternal confidence is reflected in her responsiveness toward her baby, thus promoting the baby's feeling of security (Adams & Cotgrove 1995). The father's reactions to and feelings about his baby should be afforded expression (Heath 1995, McLennan 1995). Parents may express anxiety about the possible reactions of siblings to the new arrival. A positive attitude on the part of the midwife can do much to allay fears, which are often unfounded (Gullicks & Crase 1993).

Promoting confidence and competence

It is important that the midwife does not let her own maternal feelings 'take over', thus denying the mother

opportunity to provide care for her baby. The father too should be encouraged to share in baby care. Total care should be delegated to the parents as soon as possible. In hospital especially, procedures can be rendered unnecessarily complicated for new mothers, many of who have had no previous involvement with newborn babies (Thomas 1995). Teaching the principles and discussing individual care can help to overcome these anxieties. Dressing tips, for instance pulling rather than trying to push an arm through the sleeve of a jacket, are better understood by explaining the baby's response to passive movement.

Promoting communication

The increasing interest in baby massage in recent years capitalises on the knowledge that the baby is sensitive and responsive to touch (Adamson-Macedo 1992, Lim 1996, McLintock 1995). Grapeseed or equivalent oil is used rather than baby oils, which stick to the skin. Aromatherapy oils should not be used as the extent of their absorption is not known (McLintock, personal communication, 1996). The naked baby is stroked and caressed in a leisurely manner using the fingertips and palms of the hands. Throughout this quiet time together, eye-to-eye contact is promoted by the close proximity of the baby, and the mother (or father) instinctively interacts with the baby's pleasurable responses. This assists in reinforcing the developing emotional relationship.

By applying her knowledge of the physiological and psychological capabilities and potential complications of the newborn, the midwife can ensure that optimal baby care is planned and provided and can do much to foster happy family relationships.

The foregoing discussion in this chapter have endeavoured to illustrate how the midwife can enhance the parent–baby relationship. Her teaching, support and encouragement of the mother as she learns to provide for her baby's needs is of paramount importance and should culminate in a happy, confident and competent mother being discharged from the midwife's care. The midwife can also do a great deal to encourage a father's interaction with his baby and should take every opportunity to do so. These aspects of midwifery practice are described more fully in Chapters 33 and 35.

REFERENCES

Adams L, Cotgrove A 1995 Promoting secure attachment patterns in infancy and beyond. Professional Care of Mother and Child 5(6):158–160

Adamson-Macedo E 1992 TAC-TIC therapy: the importance of systematic stroking. British Journal of Midwifery 2(6):244–269

Aronsson D D, Goldberg M J, Kling T F, Roy D R 1994 Developmental dysplasia of the hip. Pediatrics 94(2):201–208

Bacon C J 1991 The thermal environment of sleeping babies and possible dangers of overheating. In: David T J (ed) Recent advances in paediatrics. Churchill Livingstone, Edinburgh

Barclay L, Lupton D 1999 The experience of new fatherhood: a socio cultural analysis. Journal of Advanced Nursing April 29(4):1013–1020

Barclay L, Harrington A, Conroy R, Royal R, Laforgia J 1994 A comparative study of neonates' umbilical cord management. Australian Journal of Advanced Nursing 11(3):34–40

Beverley M, Nathan S 1995 Diagnosing developmental dysplasia of the hip (DDH). Maternal and Child Health 20(4):120, 122–124

Billings J R 1995 Bonding theory – tying mothers in knots? A critical review of the application of a theory to nursing. Journal of Clinical Nursing 4(4):207–211

Blackburn S T, Loper D L 1992 Maternal, fetal, and neonatal physiology: a clinical perspective. W B Saunders, Philadelphia, chs 5–12

Boyer Johnson C, 1996 Head, eyes, ears, nose, mouth and neck assessment. In: Tappero E P, Honeyfield M E (eds) Physical assessment of the newborn, 2nd edn. NICU INK, California

Brazelton T B 1984 Neonatal behavioural assessment scale, 2nd edn. Spastics International Medical Publications, Blackwell Scientific, London

Crockett M 1995 Physiology of the neonatal immune system. Journal of Obstetric, Gynecologic and Neonatal Nursing 24(7):627–634

Day M 1995 Babies at risk as maternity units fail to step up security. Nursing Times 91(28):6

DeCasper A, Fifer W 1987 Of human bonding: newborns prefer their mothers' voices. In: Oates J, Sheldon S (eds) Cognitive development in infancy. Lawrence Erlbaum Associates Open University, Hove

DoH (Department of Health) 1999 Making a Difference. Strengthening the nursing, midwifery and health visiting contribution to health and health care. Department of Health, London

Doull I J M, McCaughey E S, Bailey B J R, Betts P R 1995 Reliability of infant length measurement. Archives of Disease in Childhood 72:520–521

Downey J, Bidder R T 1990 Perinatal information on infant crying. Child: Care, Health and Development 16(2):113–121

Foundation for the Study of Infant Deaths 1996 'Feet to foot' – a new initiative to reduce sudden infant death. Press release. MIDIRS Midwifery Digest 6(1):97

Fraser Askin D 1996 Chest and lungs assessment. In: Tappero E P, Honeyfield M E (eds) Physical assessment of the newborn, 2nd edn. NICU INK, California

Fry T 1994 Monitoring children's growth: introducing the new child growth standards. Professional Care of Mother and Child 4(8):231–233

Gandy G M 1992 Examination of the neonate including gestational age assessment. In: Roberton N R C (ed) Textbook of neonatology, 2nd edn. Churchill Livingstone, Edinburgh

Gonik B, Barrett K 1995 The persistence of newborn circumcision: an American perspective. British Journal of Obstetrics and Gynaecology 102(12):940–941

Grunau R, Craig K 1987 Pain expression in neonates: facial action and cry. Pain 28:395–410

Gullicks J N, Crase S J 1993 Sibling behaviour with a newborn: parents' expectations and observations. Journal of Obstetric, Gynecologic and Neonatal Nursing 22(5):438–444

Hall D, Hill P, Elliman D 1994 The child surveillance handbook, 2nd edn. Radcliffe Medical Press, Oxford

Heath T 1995 New fatherhood. New Generation (June):11

Honeyfield M E 1996 Principles of physical assessment. In: Tappero E P, Honeyfield M E (eds) Physical assessment of the newborn, 2nd edn. NICU INK, California

Hull D, McArthur A J, Pritchard K, Goodall M 1996a Metabolic rate of sleeping infants. Archives of Disease in Childhood 75(4):282–287

Hull D, McArthur A J, Pritchard K, Oldham D 1996b Individual variation in sleeping metabolic rates in infants. Archives of Disease in Childhood 75(4):288–291

Irving V 2001 Caring for and protecting the skin of pre term neonates. Journal of Wound Care 10(7):253–256

Jethwa K 1994 Nappy rash: a pharmaceutical approach. Professional Care of Mother and Child 4(7):219–220

Jørgensen F S, Felding P, Vinther S, Andersen G 1991 Vitamin K to neonates. Per oral versus intramuscular administration. Acta Paediatrica 80:304–307

Jowitt M 1996 Birth and bonding. Midwifery Matters 69(Summer):3

Keels Conner G 1996 Abdomen assessment. In: Tappero E P, Honeyfield M E (eds) Physical assessment of the newborn, 2nd edn. NICU INK, California

Laurent C 1992 A mother's nightmare. Nursing Times 88(52):18

Lerner H 1993 Sleep position of infants: applying research to practice. Maternal and Child Nursing 18(Sept/Oct):275–277

Lim P 1996 Baby massage. British Journal of Midwifery (8):439–441

MacFarlane A 1975 Olfaction in the development of social preferences in the human neonate. In: Parent–infant interaction. CIBA Foundation Symposium 33, Elsevier, Amsterdam

MacKeith N 1995 Who should examine the 'normal' neonate? Nursing Times 91(14):34–35

McLennan I 1995 Ian's story. New Generation (June):13

McLintock F 1995 Baby massage. Connections 26(2):4–6

Michaelides S 1995 A deeper knowledge. Nursing Times 91(35)(suppl):59–61

Michie M 1996 A delicate concern: caring for neonatal skin. British Journal of Midwifery 4(3):159–163

Morley C 1992 Measuring infants' temperatures. Midwives Chronicle and Nursing Notes (Feb):26–29

Moss G D, Cartlidge P H T, Speides B D, Chambers T L 1991 Routine examination in the neonatal period. British Medical Journal 302:878–879

Mugford M, Somchiwong M, Waterhouse I 1986 Treatment of umbilical cords: a randomised trial to assess the effect of treatment methods on the work of midwives. Midwifery 2:177–186

Penny-MacGillivray T 1996 A newborn's first bath: when? Journal of Obstetric, Gynecologic and Neonatal Nursing 25(6):481–487

Perry S E 1995 Nursing care of the newborn. In: Bobak I M, Lowdermilk D L, Jensen M D (eds) Maternity nursing, 4th edn. C V Mosby, St Louis, ch 14

Rabinowitz R, Hulbert W C 1995 Newborn circumcision should not be performed without anaesthesia. Birth 22(1):45–46

RCM (Royal College of Midwives) 2000 Midwifery Practice in the Postnatal Period. Recommendations for practice. The Royal College of Midwives, London

Righard L 1995 How do newborns find their mother's breast? Birth 22(3):174–175

Roberton N R C 1992 Care of the normal term newborn baby. In: Roberton N R C (ed) Textbook of neonatology, 2nd edn. Churchill Livingstone, Edinburgh

Roberton N R C 1996 A manual of normal neonatal care, 3rd edn. Edward Arnold, London

Rose S 1994 Physical examination of the full-term baby. British Journal of Midwifery 2(5):209–213

Rush J 1990 Care of the umbilical cord. In: Alexander J, Levy V, Roch S (eds) Midwifery practice: postnatal care – a research-based approach. Macmillan, Basingstoke

Rushforth J A, Levene M I 1994 Behavioural response to pain in healthy neonates. Archives of Disease in Childhood 70(3):F174–F176

Rutter N 1992 Temperature control and its disorders. In: Roberton N R C (ed) Textbook of neonatology, 2nd edn. Churchill Livingstone, Edinburgh

Rutter M 1995 Clinical implications of attachment concepts: retrospect and prospect. Journal of Child Psychology and Psychiatry 36(4):549–571

Salariya E, Kowbus N 1988 Variable umbilical cord care. Midwifery 4:70–76

Shearer M J 1995 Vitamin K. Lancet 345(8944):229–234

Stern C M 1992 Neonatal immunology. In: Roberton N R C (ed) Textbook of neonatology, 2nd edn. Churchill Livingstone, Edinburgh

Thomas G 1995 Empowerment. The baby bath demonstration. Midwives 108(1289):178

Thomas K 1994 Thermoregulation in neonates. Neonatal Network 13(2):15–22

Thomas R, Harvey D 1992 Neonatology colour guide, 2nd edn. Churchill Livingstone, Edinburgh

UKCC (United Kingdom Central Council for Nursing, Midwifery and Health Visiting) 1998 Guidelines for records and record keeping. UKCC, London (reprinted NMC 2002)

Verber I G, Pagan F S 1993 What cord care – if any? Archives of Disease in Childhood 68(5)(Fetal and Neonatal edn):594–596

FURTHER READING

Kenner C, Wright Lott J, Flandermeyer A (eds) 1998 Comprehensive neonatal nursing: a physiologic perspective, 2nd edn. W B Saunders, Philadelphia

This book provides a comprehensive approach to neonatal care, and is an essential text for those caring for newborn babies and their families.

Klaus M H, Kennell J H 1996 Bonding: building the foundations of secure attachment and independence. Cedar, London

This book will give the midwife insight into other aspects and studies regarding the parent infant attachment and should be read to compliment the information in this chapter.

Perry S E 1995 The newborn. In: Bobak I M, Lowdermilk D L, Jensen M D (eds) Maternity nursing, 4th edn. C V Mosby, St Louis, ch 13

This book will expand on the physiology of the baby's systems at birth, which is discussed in this chapter.

Rush J, Chalmers I, Enkin M 1990 Care of the new mother and baby. In: Chalmers I, Enkin M, Keirse M J N C (eds) Effective care in pregnancy and childbirth, vol 2. Childbirth. Oxford University Press, Oxford, ch 78

This is an obstetric textbook, and a good reference source to enhance the content of this chapter.

Tappero E P, Honeyfield M E 1996 Physical assessment of the newborn. A comprehensive approach to the art of physical examination, 2nd edn. NICU INK, California

This newborn assessment book is a valuable resource for all midwives involved in the care of the newborn baby. It will also assist the midwife who has extended her role to include the final examination of the newborn baby.

Thomas R, Harvey D 1992 Neonatology Colour Guide, 2nd edn. Churchill Livingstone, Edinburgh

This is a concise text, clearly integrated with high quality colour clinical photographs; it is an essential resource for midwives involved in the examination of the newborn baby.

VIDEOTAPES

Gregg C 1979 Getting to know each other. Plymouth Medical Films, Plymouth

Morris D 1992 Babywatching. Lifetime Broadcast, distributed by Polygram Video

Watkins R 1993 Baby massage: a video for parents and carers. From birth and beyond, MIDIRS Book Service, Bristol

40 Feeding

Sally Inch

CHAPTER CONTENTS

Many hours of the mother's time, day and night for many months, will be spent feeding her baby. She should be supported in the feeding method of her choice and enabled to accomplish it with skill, knowledge, confidence and pleasure. A firm mother–baby attachment can be forged during these frequent encounters, provided that they proceed without anxiety.

When breastfeeding goes well, there is the added advantage of the mother's sense of achievement and satisfaction. For these reasons, as well as those discussed below, breastfeeding must be the ideal way to feed a baby.

The International Confederation of Midwives adopted a policy in relation to breastfeeding in 1984 that clearly defines the midwife's responsibility in this field and describes the 'unique and vital role of the midwife in the promotion of breastfeeding' (ICM 1985).

The chapter aims to consider:

- the structure and function of the female breast
- the properties and components of breastmilk
- the role of the midwife, with particular emphasis on ensuring breastfeeding success for both mother and baby
- breastmilk expression
- the different causes of difficulty with breastfeeding
- artificial feeding and the various products available
- human milk banking
- the International code of marketing of breast-milk substitutes
- the Baby Friendly Hospital Initiative.

The breast and breastmilk

In countries or cultures where the knowledge and skills of breastfeeding have been retained within society, women consider it the normal way to feed a baby. In these countries midwives will encourage mothers to breastfeed and breastfeeding will have an excellent chance of being successful. In other countries (such as the UK) where artificial feeding has come to be seen as the norm, women who do choose to breastfeed are less likely to do so successfully. The high failure rate can be attributed in part to lack of knowledge and loss of skills, both within the profession and within the community. Midwives who fully understand the importance of human milk for human babies, and the importance of lactation to a parturient woman, are likely to be more highly motivated to acquire the skills necessary to support those women who choose to breastfeed, and to avoid practices that increase breastfeeding failure.

Anatomy and physiology of the breast

The breasts are compound secreting glands composed mainly of glandular tissue, which is arranged in *lobes*, approximately 20 in number (Fig. 40.1). Each lobe is divided into lobules that consist of alveoli and ducts. The *alveoli* contain acini cells, which produce milk and are surrounded by myoepithelial cells, which contract and propel the milk out (Fig. 40.2). Small *lactiferous ducts*, carrying milk from the alveoli, unite to form larger ducts. Several large ducts (lactiferous tubules) conveying milk from one or more lobe emerge on the surface of the nipple. The lactiferous tubules are distensible. *Myoepithelial cells* are oriented longitudinally along the ducts and, under the influence of oxytocin, these smooth muscle cells contract and the tubule becomes shorter and wider (Vorherr 1974, Woolridge 1986). As the tubule distends during active milk flow it may provide a temporary reservoir for milk (while the myoepithelial cells are maintained in a state of contraction by circulating oxytocin). This is often shown diagrammatically and described as *lactiferous sinuses* (or *ampullae*). The *nipple*, composed of erectile tissue, is covered with epithelium and contains plain muscle fibres, which have a sphincter-like action in controlling the flow of milk. Surrounding the nipple is an area of pigmented skin called the *areola*, which contains Montgomery's glands. These produce a sebum-like substance, which acts as a lubricant during pregnancy and throughout breastfeeding.

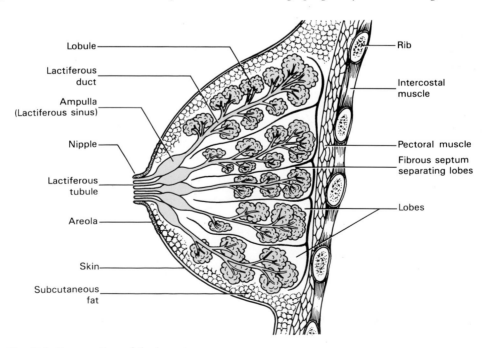

Fig. 40.1 Cross-section of the breast.

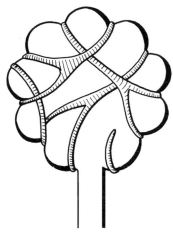

Fig. 40.2 Alveoli surrounded by myoepithelial cells, which propel the milk out of the lobule.

Breasts, nipples and areolae vary considerably in size from one woman to another.

The breast is supplied with blood from the internal and external mammary arteries and branches from the intercostal arteries. The veins are arranged in a circular fashion around the nipple.

Lymph drains freely between the two breasts and into lymph nodes in the axillae and the mediastinum.

During pregnancy, oestrogens and progesterone induce alveolar and ductal growth as well as stimulating the secretion of *colostrum*. Other hormones are also involved and they govern a complex sequence of events, which prepare the breast for lactation. Although colostrum is present from the 16th week of pregnancy, the production of milk is held in abeyance until after delivery, when the levels of placental hormones fall. This allows the already high levels of prolactin to initiate milk production. Continued production of prolactin is caused by the baby feeding at the breast, with concentrations highest during night feeds. Prolactin is involved in the suppression of ovulation, and some women may remain anovular until lactation ceases, although for others this effect is not so prolonged (Kennedy et al 1989, Romos et al 1996).

If breastfeeding (or expressing) has to be delayed for a few days, lactation can still be initiated because prolactin levels remain high, even in the absence of breast use, for at least the 1st week (Kochenour 1980). Prolactin seems to be much more important to the initiation of lactation than to its continuation. As lactation progresses, the prolactin response to suckling diminishes and milk removal becomes the driving force behind milk production (Applebaum 1970).

This is now known to be due to the presence in secreted milk of a whey protein that is able to inhibit the synthesis of milk constituents (Daly 1993, Prentice et al 1989, Wilde et al 1995). This protein accumulates in the breast as the milk accumulates and it exerts negative feedback control on the continued production of milk. Removal of this autocrine inhibitory factor (sometimes referred to as FIL – feedback inhibitor of lactation) by removing the milk allows milk production to be stepped up again. It is because this mechanism acts locally (i.e. within the breast) that each breast can function independently of the other. It is also the reason that milk production slows as the baby is gradually weaned from the breast. If necessary, it can be stepped up again if the baby is put back to the breast more often (e.g. because of illness).

Milk release is under neuroendocrine control. Tactile stimulation of the breast also stimulates the oxytocin, causing contraction of the myoepithelial cells. This process is known as the 'let-down' or 'milk-ejection' reflex and makes the milk available to the baby. This occurs in discrete pulses throughout the feed and may well trigger the bursts of active feeding.

In the early days of lactation this reflex is unconditioned. Later, as it becomes a conditioned reflex, the mother may find her breasts responding to the baby's cry (or other circumstances associated with the baby or feeding). In one small study (Ueda et al 1994), psychological stress (mental arithmetic or noise) was found to reduce the frequency of the oxytocin pulses; however, there was no effect on the amplitude of the pulse. Neither was there any effect on either prolactin levels or the amount of milk the baby received. It may be that the active removal of milk by the action of the baby's tongue and jaw plays a greater part than milk ejection in determining the quality and quantity of milk the baby receives.

Milk production and the mother

The human mother manages the process of lactation in an entirely different way from her non-primate counterpart. Much of the misinformation to which mothers are subjected derives from extrapolation from veterinary and dairy science as if 'humans were just another mammal' (Woolridge 1995). In fact, the lactating human female is able to maintain adequate milk production largely independently of her nutritional status and body mass index (Prentice et al 1994).

Not only have dietary surveys in developed countries consistently found their calorie intake to be less than the recommended amount (Butte et al 1984, Whitehead et al 1981), but controlled trials conducted in developing countries have demonstrated that giving extra food to mothers, even those who were poorly nourished, did not increase the rate of growth of their babies (Blackwell et al 1973, Delgado et al 1982, Prentice at al 1980, 1983). It has been suggested that metabolic efficiency is enhanced in lactating women, who are therefore able to conserve energy and 'subsidise' the cost of their milk production (Illingworth et al 1986). The lactational performance of the human female must become compromised when undernutrition is sufficiently severe, but it appears that this occurs only in famine or near famine conditions.

As milk production would appear to 'drive' appetite, rather than the reverse, hunger will effectively regulate the calorie intake of a breastfeeding woman, and the practice of encouraging breastfeeding mothers to eat excessively should be abandoned.

Similarly, if healthy breastfeeding women wish to undertake strenuous exercise (from 6 to 8 weeks after birth), or to lose weight (500–1000 g per week), they can be assured that neither the quality nor the quantity of their milk will be affected (Dewey et al 1994, Dusdieker et al 1994, Strode et al 1986). Exclusive breastfeeding combined with a low fat diet and exercise will result in more effective weight loss than diet and exercise alone (Dewey 1998, Hammer et al 1996).

Milk production is similarly unaffected by fluctuations in the mother's fluid intake. It has been repeatedly demonstrated that neither a significant decrease (Dearlove & Dearlove 1981) nor a significant increase (Dearlove & Dearlove 1981, Dusdieker et al 1985, Illingworth & Kilpatrick 1953, Morse et al 1992) in maternal fluid intake has any effect on milk production or the baby's weight.

Properties and components of breast-milk

Human milk varies in its composition:

- with the time of day (for example, the fat content is lowest in the morning and highest in the afternoon)
- with the stage of lactation (for example, the fat and protein content of colostrum is higher than in mature milk)
- in response to maternal nutrition (for example, although the *total amount* of fat is not influenced by diet, the *type* of fat that appears in the milk will be influenced by what the mother eats)
- because of individual variations.

The most dramatic change in the composition of milk occurs during the course of a feed. At the beginning of the feed the baby receives a high volume of relatively low fat milk. (This has come to be known as the *foremilk*.) As the feed progresses, the volume of milk decreases but the proportion of fat in the milk increases, sometimes to as much as five times the initial value (Hall 1979, Jackson et al 1987). (This has come to be known as the *hindmilk*.) The baby's ability to obtain this fat-rich milk is *not* determined by the length of time he spends at the breast, but by the quality of his attachment to the breast. The baby needs to be well attached so that he can use his tongue to maximum effect, stripping the milk from the breast, rather than relying solely on his mother's milk ejection reflex. A poorly attached baby may have difficulty in obtaining enough fat to meet his needs, and may resort to feeding very frequently in order to obtain sufficient calories from low fat feeds. A well-attached baby may, on the other hand, obtain all he needs in a very short time.

The length of the feed, provided that the baby is well attached, is thus determined by the rate of milk transfer from mother to baby. If milk transfer occurs at a high rate, feeds will be relatively short; if it occurs slowly, feeds will be longer (Woolridge et al 1982) (Fig. 40.3). Milk transfer seems to be more efficient in a second lactation than in a first (Ingram et al 2001).

Exclusive breastfeeding for the first 6 months of life

Human milk is species specific, having evolved over time to optimise the growth and development of the baby and young child. The 54th World Health Assembly, which met in Geneva in May 2001, affirmed the importance of exclusive breastfeeding for 6 months. The new resolution (ref: Agenda Item 13.1, Infant and young child nutrition, A54/45 in para. 2 (4)) urged member states to (Baby Milk Action 2001):

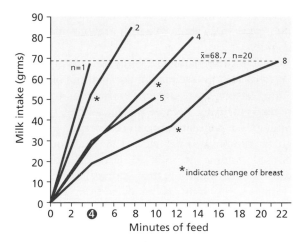

Fig. 40.3 Pattern of milk intake at a feed for 20 6-day-old babies. (From Woolridge et al 1982, with permission.)

support exclusive breastfeeding for six months as a global public health recommendation taking into account the findings of the WHO Expert Technical Consultation on optimal duration of exclusive breastfeeding and to provide safe and appropriate complementary foods, with continued breastfeeding for up to two years or beyond…

It has been known for some time that exclusively breastfed babies who consume enough breastmilk to satisfy their energy needs will easily meet their fluid requirements, even in hot dry climates (Ashraf et al 1993, Sachdev et al 1991).

Extra water will do nothing to speed the resolution of physiological jaundice, should it occur (Nicoll et al 1982, Carvahlo et al 1981). The only consistent effect of giving additional fluids to breastfed infants is to reduce the time for which they are breastfed (de Chateau et al 1977, Fenstein et al 1986, Herrera 1984, White et al 1992).

Fats and fatty acids

For the human infant, with his unique and rapidly growing brain, it is the fat and not the protein in human milk that has particular significance.

Ninety-eight per cent of the lipid in human milk is in the form of *triglycerides*: three fatty acids linked to a single molecule of glycerol. Over 100 fatty acids have so far been identified, about 46% being saturated fat and 54% unsaturated fat. There has been an explosion of interest in recent years in the unsaturated fatty acid content of human milk, particularly in the long chain polyunsaturated variety (LC-PUFAs for short), because of their role in brain growth and myelination. Two of them, arachadonic acid (AA) and docosahexanoic acid (DHA) appear to play an important role in the development of the retina and visual cortex of the newborn. Fat also provides the baby with more than 50% of his calorific requirements (Helsing & Savage King 1982). It is utilised very rapidly because *the milk itself* contains the enzyme (bile-salt-stimulated *lipase*) needed for fat digestion, but in a form which becomes active only when it reaches the infant's intestine. Pancreatic lipase is not plentiful in the newborn, so a baby who is not fed human milk is less able to digest fat.

Carbohydrate

The carbohydrate component of human milk is provided chiefly by *lactose*, which provides the baby with about 40% of his calorific requirements. Lactose is converted into galactose and glucose by the action of the enzyme lactase and these sugars provide energy to the rapidly growing brain. Lactose enhances the absorption of calcium and also promotes the growth of lactobacilli, which increase intestinal acidity thus reducing the growth of pathogenic organisms.

Protein

Human milk contains less protein than any other mammalian milk (Akre 1990a) and this accounts in part for its more 'transparent' appearance. Human milk is *whey* dominant (the whey being mainly alpha lactalbumin) and forms soft, flocculent curds when acidified in the stomach.

Allergic problems occur less frequently in breastfed babies than in artificially fed babies. This may be because the infant's intestinal mucosa is permeable to proteins before the age of 6–9 months and proteins in cow's milk can act as allergens. In particular, bovine beta lactoglobulin, which has no human milk protein counterpart, is capable of producing antigenic responses in atopic infants (Adler & Warner 1991, Bahna 1987).

Occasionally a baby may react adversely to substances in his mother's milk that come from her diet. However, this is rare and can be resolved by the mother identifying and avoiding the foods that cause the trouble so that she may continue to breastfeed.

Another bovine whey protein, bovine serum albumin, has been implicated as the trigger for the development of insulin-dependent diabetes mellitus (Paronen et al 2000, Vaarala et al 1999).

Vitamins

All the vitamins required for good nutrition and health are supplied in breastmilk, and although the actual amounts vary from mother to mother, none of the normal variations pose any risk to the infant (Worthington-Roberts 1993).

Fat-soluble vitamins.

Vitamin A. This is present in human milk as *retinol*, *retinyl esters* and *beta carotene*. Colostrum contains twice the amount present in mature human milk, and it is this that gives colostrum its yellow colour. Bile-salt-stimulated lipase (present in human milk – see fatty acids, above) assists the hydrolysation of the retinyl esters and may account for the rarity of vitamin A deficiency in breastfed babies in affluent societies (Fredrikzon et al 1978).

Vitamin D. This is the name given to two fat-soluble compounds: *calciferol* (vitamin D_2) and *cholecalciferol* (vitamin D_3). Vitamin D_3 plays an essential role in the metabolism of calcium and phosphorus in the body and prevents rickets in children. Although adults can obtain these substances from dietary sources (vitamin D_2 from irradiated yeast and vitamin D_3 from fish liver oils, butter, eggs, cheese and fortified margarine), it is not known for certain whether it is necessary to obtain any vitamin D from food as a plentiful supply of 7-dehydrocholesterol, the precursor of vitamin D_3, exists in human skin and needs only to be activated by a moderate amount of ultraviolet light (less than half an hour of sunlight) to become fully potent. For light-skinned babies, exposure to sunlight for 30 minutes per week wearing only a nappy, or 2 hours per week fully clothed but without a hat, will keep vitamin D requirements within the lower limits of the normal range (Specker et al 1985).

The babies of dark-skinned mothers living in temperate zones and preterm babies may be at risk of vitamin D deficiency, however. If a supplement is necessary it may be safer to give it to the breastfeeding mother (Pyke 1986).

Vitamin E. Although present in human milk, its role is uncertain. It appears to prevent the oxidisation of polyunsaturated fatty acids and may prevent certain types of anaemia to which preterm infants are susceptible.

Vitamin K. This vitamin (83% of which is present as *alpha tocopherol*), is essential for the synthesis of blood-clotting factors. It is present in human milk and absorbed efficiently. Because it is fat soluble, it is present in greater concentrations in colostrum and in the high fat hindmilk (Kries et al 1987), although the increased volume of milk as lactation progresses means that the infant obtains twice as much vitamin K from mature milk as he does from colostrum (Canfield et al 1991).

It has been suggested that by 2 weeks of age the breastfed baby's gut flora should be synthesising adequate amounts of vitamin K (Akre 1990b), although others maintain that the diet is the only source of vitamin K in humans (Kries et al 1987).

Babies who are at risk of haemorrhage, such as the preterm and those delivered precipitately or instrumentally, commonly receive a prophylactic dose, usually by intramuscular injection. Many paediatricians currently consider that all breastfed babies should receive vitamin K soon after birth, although there is little evidence to guide practice. Doubt currently exists as to how much and how often breastfed babies might require additional vitamin K (see Ch. 44). Recent research (Greer 1997) has confirmed earlier work suggesting that marked increases in breastmilk concentrations of vitamin K (and corresponding increases in infant blood levels) can be obtained by giving mothers oral vitamin K preparations, although whether this is necessary (since prothrombin times in infants were not altered) is still open to question. What is clear is that policies in units throughout the UK vary widely, and there is no clear consensus on which babies are at increased risk of bleeding due to vitamin K deficiency and by which route vitamin K should be given (Ansell et al 2001).

Water-soluble vitamins. Unless the mother's diet is seriously deficient, breastmilk will contain adequate levels of all the vitamins. Since most vitamins are fairly widely distributed in foods, a diet significantly deficient in one vitamin will be deficient in others as well. Thus an improved diet will be more beneficial than artificial supplements. With some vitamins, particularly vitamin C, a plateau may be reached where increased maternal intake has no further impact on breastmilk composition.

Minerals and trace elements

Iron. Normal term babies are usually born with a high haemoglobin level (16–22 g/dl), which decreases rapidly after birth. The iron recovered from haemoglobin breakdown is reutilised. They also have ample iron stores, sufficient for at least 4–6 months. Although the amounts of iron are less than those found in formulae, the bioavailability of iron in breastmilk is very much higher: 70% of the iron in breast milk is absorbed whereas only 10% is absorbed from a formula (Saarinen & Siimes 1979). The difference is due to a complex series of interactions that take place within the gut. Babies who are fed fresh cow's milk or a formula may become anaemic because of microhaemorrhages of the bowel.

Zinc. A deficiency of this essential trace mineral may result in failure to thrive and typical skin lesions. Although there is more zinc present in formulae than in human milk, the bioavailability is greater in human milk. Breastfed babies maintain high plasma zinc values compared with formula-fed infants, even when the concentration of zinc is three times that of human milk (Sandstrom et al 1983). Preterm babies may need zinc supplements.

Calcium. This is more efficiently absorbed from human milk than from breastmilk substitutes because of the higher calcium : phosphorus ratio of human milk. Infant formulas, which are based on cow's milk, inevitably have a higher phosphorus content than human milk, and this has been reported to increase the risk of neonatal tetany (Specker et al 1991).

Other minerals. Human milk has significantly lower levels of calcium, phosphorus, sodium and potassium than formulae. Copper, cobalt and selenium are present at higher levels. The higher bioavailability of these minerals and trace elements ensures that the infant's needs are met whilst also imposing a lower solute load on the neonatal kidney than do breastmilk substitutes.

Anti-infective factors

Leucocytes. During the first 10 days there are more white cells per millilitre in breastmilk than there are in blood. *Macrophages* and *neutrophils* are amongst the most common leucocytes in human milk and they surround and destroy harmful bacteria by their phagocytic activity.

Immunoglobulins. Five types of immunoglobulin have been identified in human milk: IgA, IgG, IgE, IgM and IgD. Of these the most important is *IgA*, which appears to be both synthesised and stored in the breast. Although some IgA is absorbed by the infant, much of it is not. Instead it 'paints' the intestinal epithelium and protects the mucosal surfaces against entry of pathogenic bacteria and enteroviruses. It affords protection against *Escherichia coli*, salmonellae, shigellae, streptococci, staphylococci, pneumococci, poliovirus and the rotaviruses.

Lysozyme. This kills bacteria by disrupting their cell walls. The concentration of lysozyme increases with prolonged lactation (Hamosh 1998).

Lactoferrin. This binds to enteric iron, thus preventing potentially pathogenic *E. coli* from obtaining the iron they need for survival. It also has antiviral activity (against HIV, CMV and HSV), by interfering with virus absorption or penetration, or both.

Bifidus factor. The bifidus factor in human milk promotes the growth of Gram positive bacilli in the gut flora, particularly *Lactobacillus bifidus*, which discourages the multiplication of pathogens. (Babies who are fed on cow's-milk-based formulae have more potentially pathogenic bacilli in their gut flora.)

Hormones and growth factors. *Epidermal growth factor* and *insulin-like growth factor* are among the most fully studied of the growth factors and regulatory peptides found in breastmilk and colostrum. They stimulate the baby's digestive tract to mature more quickly and strengthen the barrier properties of the gastrointestinal epithelium. Once the initially leaky membrane lining the gut matures, it is less likely to allow the passage of large molecules, and becomes less vulnerable to microorganisms. The timing of the first feed also has a significant effect on gut permeability, which drops markedly if the first feed takes place soon after birth.

Management of breastfeeding

Antenatal preparation

Breasts and nipples are altered by pregnancy (see Ch. 13). Increased sebum secretion obviates the need for cream to lubricate the nipple. Women who have inverted and non-protractile (flat) nipples often find that they improve spontaneously during pregnancy (Hytten & Baird 1958). If not, help given with attaching the baby to the breast after birth often results in successful breastfeeding (Hytten 1954). Neither the wearing of Woolwich shells nor Hoffmann's exercises are of any value (Main Trial Collaborative Group 1994) and should not be recommended, nor should any other unevaluated commercially available device. Education of the mother is likely to be more use than any physical exercises. If she understands how breast-feeding works, and has an opportunity to observe babies feeding, she will be better prepared for feeding her own.

The first feed

Unless individual circumstances dictate otherwise, the mother should have her baby with her immediately after birth. Early and extended contact will ensure the cues that indicate that the baby is ready to feed will not be missed. Early feeding contributes to the success of breastfeeding but the time of the first feed should, to a large extent, depend on the needs of the baby. Some may demonstrate a desire to feed almost as soon as they are born. Other babies may show no interest until they are an hour or so old (Righard & Alade 1990, Widström et al 1987).

The first feed should be supervised by the midwife. If it proceeds without pain and if the baby is allowed to terminate the feed spontaneously, both mother and baby will have been helped to begin the learning process necessary for good breastfeeding in a happy and positive way.

The next feed

All mothers should be offered help with the next feed also. Once the baby is feeding satisfactorily the mother should be told about the cause, and therefore preven-tion, of sore nipples (see below). She should be urged to seek help if problems do arise. She should be told about the changes that will take place in her breasts during the next few days. An explanation about the changes in the pattern of feeds and the reasons for the variation in the length of feeds will enable her to greet these changes with confidence. Helping mothers to understand that breastfeeding is a learned, not an instinctive, skill will enable them to be patient with themselves and their babies during this time (RCM 2001). It is likely that mothers who receive the right help and education at the start will require less sup-port and remedial intervention later. (The DoH-funded Best Start Breastfeeding Project (2002) tested part of this hypothesis by means of a randomised controlled trial.)

Positioning the mother

There are two main positions for the mother to adopt while she is breastfeeding. The first is *lying on her side* and this may be appropriate at different times during her lactation (see Plate 13). If she has had a caesarean section, or if her perineum is very painful, this may be the only position she can tolerate in the first few days after birth. It is likely that she will need assistance in placing the baby at the breast in this position, because she will only have one free hand. When feeding from the lower breast it may be helpful if she raises her body slightly by tucking the end of a pillow under her ribs. Once she can do this unaided she may find this a comfortable and convenient position for night feeds, enabling her to get more sleep.

The second position is *sitting up* (see Plate 14). In the early days it is particularly important that the mother's back is upright and at a right angle to her lap. This is not possible if she is sitting in bed with her legs stretched out in front of her, or if she is sitting in a chair with a deep backward-sloping seat and a sloping back.

Both lying on her side and sitting correctly in a chair (with her back and feet supported) enhance the shape of the breast and also allow ample room in which to manoeuvre the baby.

Positioning the baby

The baby's body should be *turned towards* the mother's body (Fig. 40.4) so that he is coming up to her breast at the same angle as her breast is coming down to him. Thus the more his mother's breast points down, the more on his back he needs to be (Fig. 40.5). (The advice to have the baby *tummy to tummy* may be mis-takenly taken to imply that the baby should always be lying on his side). If the baby's nose is opposite his mother's nipple before he is brought to the breast and his neck is slightly extended, the baby's mouth will be in the correct relationship to the nipple (Fig. 40.6).

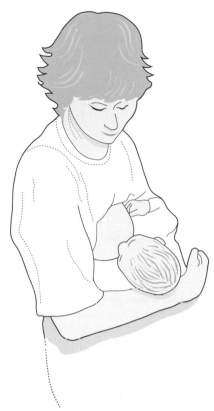

Fig. 40.4 Baby turned towards his mother's body. (From an original drawing by Hilary English.)

Attaching the baby to the breast

The baby should be supported across his shoulders, so that the slight extension of his neck can be maintained. His head may be supported by the extended fingers of the supporting hand (see Plate 15) or on his mother's forearm (see Plate 16). It may be helpful to wrap the baby in a small sheet so that his hands are by his sides (see Plate 17).

If the baby's mouth is moved gently but persistently against his mother's nipple he will open his mouth wide (see Plate 18). As he gapes (drops his lower jaw and darts his tongue down and forward) he needs to be moved quickly to the breast. The intention is to aim the bottom lip as far away from the base of the nipple as is possible. This allows the baby to draw breast tissue as well the nipple into his mouth with his tongue (see Plate 19). If correctly attached, the baby will have formed a 'teat' from the breast and the nipple. The lactiferous sinuses will now be within the

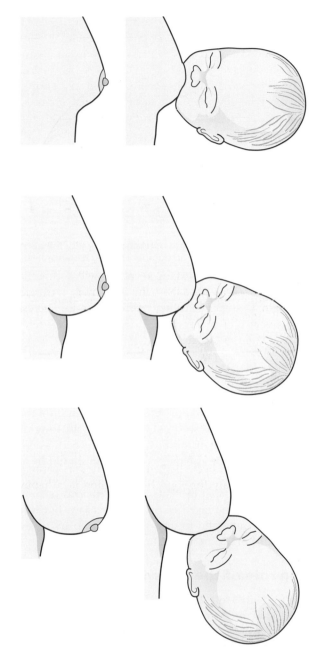

Fig. 40.5 Baby's body in relation to his mother's body, depending on the angle of the breast. (From an original drawing by Hilary English.)

baby's mouth (Fig. 40.7) (Woolridge 1986). The nipple should extend as far as the junction of the hard and soft palate. Contact with the hard palate triggers the sucking reflex. The baby's lower jaw moves up and

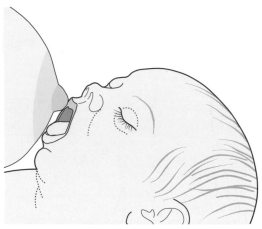

Fig. 40.6 The baby's mouth opposite the nipple, the neck slightly extended. (From an original drawing by Jenny Inch.)

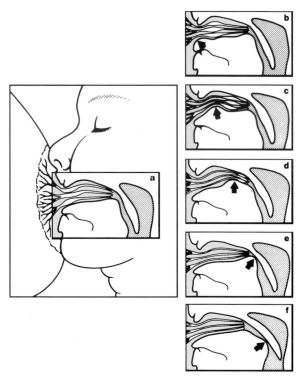

Fig. 40.7 The baby has formed a 'teat' from the breast and the nipple, which causes the nipple to extend back as far as the junction of the hard and soft palates. The lactiferous sinuses are within the baby's mouth. A generous portion of areola is covered by the bottom lip. (Reproduced from Woolridge 1986, with permission.)

down, following the action of the tongue. If the baby is well attached, minimal suction is required to hold the 'teat' within the oral cavity and the tongue can then apply rhythmical cycles of compression so that milk is stripped from the ducts. Although the mother may be startled by the physical sensation, she should not experience pain.

The baby feeds from the breast rather than from the nipple and the mother should guide her baby towards her breast without distorting its shape. The baby's neck should be slightly extended and the chin should be in contact with the breast. If the baby approaches the breast as illustrated in Plate 40.6, a generous portion of areola will be taken in by the lower jaw, but it is positively unhelpful to urge the mother to try to get 'the whole of the areola' in the baby's mouth.

The role of the midwife

The midwife's role during the first few feeds is twofold. First, she must ensure that the baby is adequately fed at the breast. Secondly, she must help the mother to develop the necessary skills so that she is able to feed her baby by herself. Newly delivered women, particularly those who have not breastfed before, need encouragement and reassurance (*emotional support*), they need to be taught the fundamentals of good attachment so that feeding is pain free (*practical support*) and they need to receive factual information about breastfeeding (*informational support*) in small, manageable chunks.

Some mothers will need more teaching and support than others; even women who have breastfed previously may require (and should be offered) help with their new babies.

Hands-on help from the midwife

Pragmatically, it may be necessary for the midwife to help attach the baby to the breast for several feeds. In this case she should think of her own comfort, as well as that of the mother and her baby, because she will be much less capable of providing skilled help if she is strained and uncomfortable. She will put less strain on her own back if she kneels (on a foam mat) beside the mother, rather than bending over her (see Plate 20).

She should also consider which hand guides the baby most skilfully and use it for preference. For example, a right-handed midwife who is helping a mother who is lying on her left side will attach the baby to the left breast with her right hand. Instead of asking the mother to turn on her right side (so that she can feed from the right breast), the midwife could raise up the baby on a pillow and attach him to the right breast, again using her right hand. Alternatively, if the mother is sitting up, she could consider placing the baby under the mother's arm on the right side, so that she can again use her right hand. (Some midwives feel more comfortable if they stand behind the mother so that they get the same view as she does.)

Once the baby has fed efficiently he is more likely to do so again and it is from this point that the mother can begin to learn how to feed her baby by herself.

If the midwife needs to give hands-on help to the mother, she should also explain what she is doing, and why, so that the mother learns from the encounter. If no explanation is given, or the midwife just attaches the baby and leaves the mother, the mother may have help with every feed and yet still be unable to attach the baby to her breast herself days later.

Feeding behaviour

When the baby first goes to the breast he feeds vigorously, with few pauses. As the feed progresses, pausing occurs more frequently and lasts longer. Pausing is an integral part of the baby's feeding rhythm and should not be interrupted. The midwife should simply encourage the mother to allow the baby to pace the feed. The change in the pattern probably relates to milk flow. The foremilk, which he obtains first, is more generous in quantity but lower in fat than the hindmilk delivered at the end, which is thus higher in calories (Woolridge & Fisher 1988). If the baby receives an excessive quantity of foremilk (owing to either poor attachment or premature breast switching – see below), it may result in increased gut fermentation causing colic, flatus and explosive stools (Woolridge & Fisher 1988).

This is the commonest cause of colic in breastfed babies and is resolved by improving attachment. Simethicone preparations, which are often prescribed for this condition, have been shown to be of no value (Metcalf et al 1994).

Finishing the first breast and finishing a feed

The baby will release the breast when he has had sufficient milk from it. His ability to know this may be controlled either by the calories he has received or by the change in the volume available. The baby *should be offered* the second breast after he has had the opportunity to bring up wind. Sometimes in the early days the baby will not need to feed from the second breast.

The baby should not be deliberately removed from the breast before he releases it spontaneously, unless he is causing pain (in which case he should be re-attached, if he is still willing). Taking the baby off the first breast before he has finished may cause two problems. First, the baby is deprived of the high calorie hindmilk; secondly, if adequate milk removal has not taken place, milk stasis may occur ultimately leading to mastitis or a reduced milk production, or both. Provided that the baby starts each feed on alternate sides, both breasts will be used equally. If the baby does not release the breast or will not settle after a feed, the most likely reason is that he had not been correctly attached to the breast and was therefore unable to strip the milk efficiently.

Other reasons for coming off the breast are:

- the baby may not have been correctly attached
- the baby may need to let go and pause if the milk flow is very fast
- the baby may have swallowed air with the generous flow of milk that occurs at the beginning of a feed and need an opportunity to burp.

There is no justification for imposing either *one breast per feed* or alternatively *both breasts per feed* as a feeding regimen.

Timing and frequency of feeds

A well, term baby knows better than anyone else how often and for how long he needs to be fed. This is described as baby-led feeding, which is a term preferable to 'demand feeding'.

It is not unusual in the 1st day or so for the baby to feed infrequently, and have 6–8 hour gaps between good feeds, each of which may be quite long (Inch & Garforth 1989, Waldenström & Swensen 1991). This is normal and provides the mother with the opportunity to sleep if she needs to. As the milk volume increases, the feeds tend to become more frequent and a little shorter. It is unusual for a baby to feed less often than six times in 24 hours from the 3rd day, and most babies ask for between six and eight feeds per 24 hours by the time they are a week old. Babies who feed infrequently may be consuming less milk than they need, or they may be unwell, or both. Babies who feed very often (10–12 feeds in 24 hours after the 1st week) may be poorly attached. The feeding technique and the weight should be monitored. However, individual mother–baby pairs develop their own unique pattern of feeding and, provided the baby is thriving and the mother is happy, there is no need to change it.

Volume of the feed

Well-grown term infants are born with good glycogen reserves and high levels of antidiuretic hormone. Consequently they do not need large volumes of milk or colostrum any sooner than these are made available physiologically. In the first 24 hours the baby takes an average of 7 ml per feed; in the second 24 hours this increases to 14 ml per feed (RCM 2001).

No precise information is available on the actual volume of breastmilk an individual baby requires in order to grow satisfactorily. Previous recommendations (150 ml per kg) were based on the requirements of *artificially fed* babies, and these can therefore be used only as a guideline.

Weight loss and weight gain

Most newborn babies lose some weight during their 1st week of life, and there is a general expectation that the baby will be back to birthweight by 10–14 days. There is less agreement about how great a weight loss is within the bounds of normal or acceptable. Although the figure of 10% is often cited as the upper limit of normal, there is little evidence to support a figure as high as this. Data from nine studies conducted between 1986 and 1999 suggest a normal range of 3%–7% (Avoa & Fischer 1990, Enzunga & Fischer 1990, Fischer & Dind 1991, Kasa & Heinonen 1993, Muskinja-montanji et al 1999, Pandove et al 1994, Tjon et al 1986, Velisavljev et al 1998, Yamauchi & Yamanouchi 1990).

Over the first 4 days of life the stools change from black meconium to the characteristic yellow stool of the baby, fed on breastmilk. A stool that is still 'changing' at 96 hours of life could indicate that further attention needs to be paid to the way the mother is feeding her baby (see Plate 21).

If the baby is difficult to attach, because he is sleepy or because the breast tissue is inelastic, the same principles ought to apply to this situation as when the baby and mother are separated by virtue of illness or prematurity – namely to teach the mother how to hand express (see below) in order to get lactation established. If this is not done, the mother's lactation will be in arrears of her baby's needs when he starts to ask for larger volumes on the 3rd/4th day.

If the mother is still not able to feed effectively as the end of the 1st week approaches, she should make expressing her milk her priority, using either her hands or an effective breast pump, so that her lactation is secured and her baby is fed. Ongoing help with improving breastfeeding will also be needed.

Expressing breastmilk

Although all breastfeeding mothers should know how to hand express milk, *routine* expression of the breasts should not be part of the normal management of lactation, even for mothers who have delivered by caesarean section (Chapman et al 2001).

Provided that no limitation is placed on either feed frequency or duration and the baby is correctly attached, the volume of milk produced will be in step with the requirements of the baby. This will prevent the occurrence of problems (such as engorgement) that would require artificial removal of milk.

The situations where expressing *is* appropriate are:

- where there is concern about the interval between feeds in the early newborn period (expressed colostrum should always be given in preference to formulae to healthy term babies)
- where there are problems in attaching the baby to the breast
- where the baby is separated from the mother, owing to prematurity or illness
- where there is concern about the baby's rate of growth, or the mother's milk supply (expressing to top up with the mother's own milk may be necessary in the short term while the cause of the problem is resolved
- later in lactation, when the mother may need to be separated from her baby for periods (occasionally, or regularly).

Manual expression of milk

This method has not been commonly practised where electric breast pumps are available but it has several advantages over mechanical pumping and should be taught to all mothers. It costs nothing and can be practised anywhere. It is the most efficient method of obtaining colostrum. Some mothers will find hand expressing superior to any breast pump (Figs 40.8 and 40.9). There are now a variety of useful teaching aids available; models, videos and leaflets (contact UNICEF-UK Baby Friendly Initiative, see Useful addresses, p. 779).

Expressing with a breast pump

If it is possible and practical, the mother should be able to experiment with a variety of breast pumps, so that she can discover what will suit her best (Auerbach & Walker 1994). Not all pumps work well for all women.

Hand pumps

Manually controlled. Most manually operated pumps are not efficient enough to allow initiation of full lactation but they can be useful when expressing is necessary in established lactation. Their major limitation is that they can be used on only one breast at a time. It is helpful to mothers to explain that the pumps function most efficiently if the vacuum phase is considerably longer than the release phase.

Electrically controlled. Some pumps provide a regular vacuum and release cycle, with variability in the strength of the suction. Some vary the frequency of the cycle as well. Double pumping is possible with most models, and this has repeatedly been shown to be of benefit, either by reducing the time for which the mother needs to pump at each session to obtain the available milk (Groh-Wargo et al 1995, Hill et al 1999), or by increasing the volume of milk obtained, for mothers of both term (Auerbach 1990) and preterm (Jones et al 2001) babies.

How much and how often?

The mothers of preterm babies who begin pumping as soon as possible after birth and pump a *minimum* of 6 times per 24 hours are more likely to sustain lactation at adequate levels than those who delay pumping or pump less frequently, or both. The earlier the mother is able to express good volumes of milk (per 24 hours) the better the outlook for continued adequate milk production.

Breast massage (Jones et al 2001) and kangaroo care (Hill et al 1999) have also been positively associated with enhanced milk production.

No time limit should be set for the length of each expressing session. The mother should be guided by the milk flow, not the clock. Expressing should continue until milk flow ceases, followed by a short break, and each breast should be expressed twice (either separately (sequential pumping) or together (double pumping)). When milk flow ceases for the second time the session should end. Frequent pumping sessions are more likely to have the desired effect than infrequent marathons.

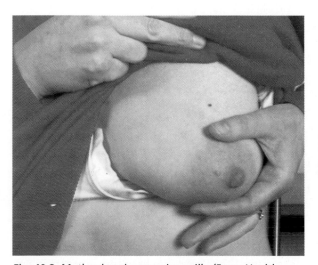

Fig. 40.8 Mother hand expressing milk. (From Health Education Board of Scotland, with permission.)

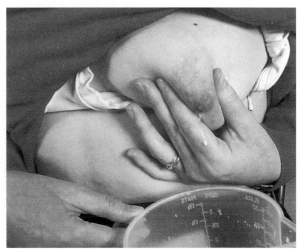

Fig. 40.9 Mother hand expressing milk. (From Health Education Board of Scotland, with permission.)

Inadequate milk volume, followed by declining production, are common problems for the mothers of preterm babies who are expressing their milk. *Prevention*, by the midwife discussing with the mother the importance of early initiation, appropriate use of the (correct size of) equipment and *frequency* (rather than regularity) of expression, is preferable to trying to rescue failing lactation pharmacologically.

Care of the breasts

Daily washing is all that is necessary for breast hygiene. The normal skin flora are beneficial to the baby. Brassieres may be worn in order to provide comfortable support and are useful if the breasts leak and breast pads (or breast shells) are used.

Breast problems

Sore and damaged nipples

These two conditions occur so commonly in developed countries that many health professionals believe them to be inevitable. The cause is almost always trauma from the baby's mouth and tongue, which results from incorrect attachment of the baby to the breast. Correcting this will provide immediate relief from pain and will also allow rapid healing to take place. Epithelial growth factor, contained in fresh human milk and saliva, may aid this process.

'Resting' the nipple also enables healing to take place but makes the continuation of lactation much more complicated because it is necessary to express the milk and to use some other means of feeding it to the baby.

Nipple shields should be used with extreme caution, and never before the mother has begun to lactate. They may make feeding less painful, but often they do not. Their use does not enable the mother to learn how to feed her baby correctly, and their longer term use may result in reduced milk transfer from mother to baby. This in turn may result in either mastitis in the mother (reduced milk removal), or slow weight gain or prolonged feeds in the baby (reduced milk transfer), or both! If mothers chose to use them, or midwives decide to suggest their use, the mother should be advised to seek help with learning to attach the baby comfortably without a nipple shield as soon as practicable.

Other causes of soreness. Infection with *Candida albicans* (thrush) can occur, although it is not common during the 1st week. The sudden development of pain when the mother has had a period of trouble-free feeding is suggestive of thrush. The nipple and areola are often inflamed and shiny, and pain typically persists throughout the feed. The baby may show signs of oral or anal thrush. Both mother and baby should receive concurrent fungicidal treatment (miconazole or nystatin; see Ch. 48) and it may take several days for the pain in the nipple to disappear.

Dermatitis

Sensitivity may develop to topical applications such as creams, ointments or sprays (including those used to treat thrush, such as clotrimazole). The mother with sore nipples should be questioned about the use of such products.

Anatomical variations

Long nipples. These can lead to poor feeding because the baby is able to latch on to the nipple without drawing breast tissue into his mouth. The mother may need to be shown how to help the baby to draw in a sufficient portion of the breast.

Short nipples. As the baby has to form a teat from both the breast and nipple, short nipples should not cause problems and the mother should be reassured of this.

Abnormally large nipples. If the baby is small, his mouth may not be able to get beyond the nipple and on to the breast. Lactation could be initiated by expressing, either by hand or by pump, provided that the nipple fits into the breast cup. (Some manufacturers now make pump kits in different sizes.) As the baby grows and the breast and nipple become more protractile, breastfeeding may become possible.

Inverted and flat nipples. If the nipple is deeply inverted it may be necessary to initiate lactation by expressing and delay attempting to attach the baby to the breast until lactation is established and the breasts have become soft and the breast tissue more protractile.

Problems with breastfeeding

Engorgement

This condition occurs around the 3rd or 4th day postpartum. The breasts are hard (often oedematous), painful and sometimes flushed. The mother may be pyrexial. Engorgement is usually an indication that the baby is not in step with the stage of lactation. Engorgement may occur if feeds are delayed or restricted (Illingworth & Stone 1952) or if the baby is unable to feed efficiently because he is not correctly attached to the breast.

Management should be aimed at enabling the baby to feed well (Box 40.1). In severe cases the only solution will be the gentle use of a pump. This will reduce the tension in the breast and *will not* cause excessive milk production. The mother's fluid intake should not be restricted, as this has no direct effect on milk production.

Deep breast pain

In most cases this responds to improvement in breastfeeding technique and is thus likely to be due to raised intraductal pressure caused by inefficient milk removal. Although it may occur during the feed it typically occurs afterwards, and thus can be distinguished from the sensation of the let-down reflex, which some mothers experience as a fleeting pain. Very rarely deep breast pain may be the result of ductal thrush infection.

Mastitis

Mastitis means inflammation of the breast. In the majority of cases it is the result of milk stasis, not infection, although infection may supervene (Thomsen et al 1984). Typically, one or more adjacent segments are inflamed (as a result of milk being forced into the connective tissue of the breast) and appear as a wedge-shaped area of redness and swelling. If milk is also forced back into the bloodstream, the woman's pulse and temperature may rise and in some cases flu-like symptoms, including shivering attacks or rigors, may occur. (The presence or absence of systemic symptoms does not help to distinguish infectious from non-infectious mastitis (WHO 2000).)

Non-infective (acute intramammary) mastitis. This condition results from milk stasis. It may occur during the early days as the result of unresolved engorgement or at any time when poor feeding technique results in the milk from one or more segments of the breast not being efficiently removed by the baby. It occurs much more frequently in the breast that is opposite the mother's preferred side for holding her baby (Inch & Fisher 1995). Pressure from fingers or

---

Box 40.1 Babies who are difficult to attach

Inelastic breast tissue, overfull or engorged breasts or deeply inverted nipples may present the baby with more of a challenge.

- If the breast is engorged, pushing away the oedema by gently manipulating the tissue that lies under the areola may be all that is required.

- Hand expression, or the use of a breast pump, may relieve fullness to the point where the baby can draw in the inner tissue to create the necessary teat from the breast.

- If attachment is still difficult, try asking the mother to lie on her side with the short edge of a pillow under her ribs to raise the breast off the bed. Use your better hand to attach the baby.

- If you are not able to attach the baby either, show the mother how to hand express and how to give her colostrum to her baby.

- It may also be necessary to show her how to use the electric pump. In the first 24–48 hours the value of the pump is mainly in its effect on the nipple and breast tissue – colostrum is usually best expressed by hand.

When attachment is difficult, the priorities should be to ensure that the baby is adequately fed on his mother's milk, and to work on making the breast tissue more elastic (both of which can be facilitated by hand or electrical expressing). Attaching the baby to the breast directly can come later.

---

clothing has been blamed for causing the condition, without any supporting evidence. It is extremely important that breastfeeding from the affected breast continues, otherwise milk stasis will increase further and provide ideal conditions for pathogenic bacteria to replicate. (An infective condition may then arise which could, if untreated, lead to abscess formation, causing much pain and distress to the mother.)

Where supervision is available, 12–24 hours could be allowed to elapse to ascertain whether the mastitis can be resolved by helping the mother to improve her feeding technique and encouraging her to allow the baby to finish the first breast first. If supervision is not available, or if no improvement occurs during that period, antibiotics (e.g. cephalexin, flucloxacillin or erythromycin) should be given prophylactically (RCM 2001, WHO 2000).

Infective mastitis. The main cause of superficial breast infection is damage to the epithelium, which allows bacteria to enter the underlying tissues. The damage results from incorrect attachment of the baby to the breast, which has caused trauma to the nipple. The mother therefore urgently needs help to improve her technique, as well as the appropriate antibiotic (see above). Multiplication of bacteria may be enhanced by the use of breast pads or shells. In spite of antibiotic therapy, abscess formation may occur. Infection may also enter the breast via the milk ducts if milk stasis remains unresolved.

Breast abscess

Here a fluctuant swelling develops in a previously inflamed area. Pus may be discharged from the nipple. Simple needle aspiration may be effective, or incision and drainage may be necessary (Dixon 1988). It may not be possible to feed from the affected breast for a few days; however, milk removal should continue and breastfeeding should recommence as soon as practicable because this has been shown to reduce the chances of further abscess formation (Benson & Goodman 1970). A sinus that drains milk may form, but it is likely to heal in time.

Blocked ducts

Lumpy areas in the breast are not uncommon – the mother is usually feeling distended glandular tissue. If they become very firm and tender (and sometimes flushed) they are often described as 'blocked ducts'. This description carries with it the image of a physical obstruction within the lumen of the duct – like 'a golf ball in a hosepipe'. This is very rarely the cause of the symptoms (see below). It is much more likely to be the case that milk removal has been somewhat uneven (as a consequence of less than optimal attachment) and that the secreted milk is now trying to occupy more space than is actually available – and thus distending the alveoli. It may subsequently be forced out into the connective tissue of the breast where it causes inflammation. The inflammatory process then narrows the lumen of the duct by exerting pressure on it from the outside as the tissue swells. A more helpful image

might therefore be that of 'compressing the hosepipe'. (This is, effectively, mastitis or incipient mastitis.) Consequently the solution is to improve milk removal (improved attachment, and possibly milk expression as well) and to treat the accompanying pain and inflammation. Massage, which is often advocated to clear the imagined 'blockage', may make matters worse by forcing more milk into the surrounding tissue.

White spots

Very occasionally, a ductal opening in the tip of the nipple may become obstructed by a white granule or by epithelial overgrowth.

White granules. These appear to be caused by the aggregation and fusion of casein micelles to which further materials become added (Cowie et al 1980). This hardened lump may obstruct a milk duct as it slowly makes its way down to the nipple, where it may be removed by the baby during a feed or expressed manually (Purves & Brown 1982).

Epithelial overgrowth. This seems to be the more common cause of a physical obstruction. A white blister is evident on the surface of the nipple, and it effectively closes off one of the exit points in the nipple, which leads from one or more milk-producing sections of the breast.

This may also be resolved by the baby feeding. Alternatively, after the baby has fed (and the skin is softened), it may be removed with a clean fingernail, a rough flannel, or a sterile needle.

True blockages of this sort tend to recur, but once the woman understands how to deal with them the progression to mastitis can be avoided.

Feeding difficulties due to the baby

Cleft lip. Provided that the palate is intact, the presence of a cleft in the lip should not interfere with breastfeeding because the vacuum that is necessary to enable the baby to attach to the breast is created between the tongue and the hard palate, not the breast and the lips.

Cleft palate. Though there are cases documented that suggest it is possible to breastfeed if the baby has a cleft of the palate, it would appear, on closer inspection, that the babies were able to obtain milk only as the result of the mother's milk ejection reflex. This would suggest that it is rarely likely to be completely successful. Because of the cleft, the baby is unable to create a vacuum and thus form a teat out of the breast and nipple. The use of an orthodontic plate is unlikely to help because the baby is unable to feel the breast against the hard palate and this is necessary to elicit the sucking response. There is no reason why the mother should be discouraged from putting the baby to the breast – for comfort, pleasure or food – provided that she is aware of the above and appreciates that it is likely that she will need to give her baby her expressed milk as well.

Many mothers have expressed their milk and used various techniques to feed it to their babies. A device called the Haberman feeder has proved useful. (These are now provided free of charge by CLAPA – see Useful addresses, p. 779.) Some mothers have maintained their lactation until the baby has had a surgical repair and have then succeeded in breastfeeding.

Tongue tie. If the baby cannot extend his tongue over his lower gum he is unlikely to be able to draw the breast deeply into his mouth, which he needs to do to feed effectively. Sometimes this is because the tongue is short, and sometimes this is because the frenulum, the whitish strip of tissue that attaches the tongue to the floor of the mouth, is preventing it. As the baby lifts his tongue, the tip becomes heart shaped as the frenulum pulls on it. Although there is much empirical evidence to suggest that tongue tie can interfere with breastfeeding (Nicholson 1991, Notestine 1990, Wiessinger & Miller 1995) and to support the value of frenotomy (surgical release of the frenulum, which takes a few seconds and is usually bloodless and painless) (Jain 1995, Marmet et al 1990, Masaitis & Kaempf 1996), there is a paucity of objective research and thus opinion as to its value can be deeply divided (Newman & Pitman 2000, Renfrew et al 2000).

Blocked nose. Babies normally breathe through their noses. If there is an obstruction, they have great difficulty with feeding because they have to interrupt the process in order to breathe. A blockage caused by mucus may be relieved with a twist of damp cotton wool, or by instilling drops of normal saline before a feed (Bollag et al 1984).

Down syndrome. Babies with this condition can be successfully breast fed, although extra help and encouragement may be necessary initially.

Prematurity. Preterm infants who are sufficiently mature to have developed sucking and swallowing reflexes may successfully breastfeed. Breastfeeding is less tiring than bottle feeding for the preterm baby (Meier & Cranston-Anderson 1987). If the reflexes are not strongly developed, the baby may tire before the feed is complete and complementary tube feeding may be necessary.

Babies who are too immature to breastfeed may be able to cup feed, as an alternative to being tube fed (Lang et al 1994). Less mature babies who are unable to suck or swallow at all will be dependent on artificial methods such as tube feeding and intravenous alimentation.

Illness or surgery. Babies recover quickly following illness or surgery. If they have never been to the breast, or if feeding has been interrupted for a long period, the mother may require skilled help to initiate or re-establish feeding.

Contraindications to breastfeeding

Drugs (see Ch. 48)

breastfeeding may have to be suspended temporarily following the administration of certain drugs or following diagnostic techniques.

Most regions have drug centres where advice may be sought about the safety of drugs for lactating women. There are also good reference books and websites available to health professionals (see Further reading, p. 777).

Cancer

If the mother has cancer, the treatment she receives will make it impossible to breastfeed without harming the baby. However, if she wishes to, she could express and discard her milk for the duration of the treatment and resume breastfeeding later. If she has had a mastectomy, she may feed successfully from the other breast. She may also be able to breast feed following a lumpectomy for cancer. She should seek advice from her surgeon.

Breast surgery

Neither breast reduction nor augmentation are an inevitable contraindication to breastfeeding, but much depends on the techniques used. Where possible, advice should be sought from the surgeon. If the nipple has been displaced, the duct system is not likely to be patent. No harm can result from testing it out by allowing the baby to go to the breast.

Breast injury

Injuries caused by scalding in childhood may cause such severe scarring that breastfeeding is impossible. Burns or other accidents may also cause serious damage.

One breast only

It is perfectly possible to feed a baby well using just one breast. If the mother has only one functioning breast, she should be reassured that in all women each breast works independently. If the baby is offered only one breast, that breast will make enough milk to feed that one baby. There are documented cases of women feeding two babies with just one breast (Nicolls 1997).

HIV infection

HIV may be transmitted in breastmilk. In developed countries, where artificial feeding is relatively safe, the mother may be advised not to breastfeed if she is HIV positive (see Ch. 21). In countries where artificial feeding is a significant cause of infant mortality, exclusive breastfeeding may be the safer option (Akre 1990c, Coutsoudis et al 1999) but research is ongoing.

Cessation of lactation

Suppression of lactation

If a mother chooses not to breastfeed or if she has a late miscarriage or stillbirth, lactation will still begin. The woman may experience discomfort for a day or two, but if unstimulated the breasts will naturally cease to produce milk. Very rarely severe discomfort with engorgement occurs. Expressing small amounts of milk once or twice can afford great relief without interfering with the rapid regression of the condition. The mother will be more comfortable if her breasts are supported but it is doubtful if binding the breasts contributes anything towards suppression.

There is no basis on which to advise the mother to restrict her fluid intake (see Engorgement, p. 762) or to seek a prescription for a diuretic, which will be equally ineffective (Hodge 1967).

These measures merely add to the woman's discomfort by making her thirsty. Pharmacological suppression of lactation with dopamine receptor agonists is effective but is not recommended for routine use. Two such drugs, bromocriptine and cabergoline, are

currently licensed for this use in the UK, although bromocriptine has now had its USA licence withdrawn. High dose oestrogens (such as stilboestrol) are no longer used because of their association with thromboembolism.

Discontinuation of breastfeeding

Stopping lactation abruptly once breastfeeding has become established may cause serious problems for the mother. She could develop engorgement or mastitis, or even a breast abscess. She should be encouraged to mimic normal weaning by expressing her breasts but reducing the frequency over several days or possibly weeks. The gradual reduction in the volume of milk removed will result in a corresponding diminution in the production of milk. Eventually she should be encouraged to express only if she feels uncomfortable. The most tragic circumstance under which this advice might be required follows the death of a baby. Cabergoline might be appropriate in this case.

Returning to work

If the breastfeeding mother returns to work, her baby will have to be fed in her absence (unless there is a crèche at work or a child minder who can bring the baby to his mother).

She may wish her baby to have her own milk at all times and she may express for this purpose.

If the mother finds it difficult to express at work, her baby could receive a formula feed (or 'solid' food if over 6 months) while she is away, but breastfeed at all other times. Midwives should help mothers to understand that returning to work does not mean that breastfeeding has to be terminated.

Weaning from the breast

When the mother or the baby decides to stop breastfeeding, feeds should be tailed off gradually. Breast feeds may be omitted, one at a time, and spaced further apart. Adding supplementary foods should not begin until about 6 months of age (see p. 767). If the mother is using solid food to give the baby 'tastes' and the experience of different textures before weaning, these should be given after the breastfeed. Solid foods given before the breastfeed (weaning) will result in the baby taking less milk from the breast and thus less will be produced.

Complementary and supplementary feeds

Complementary feeds (or 'top-ups') are feeds given *after* a breastfeed. Complementary feeds of breastmilk substitutes ('formula milk') should be given as a last resort, not as a quick fix. *Any formula at all* is enough to sensitise susceptible infants (Host 1991).

Currently 28% of babies born in UK hospitals receive breastmilk substitutes whilst in hospital (Hamlyn et al 2002). The only demonstrable effect of giving complementary feeds in hospitals is to reduce the overall duration of breastfeeding. The mothers of these babies are three times more likely to have given up breastfeeding by the time their baby is 2 weeks old, in comparison with mothers whose babies have received only breastmilk (White et al 1992).

About 10% of newborns are at risk for hypoglycaemia (see Ch. 47), and may thus need a higher intake straight from birth than their mothers are able to provide. Where possible this should be human milk – from a human milk bank (see below).

Babies who are well but sleepy (Box 40.2), jaundiced (see Ch. 46), unsettled (Box 40.3), or difficult to attach (Box 40.1), should, if necessary, be given their mother's own expressed milk in addition to being offered the breast.

If complementary feeds are clinically indicated and the mother is unable to express sufficient, donor milk from a human milk bank could be used. Donors will have been serologically tested for HIV and a negative result received before their milk can be accepted.

If the baby is very young, these additional feeds should be given by oral syringe or cup rather than in a bottle. An oral syringe (or dropper) will reduce wastage and the use of a cup would allow the baby (who will need only small amounts at this stage), to remain more in control of his intake.

If the problem (such as attachment difficulty) persists, the mother may find it quicker and more efficient to give her expressed milk by bottle. She should be reassured that there is no evidence that the baby will subsequently refuse the breast in these circumstances (Brown et al 1999, Cronenwett et al 1992, Howard C, in press, Schubiger et al 1997).

Supplementary feeds are feeds given *in place of* a breast feed. There can be no justification for their use except in extreme circumstances (such as severe illness or unconsciousness) because each breast feed missed by the baby will interfere with the establishment of lactation and damage the mother's confidence.

Box 40.2 'Sleepy' babies

Provided that the baby is otherwise well, which will be determined by checking the baby from time to time, there is no evidence that long intervals between feeds have any adverse affect. As few as three feeds in the first 24 hours life is within the normal range.

- The baby could remain in bed with his mother (in accordance with hospital guidelines). His mother will thus be able to respond immediately to her baby's feeding cues.
- The baby could be roused at intervals, possibly by changing the nappy, and offered the breast.
- The baby could be undressed down to the nappy and placed in skin contact with his mother and offered the breast.
- The mother could be shown how to hand express some colostrum, and how to give this to the baby.
- It is unnecessary to measure the baby's blood sugar (see Ch. 47).

Human milk banking

In the late 1970s and early 1980s there were over 60 human milk banks in the UK. Most of them closed in the late 1980s, driven by both the fear of HIV transmission and the rising popularity of preterm formulae. By the early 1990s there were only six milk banks left in the UK.

Slowly this number has risen, encouraged by research that demonstrated the effectiveness of pasteurisation as a means of destroying HIV (Eglin & Wilkinson 1987) and the importance of human milk in the prevention of necrotising enterocolitis (Lucas & Cole 1990). 1999 saw the publication of the second edition of the British Paediatric Association Guidelines for human milk banks. The total in 2001 stood at 14.

In the *Breastfeeding Awareness Week* of 1998, the UK Human Milk Banking Association (UKAMB) was

Box 40.3 If the baby is unsettled

An unsettled baby of any age that is crying again soon after he has been fed may not have been well attached.

- Watch what the mother is doing and, if necessary, guide her or help her directly.
- If the attachment is good, then the baby may be reacting to being removed from the closeness of his mother's body. If the mother needs to sleep, suggest that she feed lying down and help her if necessary. Use the cot-side/bed guard to ensure the safety of the baby (as per hospital guidelines for their use).
- The mother might try to express some colostrum/milk to give to the baby if she is concerned that the baby has not received all that he might from the breast.
- Some babies will appear unsettled even if they have fed well at the breast. The baby may be uncomfortable. The act of changing the nappy may help; so may wrapping the baby comfortably but securely and providing rhythmic motion, such as walking or holding the baby over the shoulder or over the forearm, both of which apply gentle pressure to the baby's abdomen.
- Show the mother what you are doing, so that she learns appropriate coping strategies from you.
- If *you* give the baby formula or a dummy to 'settle' him, that is what she will do when she goes home.
- *Do not offer* to remove the baby. Separating mother and baby – particularly removing the baby at night in the mistaken belief that the mother will benefit if she does not wake to breastfeed her baby at night – is strongly correlated with reduced breastfeeding success.
- If the mother *asks* you to – and you agree – return the baby to her when he wakes again to be fed.

launched, spearheaded by the oldest milk bank, that at Queen Charlotte's and Chelsea Hospital. Its purpose is to make human milk more readily available to preterm infants (by setting up a milk bank network) and to encourage and support the setting up of new milk banks.

Banked human milk is used predominantly for preterm and sick newborns. Occasionally, if there is sufficient, it is used for term babies whose mothers are temporarily unable to meet their babies' needs with their own (expressed) milk. Mothers who are offered donated milk for their babies should have sufficient information about the collection and screening of human milk to enable them to make an informed choice whether to accept it or not (see, for example, Box 40.4).

Feeding the baby – breast or bottle?

The part played by health professionals in assisting a mother to choose her feeding method is probably not very great (Hoddinott 1998), but in so far as the professional has an influence, it should be positive and unequivocal (Crawford 1992, Freed et al 1995).

Although the majority of women who choose to breastfeed have made this decision very early on, some may not make a final decision until after giving birth. Asking the mother to make a decision antenatally ('how do you plan to feed your baby?') is unhelpful, as it may close the door to further discussion or make the pregnant woman feel that she cannot change her mind, or both.

The subject may be more usefully raised as part of an ongoing discussion in the latter third of pregnancy. The midwife should ensure that the mother is aware of the risks of artificial feeding, and knows what the usual practice of the hospital is in relation to skin contact at birth, the management of breastfeeding, rooming-in and so on, so that the woman can make her own preferences known.

Although knowledge of the benefits of breastfeeding is important, it has been suggested that the 'decision' to bottle feed is often neither rational nor made at a specific point in time (Hoddinott 1998). Actually seeing a baby being breastfed can strongly influence the decision to breastfeed either positively or negatively, depending on the context (Hoddinott & Pill 1999). This may be of particular relevance to women from lower socioeconomic groups for whom theoretical knowledge may have less power than embodied

Box 40.4 Donated breastmilk

If you are offering a mother donated human milk for her baby for any reason, she might find the information below helpful in deciding whether to accept it.

- All human milk donors meet the same criteria as blood donors; they are in a low risk group to start with and give consent to an HIV blood test.
- All human milk donors sign a form to that effect and all have their blood tested.
- Almost all donors are currently feeding their own baby whilst donating.
- No donated milk is used for any baby until the results of the donor's blood test has been received.
- All donated milk is collected in sterilised bottles, kept in the fridge and frozen within 24 hours.
- When it arrives, still frozen, at the milk bank, it is thawed, a small sample taken for bacteriological screening and the rest pasteurised.
- After pasteurisation another small sample is taken (for postpasteurisation bacteriological screening) and the rest refrozen in a holding freezer.
- Only when the results of both samples have been received is the milk transferred to the freezer from which it can be used for preterm and term babies.
- Donors are not paid for the milk they donate – it is freely given! Quite often mothers choose to donate milk because their own babies were themselves helped in this way by the generosity of other mothers.

knowledge. It has therefore been suggested that women intending to breastfeed might benefit from an antenatal 'apprenticeship' with a known breastfeeding mother. Peer group support can influence both the initiation and the continuation of breastfeeding (Fairbank et al 2000), and introducing pregnant women to other mothers with young babies, as is often done as part of parent education classes, may be helpful.

Time should be taken during the antenatal period to talk briefly about the day-to-day progress and management of early breastfeeding. The woman should at the very least be aware that breastfeeding is a learned skill, that it should not hurt and that she may well receive conflicting advice. This does not mean that she will not need to be taught about the major details of management after the baby is born; many pregnant women find it difficult to project their thoughts forward to the time beyond the birth

The more that is known about breastfeeding, the more imperative it may seem to most midwives that all babies are breastfed. It may thus be hard to accept a woman's informed choice to do something that is not in the best interest of her baby (or herself). However, the midwife's responsibility to the woman is to ensure that her choice is 'fully informed', rather than to persuade her to breastfeed.

Conversely, many midwives will have seen women who wanted to breastfeed fail for want of appropriate help and support, and some may themselves have had negative experiences of breastfeeding. Such midwives may feel that by taking a neutral stance on the subject they will 'spare' those who are undecided the possibility of future distress. The response to this approach must again be to remind the midwife that her responsibility to the pregnant woman is to enable her to make a 'fully informed' choice. She will be unable to do this if the midwife withholds information from her.

The nutritional and immunological consequences of not breastfeeding are seen in population studies, and are to do with relative risks. It is not possible to narrow the risk down to the individual. Nevertheless all pregnant women should be made aware that, compared with a fully breastfed baby, a baby who is bottle fed from birth is:

- five times more likely to be hospitalised with gastroenteritis (within the first 3 months of life)
- five times more likely to suffer from urine infections (within the first 6 months of life)
- twice as likely to suffer from chest infections (within the first 7 years of life)
- twice as likely to suffer from ear infections (within the 1st year of life)
- twice as likely to develop atopic disease where there is a family history
- up to 20 times more likely to develop necrotising enterocolitis if born prematurely.

Additionally, the pregnant woman should know that she may increase her own risk of premenopausal breast cancer, ovarian cancer and osteoporosis if she does not breastfeed (MIDIRS 1999, UNICEF-UK 2002).

Artificial feeding

Most breastmilk substitutes (infant formulae) are modified cow's milk. Until the early 1970s they consisted of crudely modified dried cow's milk with added vitamins. Their high solute loads contributed to infantile hypocalcaemia and to hypernatraemic dehydration. As newer products were developed the older types were phased out. This included national dried milk, which was withdrawn in 1977.

Currently the minimum and maximum permitted levels of named ingredients, and named prohibited ingredients, are now laid down by statute in the Infant Formula and Follow-on Formula Regulations 1995. However, considerable variations in composition can (and do) exist within the legally permitted ranges. Over 100 changes a year are made to commercially available breastmilk substitutes (Messenger 1994).

The two main components used are *skimmed milk* (a by-product of butter manufacture) and *whey* (a by-product of cheese manufacture). Breastmilk substitutes may contain fats from any source, animal or vegetable (except from sesame and cotton seeds), provided that they do not contain more than 8% trans isomers of fatty acids. (The fat source may not always be apparent from reading the label: oleo, for example, is beef fat – unacceptable to Hindus and vegetarians; 'oils of vegetable origin' may have come from marine algae.) They may also contain, among other things, soya protein, maltodextrin, dried glucose syrup and gelatinised and precooked starch.

Formulae

There are two main types of formula: whey dominant and casein dominant. Both can be used from birth.

Whey-dominant formulae

In these a small amount of skimmed milk is combined with demineralised whey. The ratio of proteins in the formulae approximates to the ratio of whey to casein found in human milk (60 : 40). These feeds are more easily digested than the casein-dominant formulae, which will have an effect on gastric emptying times. This leads to feeding patterns that more closely resemble those of breastfed babies.

Casein-dominant formulae

These are also sold as being suitable for use from birth, but they are aimed at mothers whose babies are 'hungrier' (!) Although the proportions of the macronutrients (fat, carbohydrate, protein, etc.) are the same as is found in whey-dominant formulae, more of the protein present is in the form of casein (20 : 80). This forms large relatively indigestible curds in the stomach and is intended to make the baby feel full for longer. This will inevitably place even greater metabolic demands on the infant.

Babies intolerant of standard formulae

Predicting which babies will be prone to allergies is an inexact science. It is estimated that the likelihood of a child being predisposed to allergy is about 20–35% if one parent is affected, 40–60% if both parents are affected and 50–70% if both parents have the same allergy (Brostoff & Gamlin 1998, p. 261).

Hydrolysate formula. If breastfeeding is not possible, there are (prescription-only) alternatives that carry less risk of allergy than standard formulas – hydrolysates – some of which are designed to *treat* an existing allergy, and some of which are designed for *preventative* use in bottle-fed babies who are at high risk of developing cow's milk protein allergy (Brostoff & Gamlin 1998, p. 232). This is reflected in the British National Formulary prescribing guidelines, which require 'proven intolerance' for some hydrolysates, but not for others.

These substances are considerably more expensive than either standard or soya-based formula.

Hydrolysate formula is made of cow's milk, cornstarch and other foods, which is then treated with digestive enzymes so that the milk proteins are partially broken down. This makes them a good deal less allergenic, although they may still cause problems to babies who are highly allergenic.

Whey hydrolysates. These are made from the whey of cow's milk (rather than whole milk) and are potentially more useful for highly allergenic babies.

Amino-acid-based formula, or elemental formula. This has a completely synthetic protein base, providing the essential and non-essential amino acids, together with fat, maltodextrin, vitamins, minerals and trace elements. (It is very expensive.)

Soya-based formula. These are also covered by the Infant Formula and Follow-on Formula Regulations 1995 and are approved for use (by the Advisory Committee for Borderline Substances) as the sole source of nourishment for young infants.

They have been developed as a response to the emergence of cow's milk protein intolerance (in babies fed cow's-milk-based formulae), and they can be purchased without prescription. However, not only are many babies who are intolerant of cow's milk also intolerant of soya, but early soya formula feeding runs the risk of inducing soya protein intolerance in the child. Soya protein is much harder to avoid in the weaning diet than dairy products. There are also concerns about the possible effects of phyto-oestrogen compounds and the possibility of unavoidable high levels of manganese and aluminium (Minchin 2001). Soya formulae (as well as standard formulae) may contain genetically modified ingredients (Martyn 1999); this may be of concern to some parents.

Choosing artificial milk

It is an offence (under UK law) to sell any infant formula as being suitable from birth unless it meets the compositional and other criteria set out in the Infant Formula and Follow-on Formula Regulations 1995. Despite the claims made by formula manufacturers, there is no obvious scientific basis on which to recommend one brand over another.

There is no necessity for the mother to stick to one brand. If she finds that one brand seems to disagree with her baby, she could try switching brands. This has been made easier by the availability of ready-to-feed sachets or cartons, as, with these, mothers can experiment without having to buy large quantities.

Babies with underlying metabolic disorders, such as galactosaemia or phenylketonuria, will need the appropriate, prescribable breastmilk substitute.

Artificial milks are highly processed, factory-produced products. Inevitably there will from time to time be inadvertent errors. Recorded errors in the past include too much or too little of an ingredient, accidental contamination, incorrect labelling and foreign bodies.

(Powdered milk is not sterile and as recently as 2001, artificial milk has been contaminated with botulism.)

Mothers should be advised to inspect the contents of the tin or packet before using it – and if it looks or smells strange to return it to the place it was purchased.

Preparation of an artificial feed

The introduction of ready-to-feed formula in hospital may have saved staff time, but it has done a disservice to all mothers, as it reduces the likelihood that the mother who artificially feeds will have been shown how to prepare a bottle feed safely before she goes home (Kaufmann 1999).

All powdered formula feed available in the UK is now reconstituted using one scoopful (provided with the powder) to 30 ml of water. Clear instructions about the volumes of powder and water are also printed on the container. Nevertheless, over- and underconcentration of formula may still occur (Lucas 1991). In response to this, many of the major UK manufacturers of formula now produce ready-to-feed cartons, but the higher cost of these will preclude universal use.

A leaflet 'Preparing a bottle feed using baby milk powder' is available as a single A4 sheet of instructions (in English and other languages). This can be downloaded, free of charge, from the UNICEF UK Baby Friendly website (see Useful addresses, p. 779). A similar, companion leaflet 'Sterilisation of baby feeding equipment' is also available. These leaflets are independently produced and health care facilities can 'customise' them with their own logo if they wish.

The water supply

It is essential that the water used is free from bacterial contamination and any harmful chemicals. It is generally assumed in the UK that boiled tap water will meet these criteria, but from time to time this is shown not to be the case. In some areas of the UK, mothers who are artificially feeding their babies have to be provided with a separate supply of water because the tap water is not suitable for babies' consumption.

If bottled water is used, a still, non-mineralised variety suitable for babies must be chosen and it should be boiled as usual. Softened water is usually unsuitable.

Feeding equipment

Concern has been voiced about the nitrosamine content of rubber teats; in some countries mothers have been urged to boil the teat several times with fresh water before using. Silicone teats are now available but, as these have been known to split, the mother should be urged to check for signs of damage in order to ensure that the baby does not swallow any fragments.

It is often easier for the baby to use a simple soft long teat than industry-labelled orthodontic teats. Despite manufacturers' advertising claims, no bottle teat is like a breast. The mother should feel free to experiment, and use the type that seems to suit her baby.

Feeding bottles should meet the UK standard. This means they will be made of food-grade plastic and have relatively smooth interiors. Crevices and grooves in a bottle may make cleaning difficult. Patterned or decorated bottles may make it less easy to see whether the bottle is clean.

Sterilisation of feeding equipment

The effective cleaning of all utensils used should be demonstrated and the method of sterilisation discussed. If boiling is to be used, full immersion is essential and the contents of the pan must be boiled for 10 minutes. If cold sterilisation using a hypochlorite solution is the method of choice, the utensils must be fully immersed in the solution for the recommended time. The manufacturer's advice should be followed with regard to rinsing items that have been removed from the solution. If the item is to be rinsed, previously boiled water should be used and not water direct from the tap. Both steam and microwave sterilisation are now possible, but the mother should check that her equipment can withstand it.

Bottle teats

The size of the hole in the teat causes much anxiety to mothers. It is probably a good idea to have several teats with holes of different sizes so that the mother can experiment as necessary. A useful test for the correct hole size is to turn the bottle upside down; the feed should drip at a rate of about one drop per second.

Feeding the baby with the bottle

Mothers should be warned about the dangers of 'bottle propping', and told that the baby must never be left unattended while feeding from a bottle. They should be told about the need of the baby to relate to a small number of caregivers and that he should not be passed from person to person for feeding.

The baby is 'programmed' to feed from a breast and the mother should use the baby's innate skills when bottle feeding. The baby's lips should be touched to elicit a gape and the teat should follow the line of the baby's tongue, so that the baby uses the teat effectively. The mother should try to simulate breastfeeding conditions for the baby by holding him close, maintaining eye-to-eye contact and allowing him to determine his intake.

Modern formulae do not, when correctly prepared, cause hypernatraemia as did the older types. There is therefore no need to give the baby extra water.

The stools and vomit of a formula-fed baby have an unpleasant sour smell. The stools tend to be more formed than those of a breastfed baby and, unlike a breastfed baby, there is a real risk that the artificially fed baby may become constipated.

If in an emergency, artificial feed has to be prepared from liquid pasteurised (doorstep) milk, it should be made as follows: 2/3 full cream milk, 1/3 water and 1 level teaspoonful of sugar. The milk should be boiled for 2 minutes, so as not to overconcentrate it, before adding the previously boiled water and the sugar.

Midwives and the International code of marketing of breastmilk substitutes

In 1981, the combined forces of WHO and the United Nations Children's Fund (UNICEF) produced this Code (WHO 1981), which was adopted at the 34th World Health Assembly. The Code has major implications for the work of midwives. Although it is at present a voluntary code in most countries, some countries now have the code enshrined in law.

Recommendations in the code include:

- no advertising or promotion in hospitals, shops or to the general public (this includes posters in hospitals and advertisements in mother-and-baby books.)

- no free samples of breastmilk substitutes to be given to mothers
- no free gifts relating to products within the scope of the code to be given to mothers (including discount coupons or special offers)
- no financial or material gifts to be given to health workers for the purpose of promoting products, nor free or subsidised supplies to hospitals or maternity wards
- information provided by manufacturers to health workers should include only scientific and factual material, and should not create or imply a belief that bottle feeding is equivalent or superior to breastfeeding.
- health workers should encourage and protect breastfeeding.

The code does not prevent mothers from bottle feeding but rather seeks to contribute to safe, adequate nutrition for infants and to promote and protect breastfeeding.

The Baby Friendly Hospital Initiative

This is an initiative that was launched in 1991 by WHO and UNICEF to encourage hospitals to promote practices that are supportive of breastfeeding. It was focused around the 'ten steps' (Box 40.5), with which all hospitals who wish to achieve 'Baby Friendly' status must comply (WHO 1989). The evidence for the ten steps is contained in the WHO/UNICEF document of the same name (Vallenas and Savage 1998).

In addition, all 'Baby Friendly Hospitals' will fully implement the International code on the marketing of breastmilk substitutes. Thus if babies are born in a Baby Friendly Hospital, mothers will expect a certain standard of care.

While they are pregnant. They will expect to have a full discussion about caring for and feeding their baby, including the benefits of breastfeeding, so that they have all the facts they need to make an informed choice.

When the baby is born. They will expect:

- to be given their baby to hold against their skin straight after he is born, for as long as they want

---

Box 40.5 The ten steps

1. Have a written breastfeeding policy that is routinely communicated to all health care staff.
2. Train all health care staff in skills necessary to implement this policy.
3. Inform all pregnant women about the benefits and management of breastfeeding.
4. Help mothers initiate breastfeeding soon after birth.
5. Show mothers how to breastfeed and how to maintain lactation even if they should be separated from their infants.
6. Give newborn infants no food or drink other than breastmilk, unless medically indicated.
7. Practice rooming-in: allow mothers and infants to remain together 24 hours a day.
8. Encourage breastfeeding on demand.
9. Give no artificial teats or dummies to breastfeeding infants.
10. Foster the establishment of breastfeeding support groups and refer mothers to them on discharge from hospital or clinic.

- that a midwife will offer to help them start breastfeeding as soon as possible after the baby is born
- that their baby will stay with them at all times.

If they decide to breastfeed. They will expect:

- a midwife to show them how to hold the baby and how to help him latch on – in order to make sure he gets enough milk and that feeding is not painful
- to be given accurate and consistent advice about how to breastfeed and how to make enough milk for the baby
- that a midwife will offer to show them how to express milk by hand
- to receive information about how to get more support for breastfeeding, should they need it, once they leave hospital
- the baby *not* to be given water or artificial baby milk, unless this is needed for a medical reason.

A mother will expect that the staff will support her even if she decides that she wants to care for her baby differently or if she doesn't want the information offered. If she decides to bottle feed, she will expect to be asked if she wants to be shown how to make up a bottle feed correctly.

REFERENCES

Adler B R, Warner J O 1991 Food intolerance in children. Royal College of General Practitioners members reference book. Camden Publishing, London, p 497–502

Akre J (ed) 1990a Lactation. In: Infant feeding: the physiological basis. Bulletin of the World Health Organization 67 (1989) (suppl):25

Akre J (ed) 1990b The low birth weight infant. In: Infant feeding: the physiological basis. Bulletin of the World Health Organization 67 (1989) (suppl):79

Akre J (ed) 1990c. Health factors that may interfere with breastfeeding. In: Infant feeding: the physiological basis. Bulletin of the World Health Organization 67 (1989) (suppl):45

Ansell P, Roman E, Fear N, Renfrew M J 2001 Vitamin K policies and midwifery practice: questionnaire survey. British Medical Journal 322:1148–1152

Applebaum R M 1970 The modern management of successful breastfeeding. Paediatric Clinics of North America 17:203–205

Ashraf R N, Jalil F, Aperia A, Lindblad B S 1993 Additional water is not needed for healthy babies in a hot climate. Acta Paediatrica 82:1007–1011

Auerbach K G 1990 Sequential and simultaneous breast pumping: a comparison. International Journal of Nursing Studies 27(3):257–265

Auerbach K G, Walker M 1994 When the mother of a premature infant uses a pump: what every NICU nurse needs to know. Neonatal Network 13(4):23–29

Avoa A, Fischer P R 1990 The influence of perinatal instruction about breastfeeding on neonatal weight loss. Pediatrics 86(2):313–315

Baby Milk Action 2001 Update. No. 29(June), p 3. Online. Available: www.ibfan.org

Bahna S L 1987 Milk allergy in infancy. Annals of Allergy 59:131–136

Benson E A, Goodman M A 1970 An evaluation of the use of stilboestrol and antibiotics in the early management of acute puerperal breast abscess. British Journal of Surgery 57:258

Blackwell R Q, Chow B F, Chinn K S K, Blackwell B N 1973 Prospective maternal nutrition study in Taiwan: rationale, study design feasibility and preliminary findings. Nutrition Reports International 7:517–532

Bollag U, Albrecht E, Wingert W 1984 Medicated versus saline nose drops in the management of upper respiratory infection. Helvetica Paediatrica Acta Oct;39(4):341–345

British Paediatric Association 1999 Guidelines for human milk banks, 2nd edn. British Paediatric Association, London

Brostoff J, Gamlin L 1998 The complete guide to allergy and food intolerance. Bloomsbury Publishing, London, p 232, 261

Brown S J, Alexander J, Thomas P 1999 Feeding outcome in breast-fed term babies supplemented by cup or bottle. Midwifery 15:92–96

Butte N F, Garza C, Stuff J E, Smith E O, Bichos B J 1984 Effect of maternal diet and body composition on lactational performance. American Journal of Clinical Nutrition 39:296–306

Canfield L M, Hopkinson J M, Lima A F, Silva B, Garza C 1991 Vitamin K in colostrum and mature human milk over the lactation period – a cross sectional study. American Journal of Clinical Nutrition 53(3):730–735

Carvahlo M, Hall M, Harvey D 1981 Effects of water supplementation on physiological jaundice in breastfed babies. Archives of Disease in Childhood 56:568–569

Chapman D J, Young S, Ferris A M, Perez-Escamilla R 2001 Impact of breast pumping on lactogenesis stage II after caesarean delivery: a randomized clinical trial. Pediatrics 107(6):E94

Coutsoudis A, Pillay K, Spooner E, Kuhn L, Coovadia H M 1999 Influence of infant-feeding patterns on early mother-to-child transmission of HIV-1 in Durban, South Africa: a prospective cohort study. South African Vitamin A Study Group. Lancet 354(9177):471–476

Cowie A T, Forsyth I A, Hart I C 1980 Hormonal control of lactation. Monographs on Endocrinology, no. 15. Springer Verlag, Berlin

Crawford J 1992 Understanding our own breastfeeding experiences. JBI Newsletter no. 4, 1 June, p 1–2

Cronenwett L, Stukel T, Kearney M et al 1992 Single daily bottle use in the early weeks, postpartum and breastfeeding outcomes. Pediatrics 90(5):760–766

Daly S 1993 The short term synthesis and infant regulated removal of milk in lactating women. Experimental Physiology 78:209–220

de Chateau P, Holmberg H, Jakobsson K, Winberg J 1977 A study of factors promoting and inhibiting lactation. Developmental Medicine and Child Neurology 19:575–584

Dearlove J C, Dearlove B M 1981 Prolactin, fluid balance and lactation. British Journal of Obstetrics and Gynecology 123:845–846

Delgado H L, Marmtorell R, Klein R E 1982 Nutrition, lactation and birth interval components in rural Guatemala. American Journal of Clinical Nutrition 35:1468–1476

Dewey K G 1998 Effects of maternal caloric restriction and exercise during lactation. Journal of Nutrition 128 (2 suppl):386S–389S

Dewey K G, Lovelady C A, Nommsen-Rivers L A et al 1994 A randomised study of the effects of aerobic exercise by lactating women on breast-milk volume and composition. New England Journal of Medicine 330(7):449–453

Dixon J M 1988 Repeated aspiration of breast abscess in lactating women. British Medical Journal 297:1517–1518

Dusdieker L, Booth B, Stumbo P, Eichenberger J 1985 Effects of supplemental fluids on human milk production. Journal of Pediatrics 105:207–211

Dusdieker L B, Hemingway D L, Stumbo P J 1994 Is milk production impaired by dieting during lactation? American Journal of Clinical Nutrition 59:833–840

Eglin R P, Wilkinson A R 1987 HIV infection and pasteurisation of breastmilk. Lancet i:1093

Enzunga A, Fischer P R 1990 Neonatal weight loss in rural Zaire. Annals of Tropical Paediatrics 10:159–163

Fairbank L, Woolridge M J, Renfrew M J et al 2000 Effective health care: promoting the initiation of breastfeeding. NHS Centre for Reviews and Dissemination/University of York, vol. 6, no 2, July

Fenstein J, Berkelhamer J, Gruszka M et al 1986 Factors related to early termination of breastfeeding in an urban population. Pediatrics 78(2):210–215

Fischer P R, Dind Y 1991 Co-sleeping and neonatal weight loss. Annals of Tropical Paediatrics 11:189–191

Fredrikzon B, Hernell O, Blackberg L, Olivecrona T 1978 Bile salt-stimulated lipase in human milk: evidence of activity in vivo and of a role in the digestion of milk retinol esters. Pediatr Research 12(11):1048–1052

Freed G L, Clark S J, Sorenson J, Lohr J A, Cefalo R, Curtis P 1995 National assessment of physicians' breastfeeding knowledge and experience. Journal of the American Medical Association 273: 472–476

Greer F R 1997 Vitamin K status of lactating mothers and their infants. Acta Paediatrica (suppl) 88(430): 95–103

Groh-Wargo S, Toth A, Mahoney K, Simonian S, Wasser T, Rose S 1995 The utility of a bilateral breast pumping system for mothers of premature infants. Neonatal Network 14(8):31–36

Hall B 1979 Changing content of human milk and early development of appetite control. Keeping Abreast April/June:139

Hamlyn B, Brooker S, Oleinikova K, Wands S (2002). Infant Feeding 2000. A survey conducted on behalf of the Department of Health, the Scottish Executive, The National Assembly for Wales and the Department of Health, Social Services and Public Safety in Northern Ireland. TSO, London

Hammer R L, Babcock G, Fisher A G 1996 Low-fat diet and exercise in obese lactating women. Breastfeeding Review 4(1):29–34

Hamosh M 1998 Protective functions of proteins and lipids in human milk. Biology of the Neonate 74:163

Helsing E, Savage King F 1982 breastfeeding in practice. Oxford University Press, Oxford, p 175

Herrera A J 1984 Supplemented versus unsupplemented breastfeeding. Perinatology-Neonatology 8:70–71

Hill P, Aldag J, Chatterton R 1999 Effect of pumping style on milk production in mothers of non-nursing preterm infants. Journal of Human Lactation 15(3):209–216

Hoddinott P 1998 Why don't some women want to breastfeed and how might we change their attitudes? (MPhil thesis). University of Wales College of Medicine, Cardiff

Hoddinot P, Pill R 1999 Qualitative study of decisions about infant feeding among women in the East End of London. British Medical Journal 318(7175):30–34

Hodge C 1967 Suppression of lactation by stilboestrol. Lancet ii(7510):286–287

Host A 1991 Importance of the first meal on the development of cows' milk allergy and intolerance. Allergy Proceedings 12:227–232

Hytten F E 1954 Clinical and chemical studies in human lactation. IX breastfeeding in hospital. British Medical Journal ii:1447–1452

Hytten F E, Baird D 1958 The development of the nipple in pregnancy. Lancet i:1201–1204

ICM (International Confederation of Midwives) 1985 ICM speaks out on breastfeeding. Midwifery 1:47

Illingworth P J, Jong R T, Howie P W, Leslie P, Isles T E 1986 Diminution in energy expenditure during lactation. British Medical Journal 292:437–441

Illingworth R S, Kilpatrick B 1953 Lactation and fluid intake. Lancet ii:1175–1177

Illingworth R S, Stone D 1952 Self-demand feeding in a maternity unit. Lancet i:683–687

Inch S, Garforth S 1989 Establishing and maintaining breastfeeding. In: Chalmers I, Enkin M, Keirse M (eds) Effective care in pregnancy and childbirth. Oxford University Press, Oxford, ch 80, p 1364

Inch S, Fisher C 1995 Mastitis in lactating women. The Practitioner 239:472–476

Infant Formula and Follow-on Formula Regulations 1995. HMSO, London

Ingram J, Woolridge M, Greenwood R 2001 Breastfeeding: it is worth trying with the second baby. Lancet 358(9286):986–987

Jackson D A, Woolridge M W, Imong S M et al 1987 The automatic sampling shield: a device for sampling suckled breastmilk. Early Hum Development 15(5):295–306

Jain E 1995 Tongue-tie: its impact on breastfeeding. AARN News Letter 51(5):18. Online. Available: www.drjain@drjain.com

Jones E, Dimmock P, Spencer S A 2001 A randomised controlled trial to compare methods of milk expression after preterm delivery. Archives of Disease in Childhood, Fetal Neonatal 85:F91–F95

Kasa N, Heinonen K M 1993 Near infrared interactance in assessing superficial fat in exclusively breastfed term neonates. Acta Paediatrica 82:1–5

Kaufmann T 1999 Infant feeding: politics vs pragmatism? RCM Midwives Journal 2(8):244

Kennedy K I, Rivera R, Mcneilly A S 1989 Consensus statement on the use of breastfeeding as a family planning method. Contraception 439:477

Kochenour N K 1980 Lactation suppression. Clinical Obstetrics and Gynecology 23:1052–1059

Kries R V, Shearer M, McCarthy P T et al 1987 Vitamin K_1 content of maternal milk: influence of the stage of lactation, lipid composition, and vitamin K_1 supplements given to the mother. Pediatric Research 22(5):513–517

Lang S, Lawence C, L'E Orme R 1994 Cup feeding: an alternative method of infant feeding. Archives of Disease in Childhood 71:365–369

Lucas A 1991 Milk for babies and children (correspondence). British Medical Journal 301:350–351

Lucas A, Cole T J 1990 breastmilk and neonatal necrotising enterocolitis. Lancet 336:1519–1523

Main Trial Collaborative Group 1994 Preparing for breastfeeding: treatment of inverted and non-protractile nipples in pregnancy. Midwifery 10:200–214

Marmet C, Shell E, Marmet R 1990 Neonatal frenotomy may be necessary to correct breastfeeding problems. Journal of Human Lactation 6(3):117–121

Martyn T 1999 Soya in artificial baby milks. Practising Midwife 2(6):17–19

Masaitis N S, Kaempf J W 1996 Developing a frenotomy policy at one medical centre, a case study approach. Journal of Human Lactation 12(3):229–232

Meier P, Cranston-Anderson J 1987 Responses of small preterm infants to bottle and breastfeeding. Maternal–Child Nursing Journal 12:97–105

Messenger H 1994 Don't shoot the messenger. Health Visitor 67(5):171

Metcalf I J, Irons T G, Lawrence D S, Young P C 1994 Simethicone in the treatment of infant colic: a randomised placebo-controlled multicentre trial. Pediatrics 94:29–34

MIDIRS/NHS Centre for Reviews and Dissemination 1999. Informed choice paired leaflets for health professionals and for pregnant women. Leaflet 5: (i) Breastfeeding or bottle feeding: helping women to choose; (ii) Feeding your baby – breast or bottle? MIDIRS, Bristol

Minchin M 2001 Towards safer artificial feeding. Alma publications, Australia, Geelong. Online. Available: almapubs@netlink.com.au

Morse J M, Ewing G, Gamble D, Donahue P 1992 The effect of maternal fluid intake on breastmilk supply: a pilot study. Canadian Journal of Public Health 83(3):213–216

Muskinja-Montanji G, Molnar-Sabo I, Vekonj-Fajka G 1999 Physiologic neonatal weight loss in a 'Baby Friendly Hospital'. Medical Pregl. 52(6–8):237–240

Newman J, Pitman T 2000 Dr Jack Newman's guide to breastfeeding. Harper Collins, New York, p 160

Nicoll A, Ginsburg R, Tripp J 1982 Supplementary feeding and jaundice in newborns. Acta Paediatrica Scandinavica 71:759–761

Nicolls H 1997 Two on to one will go. Midwifery Matters 73:6–7

Nicholson W L 1991 Tongue-tie (ankyloglossia) associated with breastfeeding problems. Journal of Human Lactation 7(2):82–84

Notestine G E 1990 The importance of the identification of ankyloglossia (short lingual frenulum) as a cause of breastfeeding problems. Journal of Human Lactation 6(3):113–115

Pandove S P, Singh K, Sandhu A S 1994 Growth in term infants during neonatal period. Indian Pediatrics 31(6):675–678

Paronen J, Knip M, Savilahti E et al 2000 Effect of cow's milk exposure and maternal type 1 diabetes on cellular and humeral immunization to dietary insulin in infants at genetic risk for type 1 diabetes. Finnish Trial to Reduce IDDM in the Genetically at Risk Study Group. Diabetes 49(10):1657–1665

Prentice A M, Roberts S B, Whitehead R G 1980 Dietary supplementation of Gambian nursing mothers and lactational performance. Lancet ii:886–888

Prentice A M, Lunn P G, Watkinson M, Whitehead R G 1983 Dietary supplementation of lactating Gambian women. II. Effect on maternal health, nutritional status and biochemistry. Human Nutrition and Clinical Nutrition 37(c):65–74

Prentice A M, Addey C V P, Wilde C J 1989 Evidence for local feed-back control of human milk secretion. Biochemical Society Transactions 17:122, 489–492

Prentice A M, Goldberg G R, Prentice A 1994 Body mass index and lactational performance. European Journal of Clinical Nutrition 48 Suppl 3:S78–86, discussion S86–S89

Purves C, Browne L 1982 Blocked ducts – revisited. New Generation 1(4):16–19

Pyke M 1986 Success in nutrition. John Murray, London, p 134–137

Ramos R, Kennedy K I, Visness C M 1996 Effectiveness of lactational amenorrhoea in prevention of pregnancy in Manila, the Philippines: non-comparative prospective trial. British Medical Journal 313:909–912

RCM (Royal College of Midwives) 2001 Successful breastfeeding, 3rd edn. Churchill Livingstone, Edinburgh

Renfrew M J, Ross McGill H, Woolridge M 2000 Enabling women to breastfeed. HMSO, London

Righard L, Alade M O 1990 Effect of delivery room routines on success of first breast-feed. Lancet 336:1105–1107

Saarinen U M, Siimes M A 1979 Iron absorption from breastmilk, cow's milk and iron supplemented formula: an opportunistic use of changes in total body iron determined by hemoglobin, ferritin and body weight in 132 infants. Pediatric Research 13:143–147

Sachdev H P S, Krishna J, Puri R K 1991 Water supplementation in exclusively breastfed infants during the summer in the tropics. Lancet 337:929–933

Sandstrom B, Cederblad A, Lonnerdal B 1983 Zinc absorption from human, cows' milk and infant formula. American Journal of Diseases of Childhood 137:726

Schubiger G, Schwartz U, Tonz O 1997 UNICEF/WHO baby-friendly hospital initiative: does the use of bottles and pacifiers in the neonatal nursery prevent successful breastfeeding? European Journal of Paediatrics 156(11):874–877

Specker B L, Tsang R C, Ho M L, Landi T M, Gratton T L 1991 Low serum calcium and high para-thyroid hormone levels in neonates fed 'humanised' cows' milk based breastmilk substitutes. American Journal of Diseases of Childhood 145:941–945

Specker B L, Valanis B, Hertzberg V, Edwards N, Tsang R C 1985 Sunshine exposure and serum 25-hydroxyvitamin D concentrations in exclusively breast-fed infants. Journal of Pediatrics 107(3):372–376

Strode M A, Dewey K G, Lonnerdal B 1986 Effects of short-term caloric restriction on lactational performance of well nourished mothers. Acta Paediatrica Scandinavica 75(2):222–229

Thomsen A C, Espersen M D, Maigaard S 1984 Course and treatment of milk stasis, non-infectious inflammation of the breast, and infectious mastitis in nursing women. American Journal of Obstetrics and Gynecology 149:492–495

Tjon A, Ten W E, Kusin J A, Dewith C 1986 Early postnatal growth of Basotho infants in the Mantsonyane area, Lesotho. Annals of Tropical Paediatrics 6:195–198 (cited in Avoa & Fisher 1990)

Ueda T, Yokoyama Y, Irahara M, Aona T 1994 Influence of psychological stress on suckling-induced pulsatile oxytocin release. Obstetrics and Gynecology 84:259–262

Vaarala O, Knip M, Paronen J et al Cow's milk formula feeding induces primary immunization to insulin in infants at genetic risk for type 1 diabetes. Diabetes 48(7):1389–1394

Vallenas C, Savage F 1998 Evidence for the Ten Steps to Successful Breastfeeding. Division of Child Health and Development. WHO, Geneva

Velisavljev M, Velisavljev D, Zarkovic M 1998 (Cited in Muskinja-Montanji 1999)

Vorherr H 1974 The breast: morphology, physiology and lactation. Academic Press, New York

Waldenström U, Swensen Å 1991 Rooming-in at night in the postpartum ward. Midwifery 7:82–89

Whitehead R G, Paul A A, Black A E, Wiles S J 1981 Recommended dietary amounts of energy for pregnancy or lactation in the UK. In: Torun B, Young V R, Rang W M (eds) Protein energy requirements of developing countries: evaluation of new data. United Nations University, Tokyo, p 259–265

White A, Freith S, O'Brien M 1992 Infant feeding 1990. Survey carried out for the Department of Health by the Office of Population Censuses and Surveys. HMSO, London

WHO (World Health Organization) 1981 International code of marketing of breast-milk substitutes. WHO, Geneva

WHO (World Health Organization) 2000 Mastitis: causes and management (WHO/RCH/CAH/00.13). Dept of Child and Adolescent Health and Development, Geneva.

WHO (World Health Organization)/UNICEF 1989 Joint statement – protecting, promoting and supporting breastfeeding. WHO, Geneva

Widström A M, Ransjo-Arvidson A B, Christensson K et al 1987 Gastric suction in healthy newborn infants. Acta Paediatrica Scandinavica 76:566–578

Wiessinger D, Miller M 1995 Breastfeeding difficulties as a result of tight lingual and labial frena: a case report. Journal of Human Lactation 11(4):313–316

Wilde C J, Addey C V P, Boddy L M, Peaker M 1995 Autocrine regulation of milk secretion by a protein in milk. Biochemical Journal 305:51–58

Woolridge M W 1986 The 'anatomy' of sucking. Midwifery 2:164–171

Woolridge M W 1995 Breastfeeding: physiology into practice. In: Davis D P (ed) Nutrition in child health. Royal College of Physicians, London, p 13–31

Woolridge M W, Fisher C 1988 'Overfeeding' and symptoms of malabsorption in the breast-fed baby: a possible artefact of feed management? Lancet ii:382–384

Woolridge M W, Baum J D, Drewett R F 1982 Individual patterns of milk intake during breastfeeding. Early Human Development 7:265–272

Worthington-Roberts B 1993 Human milk composition and infant growth and development. In: Worthington-Roberts B, Williams S R (eds) Nutrition in pregnancy and lactation, 5th edn. Mosby Year Book, St Louis, p 343

Yamauchi Y, Yamanouchi I 1990 The relationship between rooming-in/not rooming-in and breastfeeding variables. Acta Paediatr Scandinavica 79:1017–1022

FURTHER READING

Akre J (ed) 1990 Infant feeding: the physiological basis. Bulletin of the World Health Organization 67(1989)(suppl)

A comprehensive and authorative summary of the biology and physiology of breastfeeding.

Henschel D, Inch S 1996 Breastfeeding – a guide for midwives. 1st edn published by Books for Midwives Press (now Butterworth Heinemann, Oxford)

A comprehensive and illustrated guide for all those involved in helping women to breastfeed, covering both the theoretical and the practical aspects of the subject. Common problems are identified and solutions suggested.

Inch S 1999 Breastfeeding update. In: Alexander J, Levy V, Roch S (eds) Midwifery practice: core topics 3. Postnatal care. Macmillan Education, Basingstoke, p 68–83

Focuses on the quality of studies that demonstrate the superiority of breastfeeding over artificial feeding, and discusses in detail the implementation of the ten steps to successful breastfeeding and the UNICEF-UK Baby Friendly Initiative.

Inch S, Fisher C 1999 Breastfeeding: into the 21st century. NT clinical monographs no 32. Emap Healthcare, London

A concise but wide-ranging review of the importance of breastfeeding, the difficulties facing midwives who want to help breastfeeding women and the ways in which these might be overcome.

Infant Formula and Follow-on Formula Regulations 1995 Stationery Office, London. Available online: www.hmso.gov.uk/si/si1995/Uksi_19950077_en_1.htm

This is the UK government's response to the European Directive 1991 (91/321/EEC OJ No. L175, 4.7.91), which sought to persuade all EU countries to adopt the International code of marketing of breastmilk substitutes. It falls short of the code in several important respects, notably in relation to advertising.

Palmer G 1993 The politics of breastfeeding, 2nd edn. Pandora Press, London

This book links biology and politics (sexual, economic and environmental) in an exploration of the consequences of women's changing role in society and the acceleration of the Industrial Revolution, which created the demand for 'artificial milks'. Health professionals are left in no doubt of the importance of their role in the promotion and establishment of breastfeeding, nor of the potential for harm in suggesting that the decision of how to feed a baby is simply a matter of choosing between two equivalent products.

Renfrew M, Fisher C, Arms S 2000 Bestfeeding, 2nd edn. Celestial Arts, Berkeley CA

Taking up where texts addressed primarily to health workers leave off, the authors blend wisdom, experience, idealism and learning to produce a clear, basic breastfeeding guide, addressed primarily to mothers. The book exudes the confidence-building conviction that breastfeeding is something that women can do, and that most problems have solutions.

Royal College of Midwives 2001 Successful breastfeeding, 3rd edn. Churchill Livingstone, London

The breastfeeding handbook of the RCM, written to help midwives and other health professionals provide more effective advice and support for the breastfeeding women in their care.

RCP 1999 Guidelines for the establishment and operation of human milk banks in the UK, 2nd edn. Royal College of Paediatrics and Child Health and United Kingdom Association for Milk Banking, London

WHO/UNICEF International code of marketing of breastmilk substitutes 1981. Available online: http://www.babymilkaction.org/regs/thecode.html

This was adopted by a resolution (WHA34.22) of the World Health Assembly in 1981. A copy of the code can also be obtained from Baby Milk Action (see Useful addresses, below).

Woolridge M W 1986 The 'anatomy' of sucking and the aetiology of sore nipples. Midwifery 2:164–171

Woolridge M W 1986 The aetiology of sore nipples. Midwifery 2:172–176

Based on cine-radiographic and ultrasound studies, these seminal, descriptive papers detail the way in which babies feed from the breast and the reason that nipples are damaged when attachment of the baby at the breast is not optimal.

WHO (World Health Organization) 1989 Protecting, promoting and supporting breastfeeding: the special role of maternity services. A joint WHO/UNICEF Statement. WHO, Geneva

This is the document which first set out the ten steps for successful breastfeeding, which formed the basis of the global Baby Friendly Hospital Initiative, and makes recommendations concerning the structure and function of (maternity) health care services. It focuses on the types of action to be taken, rather than details of the content. Obtainable also from: Stationery Office, Customer Services, 51 Nine Elms Lane, London SW8 5DR. Tel: (44) 870 600 5522, email: customer.services@theso.co.uk

USEFUL ADDRESSES

National Childbirth Trust breastfeeding line: 0870 444 8708, the enquiry line: 0870 444 8707

Breastfeeding Network helpline number: 0870 900 8787

Association of Breastfeeding Mothers helpline number: 0207 813 1481

La Leche League helpline number: 0207 242 1278

CLAPA (Cleft Lip And Palate Association) 235–237 Finchley Road London NW3 6LS Tel: 020 7431 0033

Baby Milk Action 23 St Andrew's Street, Cambridge CB2 3AX Tel: 01223 464420
www.babymilkaction.org

UNICEF UK Baby Friendly Initiative Africa House, 64–78 Kingsway, London WC2B 6NB
Tel: 020 7312 7652
www.babyfriendly.org.uk

41

The Healthy Low Birthweight Baby

Carole England

It is now generally accepted that healthy babies between 32 and 37 weeks gestation, with a birthweight of 1.7–2.5 kg, do not need automatic admission to a neonatal intensive care unit (NICU) but instead can be cared for on a postnatal ward with their mother. There is no doubt that low birthweight (LBW) babies are more vulnerable to illness compared with appropriately grown term babies, and extra monitoring may be a necessary precaution, particularly during the period of adaptation to extrauterine life and the early neonatal period. Caring for healthy LBW babies on a postnatal ward is thought to be advantageous because it removes them from the greater hazard of infection that occurs in neonatal units, prevents separation of mother and baby and, finally, eliminates the need for parents to visit the neonatal unit, which is for many, an alien and intimidating environment (Affonso et al 1992). There is growing evidence that the majority of these babies remain well, will have minimal or no illness in the neonatal period (Roberton 1999) and can be cared for by midwives as the lead professional. It therefore follows that neonatal nurses will be more able to focus their care on the critically ill, and those babies that are healthy but <1.70 kg, thus utilising neonatal nurse skills and cot resources to their best effect.

The chapter aims to:

- clarify the terminology and classifications of babies in relation to birthweight and gestational age

- detail the care of preterm babies and those who are small for their gestational age

- explore the role of the midwife in the provision of holistic care for the mother, her low birthweight baby and her family

- discuss the place and provision of care.

Introduction

Between 6 and 7% of all babies born in the United Kingdom weigh less than 2500 g at birth. In 1977, the World Health Organization (WHO 1977a) recommended that babies who weigh less than 2500 grams should be called low birthweight (LBW). Preterm babies make up about two-thirds of LBW babies. The other one-third are small for their gestational age (SGA) and 70% of these will weigh between 2000 and 2500 g. The concepts and categories that surround LBW are complex. The following classification describes the different types of LBW babies seen in practice.

Classification of babies by weight and gestation

Definitions of low birthweight are based upon weight alone and do not consider the gestational age of the baby. Likewise, definitions of gestational age disregard any considerations of birthweight.

Weight

As neonatal technology and care have become more effective, new birthweight categories have been devised to further define babies by birthweight. The low birthweight categories are:

- low birthweight (LBW) babies are those weighing below 2500 g at birth
- very low birthweight (VLBW) babies are those weighing below 1500 g at birth.
- extremely low birthweight (ELBW) babies are those who weigh under 1000 g at birth.

Gestational age

A preterm baby is one born before completion of the 37th gestational week. Gestational weeks are calculated from the first day of the last menstrual period (LMP) and have no relevance to the baby's weight, length, head circumference, or indeed any other measurement of fetal or neonatal size.

Thus, it is the *relationship* between these two separate considerations of weight (for assessment of growth) and gestational age (for assessment of maturity) that is of great importance. This relationship can be plotted on centile charts (Fig. 41.1); these charts visually demonstrate that growth is appropriate, excessive or

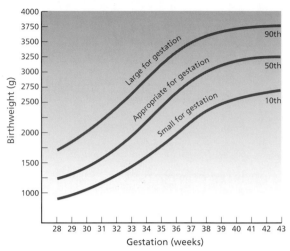

Fig. 41.1 A centile chart, showing weight and gestation. (From Simpson 1997, with permission of Baillière Tindall.)

diminished for gestational age and that the baby is either preterm, term or post-term. They are based on measurements of fetal growth that have been collected over the last 20 years, from multiple ultrasound measurements. To act as an accurate tool, growth charts should be derived from studies of local populations, because genetically derived growth differences exist between countries, cultures and lifestyles (Roberton 1999).

Various types of LBW babies can be described:

1. Babies whose rate of intrauterine growth was normal at the moment of birth: they are small because labour began before the end of the 37th gestational week. These preterm babies are appropriately grown for their gestational age (AGA).

2. Babies whose rate of intrauterine growth was slowed and who were delivered at or later than term: these term or post-term babies are undergrown for gestational age. They are small for their gestational age (SGA).

3. Babies whose rate of intrauterine growth was slowed and who, in addition, were delivered before term: these preterm babies are small by virtue of both early delivery and impaired intrauterine growth. They are small for gestational age and preterm babies.

4. Babies who are considered large for their gestational age (LGA) at any weight when they fall above the 90th centile.

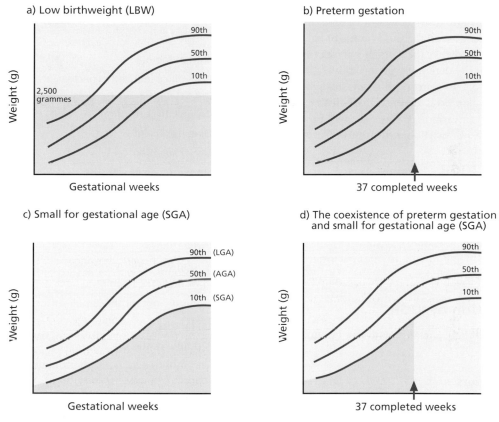

Fig. 41.2 Centile charts that illustrate how low birthweight babies are categorised by weight and gestation. (a) Low birthweight. (b) Preterm gestation. (c) Small for gestational age. (d) Coexistence of preterm gestation and small for gestational age.

Therefore, it follows that both term and preterm babies can be SGA, AGA or LGA (Fig. 41.2).

The small for gestational age baby

Expert care of newborn babies requires an understanding of intrauterine growth patterns as they relate to gestational age. A baby's clinical course following birth is in large measure, determined by these factors.

Intrauterine growth restriction (IUGR)

Anderson & Hay (1999) define IUGR as a rate of fetal growth that is less than normal for the population and for the growth potential of a specific baby.

The relationship between IUGR and SGA

In the past, the terms IUGR and SGA were used interchangeably. Although related, they are not synonymous. IUGR is a failure of normal fetal growth caused by multiple adverse effects on the fetus, whereas SGA describes a baby whose weight is lower than population norms. SGA babies are defined as having a birthweight below the 10th centile for gestational age, or <2 standard deviations below the mean (the 50th centile) for the gestational age. Thus, all IUGR babies may not be SGA and all SGA babies may not be small as a result of growth restriction (Gomella et al 1999). Indeed, Roberton (1999) contends that at least half of the SGA babies in Britain have no known aetiology. They are proportionately small; their weight, length and head circumference are all on the third centile or below. It is generally accepted that their small parents or grandparents genetically determine their smallness. They are well, healthy babies who need to be treated accordingly and do not need overzealous labelling, which may lead to unwarranted wasteful and potentially harmful interventions (Roberton 1999).

Causes of IUGR

Fetal growth is regulated by maternal, placental and fetal factors and represents a mix of genetic mechanisms and environmental influences through which growth potential is expressed. The mechanisms that appear to limit fetal growth are multifactorial and are presented in Box 41.1.

Classification of IUGR

Factors that influence fetal growth can be intrinsic or extrinsic.

Intrinsic factors

These are factors that operate from *within* the fetus, that arise from chromosomal or genetic abnormalities, or alternatively from infective agents that are transplacental in origin and act by altering the normal process of cell division.

Extrinsic factors

These are factors that influence the fetus through its intrauterine environment.

The clinical appearance and behaviour of the baby at birth can provide relevant information as to the type of growth disruption that may have been sustained and help the midwife to anticipate any future potential problems. There are two types of IUGR clinically recognised.

Asymmetric growth (sometimes called acute)

Here the fetal weight is reduced out of proportion to the length and head circumference; this is thought to be caused by extrinsic factors such as pregnancy-induced hypertension (Mupanemunda & Watkinson 1999) that adversely affect fetal nutrition during the

---

Box 41.1 Causes of intrauterine growth restriction

Maternal factors
- Pregnancy-induced hypertension, pre-eclampsia
- Chronic hypertension
- Diabetes mellitus
- Undernutrition
- Smoking, alcohol misuse
- Drugs – therapeutic (anticancer drugs) and addictive (narcotic)
- Renal disease, collagen disorders, anaemia
- Irradiation
- Young and elderly mothers
- Poor obstetric history
- Underweight mother/small stature

Fetal factors
- Multiple gestation
- Chromosomal/genetic abnormality (particularly trisomy conditions), including inborn errors of metabolism, dwarf syndromes
- Intrauterine infection – toxoplasmosis, rubella, cytomegalovirus, herpes simplex (TORCH) and syphilis

Placental factors
- Abruptio placenta
- Placenta praevia
- Chorioamnionitis
- Abnormal cord insertion
- Single umbilical artery

Sources: Anderson & Hay (1999), Blackburn & Loper (1992), Korones (1986), Mupanemunda & Watkinson (1999).

---

latter stages of gestation. The head looks disproportionately large compared with the body, but the head circumference is usually within normal parameters and brain growth is usually spared (Korones 1986). The bones are within gestational norms for length and density but the anterior fontanelle may be larger than expected, owing to diminished membranous bone formation. The abdomen looks 'scaphoid', or sunken owing to shrinkage of the liver and spleen, which surrender their stores of glycogen and red blood cell mass respectively as the fetus adapts to the adverse conditions of the uterus. Since the ratio of brain mass to liver mass is large, hypoglycaemia is more likely to be seen in such babies. There is decreased subcutaneous fat deposition and the skin is loose, which can give the baby a wizened, old appearance. The layer of vernix caseosa is frequently reduced or absent as a result of diminished skin perfusion and, in the absence of this protective covering, the skin is continuously exposed to amniotic fluid, and will begin to desquamate; thus the skin appears pale, dry and coarse and, if the baby is of a mature gestation, may be stained with meconium. Unless severely affected, these babies appear hyperactive and hungry with a lusty cry (Fig. 41.3).

Symmetric growth (chronic)

Symmetric IUGR is due either to decreased growth potential of the fetus, as a result of congenital infection or chromosomal/genetic defects (intrinsic), or to extrinsic factors that are active early in gestational life (e.g. the effects of maternal smoking, or poor dietary intake), or a combination of intrinsic and extrinsic factors (Mupanemunda & Watkinson 1999). The head circumference, length and weight are all proportionately reduced for gestational age (Gomella et al 1999). These babies are diminutive in size, do not appear wasted, have subcutaneous fat appropriate for their size and their skin is taut. They are generally vigorous and less likely to be hypoglycaemic or polycythaemic, but, because the insult began early with possible interruptions to cell division, they may suffer major congenital abnormalities and can be a source of infection to carers, as a result of transplacental infection.

Symmetric growth (genetically small). These are small normal babies and should be treated in accordance to their gestational age.

The preterm baby

This describes a baby born before the end of the 37th gestational week, regardless of birthweight. Most of these babies are appropriately grown and, whereas some are SGA, a small number are LGA (these tend to be infants of diabetic mothers). The factors that play a

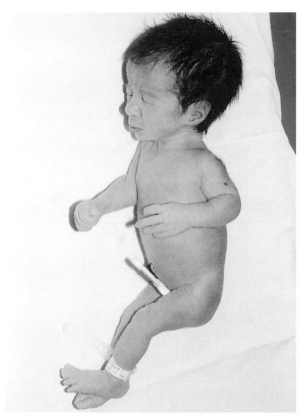

Fig. 41.3 Baby with asymmetrical growth restriction. Note the apparently large head compared with the undergrown body.

role in the initiation of preterm labour are largely unknown, are described as multifactorial and in large part overlay with factors that impair fetal growth. They are divided into those labours that start spontaneously and those where a decision is made to terminate a viable pregnancy before term (referred to as elective causes) (Box 41.2).

Characteristics of the preterm baby

The appearance at birth of the preterm baby will depend upon the gestational age. The following description will focus upon the baby born during the last trimester of pregnancy. Preterm babies rarely become large enough in utero to develop muscular flexion and fully adopt the fetal position (Young 1996) and as a result their posture appears flattened with hips abducted, knees and ankles flexed. They are generally hypotonic with a weak and feeble cry. The

Box 41.2 Causes of preterm labour

Spontaneous causes

- 40% unknown
- Multiple gestation
- Hyperpyrexia as a result of viral or bacterial infection
- Premature rupture of the membranes caused by maternal infection
- Maternal short stature
- Maternal age and parity
- Poor obstetric history; history of preterm labour
- Cervical incompetence
- Poor social circumstances

Elective causes

- Pregnancy-induced hypertension, pre-eclampsia, chronic hypertension
- Maternal disease: renal, cardiac
- Placenta praevia, abruptio placenta
- Rhesus incompatibility
- Congenital abnormality
- IUGR

Sources: Blackburn & Loper (1992), Harlow & Spencer (1999).

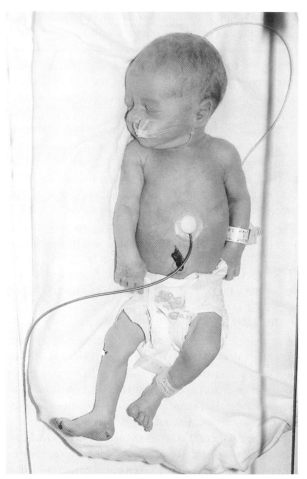

Fig. 41.4 Healthy preterm baby born at 32 weeks' gestation. Note the presence of a nasogastric tube. The thermocouple of the servo skin mode is taped to the baby's upper abdomen.

head is in proportion to the body; the skull bones are soft with large fontanelles and wide sutures. The chest is small and narrow and appears underdeveloped owing to minimal lung expansion during fetal life. The abdomen is prominent because the liver and spleen are large and abdominal muscle tone is poor (Fig. 41.4). The liver is large because it receives a good supply of oxygenated blood via the fetal circulation and is active in the production of red blood cells and erythropoiesis. The umbilicus appears low in the abdomen because linear growth is cephalocaudal (it is more apparent nearer to the head than the feet), by virtue of the fetal circulation oxygenation. Subcutaneous fat is laid down from 28 weeks' gestation, therefore its presence and abundance will affect the redness and transparency of the skin. Vernix caseosa is abundant in the last trimester and tends to accumulate at sites of dense lanugo growth (i.e. the face, ears, shoulders and sacral region) and protects the skin from amniotic fluid maceration. The ear pinna is flat with little curve, the eyes bulge and the orbital ridges are prominent. The nipple areola is poorly developed and barely visible. The cord is white, fleshy and glistening. The plantar creases are absent before 36 weeks but soon start to appear as fluid loss occurs through the skin. In girls the labia majora fail to cover the labia minora and in boys the testes descend into the scrotal sac at about the 37th gestational week.

Management at birth of the healthy LBW baby

Given the unpredictability of the LBW baby and the birth process, the role of the midwife in the delivery room is to prepare adequately the environment, staff and parents for all eventualities. This takes the form of asking the multiprofessional team (second midwife, paediatrician and neonatal nurse), to be on standby for the delivery. The incidence of perinatal asphyxia and congenital abnormality is greater in SGA babies and the baby with a scaphoid abdomen could be physically normal, but alternatively could deteriorate quickly if presenting with a diaphragmatic hernia. Current cot availability in the NICU, transitional care unit (as applicable) and postnatal ward should be known. The delivery room ambient temperature should ideally be between 23 and 25°C; the neonatal resuscitaire should be checked and ready for use.

The Apgar score is traditionally scored at 1 and 5 minutes and acts as a guide in helping staff communicate the resuscitative needs of neonates immediately after birth. Some consider it has limited usefulness in LBW babies because it was originally devised by Apgar in 1953 for term babies and does not take into account how gestational age, congenital abnormalities or sedation affect the score (Juretschke 2000). Labelling of the LBW baby is particularly important because separation of mother and baby could happen at any time if the baby's condition becomes unstable. If the baby needs admission to the NICU, the midwife may consider, on cutting the cord to size, to leave an extra length, in case access to the umbilical vessels should be necessary at a later time. A detailed but expedient examination of the baby should be conducted by the midwife in the presence of the parents and recorded accordingly. It is particularly important in SGA babies to check that the anal sphincter is patent, which could provide information on the internal integrity of the gastrointestinal system. This is a good time to allay any parental anxieties about their baby's general appearance, which may be quite different to what they were expecting (Redshaw 1997). Once it is established that the baby is healthy, the midwife may attempt to normalise the care by emphasising to the parents the importance of preventing cold stress and promoting skin-to-skin contact for a period of up to 50 minutes. The midwife should ensure that the baby is thoroughly dried before skin-to-skin contact is attempted. This will secure the baby's conductive heat transfer gains, and help him to become physically stabilised and to find the breast. If the mother chooses not to engage in skin-to-skin contact the father may wish to do so, but, if not, the baby can be dressed, wrapped and held by his parents in the normal way. The baby's axilla temperature should be maintained between 36.4 and 37°C.

Assessment of gestational age

It is generally considered essential to obtain an accurate assessment of gestational age, first to anticipate the problems a baby is more likely to develop and secondly to provide valid comparisons with respect to morbidity and mortality statistics (Philip 1996). In 1970, Dubowitz et al developed a scoring system for the assessment of gestational age in babies less than 5 days old based upon neurological and physical (external) characteristics. The purpose of the assessment, which is still used today, is to confirm the stated gestation, reveal any discrepancies and provide a reliable estimate when uncertainty exists (Philip 1996). Despite its usefulness, the accuracy of the assessment is less reliable in babies who have suffered a neurological insult such as birth asphyxia or chronic exposure to drugs. Such babies will obtain a lower score on neurological criteria. Other affected babies are those who have suffered asymmetric IUGR. Their sole creases have extra wrinkles as a result of exposure to amniotic fluid and this feature may confer upon them an enhanced maturity, whereas breast tissue formation, female external genitalia and ear cartilage will give the appearance of less maturity because of diminished amounts of adipose tissue and so they may be underscored on physical assessment, if they are near to term. Hence, gestational age assessments based on physical criteria can be misleading (Anderson & Hay 1999). Mupanemunda & Watkinson (1999) do not totally endorse the Dubowitz scoring system, believing that its margins of error are too wide. They further contend that the handling of LBW babies for the assessment is problematic because it may destabilise an otherwise well baby. With the developments of more accurate dating by antenatal ultrasound techniques, it is argued that there is less justification for a full assessment of gestational age in well LBW babies. The exception is applied when the mother deliberately conceals her pregnancy, is unable to communicate or unwilling to divulge requisite information, or is unreliable (e.g. a drug-abusing mother with unfavourable social circumstances). Therefore any assessments that are carried out should be carefully conducted, with the view that no harm should be caused as a result of the process (Anderson & Hay 1999).

Care of the healthy LBW baby

Many of the care issues relevant to the LBW baby apply to both the preterm and the SGA infant; where differences do exist, these will receive further consideration. The following areas of focus, although presented separately, do by their nature influence each other and should not be regarded as stand-alone entities.

Principles of thermoregulation

Thermoregulation is the balance between heat production and heat loss. The prevention of cold stress, which may lead to hypothermia (body temperature < 35°C), is critical for the intact survival of the LBW baby. Newborn babies are unable to shiver, move very much, or ask for an extra blanket and therefore rely upon physical adaptations that generate heat by raising their basal metabolic rate and utilising brown fat deposits. Thus, exposure to cool environments can result in multisystem physiological changes, which significantly challenge the baby's health status. As body temperature falls, tissue oxygen consumption rises as the baby attempts to raise its metabolic rate by burning glucose to generate energy and heat. Care measures should aim to provide an environment that supports thermoneutrality. This is otherwise known as the 'neutral thermal environment', a range of ambient temperatures within which the metabolic rate is minimal, the baby is neither gaining or losing heat, oxygen consumption is minimal and the core-to-skin temperature gradient is small (Blackburn & Loper 1992).

Thermoregulation and the healthy mature SGA baby

In the neonate, the head accounts for one-fifth of the total body surface area and brain heat production is thought to be 55% of total metabolic heat production. Rapid heat loss due to the large head-to-body ratio and large surface area is exaggerated, particularly in the asymmetrically grown SGA baby. Wide sutures and large fontanelles add to the heat-losing tendency. On the plus side, they have increased skin maturity but often depleted stores of subcutaneous fat, which are used for insulation. Their raised basal metabolic rate helps them to produce heat but their high energy demands in the presence of poor glycogen stores and minimal fat deposition can soon lead to hypoglycaemia and then hypothermia. Once the baby is thoroughly dried, a prewarmed hat will minimise heat loss from the head.

Thermoregulation and the healthy preterm baby

All preterm babies are prone to heat loss because their ability to produce heat is compromised by their immaturity, so factors such as their large ratio of surface area to weight, their varying amounts of subcutaneous fat and their ability to mobilise brown fat stores (which have been laid down from 28 weeks) will be affected by their gestational age. During cooling, immaturity of the heat-regulating centres in the hypothalamus and medulla oblongata fail, in different degrees, to recognise and marshall adequately coordinated homeostatic controls. In addition, preterm babies are often unable to increase their oxygen consumption effectively through normal respiratory function and their calorific intake is often inadequate to meet increasing metabolic requirements. Furthermore, their open resting postures increase their surface area and insensible water losses, which includes transepidermal water loss, render the preterm baby more susceptible to evaporative heat losses. Gestational age and the weight of the baby will influence the type of care initiated. For babies under 2.0 kg, incubator care may be necessary when the baby is not receiving skin-to-skin contact with either parent. The warm conditions in an incubator can be achieved either by heating the air to 30–32°C (air mode) or by servo-controlling the baby's body temperature at a desired set point (36°C). In servo mode, a thermocouple is taped to the upper abdomen and the incubator heater maintains the skin at that site at a preset constant (see Fig. 41.4). Babies are clothed with bedding, in a room temperature of 26°C. Most preterm babies between 2.0 and 2.5 kg will be cared for in a cot, in a room temperature of 24°C.

Hypoglycaemia

Hypoglycaemia and the healthy LBW baby

The term 'hypoglycaemia' refers to a low blood glucose concentration and in itself is not a medical condition, but a feature of illness or a failure to adapt from the fetal state of continuous transplacental glucose consumption to the extrauterine pattern of intermittent nutrient supply (WHO 1997b). It is more likely to occur in conditions where babies become cold or where the initiation of early feeding (within the first hour) is delayed. Counterregulatory mechanisms (for a more detailed account on hypoglycaemia see Ch. 47) maintain the blood glucose at safe limits to protect tissue viability; however, it is generally questioned whether LBW babies are able to counterregulate as effectively as appropriately grown term babies and some caution is recommended (WHO 1997b). The aim of management is to maintain the true blood sugar above the level considered to be the lowest level of normal, which is 2.6 mmol/dl (WHO 1997b). However, this does not mean that every LBW baby should be *routinely* screened. Well LBW babies who show no clinical signs of hypoglycaemia, are demanding and taking nutritive feeds on a regular basis and maintaining their body temperature, do not need screening for hypoglycaemia. The emphasis of care is placed upon the concept of *adequate feeding* and the cornerstone of success in this situation is the midwife's ability to assess skilfully whether the baby is feeding sufficiently well to meet energy requirements. Midwives should be guided by their local policies regarding use of reagent strips, but if a baby, despite being fed, presents with clinical signs of hypoglycaemia then a venous sample should be taken by the paediatrician to assess the true blood sugar level, and this should be dispatched to the laboratory for verification purposes. A blood glucose that remains < 2.6 mmol/dl, despite the baby's further attempts to feed by breast or colostrum by cup, may warrant transfer to the NICU, because glucose by intravenous bolus may be necessary to correct the metabolic disturbance. In addition, the midwife should consider that there may be some underlying medical condition that may call for more thorough investigation.

Hypoglycaemia and the healthy mature SGA baby

If the SGA baby does not suffer any effects of perinatal asphyxia or develop cold stress, the remaining potential problem is hypoglycaemia. Glycogen storage begins at the beginning of the third trimester and, due to altered placental transport of nutrients during this time, asymmetrically grown babies have reduced glycogen stores in liver and skeletal muscles (Ogata 1999). Their greater brain-to-body mass and a tendency towards polycythaemia increase their energy demands and, since both the brain and the red blood cells are obligatory glucose users, these factors can increase glucose requirements. Mature SGA babies with an asymmetric growth pattern will usually feed within the first half an hour of birth and will demand feeds every 2–3 hours thereafter, to make up for lost time. Feeding is thought to mature the blunted counterregulatory response, so their susceptibility to hypoglycaemia is relatively short lived and limited to the first 48 hours following birth. If the baby is taking formula milk, feeds are usually calculated at 90 ml/kg on the first day, with 30 ml increments per day.

Hypoglycaemia and the preterm baby

The preterm baby may be sleepier, and attempts to take the first feed may reflect gestational age. Total feed requirements (60 ml/kg on the first day, with 30 ml/kg increments per day) may not be taken directly from the breast and supplementary feeds can be given by cup.

Feeding the LBW baby

Both preterm and SGA babies benefit from human milk because it contains long chain polyunsaturated omega-3 fatty acids, which are thought to be essential for the myelination of neural membranes and for retinal development. Preterm breastmilk has a higher concentration of lipids, protein, sodium, calcium and immunoglobulins, a low osmolarity, and lipases and enzymes that improve digestion and absorption (Jones & Spencer 1999). The uniqueness of the mother's milk for her own baby cannot be overstated. For any mother to commit to the challenge of breastfeeding her LBW baby, and in particular the preterm baby, she should be thoroughly prepared both cognitively and emotionally by the midwife, so that her expectations are realistic as she anticipates the likely sequence of events that her baby may take her through (Lang 1997). First, she needs to understand what her baby may be able to achieve related to his development, which is based upon the combined influences of his gestational age at birth and his post-natal age. For a baby to feed for nutritive purposes, the coordination of breathing with suck and swallow reflexes is thought to reflect neurobehavioral matura-tion and organisation and is thought to occur between 32 and 36 weeks' gestation (Hepper & Shahidullah 1994, Pinelli & Symington 2001). Sucking and swal-lowing reflexes are present by 28 weeks' gestation, but the baby is unable to coordinate these activities until 34–36 weeks. Preterm babies are limited in their abil-ity to suck because of their weak musculature and flexor control, which is important for firm lip and jaw closure (Blackburn & Loper 1992). Before 32 weeks, most healthy preterm babies will need to be tube fed on a regular basis, usually on a 3-hourly regimen with preset amounts of breastmilk, hind milk or formula milk based on postnatal age and present weight, to provide the necessary calories for growth, but not at the expense of energy expenditure.

It is now common practice for parents to tube feed their own baby. Als (1986) believes that parents should be encouraged to hold their baby during tube feeds and provide physical support for his trunk and shoulders, bracing his feet and giving him something to hold. Sucking is part of the flexor pattern of devel-opment and may be enhanced by giving the baby something to grasp (Young 1996). Tube feeding has the advantage that the tube can be left in situ during a cup or breastfeed and has been shown to eliminate the need to introduce bottles into a breastfeeding regimen (Kliethermes et al 1999). However, several problems have been identified with tube feeding. First, nasal and oral gastric tubes encourage milk lipid adherence to their inside surfaces and reduce the amount of fat calo-ries available to the baby. Cup feeding is said to reduce this tendency (Lang et al 1994). Secondly, babies are preferential nose breathers and the presence of a naso-gastric tube will inevitably take up part of their avail-able airway. Finally, their prolonged use has been associated with delay in the development of sucking and swallowing reflexes simply because the mouth is bypassed. For these reasons, cup feeding has been used in favour of tube feeding in order to provide the baby with a positive oral experience, to stimulate saliva and lingual lipases to aid digestion (Lang 1997), and to accelerate the transition from naso/oral gastric feeding to breastfeeding without the introduction of bottles and teats (Jones & Spencer 1999). Oral gastric tubes

have been associated with vagal stimulation and have resulted in bradycardia and apnoea and, of the two types, most clinicians favour the nasogastric tube (Kliethermes 1999).

Certain behaviours such as licking and lapping are well established *before* sucking and swallowing (Ritchie 1998) and, when babies are given the oppor-tunity, it is not unusual to see them as early as 28 and 29 weeks, licking milk that has been expressed on to the nipple by their mother. Thus, babies between 30 and 32 weeks' gestation can be given expressed breast-milk (EBM) by cup. Lang (1994) makes the point that tongue movement is vital in the efficient stripping of the milk ducts, so cup feeding can be seen as develop-mental preparation for breastfeeding. Between 32 and 34 weeks' gestation, cup feeding can act as the main method of feeding, with the baby taking occasional complete breast feeds. Attitudes towards cup feeding vary, but initial concerns expressed by clinicians are, according to Samuel (1999), related to fear of milk inhalation and the extra time needed to give a feed. These fears have not been realised in practice because, as Samuel argues, the baby controls the pace and volume he takes; some babies are slow feeders, others more expedient, so, in general, cup feeds tend to last about the same duration as bottle feeds. More impor-tantly, however, they utilise little energy, which is a crucial factor in their favour for LBW babies.

A preterm baby of less than 35 weeks' gestation can be gently wrapped prior to a breast (or formula) feed and this is thought to provide reassurance and com-fort, not unlike the unique close-fitting tactile stimula-tion of the uterus (Sparshott 1997). A preterm baby may easily tire and the mother can be taught to start the flow of milk by hand expressing this before attach-ing him to the breast. Long pauses between sucks are to be expected. This burst–pause pattern is a signal of normal development and seems to occur earlier with breastfeeding (Blackburn & Loper 1992). The baby may appear to be asleep and a change in position may remind him of the task in hand, but it is thought to be a mistake to force a reluctant baby to feed (Sparshott 1997). If it is obvious that the baby is more interested in sleeping, the mother can complete the feed by tube.

From 35 weeks onwards, cup feeding can be gradu-ally replaced by complete breastfeeding (Lang 1997). Progress in the feeding method is often dependent upon the preterm baby, who cues his mother that he is ready to take milk from the breast. In the interim, she must express her milk so that she can maintain her milk supply and provide the milk for cup feeding as necessary. An unrushed feed can take up to an hour to complete. Any advances on this time frame should be reviewed in terms of the quality of the baby–nipple attachment (see Ch. 40), maternal milk flow (which may be affected by anxiety or other factors) and the general condition of the baby (e.g. the development of physiological jaundice). Feeding frequency can vary between 6 and 10 feeds per day. The baby should be left to establish his own volume requirements and feeding pattern. The mother should be encouraged to rely upon her own instincts and common sense so that the rhythm of total care she adopts in hospital will thoroughly prepare her for when she goes home (Lang 1997). Often the difference between early and late transfer home is more dependent upon the mother's positive attitude and skill development than the baby's maturity and inherent abilities.

The care environment: promoting health and development of the healthy LBW baby

The importance of providing an appropriate environment for the healthy LBW baby cannot be overstressed. According to Sparshott (1997) the ideal environment should resemble home, which provides a cycle of day and night, regular nourishment, rest, stimulation and loving attention. The midwife's role is to create such an environment, primarily for the physical development of the baby, but at the same time to provide psychological support for the mother and her family. The mother's desire to be involved is seen as an *essential* element in the success of caring for LBW babies on postnatal wards.

The normal sensory requirements of the developing brain depend upon subtle influences, first from the uterus and then from the breast (Reed & Freer 2000). Any disruption to this natural arrangement renders the LBW baby vulnerable to influences in the care environment that can result in poorly coordinated behaviours as a result of delays in the development of different systems (autonomic, motor, sensory, etc.). Teaching parents to support their baby's emerging developmental agenda is important in developmentally focused

care, but, as Reid (2000) believes, maternal role development depends upon the mother's self-esteem and her mastery of mothering behaviours. By attempting to adapt the care environment to be more like the intrauterine environment, the midwife can help parents to become aware of their baby's behavioural and autonomic cues and utilise them in organising care according to their baby's individual tolerance. Parents will come to know their baby, to see him as an individual, competent for his stage of development and not merely 'a baby born too early', or a dysfunctional term infant. They will be encouraged (but not cajoled) into taking a major role in their baby's emerging developmental agenda, come to understand the situation in which they find themselves, become more able to reset their expectations and thus offer more baby-led support (Reed & Freer 2000).

The emerging task of the term newborn baby is increasing alertness, with growing responsiveness to the outside world (Reed & Freer 2000). By comparison, a preterm baby is at a stage of development that is more concerned with their internal world. Term babies have stable function of the autonomic and motor systems. Preterm babies will be at different stages of this development, depending on their gestational age and health status. They will spend more time in rapid eye movement (REM) sleep or drowsy states and have difficulty in achieving deep sleep. They are unable to shut out stimulation that prevents them from sleeping and resting, and sudden noise hazards provoke stress reactions, which can adversely affect respiratory, cardiovascular and digestive stability. The term baby is able to shut out such stimuli for rest and sleep purposes. The degree to which SGA term babies have been affected by their unique intrauterine experience is difficult to assess in the short term, but hyperactivity is seen as a feature of an adaptive stress reaction. These babies, like their preterm counterparts, need an environment that supports their level of robustness. Environmental disturbances, excessive or prolonged handling and even activities like feeding may add an extra physiological burden to an already compromised state. Social contact is considered a vital element for the development of parent–child interaction, yet stereotypical notions of social contact that revolve around practical care giving and feeding may not be suitable for some babies and, when these activities are clustered together, may draw too heavily on the baby's physical resources. When the baby is overstimulated and wishes to terminate the interaction, behaviour cues such as fist clenching, furrowed brow, gaze aversion, splayed fingers and yawning may be communicated (Als 1986). Should the baby wish to initiate or continue an interaction, he may raise his brows, raise his head and engage in different degrees of eye contact with his social partner (usually the mother). Midwives can reassure parents that by paying attention to their baby's behavioural cues they can work *with* their baby's capabilities, which is crucial for maintaining a healthy status.

Handling and touch

Kangaroo care (KC) is used to promote closeness between a baby and mother and involves placing the nappy-clad baby upright between the maternal breasts for skin-to-skin contact (see Plate 22). The name is derived from similarities it bears to marsupial caregiving, in which the infant kangaroo, always born prematurely, is guided into the maternal pouch where he is kept warm, contained and close to the breast for unlimited feeding opportunities until maturation. The LBW baby remains beneath the mother's clothing for varying periods of time that suit the mother. Some mothers may have repeated contacts throughout the day, with occasional respite time; others may prefer specific periods around which they plan their day's activities. There are no rules or time limitations applied, but contact should be reviewed if there are any clinical signs of neonatal distress. Although KC appears to lessen mother and baby morbidity without any deleterious effects, much of the available evidence has been obtained from studies using different variables and modalities that have reflected the various clinical settings where the research has taken place. However, KC appears to be the central mediator for all of the crucial elements needed to maintain a healthy status in LBW babies, namely thermoregulation, effective breastfeeding and prevention of hypoglycaemia. A well-designed randomised controlled trial of KC is needed soon to strengthen this view empirically (Conde-Agudelo et al 2001). For the benefits of kangaroo care see Box 41.3.

Noise and light hazards

The time spent in a postnatal ward should be a time of rest and recuperation for both the mother and her

---

Box 41.3 The benefits of kangaroo care

- It endorses the notion of togetherness, which is far removed from the threat of separation.
- Mothers show thermal synchrony with their babies in a thermoneutral range.
- It provides a sense of containment and closeness that is reminiscent of the uterus.
- There is an increased reporting of successful lactation because of increased hormonal and sensory stimulation of the mother's milk production.
- There is promotion of early tactile, audiovisual and emotional contact for both, and the baby is given the opportunity to further his familiarity with the mother's voice, smell and heartbeat.
- It is thought to be influential in the development of strong emotional feelings to the baby.
- Mothers are more quickly adapted to the appearance of their babies.
- Mothers are more likely to become their baby's advocate.
- It is thought to strengthen the mother's confidence in gaining control over her emotions, her competency in mothering skills and her perception of herself as 'a good mother'.

Sources: Affonso et al (1989, 1992 1993); Padden & Glen (1997); Sparshott (1997); WHO (1997b).

LBW baby. Noise should be kept to a minimum. All extraneous noises should be eliminated from clinical areas such as musical toys and mobiles, harsh clattering footwear, telephones, radios, intercom systems and raised voices. Clinicians should be aware of noise hazards such as the closing of incubator portholes, use of peddle bins, ward doors and general equipment. Ward areas can be carpeted and quiet signs can be posted to remind visitors not to disrupt the peace (Young 1996). In dimmed lighting conditions, preterm babies are more able to improve their quality of sleep and alert status (Blackburn & Patteson 1991).

Reduced light levels at night will help to promote the development of circadian rhythms and diurnal cycles. Light levels can be adjusted during the day with curtains or blinds to shade windows and protect the room from direct sunlight. Screens to shield adjacent babies from phototherapy lights are essential.

Sleeping position

Preterm babies have reduced muscle power and bulk, with flaccid muscle tone, therefore their movements are erratic, weak or flailing. They exert energy to maintain their body position against the pull of gravity. Without support they may, to differing degrees, develop head, shoulder and hip flattening, which in turn can lead to poor mobility. Nesting the more immature preterm babies into soft bedding, in addition to the use of close flexible boundaries, helps to keep their limbs in midline flexion; however, it is vital that they are nursed in a supine position to prevent asphyxia. Lying the baby in the supine position is thought to be effective in promoting engagement in self-regulatory behaviours such as exploration of the face and mouth, hand and foot clasping, boundary searching, and flexion and extension of the limbs. Pressure on the occiput should over time ensure a more rounded head.

Sudden infant death syndrome (SIDS)

Placing healthy LBW babies to sleep in the prone position has been theoretically eradicated from neonatal practice since the 'back to sleep' campaign of December 1991 and various government reports that followed (DoH 1991, 1993, 1995). The side-lying position has been considered acceptable for healthy babies in hospital, for those babies that need monitoring for respiratory or cardiac function or both, but not for babies at home (Fleming et al 1996). It is now believed that *supine* should be the recommended sleeping position for *all* babies and should begin in hospital before transfer home (Hunt 1999). It is incumbent upon midwives to accustom the baby and educate the parents in adopting this approach (Willinger et al 2000). Roberts & Upton (2000) warn that, despite written information, there is a need to remind parents constantly of the risk factors and safety procedures (i.e. a feet-to-foot sleeping position, and a

smoke-free room) associated with SIDS alongside teaching parents to keep their babies warm. However, the leaflet 'Reduce the risk of cot death' (FSID 1996) may cause some confusion. The midwife needs to explain how the issues apply to individual families and take into consideration the time of year, gestational age and postnatal age when care is transferred to the community midwife. Parental training on 'what to do if my baby stops breathing' is becoming part of a routine preparation for transfer home, although this degree of preparedness can empower some parents but frighten others. The decision to receive training should be the parent's choice.

The prevention of infection

LBW babies, particularly preterm babies, are especially vulnerable to infections because of the immaturity of their host defence systems (Mupanemunda & Watkinson 1999). (See Chs 42 and 46 for further details.)

The provision of neonatal care: the question of venue and facilities

The decision to transfer a healthy LBW baby to a postnatal ward, a transitional unit or a NICU will depend upon the baby's gestational age and weight. Perhaps more influential, in these days of organisational constraints, will be the availability of facilities and level of staffing that exists at the time. Many variations exist in how specialist care is serviced (by midwives, neonatal nurses or a combination of both) and how the care is offered. Traditionally, the advantage of transitional care has been to divert medium risk babies away from the NICU, and this has been of great value (Bromley 2000). However, some would argue that part of its attraction has been to take healthy LBW babies that otherwise would have been roomed-in with their mothers on postnatal wards. It is often used as an intermediate unit where, in addition to healthy LBW babies, there are convalescing NICU graduates (Roberton 1999), term babies with congenital abnormalities, babies with feeding problems (particularly where tube feeding is required) and those babies who need antibiotic therapy. Separation from their babies

Box 41.4 The benefits and limitations of caring for healthy LBW babies on postnatal wards.

Benefits to the mother

- No separation of mother and baby
- No need for mother to visit NICU
- With rooming-in, less acquired nosocomial infections
- Less stressful environment on postnatal ward, therefore more effective communication and understanding of relevant issues and more able to overcome feelings of shock, anxiety and fear of having a LBW baby
- Rooming-in: more social and physical contact with baby
- Greater perceived sense of control; less feelings of failure
- Enhanced sense of role and identity
- More practice at mothering skills
- Better skill development and related confidence
- Care is more mother–baby focused; more holistic and 'normal'
- The mother feels part of the ward community, not just 'that mother whose baby in on the baby unit'
- More opportunity for support from peers on ward
- No 'handing over' the baby's care to a more experienced person and then 'taking back' the responsibility
- The transition to home is considered to be easier and more welcomed by the mother

Limitations that affect the mother

- The mother may not wish to commit to a prolonged and unspecified hospital stay

- The mother may not have any choice but to return home soon after birth (e.g. other caring responsibilities)
- The mother may feel ambivalence toward the birth event and her baby
- The mother may feel that the NICU is the best place for her baby
- The mother may be ill and not able to care for her baby
- There is no option for the mother who wishes after a few days to take her baby home, which may be too early

Benefits to the organisation

- More neonatal cots are made available
- Less need to close NICU (a daily concern for some maternity units)
- Less in-utero transfers of high risk women to other neonatal units
- More potential for staff development in caring for LBW babies

Organisational restraints

- Need for designated area in postnatal wards that will require a warm environment (24°C), reduced extraneous noise and subtle lighting conditions
- Longer hospital stay may block bed capacity
- Possible need for a dedicated course to provide extra education for staff
- Lack of consensus on the midwife's role and neonatal care
- Too few midwives, inadequate resourcing, skill-mix issues

Sources: Bromley (2000), Doering et al (2002), Redshaw (1997).

and lack of contact are, as reported by mothers, the worst features of having a baby that needs specialist care (Redshaw 1997). Affonso et al (1992) believe that mothers are cued by the environment in which they find themselves, so units that cater for special and intensive care imply sickness, whereas mothers with healthy babies need focused care from practitioners who provide care for healthy mothers and their healthy babies. The normalising effect of being with other postnatal women and being cared for by midwives is a powerful message that may help mothers to perceive their hospital postnatal experience as a normative life event, which will prepare them for when they go home. Indeed, midwife support should be the norm and it is recommended that postnatal visiting should *start* once the mother and her LBW baby are at home and continue for up to 6 weeks after delivery to help the mother negotiate her psychosocial transition to motherhood. (See Box 41.4 for the benefits and limitations of caring for LBW babies on postnatal wards.)

It is acknowledged that not all midwives are interested in developing their neonatology skills further and may feel unprepared to take on this new challenge, yet there are many midwives who are experienced, confident and qualified to care for these babies. The midwife's responsibility to the mother who is resident on the postnatal ward and visiting the specialist unit means that there is time and effort invested in the mother by the midwife. This time could be spent in caring for both mother and baby together. Midwives should regularly question whether imposed separations of mothers and their babies are really necessary. Mothers who are separated from their babies should, in theory, reap the benefits from support provided by both midwifery and neonatal staff; however, in reality it appears that all too often there is questionable continuity of care and a diffusion of responsibility, which may leave the mother socially isolated while in hospital. Midwives need to be ready to provide optimum maternity care for women who give birth to healthy LBW babies, to work more cohesively as part of the multiprofessional team, so as to make unnecessary separation of mother and baby a thing of the past.

REFERENCES

Affonso D D, Wahlberg V, Persson B 1989 Exploration of mother's reactions to the kangaroo method of prematurity care. Neonatal Network 7:43–51

Affonso D D, Bossque E, Wahlberg V, Brady J P 1993 Reconciliation and healing for mothers through skin to skin contact provided in an American tertiary level intensive care nursery. Neonatal Network 12(3):25–32

Affonso D D, Hurst I, Mayburry L J, Haller L, Yost K, Lynch M E 1992 Stressors reported by mothers of hospitalised premature infants. Neonatal Network 11(6):63–70

Als H 1986 A synactive model of neonatal behavioural organisation: framework for the assessment of neurobehavioural development in the premature infant and for support of infants and parents in the neonatal intensive care environment. In: Sweeney J K (ed) The high-risk neonate: development therapy perspectives. Physical and Occupational Therapy in Pediatrics Vol 314, no 6. Haworth Press, New York

Anderson M S, Hay W W 1999 Intrauterine growth restriction and the small for gestational age infant. In: Avery G B, Fletcher M A, MacDonald M G (eds) Neonatology, pathophysiology and management of the newborn. Lippincott, Williams & Wilkins, London, p 411–440

Blackburn S, Patteson D 1991 Effects of cycled lighting on activity state and cardiorespiratory function in preterm infants. Journal of Perinatal and Neonatal Nursing (4):47–54

Blackburn S T, Loper D L 1992 Maternal, fetal and neonatal physiology. A clinical perspective. W B Saunders, London

Bromley P 2000 Transitional care: let's think again. Journal of Neonatal Nursing 6(2):60–64

Conde-Agudelo A, Diaz-Rossello J L, Belizan J M 2001 Kangaroo care to reduce morbidity in low birth weight infants (Cochrane review). In: The Cochrane Library, Issue 3. Update Software, Oxford

DoH (Department of Health) 1991 Sleeping positions and the incidence of cot death. HMSO, London

DoH (Department of Health) 1993 Report of the Chief Medical Officer's Expert Group on the sleeping positions of infants and cot death. HMSO, London

DoH (Department of Health) 1995 The Confidential Enquiry into Stillbirths and Deaths in Infancy (CESDI). HMSO, London

Doering L V, Moser D K, Drapup K 2000 Correlates of anxiety, hostility, depression and psychosocial adjustment in parents of NICU infants. Neonatal Network 19(5):15–23

Dubowitz L M S, Dubowitz V, Golberg C 1970 Clinical assessment of gestational age in the newborn infant. Journal of Paediatrics 77:1–10

Fleming P J, Blair P S, Bacon C et al 1996. Confidential Enquiries into Stillbirths and Deaths regional coordinators and researchers. Environment of infants during sleep and risk of sudden infant death syndrome: results of 1993–5 case–control study for confidential enquiry into stillbirths and deaths in infancy. British Medical Journal 313:191–198

FSID (Foundation for the Study of Infant Deaths) 1996 Reduce the risk of cot death. FSID, London (available: DoH, Wetherby)

Gomella T L, Cunningham M D, Eyal F G, Zenk K E 1999 Neonatology. Appleton & Lange, Stamford, Connecticut

Harlow F D, Spencer A D 1999 Obstetrics for the neonatologist. In: Rennie J M, Roberton N R C (eds) Textbook of neonatology. Churchill Livingstone, Edinburgh, p 157–173

Hepper P G, Shahidullah S 1994 The beginnings of mind – evidence from the behaviour of the fetus. Journal of Reproductive and Infant Psychology 12(3):143–154

Hunt C E 1999 Sudden infant death syndrome. In: Avery G B, Fletcher M A, MacDonald M G (eds) Neonatology, pathophysiology and management of the newborn. Lippincott, Williams & Wilkins, London, p 569–574

Jones L, Spencer A 1999 Successful preterm breastfeeding. Practising Midwife 2(7):54–57

Juretschke L J 2000 Apgar scoring: its use and meaning for today's newborn. Neonatal Network 9(1):17–19

Kliethermes P A, Cross M L, Lanese M G, Johnson K M, Simon S D 1999 Transitioning preterm infants with nasogastric tube supplementation: increased likelihood of breastfeeding. Journal of Obstetric, Gynaecology and Neonatal Nursing 28(3):264–273

Korones S B 1986 High-risk newborn infants. The basis for intensive nursing care. C V Mosby, St Louis

Lang S 1994 Cup feeding: an alternative method. Midwives Chronicle 107:171–176

Lang S 1997 Breastfeeding special care babies. Baillière Tindall, London

Lang S, Laurence C J, Orme R L 1994 Cup feeding: an alternative method of infant feeding. Archive of Diseases in Children 71:366–369

Mupanemunda R H, Watkinson M 1999 Key topics in neonatology. Bios Scientific, Oxford

Ogata E S 1999 Carbohydrate homeostasis. In: Avery G B, Fletcher M A, McDonald M G (eds) Neonatology, physiopathology and management of the newborn. Lippincott, Williams & Wilkins, London, p 699–712

Padden T, Glen S 1997 Maternal experiences of preterm birth and neonatal care. Journal of Reproductive and Infant Psychology 15(2):121–139

Philip A G S 1996 Neonatology. A practical guide. W B Saunders, Philadelphia

Pinelli K, Symington A 2001 Non-nutritive sucking for promoting physiologic stability and nutrition in preterm infants (Cochrane review). In: The Cochrane Library, Issue 3. Update Software, Oxford

Redshaw M E 1997 Mothers of babies requiring special care: attitudes and experiences. Journal of Reproductive and Infant Psychology 15(2):109–120

Reed T, Freer Y 2000 Developmental nursing care. In: Boxwell G (ed) Neonatal intensive care. Routledge, London, p 14–38

Reid T L 2000 Maternal identity in preterm birth. Journal of Child Health Care 4(1):23–29

Ritchie J F 1998 Immature sucking response in premature babies: cup feeding as a tool in increasing maintenance of breastfeeding. Journal of Neonatal Nursing 14(2):13–17

Roberton N R C 1999 Fetal growth, intrauterine growth retardation and small for gestational age babies. In: Rennie J M, Roberton N R C (eds) Textbook of neonatology. Churchill Livingstone, London, p 389–398

Roberts H, Upton D 2000 New Mother's knowledge of sudden infant death syndrome. British Journal of Midwifery 8(3):147–150

Samuel P 1999 Cup feeding; how and when to use it with term babies. Midwifery Digest 9(2):215–217

Simpson C 1997 Small for gestational age babies. In: Sweet B (ed) Mayes' midwifery a textbook for midwives. Baillière Tindall, London, p 853

Sparshott M 1997 Pain, distress and the newborn baby. Blackwell Science, Oxford

WHO (World Health Organisation) 1977a Manual of international statistical classification of diseases, injuries and causes of death. WHO, Geneva, vol 1

WHO (World Health Organisation) 1997b Hypoglycaemia of the newborn. Review of the literature. WHO, Geneva

Willinger M K C W, Hoffman H, Kessler R, Corwin M 2000 Factors associated with caregiver's choice of infant sleep position study. Journal of the American Medical Association 283(16):2135–2142

Young J 1996 Development care of the premature baby. Baillière Tindall, London

FURTHER READING

Rennie J M, Gandy G M 1999 Examination of the newborn. In: Rennie J M, Roberton N R C (eds) Textbook of neonatology. Churchill Livingstone, Edinburgh, p. 269–287

This chapter provides a detailed account of assessment of gestational age and presents clear illustrations of the Dubowitz et al (1970) assessments. It also includes how other workers have developed revised assessment systems based on Dubowitz's original premise.

42 Recognising the Ill Baby

Jean Evelyn Bain

The length of time a mother spends in hospital with her newborn infant is ever decreasing. The focus of this chapter is to aid the midwife in the early detection of diseases in the neonate, so that appropriate action can be taken as soon as possible. The chapter design takes a systematic approach, which can be used in conjunction with the newborn examination, thus allowing the midwife to distinguish the ill from the well baby.

The chapter aims to:

- assist the midwife in the assessment and identification of the ill neonate

- provide an overview of the potential or presenting problems of the neonate

- consider the needs of the family by the integration of family-centred care in the neonatal unit.

Introduction

The majority of newborn babies are born normal and healthy; they require no intervention after delivery except to be dried with a warm towel and then to have skin-to-skin contact with their mothers. However, although the labour and birth may have been straight forward, the baby will still need to be observed at this time to ensure that the respirations are normal, there is good colour, the body temperature is stable and the baby is active and responsive.

The midwife soon becomes familiar with the appearance and behaviour of the well baby, but must also learn the signs and signals caused by illness, some of which may be subtle and non-specific. The labour and birth have an obvious effect on the well-being of the infant, but added to this are the genetic background, the mother's illnesses in pregnancy and any drugs she may have taken or received during that period (Rennie and Gandy 1999).

Parents welcome the observation of their newborn as it provides an opportunity for them to discuss any concerns they may have and the midwife can reassure them that their baby is normal and healthy. If the baby is unwell, this needs to be identified quickly and parents need to be made aware of any problem as soon as possible.

Assessment of the infant

Immediately after birth, all infants should be examined for any gross congenital abnormalities or evidence of birth trauma. They should also have their weight and gestational age plotted on a standard growth chart (see Ch. 41). Infants can then be classified as:

- appropriate for gestational age (AGA): between the 10th and 90th centile
- small for gestational age (SGA): below the 10th centile
- large for gestational age (LGA): above the 90th centile
- preterm: born before 37 weeks' gestation.

This classification allows the midwife to assess infants who may require specialised care. Infants who are preterm, SGA or LGA are at an increased risk of respiratory disease, hypoglycaemia, polycythaemia and disturbed thermoregulation. Later, usually within the next 24 hours, a more comprehensive, systematic, physical examination should take place.

Decreasing morbidity and mortality are the goal of all those involved with the care of the newborn infant. The early recognition of existing or potential problems is vital if the appropriate treatment is to be initiated as soon as possible.

Maternal health

Any disease in the mother can have an effect on the pregnancy. Some have more specific effects than others and reviewing the maternal history is an essential starting point in understanding the potential or presenting problems of the neonate. Influencing factors include:

- pregnancy-induced hypertension
- history of epilepsy
- maternal diabetes
- history of substance abuse
- history of sexually transmitted diseases.

Fetal well-being and health in pregnancy

The following are examples of significant questions that a midwife may ask herself as they may have a critical influence on the well-being of the infant:

- What was the estimated date of delivery?
- Was this a twin pregnancy?
- Was the baby presenting by the breech?
- Is the baby preterm?
- Is the infant SGA?
- Was there poor growth in utero?
- Was any evidence of congenital abnormality picked up on scanning, such as enlarged heart, or bowel obstruction?

Perinatal and delivery complications

Labour and delivery may also have an effect on the general welfare of the newborn infant. Listed below are important points that can confirm or rule out fetal compromise:

- prolonged rupture of membranes
- abnormal fetal heart rate pattern
- meconium staining
- difficult or rapid delivery
- caesarean section and the reason for this.

Over a period of a few hours the newborn baby needs to adapt to living without placental support, and it is during this time that some problems may manifest themselves. The midwife needs to be able to recognise warning signs and initiate prompt action if deterioration of the baby's condition is to be prevented.

Physical assessment

Most of the information the midwife requires for the assessment of a baby's well-being comes from observation. The baby's breathing pattern will alter depending on his level of activity but a respiratory rate above 60 breaths per minute is considered as tachypnoea. Much can be learned by observing the baby's resting position. The normal baby will lie with his limbs partially flexed and active. The skin colour should be centrally pink, indicating adequate oxygenation; there should be no rashes or skin lesions. The signs listed in Box 42.1 may indicate an underlying problem.

After the initial observation there usually follows a more systematic examination commencing at the baby's head and working gradually down towards the feet.

The skin

The skin of a neonate varies in its appearance and can often be the cause of unnecessary anxiety in the mother, midwife and medical staff. It is, however, often the first sign that there may be an underlying problem in the baby.

The presence of meconium on the skin, which is usually seen in the nail beds and around the umbilicus, is frequently associated with infants who have cardiorespiratory problems. More generally, the skin of all babies should be examined for pallor, plethora, cyanosis, jaundice and skin rashes.

Pallor

A pale, mottled baby is an indication of poor peripheral perfusion. At birth it can be associated with low circulating blood volume or with circulatory adaptation and compensation for perinatal hypoxaemia. The anaemic infant's appearance is usually pale pink, white or, in severe cases where there is vascular collapse, grey. Other presenting signs are tachycardia, tachypnoea and poor capillary refill (to assess capillary refill, press the skin briefly on the forehead or abdomen and observe how long it takes for the colour to return; this should be prompt).

The most likely causes of anaemia in the newborn period are:

- a history in the infant of haemolytic disease of the newborn

> **Box 42.1** General assessment warning signs
>
> - Pallor
> - Central cyanosis
> - Jaundice
> - Apnoea lasting longer than 20 seconds
> - Heart rate less than 110 or more than 180 beats per minute (taken during spells of inactivity)
> - Respiratory rate less than 30 or greater than 60 breaths per minute
> - Skin temperature (axilla) less than 36.2°C or above 37.2°C
> - Lack of spontaneous movement and responsiveness
> - Abnormal lying position either hypotonic or hypertonic
> - Lack of interest in surroundings

- twin-to-twin transfusions in utero (which can cause one infant to be anaemic and the other polycythaemic)
- maternal antepartum or intrapartum haemorrhage.

Pallor can also be observed in infants who are hypothermic or hypoglycaemic. Problems associated with pallor include:

- anaemia and shock
- respiratory disorders
- cardiac anomalies
- sepsis (where poor peripheral perfusion might also be observed).

Plethora

Babies who are beetroot in colour are usually described as plethoric. Their colour may indicate an excess of circulating red blood cells (polycythaemia). This is defined as a venous haematocrit greater than 70%. Newborn infants can become polycythaemic if they are recipients of:

- twin-to-twin transfusion in utero
- a large placental transfusion.

Contributing factors are delayed clamping of umbilical cord, or holding the infant below the level of the placenta, thereby allowing blood to flow into the baby and giving a greater circulating blood volume (sometimes occurring in unassisted births). Other infants at risk are:

- small for gestational age babies
- infants of diabetic mothers
- those with Down syndrome
- neonatal hypothyroidism.

Hypoglycaemia is commonly seen in plethoric infants because red blood cells consume glucose. The infant can exhibit a neurological disorder; irritability, jitteriness and convulsions can occur. Other problems that may manifest are:

- apnoea
- respiratory distress
- cardiac failure
- necrotising enterocolitis.

The diagnosis of polycythaemia is based upon haemoglobin and haematocrit level comparisons with normal values based on gestation. The treatment for symptomatic polycythaemia is to replace red blood cells by means of a partial exchange using volume expanders or plasma. Infants who are non-symptomatic show little improvement when treated and so intervention is not recommended (Bada 1992).

Cyanosis

Central cyanosis should always be taken very seriously. The mucous membranes are the most reliable indicators of central colour in all babies and if the tongue and mucous membranes appear blue this indicates low oxygen saturation levels in the blood, usually of respiratory or cardiac origin. Episodic central cyanotic attacks may be an indication that the infant is having a convulsion. Peripheral cyanosis of the hands and feet is common during the first 24 hours of life; after this time it may be a non-specific sign of illness. *Central cyanosis always demands urgent attention.*

Jaundice

Early onset jaundice (occurring in the skin and sclera within the first 12 hours of life) is abnormal and needs investigating. If a jaundiced baby is unduly lethargic, is a poor feeder, vomits or has an unstable body temperature, this may indicate infection and action should be taken to exclude this (see Ch. 46).

Other factors that affect the appearance of the skin

Preterm infants have thinner skin that is redder in appearance than that of term infants. In post-term infants the skin is often dry and cracked.

The skin is a good indicator of the nutritional status of the infant. The SGA infant may look malnourished and have folds of loose skin over the joints, owing to the lack or loss of subcutaneous fat. This can predispose the infant to problems with hypoglycaemia due to poor glycogen stores in the liver and can also cause problems with hypothermia.

If the infant is dehydrated, the skin looks dry and pale and is often cool to touch. If gently pinched, it will be slow in retracting. Other signs of dehydration are: pallor or mottled skin, sunken fontanelle or eyeball sockets and tachycardia.

Skin rashes

Skin rashes are quite common in newborn babies but most are benign and self-limiting.

Milia. These are white or yellow papules seen over the cheeks, nose and forehead. These invariably disappear spontaneously over the first few weeks of life.

Miliaria. These are clear vesicles on the face, scalp and perineum, caused by retention of sweat in unopened sweat glands. They appear on the chest and around areas where clothes can cause friction. The treatment is to nurse the infant in a cooler environment or to remove excess clothing.

Petechiae or purpura rash. These can occur in neonatal thrombocytopenia, which is a condition of platelet deficiency and usually presents with a petechial rash over the whole of the body. There may also be prolonged bleeding from puncture sites or the umbilicus, or both, and bleeding into the gut. Thrombocytopenia may be found in infants with:

- congenital infections, both viral and bacterial
- maternal idiopathic thrombocytopenia
- drugs (administered to mother or infant)
- severe Rhesus haemolytic disease.

Bruising. This can occur extensively following breech extractions, forceps and ventouse deliveries. The bleeding can cause a decrease in circulating blood volume, predisposing the baby to anaemia or, if the bruising is severe, hypotension.

Erythema toxicum. This is a rash that consists of white papules on an erythematous base; occurs in about 30–70% of infants. This condition is benign and should not be confused with a staphylococcal infection, which will require antibiotics. Diagnosis can be confirmed by examination of a smear of aspirate from a pustule, which will show numerous eosinophils (white cells indicative of an allergic response, rather than infection).

Infectious lesions (see also Ch. 46)

Thrush. This is a fungal infection of the mouth and throat. It is very common in neonates especially if they have been treated with antibiotics. It presents as white patches seen over the tongue and mucous membranes and as a red rash on the perineum.

Herpes simplex virus. If acquired in the neonatal period, this is a most serious viral infection. Transmission in utero is rare; the infection usually occurs during birth. Seventy per cent of affected infants will produce a rash, which appears as vesicles or pustules. Mortality depends on severity of the illness and when treatment commenced (Logan 1990). (see Plate 23).

Umbilical sepsis. This can be caused by a bacterial infection. Until its separation, the umbilical cord can be a focus for infection by bacteria that colonise the skin of the newborn. If periumbilical redness occurs or a discharge is noted, it may be necessary to commence antibiotic therapy in order to prevent an ascending infection.

Bullous impetigo. This is a condition which makes the skin look as though it has been scalded and is caused by streptococci or staphylococci. It presents as widespread tender erythema, followed by blisters, which break leaving raw areas of skin. This is particularly noticeable around the napkin area but can also cause umbilical sepsis, breast abscesses, conjunctivitis and, in deep infections, there may also be involvement of the bones and joints.

Respiratory system

Respiratory distress in the newborn can be a presentation of a number of clinical disorders and is the major factor in the morbidity and mortality in the neonatal period.

It is important to observe the baby's breathing when he is at rest and when he is active. The midwife should always start by observing skin colour and then carry out a respiratory inspection, taking into account whether the baby is making either an extra effort or insufficient effort to breathe.

Respiratory inspection

Respirations should be counted by watching the lower chest and abdomen rise and fall for a full minute. The respiration rate should be between 40 and 60 breaths per minute but will vary according to the level of activity. Newborn infants are primarily nose breathers and so obstructions of the nares may lead to respiratory distress and cyanosis. *Remember if suction is required at any time; always suction the mouth first and then the nose.* The chest should expand symmetrically. If there is unilateral expansion and breath sounds are diminished on one side, this may indicate that a pneumothorax has occurred. Infants at risk of pneumothorax or other air leaks are:

- preterm infants with respiratory distress
- term infants with meconium-stained amniotic fluid
- infants who require resuscitation at birth.

Increased work of breathing

If the baby's respiratory rate at rest is above 60 breaths per minute, this is described as *tachypnoea*. When observing an infant's respiratory rate the midwife must always take into consideration the environment and the temperature in which the baby is being nursed. Overheating will cause an infant to breathe faster.

Any infant with tachypnoea may be described as having respiratory distress, and the midwife should also observe the quality of the respirations, noting if there is any inspiratory pulling in of the chest wall above and below the sternum, or between the ribs (retraction). If nasal flaring is also present, this may indicate that there has been a delay in the lung fluid clearance, or that a more serious respiratory problem is developing (Dickason et al 1998).

Grunting, heard either with a stethoscope or audibly, is an abnormal expiratory sound. The grunting baby forcibly exhales against a closed glottis in order to prevent the alveoli from collapsing. These infants require help with their breathing, either by intubation or continuous positive airway pressure ventilation (CPAP) (see also Ch. 43).

Apnoea

Apnoea is defined as a cessation of breathing for 20 seconds or more. It is associated with pallor, bradycardia, cyanosis, oxygen desaturation or a change in the level of consciousness (Fanaroff & Martin 1997). Any baby having apnoeic spells needs to be admitted to a neonatal unit to have his cardiorespiratory system monitored.

The most common cause of apnoea in preterm babies is pulmonary surfactant deficiency (see Ch. 43) or the immaturity of the central nervous system control mechanism. Other disorders that may produce apnoea in the newborn are:

- hypoxia
- pneumonia
- aspiration
- pneumothorax
- metabolic disorders (e.g. hypoglycaemia, hypocalcaemia, acidosis)
- anaemia
- maternal drugs
- neurological problems (e.g. intracranial haemorrhage, convulsions, developmental disorders of the brain)
- congenital anomalies of the upper airway.

It is very important to remember that apnoea may also be induced by stimulation of the posterior pharynx by suction catheters.

Body temperature

Thermoregulation is a critical physiological function that is closely related to the survival of the infant. It is therefore essential that all those caring for newborn infants are aware of the importance of the thermal environment and understand the need for maintenance of normal body temperature (Merenstein & Gardner 1998).

A neutral thermal environment is defined as the ambient air temperature at which oxygen consumption or heat production is minimal, with body temperature in the normal range (Roncoli & Medoff-Cooper 1992).

The normal body temperature range for term infants is:

Skin temperature   36.7–37.3°C.

Environments that are outside the neutral thermal environment may result in the infant developing hypothermia or hyperthermia. Babies who are too cold or too warm will try and regulate their temperature and this action, especially in the preterm and SGA infant, can have a detrimental effect (see also Ch. 41).

Note: Intermittent temperature recordings have traditionally been taken using mercury thermometers. Recent research suggests that this practice is hazardous and should be eradicated (Smith et al 1997).

Hypothermia

Hypothermia is defined as a core temperature below 36°C (Rutter 1999). When the body temperature is below this level the infant is at risk from cold stress. This can cause complications such as increased oxygen consumption, lactic acid production, apnoea, decrease in blood coagulability and, the most commonly seen, hypoglycaemia. In preterm infants, cold stress may also cause a decrease in surfactant secretion and synthesis.

Note: *Letting infants get cold increases mortality and morbidity.*

After birth a baby's body temperature can fall very quickly. The healthy term baby will try to maintain his temperature within the normal range. If, however, he is compromised at birth by any of the following conditions, the added stress of hypothermia can be disastrous:

- severe asphyxia
- extensive resuscitation
- delayed drying at birth
- respiratory distress
- hypoglycaemia
- sepsis – septic infants often have hypothermia rather than hyperthermia

- being preterm or SGA – these infants have poor glucose stores, decreased subcutaneous tissue and little or no brown fat stores.

When a neonate is exposed to cold he will at first become very restless; then, as his body temperature falls, he adopts a tightly flexed position to try to conserve heat. The sick or preterm infant will tend to lie supine in a frog-like position with all his surfaces exposed, which maximises heat loss (Roberton 2001).

Adults can generate heat from shivering, whereas neonates perform non-shivering thermogenesis utilising their brown fat stores. During brown fat metabolism, oxygen is consumed and this may cause an alteration in the respiratory pattern, usually increasing the rate. Added to this, the baby often looks pale or mottled and may be uninterested in feeding. Hypoglycaemia is a common feature of infants with increased energy expenditure associated with thermoregulation and this can cause the infant to have jittery movements of the limbs, even though he is quiet and often limp.

Hyperthermia

Hyperthermia is defined as a core temperature above 38.0°C (Rutter 1999). The usual cause of hyperthermia is overheating of the environment but it can also be a clinical sign of sepsis, brain injury or drug therapy. If an infant is too warm, he becomes restless and may have bright red cheeks. Hyperthermia has a similar effect on the body to that of hypothermia and is equally detrimental. An infant will attempt to regulate his temperature by increasing his respiratory rate and this can lead to an increased fluid loss by evaporation through the airways. Other problems caused by hyperthermia are hypernatraemia, jaundice and recurrent apnoea.

Note: Variability in body temperature, either high or low, may be the first and only sign that a baby is unwell.

Cardiovascular system

The normal heart rate of a newborn baby is 110–160 b.p.m., with an average of 130 b.p.m. (Kozier et al 1998). The heart rate varies with respiration in the newborn; however, heart rates persistently outside this range when at rest may suggest an underlying cardiac problem. Cardiovascular dysfunction should be suspected in infants who commonly present with lethargy and breathlessness during feeding. It is often the baby's mother who first expresses concern: her baby may be slow with his feeds, and she may say he looks pale at times or that he feels very sweaty or has fast or laboured breathing.

It can be very difficult to identify infants with congenital heart disease because the clinical picture of tachycardia, tachypnoea, pallor or cyanosis may be suggestive of a respiratory problem or sepsis (Dickason et al 1998).

Problems that occur in neonatal cardiovascular function are usually caused either by congenital defects or by a failure of the transition from fetal to adult circulation. Persistent pulmonary hypertension of the newborn is usually seen in term or post-term infants who have a history of hypoxia or asphyxia at birth. The infants are slow to take their first breath or are difficult to ventilate. Respiratory distress and cyanosis are seen before 12 hours of age. Hypoxaemia is usually profound and may suggest cyanotic heart disease (see Ch. 45). Risk factors include meconium-stained amniotic fluid, nuchal cord, placental abruption, acute blood loss and maternal sedation.

Congenital heart disease affects just under 1% of newborn infants, many of whom will be asymptomatic in the neonatal period (Fowlie & Forsyth 1995). Infants who appear breathless but have little or no rib recession, are not grunting and have only a moderately raised respiratory rate may have heart disease. Cyanosis can be a prominent feature in some cardiac defects, but not all. Box 42.2 lists signs that may be indicative of congenital heart disease.

Cardiac failure may be rapid in onset; the earlier it presents, the more sinister is the cause. Delays in recognising and treating heart failure may lead to a rapid deterioration and cardiogenic shock. Cardiac shock may resemble early septicaemia, pneumonia or meningitis (David 1995). The first indication of an underlying cardiac lesion may be the presence of a murmur heard on routine examination. However, a soft localised systolic murmur with no evidence of any symptoms of cardiac disease is usually of no significance.

Central nervous system

Assessment of an infant's neurological status is usually carried out on a baby who is awake but not crying.

> **Box 42.2** Warning signs suggestive of congenital heart disease
>
> - Cyanosis (often the cyanosis is out of proportion to the degree of respiratory distress)
> - Persistent tachypnoea
> - Persistent tachycardia at rest
> - Poor feeding: infants may be breathless and sweaty during the feed or after feeding; they may not complete their feeds and subsequently fail to thrive
> - A sudden gain in weight leading to clinical signs of oedema; this is usually noted as the baby having puffy feet or eyelids and, in males, the scrotum being swollen
> - A very loud systolic murmur is invariably significant
> - Evidence of cardiac enlargement on X-ray, persisting beyond 48 hours of life
> - Enlargement of the liver

Abnormal postures, which include neck retraction, frog-like postures, hyperextension or hyperflexion of the limbs, jittery or abnormal involuntary movements and a high-pitched or weak cry, could be indicative of neurological impairment and a need for investigation (Rennie & Gandy 1999).

Neurological disorders

Neurological disorders found at or soon after birth may be either prenatal or perinatal in origin. They include:

- congenital abnormalities: hydrocephaly, microcephaly, encephalocele, chromosomal anomalies
- hypoxic–ischaemic cerebral injuries
- birth traumas: skull fractures, spinal cord and brachial plexus injuries, subdural and subarachnoid haemorrhage
- infections passed on to the fetus (toxoplasmosis, rubella, cytomegalovirus (CMV), syphilis).

Neurological disorders that appear in the neonatal period need to be recognised promptly in order to minimise brain damage. These include:

- infection: meningitis, herpes simplex, viral encephalitis
- hypoxia: birth asphyxia, respiratory distress, apnoeic episodes
- metabolic: acidosis, hypoglycaemia, hyponatraemia, hypernatraemia, hypothermia, hypocalcaemia, hypomagnesaemia
- drug withdrawal: narcotics, barbiturates, general anaesthesia
- intracranial haemorrhage or intraventricular haemorrhage (IVH)
- secondary bleeding: intracranial haemorrhage from thrombocytopenia or disseminated intravascular coagulation (DIC).

Cerebral hypoxia and bacterial infections are of prime importance. Prompt diagnosis, investigation and treatment are vital as delay can have a significant impact on neurological development (Rennie 1999).

Terminology

Terminology that describes abnormal movement in babies is very variable and includes 'fits', 'convulsions', 'seizures', 'twitching', 'jumpy' and 'jittery'. In contrast, a baby with poor muscle tone is described as 'floppy.' It is often very difficult to distinguish a seizure from jitteriness or irritability. The jittery baby has tremors, rapid movement of the extremities or fingers that are stopped when the limb is held or flexed. Jitteriness can be normal but is more often seen in infants who are affected by drug withdrawal or in infants with hypoglycaemia.

Seizures

Seizures in the newborn period can be extremely difficult to diagnose as they are often very subtle and easily missed (Table 42.1).

The most common causes of seizure activity are:

- asphyxia
- metabolic disturbance
- intracranial or intraventricular haemorrhage
- infection
- malformation or genetic defect.

Hypotonia (floppy infant)

The term *hypotonia* or 'floppy baby' describes the loss of body tension and tone. As a result, the infant adopts an abnormal posture that is noticeable on handling.

Table 42.1 Neonatal seizure chart (Data modified from Volpe & Hill 1994)

Type	Affected infants
Subtle Apnoea usually seen with abnormal eye movements, tonic horizontal deviation, blinking, fluttering eyelids, jerking, drooling, sucking, tonic posturing or unusual movements of limbs (rowing, peddling or swimming)	Most frequent type and most common in preterm infants
Clonic Jerking activity	
Multifocal: movements of one body part followed by encephalopathy or inborn errors of metabolism	Term infants: hypoxic–ischaemic
Focal: movement of one part	Disturbance of the entire cerebrum
Tonic Posturing similar to decerebrate posture in adults	Preterm infants with intraventricular haemorrhage
Myoclonic Single or multiple jerks of upper and lower extremities	Possible prediction of myoclonic spasms in early infancy

Preterm infants below 30 weeks' gestation have a resting position that is usually characterised as hypotonic. By 34 weeks their thighs and hips are flexed and they lie in a frog-like position, usually with their arms extended. At 36–38 weeks' gestation, the resting position of a healthy newborn baby is one of total flexion with immediate recoil. Hypotonia in a term infant is not normal and requires investigation. It is also important to determine whether the hypotonia is associated with weakness or normal power in the infant's limbs. The causes of hypotonia include:

- maternal sedation
- birth asphyxia
- prematurity
- infection
- Down syndrome
- metabolic problems (e.g. hypoglycaemia, hyponatraemia, inborn errors of metabolism)
- neurological problems (e.g. spinal cord injuries (sustained by difficult breech or forceps delivery), myasthenia gravis related to maternal disease, myotonic dystrophy)
- endocrine (e.g. hypothyroidism)
- neuromuscular disorders.

Renal and genitourinary system

Urinary infections in the newborn period are quite common, especially in males. The baby typically presents with lethargy, poor feeding, increasing jaundice and vomiting. Urine that only dribbles out, rather than being passed forcefully, may be an indication of a problem with posterior urethral valves. Urine that is cloudy in appearance or smelly may be an indication of a urinary tract infection.

The genitourinary tract has the highest percentage of anomalies, congenital or genetic, of all the organ systems. Prenatal diagnosis is possible with ultrasound and aids the early assessment and intervention, which is essential if kidney damage is to be prevented. Renal problems may present as a failure to pass urine. The normal infant usually passes urine 4–10 hours after birth (Dickason et al 1998). Normal urine output for a term baby in the first day of life should be 2–4 ml/ kg/h. A urine output of less than 1 ml/kg/h (oliguria) should be investigated (Beresford & Boxwell 2001). Urinalysis using reagent strips will give information that may be helpful in diagnosis (Table 42.2).

Common causes of reduced urine output include:

- inadequate fluid intake
- increased fluid loss due to hyperthermia, use of radiant heaters and phototherapy units
- birth asphyxia
- congenital abnormalities
- infection.

Care should be taken, of course, that urine output does not go unnoticed by the midwife when the infant is on the labour ward or elsewhere.

Table 42.2 Information obtainable from urinalysis with reagent strips

Test	Significance
Urine pH	Failure to acidify the urine may indicate a dysfunction of the renal tubular system, which plays a primary role in the regulation of bicarbonate concentration
Specific gravity	Indicates urine concentration
Blood	Is suggestive of trauma or inflammation of the genitourinary tract
Protein	May suggest renal disease

Gastrointestinal tract

Some congenital abnormalities of the gastrointestinal tract can now be diagnosed antenatally by ultrasound. This knowledge allows for time to prepare for an affected infant, which is vital when dealing with exposed organs as in the disorder of gastroschisis or omphalocele. Parents can also have a clear understanding of the condition and are able to prepare themselves for the events that will follow after the birth. Other defects, however, may not be suspected until the infant becomes unwell.

Structural deformities of the oesophagus or intestine can be life threatening in the newborn period. Oesophageal atresia can be diagnosed antenatally because the fetus is unable to swallow the amniotic fluid, giving rise to polyhydramnios in the mother. However, if the condition is not identified antenatally, the infant usually presents with copious saliva, which causes gagging, choking, pallor or cyanosis. If such babies are inadvertently fed milk this may cause a severe respiratory arrest due to milk aspiration.

Intestinal obstructions may be caused by atresias, malformations or structural damage anywhere below the stomach. In the newborn period, gastrointestinal disorders often present with vomiting, abdominal distension, a failure to pass stools, or diarrhoea with or without blood in the stools. However, vomiting in the postnatal period can be caused by factors other than gastrointestinal obstructions. The midwife should distinguish between posseting, which occurs with winding and overhandling after feeding, and vomiting due to overfeeding, infection or intestinal abnormalities.

Early vomiting may be caused by the infant swallowing meconium or maternal blood at delivery. This can cause a gastritis, which will eventually settle. Some infants may require a gastric lavage if the symptoms are severe.

All vomit should be checked for the presence of bile or blood. Observe the infant for other signs such as abdominal distension, watery or bloodstained stools and temperature instability.

The normal term baby usually passes about eight stools a day. Breastfed babies' stools are looser and more frequent than those of bottle-fed infants and the colour varies more and sometimes appears greenish. The infant who has an infection can often display signs of gastrointestinal problems, usually poor feeding, vomiting or diarrhoea, or both. Diarrhoea caused by gastroenteritis is usually very watery and may sometimes resemble urine. The cause is either bacterial or viral. Infants with this condition must be isolated and scrupulous hand washing adhered to (Isaacs & Moxon 2000). Loose stools can also be a feature of infants being treated for hyperbilirubinaemia with phototherapy.

Some of the more commonly seen gastrointestinal problems include: duodenal atresia, malrotation of the gut, volvulus, meconium ileus, necrotising enterocolitis, imperforate anus, rectal fistulas and Hirschsprung's disease.

Duodenal atresia

Duodenal atresia usually presents with bile-stained vomiting within 24 hours of birth. Abdominal distension is not usually present, but often visible peristalsis is seen over the stomach. Insertion of a nasogastric tube may reveal a large amount of bile in the stomach and there is usually a history of polyhydramnios and a delay in passing meconium. Antenatal diagnosis is possible. The most commonly associated anomaly is Down syndrome, which occurs in 30% of cases (Davis & Young 1999).

Malrotation of the gut

Malrotation may present as a mechanical bowel obstruction caused by abnormal attachments (Ladd's bands). The infant usually has no problems in the first few days of life, but then presents with bilious vomiting and abdominal distension.

Volvulus

Volvulus can occur in infants who have an incomplete rotation of the gut. Diagnosis can be delayed because the obstruction is intermittent, twisting enough to cause obstruction, then untwisting causing relief. As a result of venous impairment and mucosal injury, there may be blood passed per rectum. Bilious vomiting also occurs. These babies are commonly gravely ill.

Meconium ileus

The baby with meconium ileus often has cystic fibrosis. Clinical signs include marked abdominal distension. Meconium is not passed, but occasionally small pellet-type stools, pale in colour, are mistakenly identified as bowel action. Vomiting gradually increases, mainly of gastric secretions and feed, but later becomes bilious.

Necrotising enterocolitis (NEC)

NEC is an acquired disease of the small and large intestine caused by ischaemia of the intestinal mucosa. It occurs more often in preterm babies, but may also occur in term babies who have been asphyxiated at delivery or babies with polycythaemia and hypothermia (commonly found in SGA babies). NEC may present with vomiting or, if gastric emptying is being monitored, the aspirate is large and bile stained. The abdomen becomes distended (see Plate 24), stools are loose and may have blood in them. In the early stages of NEC, the baby can display non-specific signs of temperature instability, unstable glucose levels, lethargy and poor peripheral circulation. As the illness progresses, the baby becomes apnoeic and bradycardic and may need ventilating. (See also Chs 43 and 46.)

Imperforate anus

All babies should be checked at birth for this.

Rectal fistulas

The midwife should look for the presence of meconium in the urine or, in female babies, meconium being passed from the vagina.

Hirschsprung's disease

Hirschsprung's disease should be suspected in term babies with delayed passage of meconium, certainly after the first 24 hours of life. It is caused by an absence of ganglion cells in the distal rectum. The area of aganglionosis varies and may include the lower rectum, colon and small intestine. An incomplete obstruction occurs above the affected segment. Abdominal distension and vomiting are clinical signs, with the vomit becoming bile stained if meconium is not passed.

Metabolic disorders

Metabolic disorders, such as galactosaemia and phenylketonuria, present in the newborn period with vomiting, weight loss, jaundice and lethargy (see Ch. 47).

Meeting the needs of the ill baby and the family

The baby

Babies who are clearly unwell, distressed or less than 1800 g at birth require admission to a neonatal unit (NNU). Early separation of mother and baby is very

Table 42.3 Commonly used drugs to treat neonatal sepsis		
Drug	**Some possible neonatal infections**	**Organism**
Acyclovir	Rous sarcoma virus, chicken pox	Virus
Ceftriaxone	Meningitis	Gram – ve cocci
Ceftazidime	Meningitis	Gram – ve cocci
Clarithromycin	Chlamydia	Gram + ve and Gram – ve cocci
Co-amoxclav	Otis media, lower respiratory infections	Gram – ve and Gram + ve cocci
Flucloxacillin	Skin infections, *Staphylococcus aureus*	Gram – ve cocci
Gentamicin	*Escherichia coli, Klebsiella*	Gram – ve cocci
Metronidazole	Necrotising enterocolitis	Anaerobes
Penicillin G and V	Group B *Streptococcus*	Gram + ve cocci
Vancomycin	*Staphylococcus epidermidis, S. aureus*	Gram + ve cocci

damaging and should be avoided unless absolutely necessary. Asymptomatic babies above 1800 g, irrespective of gestation, should be able to stay with their mother either on a ward, or for infants with minor problems only, in a transitional care unit. Managing these babies can be challenging for midwives as some of them may require tube feeding, monitoring of their blood glucose levels and antibiotic therapy. Drug administration is playing an ever-increasing role in the management of the ill baby. Table 42.3 lists some antibiotic drugs commonly used to treat suspected neonatal sepsis.

Drug administration

Antibiotics are the most common drugs used in NNUs. Premature babies have very little immunity to infections that can be acquired congenitally. Suspected infections are always treated with antibiotics, immediately after blood cultures have been taken. Once the result of the blood cultures are known, antibiotics may be continued or stopped.

Drugs can be given to neonates orally, intramuscularly, intravenously, topically or rectally. The most efficient and effective route to administer drugs to a sick baby is by the intravenous route; this is because the absorption of drugs via the stomach is dependent on factors in the baby, relating to gastric emptying time and gastric and duodenal pH. Intramuscular administration is often a painful route and absorption is dependent on blood flow to the muscle, which can be compromised in a baby who is poorly perfused.

Whichever route is used, all drugs must be administered safely in accordance with unit/ward/hospital policy and meet the Midwives' rules and code of practice (UKCC 1998). Many drugs will need to be diluted prior to administration to allow for accurate measurement of the required dose (Northern Network 1998). Unfortunately, mistakes in drug administration are not uncommon, and having two nurses/midwives calculate and check the dose will decrease the risk of an error occurring.

Before administering any drugs to a baby the midwife should always check that it is:

- the right drug
- the right baby
- the right route
- the right dose
- the right time.

Drug calculations

To avoid misinterpretation of doses prescribed, only approved abbreviations should be used:

- milligram = mg
- millilitre = ml (or mL)
- microgram(s) should always be written out in full.

Before calculating the volume required to give the correct dose, the midwife should write down the strength of the drug in the ampoule or vial; for example, ampoules of gentamicin (paediatric) contain 20 mg of gentamicin diluted in 2 ml of water. If the dose prescribed is 8 mg the calculation is as follows:

(Dose you require) *times* (the volume of the gentamicin) *divided by* (the amount of gentamicin in the vial) which in this case is: (8 mg) × (2 ml)/ 20 mg = 0.8 ml therefore, *0.8 ml is to be administered to the infant.*

Once you have the answer, ask yourself *Does it make sense?*

Developmentally focused, family-centred care

For parents, the birth of a baby is a mixture of joy, emotional exhilaration and relief. Most newborn babies are normal and healthy and few parents ever expect or consider the possibility of having a baby that is less than perfect (Cameron 1996). Neither will they have considered the implications of separation if their baby has to be admitted to the NNU. So when a baby requires medical assistance, because of prematurity, illness or congenital malformations, the effect on the parents can be significant and force the family into a crisis that can be as devastating as a bereavement. The parents' ability to resolve the crisis will depend on how realistically they perceive their baby's problems.

The period immediately after the birth is a very sensitive time for mother and baby where the attachment process, which began during the prenatal period, is built upon and strengthened. Separation of mother and baby, even if it is for a short while, may increase the risk of the parents developing parental difficulties, with effects on their pattern of behaviour and general responses towards their baby (Coffman 1992).

The environment of the NNU, however thoughtful the layout and design, is an alarming place to enter.

With the emphasis on modern technology, babies are wired up to machines that bleep and alarm continuously (see Plates 25 and 26). Entering the NNU following the admission of their baby is a first time experience for many parents; therefore it is of utmost importance that midwives, nurses and medical staff learn skills that enable them to reduce the level of anxiety that parents feel and emphasise the importance of them becoming partners in care.

NNUs should be bright, friendly and welcoming. Walls should be decorated with appropriate, coloured pictures and parents should be encouraged to bring in brightly coloured toys and mobiles for their babies; one or two of these can be placed in the incubator or cot. In most NNUs, a sitting room, often with kitchen facilities, is provided for parents and children. This is a place of retreat, away from the stresses and strains of busy nurseries. The provision of bedrooms or family rooms, or both, where parents can stay if their baby is critically ill, or a place where they can be alone with their baby if sadly he has died, is of crucial importance (see Ch. 37).

If it is known in advance that a baby may require admission to the NNU, parents should be given the opportunity to visit and meet some of the staff. They can be shown the room or area where their baby will be admitted, and a brief explanation of the various items of monitoring equipment may help to alleviate some of their fears about what will happen to their baby after it has been born. Following the delivery and if it is at all possible, the parents should be allowed to hold or touch their baby, even if it is for just a few moments, before he is taken to the NNU.

On admission to the NNU, a photograph should be taken. This photograph must be given to the parents as soon as possible, as this will go some way towards reassuring them that their baby is safe and alive (Slade 1988). Parents should be encouraged to visit their baby in the NNU as soon they are able. When discussing the baby with the parents, the midwife should try always to use the name that they have given their child as this establishes the baby's identity and makes the conversation more personalised.

The preterm infant may require a lengthy stay in the NNU, in which case parenting roles may be difficult to establish owing to the physical condition of the baby who may be on a ventilator, being fed intravenously, or be under phototherapy lights. All of these act as a barrier between the baby and the parents and undermine their confidence. Even parents who know their baby is to be admitted to the NNU will experience shock and grief at being separated. They may look for areas of baby care with which they are familiar, and will often adopt a passive role and concentrate on family routines in order to cope (Redshaw & Harris 1993). It is during this time of crisis, when parents are at their most vulnerable, that they will look to staff to provide information and support. Communication at this time must be on a basic level and backed up with information leaflets in a language they can understand (Taylor 1996).

The most important visual aid for any baby is the human face, especially the talking face, which stimulates both visual and auditory pathways. Parents and siblings should be encouraged to communicate with their baby even if it has to be through the porthole window of the incubator (Gardner & Lubchenco 1998).

Involving the parents as partners in care should be encouraged as soon as the baby's condition and tolerance to handling permits. This early involvement will strengthen their understanding of the baby belonging to them and increase their confidence in their ability to provide care. A supportive environment, in which the parents gain confidence in assuming the role of caregivers, is of fundamental importance to the general well-being of the baby. In order to reinforce the parents' involvement in the care of their baby, it is important to discuss whether the baby is to be breast or bottle fed. Midwives and neonatal nurses should encourage mothers to breast feed their babies, or to express their breastmilk, as it provides a greater protection against infection. breastfeeding or expressing milk may help the mother feel closer to her baby and may also make her feel that she is contributing to her baby's care in a way that nobody else can.

Minimal handling

Care should be individualised for each baby and not be performed routinely. At the start of each work shift, the midwife should determine what the needs of the baby are and carry out the required care all at one time, instead of repeatedly disturbing the baby. Questions should be asked about performing unnecessary procedures such as repeated heel stabs. Painful, invasive procedures that are not vital to the individual baby's needs are stress-producing events and should be eliminated. Studies by Sparshott (1991) and Becker et al (1993) have shown that babies' responses to their environment can be directly linked to their experiences. Often the best care for the sick baby is rest and recuperation (Carter 1994). Increasingly, NNUs are introducing a system of individualised developmental care for preterm babies aimed at reducing their stress levels. This innovative care programme is based on the studies by Als et al (1994). A lot of noises that occur in the NNU are unnecessary and could be eliminated if more thought were given (see Ch. 41). Day and night cycles should be recognised, lights should be dimmed at nighttime and noise further reduced, remembering though that it is essential that ill babies are observed; when monitor alarms are cancelled they need to be reset.

Sibling relationships

Encouraging brothers and sisters to visit their new baby is important. Parents are often anxious about the effect an ill baby may have on the family. However, this may cause anxiety in the siblings and they may feel worried, rejected and left out, causing them to demonstrate behavioural problems.

Discharge home

Effective discharge planning should commence as soon as the baby is admitted to the NNU. Encouraging parents to participate in the care of their baby from the beginning enables them eventually to be the sole caregivers and resume total charge.

Every parent should learn how to feed, bathe, dress and generally care for their baby. If the baby has special needs like tube feeding or stoma care, training needs may span several weeks and must be backed up with written information. The parents must feel comfortable about caring for their baby before going home.

REFERENCES

Als H, Lawhon G, Duffy F H 1994 Individualised developmental care for the very low birth weight preterm infant. Journal of the American Medical Association 272(11):853–858

Bada H S 1992 Asymptomatic syndrome of polycythaemia hypoviscosity, effects of a partial plasma exchange transfusion. Journal of Pediatrics 120:579

Becker P T, Grunwald P C, Moorman J 1993 Effects of developmental care on behavioural organisation in very low birth weight infants. Nursing Research 42(4):214–220

Beresford D, Boxwell G 2001 In: Boxwell G (ed) Neonatal intensive care nursing. Routledge, London, ch 10, p 211–233

Cameron J 1996 Parents as partners in care. British Journal of Midwifery 4(4):218–219

Carter B 1994 Child and infant pain: principles of nursing care and management. Chapman & Hall, London

Coffman S 1992 Parent and infant attachment: review of nursing research 1981–1990. Paediatric Nurse 18(4):421–425

David T J 1995 Symptoms of disease in childhood. Blackwell Science, Oxford, ch 4, p 92–94

Davis C F, Young D G 1999 Congenital defects and surgical problems. In: Rennie J, Roberton N C R (ed) Textbook of neonatology, 3rd edn. Churchill Livingstone, Edinburgh, p 765–793

Dickason E J, Kaplan J A, Silverman L 1998 Maternal infant nursing care, 5th edn. C V Mosby, St Louis

Fanaroff A A, Martin J M 1997 Neonatal perinatal medicine. C V Mosby, St Louis

Fowlie P, Forsyth J S 1995 Examination of the newborn infant. Modern Midwife 4(12):15–17

Gardner S L, Lubchenco L O 1998 The neonate and the environment: impact on development. In: Merenstein G V, Gardner S L (eds) Handbook of neonatal intensive care, 4th edn. CV Mosby, St Louis, p 197–242

Isaacs D, Moxon R 2000 Handbook of neonatal infections; a practical guide. W B Saunders, London, ch 19, p 423–434

Kozier B, Erb G, Blais K, Wilkinson J 1998 Fundamentals of nursing, 5th edn. Addison Wesley, New York

Logan S 1990 Viral infections in pregnancy. In: Chamberlain G L (ed) Modern ante-natal care of the fetus. Blackwell Scientific, Oxford, p 201–221

Merenstein G V, Gardner S L 1998 Handbook of neonatal intensive care, 4th edn. CV Mosby, St Louis

Northern Network 1998 The neonatal formulary. BMJ Books, London

Redshaw M, Harris A 1995 Maternal perceptions of neonatal care. Acta Paedratrica 84:593–598

Rennie J 1999 Seizures in the newborn part 2. In: Rennie J, Roberton N C R (eds) Textbook of neonatology, 3rd edn. Churchill Livingstone, Edinburgh, p 100–107

Rennie J, Gandy G 1999 Examination of the newborn. In: Rennie J, Roberton NCR (eds) Textbook of neonatology, 3rd edn. Churchill Livingstone, Edinburgh, p 269–288

Roberton N C R 2001 A manual of neonatal intensive care. Edward Arnold, London

Roncoli M, Medoff-Cooper B 1992 Thermoregulation in low birth weight infants NAACOG. Clinical Issues 3(1):25–33

Rutter N 1999 Thermo-regulation. In: Rennie J, Roberton N C R (eds) Textbook of neonatology, 3rd edn. Churchill Livingstone, Edinburgh, p 289–301

Slade P 1988 A psychologist's view of a special care baby unit. Maternal and Child Health 13(8):208–212

Smith S R, Jaffe D M, Skinner M 1997 A case report of metallic mercury injury. Paediatric Emergency Care 13(2):114–116

Sparshott M 1991 This is your baby. Southern Western Regional Health Authority, Plymouth

Taylor B 1996 Parents as partners in care. Paediatric Nursing 8(4):4–7

UKCC (United Kingdom Central Council for Nursing, Midwifery and Health Visiting) 1998 Standards for the administration of medicines. UKCC, London

Volpe J J, Hill A 1994 Neurologic disorders. In: Avery G, Fletcher M A, MacDonald M G (eds) Neonatology, pathophysiology and management of the newborn, 4th edn. J B Lippincott, Philadelphia, p 1119

FURTHER READING

Beachy P, Deacon J 1999 Core curriculum for neonatal intensive care nurses. W B Saunders, Philadelphia

This book outlines the broad scope of neonatal intensive care. Its easy reference format covers all aspects of obstetrical care, common disorders of the sick infant, family care and current issues in neonatal care.

Crawford D, Morris M 1994 Neonatal nursing. Chapman & Hall, London

Neonatal nursing is written in a style that is easily understood by practising midwives, neonatal nurses and students. It covers all aspects of the nursing and medical management of the sick infant.

Yeo H (ed) 1998 Nursing the neonate. Blackwell Science, Oxford

This comprehensive book covers all aspects of neonatal nursing and its well-written text is aimed at students as well as practising midwives. It addresses issues of discharge planning, stress, transculture nursing and ethics.

43 Respiratory Problems

Alison Gibbs

Respiratory compromise in the newborn is a common presentation for a variety of diseases, not all of which may be respiratory in origin. To ascertain the exact nature of any respiratory disease some further investigation will be needed. This chapter offers a review of the signs and symptoms of respiratory compromise and an examination of some of the common causes of respiratory distress.

The second part of the chapter describes the typical nursing care for a baby that needs intensive care support for a respiratory disease. This overview includes some of the pertinent debates presently being explored in neonatal care.

The chapter aims to:

- list the signs of respiratory distress

- describe some of the common neonatal respiratory conditions

- identify the pertinent anatomical features that contribute to neonatal respiratory distress

- discuss neonatal respiratory and cardiovascular support

- define the effects of the environment upon the neonate

- explain the options for maintaining nutrition and hydration

- propose measures to support the parents with a baby in the neonatal unit.

Pathophysiology

Anatomical influences

Neonates are susceptible to respiratory compromise, for a number of reasons. First, this may be a result of their stage of lung development and contributing lack of maturation in the other body systems. The gestation of the baby at birth has implications for the susceptibility to disease processes like hyaline membrane disease (HMD), where surfactant production is inhibited.

The stages of lung development are, in summary:

Embryonic phase. This lasts until the 5th week of gestation. In this phase the proximal airways develop.

Pseudoglandular phase. This lasts from the 5th to the 16th week of gestation. During this phase there is development of the lower conducting airways, bronchi and large bronchioles.

Canalicular phase. This lasts from the 17th to the 24th week of gestation. It is the period for the development of the gas exchanging bronchioles.

Terminal sac phase. This takes place between the 24th week and the 36th week of gestation. Surfactant production begins with increasing efficiency as the alveolar ducts develop.

Alveolar phase. This is ongoing from the 37th week of gestation until the 8th year of life. During this phase alveoli increase in number and there is maturation of the surfactant production.

Secondly, neonates experience an increased work of breathing owing to the high compliance of the neonatal lung, which results from the cartilaginous nature of the rib structure. This flexibility allows for some collapse of the airways with each breath, which would not occur with a rigid rib structure. Subsequently, with each breath, the baby needs to generate larger pressures within the lung to prevent respiratory compromise through airway collapse.

Thirdly, neonates also have a different diaphragmatic muscle structure to adults. The neonatal diaphragm is more susceptible to fatigue owing to the composition and the location of the muscle within the neonatal chest.

Fourthly, the size of neonatal airways is smaller, which generates higher resistance to air flow and a smaller area through which perfusion can occur.

A final contributing factor is the tendency for pulmonary blood flow to bypass areas of hypoxia, across the alveolar bed, consequently reducing the alveoli perfusion.

Signs of respiratory compromise

Grunting

Grunting is an audible noise heard on expiration. The sound appears when there is partial closure of the glottis as the breath is expired. The baby is attempting to preserve some internal lung pressure and prevent the airways from collapsing at the end of the breath.

Retractions

Chest distortions occur due to an increase in the need to create higher inspiratory pressures in a compliant chest. They appear as intercostal, subcostal or sternal recession across the thorax.

Asynchrony

Here the breathing has a 'see-saw' pattern as the abdominal movements and the diaphragm work out of unison. This is a result of increased muscle fatigue and the compliant chest wall.

Tachypnoea

This is a compensatory rise in the respiratory rate initiated from the respiratory centre. It is described as a rate above 60, the aim of which is to remove the hypoxia and hypercarbia.

Nasal flaring

This is an attempt to minimise the effect of the airways resistance by maximising the diameter of the upper airways. The nares are seen to flare open with each breath.

Apnoea

Apnoea occurs as the conclusion of increasing respiratory fatigue in the term baby. The preterm baby may experience apnoea of prematurity due to the immature respiratory centre, as well as apnoea from respiratory fatigue.

Common respiratory problems

Pneumothorax

Pneumothoraces are known to occur spontaneously in 1% of the newborn population either during or after delivery; however, only a tenth of this 1% will be symptomatic (Steele et al 1971). A pneumothorax at birth is caused by the large pressures generated by the baby's first breaths. These may be in the range of up to 40–80 cm of water. This leads to alveoli distension and rupture, which allows air to leak to a number of sites of which the potential space between the lung pleura is one.

Babies receiving assisted ventilation also have an increased susceptibility to a pneumothorax. This may be due to maldistribution of the ventilated gas in the lungs, high ventilation settings or baby–ventilator breathing interactions.

Term babies may present with symptoms of respiratory distress on the postnatal ward. Although it is difficult to diagnose a pneumothorax in the absence of a chest X-ray, there may be reduced breath sounds on the affected side, displaced heart sounds and a distorted chest/diaphragm movement with respiration and distension of the chest on the affected side. These signs become harder to detect in the baby with bilateral pneumothoraces, as seen in 15–20% of cases (Greenough 1996).

A baby with a suspected pneumothorax needs a paediatric consultation with the view to an emergency procedure. The procedure will be either a needle aspiration or the placement of a chest drain. This will drain the air leak and prevent a further accumulation of the air. The placement of a chest drain is a painful procedure and the baby will need some sedation along with nursing on the neonatal unit.

Transient tachypnoea of the newborn

The recorded incidence of transient tachypnoea of the newborn (TTN) varies widely; this is partly a result of the variety of recording methods, differences in radiological interpretation and clear diagnostic features. It is frequently seen as a diagnosis of exclusion of other possible respiratory causes. Nevertheless the chest X-ray may show a streaky appearance with fluid apparent in the horizontal fissure, which confirms the diagnosis and also accounts for the colloquialism of 'wet lung'.

These infants present with respiratory distress normally restricted to tachypnoea alone, with rates up to 120 breaths per minute. Occasionally supplemental oxygen is required, but during the 12 to 24 hours following birth the condition normally resolves. The most common predisposing factor for TTN is a caesarean section because the thorax has not been squeezed whilst the baby descends along the birth canal. This results in lower thoracic pressures after delivery. Although these babies require initial care on a neonatal unit, their stay is usually of a short duration with the provision of oxygen and observation.

Infection/pneumonia

A number of infectious disease processes present with symptoms of respiratory distress in the newborn. The mortality from neonatal infection is reported to be 20% (Gerdes 1991); however, as strides continue to be made in neonatalogy the aim of any management is to reduce this figure. All babies presenting with respiratory distress need to be treated for infection until there is proof to the contrary.

Pneumonia in the neonate is difficult to diagnose as secretions are difficult to obtain and the radiological appearances can be hard to distinguish. However, pneumonia presenting before 48 hours of age has normally been acquired either at or before birth whereas presentation after 48 hours indicates infection resulting from hospitalisation. All infants with infection require antibiotics but their length of stay on a neonatal unit will vary depending upon the nature of the infection, their symptoms and their antibiotic course.

Meconium aspiration syndrome

Greenough & Roberton (1999) report the incidence for meconium aspiration syndrome in one UK hospital as 0.2 per 1000 live births; however, this incidence is low and other countries such as the USA have higher rates of the disease (Greenough & Roberton 1999). The initial difficulty of fetal asphyxia causes the passage of meconium into the liquor. This meconium is unproblematic unless the baby gasps or breathes in amniotic fluid, in which case the meconium is inhaled simultaneously. Consequently it is the babies showing symptoms of fetal hypoxia, a deranged heart rate or a lowered cord gas pH who present most frequently. A baby can develop meconium aspiration syndrome if stimulated to breath or gasp, either before or after birth, if there is meconium in the airway that could be inhaled. The passage of meconium into the liquor is rarely seen prior to 34 weeks and Matthews suggests this is due to the immaturity of the preterm gastrointestinal tract (Matthews & Warshaw 1979). Nevertheless, although a large number of births have meconium-stained liquor, only a few will cause the severe meconium aspiration syndrome, with its associated mortality, that is seen in the NNU. In the majority there is a milder disease process that requires initial supportive treatment but quickly resolves over 24 to 48 hours.

The initial respiratory distress may be mild, moderate or severe with a gradual deterioration over the first 12 to 24 hours in the moderate or severe cases. The baby may present with cyanosis, increased work of breathing and a barrel-shaped chest. This chest appearance occurs as a result of gas being trapped, leading to hyperexpansion of the lung fields. The meconium becomes trapped in the airways and causes a ball-valve effect: although air can enter the lung during inhalation, the meconium then blocks the airway during expiration so that air accumulates behind the blockage. This accumulation can then lead to the rupture of the alveoli and cause the baby to develop a pneumothorax. Where the meconium has contact with the lung tissue a pneumonitis occurs and a fertile site for infection is created. The surfactant is also broken down in the presence of meconium.

These factors in a previously hypoxic infant combine to produce a severe disease process. The external respiration across the alveoli is inhibited, areas of hypoxic lung are bypassed as blood flow shunts away from them and the pattern of fetal circulation across the arterial duct is difficult to break owing to high pulmonary vascular resistance. These infants will need full intensive care and ventilation to prevent further deterioration. Recent modalities such as ECMO (extracorporeal membrane oxygenation) have been shown to increase survival for these infants by 50% (UK Collaborative ECMO Trial Group 1996) whilst the introduction of nitric oxide therapy will further assist these severely compromised infants. A number of the more severely affected infants will be symptomatic for some months with ongoing residual symptoms during early childhood.

Respiratory distress syndrome

The term respiratory distress syndrome (RDS) is used interchangeably with the diagnosis of HMD in the neonatal culture. The diagnosis of HMD is derived from the presence of hyaline membranes in the airways resulting from the damaged epithelium. RDS refers to the clinical disease process. The disease occurs as a result of the insufficient production of surfactant and is seen most frequently after a premature birth; however, other disorders such as maternal diabetes or meconium aspiration syndrome can also inhibit surfactant production. The majority of babies born before 30 completed weeks of gestation will experience RDS; Greenough et al (1996) suggest that 1.12% of all newborn babies may experience severe RDS.

Surfactant is produced by the type II epithelial cells (Tortora & Grabowski 2000) to reduce the surface tension within the alveoli, preventing their collapse at the end of exhalation. Collapsed alveoli require much greater pressure and exertion to reinflate than do partially collapsed alveoli. The introduction of surfactant therapy into neonatal care has significantly decreased the mortality and morbidity previously seen in RDS. Surfactant itself consists of several different types of proteins and phospholipids, which play a further role in the prevention of infection and in the production of more surfactant.

Preterm babies are born with a small amount of surfactant but, as the time from birth increases, the demands outstrip the supply. This gives a clinical picture of an infant with progressive respiratory distress, in which it may be 4 hours before there is a significant presentation. The X-ray has a ground-glass appearance across the lung fields, whilst severe disease is represented by a 'white-out'. This appears like a snowstorm within the lungs, the density of the 'blizzard' corresponding to the severity of the disease (Fig. 43.1). The infant has an increasing respiratory distress and work in breathing; it may take 48 to 72 hours to reach the peak of the disease without the administration of surfactant. Resolution of the associated inflammation and the hyaline membrane formation may take up to 7 days in the unventilated baby.

Treatment includes oxygen therapy, administration of surfactant directly into the lungs and, for the more significant disease, whether actual or anticipated by virtue of the gestation, ventilatory support. The length of stay on the NNU is dependent upon the severity of the disease and the gestational age of the baby.

It could be anticipated that a baby will remain in the NNU for the equivalent number to the number of weeks he is born preterm. This allows the midwife to give the parents a ballpark figure to enable them to adjust accordingly, e.g.: 'your baby is 16 weeks early so you can anticipate a stay on the NNU of 16 weeks'.

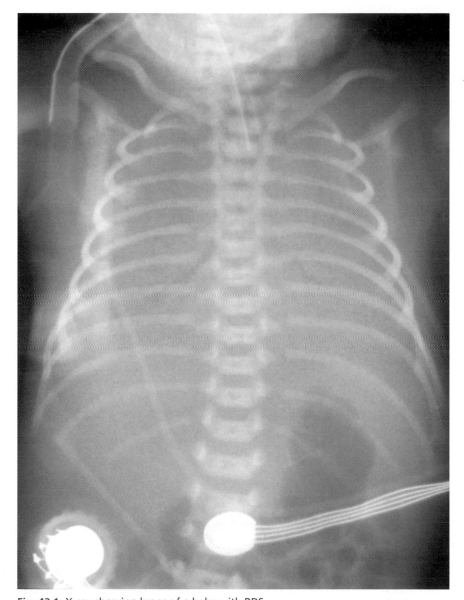

Fig. 43.1 X-ray showing lungs of a baby with RDS.

Cardiac disease

Cardiac disease, although not a respiratory disease, presents with respiratory symptoms and, as it accounts for 30% of congenital defects (Jordan & Scott 1989), will be considered here. Cardiac defects can be divided into left-sided and right-sided defects to aid identification (see also Ch. 45).

Right-sided lesions

The most frequently seen lesions are transposition of the great arteries, tetralogy of Fallot and pulmonary atresia or stenosis (p. 850). These babies typically present as a 'blue' baby. On examination there is little to note other than the presence of cyanosis. Their respiratory distress, if present, is mild and consists of tachypnoea alone. These babies will remain cyanotic in the presence of 100% oxygen.

Left-sided lesions

These frequently present with neonatal heart failure. Initially the baby may appear irritable, lethargic, sweaty and not interested in feeding. The presence of 'effortless' tachypnoea may be seen. This tachypnoea is characterised by the lack of any other sign of respiratory compromise; for example, no grunting is heard and there is no head bobbing or minimal recession. As the heart failure progresses the infant shows signs of cardiogenic shock and will go on to require full resuscitative measures if left unsupported. The most frequently seen left-sided lesions are hypoplastic left heart syndrome and coarctation of the aorta (see p. 851).

When a cardiac condition is suspected the majority of infants will require confirmation of the diagnosis from a cardiologist. A postnatal transfer to a cardiac centre may be necessary for treatment. Parents need clear explanations to enable them to feel supported during this time of anxiety. Prior to departure any resuscitation and stabilisation will be managed depending on the advice received from the cardiac centre and the nature of the defect.

Common practice involves the administration of an infusion of prostaglandin to maintain the patency of the arterial duct. This may then necessitate the elective intubation and ventilation of a baby who has previously appeared to be breathing adequately without assistance. This assisted mechanical ventilation is provided without oxygen, even if the saturation monitor records saturations in the eighties or seventies, as additional oxygen can stimulate the arterial duct to close. The patency of the arterial duct is needed to keep the blood flowing through the heart and around the peripheral circulation.

Cardiac surgery is complex and some defects require a number of procedures to optimise the baby's future. It is not possible to treat all the different cardiac defects and for a few there is a very poor prognosis. However, advances are continuously being made in the management of some of the defects that previously have been fatal – hypoplastic left heart syndrome, for example.

What to anticipate in the NNU

The parents will be confronted with a technological environment with an array of buzzers, bleeps, flashing lights and alarms. It is easy to lose sight of the baby behind the technology, as Plate 25 demonstrates. However, all these machines and alarms will have a role to play in the care of the baby. The second part of the chapter explores the environment of the NNU and examines some of the technological and therapeutic support available in the neonatal intensive care unit (NICU).

Respiratory care

Babies showing the signs of respiratory compromise require a further assessment by a paediatrician. This may necessitate an admission to the NNU for continuous supervision and observation of their respiratory status. They require the skills of a practitioner who is able to maintain their airway, recognise critical changes in status and implement the care that is required. To assist in these observations the use of saturation monitors, transcutaneous monitors and arterial catheter readings are recorded. When satisfactory oxygenation is not being achieved the baby may need additional oxygen. This can be delivered via a nasal cannula into the incubator or into a headbox creating an oxygen-enriched microenvironment.

Some babies will need ventilation to assist the maintenance of an adequate airway or to maximise their external respiration. Present options for ventilation are all pressure controlled, but there is a variety of ventilation styles to choose from. These include high frequency oscillation (HFOV), conventional ventilation (CMV) and continuous positive airway pressure (CPAP). Figure 43.2 shows a neonatal ventilator that offers all three of these.

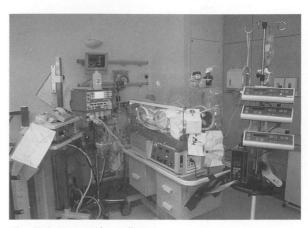

Fig. 43.2 Neonatal ventilator.

HFOV. This is commonly used for extreme prematurity, as a rescue therapy or in combination with nitric oxide. When babies are being oscillated they are seen to 'vibrate', whilst some continue to breathe in addition to the ventilation. Pressure is used to reach optimal lung expansion and 'bounce' or oscillations are added to help the distribution of the gases.

CMV. Conventional ventilation techniques are increasingly being delivered in ways similar to the natural breathing patterns. During the critical phase of the illness the ventilator may deliver preset rates and pressures only. However, as the baby stabilises and improves, ventilators are now able to mimic the babies' individual rates, pressures or lung volumes thereby minimising the associated lung trauma.

CPAP. Nasal continuous positive airway pressure (NCPAP) is used either as a therapy for moderate disease or as weaning tool. Pressure is delivered to the nares or the oropharynx which, when transmitted through the bronchial tree, distends the alveoli at the end of respiration preventing their collapse. The aim is to avoid the trauma of an endotracheal tube and the bronchiolar damage from ventilation. Figure 43.3 shows a 'CPAP driver'.

Recent research (e.g. Johnson et al 2002) suggests that all three types of ventilation described are appropriate for neonatal care.

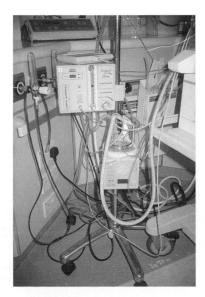

Fig. 43.3 Nasal CPAP driver.

Some ventilation techniques are available at specialised centres only. This includes continuous negative end expiratory pressure (CNEEP) and ECMO. Liquid ventilation is not routinely available in Britain at the time of writing.

ECMO. This involves the oxygenation of the blood supply outside the body. Large cannulae are inserted to remove and reintroduce the blood to the baby. The procedure uses technology similar to cardiac bypass support for the oxygenation of the blood. During this time the lungs are allowed to rest and heal. This type of ventilation is governed by strict criteria and babies need to be at least 34 gestational weeks and weigh more than 1.8 kg.

CNEEP. This is unsuitable for newly delivered premature babies as the tight fixation around the baby's neck may lead to an increased risk of IVH. However, in those babies for whom this risk has passed, CNEEP works using similar principles to the technology of the iron lung.

Box 43.1 is a list of key points relating to respiratory support.

Cardiovascular support

Cardiac failure in a neonate is rare, as the majority of arrests are respiratory in origin. However, neonates may require support to maintain a normal heart rate or stroke volume. Continuous observation and supervision of the cardiac parameters will be needed, which can be achieved using either an indwelling catheter or non-invasive monitoring. Maintenance of an adequate blood pressure, for example the mean equivalent to the gestational age, may need pharmaceutical support. A bradycardia (a heart rate below 80) may be a sign of various influences such as a blocked endotracheal tube or sepsis.

Occasionally the transition from a fetal to an adult circulation is compromised and the baby develops persistent pulmonary hypertension of the newborn.

> **Box 43.1** Key points – respiratory support
>
> - Respiratory support is frequently provided by conventional ventilation, HFOV or CPAP
> - Other options are available for suitable infants

The compromise may be due to a primary defect in the pulmonary vasculature or secondary to other factors that raise the pulmonary vascular resistance, such as meconium aspiration syndrome. This condition has previously been called 'persistent fetal circulation', which describes the tendency of the blood flow to mimic the circulation within the fetus. The use of nitric oxide as the vasodilator, delivered with the ventilation gases, works directly upon the pulmonary vessels with minimal effect to the systemic circulation. Nitric oxide reduces the need to refer neonates for ECMO and has impacted upon the mortality associated with persistent pulmonary hypertension (Neonatal Inhaled Nitric Oxide Study Group 1997). However, the role of nitric oxide in the preterm neonate remains unclear (Franco-Belgium Collaborative NO Trial Group 1999).

Box 43.2 is a key point relating to cardiovascular support.

Nutrition and hydration

The role of breastmilk and its associated benefits has been clearly established (see Ch. 40). These benefits are of an increased value in the preterm baby, for whom an immature gut can give rise to feeding difficulties. A preterm baby has little nutritional reserves and will need supplementation soon after birth to meet the continual demand for glucose from the brain. Although the ideal would be to establish oral breastmilk feeding, for a sick neonate this is not possible as the presence of the endotracheal tube or the absence of a suck reflex prevents oral feeding.

The majority of such babies will receive a glucose-based intravenous infusion. This allows the practitioner to give milk feeds via a nasogastric, orogastric or nasojejunal tube and increase the volumes as the baby's condition allows. Opinions vary concerning the method of administration and the frequency of these early feedings (Grant & Denne 1991, Lucas et al 1986, Newell 1998). Nevertheless sick or immature babies need a cautious introduction to milk, whether expressed breastmilk or formula feeds, as these infants are susceptible to necrotising enterocolitis (NEC; see below).

When a baby is expected to take more than 4 to 5 days before full feeding is established then total parenteral nutrition (TPN) is needed to ensure that all

> **Box 43.2** Key point – cardiovascular support
>
> - Neonates may need additional cardiovascular support through medication

nutritional requirements can be met. TPN is normally administered through a central line, either a longline or umbilical catheter. The strength and irritability of the solution necessitate its delivery into a large vein. Weak TPN solutions can be started on the 1st day of life. TPN typically contains amino acids, fats, carbohydrates, minerals, vitamins and trace elements. All help to prevent the depletion of these essential components, which is easily exhibited in the preterm baby. The strength and composition of the TPN can be built up over a few days as the baby demonstrates its ability to tolerate the solution. Although some babies may need TPN for many weeks, it can have some undesirable side-effects upon the liver, giving rise to a conjugated hyperbilirubinaemia or cholestasis. Prolonged TPN is sometimes needed in very immature babies, infants with gastroschisis and those with NEC.

Necrotising enterocolitis

NEC is a disease seen in the neonatal population only and its causes are multifactorial. Prior to birth the gut mucosa is sterile; consequently during the first few days and weeks of life colonisation with the normal bacterial flora must occur. This normal process can be altered by delaying feeding. A delay could occur when a baby is unwell and the effect of this is a lowered immune response to potential pathogens.

The administration of antibiotics can alter the dominant gut flora, as can formula milk. This can lead to a proliferation of anaerobes and bacterial invasion into the gut wall. Bacterial infection can also occur following episodes of hypoxia or other conditions such as polycythaemia that reduce the arterial blood flow through the mesenteric circulation. This causes mucosal ischaemia, which when reperfused leads to oedema, haemorrhage, ulceration and necrosis.

The baby may present with mild symptoms of the disease, a painful distended abdomen, blood in the stool and poor food tolerance. Or there may be more acute pathology; symptoms may include air within the gut wall, leading to a perforation, hypovolaemic shock or disseminated intravascular coagulation.

Treatment is initially with antibiotics and medical management. However, surgery is needed if there is a perforation or a failure to respond to the medical therapy. The long term problems for those who do recover can be short gut syndrome and gut stenosis. (See also Chs 42 and 46.)

Box 43.3 is a list of key points relating to nutrition.

A safe environment

Neonatal infection

A neonate has an increased susceptibility to infection owing to the immaturity of the neonatal defence mechanisms. These limitations decrease as gestational age lengthens; nevertheless a term baby still has not achieved the immunity of an adult. Neonates, and preterm babies especially, experience reduced immunoglobulin protection. Their responses to infection take longer as the organisms are new and not recognised by the memory cells. Consequently there is a delay in response time, as fresh responses are required to each new organism. The complement cascade, a supplementary defence mechanism of plasma proteins, remains inefficient. The phagocytic cells are restricted in their role whilst the external defences like the skin are immature. Consequently the neonate has a reduced ability to fight infection, whether contracted prior to birth or after.

The uterus is a sterile environment, which cannot be replicated on the neonatal unit. However, strict infection control measures can be exercised. These include the request that hands are washed by all caregivers, restriction of handling to a few individuals and thorough cleaning of all equipment. Nursing a baby in an incubator provides a microenvironment that is easier to manage. However, neonatal infection, whether prenatal or postnatal, continues to contribute to neonatal mortality and the use of prophylactic antibiotics is widespread throughout Britain.

Box 43.4 is a key point relating to infection.

Thermoneutral environment

A baby requires an environment that is going to need minimal metabolic activity to maintain internal temperature stability. Babies born at the extremes of viability have immature skin owing to reduced keratin in the epidermis, hence heat and water is easily lost. This, along with their immature responses to cold stress, makes neonates vulnerable to the effects of a cool environment.

The use of heated boxes has developed into the use of the sophisticated incubators and overhead heaters, as shown in Figure 43.4. These provide an environment where heat can be controlled and a humidified microclimate can be created for the most immature. Continuous attention to thermoregulation can be made with the use of temperature probes placed upon the skin.

A stress-free environment

The neonate experiences a number of stressors within the neonatal environment (Plate 26). Even when analgesia and sedation have already been administered the baby may still be showing signs of distress and agitation.

Box 43.3 Key points – nutrition

- Whilst nutrition is essential for the neonate, feeding needs to be introduced cautiously
- TPN may be given until feeding is established
- NEC remains a serious neonatal disease of the gut

Box 43.4 Key point – infection

- Neonates have immature defence mechanisms for fighting disease

---

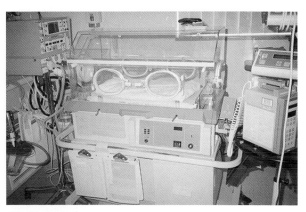

Fig. 43.4 Incubator.

The use of opiates for pain relief and sedation has become routine in neonatal care. The possibility of pain relief from sucking sucrose from a dummy continues to be debated (Noerr 2001). The recognition of pain in the neonate has prompted a number of pain assessment tools to aid its identification as their behavioural responses may not reflect the severity of the pain.

- CRIES is a tool that assesses crying, saturation, vital signs, expression and sleeping and has particular benefit for postoperative pain in the term baby (Krechel & Bildner 1995).
- The preterm baby may show altered responses owing to the immaturity of the musculoskeletal system and consequently the Premature Infant Pain Profile may reflect the needs of the preterm infant more appropriately (Stevens et al 1996).

The preterm baby can also find other 'routine' stimuli noxious – for example the lighting and the noise levels, the superfluous handling and the sleep deprivation associated with the delivery of intensive care.

Neonates who are being ventilated need pharmacological support for their pain and distress. However, simple comforting measures can be effective for short term use, especially for the non-ventilated baby. These actions include swaddling, nesting, positioning and non-nutritive sucking from a pacifier. These measures can be learnt by the family to aid the attachment process, as some babies demonstrate disorganised behaviour when presented with the usual parental interactions like cuddling and play. Consideration for the environmental stimuli should also be made by lowering the lighting and minimising the noise levels.

Box 43.5 is a key point relating to stimuli.

Parents

The importance of attachment for the future relationship between the parents and their baby has been recognised for a number of years from the work of people like Klaus & Kennell (1989). Bonding would normally occur as the mother interacts with her baby. Some mothers bond instantaneously, whilst for others the process occurs more slowly as they meet their baby's needs. However, when this normal maternal role and interaction is denied, the process of attachment can be delayed and difficult (Bialoskurski et al 1999). It is now common for the parents to be given photographs and mementoes to aid the attachment process, and recently the importance of this communication for the parents has been revisited by Cox & Bialoskurski (2001). Consequently the midwife has a significant role to play in supporting the parents following the birth of a baby for whom intensive care is required.

For the majority of parents the question of survival will be paramount. This fear will be intensified with increasing prematurity. The EPICure study data (Costello et al 2000) gives the exact data for the outcome of births on the edge of viability. An easily remembered guide suggested by these data is that deliveries at 25 weeks of gestation have a 50% mortality rate, and the surviving babies have a 50% morbidity rate. The survival of their baby is the initial concern for parents, but once there is less of a danger the need for ongoing daily communication should continue as it helps the parents 'feel' for their babies. The mothers rely on this information to help them facilitate an attachment with their baby.

Cox & Bialoskurski (2001) found that, for 99% of mothers, the information regarding their baby's status was the most important maternal concern during their stay on the NNU. This was paramount – ranking above their own maternal, emotional and social needs. The information that was the most valuable needed to be current and reliable. Further factors that affected the attachment process were the separation away from the baby, which made the baby seem unreal, the fear of attachment and a prolonged stay in the neonatal unit.

Cox & Bialoskurski (2001) identified some maternal factors that hindered the attachment process. The midwife and nursing team can assist the parents to overcome difficulties by improving their quality of communication, identifying the support structures that are available for parents and by facilitating the parents' easy and frequent access to their baby.

Box 43.6 is a key point relating to parents.

> **Box 43.5** Key point – stimuli
>
> - The environment contains a variety of distressing stimuli for the neonate

> **Box 43.6** Key point – parents
>
> - The midwife can augment the parental growth in attachment with effective communication

REFERENCES

Bialoskurski M, Cox C, Hayes J 1999 The nature of attachment in the neonatal intensive care unit. Journal of Perinatal and Neonatal Nursing 13(1):66–77

Costello K, Hennessy E, Gibson A, Marlow N, Wilkinson A 2000 The EPICure study: outcomes to discharge from hospital for babies born at the threshold of viability. Pediatrics 106:659–671

Cox C L, Bialoskurski M 2001 Neonatal intensive care: communication and attachment. British Journal of Nursing 10:668–676

Franco-Belgium Collaborative NO Trial Group 1999 Early compared with delayed inhaled nitric oxide in moderately hypoxaemic neonates with respiratory failure: a randomised controlled trial. Lancet 354:1066–1071

Gerdes J S 1991 Clinico-pathologic approach to the diagnosis of neonatal sepsis. Clinical Perinatology 18:361–390

Grant J, Denne S C 1991 Effect of intermittent versus continuous enteral feeding on energy expenditure in premature infants. Journal of Pediatrics 118:928–932

Greenough A 1996 Airleak. In: Greenough A, Milner A, Roberton N R C (eds) Neonatal respiratory disorders. Arnold, London, p 334–354

Greenough A, Roberton N R C 1996 Respiratory distress syndrome. In: Greenough A, Milner A, Roberton N R C (eds) Neonatal respiratory disorders. Arnold, London, p 238–279

Greenough A, Roberton N R C 1999 Acute respiratory distress in the newborn. In: Rennie J M, Roberton N R C (eds) Textbook of neonatology, 3rd edn. Churchill Livingstone. Edinburgh, p 481–607

Greenough A, Milner A, Roberton N R C (eds) 1996 Neonatal respiratory disorders. Arnold, London

Johnson A, Peacock J, Greenough A, Marlow N, Limb E, Marston L, Calvert S United Kingdom Oscillation Study Group 2002 High-frequency oscillatory ventilation for the prevention of chronic lung disease of prematurity. New England Journal of Medicine 347(9):663–642

Jordan S C, Scott O 1989 Heart disease in paediatrics, 3rd edn. Butterworth-Heinemann, Oxford, p 3

Klaus M H, Kennell J H 1989 Parent–infant bonding, 3rd edn. C V Mosby, St Louis

Krechel S, Bildner J 1995 CRIES: a new neonatal post-operative pain measurement score: initial testing of validity and reliability. Paediatric Anaesthesia 5(1):53–61

Lucas A, Bloom S, Aynsley-Green A 1986 Gut hormones and 'minimal enteral feeding'. Acta Paediatrica Scandinavica 75:719–723

Matthews T G, Warshaw J B 1979 Relevance of the gestational age on distribution of meconium passage in utero. Pediatrics 64:30–31

Neonatal Inhaled Nitric Oxide Study Group 1997 Inhaled nitric oxide in full term and nearly full-term infants with hypoxic respiratory failure. New England Journal of Medicine 336:597–604

Newell S 1998 Enteral nutrition. In: Campbell A G M, McIntosh N (eds) Forfar and Arneil's textbook of pediatrics, 5th edn. Churchill Livingstone, New York, p 152–155

Noerr B 2001 Sucrose for neonatal procedural pain. Neonatal Network 20(7):63–67

Steele R W, Metz J R, Bass J W, du Bois J J 1971 Pneumothorax and pneumomediastinum in the newborn. Radiology 98:629–632

Stevens B, Johnston C, Petryshen P, Taddio A 1996 Premature infant pain profile: development and initial validation. Clinical Journal of Pain 12:13–22

Tortora G, Grabrowski S 2000 Principles of anatomy and physiology, 9th edn. John Wiley, New York

UK Collaborative ECMO Trial Group 1996 UK collaborative randomised trial of neonatal extracorporeal membrane oxygenation. Lancet 348:75–82

FURTHER READING

Merenstein G, Gardner S 1998 Handbook of neonatal intensive care, 4th edn. CV Mosby, St Louis

A good authority for a combination of pertinent nursing and medical issues. The book covers topics more relevant for holistic management of babies needing intensive care. Although the work is American the balanced approach to all aspects of neonatology ensures the book retains its recommendation as a resource in Britain.

Rennie J, Roberton N R C (eds) 1999 Textbook of neonatology, 3rd edn. Churchill Livingstone, Edinburgh

A comprehensive coverage of all aspects of neonatology. This book provides an invaluable resource for British neonatologists. It covers an extensive range of medical topics and yet retains an easy to read reference approach.

Rennie J, Roberton N R C 2002 A manual of neonatal intensive care, 4th edn. Arnold, London

A succinct version of their Textbook of neonatology for neonatal intensive care. The book provides essential information for the daily management of infants needing extra care. Ideal as a straightforward reference source.

44 Trauma during Birth; Haemorrhage and Convulsions

Claire Greig

CHAPTER CONTENTS

This chapter offers the opportunity to learn about complications that occur in specifically vulnerable babies; the midwife's awareness of this vulnerability may prevent such complications. However, if the complications occur, the midwife's role is to detect them and facilitate and assist with treatment.

The chapter aims to present information on:

- trauma that can occur during birth to skin and superficial tissues, muscle, nerves and bones

- major types of neonatal haemorrhage due to trauma, disruptions in blood flow, coagulopathies and other causes

- neonatal convulsions

- specific interventions with parents.

Following reading of this chapter, further study and experience in relation to these complications, it is expected the midwife will be able to:

- employ, when possible, preventive strategies

- detect signs

- facilitate and assist with effective treatment

- understand possible sequelae.

Trauma during birth

Trauma during birth includes:

- trauma to skin and superficial tissues
- muscle trauma
- nerve trauma
- fractures.

Despite the skilled midwifery and obstetric care in developed, Western societies and a reduction in the incidence, birth trauma does still occur. It is important that the midwife understands the cause and nature of the main traumas to which a baby can be subjected, in order that attempts can be made to prevent their occurrence perinatally. However, if trauma does occur, the midwife's role is to detect it and facilitate and assist with effective treatment.

Trauma to skin and superficial tissues

Skin

Damage to the skin is often iatrogenic, resulting, for example, from forceps blades (Plate 27), vacuum extractor cups, scalp electrodes and scalpels. Poorly applied forceps blades or vacuum extractor cup can result in abrasion of the scalp (Plate 28), although fewer problems occur with the use of softer vacuum extractor cups. Forceps blades can cause bruising or superficial fat necrosis. Scalp electrodes cause puncture wounds, as do fetal blood sampling techniques. Occasionally, during incision of the uterus at caesarean section, laceration of the baby's skin can occur.

All of these injuries, except superficial fat necrosis, should be detected during the midwife's detailed physical examination of the baby immediately after birth.

Superficial fat necrosis is not evident until several days after the birth, at which time the well-defined areas of induration where pressure was applied can be detected.

Abrasions and lacerations should be kept clean and dry. If there are signs of infection, medical advice should be sought. Antibiotics may be required. Deeper lacerations may require closure with butterfly strips or sutures. There is no specific management for fat necrosis. Healing is usually rapid with no residual scarring.

Superficial tissues

Trauma to soft tissue involves oedematous swellings or bruising, or both. During labour the part of the fetus overlying the cervical os can be subjected to pressure, a 'girdle of contact'. This leads to obstruction of the venous return; congestion and oedema result. The oedema consists of serum and blood (serosanguineous fluid).

Caput succedaneum. If the presentation was cephalic, there may be oedematous swelling under the scalp and above the periosteum, called a caput

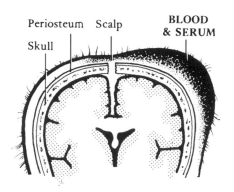

Fig. 44.1 Caput succedaneum.

succedaneum (Fig. 44.1). In the occipitoanterior position, one caput succedaneum may be present. In an occipitoposterior position, a caput succedaneum may form, but then if the occiput rotates anteriorly a second caput succedaneum can develop. A second caput succedaneum may also form if, during the second stage of labour, the birth of the head is delayed and the perineum acts as another 'girdle of contact'. A 'false' caput succedaneum can also occur if a vacuum extractor cup is used; because of its distinctive shape, the resulting oedematous deformity is known as a 'chignon' (Plate 28).

A caput succedaneum is present at birth, does not usually enlarge, can 'pit' on pressure, can cross a suture line and the oedema may move to the dependent area of the scalp (Furdon & Clark 2001). The baby will usually experience some discomfort and, although care continues as normal, gentle handling or dressing is appropriate. Abrasion of the chignon is possible and the interventions for abrasions should be employed.

The caput succedaneum usually resolves by 36 hours of life, with no longer term consequences. An abraded chignon usually heals rapidly if the area is kept clean, dry and is not irritated.

Other injury. The cervical os may restrict venous return when the fetal presentation is not cephalic. When the face presents, it becomes congested and bruised and the eyes and lips become oedematous. In a breech presentation the fetus will develop bruised and oedematous genitalia and buttocks.

This type of trauma is apparent at birth. The baby experiences discomfort and pain; therefore extreme care must be taken when handling, changing nappies or dressing the baby. Maintaining nappy area hygiene is important and needs to be accomplished without inflicting trauma to the skin. The early and repeated gentle application of barrier ointment or cream may be required if disposable nappies designed to limit the contact of urine and faecal fluid with the skin are not available. If skin excoriation does occur, the possibility of infection increases and consultation with a wound care specialist nurse may be required to ensure best skin care practice.

Uncomplicated oedema and bruising usually resolve within a few days of life. However, if there is significant trauma during a vaginal breech birth there can be serious complications that require specific treatment and thus take longer to resolve. These complications include excessive red cell breakdown resulting in hyperbilirubinaemia; excessive blood loss resulting in hypovolaemia, shock, anaemia and disseminated intravascular coagulation (DIC); and damage to muscles resulting in difficulties with micturition and defecation.

Muscle trauma

Injuries to muscle result from tearing or when the blood supply is disrupted.

Torticollis

The most commonly damaged muscle is the sternomastoid muscle. The right and left sternomastoid muscles run from the respective side of the top of the sternum, along the right or left side of the neck and are inserted into the mastoid process of the right or left temporal bone (Tortora & Grabowski 2000). When contracted simultaneously, these muscles allow the head to flex. When contracted separately, each turns the head to the opposite side.

Excessive traction or twisting causing tearing to one of these muscles can occur during the birth of the anterior shoulder of a fetus with a cephalic presentation, or during rotation of the shoulders when the fetus is being born by vaginal breech. A small lump, consisting of blood and fibrous tissue, can be felt on the affected sternomastoid muscle. It appears to be painless for the baby. The muscle length is shortened, therefore the neck is twisted on the affected side: a torticollis or wry neck. If the techniques for assisting at these stages of birth are correctly applied, torticollis can be prevented.

The management of torticollis involves stretching of the affected muscle, which is achieved by laying the baby on the unaffected side and by using muscle-stretching exercises under the guidance of a physiotherapist. The swelling will usually resolve over several weeks.

Nerve trauma

Commonly there is trauma to the facial nerve or to the brachial plexus nerves.

Facial nerve

Damage to the facial nerve usually results from its compression against the ramus of the mandible by a forceps blade, resulting in a unilateral facial palsy. The eyelid on the affected side remains open and the mouth is drawn over to the normal side (Plate 29). If the baby cannot form an effective seal on the breast or teat, there may be some initial feeding difficulties.

There is no specific treatment. If the eyelid remains open, regular instillation of methyl cellulose eye drops can help lubricate the eyeball. Feeding difficulties are usually overcome by the baby's own adaptation, although alternative feeding positions can be tried. Spontaneous resolution usually occurs within 7–10 days.

Brachial plexus

Nerve roots exiting from the spine at the level of the fifth, sixth, seventh and eighth cervical vertebrae and the first thoracic vertebra form a matrix of nerves in the neck and shoulder, known as the brachial plexus (Tortora & Grabowski 2000). Trauma to this group of nerves usually results from excessive lateral flexion, rotation or traction of the head and neck during vaginal breech birth or when shoulder dystocia occurs.

There are three main injuries: Erb's palsy, Klumpke's palsy and total brachial plexus palsy, with an incidence of between 0.3 and 2 per 1000 births (Laurent 1997). These injuries can be unilateral or bilateral.

Erb's palsy. Here there is damage to the upper brachial plexus involving the fifth and sixth cervical nerve roots. The baby's affected arm is inwardly rotated, the elbow is extended, the wrist is pronated and flexed and the hand is partially closed. This is commonly known as the 'waiter's tip position'. The arm is limp, although some movement of the fingers and arm is possible (Plate 30).

Klumpke's palsy. Here there is damage to the lower brachial plexus involving the seventh and eighth cervical and the first thoracic nerve roots. The upper arm has normal movement but the lower arm, wrist and hand are affected. There is wrist drop and flaccid paralysis of the hand with no grasp reflex.

Total brachial plexus palsy. Here there is damage to all brachial plexus nerve roots with complete paralysis of the arm and hand, lack of sensation and circulatory problems. If there is bilateral paralysis, spinal injury should be suspected.

All types of brachial plexus trauma will require further investigations such as X-ray and ultrasound scanning (USS) of the clavicle, arm, chest and cervical spine, and assessment of the joints. Passive movements of the joints and limb can then be initiated under the direction of a physiotherapist. At approximately 1 month of age, magnetic resonance imaging can offer specific data on nerve damage.

Spontaneous recovery within days to weeks is expected for 80% of babies, with Erb's palsy tending to resolve more quickly than the other forms. Follow-up is recommended. Babies with no functional recovery by 4 months of age (approximately 2 in 10 000 births) may require surgical repair by 6 months of age to achieve full function (Laurent 1997).

Fractures

Fractures are rare but the most commonly affected bones are the clavicle, humerus, femur and those of the skull. With all such fractures, a 'crack' may be heard during the birth.

Clavicle

Fractures can occur if there is shoulder dystocia or during a vaginal breech birth. The affected clavicle is usually the one that was nearest the maternal symphysis pubis.

Humerus

Midshaft fractures can occur if there is shoulder dystocia or during a vaginal breech birth as the extended arm is brought down and born.

Femur

Midshaft fractures can occur during vaginal breech birth as the extended legs are brought down and born.

With fractures, distortion or deformity is usually evident on examination; crepitus may also be felt, and the baby feels pain and is reluctant to move the affected area. An X-ray examination can usually confirm the diagnosis.

The baby requires careful handling, cleansing and dressing to avoid further pain, and, for some babies, mild analgesia such as paracetamol is appropriate (Northern Neonatal Network 1998). Positioning the baby on the back or unaffected side is likely to be more comfortable and assist healing.

Fractures of the clavicle require no specific treatment. Immobilisation of a fractured humerus is achieved by placing a pad in the axilla and splinting the arm to the chest with a bandage. Application should be firm but should not embarrass respiration. Immobilisation of a fractured femur is relatively easy using a splint and a bandage.

Stable union of a fractured clavicle usually occurs in 7–10 days, while the humerus and the femur take 2–3 weeks.

Skull

Although rare, these fractures can occur during prolonged or difficult instrumental births, and are usually linear or depressed. Although there may be no signs, an overlying cephalhaematoma, or signs of associated complications such as intracranial haemorrhage, raised intracranial pressure, neurological disturbances, leakage of cerebrospinal fluid (CSF) or seizures, can lead to the detection of a fracture.

X-ray examination can confirm the diagnosis. Linear fractures usually require no treatment. Depressed fractures may require surgical intervention. If there is leakage of CSF through the ear or nose, antibiotic therapy is indicated. Treatment of associated complications is necessary.

Linear skull fractures usually heal quickly with no sequelae. Depressed fractures have a similarly optimistic outcome except if complications occur, when permanent neurological damage is likely (McCulloch 1999).

Haemorrhage

Haemorrhages can be due to:

- trauma
- disruptions in blood flow

or can be related to:

- coagulopathies
- other causes.

Blood volume in the term baby is approximately 80–100 ml/kg and in the preterm baby 90–105 ml/kg; therefore even a small haemorrhage can be potentially fatal. In this section, newborn haemorrhages are discussed according to their principal cause, (i.e. trauma, disruptions in blood flow, coagulopathies and other causes).

Haemorrhage due to trauma

Cephalhaematoma

A cephalhaematoma (or cephalohaematoma) is an effusion of blood under the periosteum that covers the skull bones (Fig. 44.2). During a vaginal birth, if there is friction between the fetal skull and the maternal pelvic bones, such as in cephalopelvic disproportion or precipitate labour, the periosteum is torn from the bone, causing bleeding underneath. Cephalhaematomas can also be caused during vacuum-assisted births. Because the fetal or newborn skull bones are not fused, and as the periosteum is adherent to the edges of the skull bones, a cephalhaematoma is confined to one bone. However, more than one bone may be affected; therefore multiple cephalhaematomas may develop. A double cephalhaematoma is usually bilateral (Fig. 44.3).

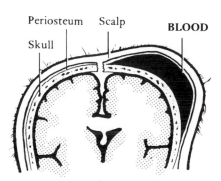

Fig. 44.2 Cephalhaematoma.

A cephalhaematoma is not present at birth but the swelling appears after 12 hours, grows larger over subsequent days and can persist for weeks. The swelling is circumscribed, firm, does not pit on pressure, does not cross a suture and is fixed (Furdon & Clark 2001).

No treatment is necessary and the swelling subsides when the blood is reabsorbed. Erythrocyte breakdown in the extravasated blood may result in hyperbilirubinaemia. A ridge of bone may later be felt round the periphery of the swelling, owing to the accumulation of osteoblasts.

Subaponeurotic haemorrhage

A subaponeurotic (or subgaleal) haemorrhage is rare. Under the scalp, the epicranial aponeurosis, a sheet of fibrous tissue that covers the cranial vault allowing for muscles to attach to the bone, provides a potential space above the periosteum through which many veins travel. Excessive traction on these veins results in haemorrhage, the epicranial aponeurosis is pulled away from the periosteum of the skull bones and swelling is evident (Fig. 44.4). Subaponeurotic haemorrhage can occur with any type of birth but more often it is associated with vacuum-assisted births, primiparous women, severe dystocia, occipitolateral or posterior head positions, preterm babies, precipitate births, macrosomia, coagulopathies and male baby gender (Katz & Nishioka 1998).

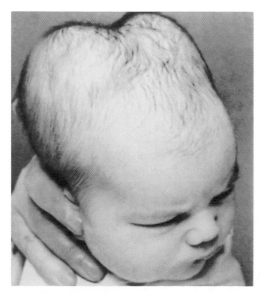

Fig. 44.3 Bilateral cephalhaematoma.

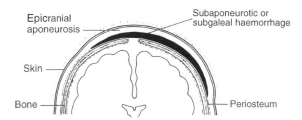

Fig. 44.4 Subaponeurotic haemorrhage.

The swelling is present at birth, increases in size and is a firm, fluctuant mass. The scalp is movable rather than fixed. The swelling can cross sutures and extend into the subcutaneous tissue of neck and eyelids. The baby experiences pain when there is head movement or the swelling is handled.

The incidence of subaponeurotic haemorrhage is estimated to be 1 in 2500 births. There is a risk of excessive haemorrhage into this potential space and, if this occurs, the baby shows signs of severe shock. Management of this emergency requires medical assistance; stabilisation and full supportive care, including blood transfusion, will be required. Subaponeurotic haemorrhage is associated with a mortality rate of 22% (Furdon & Clark 2001).

With a smaller haemorrhage and in the babies who survive larger haemorrhages, bruising is evident for days and sometimes weeks. The blood is reabsorbed and the swelling resolves over 2–3 weeks. Hyperbilirubinaemia may complicate the baby's recovery.

Subdural haemorrhage

A sickle-shaped, double fold of dura mater known as the falx cerebri dips into the fissure between the cerebral hemispheres. Attached at right angles to the falx cerebri, between the cerebrum and the cerebellum, is a horseshoe-shaped fold of dura mater known as the tentorium cerebelli. Within these folds of dura run the large venous sinuses draining blood from the brain.

Normally moulding of the fetal skull bones and stretching of the underlying structures during birth is well tolerated. Trauma to the fetal head, such as excessive compression or abnormal stretching, can result in tearing of the dura, rupture of the venous sinuses and a subdural haemorrhage. Predisposing traumatic circumstances include those in which the moulding is rapid, abnormal or excessive, such as precipitate labour or rapid birth, malpositions, malpresentations, cephalopelvic disproportion or undue compression during forceps manoeuvres. A tentorial tear is the most common lesion and is most often experienced by term babies (Korones 1986).

A baby with a large subdural haemorrhage is likely to be severely asphyxiated and be difficult to resuscitate. However, if the haemorrhage is initially smaller, the signs develop over several days. As blood accumulates, there is cerebral irritation, cerebral oedema and raised intracranial pressure. The baby is likely to vomit, be non-responsive, and have a bulging anterior fontanelle, abnormal eye movements, apnoea, bradycardia and convulsions.

Diagnosis is confirmed by cranial USS. Supportive treatment is geared towards controlling the consequences of asphyxia and raised intracranial pressure. Subdural taps may be required to drain large collections of blood. This type of haemorrhage can be fatal.

Haemorrhage due to disruptions in blood flow

Subarachnoid haemorrhage

A primary subarachnoid haemorrhage involves bleeding directly into the subarachnoid space. Preterm babies, those who suffer hypoxia at birth, resulting in disruption of cerebral blood flow, and those term babies who suffer traumatic births are vulnerable (Korones 1986, Levene et al 2000). A secondary haemorrhage involves the leakage of blood into the subarachnoid space from an intraventricular haemorrhage (IVH) (Levene et al 2000).

The baby may have generalised convulsions from the second day of life, preterm babies may have apnoeic episodes, but otherwise the baby appears normal and some babies exhibit no signs. Subarachnoid haemorrhage is difficult to see on USS, although computerised tomography scanning can demonstrate the haemorrhage. If a lumbar puncture is performed, the CSF will be uniformly bloodstained. Management involves control of the consequences of asphyxia and of convulsions. The condition is usually self-limiting.

Posthaemorrhagic hydrocephalus, demonstrated on serial cranial USS, can complicate the baby's recovery. Drainage of the hydrocephaly is usually not required and the prognosis for recovery is usually favourable (Levene et al 2000).

Periventricular/intraventricular haemorrhage

Periventricular/intraventricular haemorrhage (PVH/IVH) is the most common and serious of all intracranial haemorrhages and primarily affects babies of less than 32 weeks' gestation and those weighing less than 1500 g, although term babies can be affected (Heuchan 1999, Horbar 1992). In recent years, the incidence of PVH/IVH appears to be falling, with a 40% incidence reported in the 1970s for at-risk babies (Papile et al 1978), decreasing to an incidence of 15% for at-risk babies in the 1990s (Heuchan 1999).

The stage of brain development is a crucial factor in the aetiology of PVH/IVH. The two lateral ventricles are lined with ependymal tissue. Tissue lying immediately next to the ependyma is the germinal matrix, sometimes also known as the subependymal layer. From 8 to 28 weeks' gestation, the germinal matrix is responsible for producing neuroblasts that migrate to become the cerebral cortex. During this period, a rich blood supply is provided to the germinal matrix through fragile immature capillaries that lack supporting muscle or collagen fibres. These vessels are particularly vulnerable to increases in cerebral blood flow as they can easily rupture causing haemorrhage. After 32 weeks' gestation the germinal matrix becomes less active and by term has almost completely involuted. At the same time the capillaries become more stable; therefore PVH/IVH in more mature babies is less common than in those less than 32 weeks' gestation (Heuchan 1999).

In the baby of less than 32 weeks' gestation, the arterial supply to the area around the lateral ventricles is limited, with arteries still to make growth and interconnections. These arteries form an end zone or watershed, a boundary zone between arteries that is relatively poorly supplied with blood. When cerebral blood flow is reduced, this area is vulnerable to ischaemic damage; with reperfusion a haemorrhage can result.

The venous drainage from white matter and the deep areas of the brain, including the lateral ventricles, involves the blood following a peculiar U-turn route in the area of the germinal matrix. Disruptions to venous flow lead to congestion, with a risk of haemorrhage or ischaemia (Cullens 2000).

Throughout the perinatal period there are multiple factors that can affect cerebral haemodynamics and result in PVH/IVH. Early factors include obstetric haemorrhage, lack of antenatal steroids, birth outside a regional unit, chorioamnionitis, low 1 minute apgar score, bruising at birth and low umbilical artery pH. Later risk factors include acidosis, hypotension, hypertension, respiratory distress syndrome (RDS) requiring mechanical ventilation, rapid volume expansion, rapid administration of sodium bicarbonate or other hyperosmolar solutions, pneumothorax and patent ductus arteriosus (Heuchan 1999). Also implicated are excessive handling of the baby, exposure to light and noise, lateral flexion of the head and crying (Deitch 1993).

With a significant haemodynamic insult in an at-risk baby, there may be haemorrhage into the germinal matrix. This is a PVH that is also known by three synonyms: subependymal, germinal matrix and grade 1 haemorrhage. If there is extension of the haemorrhage into the lateral ventricle(s), this is known as an intraventricular haemorrhage or grade 2 haemorrhage. The choroid plexus of the lateral ventricles normally produces CSF. If there is blockage to the outflow of CSF, posthaemorrhagic hydrocephalus develops and the ventricles dilate; this is a grade 3 IVH. A grade 3 haemorrhage can also extend into the cerebral tissue, giving rise to a parenchymal haemorrhage, which is also known as a grade 4 haemorrhage (Papile et al 1978).

More recently, Volpe (1997) proposed that the intraventricular clot in the grade 3 haemorrhage disrupts venous drainage, causing stasis and then infarction. With reperfusion of the area, there is haemorrhage into the area of infarction leading to necrotic damage of the white matter. Volpe (1997) therefore suggested that a grade 4 haemorrhage should be regarded as a complication of a grade 3 PVH/IVH and should be referred to as a periventricular haemorrhagic infarction (PHI). This venous haemorrhagic infarction can be viewed on USS and is usually unilateral, or if bilateral is asymmetric. As the necrosis of the white matter progresses, large cyst formations persist and are visible on USS (Volpe 1997).

Approximately 30% of PVH/IVH will be apparent within the first 6 hours of life, indicating a prenatal or intranatal insult (Heuchan 1999). A further 20% will have occurred by the end of the 1st day and 90% have occurred within 3 days of birth (Horbar 1992). A small PVH can have a 'silent' onset, and is detectable only on USS. If the haemorrhage is larger or extends, the clinical features may gradually appear and worsen. These may include apnoeic episodes, which become more frequent and severe, episodes of bradycardia, pallor, falling haematocrit, tense anterior fontanelle, metabolic acidosis and convulsions. The baby may be limp or unresponsive. If the PVH/IVH is large and sudden in onset, the baby may present with apnoea and circulatory collapse (Cullens 2000).

At-risk babies are usually screened by 7 days of life for PVH/IVH using cranial USS. Earlier scanning may be done on the basis of the clinical condition. If a haemorrhage is detected, serial scanning can determine any increase, extension or complication.

The care of at-risk babies is focused on prevention of PVH/IVH. Prenatally, the administration of steroids to the mother to stimulate the maturation of surfactant may have a neuroprotective effect; when followed by the administration of artificial surfactant postnatally, there is a reduction in the incidence of PVH/IVH (Heuchan 1999, Jobe et al 1993). Antibiotic therapy in the management of preterm premature rupture of the membranes has also reduced the incidence of PVH/IVH (Mercer & Arheart 1995).

To help at-risk babies remain haemodynamically stable and reduce the likelihood of PVH/IVH occurring or extending, the birth should be in a regional obstetric unit with intensive neonatal facilities. Haemodynamic stability is the aim of all postnatal care, as is the prevention of the many complications that can develop. The at-risk baby's needs related to respiration and acid–base balance, circulation and blood pressure, temperature control, nutrition and elimination must be carefully assessed and meticulously met, with continuing evaluation and appropriate adjustments to care. Sophisticated monitoring equipment and the judicious use of analgesic, sedative and inotropic drugs can assist in achieving and maintaining stability (Northern Neonatal Network 1998). If complications develop, such as pneumothorax or patent ductus arteriosus, these should be quickly detected and effectively treated (Heuchan 1999). The baby's neurodevelopmental needs should be met, particularly in relation to supportive positioning, adjustment to lighting, a quiet, undisturbed environment and appropriate interaction with parents and others (Wyly 1995).

Despite preventative measures, babies do develop PVH/IVH and the outcome depends on the nature of the haemorrhage. The neurological prognosis for babies with grade 1 and 2 haemorrhages is usually good. Even in a grade 3 haemorrhage, the ventricular dilatation can resolve spontaneously with no long term consequences. However, if there is a large grade 3 haemorrhage, the accumulating CSF may require temporary drainage using ventricular taps or external ventricular drainage. Some babies may require permanent CSF drainage via a 'shunt'. For this a drainage tube is surgically inserted into the ventricular system and is connected to a one-way valve placed subcutaneously behind the ear. The outflow tube from the valve is attached to a catheter allowing drainage of the CSF into a large vein in the neck, or into the peritoneum, where it is subsequently reabsorbed and eliminated (Heuchan 1999).

Babies who suffer a massive haemorrhage may die within 48 hours of the onset and those who survive are likely to develop significant neurological and intellectual impairment. Long term follow-up is necessary and parents need much support. Of the 85% of the babies at risk of PVH/IVH who survived in the USA, Volpe (1997) suggested an incidence of spastic motor deficits in 5–15%. These deficits included spastic diplegia and spastic hemiparesis, with or without intellectual deficits. The main causes of this morbidity were periventricular leucomalacia and periventricular haemorrhagic infarction (Volpe 1997, Weindling 1995).

Periventricular leucomalacia

Although not strictly a haemorrhage, periventricular leucomalacia (PVL) is included because of its association with PVH/IVH (Zupan et al 1996). Between 27 and 30 weeks' gestation, the area of white matter around the lateral ventricles and within the watershed area of the deep cerebral arteries is undergoing considerable development. It is very sensitive to any insult that results in reduced cerebral perfusion, such as those insults associated with PVH/IVH (Levene et al 2000), and intrauterine infection with or without ruptured membranes (Heuchan 1999, Zupan et al 1996). Reduced perfusion results in areas of ischaemia and degeneration of the nerve fibre tracts, disrupting nerve pathways between areas of the brain and between the brain and spinal cord. This softening and necrosis of tissue is PVL and is visible on USS. The areas can become cystic cavities, porencephalic cysts; unlike the cystic formation in PHI, however, the cysts of PVL can regress (Levene et al 2000).

Similar pathogenesis is seen in the older preterm and term baby, but the lesion occurs in the subcortical region rather than the periventricular region. This is because the watershed moves away from the ventricles to the cortex once the germinal matrix involutes. These lesions are known as subcortical leucomalacia.

Care instituted to reduce the incidence of PVH/IVH can also reduce the incidence of PVL or the severity of the related ischaemic damage.

Haemorrhage related to coagulopathies

These haemorrhages occur because of a disruption in the baby's blood-clotting abilities.

Vitamin K deficiency bleeding

Vitamin K deficiency bleeding (VKDB) can occur up to 12 months of age, although it more commonly occurs between birth and 8 weeks of life. It was previously known as haemorrhagic disease of the newborn (HDN). Several proteins – factor II (prothrombin), factor VII (proconvertin), factor IX (plasma thromboplastin component) and factor X (thrombokinase) – require vitamin K to convert them into active clotting factors. A deficiency of vitamin K, as in VKDB, leads to a deficiency of these clotting factors and resultant bleeding.

Vitamin K_1 (phytonadione/phylloquinone) is poorly transferred across the placenta; therefore the fetus has low stores. Any stores are quickly depleted after birth and so, to enable normal clotting to occur, the baby must receive dietary vitamin K_1, the absorption of which requires fat and bile salts. Vitamin K_2 (menaquinone) is synthesised by bowel flora and may assist in the conversion of proteins to active clotting factors. Because the neonate's bowel is sterile, vitamin K_2 production is restricted until colonisation has occurred. Therefore all newborns are deficient in vitamin K and vulnerable to VKDB. The incidence of VKDB in babies with no additional risk factors is 10 per 100 000 (Tripp & McNinch 1998, 1999).

There are three forms of VKDB, which were first described by Lane & Hathaway (1985):

- 'early' (0–24 hours)
- 'classical' (1–7 days)
- 'late' (1–12 months, although the peak onset is before 8 weeks).

Early VKDB is rare and principally affects babies born to women who, during pregnancy, have taken warfarin, phenobarbital or phenytoin for treatment of their medical conditions. These drugs interfere with vitamin K metabolism (Anonymous 1998). If such women take vitamin K_1 supplements during the last 2 weeks of pregnancy, early VKDB is preventable (Lane & Hathaway 1985).

The babies who are more susceptible to developing classical VKDB are those with birth trauma, asphyxia, postnatal hypoxia and those who are preterm, or of low birthweight. These babies are more likely to spontaneously bleed or have invasive interventions resulting in bleeding that cannot be controlled owing to lack of clotting factors. Disruptions to the colonisation of the bowel due to antibiotic therapy, or lack of or poor enteral feeding, can also result in classical VKDB. Breastfed babies produce bifidobacteria in their bowel that inhibit the production of menaquinones. Serum menaquinone is naturally low in the newborn breastfed baby, resulting in increased susceptibility to VKDB, although there are doubts as to the role of the menaquinones produced in the bowel, emphasising the importance of the dietary source of vitamin K_1 (Gasking 1998).

The amount of vitamin K_1 in breastmilk is naturally low, although colostrum and hindmilk do contain higher levels than foremilk (WHO 1989). The low levels of vitamin K_1 in breastmilk have been considered insufficient for the exclusively breastfed newborn (Greer 1999). Cow's milk has higher concentrations of vitamin K_1 than breastmilk, although the levels are still low (Tripp 1997). Artificial infant formulae are fortified with vitamin K_1, offering some prophylaxis against VKDB.

Late VKDB occurs almost exclusively in breastfed babies. However, babies who have liver disease or a condition that disrupts vitamin K_1's absorption from the bowel, for example cystic fibrosis, may develop late VKDB.

Bleeding may be evident superficially as bruising; or there may be blood loss from the umbilicus, puncture sites, the nose or the scalp. Severe jaundice for more than 1 week and persistent jaundice for more than 2 weeks are also warning signs. Gastrointestinal bleeding is manifested as melaena and haematemesis. In early and late VKDB, there may be serious extracranial and intracranial bleeding. With severe haemorrhage, circulatory collapse occurs. Late VKDB has a reported incidence of 40–100 per million livebirths and is associated with higher mortality and morbidity (Anonymous 1998). Diagnosis is confirmed if blood tests reveal prolonged prothrombin and partial thromboplastin times, a normal platelet count and raised levels of proteins induced in vitamin K absence, like factor II (PIVKA II) now known as descarboxy prothrombin (Gasking 1998).

Babies who have VKDB require careful investigation and monitoring to assess their need for treatment. With all forms of VKDB, the baby will require administration of vitamin K_1, 1–2 mg intramuscularly. In severe cases, when coagulation is grossly abnormal and there is severe bleeding, replacement of deficient clotting factors is essential. If circulatory collapse and severe anaemia occur, blood transfusion or exchange transfusion may be required. Affected babies usually require other supportive therapy to assist in their recovery.

VKDB is a potentially fatal condition; therefore prophylactic administration of vitamin K became the norm in many countries, including the UK. Various types, routes and doses were used, but vitamin K_1 1 mg given intramuscularly within the 1st hour after birth became the most effective practice, despite some disquiet over the invasive nature of the prophylaxis (Soin & Katesmark 1993).

Controversy over this prophylaxis was heightened when results of two case–control studies suggested an association between intramuscular vitamin K_1 administration and the development of childhood cancers (Golding et al 1990, 1992). This finding has not been confirmed in subsequent case–control studies (Ansell et al 1996, Ekelund et al 1993, Klebanoff et al 1993, McKinney et al 1998, von Kries et al 1996). However, one large retrospective case–control study reported a significant association between the administration of vitamin K_1 intramuscularly and the development of acute lymphoblastic leukaemia in 1–6 year olds, although not with other cancers (Parker et al 1998).

These studies have been limited by their design and unreliable record keeping in terms of the route and dose of vitamin K_1. The statistical association reported in the studies by Golding et al (1990, 1992) and Parker et al (1998) indicates that the children with childhood cancers were more likely to have been given vitamin K_1 intramuscularly at birth, but not that the

vitamin K_1 *caused* the cancer. Indeed, none of the studies has reported that vitamin K_1 given intramuscularly at birth caused childhood cancer. However, just because a causal link has not been identified does not mean that the causal link does not exist. A randomised controlled trial would be more likely to identify any causal link, but this would be very difficult to design and the sample would need to be very large (Wariyar et al 2000).

The concerns about vitamin K and cancer resulted in a reassessment of vitamin K_1 prophylaxis in the early 1990s and a variety of regimens emerged. Most authorities agreed that vitamin K_1 1 mg intramuscularly given within 1 hour of birth is essential for the babies particularly at risk of VKDB. This dose and route give a transient peak serum concentration, reducing the risk of early VKDB. Some vitamin K_1 also remains within the muscle and acts as a slow release depot, providing prophylaxis for classical and late VKDB (Loughnan & McDougall 1995, Wariyar et al 2000). However, there is debate about the need for vitamin K_1 prophylaxis for 'normal risk' babies and the most appropriate route (Tyler 1996, Wariyar et al 2000). There is also continuing controversy about the administration of vitamin K_1 to breastfed babies (Greer 1999). As this controversy may undermine the efforts of health professionals to promote breastfeeding, it is important to continue to research the relationship between breastmilk and VKDB (Jackson 1993, Magill-Cuerden 1997, Tyler 1996).

A licensed oral preparation of vitamin K_1 became available in August 1996 and other oral preparations are now available. These can be used as an alternative to intramuscular injection. The intramuscular preparation should not be given orally (RCM 1996).

Because the understanding of the role of vitamin K in the fetus and newborn is still incomplete, especially in relation to breastfed babies, Zipursky (1999), in a review of the available evidence, suggested that all babies should be given intramuscular vitamin K_1 prophylaxis. Greer (1999) suggested that intramuscular or oral prophylaxis could be offered to all babies. Regimens of prophylaxis continue to be investigated. Current evidence indicates that, if a single 1 mg dose of vitamin K_1 is not given to the baby at birth, an oral prophylaxis regimen should be instituted. This will involve oral administration on the 1st day and between 4 and 7 days of life. If the baby is breastfed, a further dose is required at 30 days. This regimen has been shown to be effective in protecting against all forms of VKDB; however, this is dependent on the involvement, motivation and compliance of health care professionals and parents. Further research is required to establish the optimal dose and frequency of administration for breastfed babies (Wariyar et al 2000).

Greer et al (1997) and Bolisetty et al (1998) demonstrated that administration of vitamin K_1 to lactating women increased the levels of vitamin K_1 in the maternal serum and breastmilk. Their babies had higher serum levels of vitamin K_1, giving some VKDB prophylaxis. However, some of these babies were also given intramuscular vitamin K_1, thus affecting their serum levels of vitamin K_1. Wariyar et al (2000) concluded that, while maternal prophylaxis during breastfeeding was a possible alternative to prophylaxis for the baby, it was a more complicated strategy.

All parents should be given the opportunity to discuss vitamin K_1 prophylaxis during pregnancy and agree on their choice for their baby; they should also understand the signs and treatment of VKDB, especially if their baby has one or more of the risk factors.

Thrombocytopenia

Thrombocytopenia is a low count of circulating platelets, less than 100 000 per microlitre (Sola et al 2000); it results from either a decreased rate of formation of platelets or an increased rate of consumption. In the general neonatal population, thrombocytopenia is rare – a level of 0.7% (Uhrynowska et al 1997). However, it occurs in 20–35% of preterm and sick babies admitted to neonatal units (Sola et al 2000). Babies who are at risk of developing thrombocytopenia include those:

- who have a severe congenital or acquired infection (e.g. syphilis, cytomegalovirus, rubella, toxoplasmosis, bacterial infection)
- whose mother has idiopathic thrombocytopenia, purpura, systemic lupus erythematosus or thyrotoxicosis
- whose mother takes thiazide diuretics
- who have isoimmune thrombocytopenia
- who have inherited thrombocytopenia.

Thrombocytopenia in an ill infant is also associated with DIC (see below) (Johnson et al 1998). In up to 60% of babies with thrombocytopenia, no cause can be determined (Sola et al 2000).

A petechial rash appears soon after birth, presenting in a mild case with a few localised petechiae. In a severe case there is widespread and serious haemorrhage from multiple sites. Diagnosis is based on history, clinical examination and the presence of a reduced platelet count. It is differentiated from other haemorrhagic disorders because coagulation times, fibrin degradation products and red blood cell morphology are normal. In mild cases no treatment is required. In immune-mediated thrombocytopenia, intravenous immunoglobulin administration is helpful. In severe cases where there is haemorrhage and a very low platelet count, transfusion of platelet concentrate may be required.

Recombinant interleukin-II is a haematopoietic growth factor that stimulates platelet production. Recombinant Tpo regulates platelet production. Both substances have been effective in increasing the platelet count in animal models, but further research is required to determine which thrombocytopenic babies would benefit from their administration (Sola et al 2000).

Disseminated intravascular coagulation (consumptive coagulopathy)

Disseminated intravascular coagulation (DIC) is an acquired coagulation disorder associated with the release of thromboplastin from damaged tissue, stimulating abnormal coagulation and fibrinolysis. This results in widespread deposition of fibrin in the microcirculation and the excessive consumption of clotting factors and platelets (Dent 2000, Emery 1992).

DIC is a condition secondary to other primary conditions. Maternal causes include pre-eclampsia, eclampsia and placental abruption. Fetal causes include severe fetal distress, the presence of a dead twin in the uterus and a traumatic birth. Neonatal causes include conditions resulting in hypoxia and acidosis, severe infections, hypothermia, hypotension and thrombocytopenia.

As clotting factors and platelets are depleted and fibrinolysis is stimulated, the baby will develop a generalised purpuric rash and bleed from multiple sites, including internally. With stimulation of the clotting cascade, multiple microthrombi appear in the circulation. These can occlude vessels, leading to organ and tissue ischaemia and damage, particularly affecting the kidneys, resulting in haematuria and reduced urine output. The baby will also become anaemic owing both to the haemorrhage and to fragmentation of red cells by the fibrin deposits in blood vessels (Emery 1992).

As well as the clinical signs, the diagnosis is made from laboratory findings, which show a low platelet count, low fibrinogen level, distorted and fragmented red blood cells, low haemoglobin and raised fibrin degradation products (FDPs) with a prolonged prothrombin time (PT) and partial thromboplastin time (PTT) (Dent 2000).

Treatment includes correction of the underlying cause if possible and full supportive care. To try to control DIC, transfusions of concentrated clotting factors and platelets are required. When the baby also has anaemia, transfusions of whole blood or red cell concentrate are required. Occasionally an exchange transfusion of fresh heparinised blood may be performed, to remove FDPs while replacing the clotting factors (Dent 2000, Emery 1992).

If treatment of the primary disorder or replacement of clotting factors, or both, is ineffective, heparin can be administered to try to reduce fibrin deposition. An initial dose is given, followed by a continuous infusion, the dose of which is titrated to maintain a PTT of 60–70 seconds (Glass 1999).

The prognosis depends on the severity of the primary condition, as well as of the DIC, and the response to treatment.

Inherited coagulation factor deficiencies

X-linked recessive conditions such as haemophilia (factor VIII deficiency) and Christmas disease (factor IX deficiency) rarely cause problems in the neonatal period but may present with excessive bleeding after birth trauma or surgical intervention such as circumcision. Diagnosis is confirmed by a prolonged PTT and a normal PT, with decreased levels of the specific factors. Replacement transfusions are required. An affected baby requires follow-up by haematologists. If there is no previous experience of the condition in the family, there may be a requirement for education, genetic counselling and support.

Haemorrhage related to other causes

Umbilical haemorrhage

This usually occurs as a result of a poorly applied cord ligature. The use of plastic cord clamps has almost eliminated this type of haemorrhage, although it is essential to avoid catching or pulling the clamp. Tampering with partially separated cords before they are ready to separate is discouraged. Cord haemorrhage is a potential cause of death. A purse-string suture should always be inserted if umbilical bleeding does not stop after 15 or 20 minutes.

Vaginal bleeding

A small temporary discharge of bloodstained mucus occurring in the first days of life, and often referred to as pseudomenstruation, is due to the withdrawal of maternal oestrogen. Parents need to know that this is a possibility, is normal and is self-limiting. Continued or excessive bleeding warrants further investigation to exclude a pathological cause.

Haematemesis and melaena

These signs usually present when the baby has swallowed maternal blood during delivery, or from cracked nipples during breastfeeding. The diagnosis must be differentiated from VKDB, from other causes of haematemesis, which include oesophageal, gastric or duodenal ulceration, and from other causes of melaena, which include intestinal duplications, gut haemangiomas, necrotising enterocolitis and anal fissures.

If the cause is swallowed blood, the condition is self-limiting and requires no specific treatment. However, if the cause is cracked nipples, appropriate treatment for the mother must be implemented.

Haematuria

Haematuria can be associated with coagulopathies, urinary tract infections and structural abnormality of the urinary tract. Birth trauma may cause renal contusion and haematuria. Occasionally, after suprapubic aspiration of urine, transient mild haematuria may be observed. Treatment of the primary cause should resolve the haematuria.

Bleeding associated with intravascular access

Some sick or preterm babies require the insertion of catheters, lines or cannulae into central or peripheral arteries or veins, or both, to provide routes for the infusion of fluids and drugs. However, there is a risk of severe external haemorrhage if there is dislodgement of these from the vessel or accidental disconnection from the infusion equipment, and of severe haemorrhage if a central vessel is punctured internally.

Skilled technique, close observation and careful handling of babies with intravascular access are imperative to prevent these potentially fatal haemorrhages. If an external haemorrhage does occur, continuous pressure should be applied to the site until natural haemostasis occurs or until haemostatic sutures are inserted. If there is external bleeding from an umbilical vessel, the cord stump should be squeezed between the fingers until haemostasis occurs. A replacement transfusion of whole blood or packed red cells may be required. Internal haemorrhage may require surgical intervention.

Convulsions

A convulsion is a sign of neurological disturbance, not a disease. Because the newborn brain lacks organisation and development of neuronal contacts and myelination, convulsions (seizures, fits) can present quite differently in the neonate and can be more difficult to recognise than those of later infancy, childhood or adulthood. The incidence of convulsions is suggested as 5–8 per 1000 live births (Levene et al 2000).

Convulsive movement can be differentiated from jitteriness or tremors in that, with the latter two, the movements are rapid, rhythmic, equal, are often stimulated or made worse by disturbance and can be stopped by touching or flexing the affected limb. They are normal in an active, hungry baby and are usually of no consequence, although their occurrence should be documented. Convulsive movements tend to be slower, less equal, are not necessarily stimulated by disturbance, cannot be stopped by restraint and are always pathological (Ballweg 1991).

If a baby demonstrates abnormal, sudden or repetitive movements of any part of the body, investigations of possible convulsions should be undertaken. However, Ballweg (1991) suggests that the type of movement can help classify the convulsion as subtle, tonic, multifocal clonic, focal clonic or myoclonic. The specific appearance of these convulsions is as follows.

Subtle convulsions include movements such as blinking or fluttering of the eyelids, staring, clonic movements of the chin, horizontal or downward movements of the eyes, sucking, drooling, sticking the tongue out, cycling movements of the legs and apnoea. Both term and preterm babies can experience subtle convulsions. These movements should be differentiated from the normal movements associated with rapid eye movement (REM) sleep.

If the baby has *tonic convulsions*, there will be extension or flexion of the limbs, altered patterns of breathing and maintenance of eye deviations. Tonic convulsions are more common in preterm babies.

Term babies demonstrate *multifocal clonic convulsions* and the movements include random jerking movements of the extremities.

Term babies also experience *focal clonic convulsions*, in which localised repetitive clonic jerking movements are seen. An extremity, a limb or a localised muscle group can be affected.

Myoclonic convulsions are the least common; they affect both term and preterm babies. The movements are single or multiple flexion jerks of the feet, legs, hands or arms, which should not be confused with similar movements in a sleeping baby.

During a convulsion the baby may have tachycardia, hypertension, raised cerebral blood flow and raised intracranial pressure, all of which predispose to serious complications.

There are many conditions that cause newborn convulsions; they are classified into central nervous system causes, metabolic causes, other causes and idiopathic causes (Table 44.1).

Treatment

Immediate treatment of a convulsion necessitates obtaining assistance from a doctor while ensuring that the baby has a clear airway and adequate ventilation, either spontaneously or mechanically. The baby can be turned to the semiprone position, with the head neither hyperflexed nor hyperextended. Gentle oral and nasal suction may be required to remove any milk or mucus. If the baby is breathing spontaneously but is cyanosed, facial oxygen is given. Resuscitation is required if apnoea occurs and cyanosis persists. The

Table 44.1 Selected causes of neonatal convulsions

Category	Selected causes
Central nervous system	Intracranial haemorrhage Intracerebral haemorrhage Hypoxic–ischaemic encephalopathy Kernicterus Congenital abnormalities
Metabolic	Hypo- and hyperglycaemia Hypo- and hypercalcaemia Hypo- and hypernatraemia Inborn errors of metabolism
Other	Hypoxia Congenital infections Severe postnatally acquired infections Neonatal abstinence syndrome Hyperthermia
Idiopathic	Unknown

baby should not be handled unnecessarily. If the baby is nursed in an incubator without covering blankets, yet dressed and well supported, observation and maintenance of a neutral thermal environment can be achieved.

It is important that observations of a convulsion are documented, noting the type of movement, the areas affected, its length, any colour change, any change in heart rate, respiratory rate or blood pressure and any immediate sequelae.

If a convulsion is suspected, a complete history and physical and laboratory investigations would be undertaken, related to the possible causes.

An electroencephalogram (EEG) can help detect the abnormal electrical brain activity associated with convulsions, and guide treatment. The aims of care are to treat the primary cause and control the convulsions. The pharmacological treatment of convulsions is controversial in respect of which anticonvulsant to use, at what dose and for how long treatment should continue (Ballweg 1991, Levene et al 2000).

The drug most commonly used is phenobarbital, given intravenously (IV) as a loading dose followed by a maintenance dose given IV or orally (Northern Neonatal Network 1998). Phenytoin can help control convulsions and is usually given IV as a loading dose, followed by a maintenance dose (Northern Neonatal Network 1998).

Other anticonvulsants such as clonazepam, paraldehyde and diazepam have been effective, but their side-effects limit their use (Levene et al 2000). Anticonvulsant therapy may be discontinued when convulsions cease, preferably before the baby is discharged home, although some babies continue to need therapy for 3–6 months (Anonymous 1989).

The outcome for babies who have convulsions is also controversial and statistics vary remarkably. Ballweg (1991) suggests that the prognosis depends on the cause of convulsion, the type of convulsion and the EEG tracing. Babies with congenital malformations of the brain, hypoxic–ischaemic encephalopathy, PVH/IVH of grade 3 or grade 4/PHI or types of bacterial meningitis tend to have a higher mortality or a poor neurological outcome. However, babies with late hypocalcaemia, hyponatraemia, benign familial neonatal seizures or primary subarachnoid haemorrhage are more likely to survive neurologically intact (Moe & Paige 1998).

Babies with subtle, generalised tonic and some myoclonic convulsions have a poorer neurological outcome than babies experiencing other types of convulsions. Abnormal EEG tracings generally indicate a poor prognosis (Ballweg 1991, Blackburn 1993). The need for well-conducted randomised controlled trials to determine the most effective treatment remains.

Parents

When their baby suffers trauma during birth, or haemorrhage or convulsions, parents are likely to be extremely shocked. Although the care of parents is more comprehensively discussed elsewhere, it is important to summarise their care under these circumstances.

Although the extent of the contact with parents will depend on circumstances, all parents are entitled to be given honest, clear information about their baby's condition as soon as possible after detection. It is recommended that parents receive such bad news when they are together and from someone who is known to them (Richards & Reed 1991). Involvement of the neonatologist is advisable. Uninterrupted time for giving information is essential, as is time for questions, which the parents should be encouraged to ask. Follow-up discussions are essential and all verbal interaction should be documented so other staff not intimately involved can understand what the parents have been told and so do not give conflicting information. Parental involvement in their baby's care is essential.

Continuing supportive care for parents is usually required and help may be available from specialised outside agencies if parents consider this helpful to them (Price 1994, Richards & Reed 1991, Sablewicz et al 1994).

REFERENCES

Anonymous 1989 Neonatal seizures. Lancet 8655:135–137

Anonymous 1998 Which vitamin K preparation for the neonate. Drug and Therapeutics Bulletin 36(3):17–19

Ansell P, Bull D, Roman E 1996 Childhood leukaemia and intramuscular vitamin K: findings from a case control study. British Medical Journal 313:204–205

Ballweg D D 1991 Neonatal seizures: an overview. Neonatal Network 10(1):15–21

Blackburn S T 1993 Assessment and management of neurological dysfunction. In: Kenner C, Brueggemeyer A, Gunderson L P (eds) Comprehensive neonatal nursing. W B Saunders, Philadelphia, ch 29, p. 564–607

Bolisetty S, Gupta J M, Graham G G et al 1998 Vitamin K in preterm breastmilk with maternal supplementation. Acta Paediatrica 87(9):960–962

Cullens V 2000 Brain injury in the premature infant. In: Boxwell G (ed) Neonatal intensive care nursing. Routledge, London, ch 7, p 152–163

Deitch J S 1993 Periventricular–intraventricular hemorrhage in the very low birth weight infant. Neonatal Network 12(1):7–16

Dent J 2000 Haematological problems In: Boxwell G (ed) Neonatal intensive care nursing. Routledge, London, ch 8, p. 164–187

Ekelund H, Finnström O, Gunnarskog J et al 1993 Administration of vitamin K to newborn infants and childhood cancer. British Medical Journal 307:89–91

Emery M L 1992 Disseminated intravascular coagulation in the neonate. Neonatal Network 11(8):5–14

Furdon S, Clark D 2001 Differentiating scalp swelling in the newborn. Advances in Neonatal Care 1(1):22–27

Gasking D 1998 Vitamin K: implications for prophylaxis. Journal of Neonatal Nursing 4(1):29–33

Glass S M 1999 Haematological disorders. In: Deacon J, O'Neill P (eds) Core curriculum for neonatal intensive care nursing, 2nd edn. W B Saunders, London, ch 16, p 383–412

Golding J, Patterson M, Kinlen L J 1990 Factors associated with childhood cancer in a national cohort study. British Journal of Cancer 62:304–308

Golding J, Greenwood R, Birmingham K et al 1992 Childhood cancer, intramuscular vitamin K and pethidine given during labour. British Medical Journal 305:341–346

Greer F R 1999 Vitamin K status of lactating mothers and their infants. Acta Paediatrica 88(430):95–103

Greer F R, Marshall S P, Foley A L et al 1997 Improving the vitamin K status of breastfeeding infants with maternal vitamin K supplements. Pediatrics 99(1):88–92

Heuchan A-M 1999 Intraventricular haemorrhage. Online. Available: www.cs.nsw.gov.au/rpa/neonatal/html/newprot/ivh.htm 11/01

Horbar J D 1992 Prevention of periventricular–intraventricular hemorrhage. In: Sinclair J C, Bracken M B (eds) Effective care of the newborn infant. Oxford University Press, Oxford, ch 23, p 562–589

Jackson S 1993 Vitamin K prophylaxis in infancy. British Journal of Midwifery 1(3):128–132

Jobe A H, Mitchell B R, Gunkel J H 1993 Beneficial effects of the combined use of prenatal corticosteroids and postnatal surfactant on preterm infants. American Journal of Obstetrics and Gynecology 168:508–513

Johnson M, Rodden D, Collins S 1998 Newborn hematology. In: Merenstein G B, Gardner S L (eds) Handbook of neonatal intensive care, 4th edn. C V Mosby, St Louis, ch 19, p 367–392

Katz K, Nishioka E 1998 Neonatal assessment. In: Kenner C, Lott J W, Flandermeyer A A (eds) Comprehensive neonatal nursing: a physiologic perspective. W B Saunders, Philadelphia, ch 17, p 223–251

Klebanoff M A, Read J S, Mills J L et al 1993 The risk of childhood cancer after neonatal exposure to vitamin K. New England Journal of Medicine 329(13):905–908

Korones S B 1986 High-risk newborn infants, 4th edn. C V Mosby, St Louis

Lane P A, Hathaway W E 1985 Vitamin K in infancy. Journal of Pediatrics 106:351–359

Laurent D P 1997 Brachial plexus injury. Online. Available: http://nyneurosurgery.org/cfr/brachial plexus.htm 11/01

Levene M I, Tudehope D, Thearle M J 2000 Essentials of neonatal medicine, 3rd edn. Blackwell Science, Oxford

Loughnan P M, McDougall P N 1995 The duration of vitamin K_1 efficacy: is intramuscular vitamin K_1 acting as a depot preparation? Vitamin K in infancy: international symposium. Hoffman-La Roche, Switzerland

McCulloch M 1999 Neurological disorders. In: Deacon J, O'Neill P (eds) Core curriculum for neonatal intensive care nursing, 2nd edn. W B Saunders, London, ch 19, p 474–509

McKinney P A, Jaszczak E, Findlay E et al 1998 Case–control study of childhood leukaemia and cancer in Scotland: findings for neonatal intramuscular vitamin K. British Medical Journal 316:173–179

Magill-Cuerden J 1997 Vitamin K unresolved. Modern Midwife 7(2):4

Mercer B M, Arheart K L 1995 Antimicrobial therapy in expectant management of preterm premature rupture of the membranes. Lancet 8985(346):1271–1279

Moe P, Paige P L 1998 Neurologic disorders. In: Merenstein G B, Gardner S L (eds) Handbook of neonatal intensive care, 4th edn. CV Mosby, St Louis, ch 25, p 571–603

Northern Neonatal Network 1998 Neonatal formulary, 10th edn. BMJ Books, London

Papile L A, Burnstein J, Burnstein R et al 1978 Incidence and evolution of subependymal and intraventricular hemorrhage: a study of infants with birth weights less than 1500 gm. Journal of Pediatrics 92:529–534

Parker L, Cole M, Craft A W et al 1998 Neonatal vitamin K administration and childhood cancer in the north of England: retrospective case–control study. British Medical Journal 305:341–346

Price W R 1994 What do families need and what can we do to meet their needs? Neonatal Network 13(5):70

RCM (Royal College of Midwives) 1996 Position paper no 13. The midwife's role in the administration of vitamin K. RCM, London

Richards C, Reed J 1991 Your baby has Down's syndrome. Nursing Times 87(46):60–61

Sablewicz P, Kershaw B, Mangan P 1994 Breaking bad news: the role of the nurse. Nursing Times 90(11) (unit 2):5–8

Soin H, Katesmark M 1993 By muscle or mouth. Nursing Times 89(42):32–33

Sola M C, Del Vecchio A, Rimsza L M 2000 Evaluation and treatment of thrombocytopenia in the neonatal intensive care unit. Clinics in Perinatology 27(2):655–679

Thomas R, Harvey D 1997 Colour guide: neonatology, 2nd edn. Churchill Livingstone, Edinburgh

Tortora G J, Grabowski S R 2000 Principles of anatomy and physiology, 9th edn. John Wiley, New York

Tripp J 1997 Vitamin K: mandatory prevention for breast fed babies. Modern Midwife 7(10):22–25

Tripp J H, McNinch A W 1998 The vitamin K debacle: cut the Gordian knot but first do no harm. Archives of Disease in Childhood 79:295–299

Tripp J H, McNinch A W 1999 Letter – the vitamin K debacle: cut the Gordian knot. Archives of Disease in Childhood 81:372

Tyler S 1996 Catching up with vitamin K. Midwives 109(1305):273

Uhrynowska M, Maslanka K, Zupanska B 1997 Neonatal thrombocytopenia: incidence, serological and clinical observations. American Journal of Perinatology 14:415–418

Volpe J J 1997 Brain injury in the premature infant. Clinics in Perinatology 24(3):567–587

von Kries R, Gobel U, Hachmeister A et al 1996 Vitamin K and childhood cancer: a population-based case–control study in Lower Saxony, Germany. British Medical Journal 313:199–203

Wariyar U, Hilton S, Pagan J et al 2000 Six years' experience of prophylactic oral vitamin K. Archives of Disease in Childhood Fetal and Neonatal Edition 82:F64–F68

Weindling M 1995 Periventricular haemorrhage and periventricular leukomalacia. British Journal of Obstetrics and Gynaecology 102(4):278–281

WHO (World Health Organisation) 1989 Infant feeding: the physiologic basis. Bulletin 67 (suppl):28–29

Wyly M 1995 Premature infants and their families. Singular Publishing, San Diego

Zipursky A 1999 Prevention of vitamin K deficiency bleeding in newborns. British Journal of Haematology 104(3):430–437

Zupan V, Gonzalez P, Lacaze-Masmonteil T et al 1996 Periventricular leukomalacia: risk factors revisited. Developmental Medicine and Child Neurology 38(12):1061–1067

FURTHER READING

Boxwell G (ed) 2000 Neonatal intensive care nursing. Routledge, London

This book is primarily written for neonatal nurses and teachers. Student midwives and midwives would benefit from the additional more detailed information about many of the conditions addressed in this chapter. Chapters 2, 7, 8, 9, 17 and 19 are recommended.

Clark D A, Thompson J E, Barkemeyer B M 2000 Atlas of neonatology. W B Saunders, Philadelphia, ch 1

This illustrative companion to Avery's Diseases of the newborn is designed using a systems approach to give examples of fetal and neonatal conditions. The illustrations in Chapter 1 supplement those given in this chapter.

Gasking D 1998 Vitamin K: implications for prophylaxis. Journal of Neonatal Nursing 4(1):29–33

Written by a neonatal nurse, this article presents a clear discussion of some of the issues related to vitamin K. The need for more research into the nature and role of vitamin K in the newborn is emphasised.

45 Congenital Abnormalities

Tom Turner

CHAPTER CONTENTS

Looking forward to the arrival of a healthy baby is every prospective parent's dream. Sadly for some this dream is shattered when the presence of some form of abnormality is recognised prenatally, at birth or in the neonatal period. According to Modell & Modell (1992) the incidence of major congenital abnormalities is 2–3% of all births. This figure is of course subject to familial, cultural and geographic variations for certain abnormalities. It is therefore very likely that every practising midwife will at some time be confronted with the challenge of providing appropriate care and support for such babies and their families.

The chapter aims to:

- describe and explain specific congenital abnormalities
- explore the complementary roles of the midwife and paediatrician in providing care
- address issues such as who should tell the parents and how and when they should be told
- consider the psychological impact on staff and the strategies that could be put in place to minimise the accompanying stress.

Definition and causes

By definition, a congenital abnormality is any defect in form, structure or function. Identifiable defects can be categorised in four ways:

- chromosome and gene abnormalities
- teratogenic causes
- multifactorial causes
- unknown causes.

Chromosome and gene abnormalities

Each human cell carries a blueprint for reproduction in the form of 44 chromosomes (autosomes) and two sex chromosomes. Each chromosome comprises a number of genes, which are portions of DNA coded for a particular protein. The fertilised zygote should have 22 autosomes and one sex chromosome from each parent. Should a fault occur in either the formation of the gametes or following fertilisation, an excess or deficit of chromosomal material will result. Each abnormal chromosomal pattern has a different clinical presentation. Only the most common of these will be discussed.

Genetic disorders (Mendelian inheritance)

Genes are composed of DNA and each is concerned with the transmission of one specific hereditary factor. Genetically inherited factors may be dominant or recessive.

A *dominant* gene will produce its effect even if present in only one chromosome of a pair. An autosomal dominant condition can usually be traced through several generations. Achondroplasia, osteogenesis imperfecta, adult polycystic kidney disease and Huntington's chorea are examples of dominant conditions.

A *recessive* gene needs to be present in both chromosomes before producing its effect. Examples of autosomal recessive conditions are cystic fibrosis or phenylketonuria.

Some congenital abnormalities are a consequence of single gene defects. In a dominantly inherited disorder the risk of an affected fetus is 1 : 2 (50%) for each and every pregnancy. In a recessive disorder the risk is 1 : 4 (25%) for each and every pregnancy. In an X-linked recessive inheritance the condition effects almost exclusively males, although females can be carriers. X-linked recessive inheritance is responsible for conditions such as haemophilia A and B and Duchenne muscular dystrophy. Spontaneous mutations commonly arise in X-linked recessive disorders. When a woman is a carrier of an X-linked condition, there is a 50% chance of each of her sons being affected and an equal chance that each of her daughters will be carriers.

The recent work on the human genome is likely to clarify further some of these disorders and may offer a way into treatment in the future; for example, polycystic kidney disease (see later) arises from a mutation on chromosome 6 and cystic fibrosis is due to a defect on chromosome 7.

Teratogenic causes

A teratogen is any agent that raises the incidence of congenital abnormality. The list of known and suspected teratogens is continually growing but includes: prescribed drugs (e.g. anticonvulsants, anticoagulants and preparations containing large concentrations of vitamin A such as those prescribed for the treatment of acne), drugs used in substance abuse (e.g. heroin, alcohol and nicotine), environmental factors such as radiation and chemicals (e.g. dioxins, pesticides), infective agents (e.g. rubella, cytomegalovirus) and maternal disease (e.g. diabetes). It should be borne in mind that several factors influence the effect(s) produced by any one teratogen, such as gestational age of the embryo or fetus at the time of exposure, length of exposure and toxicity of the teratogen. Direct cause and effect is sometimes difficult to establish.

Multifactorial causes

These are due to a genetic defect in addition to one or more teratogenic influences.

Unknown causes

In spite of a growing body of knowledge, the specific cause of around 80% of abnormalities remains unspecified.

The role of preconception advice

Although the midwife may advise on modulation of behaviour or diet during pregnancy, by the time the majority of women present for a booking visit the damage has been done. The burden of prevention therefore lies with dissemination of information and appropriate counselling in preconception clinics. The increasing awareness and availability of preconception advice has helped reduce the incidence of some categories of abnormality, notably those associated with poorly controlled diabetes and neural tube defects. Whyte (1995) cites a 72% decrease in neural tube defects as a result of folic acid supplements being taken prior to conception.

Prenatal screening and diagnosis

Improved prenatal screening and diagnostic techniques have led to increased recognition of abnormality, particularly in early pregnancy. This has resulted in some families making the decision to have their pregnancy terminated, whilst allowing many others time to adjust and try to come to terms with the news that their baby will be born with a particular problem. One advantage of prenatal diagnosis is that, if necessary, arrangements can be made for the mother to have prenatal transfer to a unit where neonatal surgical or intensive care facilities are available. The disadvantage of transfer is that the mother may then be separated from family, friends and the support of the midwives she knows best. This makes it all the more imperative that the staff in these units are sensitive to the needs of such women.

Breaking the news

It is often the midwife who first notices an abnormality in the baby either during the process of the birth or during the subsequent examination of the baby. All abnormalities, identified or suspected, should be notified to medical staff but there is sometimes a difference of opinion as to who should break the news to the parents.

There is a very strong argument for suggesting that this should be done by the midwife present at the delivery. The midwife–client relationship is or ought to be one of mutual trust and respect. Honesty is an implicit tenet of such a relationship. It is well recognised that one of the first questions a mother will ask of the midwife after the birth is 'is the baby all right?' For the midwife to be non-committal or economical with the truth is to betray that trust. It is preferable that the midwife tell the mother (and if possible the father

at the same time), albeit sensitively but honestly, and show her any obvious abnormality in the baby.

Where there is doubt in the midwife's mind, for example in cases of suspected chromosomal abnormalities, it could be argued that the issue is less clear cut. Discretion could therefore be exercised in the precise form of words used, but the intention of inviting a second opinion should be made clear to the parents. It is advisable that both the parents and the midwife be present when the paediatrician examines the baby and that the midwife be present during any dialogue between the parents and medical staff so that she is aware of exactly what has been said. She is then in a position to be able to clarify, explain or repeat any points not fully understood. Opportunities for repeat consultation with the paediatrician should be offered as and when the parents desire. Patience, tact and understanding are prerequisites for midwives caring for these families.

Some abnormalities are slight and cause no further problems for the parents or child, whereas others are profound and cause the subsequent daily care to be fraught with difficulties. Unlike most others, abnormalities involving the face cannot be disguised or hidden and therefore must rate amongst the most distressing for parents. This is confirmed by Wirt et al (1992) who claim that congenital defects of the head, face and neck often precipitate a major family crisis. The psychological impact on parents of being told or shown, or both, that their baby has a congenital abnormality is often not dissimilar to the grieving process discussed in Chapter 37. Great sensitivity is required on the part of the midwife when showing the baby to the parents for the first time.

Since a comprehensive discussion of every abnormality is clearly not possible, selection has been made of those the midwife is most likely to encounter.

Fetal alcohol syndrome

This topic has been chosen to open the discussion on congenital abnormalities since the direct link between the abuse of alcohol and this condition is established. Preconception preparation for pregnancy advice on alcohol intake, if heeded, could dramatically reduce the incidence of this phenomenon. Health promotion objectives and successful outcomes are, however, rarely totally synchronous.

The midwife may be alerted to the possibility of a baby being born with this syndrome prenatally if, in addition to psychosocial markers, clinical intrauterine growth restriction is evident. Postnatally the following characteristics are recognisable: a growth-restricted infant with microcephaly, flat facies, close-set eyes, epicanthic folds, small upturned nose, thin upper lip and low set ears. According to Spohr et al (1993) most of these features become less pronounced as the child grows. Microcephaly, small stature and mental retardation remain. The baby will probably experience acute withdrawal symptoms and require appropriate supportive therapies. The midwife will need to exercise counselling skills to provide much-needed support for the mother. Collaboration with social services is usually called for to ensure that the care options decided are in the best interests of the family.

Establishing such a direct link between a teratogen and such a complex clinical pattern is the exception rather than the rule.

Gastrointestinal malformations

Most of the abnormalities affecting this system call for prompt surgical intervention, for example atresias, gastroschisis and exomphalos. With the increasing use of routine ultrasound screening at 18–20 weeks' gestation many are likely to be diagnosed prenatally. If prenatal diagnosis has been made, the parents will be at least partially prepared. In this event, where possible, the paediatric team of neonatal paediatrician and paediatric surgeon should speak to the parents before delivery of the baby to explain the probable sequence of events. Once the baby is born, prior to obtaining their consent for surgery, the paediatric surgeon should have a full discussion with the parents. If the baby's condition allows, the parents should be encouraged to hold the baby and photographs should be taken.

Gastroschisis and exomphalos

Gastroschisis (Fig. 45.1) is a paramedian defect of the abdominal wall with extrusion of bowel that is not covered by peritoneum, thus making it very vulnerable to infection and injury. Surgical closure of the defect is usually possible; the size of the defect will determine whether primary closure is possible or whether a temporary silo made from synthetic materials

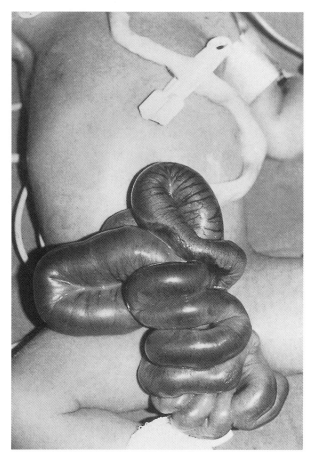

Fig. 45.1 Gastroschisis showing prolapsed intestine to the right of umbilical cord. (From Rennie & Roberton 1999, with permission of Churchill Livingstone.)

(e.g. Silastic) is necessary until the abdominal cavity is able to contain all the abdominal organs.

Exomphalos or omphalocele (Fig. 45.2) is a defect in which the bowel or other viscera protrude through the umbilicus. Very often these babies have other abnormalities, for example heart defects, which could be a contraindication to surgery in the immediate neonatal period. Closure of the defect may consequently be delayed as long as 1 or even 2 years.

The immediate management of both the above conditions is to cover the herniated abdominal contents with clean cellophane wrap (e.g. Clingfilm) or warm sterile saline swabs to reduce fluid and heat losses and to give a degree of protection. Stomach contents should be aspirated. It is important to reduce heat losses in these babies by either appropriate wrapping

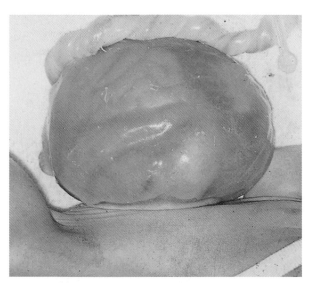

Fig. 45.2 Omphalocele defect with bowel visible through sac in the lower part and abnormally lobulated liver in the sac in the upper part. (From Rennie & Roberton 1999, with permission of Churchill Livingstone.)

or incubator care, or both. Transfer of the baby to a surgical unit is then expedited.

Atresias

Oesophageal atresia

Oesophageal atresia (Fig. 45.3) occurs when there is incomplete canalisation of the oesophagus in early intrauterine development. It is commonly associated with tracheo-oesophageal fistula, which connects the trachea to the upper or lower oesophagus, or both. The commonest type of abnormality is where the upper oesophagus terminates in a blind upper pouch and the lower oesophagus connects to the trachea. This abnormality should be suspected in the presence of maternal polyhydramnios and should be screened for after birth in all such affected pregnancies. At birth the baby has copious amounts of mucus coming from the mouth. Early detection is essential. The midwife should attempt to pass a wide orogastric tube but it may travel less than 10–12 cm. Radiography will confirm the diagnosis. The baby must be given no oral fluid but a wide bore oesophageal tube should be passed into the upper pouch and connected to gentle continuous suction apparatus. Usually a double lumen 10 fg (replogle) tube is used and the baby nursed head up. He should be transferred immediately

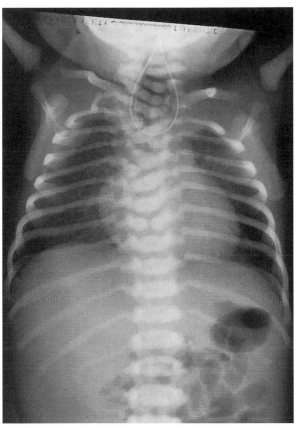

Fig. 45.3 Oesophageal atresia. Coiled feeding tube in proximal pouch. Note vertebral and rib abnormalities. Distal gas confirms a tracheo-oesophageal fistula. (From Rennie & Roberton 1999, with permission of Churchill Livingstone.)

to a paediatric surgical unit, ensuring that continuous suction is available throughout the transfer. It may be possible to anastomose the blind ends of the oesophagus. If the gap in the oesophagus is too large a series of bouginages can be carried out in an attempt to stretch the ends of the oesophagus, stimulate growth and thereby eventually facilitate repair by end-to-end anastomosis. Alternatively transplant of, for example, a section of colon may be needed at a later date. Rarely, if the repair is delayed, cervical oesophagostomy may be performed to allow drainage of secretions. Meanwhile the baby will need to be fed via a gastrostomy tube. This method of feeding obviously deprives the baby of oral stimuli. Such a baby may be given 'sham' feeds to allow him to taste the milk and to promote sucking, swallowing and normal development of the mandible.

Duodenal atresia

Atresia may occur at any level of the bowel but the duodenum is the most common site. If this has not already been diagnosed in the prenatal period, persistent vomiting within 24–36 hours of birth will be the first feature encountered. The vomit will often contain bile unless the obstruction is proximal to the entrance of the common bile duct. Abdominal distension may not be present and the baby may pass meconium. A characteristic double bubble of gas may be seen on radiological examination (Fig. 45.4). Treatment is by surgical repair. Prognosis is good if the baby is otherwise healthy, but this abnormality is often associated with others; 30% of cases occur in children with Down syndrome, according to Roberton (1993).

Rectal atresia and imperforate anus

Careful examination of the perineum is an important aspect of any newborn examination. An imperforate anus should be obvious at birth on examination of the baby, but a rectal atresia might not become apparent until it is noted that the baby has not passed meconium. Occasionally, for the unwary, the passage of meconium through a rectovaginal fistula may mask an imperforate anus. Whatever the anatomical arrangement, all babies should be referred for surgery.

Should a baby fail to pass meconium in the first 24 hours, three other possibilities should be considered:

- malrotation/volvulus
- meconium ileus (cystic fibrosis)
- Hirschsprung's disease.

Malrotation/volvulus

This is a developmental abnormality where incomplete rotation of the small bowel has taken place, giving rise to signs of obstruction. There is often bilious vomiting and abdominal distension.

Surgical assessment and correction are necessary. Because of the risks of severe bowel damage secondary to the obstruction of blood flow in the mesentery in unrecognised malrotation, any newborn infant with bile-stained vomiting requires urgent medical assessment.

Meconium ileus (cystic fibrosis)

Fifteen percent of children with cystic fibrosis present with meconium ileus in the neonatal period. Cystic fibrosis is an autosomal recessive condition affecting 1

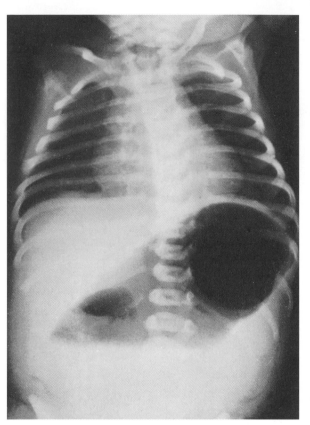

Fig. 45.4 Double bubble of duodenal atresia. The stomach is overlapping the duodenum with the second bubble being seen through the stomach. (From Rennie & Roberton 1999, with permission of Churchill Livingstone.)

in 2500 births. In the past, the majority of cases were not diagnosed until later in infancy or childhood when the child failed to thrive or had repeated chest infections. In meconium ileus the meconium is particularly viscous and causes intestinal obstruction. There is accompanying abdominal distension and bile-stained vomiting. Intravenous fluids and a gastrografin enema may relieve the obstruction. Definitive diagnosis may be difficult initially, but the presence of a raised immunoreactive trypsin level (IRT) and of markers in the serum using the polymerase chain reaction (PCR) may demonstrate the $\Delta F508$ deletion in both copies of the cystic fibrosis gene on chromosome 7. Histology of any resected bowel may also indicate the likelihood of cystic fibrosis, but a definitive diagnosis is not usually possible until a sweat test has been carried out at 4–6 weeks of age. Treatment of cystic fibrosis is supportive rather than curative and involves administration of pancreatic enzymes and a rigorous programme of chest physiotherapy and antibiotics as indicated by bacteriological evidence.

Hirschsprung's disease

In this disease, which has an incidence of 1 in 5000 births, an aganglionic section of the large bowel is present. This means that peristalsis does not occur and the bowel therefore becomes obstructed. The baby develops abdominal distension and bile-stained vomiting. Definite diagnosis is made by carrying out a rectal biopsy. Resection of the aganglionic segment of bowel is indicated.

Pyloric stenosis

Pyloric stenosis arises from a genetic defect that causes hypertrophy of the muscles of the pyloric sphincter. The characteristic clinical presentation is projectile vomiting usually at around 6 weeks of age, but it may occur earlier and hence is included in this section. There is a gender-related predominance in that it is usually boys who are affected. Surgical repair is effected by pyloromyotomy (Ramstedt's operation), which involves partial splitting of the hypertrophied pyloric muscle along its length.

The remaining abnormalities of the gastrointestinal system, while amenable to surgery, do not usually necessitate immediate action.

Cleft lip and cleft palate

The incidence of cleft lip occurring as a single deformity is 1.3 in 1000. This defect may be unilateral or bilateral. Since it is very often accompanied by cleft palate, both will be considered together.

Clefts in the palate may affect the hard palate, soft palate, or both. Some defects will include alveolar margins and some the uvula. It is recommended that, during the initial examination of the baby, the palate be examined by means of a good light source rather than by digital palpation. The greatest problem for these babies initially is feeding. If the defect is limited to unilateral cleft lip, mothers who had intended to breastfeed should be encouraged to do so. Where there is the additional problem of cleft palate, arranging for the baby to be fitted with an orthodontic plate may facilitate breastfeeding but this obviously does not afford the same stimulus as nipple-to-palate contact.

Middle ear infection is a concomitant risk for babies with cleft palate. Repeated infections of this type could impede hearing and subsequent development of speech.

Danner (1992) suggests that breastfeeding be encouraged since passive immunity may protect these babies from the infections to which they are prone. Expressed breastmilk may of course be given. Cup or spoon feeding is an alternative method but for those who wish to bottle feed there is a wide variety of specially shaped teats available to accommodate the different sizes and positions of palate defects. Above all else, an unending supply of patience is required. The midwife should encourage the mother and father to find the most successful technique rather than 'taking over' since this may compound any feelings of guilt or inadequacy the parents may feel. Early referral to the cleft team of paediatric or plastic surgeon and orthodontists should be arranged. These teams may also include specialist nursing staff, speech and language therapists and audiologists.

Corrective surgery will be carried out at some stage but there is some debate as to the most appropriate time to carry out these procedures. Sullivan (1996) examines the arguments for both early and late repair of a cleft lip. He explains that some surgeons advocate effecting closure of the cleft lip within 2 weeks of birth in order to capitalise on the increased tissue-healing properties that are present as a short-lived legacy of intrauterine existence. They also argue that an early repair will be instrumental in encouraging healthy attachment between mother and baby. Advocates of later intervention suggest cleft lip repair at the age of 3–4 months because cleft lip often occurs as a feature of other medical conditions that may not be detected immediately. Surgery in the early neonatal period for such a baby may be too hazardous. Closure of the palate defect is suggested at around the age of 12–15 months. One of the main reasons for this apparently long delay is to allow sufficient growth to take place, which may result in reducing the size of the defect thus increasing the possibility of a more satisfactory repair. Some children have a series of cosmetic operations at some time after the initial repairs are carried out. It is often helpful for the midwife to show families 'before and after' photographs of babies for whom surgery has been a success (Fig. 45.5A and B).

Clearly, although the midwife may offer valuable support in these early days, she is limited in the length of time she has available to help these families. Giving the parents the address of a support group such as the Cleft Lip And Palate Association (CLAPA) is useful (see Useful addresses, p. 861).

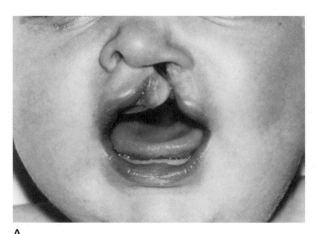
A

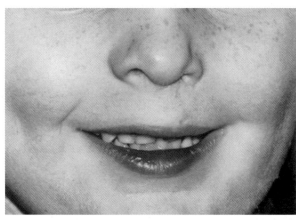
B

Fig. 45.5 A, B (A) Cleft lip and palate. (B) The repaired cleft. (From Raine 1994, with permission of Churchill Livingstone.)

Pierre Robin syndrome

Pierre Robin syndrome is characterised by micrognathia (hypoplasia of the lower jaw), abnormal attachment of muscles controlling the tongue, which allows it to fall backward and occlude the airway, and a central cleft palate. This triad of abnormalities presents a challenge for nursing care. Maintenance of a clear airway is paramount. In order to achieve this the baby will need to be nursed prone and some may require the insertion of an oral airway. Nasal and nasopharyngeal constant positive airways pressure may be necessary for some time after birth. This is one of the few exceptions to the 'Back to sleep' campaign aimed at reducing cot deaths. Feeding can be problematic. There is a high risk of aspiration occurring. Suction catheter and oxygen equipment should be ready to hand. Some of these babies may be fitted with an orthodontic plate to facilitate feeding. The action of sucking will encourage development of the mandible. Parents will need considerable support during what may for some babies be a protracted period of hospitalisation. Discharge will be when the lower jaw has grown sufficiently or when the parents feel comfortable about taking the baby home. Habel et al (1996) suggest that some of these babies can have an earlier transfer home if a shortened endotracheal tube is in place to ensure a patent nasopharyngeal airway. They recommend replacing the tube every 2 weeks until adequate mandibular development has taken place. Despite this, there remains a small risk of sudden death in these infants.

Abnormalities relating to respiration

Making a successful transition from fetus to neonate includes being able to establish regular respiration. Any abnormality of the respiratory tract or accessory respiratory muscles is likely to hamper this process.

Diaphragmatic hernia

This abnormality consists of a defect in the diaphragm that allows herniation of abdominal contents into the thoracic cavity (Fig. 45.6). The extent to which lung development is compromised as a result depends on the size of the defect and the gestational age at which herniation first occurred. The condition is increasingly diagnosed antenatally by ultrasound; where there is prenatal diagnosis, delivery in a specialist unit is advisable. At birth, the condition may be suspected if the baby is cyanosed and difficulty is experienced in resuscitation. In addition, since the majority of such defects are left sided, heart sounds will be displaced to the right. The abdomen may have a flat or scaphoid appearance. Chest X-ray will confirm the diagnosis. Continuous gastric suction should be commenced. Surgical repair of the defect is necessary, but this is not urgent. It's more important to stabilise the baby's general condition before surgery. It is especially critical to deal with the problem of persistent pulmonary hypertension and right-to-left shunting of blood within the heart. This may necessitate the use of newer ventilation techniques and pharmacological

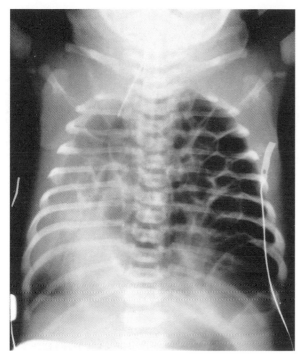

Fig. 45.6 Chest radiograph of infant at 1 hour of life, showing left diaphragmatic hernia, displacement of air-filled viscera into the hemithorax and a marked shift of mediastinum and heart. (From Rennie & Roberton 1999, with permission of Churchill Livingstone.)

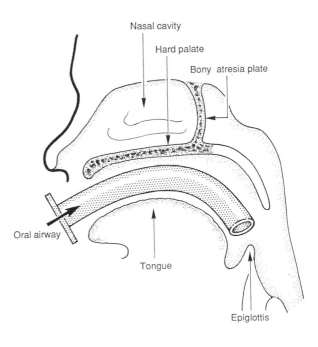

Fig. 45.7 Choanal atresia. A bony plate blocks the nose. (From Rennie & Roberton 1999, with permission of Churchill Livingstone.)

agents such as nitric oxide. Prognosis relates to the degree of pulmonary hypoplasia. There is also the possibility of coexistent abnormalities such as cardiac defects or skeletal anomalies. The incidence is 1 in 2000 births.

Choanal atresia

Choanal atresia describes a unilateral or bilateral narrowing of the nasal passage(s) with a web of tissue or bone occluding the nasopharynx (Fig. 45.7). Tachypnoea and dyspnoea are cardinal features, particularly when a bilateral lesion is present. The diagnosis is made relatively easily by noting that the baby mouth breathes and finds feeding impossible without cyanosis. In addition, nasal catheters cannot be passed into the pharynx and if a mirror or cold spoon is held under the nose no vapour will collect. A helpful diagnostic aid is that the baby's colour will improve with crying (Bagwell 1993). Maintaining a clear airway is obviously essential and an oral airway may have to be used to effect this. *A unilateral defect may not be noticed until the baby feeds for the first time. The midwife should therefore bear in mind the possibility of this problem if respiratory difficulty and cyanosis occur at this time.* Surgery will be required to remove the obstructing tissue. The incidence is 1 in 8000. Occasionally choanal atresia is associated with other abnormalities such as 'Charge' syndrome, a syndrome in which there are defects found in the eye (coloboma), the heart, the ear, occasionally oesophageal atresia and usually growth retardation.

Laryngeal stridor

This is a noise made by the baby, usually on inspiration and exacerbated by crying. Most commonly the cause is laryngomalacia, which is due to laxity of the laryngeal cartilage. Although it sounds distressing, the baby generally is not at all upset. It is the parents who require comforting and reassurance (often repeatedly). It should be explained to them that the stridor may take some time to resolve, perhaps up to 2 years. If, however, the stridor is accompanied by signs of dyspnoea or feeding problems, further investigations such as bronchoscopy or laryngoscopy would become necessary to rule out a more sinister cause.

Congenital cardiac defects

Babies born with congenital heart defects comprise the second largest group of babies born with abnormalities, according to Nixon & O'Donnell (1992). Approximately 8 in 1000 livebirths have some degree of congenital heart disease and about one-third of babies will be symptomatic in early infancy.

Causes

Approximately 90% of cardiac defects cannot be attributed to a single cause, chromosomal and genetic factors account for 8%, and a further 2% are reckoned to be caused by teratogens. The critical period of exposure to teratogens in respect of embryological development of cardiac tissue is from the 3rd to the 6th week.

Prenatal detection

An increasing number of cardiac problems are being identified by means of detailed ultrasound scanning (see Ch. 23). However, the detection of many defects is still dependent upon accurate observations and examination during the neonatal period.

Postnatal recognition

Clinically, babies with cardiac anomalies can be divided into two groups: those with central cyanosis and those without, i.e. cyanotic and acyanotic congenital heart disease.

Cardiac defects presenting with cyanosis

Defects included in this group are in order of frequency:

- transposition of the great vessels
- pulmonary atresia
- Fallot's tetralogy
- tricuspid atresia
- total anomalous pulmonary venous drainage
- univentricular/complex heart.

The persistence of central cyanosis (i.e. cyanosis of the lips and mucous membranes), tachypnoea and tachycardia may be the first signs that a cardiac defect is present. If cyanosis is present, administration of oxygen to these babies will be ineffective in improving their colour and oxygen saturation monitoring will show no improvement. Indeed, giving 100% oxygen may encourage closure of the ductus arteriosus, the patency of which, as Paul (1995) remarks, is literally a lifeline for some of these babies. If 100% oxygen therapy does not lead to improvement within 10 minutes of starting, the midwife should not persist at that concentration without seeking medical advice. Chest X-ray should be carried out to exclude abnormalities of the respiratory tract, respiratory disease and diaphragmatic hernia. The precise nature of the cardiac anomaly will need to be further explored by electrocardiography and echocardiography.

The baby with transposition of the great arteries is worthy of special mention since early detection allows intervention, which will be life saving. This is a condition wherein the aorta arises from the right ventricle and the pulmonary artery from the left ventricle (Fig. 45.8). Consequently, oxygenated blood is circulated back through the lungs and deoxygenated blood back into the systemic circuit. It is apparent therefore that unless there is an opportunity for oxygenated blood to access the systemic circulation, either by means of a patent ductus arteriosus or through accompanying septal defects, such a baby will die. Maintaining the patency of the ductus arteriosus is essential.

Prostaglandin infusion should be commenced to achieve this, but many babies develop apnoea with this treatment and may require ventilatory support. Arrangements should be made to transfer the baby to a unit where an atrial septostomy (Rashkind) can be performed. This procedure involves enlarging the foramen ovale with a balloon catheter to allow oxygenated blood to cross at atrial level and hence into the systemic circulation. Corrective surgery is then carried out, usually within a few weeks of birth.

Pulmonary atresia usually produces early central cyanosis and responds well to prostaglandin therapy to keep the duct open while surgery (usually a palliative shunt, Blalock) is planned.

Tricuspid atresia usually occurs with a ventricular septal defect or an atrial septal defect, or both, allowing mixing of the circulation.

Potentially more distressing for the parents are the defects that do not initially present with marked

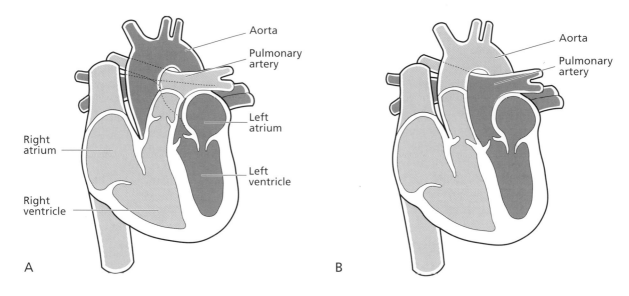

Fig. 45.8 Transposition of the great arteries. (A) Normal. (B) Transposition.

cyanosis. These babies may for a time be considered to be healthy.

Tetralogy of Fallot (Fig. 45.9) is a good example of this. In this condition there is pulmonary outflow tract obstruction, a ventricular septal defect, right ventricular hypertrophy and an overriding aorta. It seldom presents in the immediate newborn period, but produces problems a few weeks after birth with increasing cyanosis and heart failure. Corrective surgery is available.

'Acyanotic' cardiac defects

Anomalies subsumed under this heading include in order of frequency:

- patent ductus arteriosus
- ventricular or atrial septal defects
- coarctation of the aorta
- hypoplastic left heart syndrome.

Close observation of each baby in her care is part of the midwife's role. Astute observers may detect in these babies the first signs of cardiac failure, that is tachypnoea, tachycardia and incipient cyanosis, especially following the exertion of crying or feeding. These signs will become more evident, sometimes dramatically so,

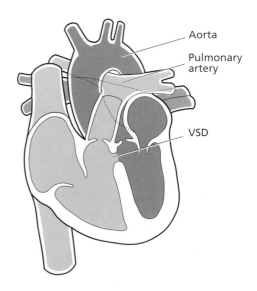

Fig. 45.9 Tetralogy of Fallot. (VSD = ventrical septal defect)

with the closure of the ductus arteriosus if either coarctation of the aorta or hypoplastic left heart syndrome is present. Detailed examination may disclose heart murmurs and diminution or absence of femoral pulses in both conditions. In this event resuscitation with prostaglandin usually stabilises the baby and allows time for further assessment. While coarctation of the aorta is usually amenable to surgical correction, hypoplastic left heart syndrome is still a major surgical challenge with a poor long term outcome. There is a substantial psychological impact on the parents following confirmation of such a diagnosis, which calls for particularly supportive management.

Patent ductus arteriosus, ventricular septal defects (Fig. 45.10) and atrial septal defects seldom require medical or surgical intervention in early neonatal life, but do require careful follow-up for signs of developing heart failure and may require surgery or interventional cardiology at a later stage.

Changing patterns of postnatal care often mean early discharge home. Ideally each baby should be examined by a competent practitioner before going home. It is equally important to realise, however, that not all heart murmurs heard at this time are significant. There is therefore increased responsibility on community midwives to be observant and to communicate effectively with parents. Parents who report any changes in the baby's behaviour such as breathlessness or cyanosis should never be ignored, but rather encouraged to seek medical advice promptly.

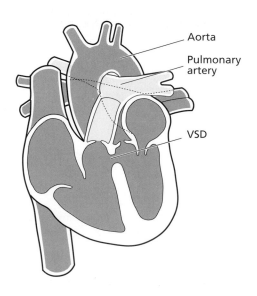

Fig. 45.10 Ventricular septal defect (VSD).

Aorta

Pulmonary artery

VSD

Central nervous system abnormalities

Ingestion of folic acid supplements prior to conception and during the early stages of pregnancy has helped prevent such abnormalities. In addition, the ability to recognise these anomalies prenatally (see Ch. 23) has resulted in some parents choosing selective termination of pregnancies where severe neural tube defects are found. All of these measures have combined to reduce the number of babies born with abnormalities of the central nervous system.

Anencephaly

This major abnormality describes the absence of the forebrain and vault of the skull. It is a condition that is incompatible with sustained life but occasionally such a baby is born alive. The midwife should wrap the baby carefully before showing him to the mother. It is recognised that seeing and holding the baby will facilitate the grieving process. It may be beneficial for the parents then to see the full extent of the abnormality, unpleasant though it is. Seeing the whole baby will help them to accept the reality of the situation and prevent imagination of an even more gruesome picture.

Spina bifida aperta

Spina bifida aperta results from failure of fusion of the vertebral column. There is no skin covering the defect, which allows protrusion of the meninges, hence the term *meningocele* (Fig. 45.11). The meningeal membrane may be flat or appear as a membranous sac, with or without cerebrospinal fluid, but it does not contain neural tissue. *Meningomyelocele*, on the other hand, does involve the spinal cord (Figs 45.11, 45.12 and Plate 31). This lesion may be enclosed, or the meningocele may rupture and expose the neural tissue. Meningomyelocele usually gives rise to neural damage, producing paralysis distal to the defect, and impaired function of urinary bladder and bowel. The lumbosacral area is the most common site for these to present, but they may appear at any point in the vertebral column. When the defect is at base of skull level it is known as an *encephalocele*. The added complication here is that the sac may contain varying amounts of brain tissue. Normal progression of labour may be impeded by a large lesion of this type.

Immediate management involves covering open lesions with a non-adherent dressing. Babies with enclosed lesions should be handled with the utmost care in an attempt to preserve the integrity of the sac. This will limit the risk of meningitis occurring. A paediatric surgeon or neurosurgeon should be contacted. Surgical intervention for myelomeningocele carries a high rate of success of skin closure, but has no impact on any damage already present in the cord or more distally. There is usually associated hydrocephalus (see below), which requires surgical shunting to prevent a rapid increase in the intracranial pressure. Nixon & O'Donnell (1992) suggest that it is no longer necessary to close the back within 24 hours of birth. Following examination of the baby, discussion with the parents will allow them to make an informed choice about whether or not they wish their baby to have surgery.

Spina bifida occulta

Spina bifida occulta (see Fig. 45.11) is the most minor type of defect where the vertebra is bifid. There is usually no spinal cord involvement. A tuft of hair or sinus at the base of the spine may be noted on first examination of the baby. Ultrasound investigation will confirm the diagnosis and rule out any associated spinal cord involvement.

Parents who have a baby with a neural tube defect should be offered genetic counselling since the risk of recurrence is 1 in 25.

Hydrocephalus

This condition arises from a blockage in the circulation and absorption of cerebrospinal fluid, which is produced from the choroid plexuses within the lateral ventricles of the brain. The large lateral ventricles increase in size and eventually compress the surrounding brain tissue. It is a not infrequent accompaniment to the more severe spina bifida lesions because of a structural defect around the area of the foramen magnum known as the Arnold–Chiari malformation. Consequently, hydrocephalus may either be present at birth or develop following surgical closure of a myelomeningocele. In the absence of myelomeningocele, aqueduct stenosis is the commonest cause of hydrocephalus. The risk of cerebral impairment may be minimised by the insertion of a ventriculoperitoneal shunt. As the baby grows, this will need to be

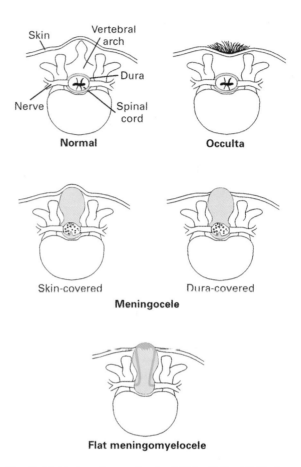

Flat meningomyelocele

Fig. 45.11 Various forms of spina bifida. (After Wallis & Harvey 1979, with permission of Nursing Times.)

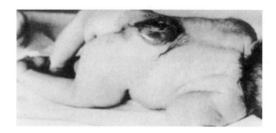

Fig. 45.12 Baby with meningomyelocele.

replaced. Attendant risks with these devices are that the line blocks and that the shunt is a portal for infection leading to meningitis. The midwife must be alert for the signs of increased intracranial pressure:

- large tense anterior fontanelle
- splayed skull sutures

- inappropriate increase in occipitofrontal circumference
- sun-setting appearance to the eyes
- irritability, or abnormal movements.

Microcephaly

This is where the occipitofrontal circumference is more than two standard deviations below normal for gestational age. The disproportionately small head may be the result of intrauterine infection (e.g. rubella), a feature of fetal alcohol syndrome, or part of a number of defects in some trisomic disorders. Most babies will have learning difficulties with evidence of cerebral palsy and often seizures.

Musculoskeletal deformities

These range from relatively minor anomalies, for example an extra digit, to major deficits such as absence of a limb.

Polydactyly and syndactyly

Careful examination including separation and counting of the baby's fingers and toes during the initial examination is important, otherwise anomalies such as syndactyly (webbing) and polydactyly (extra digits) may go unnoticed.

Syndactyly more commonly affects the hands. It can appear as an independent anomaly or as a feature of a syndrome such as Apert's syndrome; this is a genetically inherited condition in which there is premature fusion of the sutures of the vault of the skull, cleft palate and complete syndactyly of both hands and feet. Whether or not any surgical division needs to be carried out depends on the degree of webbing or fusion.

In *polydactyly* the extra digit(s) may be fully formed or simply extra tissue attached by a pedicle. Even where there is a rudimentary digit without bone involvement, better cosmetic results are obtained if the offending digit is surgically excised and this is mandatory in more complex cases.

Where there is a family history of either of these defects and this is common, the mother will be anxious to examine the baby for herself.

Limb reduction anomalies

Over the years various suggestions have been postulated with regard to the cause(s) of limb reduction anomalies. *Amniotic band syndrome* (see Plate 32) was the reason most often given for a baby being born with a limb deficit. It was thought that the amnion ruptured, then wrapped itself around a developing limb causing strangulation and necrosis. Although this may account for some instances, it cannot explain all of them. Clustering of cases in certain geographical areas, for example in close proximity to chemical waste plants, has provoked research in an attempt to identify environmental teratogens, as yet to no avail. One possibility being mooted is an iatrogenic cause – namely damage inflicted at the time of chorionic villus sampling (Carr & Lui 1994).

Limb reduction defects, which may be due to failure of formation (arrest of development), comprise a wide range of possibilities. In some either a hand or a foot will be completely missing, whereas in others a normal hand or foot will be present on the end of a shortened limb (longitudinal arrest). Thalidomide has been proven to be teratogenic in this context.

Although, as with any deviation from normal, the parents of a child with a limb defect will grieve for the loss of their perfect child, the child is not ill and will not be upset by the defect. Children usually prove themselves to be most adaptable and able to cope (Fig. 45.13). For those who require them, different types of prostheses are available and can be fitted as early as 3 months of age. Innovative surgical techniques such as the transferring of toe(s) to hand to serve as substitute finger(s) are proving successful for some children. Once again one of the most helpful things the midwife can do in these early days of parental adjustment is to offer the address of a support group such as Reach (see Useful addresses, p. 861). This appropriately named support group for parents of children with upper limb deformities has branches throughout the UK.

Talipes

Talipes equinovarus (TEV, club foot) is the descriptive term for a deformity of the foot where the ankle is bent downwards (plantarflexed) and the front part of the foot is turned inwards (inverted). Talipes calcaneovalgus describes the opposite position where the foot is dorsiflexed and everted. It is thought that these deformities are more likely to occur when intrauterine space has been at a premium, for example in multiple pregnancy, macrosomic fetus or oligohydramnios. TEV is also more likely to occur in conjunction with spina bifida deformities. They may be unilateral or bilateral. There is, in some instances, a family history of the defect. Statistically more boys than girls are born with talipes. In the mildest form the foot may easily be turned to the correct position. The midwife should encourage the mother to exercise the baby's foot in this way several times a day. More severe forms will require one or more of manipulation, splinting, or surgical correction. The advice of an orthopaedic surgeon should be sought as soon as possible after birth as early treatment with manipulation or splinting may enhance results. Care should be taken to ensure that, for babies who have splints applied, the strapping is not too tight and that the baby's toes are well perfused.

Developmental hip dysplasia

Congenital hip dysplasia is an abnormality more commonly found where there has been a history of oligohydramnios or breech presentation. It most often occurs in primigravida pregnancies and there is a higher percentage of girls than boys born with this defect. The left hip is more often affected than the right. The dysplastic hip may present in one of three ways: dislocated, dislocatable or with subluxation of the joint. Prenatal diagnosis by ultrasound is possible; most, however, are diagnosed in the neonatal period. Examination of the hip should be carried out by an experienced practitioner with the baby lying relaxed on a firm surface. It will depend on individual unit policies whether this is a midwife, paediatrician or GP. Repeated examinations by inexperienced people may compound any pre-existing damage to the joint. Either Ortolani's test or Barlow's test is employed (Ch. 39). Any abnormal findings should be reported and the baby referred for an orthopaedic opinion or ultrasound scan of the hips, or both. Where the diagnosis is confirmed it is usual for the baby to have a splint or harness such as the Pavlik harness (Fig. 45.14)

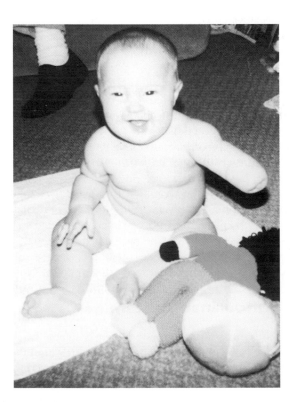

Fig. 45.13 A baby with a limb reduction defect quickly learns to adapt. (Photograph courtesy of Reach.)

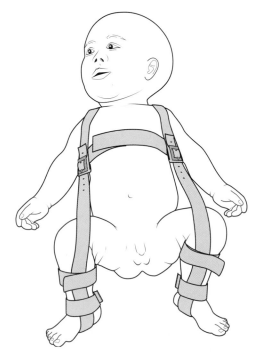

Fig. 45.14 Pavlik harness for congenital dislocation of hip. (From Barr 1992, with permission of Churchill Livingstone.)

applied, which will keep the hips in a flexed and abducted position of about 60%. The splint should not be removed for napkin changing or bathing (Le Maistre 1991). Parents will require additional support in learning how to handle and care for their baby. Particular attention should be paid to skin care and checking for signs of chafing or excoriation.

Achondroplasia

Achondroplasia is an autosomal dominant condition where the baby is generally small with a disproportionately large head and short limbs. Eighty per cent of cases are new mutations and hence these families may have no anticipation of the disorder unless an antenatal diagnosis has been made. These babies often develop a marked lordosis. Cognitive development is not usually impaired.

Osteogenesis imperfecta

This autosomal dominant disorder of collagen production has at least four forms and leads to unduly brittle bones in the affected fetus and infant. In some types (II–IV) it can cause either lethal multiple fractures of the skull, ribs and long bones in utero or neonatal long bone fractures. Recognition and genetic counselling are important for future pregnancies.

Abnormalities of the skin

Vascular naevi

These defects in the development of the skin can be divided into two main types, which commonly overlap.

Capillary malformations

These are due to defects in the dermal capillaries. The most commonly observed are 'stork marks'. These are usually found on the nape of the neck. They are generally small and will fade. No treatment is necessary.

Port wine stain

This is a purple-blue capillary malformation affecting the face. It occurs in approximately 1 in 3000 births and is twice as common in girls as in boys. This type of birthmark does not regress with time. However, laser

treatment and the skillful use of cosmetics will help to disguise the problem. The parents, and later the child, will need substantial psychological support.

Should the malformation appear to mimic the distribution of a branch of the trigeminal nerve, it can be suspected that there will be further malformations in the meninges. This is known as Sturge–Weber syndrome.

Capillary haemangiomata ('strawberry marks')

Capillary haemangiomata are not usually noticeable at birth but appear as red, raised lesions in the first few weeks of life. These lesions are particularly common in preterm infants and especially in girls. They can appear anywhere in the body but cause particular distress to the parents when they appear on the face. However, parents may be reassured that, although the lesion will grow bigger for the first few months (see Plate 33), it will then regress and usually disappears completely by the age of 5 to 6 years. No treatment is normally required unless the haemangioma is situated in an awkward area where it is likely to be subject to abrasion, such as on the lip. Treatment with steroids or pulsed laser therapy is possible.

Pigmented (melanocytic) naevi

These are brown, sometimes hairy, marks on the skin that vary in size and may be flat or raised. A percentage of this type of birthmark may become malignant. Surgical excision may be recommended to pre-empt this.

It is unlikely that treatment for any of these birthmarks will be carried out in the immediate neonatal period except in the case of larger pigmented naevi (see Plate 34). The midwife's responsibilities are therefore to notify appropriate medical staff and offer parents general emotional support.

Genitourinary system

At birth the first indication that there is an abnormality of the renal tract may be finding a single umbilical artery in the umbilical cord, or alternatively recognising the abnormal facies associated with Potter's syndrome (discussed later). Attention should be paid at the time of delivery to see whether the baby passes urine. If no urine is passed within 24 hours, the baby is noted to be dribbling urine constantly, or the urine stream seems poor, the paediatrician should be informed. Dribbling of urine is a sign of nerve damage such as occurs with neural tube defects, as previously discussed, whereas a poor urine stream may indicate lower urinary tract obstruction (posterior urethral valve).

Posterior urethral valve(s)

This is an abnormality affecting boys. The presence of valves in the posterior urethra prevents the normal outflow of urine. As a result the bladder distends, causing back pressure on the ureters and to the kidneys. This will ultimately cause hydronephrosis. Prenatal diagnosis and intervention by intrauterine fetal bladder catheterisation is possible. Failing this, early diagnosis in the neonatal period is clearly important but severe renal damage may already have been sustained. Different treatment strategies are possible with surgical procedures featuring prominently.

Polycystic kidneys

It is likely that problems may arise in delivering a baby with polycystic kidneys because of an increase in abdominal girth. On abdominal examination the kidneys will be palpable. Radiological or ultrasound investigations will be carried out to confirm the diagnosis. Unfortunately the prognosis is poor, as renal failure is the likely outcome. The severest forms of polycystic kidney disease are usually linked to an autosomal recessive inheritance, but an autosomal dominant variety also occurs with a less gloomy prognosis.

Hypospadias

Examination of a baby boy may reveal that the urethral meatus opens on to the undersurface of the penis. The meatus can be placed at any point along the length of the penis and in some cases will open on to the perineum. This abnormality often coexists with chordee, in which the penis is short and bent and the foreskin is present only on the dorsal side of the penis. It is anticipated that some babies will require surgery in the neonatal period to 'release' the chordee and enlarge the urethral meatus. It is important that the parents are made aware that circumcision should be deferred until consultation with the paediatric surgeon is completed.

Cryptorchidism

Undescended testes may be unilateral or bilateral and occur in 1–2% of male infants. If on examination of the baby after delivery the scrotum is empty, the undescended testes may be found in the inguinal pouch. Sometimes the testis in this position can be manipulated into the scrotal pouch. This augurs well for future normal development. Testes that are found too high in the inguinal canal to manipulate into the scrotum may be malformed. Parents are encouraged to have the baby examined at regular intervals. If descent of the testis has not occurred by the time the child is 2 years old, arrangements for orchidopexy may be made.

Ambiguous genitalia

Parents are usually invited to identify the baby's sex for themselves at delivery. On some occasions the midwife may be asked to clarify this and if there is any doubt should decline to assign a gender to the baby. Examination of the baby may reveal any of the following: a small hypoplastic penis, chordee, bifid scrotum, undescended testes (careful examination should be made to detect undescended testes in the inguinal canal) or enlarged clitoris, incompletely separated or poorly differentiated labia. There are a number of causes of ambiguous genitalia, all of which need expert clarification.

Congenital adrenal hyperplasia

One of the reasons for ambiguous genitalia is an autosomal recessive condition called congenital adrenal hyperplasia. In this condition the adrenal gland is stimulated to overproduce androgens because of a deficiency of an enzyme called 21-hydroxylase, which is necessary for normal production of steroid from cholesterol. If aldosterone production is reduced then these babies will rapidly lose salt. Urea and electrolyte levels, blood glucose and 17-hydroxy progesterone concentrations should be measured and appropriate fluid replacement given. In the process of eliminating or confirming the cause, a 24 hour urine collection may be requested. It is necessary to ensure that the urine bag is correctly placed to avoid faecal contamination. Placing one end of a catheter or feeding tube in the urine bag and aspirating the contents at regular intervals will help to prevent spillage and the unnecessary trauma to the baby of repeated applications of urine bags. Babies with this condition may require later cosmetic surgery. The condition is not always recognised in boys in the neonatal period.

Intersex

This is where the internal reproductive organs are at variance with the external appearance of the genitalia. Ultrasound examination will help to identify the nature of the internal reproductive organs. True hermaphroditism is extremely rare. The decision of gender attribution is made following chromosomal studies to determine genetic make-up, hormone assays and consideration of the potential for cosmetic surgery.

Clearly, this time of waiting for results of investigations is a time of great concern for parents because they cannot tell relatives and friends the gender of the baby. Delay in naming the baby is an additional pressure. Some parents in this invidious position elect to give the baby a name that would suit either a boy or a girl. It is, however, more common for a child of truly ambiguous gender to be raised as a girl.

Commonly occurring syndromes

Box 45.1 provides definitions of terms used in this section.

Trisomy 21 (Down syndrome)

The classic features of what is now known as Down syndrome were first described in 1866 by physician John Down (Fig. 45.15). He recognised a commonly occurring combination of facial features amongst mentally subnormal individuals. His description included features such as widely set and obliquely slanted eyes, small nose and thick rough tongue (Toliss 1995). In addition to these, it is now accepted that other signs are evident: a small head with flat occiput, squat broad hands with an incurving little finger, a wide space between the thumb and index finger, a single palmar (simian) crease, Brushfield spots in the eyes, and generalised hypotonia. Not all of these manifestations need be present and any of them can occur alone without implying chromosomal aberration. Babies born with Down syndrome also have a higher incidence of cardiac anomalies, leukaemia and hypothyroidism. Intelligence quotient is below average, at 40–80.

Although there may be little doubt in the midwife's mind that a baby has Down syndrome, she should be careful not to make any definitive statements. Family likeness alone may explain some babies' appearance. Parents themselves may voice their suspicions. If they do not, a sensitive but honest approach should be made by either the midwife or paediatrician to alert them to the possibility and to request permission to conduct further investigations. It is inappropriate to transfer the baby to the special care nursery in order to carry out these investigations under guise of the baby being cold or sleepy. Investigations indicated include the karyotype and echocardiography, because of the increased risk of congenital heart disease. Some centres offer diagnosis using fluorescent in situ hybridisation (FISH) techniques (see Ch. 23), which provide an answer within 2 rather than the standard 5–7 days.

Box 45.1 Glossary of terms

Karyotyping The process of identifying chromosomes by size

Meiosis The type of cell division that occurs in the formation of gametes, in which one of each chromosome pair is reduced or 'lost'

Mitosis The type of cell division that occurs in somatic cells

Non-disjunction Failure of a chromosome pair to separate during meiosis or paired chromatids during mitosis

Trisomy A situation where a particular chromosome is represented three times in the nucleus

Deletion Breaking off or loss of part of a chromosome

Translocation Transfer of material from one chromosome to another of a different kind. Should this occur during mitosis, the result will be a balanced or reciprocal translocation where the total chromosomal complement is normal. This would be discovered only during karyotyping; there is no clinical manifestation. If, however, translocation happens during meiosis an unbalanced translocation will result in either an excess or deficit of chromosomal material in the gamete formed

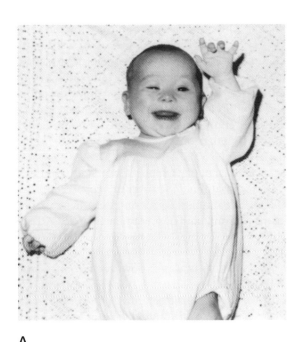

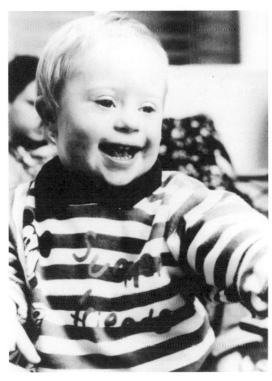

A   B

Fig. 45.15 (A) Baby with Down syndrome: note slant of eyes and incurving little finger. (B) With good parental involvement and stimulus these infants can reach maximum potential. (Photographs courtesy of Scottish Down's Syndrome Association.)

Down syndrome arising as a result of a non-disjunction process occurs in 95% of cases. Unbalanced translocation occurs in 2.5% of cases, usually between chromosomes 14 and 21. Mosaic forms also occur. There is no difference between the types in clinical appearance. Parents who have a baby with Down syndrome, therefore, should be offered genetic counselling to establish the risk of recurrence. The overall incidence of Down syndrome is 1 in 700.

An individual baby's needs will vary depending on whether there are any coexisting abnormalities. Apart from any emotional support the mother may require, the midwife may also offer help with feeding. Problems are likely to be encountered because of the baby's generalised hypotonia. Breastfeeding should be encouraged if the mother had so planned. Providing a videotape or reading material about Down syndrome for the parents may be helpful, or the address of the local branch of the Down Syndrome Association (see Useful addresses, p. 861).

Trisomy 18 (Edwards syndrome)

This condition is found in about 1 in 5000 births. An extra 18th chromosome is responsible for the characteristic features. The lifespan for these children is short and the majority die during their 1st year. The head is small with a flattened forehead, a receding chin and frequently a cleft palate. The ears are low set and maldeveloped.

The sternum tends to be short, the fingers often overlap each other and the feet have a characteristic rocker-bottom appearance. Malformations of the cardiovascular and gastrointestinal systems are common.

Trisomy 13 (Patau syndrome)

An extra copy of the 13th chromosome leads to multiple abnormalities. These children have a short life. Only 5% live beyond 3 years. Affected infants are small and are microcephalic. Midline facial abnormalities such as cleft lip and palate are common and limb abnormalities are frequently seen. Brain, cardiac and renal abnormalities may coexist with this trisomy.

Potter syndrome

This collection of features in a series of stillborn infants was first described by Edith Potter, a perinatal pathologist, in 1946. It is due to the compressive effects of oligohydramnios in renal agenesis or severe hypoplasia.

The baby's face will have a flattened appearance, low set ears, an antimongoloid slant to the eyes, with deep epicanthic folds, and a beaked nose. These babies are usually severely asphyxiated at birth because they have lung hypoplasia. It is a syndrome incompatible with sustained life.

Turner syndrome (XO)

In this monosomal condition, only one sex chromosome exists: an X. The absent chromosome is indicated by 'O'. The child is a girl with a short, webbed neck, widely spaced nipples and oedematous feet. The genitalia tend to be underdeveloped and the internal reproductive organs do not mature. The condition may not be diagnosed until puberty fails to occur. Congenital cardiac defects may also be found. Mental development is usually normal.

Klinefelter syndrome (XXY)

This is an abnormality affecting boys but it is not normally diagnosed until pubertal changes fail to occur.

Support for the midwife

Caring for a mother whose baby has some major congenital abnormality places extra demands on the midwife. This stress is compounded if the abnormality was not anticipated prior to delivery or if the midwife has not previously encountered the particular problem. The exercising of effective counselling and communication skills is invaluable in helping the family to adjust and in facilitating appropriate lines of support. The extra effort expended can be costly in terms not only of time but of the emotional stress the midwife may experience.

It is important that support is available for midwives in these situations (e.g. from her supervisor of midwives). Preparatory courses on grief and bereavement counselling are also of some benefit as many parents with affected babies will experience many of these emotions. Midwives who have acquired experience in this realm should not, however, automatically be targeted as the experts and always be called upon to fulfil this role. Conversely, student midwives ought not to be deliberately shielded from being involved in caring for such families. The provision of quality care for parents who have a child with a congenital abnormality is contingent upon meeting the needs of the carers.

REFERENCES

Bagwell C E 1993 Surgical lesions of pediatric airways and lungs. In: Koff P B, Eitzman D, Neu J (eds) Neonatal and pediatric respiratory care, 2nd edn. Mosby Year Book, St Louis, ch 8, p 132

Barr D G D 1992 Disorders of bone. In: Campbell A G M, McIntosh N (eds) Forfar and Arneil's textbook of paediatrics. Churchill Livingstone, Edinburgh, ch 23, p 1628

Carr A J, Lui D T Y 1994 Chorionic villus sampling. Advantages and disadvantages for prenatal diagnosis. Midwives Chronicle 107(1279):284–287

Danner S C 1992 breastfeeding the infant with a cleft defect. NAACOGs Clinical Issues in Perinatal and Women's Health Nursing 3(4):634–639

Habel A, Sell D, Mars M 1996 Management of cleft lip and palate. Archives of Disease in Childhood 74(4):360–366

Le Maistre G 1991 Ultrasound and dislocation of the hip. Paediatric Nursing 64:13–16

Modell B, Modell M 1992 Towards a healthy baby. Oxford University Press, Oxford, ch 1, p 5

Nixon H, O'Donnell B 1992 Essentials of paediatric surgery, 4th edn. Butterworth Heinemann, Oxford, ch 8, p 57–69

Paul K 1995 Recognition, stabilisation and early management of infants with critical congenital heart disease presenting in the first days of life. Neonatal Network 14(5):13–25

Raine P 1994 Cleft lip and palate. In: Freeman N V, Burge D M, Griffiths M, Malone P S J (eds) Surgery in the newborn. Churchill Livingstone, Edinburgh, ch 34, p 375

Roberton N R C 1993 Neonatal intensive care, 3rd edn. Edward Arnold, London, ch 16, p 271

Sphor H L, Wilms J, Sternhausen H C 1993 Prenatal alcohol exposure and longterm developmental consequences. Lancet 341(8850):907–910

Sullivan G 1996 Parental bonding in cleft lip and palate repair. Paediatric Nursing 8(1):21–24

Toliss D 1995 Who was Down? Nursing Times 91(5):61

Wallis S, Harvey D 1979 Disorders in the newborn – 1. Nursing Times 75:1315–1327

Whyte A 1995 Folic acid fortifying the pregnancy message. Health Visitor 68(10):397–398

Wirt S, Algren C L, Arnold S L 1992 Cleft lip and palate: a multidisciplinary approach. Plastic Surgical Nursing 12(4):140–145

USEFUL ADDRESSES

Association for Spina Bifida and Hydrocephalus (ASBAH)
ASBAH House
42 Park Road
Peterborough PE1 2UQ

Cleft Lip and Palate Association (CLAPA)
138 Buckingham Palace Road
London SW1 9SA

Cystic Fibrosis Research Trust (CF)
11 London Road
Bromley
Kent BR1 1BY

Down Syndrome Association
155 Mitcham Road
London SW17 9BR

Scottish Down's Syndrome Association (SDSA)
158–160 Balgreen Road
Edinburgh EH11 3AU

Reach: The Association for Children with Hand or Arm Deficiency
12 Wilson Way
Earls Barton
Northamptonshire NN6 0NZ

STEPS (National Association for Children with Lower Limb Abnormalities)
11 Eagle Brow
Lymm
Cheshire WA13 0LP

Support around Termination for Abnormality (SATFA)
71–75 Charlotte Street
London W1P 1LB

46 Jaundice and Infection

Patricia Percival

As a result of the transition from intrauterine to extrauterine physiology, all neonates have a transient rise in serum bilirubin in the 1st week of life and about 50% of term babies become visibly jaundiced. Jaundice is, by definition, the yellow discoloration of the skin and sclera that results from raised levels of bilirubin in the blood (hyperbilirubinaemia). In neonates jaundice is considered to be either physiological or pathological. Physiological jaundice appears about 48 hours after birth and usually settles within 10–12 days. Jaundice that appears earlier, is persistent or associated with high bilirubin levels can have a number of pathological causes, which include increased haemolysis, metabolic and endocrine disorders and infection. The role of the midwife is to detect and differentiate between physiological and pathological jaundice by the timing, clinical presentation and neonatal behaviour, and to instigate appropriate management. It is also vital that the family is kept fully informed of events and progress.

The newborn baby is very vulnerable to infection, defence mechanisms are immature and the skin is thin and easily damaged. Infections may be acquired before, during or soon after birth and, while some may be minor, others are potentially damaging or life threatening.

The chapter aims to:

- consider the physiological basis of neonatal jaundice and the causes and consequences of pathological jaundice
- emphasise the role of the midwife in the prevention of Rhesus isoimmunisation
- discuss the management of jaundice
- discuss the role of the midwife in the prevention, assessment, diagnosis and treatment of infection
- review infections that may be acquired by the neonate before, during and shortly after birth.

Conjugation of bilirubin

Bilirubin is a waste product from the breakdown of haem, most of which is found in red blood cells (RBCs). Ageing, immature or malformed RBCs are removed from the circulation and broken down in the reticuloendothelial system (liver, spleen and macrophages) and haemoglobin is broken down to the by-products haem, globin and iron.

- *Haem* is converted to biliverdin and then to unconjugated bilirubin.
- *Globin* is broken down into *amino acids*, which are reused by the body to make proteins.
- *Iron* is stored in the body or used for new RBCs.

Two main forms of bilirubin are found in the body:

- *Unconjugated bilirubin* is fat soluble and cannot be excreted easily either in bile or urine.
- *Conjugated bilirubin* has been made water soluble in the liver and can be excreted either in faeces or urine.

Three stages are involved in the process of bilirubin conjugation: transport, conjugation and excretion (Fig. 46.1).

Transport of bilirubin

Unconjugated bilirubin is transported in the plasma to the liver bound to the plasma protein albumin. If not attached to albumin it can be deposited into extravascular fatty and nerve tissues in the body. Staining of the skin (jaundice) and the brain are the two most common sites. Damage to the brain as a result of bilirubin staining and toxicity is known as *kernicterus* (Box 46.1).

Conjugation

Once in the liver bilirubin is detached from albumin and transported by intracellular carrier proteins Y and Z to the smooth endoplasmic reticulum of the liver. Here bilirubin is combined with glucose and *glucuronic acid* and conjugation occurs in the presence of oxygen. *Uridine diphosphoglucuronyl transferase* (*UDP-GT*, or *glucuronyl transferase*) is the major enzyme involved in bilirubin conjugation. The conjugated bilirubin is now water soluble and available for excretion.

Excretion

The conjugated bilirubin is excreted via the biliary system into the small intestine where it is catabolised by normal intestinal bacteria to form urobilinogen, then oxidised into orange-coloured urobilin. Most of the conjugated bilirubin is excreted in the faeces but a small amount is excreted in urine (Blackburn 1995, Gartner & Lee 1999, Hintz et al 2001, Wheeler 2000).

Jaundice

Jaundice results from deposits of bilirubin in the skin. In term neonates it appears when serum bilirubin concentrations reach 85–120 µmol/L (5–7 mg/dl) with a cephalo-caudal progression as levels increase (Manzar 1999). Asian and Native American babies usually have higher bilirubin levels than caucasian infants, whereas babies of African origin have lower levels. Preterm babies are also more likely to develop jaundice. Plate 35 shows a caucasian baby with jaundice who required 24 hours of fibreoptic phototherapy. Plate 36 demonstrates the difference in skin tone between the jaundiced baby and her mother.

Physiological jaundice

Neonatal physiological jaundice is a normal transitional state that affects up to 50% of term babies who have a *progressive rise* in unconjugated bilirubin levels and jaundice on day 3. Physiological jaundice *never* appears before 24 hours of life, *usually* fades by one week of age and bilirubin levels *never* exceed 200–215 µmol/L (12–13 mg/dl).

Causes

Neonatal physiological jaundice is the result of a *discrepancy* between RBC breakdown and the baby's ability to transport, conjugate and excrete unconjugated bilirubin.

Increased red cell breakdown. Newborn bilirubin production is more than twice that of normal adults per kilogram of weight. In the hypoxic environment of the uterus the fetus relies on haemoglobin F (fetal haemoglobin), which has a greater affinity for oxygen than does haemoglobin A (adult haemoglobin). At birth, when the pulmonary system becomes functional, the large red cell mass removed by haemolysis

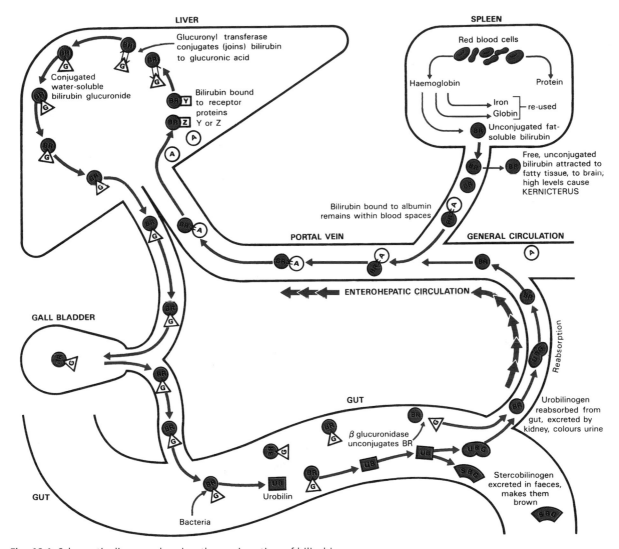

LIVER

Glucuronyl transferase conjugates (joins) bilirubin to glucuronic acid

Conjugated water-soluble bilirubin glucuronide

Bilirubin bound to receptor proteins Y or Z

SPLEEN

Red blood cells

Haemoglobin — Protein

Iron ⎤ re-used
Globin ⎦

Unconjugated fat-soluble bilirubin

Free, unconjugated bilirubin attracted to fatty tissue, to brain, high levels cause KERNICTERUS

Bilirubin bound to albumin remains within blood spaces

PORTAL VEIN

GENERAL CIRCULATION

ENTEROHEPATIC CIRCULATION

GALL BLADDER

Reabsorption

Urobilinogen reabsorbed from gut, excreted by kidney, colours urine

GUT

β glucuronidase unconjugates BR

Stercobilinogen excreted in faeces, makes them brown

GUT

Urobilin

Bacteria

Fig. 46.1 Schematic diagram showing the conjugation of bilirubin.
Key: BR   bilirubin
= bound to
A albumin
G glucuronic acid
UB urobilin
UBG urobilinogen
SBG stercobilinogen

creates the bulk of the bilirubin, which can potentially overload the system.

Decreased albumin-binding capacity. The transport of bilirubin to the liver for conjugation is reduced by lower albumin concentrations in preterm babies, decreased albumin-binding capacity (which may occur if the baby is acidotic) and possible competition for albumin-binding sites from some drugs. As available binding sites on albumin are used, levels of unbound, unconjugated, fat-soluble bilirubin in the blood rise and will find tissues with fat affinity, such as the skin and brain.

Box 46.1 Kernicterus (bilirubin toxicity)

Kernicterus is an encephalopathy caused by deposits of unconjugated bilirubin in the basal nuclei of the brain. The early reversible signs of bilirubin toxicity include lethargy, changes in muscle tone and a high-pitched cry. In some babies these signs may progress to irritability, muscle hypertonia and death. In surviving babies, the long term clinical features of kernicterus may become apparent during the 1st year of life. Deafness, blindness, cerebral palsy, developmental delay, learning difficulties and extrapyramidal disturbances such as athetosis, drooling, facial grimace, chewing and swallowing difficulties can result from kernicterus (Stanley 1997, Wolf et al 1997).

Kernicterus is usually associated with serum bilirubin levels greater than 340 μmol/L (20 mg/dl). However, despite recent advances in the effects of bilirubin on the brain, doubt remains as to the critical threshold of bilirubin in terms of long term morbidity (see Wheeler 2000 for a review of the pathology of kernicterus). It has been hypothesised that in the presence of anoxia, infection, hypothermia and dehydration, the blood–brain barrier allows bilirubin to enter the brain. These factors are more likely in preterm and sick term infants (Newman et al 2000, Rose 2000).

Kernicterus rarely occurs in healthy, term breastfed babies. However, what is important for midwives is that *it does* occur. In one group of six infants with kernicterus no cause was found for the hyperbilirubinaemia other than breastfeeding (Maisels & Newman 1995). It has been speculated that inadequate establishment of breastfeeding may play a role in hyperbilirubinaemia in some infants with kernicterus (Harris et al 2001). Bertini et al (2001) also found a small subpopulation of breastfed infants with jaundice, who were particularly susceptible to bilirubin encephalopathy if starved.

If kernicterus is suspected, a complete neurodevelopmental examination is undertaken and diagnostic testing may include MRI and brain stem auditory-evoked response (BAER). Treatment of kernicterus is usually aggressive and can include phototherapy, intravenous fluids and exchange transfusion. Ongoing follow-up is essential, including complete neurodevelopmental examinations, repeat MRIs, and behavioural hearing evaluations (Harris et al 2001, Wheeler 2000, Wolf et al 1997). A joint international effort is required to secure adequate funding for basic and applied research into the mechanisms of kernicterus that will help identify babies most at risk (Hansen 2001a).

Enzyme deficiency. Lower levels of UDP-GT enzyme activity during the first 24 hours after birth reduce bilirubin conjugation. Although levels increase after the first 24 hours, adult levels are not reached for 6–14 weeks.

Increased enterohepatic reabsorption. This process is increased in the newborn bowel as neonates lack the normal enteric bacteria that break down bilirubin to urobilinogen; they also have increased *beta-glucuronidase* enzyme activity, which hydrolyses conjugated bilirubin back into the unconjugated state (when it is absorbed back into the system). If feeding is delayed then bowel motility is also decreased, further compromising excretion of unconjugated bilirubin. Asian babies have enhanced enterohepatic circulation of bilirubin, higher peak bilirubin concentrations and more prolonged jaundice (Bertini et al 2001, Blackburn 1995, Coe 1999, Wheeler 2000).

Exaggerated physiological jaundice in breastfed infants

Current evidence suggests that two different processes cause jaundice in the breastfeeding baby, although the exact mechanisms are unknown:

1. *Breast-feeding or early onset jaundice* – it is thought that low fluid and calorie intake during colostrum production causes a slower intestinal transit time, which increases exposure to beta glucuronidase, which adds more unconjugated bilirubin to the system.
2. *Breastmilk or later onset jaundice* – research into lipoprotein lipase, beta glucuronidase and free fatty acids is attempting to shed light on this form of prolonged jaundice.

Breastfeeding jaundice and breastmilk jaundice are different, but possibly overlapping syndromes that are an exaggeration of normal physiological mechanisms (see Gartner & Lee 1999 for a review that emphasises the differences between the two).

Research findings about jaundice in breastfed babies are conflicting, with some researchers finding a significant relationship between breastfeeding and hyperbilirubinaemia or jaundice. In one study, neonates fed with two different artificial milks had significantly lower jaundice levels than breastfed infants on days 13 to 19 (using a transcutaneous measurement of jaundice) (Gourley et al 1999). In two further samples of 51 387 and 1177 healthy term newborns, one of the predictors of hyperbilirubinaemia or jaundice was also exclusive breastfeeding (Newman et al 2000, Seidman et al 1999).

In a further multicentre study, the serum bilirubin level was significantly higher in exclusively breastfed babies at 72 ± 12 h of age; however, treatment needs were the same (Hintz et al 2001). Of the 3661 babies in Crofts et al's (1999) study, 127 were jaundiced at 28 days of age. Of these, 125 were breastfed, with many having abnormal liver function tests (no baby had abnormal stool or urine colour and none was found to have liver disease). The researchers concluded that jaundiced breastfed babies who are well are unlikely to have serious disease, and further that elevated liver function tests are compatible with a diagnosis of breastmilk-related jaundice.

Conversely, early researchers (Rubaltelli & Griffith 1992) found no significant difference in the serum bilirubin concentrations of 1454 breast- or formula-fed neonates. Also, breastfed neonates in Bertini et al's (2001) research of 2174 babies (≥ 37 weeks) did not have more hyperbilirubinaemia in the first days of life.

These evidence-based differences can lead to clinical dilemmas, and a need for further research (Hansen 2001b) but stopping breastfeeding is not necessary. However, although very rare, classic kernicterus can occur in apparently healthy, term, breastfed newborns (Maisels & Newman 1995), particularly if they are starved (Bertini et al 2001), or if inadequate establishment of breastfeeding occurs (Harris et al 2001) (see Box 46.1).

Exaggerated physiological jaundice in preterm babies

This is characterised by bilirubin levels of 165 μmol/L (10 mg/dl) or greater by day 3 or 4, with peak concentrations on day 5 to 7 that return to normal over several weeks. Preterm babies are more at risk of kernicterus (see Box 46.1), so management is particularly important. Contributing factors include:

- a delay in the expression of the enzyme UDP-GT
- shorter red cell life
- complications such as hypoxia, acidosis and hypothermia, which can interfere with albumin-binding capacity (Newman et al 2000, Rose 2000).

Midwifery practice and physiological jaundice

Jaundice in newborns is a challenge for midwives as it is important to distinguish between healthy babies with a normal physiological response who need no active treatment and those who require serum bilirubin testing (see Management of jaundice) (Smith et al 1997). For example, a moderately jaundiced 4-day-old baby with a good urinary output, who is not sleepy but wakes regularly and feeds well, does not need invasive blood tests. However, a 1-day-old baby with mild jaundice requires further investigation. Family involvement can maximise midwifery time, as parents can actively contribute to their baby's assessment if they are aware of the importance of such things as excessive sleepiness, reluctance to feed and a decrease in the number of wet nappies. Families also need to be told in a positive manner about the possible time scale of the jaundice in some breast-fed babies and can be asked to report pale stools and yellow or orange urine (these may indicate cholestatic liver disease). In formula-fed babies prolonged jaundice and persistent pallor of stools or yellow or orange urine are rare, and merit immediate investigation (Crofts et al 1999).

One way of using evidence-based practice to manage hyperbilirubinaemia is to help women effectively feed their babies from birth. Early, frequent feeding assists newborns to cope with an increased bilirubin load by reducing the factors that cause physiological jaundice (particularly decreased albumin-binding capacity, enzyme deficiency and increased enterohepatic reabsorption). Effective feeding supplies glucose to the liver, encourages bowel colonisation with normal flora and increases bowel motility. In turn, this helps production of the enzymes needed for conjugation and also decreases enterohepatic reabsorption. As well as reducing jaundice, being with women while they learn to breastfeed also extends midwives' partnership role with women well beyond the birth.

Pathological jaundice

Pathological jaundice in newborns usually appears within 24 hours of birth, and is characterised by a *rapid* rise in serum bilirubin. Criteria include:

- jaundice within the first 24 hours of life
- a rapid increase in total serum bilirubin > 85 μmol/L (5 mg/dl) per day
- total serum bilirubin > 200 μmol/L (12.9 mg/dl)
- conjugated (direct-reacting) bilirubin > 25–35 μmol/L (1.5–2 mg/dl)

- persistence of clinical jaundice for 7–10 days in term or 2 weeks in preterm babies.

Causes

The underlying aetiology of pathological jaundice is some *interference* with bilirubin production, transport, conjugation or excretion (Fig. 46.2). Any disease or disorder that increases bilirubin production or that alters the transport or metabolism of bilirubin is superimposed upon normal physiological jaundice.

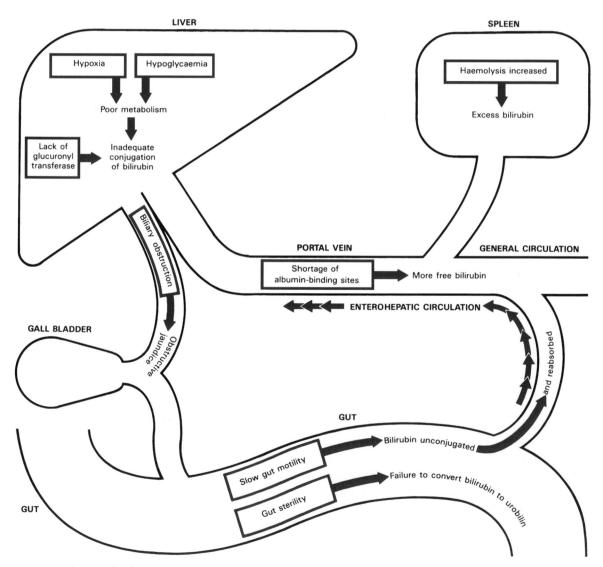

Fig. 46.2 Sites of events leading to jaundice.

Production. Factors that increase haemoglobin destruction also increase bilirubin levels. Causes of increased haemolysis include:

- *blood type/group incompatibility* – Rhesus anti-D, anti-A, anti-B and anti-Kell, also ABO
- *haemoglobinopathies* – sickle cell disease and thalassaemia (affects babies of African and Mediterranean descent)
- *enzyme deficiencies* – *glucose-6-phosphate dehydrogenase (G6PD)* maintains the integrity of the cell membrane of RBCs and a deficiency results in haemolysis (it is an X-linked genetic disorder carried by females that affects male infants of African, Asian and Mediterranean descent – see Ch. 19)
- *spherocytosis* – fragile RBC membrane
- *extravasated blood* – cephalhaematoma and bruising
- *sepsis* – can lead to increased haemoglobin breakdown
- *polycythaemia* – blood contains too many red cells as in maternofetal or twin-to-twin transfusion.

Transport. Factors that lower blood albumin levels or decrease albumin-binding capacity include:

- hypothermia, acidosis or hypoxia can interfere with albumin-binding capacity
- drugs that compete with bilirubin for albumin-binding sites (e.g. aspirin, sulphonamides and ampicillin).

Conjugation. As well as immaturity of the neonate's enzyme system, other factors can interfere with bilirubin conjugation in the liver including:

- dehydration, starvation, hypoxia and sepsis (oxygen and glucose are required for conjugation)
- TORCH infections (toxoplasmosis, others, rubella, cytomegalovirus, herpes)
- other viral infections (e.g. neonatal viral hepatitis)
- other bacterial infections, particularly those caused by *Escherichia coli* (*E. coli*)
- metabolic and endocrine disorders that alter UDP-GT enzyme activity (e.g. Crigler–Najjar disease and Gilbert's syndrome)
- other metabolic disorders such as hypothyroidism and galactosaemia.

Excretion. Factors that can interfere with bilirubin excretion include:

- hepatic obstruction caused by congenital anomalies such as extrahepatic biliary atresia
- obstruction from `bile plugs' from increased bile viscosity (e.g. cystic fibrosis, total parenteral nutrition, haemolytic disorders and dehydration)
- saturation of protein carriers needed to excrete conjugated bilirubin into the biliary system
- infection, other congenital disorders, and idiopathic neonatal hepatitis, which can also cause an excess of conjugated bilirubin.

After processing by the liver, most of the bilirubin is conjugated so babies are at less risk of kernicterus. However, they may require urgent treatment for other serious conditions (Hannam et al 2000, Hintz et al 2001, Rose 2000, Seidman et al 1999).

Haemolytic jaundice

As previously discussed, factors that increase haemoglobin destruction also increase bilirubin production and in turn cause pathological jaundice. In the following section Rhesus (RhD) isoimmunisation is emphasised because of the midwife's role in prevention. This condition causes haemolytic disease of the newborn (HDN), which usually requires some form of obstetric intervention. Few antibodies to blood group antigens other than those in the Rh system cause severe HDN; fetal transfusion is unusual for multiple maternal antibody isoimmunisation without anti-D. ABO incompatibility is also emphasised, as it is possibly the most frequent cause of mild to moderate haemolysis in neonates (Craig et al 2000, Filbey et al 1995, Spong et al 2001).

RhD incompatibility

RhD incompatibility can occur when a woman with Rh negative blood type is pregnant with a fetus with a Rh positive but not Rh negative blood type. This condition is commonest among caucasians, about 15% of whom are Rh negative, compared with 8% of African and 1% of Asian populations (Gunston 1993).

The placenta usually acts as a barrier to fetal blood entering the maternal circulation (Fig. 46.3). However, as shown in Figure 46.4, during pregnancy or birth, fetomaternal haemorrhage (FMH) can occur (small amounts of fetal Rh positive blood cross the placenta and enter the circulation of the mother with Rh negative blood). The woman's immune system reacts by producing anti-D antibodies that cause sensitisation (Fig. 46.5). In subsequent pregnancies these maternal antibodies can cross the placenta and destroy fetal erythrocytes (Fig. 46.6). This haemolytic disease of the fetus and newborn caused by Rh isoimmunisation can occur during the first pregnancy, but usually sensitisation during the first pregnancy or birth leads to extensive destruction of fetal red blood cells during subsequent pregnancies. Rh isoimmunisation can result from any procedure or incident where maternal blood leaks across the placenta or from the inadvertent transfusion of Rh positive blood to the woman.

Before the introduction of anti-D immunoglobulin (anti-D Ig) this condition resulted in haemolytic disease of the fetus and newborn in about 10% of pregnancies. Rh isoimmunisation was previously a major cause of perinatal morbidity and mortality, the effect on the fetus and neonate depending on the severity of the haemolysis (American College of Obstetricians and Gynaecologists 1999).

Prevention of RhD isoimmunisation

Midwives play an important preventive role with families who have Rh incompatibility. Most cases of Rh isoimmunisation can now be prevented by the administration of anti-D Ig (to mothers with non-sensitised Rh negative blood type who have a baby with Rh positive

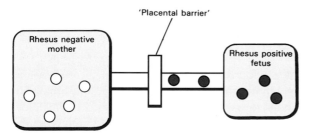

Fig. 46.3 Normal placenta with no communication between maternal and fetal blood.

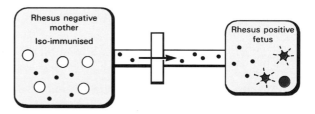

Fig. 46.6 In a subsequent pregnancy maternal Rhesus antibodies cross the placenta, resulting in haemolytic disease of the newborn.

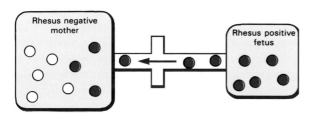

Fig. 46.4 Fetal cells enter maternal circulation through 'break' in 'placental barrier', e.g. at placental separation.

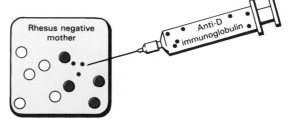

Fig. 46.7 Anti-D immunoglobulin administered within 72 hours of birth or other sensitising event.

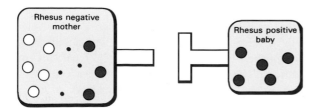

Fig. 46.5 Maternal production of Rhesus antibodies following introduction of Rhesus positive blood.

Figs 46.3–46.8 Rhesus isoimmunisation and its prevention.

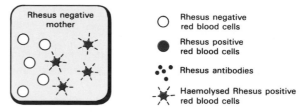

Fig. 46.8 Anti-D immunoglobulin has destroyed fetal Rhesus positive red cells and prevented isoimmunisation.

blood type) within 72 hours of birth or any other sensitising event (Fig. 46.7). Anti-D Ig is a human plasma-based product that has been used since at least the 1970s to prevent the production of anti-D antibodies by the mother. It does not, however, protect against the development of other antibodies that can cause haemolytic disease of the newborn (e.g. anti-A, anti-B and anti-Kell).

Postnatal prophylaxis. In the UK postnatal immunoprophylaxis with anti-D Ig began in 1969 and most cases of HDN have been prevented by its use following birth and other sensitising events. A systematic review of six eligible trials of over 10 000 women found that, when given within 72 hours of birth (and other antenatal sensitising events), anti-D Ig lowered the incidence of Rh isoimmunisation 6 months after birth and in a subsequent pregnancy, regardless of the ABO status of the mother and baby (Crowther & Middleton 2001). At the present time in England and Wales there are about 500 cases of haemolytic disease of the fetus and newborn caused by Rh isoimmunisation each year, with an estimated 25 to 30 deaths (NICE 2002).

Prophylaxis following other sensitising events. Available evidence (Allaby et al 1999, Crowther & Middleton 2001, McSweeney et al 1998, RCOG 1999) suggests that anti-D Ig prophylaxis should be given to all non-sensitised Rh-negative women within 72 hours of the following:

- any threatened, complete or incomplete or missed abortion *after* 12 weeks of pregnancy (if bleeding continues intermittently after 12 weeks' gestation, anti-D Ig should be given at 6 week intervals)
- any spontaneous miscarriage before 12 weeks that requires surgical intervention to evacuate the uterus (some evidence suggests that significant FMH does not occur after complete spontaneous or threatened abortion without surgical intervention when bleeding ceases by 12 weeks; however, in McSweeney et al's (1998) audit of 20 women who developed anti-D antibodies, 13 had therapeutic or spontaneous abortions before 20 weeks of gestation)
- therapeutic termination of pregnancy by surgical or medical methods regardless of gestational age
- ectopic pregnancy

- amniocentesis, cordocentesis, chorionic villus sampling, fetal blood sampling or any other invasive intrauterine procedure such as shunt insertion
- external cephalic version of the fetus
- fetal death in utero or stillbirth
- abdominal trauma and antepartum haemorrhage
- any other instance of inadvertent transfusion of Rh positive red blood cells (e.g. incorrect blood transfusion of Rh positive blood or platelets or drug use).

Antenatal prophylaxis. Despite the anti-D Ig prophylaxis outlined above, about 1.5% of Rh negative women still develop anti-D antibodies following a first Rh positive pregnancy. A meta-analysis (Allaby et al 1999) and Cochrane review (Crowther & Keirse 1999) showed the antenatal sensitisation rate was further reduced by routine antenatal prophylaxis. In the UK since 2002, routine antenatal anti-D prophylaxis (in doses of at least 500 i.u. at 28 and 34 weeks' gestation) for all non-sensitised Rh negative women has been recommended by NICE in an attempt to reduce further the incidence of HDN.

However, it is important to note some cases of Rh isoimmunisation are due to failure to follow already established protocols, particularly during pregnancy. Specific examples of failure to adhere to recommendations for the administration of anti-D Ig include:

- not testing the size of a FMH to ensure an appropriate dose of anti-D Ig was given (Vause et al 2000)
- not administering anti-D Ig appropriately, or women not attending for treatment of bleeding in pregnancy (Portmann et al 1997)
- administering anti-D Ig for abdominal trauma in only 20% of cases (Howard et al 1997)
- using an inadequate dose of anti-D Ig following antepartum haemorrhage after 20 weeks of gestation (Howard et al 1997)
- not managing miscarriages and medical terminations of pregnancy (McSweeney et al 1998)
- not managing sensitising events occurring after 20 weeks' gestation according to the guidelines (Howard et al 1997, Morrison 2000)

- not understanding Kleihauer test results, with a `negative' result interpreted as a reason not to give anti-D immunoglobin (Howard et al 1997)
- postnatal omissions resulting from confusion with women who had recently received antenatal treatment with anti-D Ig (Howard et al 1997).

Administration of anti-D Ig. Anti-D Ig is administered to Rh negative women who are pregnant with, or have given birth to, an Rh positive baby. It destroys any fetal cells in the mother's blood (Fig. 46.8) before her immune system produces antibodies. Anti-D Ig should *not* be given to women who are Rh sensitised, as they have already developed antibodies. The process for non-sensitised women is as follows (Fung et al 1998, Maayan-Metzger et al 2001, RCOG 1999):

1. During pregnancy blood is grouped for ABO and Rh type, and women who are Rh negative are screened for Rh antibodies (indirect Coombs' test). A negative test shows an *absence* of antibodies or sensitisation.
2. Blood is retested at 28 weeks of pregnancy. In countries where antenatal prophylaxis is routine (at 28 and 34 weeks' gestation), the first injection of anti-D Ig is given just after this blood sample is taken.
3. Where a policy of routine antenatal anti-D Ig prophylaxis is *not* in place, blood is retested for antibodies at 34 weeks of pregnancy.
4. When anti-D Ig prophylaxis is given at 28 weeks, blood is not retested as it is difficult to distinguish passive anti-D Ig from immune anti-D (enzyme or antiglobulin techniques can detect passive anti-D Ig for 6 weeks or longer after the administration of antenatal or postnatal anti-D Ig).
5. Following the birth, cord blood is tested for confirmation of Rh type, ABO blood group, haemoglobin and serum bilirubin levels and the presence of maternal antibodies on fetal red cells (direct Coombs' test). Again, a negative test indicates an absence of antibodies or sensitisation. However, 20% of Rh positive babies born to mothers given two doses of antenatal anti-D Ig have a *positive* direct Coombs' test from passive anti-D Ig (Maayan-Metzger et al 2001). The postnatal dose of anti-D Ig *is still given* if passive anti-D Ig is present.
6. A Kleihauer acid elution test is also carried out on an anticoagulated maternal blood sample as soon as possible, and within 2 hours after the birth. This test detects fetal haemoglobin and estimates the number of fetal cells in a sample of maternal blood (see Dose of anti-D Ig, below).
7. Anti-D Ig must always be given as soon as possible, and within 72 hours of any sensitising event and the birth (although successful immunoprophylaxis requires anti-D Ig be given within 72 hours, some protection may occur when given within 9–10 days (RCOG 1999)). Anti-D Ig is injected into the deltoid muscle from which absorption is optimal. Absorption may be delayed if the gluteal region is used.

Dose of anti-D Ig. To prevent isoimmunisation in subsequent pregnancies it is vital that an adequate amount of anti-D Ig is given. However, research evidence on the optimal dose is still limited (Crowther & Middleton 2001). The dose of anti-D Ig, and the requirement for a test to identify the size of FMH, varies in different countries (RCOG 1999). The best available evidence suggests an intramuscular dose of 100 μg (500 i.u.) of anti-D Ig will suppress the immunisation that could occur following a FMH of 4–5 ml of RhD positive red cells (most women have a FMH less than 4 ml at the birth) (cited in RCOG 1999). The following doses of anti-D Ig are recommended:

- 100 μg (500 i.u.) anti-D Ig at 28 and 34 weeks' gestation for women in their first pregnancy
- at least 500 i.u. for all non-sensitised Rh negative woman following the birth of a Rh positive infant
- 250 i.u. following sensitising events *up to* 20 weeks' gestation
- at least 500 i.u. following sensitising events *after* 20 weeks' gestation
- larger doses for traumatic events and procedures such as caesarean birth, stillbirths and intrauterine deaths, abdominal trauma during the third trimester, or manual removal of the placenta (dose calculated on 500 i.u. of anti-D Ig suppressing immunisation from 4 ml of RhD positive red blood cells)
- larger doses for any other instance of inadvertent transfusion of Rh positive red blood cells (e.g. from an incorrect blood transfusion of Rh positive blood platelets).

Even with routine antenatal prophylaxis, a large FMH can still result in women producing anti-D antibodies. To ensure an adequate dose, when anti-D Ig is given after 20 weeks, a test is required to estimate the size of any FMH (Kleihauer acid elution test or more recently flow cytometry). Additional anti-D Ig is needed if the Kleihauer test indicates that higher levels of fetal cells are present in maternal blood (above 50 fetal cells per 50 low power fields). In such cases a further blood test is also ordered to ensure that an adequate amount of anti-D Ig has been given. In some hospitals or community settings, follow-up Kleihauer and further antibody screens are performed 48 hours after injection of anti-D Ig, regardless of the fetal cell count (Allaby et al 1999, Crowther & Keirse 1999, Crowther & Middleton 2001, Fung et al 1998, RCOG 1999).

Ethical and legal issues. A number of ethical, moral, legal and safety issues surround anti-D Ig, a human plasma-based product, and several writers discuss these (see Coombes 1999, NICE 2002, Wickham 1999a, b, 2001, Wray & Benbow 1999). To assist midwives further in their discussions with families, a number of anti-D Ig information and resources are provided in the annotated bibliography. Midwives also need to be aware of the content of consumer information leaflets available nationally and locally. To give informed consent, women need to know the possible consequences of treatment versus non-treatment with anti-D Ig.

For example, women in the UK must be informed that, because of the hypothetical risk of transmitting new variant Creutzfeldt–Jakob disease to pregnant women, anti-D Ig is now mainly derived from paid donors in the USA. They also have the right to refuse anti-D Ig and, although this may create a dilemma for the midwife, women's informed choices must be respected (NICE 2002). Wickham (1999a, b) documents a case study of a pregnant woman (Rh negative) who chose not to have anti-D following the birth of her baby (Rh positive). Midwives also have rights with respect to anti-D Ig, which they usually administer. In particular, they have a right to be involved in policy decisions that affect anti-D Ig protocols.

Management of RhD isoimmunisation

Effects of RhD isoimmunisation. Destruction of fetal RBCs results in a deficiency of mature red cells and the production of erythroblasts or immature red cells that cannot adequately carry oxygen to fetal tissue. The fetus becomes more anaemic and can develop

oedema and congestive cardiac failure. Fetal bilirubin levels also increase as more red cells are destroyed, with possible neurological damage as bilirubin is deposited in the brain. Lesser degrees of destruction result in haemolytic anaemia, whereas extensive haemolysis can cause hydrops fetalis and death in utero.

Mild to moderate haemolytic anaemia and hyperbilirubinaemia occur in about 25–30% of fetuses and neonates, hydrops fetalis in about 25% and fetal and neonatal death in up to 30%. Reports of fetal survival rates in severe cases are about 90% (Portmann et al 1997), reducing to 70% with hydrops fetalis (Cheong et al 2001). In the UK, recording of early fetal deaths as 'abortions' rather than as HDN results in systematic underreporting (Urbaniak 1998).

Antenatal monitoring and treatment of RhD isoimmunisation. Once Rh isoimmunisation has occurred, the primary focus is on reducing the effects of the haemolyis. Intensive fetal monitoring is usually required, and often a high level of intervention throughout the pregnancy. In one group of women (31 pregnancies) a total of 30 amniocenteses, 8 cordocenteses and 54 fetal blood transfusions were performed (Cheong et al 2001). In another group the median number of intrauterine transfusions for each patient was 3 (range 2–8) from 22 to 37 weeks' gestation (Goodrum et al 1997). Depending on the severity of Rh isoimmunisation, monitoring and treatment can include the following (Cheong et al 2001, Deka et al 1996, Goodrum et al 1997, Ismail et al 2001, Portmann et al 1997, Voto et al 1997):

1. In early pregnancy blood is grouped for Rh type, and women who are Rh negative are screened for Rh antibodies (indirect Coombs' test). A positive test indicates the *presence* of antibodies or sensitisation.
2. RBCs obtained by chorionic villus sampling (using an immune rosette technique) can be Rh phenotyped as early as 9 to 11 weeks' gestation.
3. Maternal blood is retested frequently to monitor any increase in antibody titres. Weak antibody titres should be detected using enzyme-treated red cells as, even with low anti-D levels, sudden and unexpected rises in serum anti-D levels can result in hydrops fetalis.
4. If antibody titres remain stable, ongoing monitoring is continued.

5. If antibody titres increase, amniocentesis is used to evaluate changes in the optical density of amniotic fluid. Elevated optical density measurements indicate a worsening of the isoimmunisation.

6. High concentrations of anti-D antibodies in the mother, in the fetus and in the amniotic fluid indicate an active transport across the placenta and passive excretion into the amniotic fluid.

7. Changes in fetal serum bilirubin levels are observed.

8. The fetus is closely monitored by ultrasonography for oedema and hepatosplenomegaly.

9. Intravenous immunoglobulin (IVIG) has the potential to maintain the fetus until intrauterine fetal transfusion (IUT) can be performed. IVIG works by blocking Fc-mediated antibody transport across the placenta, hence blocking fetal red cell destruction and reducing maternal antibody levels.

10. IUT can be used from about 20 weeks of gestation to reduce the effects of haemolysis until the fetus is capable of survival outside the uterus. With improved sonographic equipment in recent years, intravascular rather than intraperitoneal transfusions are more likely.

11. Depending upon the ongoing severity of the haemolysis and the condition of the fetus, the pregnancy may be allowed to continue or delivery of the baby discussed with the parents.

Postnatal treatment of RhD isoimmunisation. As with the fetus, treatment depends upon the baby's condition. Those with mild to moderate haemolytic anaemia and hyperbilirubinaemia may require careful monitoring but less aggressive management. Severely affected babies often require admission to intensive care units. Babies with hydrops fetalis are pale, have oedema and ascites and may be stillborn. Management aims to prevent further haemolysis, reduce bilirubin levels, remove maternal Rh antibodies from the baby's circulation and combat anaemia. In some cases phototherapy can be effective but exchange transfusion is often required, and packed cell transfusion may be needed to increase haemoglobin levels. Babies are at risk of ongoing haemolytic anaemia. A recent trial of 34 newborn babies with Rh haemolytic disease (Tanyer et al 2001) suggests IVIG treatment can be effective at blocking ongoing haemolysis in babies, who then require shorter duration of phototherapy and less exchange transfusions (Cheong et al 2001, Goodrum et al 1997, Portmann et al 1997, Voto et al 1997).

ABO incompatibility

ABO isoimmunisation usually occurs when the mother is blood group O and the baby is group A, or less often group B (type O women are 5.5 times more likely to have sensitisation than those with type A or B (Ozolek et al 1994)). Blood of types A and B has a protein or antigen not present in type O blood. Individuals with type O blood develop antibodies throughout life from exposure to antigens in food, Gram-negative bacteria or blood transfusion, and by the first pregnancy may already have high serum anti-A and anti-B antibody titres. Some women produce IgG antibodies that can cross the placenta and attach to fetal red cells and destroy them (see Effects of Rh isoimmunisation). First and subsequent babies are at risk; however, the destruction is usually much less severe than with Rh incompatibility. ABO incompatibility is also thought to protect the fetus from Rh incompatibility as the mother's anti-A and anti-B antibodies destroy any fetal cells that leak into the maternal circulation.

Antibody titres are monitored throughout the pregnancy, but a high level of antenatal intervention is not usually required. In most cases haemolysis is fairly mild; however, in subsequent pregnancies it can become more severe from previous exposure to the fetus' type O antigens. ABO erythroblastosis can, rarely, cause severe fetal anaemia and hydrops. The condition is more severe in individuals of African descent than in caucasions, with McDonnell et al (1998) reporting two cases of hydrops fetalis in this group (from anti-B haemolysis).

Postnatal management depends on the severity of haemolysis and, as with Rh isoimmunisation, aims to prevent further haemolysis, reduce bilirubin levels and combat any anaemia. After the birth, cord blood can be tested to confirm blood type, check haemoglobin and serum bilirubin levels and identify the presence of maternal antibodies on fetal red cells (direct Coombs' test). A positive direct Coombs test result is a better indicator of significant hyperbilirubinaemia than a positive indirect Coombs test or a positive result on both antiglobulin tests (Ozolek et al 1994). If antibodies are present, the baby is monitored closely for jaundice.

As with other causes of haemolysis, if infants require phototherapy it is usually commenced at a lower range of serum bilirubin levels (140–165 µmol/L or 8–10 mg/dl). In rare cases, babies with high serum bilirubin level require exchange transfusion (Craig et al 2000, Spong et al 2001).

Management of jaundice

The management of neonatal jaundice continues to be controversial. On the one hand, there are more than 50% of term and 80% of preterm infants whose jaundice is a normal physiological response. On the other, there are the 1 in 500 newborn babies with liver disease, and those who may be at risk of kernicterus from hyperbilirubinaemia. Diagnosis of the latter must be balanced against the risks of aggressive management of the former. Some feel that neonatal jaundice is a normal physiological event that is treated pathologically, with treatment based on historical fears of bilirubin-associated brain damage (kernicterus) and not on available evidence (Coe 1999, Smith 1997). However, case reports of kernicterus have followed calls for less aggressive treatment protocols (Newman & Maisels 2000).

Some argue that guidelines for the management of neonatal jaundice do not satisfy the requirements of evidence-based medicine. When limited evidence exists, a wider range of treatment options are needed, and the midwife's individual assessment skills are even more essential in managing neonatal jaundice. Management protocols must emphasise both a careful, individual assessment of each case and a range of therapeutic and diagnostic options (Coe 1999, Hansen 2001a, Newman & Maisels 2000).

In countries such as the UK, Australia, New Zealand and many European countries, midwives have an important role in the diagnosis and treatment of jaundice. During the first weeks of the baby's life, midwives can identify at risk newborns, make follow-up visits when women are discharged from hospital or birth at home, arrange home phototherapy and inform and teach parents. This is particularly so in the UK where midwives are encouraged to extend their public health role and work with women for up to 6 weeks after the birth. As part of this role it is also expected that midwives will be responsible for referrals and communication with other agencies during the first 6 weeks. Jaundice persisting beyond 14 days of age can be a sign of serious underlying liver disease (Hannam et al 2000) so babies with prolonged jaundice may need a number of laboratory investigations and referrals, particularly if formula fed.

Assessment and diagnosis

When evaluating neonatal jaundice two initial questions are considered:

- Does the jaundice result from the physiological breakdown of bilirubin or the presence of another underlying factor?
- Is the baby at risk of kernicterus (bilirubin toxicity)?

Individual risk factors for jaundice

Individual assessment of each infant includes identifying any particular risk factors for jaundice. These include any disease or disorder that increases bilirubin production, or that alters the transport or excretion of bilirubin (see above and Fig. 46.2). For example:

- Does the baby have any birth trauma or evident bruising?
- Was feeding or meconium passage delayed?
- Is the baby preterm and therefore at greater risk?
- Is there a family history of significant haemolytic disease or jaundiced siblings, or an ethnic predisposition to jaundice or inherited disease?
- Did the jaundice appear within the first 24 hours (suggesting haemolysis), or is it prolonged (possibly indicating serious disease such as hypothyroidism or obstructive jaundice)?

Physical assessment. This includes observation of:

- the extent of changes in skin and scleral colour
- the cephalo-caudal progression of jaundice
- other clinical signs such as lethargy and decreased eagerness to feed
- dark urine or light stools
- the presence of dehydration, starvation, hypothermia, acidosis or hypoxia
- vomiting, irritability or a high-pitched cry.

Laboratory investigations. These may include (Crofts et al 1999, Hannam et al 2000, Manzar 1999):

- serum bilirubin to determine levels and whether the bilirubin is unconjugated or conjugated
- direct Coombs' test to detect the presence of maternal antibodies on fetal RBCs
- indirect Coombs' test to detect the presence of maternal antibodies in serum
- reticulocyte count – elevated as a result of haemolysis when new RBCs are being produced
- ABO blood group and Rh type for possible incompatibility
- haemoglobin/haematocrit estimation to assess anaemia
- peripheral blood smear – red cell structure for abnormal cells
- white cell count to detect infection
- serum samples for specific immunoglobulins for the TORCH infections
- glucose-6-phosphate dehydrogenase (G6PD) assay
- urine for substances such as galactose.

In recent years, transcutaneous bilirubinometry has reduced the number of blood tests in neonates. In home and hospital settings this method provides a digital assessment of skin pigmentation, with an estimate of plasma bilirubin derived from the number displayed by the meter.

Treatment strategies

Phototherapy

Phototherapy is used to prevent the concentration of unconjugated bilirubin in the blood from reaching levels where neurotoxicity may occur. The neonate's skin surface is exposed to high intensity light, which photochemically converts fat-soluble unconjugated bilirubin into water-soluble bilirubin that can be excreted in bile and urine. Treatment may be intermittent, or continuous with phototherapy interrupted only for essential care.

Types of phototherapy. These include:

- *Conventional phototherapy systems* – these use high intensity light from white and more recently blue fluorescent phototherapy lamps. Blue lamps have an emission spectrum almost identical to the bilirubin absorption spectrum (Sarici et al 1999), are as effective as white at similar light intensities and have the future potential to provide much higher irradiance and improved results (Seidman et al

2000). The baby is usually placed about 45–60 cm from the light with the entire skin exposed. The eyes must be protected.
- *Fibreoptic light systems* – these use a woven fibreoptic pad (such as the Biliblanket – see Plate 37) that delivers high intensity light with no ultraviolet or infrared irradiation. The tungsten–halogen lamp of fibreoptic phototherapy has a broad emission through the blue and green phototherapy group, mainly in the green spectrum (Sarici et al 1999). The device is placed around the baby, under the clothing, again with the entire skin exposed to light.

Indications for phototherapy. The commencement of phototherapy is based on serum bilirubin levels and the individual condition of each baby, particularly when jaundice occurs within the first 12–24 hours:

- *for preterm infants < 1500 g* – between 85 and 140 µmol/L (5 and 8 mg/dl)
- *for preterm infants > 1500 g, sick infants and those with haemolysis* – between 140 and 165 µmol/L (8 and 10 mg/dl)
- *for healthy term infants jaundiced after 48 hours* – between 280 and 365 µmol/L (17 and 22 mg/dl).

The above individual factors, and serum bilirubin levels below 215 µmol/L (13 mg/dl), are usually accepted as necessary for stopping phototherapy. Although bilirubin levels can rise following phototherapy, healthy babies do not require further testing solely to identify this rebound effect.

Side-effects of phototherapy. Side-effects of conventional white and blue fluorescent phototherapy can include:

- hyperthermia, increased fluid loss and dehydration
- damage to the retina from the high intensity light
- lethargy or irritability, decreased eagerness to feed, loose stools
- skin rashes and skin burns
- alterations in a baby's state and neurobehavioural organisation
- isolation and lack of usual sensory experiences, including visual deprivation
- a decrease in calcium levels leading to hypocalcaemia
- low platelet counts and increased red cell osmotic fragility
- bronze baby syndrome, riboflavin deficiency and DNA damage.

Although some authors claim fibreoptic systems are less effective than conventional phototherapy lamps (Sarici et al 1999, Seidman et al 2000), they may be more comfortable for babies and allow easier accessibility and handling (Sarici et al 1999) and eye protection is not required. Plate 37 shows the ease with which families can care for their baby during fibreoptic phototherapy, either at the mother's bedside in hospital or at home.

Midwifery practice and phototherapy. Depending upon individual circumstances, phototherapy can be given in hospital or at home, with midwives and family usually responsible for infant care. With both systems, but particularly with conventional phototherapy, babies need to be carefully monitored.

Temperature. The baby is maintained in a warm thermoneutral environment and observed for any hypo- or hyperthermia. If nursed in an incubator, servocontrol can be used.

Eyes. Eye shields or patches are closely monitored to ensure they cover the eyes without occluding the nose and are not tight or causing eye discharge or weeping.

Skin. Skin is cleaned with warm water and observed frequently for rashes, dryness and excoriation. Creams and lotions are not used.

Hydration. Fluid intake and stool and urine output are monitored. Demand feeding is continued and routine supplements are not usually required. Extra fluids may be required for severely ill or dehydrated babies.

Neurobehavioural status. Monitoring of the baby's neurobehavioural status is important, and should include sleep and wake states, feeding behaviours, responsiveness, response to stress, and interaction with parents and other carers. To reduce sensory and visual deprivation and the effects of isolation, phototherapy is discontinued for feeding and parents are encouraged to hold and feed their baby.

Calcium levels. In neonates, hypocalcaemia is defined as a total serum of <1.7 mmol/L (7 mg/dl). Signs include jitteriness, irritability, rash, loose stools, fever, dehydration and convulsions.

Bilirubin levels. The reduction in bilirubin levels appears to be greatest in the first 24 hours of phototherapy and bilirubin levels are usually estimated daily.

Parent support. Whether at home or in hospital, in most cases parents will be caring for their baby; they are active partners with the midwife and need adequate information, support and reassurance to enable them to make decisions and assume this role. To give informed consent, parents must know the side-effects of phototherapy versus the possible risks of not treating their baby. If they feel able to ask questions this may help reduce any fear and distress they may experience.

Exchange transfusion

Excess bilirubin is removed from the baby during a blood exchange transfusion. With HDN sensitised erythrocytes are replaced with blood compatible with both the mother's and the infant's serum.

Indications for exchange transfusion. In recent years, cord blood screening and advances in phototherapy have reduced exchange transfusion for infants with many haemolytic and enzyme deficiency diseases. With the exception of very premature babies and Rh incompatibility, exchange transfusion may now be used only when phototherapy has failed, or there is a risk of kernicterus. As with phototherapy, the timing of exchange transfusion is not only based on serum bilirubin levels. With smaller, sick or very preterm babies, those with haemolysis or where jaundice occurs within the first 12–24 hours, exchange transfusion may be considered at a lower range of serum bilirubin levels:

- 255 µmol/L (15 mg/dl) for preterm babies < 1500 g
- 300–400 µmol/L (17–23 mg/dl) for sick and preterm babies > 1500 g, and those with haemolysis
- 400–500 µmol/L (23–29 mg/dl) for healthy term babies

Side-effects of exchange transfusion. Complications can result from the procedure and from the blood products. In one sample of 106 babies, 2% died (Jackson 1997) following exchange transfusion. Babies with other medical problems were more likely to have severe complications such as hypocalcaemia, thrombocytopenia and a higher death rate (12%). Necrotising enterocolitis (NEC) also increases with exchange transfusions (see Ch. 42). Jackson (1997) concluded that, in ill infants, exchange transfusion should be delayed until the risk of kernicterus is as high as the risks of the procedure.

Exchange transfusion is usually carried out in a neonatal intensive care unit (refer to individual hospital protocols). If midwives are involved in the consent process they need to inform families of the available evidence and the possible consequences of the procedure (Cheong et al 2001, Goodrum et al 1997, Jackson 1997, Portmann et al 1997, Voto et al 1997).

Drug treatments

Recently metalloporphyrins (tin–mesoporphyrin or SnMP, and tin–protoporphyrin or SnPP) are being used experimentally to prevent and treat neonatal hyperbilirubinaemia (Kappas et al 2001, Steffensrud 1998). Unlike other treatments that seek to remove excess bile pigment, these drugs prevent bilirubin formation. SnMP is a potent inhibitor of haem oxygenase activity, and thus bilirubin production, and has been found to be particularly valuable in treating babies with G6PD deficiency. In a clinical trial Kappas et al (2001) administered a single dose of SnMP to 172 newborns with G6PD-deficiency on the 1st day of life. None of those treated required phototherapy, compared with control group rates of 15% of 168 G6PD-normal and 31% of 58 G6PD-deficient newborns.

Neonatal infection

Modes of acquiring infection

Babies may acquire infections through the placenta (transplacental infection) from amniotic fluid as they traverse the birth canal, or after birth from sources such as carers' hands, contaminated objects or droplet infection.

Vulnerability to infection

Compared with older children and adults, newborns are immunodeficient and prone to a higher incidence of infection. Preterm babies are even more vulnerable as they have less well-developed defence mechanisms at birth (transfer of IgG mainly occurs after 32 weeks' gestation), and are more likely to experience invasive procedures. Full immunocompetence requires both innate and acquired immune responses.

Innate immunity. Innate (natural) responses do not require previous exposure to microorganisms and act as a first line of defence against infection. These responses include intact skin, mucous membranes and gastric acid and digestive enzymes. However, immediately after birth, skin is more easily irritated and damaged and the baby's bowel is not immediately colonised with normal protective flora.

Acquired immunity. Acquired (specific immune) responses develop and improve with ongoing exposure to a pathogen or organism. At birth the baby has some immune protection from the mother, but immunoglobulins are deficient. Maternal exposure and transfer of IgG across the placenta limit antibody levels, and to a large extent this immune response must be actively acquired after birth. Breastfeeding increases the baby's immune protection through the transmission of secretory IgA in breastmilk (see Ch. 40). During the early weeks of life the baby also has deficiencies in both the quantity and the quality of neutrophils (Askin 1995, Lawson 2001, Yancey et al 1996).

Management of infection

The midwife's role in the management of fetal and neonatal infection includes the prevention, diagnosis and treatment of infection in the mother, baby and midwife. Meeting these individual needs may involve a high level of interprofessional and interagency collaboration.

Prevention of infection in the mother

Before, during and after pregnancy, good midwifery practice involves an evidence-based primary prevention role that informs each woman of potential sources of infection that may harm her or her child. Antenatal health education includes informing women of such things as the importance of avoiding high risk foods, countries or areas with a high prevalence of some infections and contact with individuals with infectious diseases. It is also important to manage appropriately any infection that occurs during pregnancy. Prevention or treatment of infection in the mother during pregnancy can often prevent or reduce both short and long term sequelae in the child.

Prevention of infection in the newborn

Provision of a safe environment for newborns is of central importance, particularly in hospital where babies are at risk of cross-infection. Careful and frequent hand washing with soap or alcohol remains the single most important method of preventing infection. In busy situations cleansing with an alcohol-based hand-rub solution is the most practical means of improving staff compliance, and wearing gloves further reduces contamination. Other evidence-based midwifery strategies that help reduce infection in all environments include:

- encouraging and assisting women with breast feeding, thus increasing the baby's immune protection
- discouraging visitors who have infections, or who have been exposed to a communicable disease
- avoiding any irritation or trauma to the baby's skin and mucous membranes
- early diagnosis and treatment of infection
- ongoing education to ensure infection control practice is evidence based.

In hospital they include (Bott 1999, Lawson 2001, Senior 2001):

- having the baby rooming in with the mother
- adequately spacing cots if babies are in the nursery
- always using individual equipment for each baby
- isolating infected babies when absolutely essential.

Prevention of infection in the midwife

This is an important midwifery practice issue, as all health professionals are increasingly at risk of exposure to bloodborne infections. Universal precautions are based on the *routine* use of techniques that reduce exposure to blood, other body fluids and tissue that may contain bloodborne pathogens, and *every* client is considered a possible source of infection. The Department of Health (DoH 1998) recommends the following precautions to avoid exposure to body fluids:

1. wearing gloves, masks, goggles, gowns and protective footwear if there is any risk of exposure to body fluids (e.g. blood)
2. covering all skin lesions
3. changing gloves between patients and washing hands when gloves are changed
4. disinfecting all blood splashes and spillage
5. disposing safely of sharp instruments and waste
6. vaccination against hepatitis B.

One recent UK study suggests compliance with universal precautions does not always occur, however (Bott 1999). Reasons include problems with poorly fitting, uncomfortable, impractical or even unsafe equipment, such as goggles steaming up during the birth and overshoes that caused midwives to slip. In some instances wearing of goggles and gowns was seen as detrimental to the relationship between woman and midwife.

Diagnosis

Midwives play a central role in the diagnosis and treatment of infection in both mother and baby. In the newborn, early signs of infection may be subtle and difficult to distinguish from other problems; the mother or midwife may simply feel the baby is `off colour'.

Individual risk factors for infection. These include:

- a maternal history of prolonged rupture of membranes
- chorioamnionitis
- pyrexia during birth
- offensive amniotic fluid.

Physical assessment. This can include observation of:

- temperature instability
- lethargy or poor feeding, dehydration, starvation, hypothermia, acidosis or hypoxia
- bradycardia or tachycardia, and any apnoea
- urine and stool output and any vomiting
- central nervous system signs that require a complete neurodevelopmental examination.

Investigations. These may include:

- a complete blood cell count
- testing of specimens of urine and meconium for specific organisms
- swabs from the nose, throat and umbilicus, and from any skin rashes, pustules or vesicles to test for specific organisms
- MRI, CT scans and chest X-rays
- a lumbar puncture to enable examination of CSF
- testing of amniotic fluid, placental tissue and cord blood for specific organisms.

Treatment

The overall aim of management is to provide prompt and effective treatment that reduces the risk of septicaemia and life-threatening septic shock in this vulnerable group. Good management includes (Askin 1995, Wright Lott et al 1994):

1. caring for the baby in a warm thermoneutral environment and observing for temperature instability
2. good hydration and the correction of electrolyte imbalance, with demand feeding if possible and intravenous fluids as required
3. prompt systemic antibiotic or other drug therapy and local treatment of infection
4. ongoing monitoring of the baby's neurobehavioural status
5. reducing separation of mother and baby; if the baby requires admission to a neonatal intensive care unit then the midwife should encourage parents to be with their baby
6. providing evidence-based information, support and reassurance to parents
7. encouraging breast feeding, or expressing of milk, and informing women of the important role of breastmilk in fighting infection.

Infections acquired before or during birth

A number of infections may be acquired through the placenta, from amniotic fluid, or from the birth canal. The effects of sexually transmissible and reproductive tract infections, and the specific maternal and infant treatment of these infections, are presented in Ch. 21. Other infections are discussed below, with emphasis on those where midwives have an important preventive role.

Toxoplasmosis

Toxoplasmosis is caused by *Toxoplasma gondii (T. gondii)* a protozoan parasite found in uncooked meat and cat and dog faeces. Risk factors predicting an acute infection during pregnancy include eating undercooked meats, having a pet cat, poor hand hygiene, contact with soil, travel outside Europe and the USA and Canada and frequent consumption of raw vegetables outside the home (Baril et al 1999, Cook et al 2000). Some women are seropositive for *T. gondii* before pregnancy, with a first trimester IgG positive serum sample indicating previous maternal infection (Lebech et al 1999). Adults are often asymptomatic, or experience some malaise and lymphadenopathy and do not recall the infection. A survey of 13 000 pregnant women in eastern England found only 7–18% of them were

seropositive (rates increasing with age), which left up to 90% at risk of primary infection during pregnancy (Allain et al 1998).

Incidence and effects during pregnancy. Toxoplasmosis is far more common in pregnancy than rubella, or salmonella. Overall, in the UK, 640 babies are infected each year (Toxoplasmosis Trust 1998), and in eastern England a fetal infection rate of 3–16 per 10 000 women was reported, with significantly more first trimester infections (Allain et al 1998). Of particular relevance for midwives is the finding that France has a high rate of 4900 cases of primary infection during pregnancy each year (Baril et al 1999), whereas Brazil possibly has the highest reported prevalence of congenital toxoplasmosis (Neto et al 2000).

When primary infection occurs during pregnancy the reported maternal–fetal transmission rates vary from 19% (Lebech et al 1999) to 44% (Foulon et al 1999a). Risks for the infected fetus include intrauterine death, low birthweight, enlarged liver and spleen, jaundice and anaemia, hydrocephalus and chorioretinitis. Infected neonates may be asymptomatic at birth, but can later develop retinal and neurological disease. Those with subclinical disease at birth can develop seizures, significant cognitive and motor deficits and reduced cognitive function over time (Foulon et al 2000, Lebech et al 1999, Roizen et al 1995).

Diagnosis and treatment. It may not be possible to identify all cases of congenital toxoplasmosis. Antenatally a combination of *T. gondii* polymerase chain reaction (PCR) and mouse innoculation of amniotic fluid most accurately predicts the infection, with a sensitivity of 91% (Foulon et al 1999b). A negative PCR alone *does not* rule out congenital infection (Romand et al 2001). After birth, specific *T. gondii* IgA antibodies (sensitivity 64% in cord blood and 66% in neonatal blood) are more frequently detected than IgM (sensitivity of 41% in cord blood and 42% in neonatal blood) (Naessens et al 1999).

In one cohort of 144 women, antenatal antibiotic therapy resulted in a significant reduction in the number of severely affected infants. Although the drugs did not reduce the fetomaternal transmission rate, early treatment was associated with more positive outcomes in congenitally infected babies (Foulon et al 1999a). Roizen et al (1995) also found significantly better cognitive and motor outcomes in a group of 36 infants with congenital toxoplasmosis who were treated with pyrimethamine and sulfadiazine for one year, compared with those reported for untreated children, or those treated for only one month. However, despite a large amount of research, the effectiveness of antenatal treatment (for pregnant women with presumed toxoplasmosis) in reducing the congenital transmission of *T. gondii* is not proven (Peyron et al 2001, Wallon et al 1999).

Prevention. Providing information about toxoplasmosis is the most effective preventive strategy, as health education can decrease the incidence of primary infection during pregnancy (Baril et al 1999) by as much as 60% (Foulon et al 2000). In the UK, the Toxoplasmosis Trust's (1998) `daisy chain' campaign educates health professionals and the public (a handbook for midwives is available from the trust). Appropriate information includes advising women about washing kitchen surfaces following contact with uncooked meats, stringent hand washing and avoiding contact with cat and dog faeces. Preventive strategies should also aim to reduce the prevalence of the protozoan parasite *T. gondii* in meat (Baril et al 1999, Cook et al 2000, Foulon et al 2000).

A further possible preventive strategy is serologic screening during pregnancy (Foulon et al 2000). In France, all pregnant women at risk of toxoplasmosis must have monthly testing (Baril et al 1999) and, in some regions of the UK, proponents claim repeated screening would detect and possibly prevent infection in about 10 neonates per 10 000 women (Allain et al 1998). However, routine antenatal screening assumes that treatment during pregnancy can reduce the fetomaternal transmission rate and result in improved infant outcomes (Foulon et al 2000). In countries where screening is not routine, some argue it should be introduced only as part of clinical trials that evaluate screening and treatment (Peyron et al 2001, Wallon et al 1999).

Varicella zoster

Varicella zoster virus (VZV) is a highly contagious DNA virus of the herpes family transmitted by respiratory droplets and contact with vesicle fluid that causes varicella (chickenpox). It has an incubation period of 10–20 days and is infectious for 48 hours before the rash appears until vesicles crust over. After the primary infection the virus remains dormant in sensory nerve root ganglia, with any recurrent infection resulting in herpes zoster (shingles). In adults varicella can be more severe and may be complicated by pneumonia, hepatitis and encephalitis. Before pregnancy, up to 90% of women are seropositive for VZV immunoglobulin G (IgG) antibodies (O'Riordan et al 2000), with lower rates in most tropical and subtropical areas.

Incidence and effects during pregnancy. A UK confidential enquiry into maternal deaths in the UK between 1985 and 1997 reported seven maternal deaths associated with varicella infection during pregnancy (cited in Heuchan & Isaacs 2001). Fetal sequelae from primary maternal infection vary with the gestation at the time of the infection.

With maternal infection during the first 20 weeks of pregnancy the baby has about a 2% risk of fetal varicella syndrome (FVS) (previously known as congenital varicella syndrome or CVS) (Pastuszak et al 1994). Symptoms can include skin lesions and scarring in a dermatomal distribution, eye problems, such as chorioretinitis and cataracts, and skeletal anomalies, in particular limb hypoplasia. Severe neurological problems may include encephalitis, microcephaly and significant developmental delay. About 30% of babies born with skin lesions die in the first months of life (Sauerbrei & Wutzler 2000).

Maternal chickenpox from 20 weeks' gestation up to almost the time of birth can result in milder forms of neonatal varicella that do not result in negative sequelae for the neonate. The child may have shingles during the first few years of life. However, maternal infection after 36 weeks, and particularly in the week before the birth (when cord blood VZV IgG is low) to 2 days after, can result in infection rates of up to 50%. About 25% of those infected will develop neonatal clinical varicella (or varicella infection of the newborn). Newborns are also at risk of contracting varicella from mothers or siblings in the postnatal period. Most affected babies will develop a vesicular rash and about 30% will die. Other complications of neonatal varicella include clinical sepsis, pneumonia, pyoderma and hepatitis (Singalavanija et al 1999).

Diagnosis and treatment. Diagnosis of FVS can include a recent history of maternal varicella and laboratory evidence of in utero infection following cordocentesis and amniocentesis for VZV DNA in amniotic fluid. PCR is more sensitive than cell culture in detecting the virus. Structural changes in the fetus may be confirmed with ultrasonography 5 weeks or more after the primary infection. Skin lesions in a dermatomal distribution are present in 76% of infants with FVS and neonatal clinical varicella. However, diagnosis is not always conclusive. In one cohort of 107 women the risk of transplacental passage before 24 weeks of pregnancy was 8.4%, but only four of the nine women gave birth to babies with FVS. No case of FVS occurred when amniocentesis was negative for VZV DNA (Mouly et al 1997, Sauerbrei & Wutzler 2000).

Varicella seronegative pregnant women who have appreciable exposure to chickenpox (defined as living in the same house, or having face to face contact for at least 5 minutes) should be offered varicella zoster immune globulin (VZIG), ideally within 72 hours of contact with the infectious person, and always within 10 days. Some evidence suggests passive immunisation may prevent or reduce the severity or infection in women who have not already had chickenpox. With parental permission, VZIG should also be given to a baby whose mother develops chickenpox between 7 days before and 28 days after the birth, or whose siblings at home have chickenpox (if the mother is seronegative) (Heuchan & Isaacs 2001). Informed consent is essential as VZIG is a blood product obtained from human volunteers.

Although at the present time no clinical trials have confirmed that antiviral chemotherapy prevents CVS (Sauerbrei & Wutzler 2000), the antiviral drug acyclovir appears to reduce the mortality and risk of severe disease in some groups. Oral acyclovir can be offered to pregnant women with appreciable exposure to chickenpox (who did not receive VZIG), particularly those in high risk groups. Intravenous acyclovir is recommended for pregnant women with severe complications, and also for newborns with chickenpox during the first 2 weeks of life if they are unwell or have added risk factors (e.g. prematurity or corticosteroid therapy). Although the mother and baby should be isolated from other neonates, they should always be kept together (Heuchan & Isaacs 2001, Kesson et al 1996).

Prevention. At the present time, particularly in the UK the most effective preventive strategy for midwives is health education. Many pregnant women are unaware of the need to avoid and immediately report significant contact with varicella infection, particularly when serologic status is uncertain. Nearly half of all chickenpox cases during pregnancy could be prevented by routinely serotesting all pregnant women, or by selectively testing those without a known history of varicella. However, antenatal screening is only cost effective as part of a screening and vaccination programme (or for groups of women with increased exposure) (Glantz & Mushlin 1998, Smith et al 1998).

Although an attenuated live-virus vaccine is available for children and adults, in the UK at the present time the vaccine is not available routinely for seronegative women. Where available, midwives can encourage seronegative women to be vaccinated before and after, but *not during* pregnancy until safety has been proven (Huang et al 1999). In one small group of 58 women inadvertently given varicella vaccine during the first or second trimester, no cases of FVS were identified (Shields et al 2001). However, one case of a woman with primary varicella infection at 39 weeks of gestation (confirmed by serologic studies) was reported whose only VZV exposure was to her two children who were vaccinated with the varicella zoster vaccine 8 days before (Huang et al 1999).

Rubella

For most immunocompetent children and adults (including pregnant women), the rubella virus causes a mild and insignificant illness that is spread by droplet infection. Rubella seropositive rates before pregnancy are high in some countries (usually due to vaccination) but low in others. Rubella vaccine is used in 92% of industrialised countries, 36% of those with economies in transition and 28% of developing countries (United Nations country classification) (Robertson et al 1997). Women born in the UK, Australia and New Zealand are nearly 16 times more likely to be vaccinated against rubella (Marsack et al 1995). However, the rates are much lower for women in these countries who were born elsewhere, particularly Asia (Cheffins et al 1998, Miller et al 1993). In England, a woman recently arrived from Asia gave birth to a baby with congenital rubella syndrome (CRS) (Sheridan et al 2002), and in Scotland a case of CRS was linked to an outbreak of rubella in Greece (Tookey et al 2000).

Incidence and effects during pregnancy. Since 1988, in most industrialised countries the measles, mumps and rubella (MMR) vaccine has reduced rubella incidence to a low endemic level (Miller et al

1993). However, other countries still report rates similar to those of industrialised countries during the prevaccination era (Cutts et al 1997). If primary rubella infection occurs during the first 12 weeks of pregnancy, maternal–fetal transmission rates are as high as 85%. Intrauterine infection is unlikely when the mother's rash appears before, or within 11 days after the last menstrual period, and with proven infection later than the 16th week the risk of severe fetal sequelae is less (Enders et al 1988, Munro et al 1987). First trimester infection can result in spontaneous abortion, and in surviving babies a number of serious and permanent consequences are associated with CRS. These include cataracts, sensorineural deafness, congenital heart defects, microcephaly, meningoencephalitis, dermal erythropoiesis, thrombocytopenia and very significant developmental delay (Cutts et al 1997).

Diagnosis and treatment. Diagnosis of congenital rubella can include (Aboudy et al 1997, Munro et al 1987, Tanemura et al 1996):

1. a maternal history of a rash or contact with rubella
2. serological screening of women for rubella-specific IgG and IgM antibodies
3. cordocentesis to establish the presence of rubella IgM antibody in umbilical cord blood
4. the detection of viral ribonucleic acid in chorionic villi, amniotic fluid, or fetal blood
5. ultrasonic examination of the fetus and neonate
6. specific antibody detection in cord blood at birth
7. isolation of the rubella virus from the throat, urine and CSF of the neonate
8. ongoing physical examinations during early childhood.

Most women with a first trimester infection require a great deal of information and support and some may request termination of pregnancy. Following the birth, management is mainly symptomatic with an emphasis on support for the parents and appropriate referrals to ensure best outcomes for the baby. Infants with CRS are highly infectious and should be isolated from other infants and pregnant women (but not from their own mothers). Babies should always be followed up for several years, as some problems may not become apparent until they are older.

Prevention. At the present time in the UK a number of factors contribute to CRS. These include immigration from countries where rubella vaccination is not routine or has only recently been introduced, maternal reinfection and missed opportunities for immunisation at school or after the birth (Miller et al 1993). The best protection against CRS is a strategy that targets all children, and also offers the vaccine to susceptible schoolgirls or women before pregnancy, or both groups (Robertson et al 1997). As part of their extended public health role, midwives can encourage vaccination for seronegative women before and after, but *not* during pregnancy, and also discuss the importance of vaccinating their children. Targeted immunisation for at-risk groups is also recommended (Sheridan et al 2002). Susceptible individuals who work with pregnant women can also be offered rubella vaccination. As with chickenpox, midwives need to emphasise the importance of avoiding contact with rubella during pregnancy, as reinfection during pregnancy has been reported despite previous vaccination (Aboudy et al 1997).

Ophthalmia neonatorum

Ophthalmia neonatorum is a notifiable condition, defined in England as any purulent discharge from the eyes of an infant within 21 days of birth, and in Scotland as any inflammation that occurs in the eyes of an infant within 21 days of birth that is accompanied by a discharge. The condition is usually acquired during vaginal delivery and causative organisms include *Staphylococcus aureus*, *Streptococcus pneumoniae*, *Haemophilus influenzae*, *E. coli*, *Klebsiella*, *Pseudomonas*, *Chlamydia trachomatis* and *Neisseria gonorrhoeae*.

A swab must be taken for culture and sensitivity testing, and a doctor notified immediately. Differential diagnosis of the organism is essential, particularly for chlamydial and gonococcal infections (see Ch. 21), as these organisms can cause conjunctival scarring, corneal infiltration, blindness and systemic spread. Other causes of inflammation must also be excluded. Treatment includes local cleaning and care of the eyes with normal saline, and appropriate drug therapy for the baby and also the mother if required (Hammerschlag 1993, O'Hara 1993.)

Candida

Candida is a Gram-positive yeast fungus that has a number of strains including *C. albicans*, *C. parapsilosis*, *C. tropicalis* and *C. lusitainiae*. *C. albicans* is responsible for most fungal infections, including thrush in infants.

Infection can affect the mouth (oral candidiasis), skin (cutaneous candidiasis) and other organs (systemic candidiasis).

Oral candidiasis. Oral candidiasis or thrush presents as white patches on the baby's gums, palate and tongue. It can be acquired during birth and also from caregivers' hands or feeding equipment (see Ch. 42). Raw areas on the edge of the tongue (removed by the infant sucking) may be a valuable aid to diagnosis. Breast-feeding women may also have infected breasts, with such symptoms as persistently sore and red nipples and a burning, itching or stabbing pain in the breasts. Nystatin is the most effective and least expensive treatment: oral for the baby and topical breast application for the mother (Amir et al 1996, MacDonald 1995).

Cutaneous candidiasis. Cutaneous candidiasis presents as a moist papular or vesicular rash, usually in the region of the axillae, neck, perineum or umbilicus. Management includes keeping the area as dry as possible and applying topical nystatin. Oral nystatin may also be needed to reduce the yeast population as neonatal candidal meningitis has been reported with congenital cutaneous candidiasis in a term baby (Barone & Krilov 1995). In preterm babies the thin cutaneous barrier may contribute to the early onset of systemic *Candida* infection (Melville et al 1996).

Disseminated candidiasis. Systemic colonisation with *Candida* occurs frequently in very low birthweight babies, with progression from colonisation to systemic infection more common in the smallest neonates. Complications can include meningitis, endocarditis, pyelonephritis, pneumonia and osteomyelitis (Barone & Krilov 1995). Intravenous amphotericin B drug therapy is usually required and oral flucytosine (a fungistatic agent) may also be given (Weisse et al 1993). Prompt management is essential as the condition can be life threatening; for instance, in one cohort 9 out of 19 patients infected with *C. parapsilosis* and 5 out of 15 patients infected with *C. albicans* died of fungaemia. Neonates with candidiasis also had a history of greater exposure to systemic steroids, catecholamine infusions and antibiotics (particularly prolonged use of third generation cephalosporin) (Benjamin et al 2000).

Some infections acquired after birth

After the birth the most common routes for neonatal infection are the umbilicus, broken skin, the respiratory tract and those that result from invasive procedures and devices (Askin 1995). Infections acquired after birth are also discussed in Chapters 42 and 43.

Eye infections

Mild eye infections are common in babies and can be treated with routine eye care and antibiotics if required. Other more serious conditions must be excluded, such as ophthalmia neonatorum (see above), trauma, foreign bodies, congenital glaucoma and nasolacrimal duct obstruction (Hammerschlag 1993, O'Hara 1993).

Skin infections

Most neonatal skin infections are caused by *S. aureus*. In newborn babies the most likely skin lesions are septic spots or pustules found either as solitary lesions or clustered in the umbilical and buttock areas. For the well neonate with limited pustules, management includes regular cleansing with an antiseptic solution and antibiotic therapy for more extensive pustules (Wright Lott et al 1994) (see Ch. 42).

Meningitis

Neonatal meningitis is an inflammation of the membranes lining the brain and spinal column; it is caused by organisms such as *E. coli*, group B streptococci and *Listeria monocytogenes*, and more unusually *Candida* and herpes. Very early signs may be non-specific, followed by those of meningeal irritation and raised intracranial pressure such as irritability, bulging fontanelle, increasing lethargy, crying, tremors, twitching, severe vomiting, alterations in consciousness and diminished muscle tone. Babies may also present with hemiparesis, horizontal deviation and decreased pupillary reaction of the eye, decreased retinal reflex and an abnormal Moro reflex. Early diagnosis and treatment are vital to prevent collapse and death. Diagnosis is usually confirmed by examination of CSF.

Very ill babies will require intensive care, intravenous fluids and antibiotic therapy. Long term neurological complications can occur in surviving infants (Adhikari et al 1995, Barone & Krilov 1995, Synnott et al 1994).

Respiratory infections

These may be minor (nasopharyngitis and rhinitis) or more severe such as pneumonia (see Chs 42 and 43).

Gastrointestinal tract infections

In the newborn these can include gastroenteritis or the more severe NEC (see Chs 42 and 43). Causative organisms for gastroenteritis include rotavirus, *Salmonella*, *Shigella* and a pathogenic strain of *E. coli*. The secretory IgA in breastmilk offers important protection against these organisms, particularly rotavirus. Treatment depends upon the severity of symptoms. The correction of fluid and electrolyte imbalance is an urgent priority, as nausea and vomiting can rapidly cause dehydration in neonates.

Umbilical infection

Signs can include localised inflammation and an offensive discharge. Untreated infection can spread to the liver via the umbilical vein and cause hepatitis and septicaemia. Treatment may include regular cleansing, the administration of an antibiotic powder and appropriate antibiotic therapy (see Ch. 42).

Urinary tract infections

Urinary tract infections can result from bacteria such as *E. coli*, or less often from a congenital anomaly that obstructs urine flow. The signs are usually those of an early non-specific infection, and diagnosis is usually confirmed through laboratory evaluation of a urine sample (see Ch. 42).

REFERENCES

Aboudy Y, Fogel A, Barnea B et al 1997 Subclinical rubella reinfection during pregnancy followed by transmission of virus to the fetus. Journal of Infection 34(3):273–276

Adhikari M, Coovadia Y M, Singh D 1995 A 4 year study of neonatal meningitis: clinical and microbiological findings. Journal of Tropical Pediatrics 41(2):81–85

Allaby M, Forman K, Touch S et al 1999 The use of routine anti-D prophylaxis antenatally to Rhesus negative women. Trent Institute for Health Services Research, Universities of Leicester, Nottingham and Sheffield, ref 99/04.

Allain J P, Palmer C R, Pearson G 1998 Epidemiological study of latent and recent infection by toxoplasma gondii in pregnant women from a regional population in the UK. Journal of Infection 36:189–196

American College of Obstetricians and Gynaecologists 1999 Prevention of Rh D alloimmunization: clinical management guidelines for obstetricians and gynecologists. International Journal of Gynecology and Obstetrics 66(1):63–70

Amir L H, Garland S M, Dennerstein L et al 1996 *Candida albicans*: is it associated with nipple pain in lactating women? Gynecologic and Obstetric Investigation 41(1):30–34

Askin D F 1995 Bacterial and fungal infections in the neonate. Journal of Obstetric, Gynecologic and Neonatal Nursing 24(7):635–643

Baril L, Ancelle T, Goulet V 1999 Risk factors for toxoplasma infection in pregnancy: a case–control study in France. Scandinavian Journal of Infectious Diseases 31(3):305–309

Barone S R, Krilov L R 1995 Neonatal candidal meningitis in a full-term infant with congenital cutaneous candidiasis. Clinical Pediatrics 34(4):217–219

Benjamin D K, Ross K, McKinney R E et al 2000 When to suspect fungal infection in neonates: a clinical comparison of *Candida albicans* and *Candida parapsilosis* fungemia with coagulase-negative staphylococcal bacteremia. Pediatrics 106(4):712–718

Bertini G, Dani C, Tronchin M et al 2001 Is breastfeeding really favoring early neonatal jaundice. Pediatrics 107(3):E41

Blackburn S 1995 Hyperbilirubinemia and neonatal jaundice. Neonatal Network 14(7):15–25

Bott J 1999 HIV risk reduction and the use of universal precautions. British Journal of Midwifery 7(11):671–675

Cheffins T, Chan A, Keane R J et al 1998 The impact of rubella immunisation on the incidence of rubella, congenital rubella syndrome and rubella-related terminations of pregnancy in South Australia. British Journal of Obstetrics and Gynaecology 105(9):998–1004

Cheong Y C, Goodrick J, Kyle P M et al 2001 Management of anti-rhesus-D antibodies in pregnancy: a review from 1994 to 1998. Fetal Diagnosis and Therapy 16(5):294–298

Coe L 1999 Pathology and physiology of neonatal jaundice. British Journal of Midwifery 7(4):240–243

Cook A J C, Gilbert R E, Buffolano W et al 2000 Sources of toxoplasma infection in pregnant women: European multicentre case–control study. British Medical Journal 321(7254):142–147

Coombes R 1999 Midwives cautioned over risks of using untested blood product. Nursing Times 95(24):7

Craig S, Morris K, Tubman T et al 2000 The fetal and neonatal outcomes of rhesus D antibody affected pregnancies in Northern Ireland. Irish Medical Journal 93(1):17–18

Crofts D J, Michel V J M, Rigby A S et al 1999 Assessment of stool colour in community management of prolonged jaundice in infancy. Acta Paediatrica 88(9):969–974

Crowther C, Middleton P 2001 Anti-D administration after childbirth for preventing Rhesus alloimmunisation. In: Cochrane Library, Issue 3. Update Software, Oxford

Crowther C A, Keirse M J N C 1999 Anti-D administration during pregnancy for preventing Rhesus alloimmunisation (Cochrane review). In: Cochrane Library, Issue 2. Update Software, Oxford

Cutts F T, Robertson S E, Diaz-Ortega J L et al 1997 Control of rubella and congenital rubella syndrome (CRS) in developing countries, part 1: burden of disease from CRS. Bulletin of the World Health Organization 75(1):55–68

Deka D, Buckshee K, Kinra G 1996 Intravenous immunoglobulin as primary therapy or adjuvant therapy to intrauterine fetal blood transfusion: a new approach in the management of severe Rh-immunization. Journal of Obstetrics and Gynaecology Research 22(6):561–567

DoH (Department of Health) 1998 Guidance for clinical health care workers: protection against infection with blood-borne viruses. Recommendations of the Expert Advisory Group on AIDS and the Advisory Group on Hepatitis. DoH, London

Enders G, Pacher U N, Miller E et al 1988 Outcome of confirmed periconceptional maternal rubella. Lancet 1(8600):1445–1446

Filbey D, Hanson U, Wesstrom G 1995 The prevalence of red cell antibodies in pregnancy correlated to the outcome of the newborn: a 12 year study in central Sweden. Acta Obstetricia et Gynecologica Scandinavica 74(9):687–692

Foulon W, Villena I, Stray-Pedersen B 1999a Treatment of toxoplasmosis during pregnancy: a multicenter study of impact on fetal transmission and children's sequelae at age 1 year. American Journal of Obstetrics and Gynecology 180(2):410–415

Foulon W, Pinon J M, Stray-Pedersen B et al 1999b Prenatal diagnosis of congenital toxoplasmosis: a multicenter evaluation of different diagnostic parameters. American Journal of Obstetrics and Gynecology 181(4):843–847

Foulon W, Naessens A, Ho-Yen D 2000 Prevention of congenital toxoplasmosis. Journal of Perinatal Medicine 28(5):337–345

Fung K A F K, Giulivi A, Chisholm J et al 1998 Clinical usefulness of flow cytometry in detection and quantification of fetomaternal hemorrhage. Journal of Maternal-Fetal Investigation 8(3):121–125

Gartner L M, Lee K S 1999 Jaundice in the breastfed infant. Clinics in Perinatology 26(2):431–445

Glantz C, Mushlin A I 1998 Cost-effectiveness of routine antenatal varicella screening. Obstetrics and Gynecology 91(4):519–528

Goodrum L A, Saade G R, Belfort M A et al 1997 The effect of intrauterine transfusion on fetal bilirubin in red cell alloimmunization. Obstetrics and Gynecology 89(1):57–60

Gourley G R, Kreamer B, Cohnen M et al 1999 Neonatal jaundice and diet. Archives of Pediatrics and Adolescent Medicine 153(2):184–188

Gunston K D 1993 Severity of fetal haemolysis in different racial groups in relation in predelivery anti-D (rhesus) titres. South African Medical Journal 83(5):366

Hammerschlag M R 1993 Neonatal conjunctivitis. Pediatric Annals 22(6):346–351

Hannam S, McDonnell M, Rennie J M 2000 Investigation of prolonged neonatal jaundice. Acta Paediatrica 89(6):694–697

Hansen T W R 2001a Guidelines for treatment of neonatal jaundice: is there a place for evidence-based medicine? Acta Paediatrica 90(3):239–241

Hansen T W R 2001b Bilirubin production, breast-feeding and neonatal jaundice. Paediatric and Perinatal Epidemiology 90(7):716–723

Harris M C, Bernbaum J C, Polin R J et al 2001 Developmental follow-up of breastfed term and near-term infants with marked hyperbilirubinemia. Pediatrics 107(5):1075–1080

Heuchan A M, Isaacs D 2001 The management of varicella-zoster virus exposure and infection in pregnancy and the newborn period. Medical Journal of Australia 174(6):288–292

Hintz S R, Gaylord T D, Oh W et al 2001 Serum bilirubin levels at 72 hours by selected characteristics in breastfed and formula-fed infants delivered by cesarean section. Acta Paediatrica 90(7):776–781

Howard H L, Martlew V J, McFadyen I R et al 1997 Preventing Rhesus D haemolytic disease of the newborn by giving anti-D immunoglobulin: are the guidelines being adequately followed? British Journal of Obstetrics and Gynaecology 104(1):37–41

Huang W, Hussey M, Michel F 1999 Transmission of varicella to a gravida via close contacts immunized with varicella-zoster vaccine: a case report. Journal of Reproductive Medicine 44(10):905–907

Ismail K M K, Martin W L, Ghosh S 2001 Etiology and outcome of hydrops fetalis. Journal of Maternal–Fetal Medicine 10(3):175–181

Jackson J C 1997 Adverse events associated with exchange transfusion in healthy and ill newborns. Pediatrics 99(5):E7

Kappas A, Drummond G S, Valaes T 2001 A single dose of Sn-mesoporphyrin prevents development of severe hyperbilirubinemia in glucose-6-phosphate dehydrogenase-deficient newborns. Pediatrics 108(1):25–30

Kesson A M, Grimwood K, Burgess M A 1996 Acyclovir for the prevention and treatment of varicella zoster in children, adolescents and pregnancy. Journal of Paediatrics and Child Health 32(3):211–217

Lawson L G 2001 Handwashing: a neonatal perspective. Journal of Neonatal Nursing 7(2):42–46

Lebech M, Andersen O, Christensen N C et al 1999 Feasibility of neonatal screening for toxoplasma infection in the absence of prenatal treatment. Lancet 353(9167):1834–1837

Maayan-Metzger A, Schwartz T, Sulkes J et al 2001 Maternal anti-D prophylaxis during pregnancy does not cause neonatal haemolysis. Archives of Disease in Childhood: Fetal and Neonatal Edition 84(1):F60–F62

MacDonald H 1995 Candida: the hidden deterrent to breastfeeding. Canadian Nurse 91(9):27–30

McDonnell M, Hannam S, Devane S P 1998 Hydrops fetalis due to ABO incompatibility. Archives of Disease in Childhood: Fetal and Neonatal Edition 78(3):F220–F221

McSweeney E, Kirkham J, Vinall P, Flanagan P 1998 An audit of anti-D sensitisation in Yorkshire. British Journal of Obstetrics and Gynaecology 105:1091–1094

Maisels M J, Newman T B 1995 Kernicterus in otherwise healthy, breast-fed term newborns. Pediatrics 96(4):730–733

Manzar S 1999 Cephalo-caudal progression of jaundice: a reliable, non-invasive clinical method to assess the degree of neonatal hyperbilirubinaemia. Journal of Tropical Pediatrics 45(5):312–313

Marsack C R, Alsop C L, Kurinczuk J J et al 1995 Pre-pregnancy counselling for the primary prevention of birth defects: rubella vaccination and folate intake. Medical Journal of Australia 162(8):403–406

Melville C, Kempley S, Graham J et al 1996 Early onset systemic Candida infection in extremely preterm neonates. European Journal of Pediatrics 155(10):904–906

Miller E, Waight P A, Vurdien J E 1993 Rubella surveillance to December 1992: second joint report from the PHLS and National Congenital Rubella Surveillance Programme CDR (Communicable Disease Report) Review 3(3):R35–R40

Morrison J 2000 Audit of anti-D immunoglobin administration to pregnant Rhesus D negative women following sensitising events. Journal of Obstetrics and Gynaecology 20(4):371–373

Mouly F, Mirlesse V, Meritet J F et al 1997 Prenatal diagnosis of fetal varicella-zoster virus infection with polymerase chain reaction of amniotic fluid in 107 cases, American Journal of Obstetrics and Gynecology 177(4):894–898

Munro N D, Sheppard S, Smithells R W et al 1987 Temporal relations between maternal rubella and congenital defects. Lancet ii(8552):201–204

Naessens A, Jenum P A, Pollak A et al 1999 Diagnosis of congenital toxoplasmosis in the neonatal period: a multicenter evaluation. Journal of Pediatrics 135(6):714–719

Neto E C, Anele E, Rubim R et al 2000 High prevalence of congenital toxoplasmosis in Brazil estimated in a 3-year prospective neonatal screening study. International Journal of Epidemiology 29(5):941–947

Newman T B, Maisels M J 2000 Less aggressive treatment of neonatal jaundice and reports of kernicterus: lessons about practice guidelines. Pediatrics 105(1):242–245

Newman T B, Xiong B, Gonzales V M et al 2000 Prediction and prevention of extreme neonatal hyperbilirubinemia in a mature health maintenance organization. Archives of Pediatrics and Adolescent Medicine 15(11):1140–1147

NICE (National Institute for Clinical Excellence) 2002 Guidance on the use of routine antenatal anti-D prophylaxis for RhD-negative women. Technology appraisal guidance no 41, ref. NOO92. NICE, London. Online. Available: www./nice.org.uk

O'Hara M A 1993 Ophthalmia neonatorum. Pediatric Ophthalmology 40(4):715–725

O'Riordan M, O'Gorman C, Morgan C et al 2000 Sera prevalence of varicella zoster virus in pregnant women in Dublin. Irish Journal of Medical Science 169:288

Ozolek J A, Watchko J F, Mimouni F 1994 Prevalence and lack of clinical significance of blood group incompatibility in mothers with blood type A or B. Journal of Pediatrics 125(1):87–91

Pastuszak A L, Levy M, Schick B et al 1994 Outcome after maternal varicella infection in the first 20 weeks of pregnancy. New England Journal of Medicine 330(13):901–905

Peyron F, Wallon M, Liou C et al 2001 Treatments for toxoplasmosis in pregnancy (date of most recent substantive amendment 10 May 1999). Cochrane Library Issue 3. Update Software, Oxford.

Portmann C, Ludlow J, Joyce A 1997 Antecedents to and outcomes of Rh(D) isoimmunization: Mater Mothers Hospital, Brisbane, 1988–1995. Australian and New Zealand Journal of Obstetrics and Gynaecology 37(1):12–16

RCOG (Royal College of Obstetricians and Gynaecologists) 1999 Use of anti-D immunoglobulin for Rh prophylaxis. Clinical `green top' guidelines. RCOG, London. Online. Available: www.rcog.org.uk/guidelines/antid.html

Robertson S E, Cutts F T, Samuel R et al 1997 Control of rubella and congenital rubella syndrome (CRS) in developing countries, part 2: vaccination against rubella. Bulletin of the World Health Organization 75(1):69–80

Roizen N, Swisher C N, Stein M A et al 1995 Neurologic and developmental outcome in treated congenital toxoplasmosis. Pediatrics 95(1):11–20

Romand S, Wallon M, Franck J et al 2001 Prenatal diagnosis using polymerase chain reaction on amniotic fluid for congenital toxoplasmosis. Obstetrics and Gynecology 97(2):296–300

Rose F M 2000 Monitoring bilirubin. Journal of Neonatal Nursing 6(5): separately paginated insert

Rubaltelli F F, Griffith P F 1992 Management of neonatal hyperbilirubinaemia and prevention of kernicterus. Practical Therapeutics 43(6):864–872

Sarici S U, Alpay F, Unay B et al 1999 Comparison of the efficacy of conventional special blue light phototherapy and fiberoptic phototherapy in the management of neonatal hyperbilirubinaemia. Acta Paediatrica 88(11):1249–1253

Sauerbrei A, Wutzler P 2000 The congenital varicella syndrome. Journal of Perinatology 20(8):548–554

Seidman D S, Ergaz Z, Paz I et al 1999 Predicting the risk of jaundice in fullterm healthy newborns: a prospective population-based study. Journal of Perinatology 19(8):564–565

Seidman D S, Moise J, Ergaz Z et al 2000 A new blue light-emitting phototherapy device: a prospective randomized controlled study. Journal of Pediatrics 136(6):771–774

Senior K 2001 Can we keep up with hospital-acquired infections? Lancet (Infectious Diseases) April:8

Sheridan E, Aitken C, Jeffries D et al 2002 Congenital rubella syndrome: a risk in immigrant populations. Lancet 359(9307):673–674

Shields K E, Galil K, Seward J 2001 Varicella vaccine exposure during pregnancy: data from the first 5 years of the pregnancy registry. Obstetrics and Gynecology 98(1):14–19

Singalavanija S, Horpoapan S, Limpongsanurak W et al 1999 Neonatal varicella: a report of 26 cases. Journal of the Medical Association of Thailand 82(10):957–962

Smith M G 1997 Hyperbilirubinaemia in healthy breastfed infants. British Journal of Midwifery 5(6):340–343

Smith W J, Jackson L A, Watts D H 1997 Prevention of chickenpox in reproductive-age women: cost-effectiveness of routine prenatal screening with postpartum vaccination of susceptibles. Obstetrics and Gynecology 92(4):535–545

Spong C Y, Porter A E, Queenan J T 2001 Management of isoimmunization in the presence of multiple maternal antibodies. American Journal of Obstetrics and Gynecology 185(2):481–484

Stanley T V 1997 A case of kernicterus in New Zealand: a predictable tragedy? Journal of Paediatrics and Child Health 33:451–453

Steffensrud S 1998 Tin-metalloporphyrins: an answer to neonatal jaundice? Neonatal Network 17(5):11–17

Synnott M B, Morse D L, Hall S M 1994 Neonatal meningitis in England and Wales: a review of routine national data. Archives of Disease in Childhood 71(2):75–80

Tanemura M, Suzumori K, Yagami Y 1996 Diagnosis of fetal rubella infection with reverse transcription and nested polymerase chain reaction: a study of 34 cases diagnosed in fetuses. American Journal of Obstetrics and Gynecology 174(2):578–582

Tanyer G, Siklar Z, Dallar Y et al 2001 Multiple dose IVIG treatment in neonatal immune hemolytic jaundice. Journal of Tropical Pediatrics 47(1):50–53

Tookey P, Molyneaux P, Helms P 2000 UK case of congenital rubella can be linked to Greek cases. British Medical Journal 321(7263):766–767

Toxoplasmosis Trust 1998 Toxoplasmosis survey reveals ignorance and misconceptions: daisy chain campaign aims to end an avoidable tragedy. Toxoplasmosis Trust London, 18 March

Urbaniak S J 1998 The scientific basis of antenatal prophylaxis. British Journal of Obstetrics and Gynaecology 105(suppl 18):11–18

Vause S, Wray J, Bailie C 2000 Management of women who are Rhesus D negative in Northern Ireland. Journal of Obstetrics and Gynaecology 20(4):374–377

Voto L S, Mathet E R, Zapaterio J L 1997 High-dose gammaglobulin (IVIG) followed by intrauterine transfusions (IUTs): a new alternative for the treatment of severe fetal hemolytic disease. Journal of Perinatal Medicine 25(1):85–88

Wallon M, Liou C, Garner P 1999 Congenital toxoplasmosis: systematic review of evidence of efficacy of treatment in pregnancy. British Medical Journal 318(7197):1511–1514

Weisse M E, Person D A, Berkenbaugh J T 1993 Treatment of Candida arthritis with flucytosine and amphotericin B. Journal of Perinatology 13(5):402–404

Wheeler B J 2000 Kernicterus: ancient history or ongoing threat? Mother Baby Journal 5(2):21–30

Wickham S 1999a Anti-D: an informed choice? Part 1. Practising Midwife 2(5):18–19

Wickham S 1999b Anti-D Part 2: risks and benefits. Practising Midwife 2(6):38–39

Wickham S 2001 Anti-D in midwifery: panacea or paradox? Books for Midwives, Oxford

Wolf M J, Beunen G, Casaer P 1997 Extreme hyperbilirubinaemia in Zimbabwean neonates: neurodevelopmental outcome at 4 months. European Journal of Pediatrics 156(10):803–807

Wray J, Benbow 1999 A current debate and issues surrounding anti-D immunoglobulin. MIDIRS Midwifery Digest 9(4):517–519

Wright Lott J, Kenner C, Polak J D 1994 Common neonatal infections and complications. In: Wright Lott J (ed) 1994 Neonatal infection: assessment, diagnosis and management. Nicu, California, p 36–63

Yancey M K, Duff P, Kubilis P et al 1996 Risk factors for neonatal sepsis. Obstetrics and Gynecology 87(2):188–194

FURTHER READING

American College of Obstetricians and Gynecologists 1999 Prevention of Rh D alloimmunization: clinical management guidelines for obstetricians and gynecologists. International Journal of Gynecology and Obstetrics 66(1):63–70

Provides direction for health professionals in the USA on the management of women at risk of Rh alloimmunisation.

National Health and Medical Research Council 1999 (Australia) Guidelines on the prophylactic use of Rh D immunoglobulin (anti-D) in obstetrics. Online. Available: www.health.gov.au: 80/nhmrc/publications/synopses/wh27syn.htm

Provides information for health professionals on the use of anti D Ig in Australia.

NICE (National Institute for Clinical Excellence) 2002 Guidance on the use of routine antenatal anti-D prophylaxis for RhD-negative women. Technology appraisal guidance no. 41, ref. NOO92. NICE, London. Online. Available: www./nice.org.uk

NICE make updated recommendations for midwives on routine antenatal anti-D prophylaxis in the UK.

RCOG (Royal College of Obstetricians and Gynaecologists) 1999 Use of anti-D immunoglobulin for Rh prophylaxis. Clinical `green top' guidelines. RCOG, London.

Online. Available: www.rcog.org.uk/guidelines/antid.html, or from 27 Sussex Place, London NW1 4RG.

The RCOG (1999) recommend routine antenatal anti-D prophylaxis, and also discuss antenatal and postnatal prophylaxis, prebirth sensitising events and procedures, tests for FMH, anti-D Ig preparations and administration and dose of anti-D Ig.

47 Metabolic Problems, Endocrine Disorders and Drug Withdrawal

Stephen P. Wardle

CHAPTER CONTENTS

Acquired metabolic disorders, inborn errors of metabolism, endocrine disorders and the effects of maternal drug abuse all have the potential to cause long term developmental abnormalities in the newborn. This chapter attempts to summarise the monitoring, detection and management of some of these complex problems in the newborn period.

The chapter aims to:

- review the most common acquired metabolic disturbances in the newborn, and describe the normal mechanisms of control and abnormalities that can occur in electrolyte, fluid and particularly glucose balance in the newborn infant. The emphasis is placed on the normal infant, although obviously many of these problems are more common in growth-restricted or preterm infants

- describe the presentation, detection and management of inborn errors of metabolism and describe a few specific inherited metabolic abnormalities, most of which are rare

- describe the range of endocrine disorders in the newborn, including the presentation and management of abnormalities of hormonal control in the newborn

- describe the effects of fetal exposure to drugs and the effects of this on the newborn, its treatment and prognosis.

Metabolic disturbances in the newborn

Many metabolic abnormalities can occur in the newborn, particularly in preterm or growth-restricted infants. By far the most common problem is hypoglycaemia. Some other common problems are also highlighted here.

Glucose homeostasis

In utero the healthy fetus has a constant supply of glucose via the placenta. Following birth this supply of nutrient ceases and there is a fall in glucose concentration (Srinivasan et al 1986). However, at the same time endocrine changes (a decrease in insulin, a surge of catecholamines and release of glucagon) result in an increase in glycogenolysis (the breakdown of glycogen stores to provide glucose), gluconeogenesis (glucose production from the liver), ketogenesis (production of ketones, an alternative fuel) and lipolysis (release of fatty acids from adipose tissue) bringing about an increase in glucose and other metabolic fuel. Problems arise in the newborn when there is either a lack of glycogen stores to mobilise (in preterm and growth-restricted infants) or excessive insulin production (infants of diabetic mothers), or when infants are sick and have a poor supply of energy but increased requirements.

Low glucose concentrations are a potential problem in the newborn infant because if there is a lack of fuel or nutrient available for the brain then cerebral dysfunction, and potentially brain injury, may occur. The problem for those caring for newborn infants is not only to identify infants who are at risk and treat them appropriately but also to avoid excessive treatment and investigation in infants who are normal and where intervention is not required.

Hypoglycaemia

Definition of hypoglycaemia. The definition of hypoglycaemia is controversial and many different definitions can be found in the literature (Koh et al 1988a). The problem is that defining a specific level of blood glucose is unhelpful because an infant's ability to compensate and use alternative fuels may be as important as the specific glucose concentration. However, pragmatically a specific level is helpful for management purposes. The consensus would appear to favour a cut-off value in the newborn of 2.6 mmol/L. This figure comes mainly from two studies (Koh et al 1988b, Lucas et al 1988). Koh et al demonstrated abnormal sensory-evoked brain stem potentials in a

small number of term infants. This did not occur in any infants where the blood glucose was above 2.6 mmol/L whether or not symptoms were present (Koh et al 1988b). In addition, and perhaps more importantly, in a retrospective study of preterm infants the neurological outcome was less good if the blood glucose concentration had been below 2.6 mmol/L on 5 or more days during the neonatal period (Lucas et al 1988). These studies suggest that levels of blood glucose concentration above 2.6 mmol/L are likely to be safe but they do not take into account infants' ability to compensate for low glucose concentrations. Lower values may be safe in some infants.

Symptoms of hypoglycaemia. Any infant who has symptomatic hypoglycaemia has a glucose concentration that is too low and this should be treated whatever the exact glucose level. The symptoms of hypoglycaemia are lethargy, poor feeding, seizures and decreased consciousness level. Jitteriness is commonly ascribed to hypoglycaemia but is a common symptom in the newborn and alone should not be used as an indication for measuring blood glucose concentration.

Normal term infants. It is likely that healthy term infants are able to tolerate low blood glucose concentrations using compensatory mechanisms and alternative fuels such as ketone bodies, lactate or fatty acids (Hawdon et al 1992). These infants may have blood glucose concentrations as low as 2.0 mmol/L without any ill effects because, if responding normally, they are likely to have increased ketone body concentrations so fuel is available for the brain (Hawdon et al 1992). Term infants who are breastfed are a group who are particularly likely to have low blood glucose concentrations, probably because of the low energy content of breastmilk in the first few postnatal days. However, these infants have higher ketone body concentrations to compensate (Hawdon et al 1992) and they are unlikely therefore to suffer any ill effects. Unfortunately routine measurements of ketone body concentrations are not readily available and when glucose measurements are made in these infants it becomes difficult for practitioners to resist giving treatment that may involve supplementary formula feeding or even intravenous dextrose. This should obviously be avoided unless there are other clinical indications for intervention.

Because of the ability to compensate, clinically well appropriately grown term infants who are feeding do not require monitoring of their glucose concentration.

Doing so would result in many infants being inappropriately treated.

Infants at risk of neurological sequelae of hypoglycaemia. Infants where monitoring and treatment should be considered are those in whom counter-regulation may be impaired for some reason. These groups of infants are:

- *Preterm infants (less than 37 weeks) and growth-restricted infants (less than third centile for gestation)* – preterm and growth-restricted infants have lower glycogen stores and cannot therefore mobilise glucose as rapidly as normal term infants during the immediate post-natal period. In addition they also have immature hormone and enzyme responses and are less likely to be enterally fed at an early stage
- *Infants of diabetic mothers* – these infants frequently have low blood glucose concentrations because of an excess of insulin. This is produced by the fetal pancreatic gland as a result of stimulation by increased maternal glucose concentrations. This excess of insulin also acts as a growth factor and brings about excessive fat and glycogen deposition. This is why these infants have a characteristic appearance and are relatively macrosomic (see Plate 37).
- *Sick term infants* e.g. septic or following perinatal hypoxia–ischaemia – there may also be low substrate stores, but there are frequently feeding difficulties that add to the problem.
- *Infants with inborn errors of metabolism.*

Diagnosis, prevention and management of hypoglycaemia. *Term infants who are admitted to the postnatal ward and are feeding should not have measurements of blood glucose unless they are symptomatic.* In particular breastfeeding advice and intervention should not be based on blood glucose concentrations.

Infants at risk of neurological complications of hypoglycaemia can be easily identified from the above categories and the following infants should be monitored:

1. infants less than 37 weeks' gestation
2. and/or less than 2.5 kg
3. infants of diabetic mothers
4. infants with sepsis or following perinatal hypoxia.

Prevention is important in these infants and they should therefore have:

1. adequate temperature control – keep warm
2. early feeding (within 1 hour of birth) with 100 ml/kg/day if formula feeding
3. frequent feeding (every 3 hours or less)
4. blood glucose check immediately before the second feed and then every 4–6 hours.

There is no advantage to checking the blood glucose concentration earlier than this as long as there are no symptoms; it is likely to be low and the appropriate treatment at that stage is to feed the baby. If there are symptoms the glucose should be checked and treatment given immediately. Breastfed infants are particularly difficult in this situation as it is important to avoid supplemental feeding with formula to promote successful breastfeeding, but the risks associated with significant hypoglycaemia in at risk infants outweigh this advantage.

If the blood glucose concentration is < 2.6 mmol/L then feed should be given at an increased volume and decreased frequency (every 2 hours, or even every hour). This may require supplementary feeding with formula milk in infants who are breastfed or nasogastric tube (NGT) feeding, or both. Breastmilk can also be expressed to give via an NGT.

If the blood glucose concentration remains low despite these measures and there is an adequate feed volume intake then intravenous treatment with dextrose is required. It is important in this situation that enteral feeding is continued as feeding contains much more energy than 10% glucose, it promotes ketone body production and metabolic adaptation.

If the blood glucose concentration is > 2.6 mmol/L before the second and the third feed then glucose monitoring can be discontinued but feeding should continue at 3 hour intervals.

In infants where enteral feeding is contraindicated for some reason then intravenous 10% dextrose, at least 60 ml/kg day, should commence.

Hyperglycaemia

Hyperglycaemia is much less of a clinical problem than hypoglycaemia; it occurs predominantly in preterm and severely growth-restricted infants. It is also seen in term infants in response to stress especially following perinatal hypoxia–ischaemia, surgery or drugs (especially corticosteroids). In general, no treatment is required.

In preterm infants it is usually a transient phenomenon related to the infant's immature glucoregulation or inability to deal with excessive glucose intakes. In general, treatment is not required unless there is significant loss of glucose in the urine, which may cause an osmotic diuresis. If treatment is required the rate of glucose infusion can be decreased but there may be some advantages in this situation of giving an intravenous insulin infusion. This allows glucose input to continue and sufficient calories to continue to be given and may result in better weight gain (Collins et al 1991).

Electrolyte imbalances in the newborn

Postnatal weight loss, fluid and electrolyte changes

In the first few days after birth all babies lose weight owing to a loss of extracellular fluid. This diuresis and loss of weight are associated with cardiopulmonary adaptation; they occur rapidly in healthy babies but may be delayed in those with respiratory distress syndrome. As extracellular fluid is lost there is a net loss of both water and sodium over these first few days after birth, although the infant's serum sodium should remain within the normal range. The normal infant should lose up to 10% of its birthweight. This weight loss is physiological and should be expected.

In general many infants are not weighed during this period. Mothers who are breastfeeding can be discouraged by the fact that their infant has lost weight despite a good technique; this can serve to undermine breastfeeding no matter how carefully the physiology of the phenomenon is explained. Additionally (particularly in primiparous mothers) lactogenesis is only just becoming established between 48 and 72 hours. Thus the volume of milk transferred to the infant is still rising sharply between 72 and 96 hours of age. However, weighing babies during this period can be very useful when a baby is unwell or if there are concerns about intake and fluid and electrolyte balance.

Sodium

Sodium is normally excreted via the kidney, controlled by the renin–angiotensin system (see Fig. 13.9, p. 201).

This control mechanism is functional in the preterm infant, but loss of sodium may occur in preterm infants because of renal tubule unresponsiveness. Term breastmilk has relatively little sodium (< 1 mmol/kg/day) showing that the normal newborn can preserve sodium via the kidney in order to maintain growth. Normal sodium requirements are 1–2 mmol/kg/day in term infants and 3–4 mmol/kg/day in preterm infants.

Changes in serum sodium reflect changes in sodium and water balance. In order to assess changes in sodium concentration it is important to know an infant's weight. Hypernatraemia in the presence of a loss of weight suggests dehydration, whereas when there is weight gain it is due to fluid and sodium overload. Hyponatraemia in the presence of weight gain represents fluid overload, whereas a low sodium with inappropriate weight loss represents sodium depletion. The normal serum sodium concentration is 133–146 mmol/L (Green & Keffler 1999).

Hyponatraemia. Hyponatraemia is due to either fluid overload or sodium depletion. The latter may be a result of inadequate intake or excessive losses.

Fluid overload. In the first few days after birth this is the commonest cause of a low sodium concentration. It is commonly seen in infants receiving intravenous fluids or in infants with oliguric renal failure.

Causes include:

- excessive intravenous fluid administration (to mother or infant)
- oliguric renal failure
- drugs (e.g. indometacin) given to preterm infants.

Appropriate treatment is to limit the fluid intake whilst maintaining normal sodium intake with appropriate intravenous fluids.

Sodium depletion. This is commonest in preterm infants after the first few days after birth, owing to renal losses, but is also common in term infants on diuretics (usually for cardiac failure).

Causes include:

- renal loss in preterm infants – this is treated by increasing sodium intake to cope with the losses; some preterm infants may require a very large daily intake of intravenous sodium with their intravenous fluids when losses are high

- loss into the bowel due to ileus (intestinal obstruction, sepsis or prematurity) or severe vomiting
- drugs (e.g. diuretics)
- adrenocortical failure – this is rare but may be due to congenital adrenal hyperplasia, hypoplasia or adrenal haemorrhage in a sick infant

Hypernatraemia. Increased sodium concentration is almost always due to water depletion and loss of extracellular fluid but can also rarely be due to an excessive sodium intake. These causes can again be easily differentiated by weighing an infant to assess the change since birth.

Water depletion. This is rare in term babies but does occur occasionally in infants with an inadequate intake of breastmilk. It is more common in preterm infants.

Causes include:

- transepidermal water loss in preterm infants – this occurs particularly in infants of less than 28 weeks' gestation; it can be prevented by adequate environmental humidity and regular weighing to gauge fluid loss and predict fluid requirements
- excessive urine output in preterm infants during recovery from respiratory distress syndrome
- high rates of fluid loss during vomiting, diarrhoea or bowel obstruction
- inadequate lactation.

For the midwife the last is perhaps the most important cause of hypernatraemia. The incidence has been estimated as 2.5 per 10 000 livebirths and it typically occurs in term infants of breastfeeding primiparous mothers (Oddie et al 2001). It can be associated with significant morbidity and even mortality (Edmondson et al 1997). However, it can be prevented with sufficient assistance and supervision of feeding. Babies typically present at 5–9 days of age with lethargy and poor feeding. They have lost more than 15% of their birthweight and are usually significantly jaundiced. The serum sodium concentration can be between 150 and 200 mmol/L.

The infant's fluid deficit can be calculated from the loss in weight and this is then replaced by gradual rehydration over 24–48 hours. Feeding can continue but intravenous treatment is often required with normal saline and dextrose. Assistance with lactation can then be given to continue to promote breastfeeding.

Excessive sodium intake. In general this is rare in term infants, although it may be seen in sick preterm infants owing to excessive bicarbonate and other sodium-containing fluids.

Causes include:

- incorrect fluid prescription
- excessive administration of sodium bicarbonate
- incorrectly formulated powdered feeds
- Munchausen's syndrome by proxy – intentional administration of salt to an infant (Meadow 1993).

Potassium

Potassium is the major intracellular cation. A low serum concentration therefore implies significant potassium depletion. Abnormalities in serum potassium concentration are important because they can cause significant arrhythmias. Potassium concentrations can be severely affected by measurement technique; any haemolysis of the blood sample especially from capillary sampling is likely to lead to a falsely high value.

Hyperkalaemia. Causes include:

- acidosis
- acute renal failure
- congenital adrenal hyperplasia.

The treatment is to remove all potassium supplements from intravenous fluids, and to consider giving calcium resonium rectally, intravenous calcium gluconate, sodium bicarbonate to increase pH, and intravenous glucose and insulin. In general these measures will be required only where there is a serum potassium that is very high (> 8 mmol/L), or evidence of an abnormal ECG/arrhythmias, or both.

Hypokalaemia. Causes include:

- inadequate intake of potassium
- bowel losses (vomiting or diarrhoea)
- diuretic therapy
- hyperaldosteronism.

Hypokalaemia is treated by adding potassium to intravenous infusion fluids or orally. The normal daily requirement of potassium is 2 mmol/kg/day.

Calcium

Calcium metabolism is closely linked to phosphate metabolism and these are very important minerals in relation to bone development. This is of particular importance in the preterm infant; preterm infants need much higher concentrations of phosphate and calcium. These are given as intravenous supplements, by supplementing breastmilk with fortifier (Lucas et al 1996) or by giving specific preterm milk formula rather than term formula.

High serum calcium concentrations are unusual; however, there are rare but important causes of low serum calcium. The normal serum concentration is 2.2–2.7 mmol/L, although this must be interpreted along with the serum albumin concentration as the serum calcium is bound to albumin. Therefore a low albumin concentration will lead to a falsely low serum value.

Calcium concentrations fall within 18–24 hours of birth as the infant's supply of placental calcium ceases but accretion into bone continues. In the past, hypocalcaemia during the first week after birth used to be caused by giving unmodified cow's milk. This has a high phosphate concentration and a relatively low calcium concentration that depresses the serum calcium concentration and causes seizures. With the advent of modern formula feeds this is now rarely seen.

Hypocalcaemia can cause seizures, tremors, jitteriness, lethargy, poor feeding and vomiting. Severe symptoms can be treated by intravenous replacement of calcium. Longer term management depends on the cause.

Hypocalcaemia can be caused by:

- prematurity
- significant hypoxia–ischaemia
- renal failure
- hypoparathyroidism including DiGeorge syndrome (see later)
- maternal diabetes mellitus.

Inborn errors of metabolism

Background/incidence

Inborn errors of metabolism (IEM) are rare inherited disorders occurring in approximately 1 in 5000 births. They result mainly from enzyme deficiencies in metabolic pathways leading to an accumulation of substrate, resulting in toxicity. In utero the placenta provides an effective dialysis system for most disorders, removing toxic metabolites. Most affected babies are therefore initially born in good condition with normal birthweight. A high index of suspicion is needed when evaluating an acutely ill neonate, as many disorders are treatable and early diagnosis and institution of therapy can reduce morbidity. It has been estimated that 20% of infants presenting with sepsis in the absence of risk factors have an inborn error of metabolism.

Patient group

The mode of inheritance is usually autosomal recessive, therefore family history is crucial and the following features should be sought:

- affected sibling
- previous stillbirth or neonatal death
- parental consanguinity
- symptoms associated with feeding, fasting or a surgical procedure
- improvement when feeds stopped and relapse on restarting.

Clinical examination, however, is usually normal. The following features may be seen in isolation with many diagnoses. However, multiple features indicate that an underlying IEM should be seriously considered.

- septicaemia
- hypoglycaemia
- metabolic acidosis
- convulsions
- coma
- cataracts
- cardiomegaly
- jaundice or liver disease
- severe hypotonia
- unusual body odour
- dysmorphic features
- abnormal hair
- hydrops fetalis
- diarrhoea.

Diagnosis

The following tests are a basic first step in investigation:

- full blood count
- septic screen
- creatinine, urea and electrolytes (including chloride)

- liver enzymes
- blood gas
- blood glucose and lactate concentration
- urine reducing substances
- urine ketones (dipstick)
- plasma ammonia concentration
- coagulation tests.

Many other investigations may be necessary and useful but, in general, investigations need to be discussed with a consultant biochemist or pediatrician with an interest in metabolic disorders.

Principles of emergency management are to reduce the load on affected pathways by removing toxic metabolites and stimulating residual enzyme activity. Hypoglycaemia is corrected, adequate ventilatory support and hydration are maintained, convulsions are treated and significant metabolic acidosis is treated with intravenous sodium bicarbonate, and electrolyte abnormalities are corrected. In general, antibiotics are frequently given as infection may have precipitated metabolic decompensation, Occasionally dialysis may also be required (Wraith & Walker 1996).

Phenylketonuria

Phenylketonuria (PKU) is important, first because it is a treatable cause of brain injury and secondly because it is possible to screen successfully for it during the first week of life in order to identify affected individuals, These can then be treated appropriately to produce a favourable outcome.

PKU is an autosomal recessive disorder that has an incidence of approximately 1 in 10 000 in the UK. Babies with PKU are born in good condition but begin to be affected by their condition during the first few weeks or months after birth. If untreated PKU leads to severe mental retardation (IQ < 30). However, if it is identified early (within the first 3 weeks) it can be treated by a diet specifically restricted in phenylalanine. The common type is caused by the absence of, or reduction in, an enzyme in the liver that converts phenylalanine to tyrosine (phenylalanine hydroxylase). This leads to a build-up of phenylpyruvic acid, which is toxic to the brain.

PKU is particularly suitable for mass screening because there is a simple widely available diagnostic test and because treatment is effective. Midwives or health visitors collect the blood sample for PKU screening in the UK between days 5 and 8 after birth. It is commonly collected on the Guthrie card, along with a sample for screening for congenital hypothyroidism (see later). The level of phenylalanine is analysed and babies with increased levels need to be prescribed a low phenylalanine diet and have further assessment to determine whether they are affected by the 'classic' type or other variants.

If it is treated early the prognosis for PKU is good and normal intelligence can result. In females, a return to a low phenylalanine diet is essential prior to conception and during pregnancy. This is because fetal brain injury may result from exposure to high concentrations of phenylalanine and its metabolites in the mother.

Galactosaemia

Galactosaemia is a disorder of carbohydrate metabolism that is autosomal recessive in inheritance and has an incidence of 1 in 60 000. It is caused by an absence or severe deficiency of the enzyme galactose-1-phosphate uridyltransferase (often referred to as Gal-I-P UT). This enzyme is important for converting galactose to glucose. Since milk's main sugar, lactose, is a disaccharide containing glucose and galactose, infants with this condition rapidly become affected when fed either human breastmilk or cow's milk formulae. The metabolite that builds up and is harmful is galactose-1-phosphate.

The clinical signs and symptoms of the disorder are those of liver failure and renal impairment. Babies tend to present with vomiting, hypoglycaemia, jaundice, bleeding, acidosis, failure to gain weight and hypotonia during the first few days after birth. Another important clinical feature sometimes present is cataracts. Affected babies may also present with septicaemia (particularly *E. coli*) caused by damage to intestinal mucosa from the high levels of galactose in the gut. Galactosaemia is an important differential diagnosis to consider when dealing with an infant with unresponsive hypoglycaemia and prolonged or severe jaundice.

Infants with galactosaemia will have galactose but not glucose in their urine. The diagnosis can therefore be made by looking for urine reducing substances (i.e. galactose) using a Clinitest, whereas a urine test for glucose will be negative. Confirmation of the diagnosis is by assay of the enzyme level (Gal-I-P UT) within red blood cells.

Treatment is with a lactose-free milk formula, which must be commenced as soon as the diagnosis is suspected. This results in a rapid correction of the abnormalities. However, cataracts and mild brain injury have occurred even when galactosaemic infants have been fed lactose-free milk from birth.

Screening for this disorder is possible but many infants will have presented before the screening test is available. There is little evidence to suggest that diagnosis at or soon after birth gives a better long term outlook than diagnosis by rapid screening of the symptomatic neonate.

Endocrine disease in the newborn

Endocrine problems in the newborn are relatively rare but may be serious, even life threatening; however, they are nearly always treatable so identification and diagnosis are important. Disorders of blood glucose homeostasis have already been described so this section will concentrate on other endocrine abnormalities that may present in the newborn.

Thyroid disorders

The thyroid gland produces hormones that have an effect on the metabolic rate in most tissues. They are also essential for normal neurological development. TSH is produced by the anterior pituitary gland and this stimulates production of T_3 and T_4 by the thyroid gland, with a feedback mechanism to the anterior pituitary (see Ch. 13).

Hypothyroidism

The incidence of hypothyroidism in the newborn is 1 in 3500. There are several possible causes for hypothyroidism in the newborn, including abnormalities in gland formation (thyroid dysgenesis), defects in hormone synthesis (dyshormonogenesis) and rarely secondary pituitary causes. The last of these causes a decrease or lack of TSH, whereas primary (thyroid) causes result in very high TSH values. The presentation is the same, although this has implications for screening.

Infants with hypothyroidism tend to be large, postmature and have a large posterior fontanelle. They have coarse features and often an umbilical hernia. These features are often missed, however; this is why screening for this disorder is so important. Untreated infants develop impaired motor development with growth failure, a low IQ, impaired hearing and language problems. With treatment the physical signs of hypothyroidism do not appear. However, the intellectual and neurological prognosis is poor unless treatment is started within the first few weeks of life – but this should always occur when infants are detected by screening.

Screening. Screening for hypothyroidism involves measuring TSH on a blood spot taken along with the screening test for PKU at 5–8 days of age. This method detects almost all cases, although it cannot detect cases caused by secondary (pituitary) hypothyroidism that will have a low TSH. This condition is, however, much less common with an incidence of 1 in 60–100 000 (Fisher et al 1979).

Hyperthyroidism

Graves disease is an autoimmune disorder that causes hyperthyroidism. Neonatal hyperthyroidism occurs relatively rarely but is possible when the mother has or has had Graves disease. It occurs not because of neonatal autoantibodies but as a result of the transfer of maternal thyroid-stimulating immunoglobulins. These are autoantibodies that are produced and act in the same way as TSH. This can occur when a mother has active, inactive or treated Graves disease (Teng et al 1980). Thyrotoxicosis in the fetus can lead to preterm labour, low birthweight, stillbirth and fetal death, but only a small percentage of infants of mothers with Graves disease become symptomatic.

In the neonate the symptoms are irritability, jitteriness, tachycardia, prominent eyes, sweating, excessive appetite and weight loss. These symptoms may be present immediately after birth, or presentation may be delayed for as long as 4–6 weeks (Skuza et al 1996). Infants therefore need to be observed for this period and treatment will be required with antithyroid medication if there are symptoms.

Adrenal disorders

The adrenal glands are vital for normal function of many systems within the body. They are divided into a medulla and a cortex. The medulla produces catecholamines; these help to maintain blood pressure and are produced at times of stress. Abnormalities of function of the adrenal medulla are not described in the newborn. The adrenal cortex produces three groups of hormones: glucocorticoids, mineralocorticoids and sex hormones, which have distinct functions. Glucocorticoids regulate the general metabolism of carbohydrates, proteins and fats on a long term basis. They have a particular role in modifying the metabolism in times of stress. Mineralocorticoids regulate sodium, potassium and water balance. The sex hormones are responsible for normal development of the genitalia and reproductive organs. Abnormalities in function of the glands represent the functions of these different groups of hormones.

Adrenocortical insufficiency

This is caused by congenital hypoplasia, adrenal haemorrhage or enzyme defects, or can be secondary to pituitary problems. It generally presents with symptomatic hypoglycaemia, poor feeding, vomiting, poor weight gain and even prolonged jaundice. Infants may have hyponatraemia, hypoglycaemia, hyperkalaemia and acidosis. Treatment is by intravenous therapy with glucose and electrolytes; replacement of corticosteroid and mineralocorticoid hormones is then required.

Adrenocortical hyperfunction

This may occur in the form of congenital adrenal hyperplasia (CAH) – the name given to a group of inherited disorders that are due to deficiency of the enzymes responsible for hormone production within the adrenal glands. The most common enzyme deficiency results in an excess of androgenic hormones, but a deficiency of glucocorticoid and mineralocorticoids often also occurs. These disorders can cause abnormalities in the formation of the genitalia leading to ambiguous genitalia (virilisation of females or inadequate virilisation of males), and symptoms of adrenal insufficiency (vomiting, diarrhoea, vascular collapse, hypoglycaemia, hyponatraemia or hyperkalaemia) (Fig. 47.1).

It is important to make a prompt diagnosis. The genetic sex must be determined (chromosome analysis) and it is important not to assign a sex until the diagnosis has been established. The biochemical diagnosis is made by analysing urine and plasma

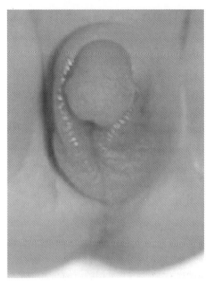

Fig. 47.1 Female infant with ambiguous genitalia due to congenital adrenal hyperplasia.

for steroid hormone metabolites. Treatment is as for adrenocortical insufficiency, by replacement of glucocorticoid and mineralocorticoid hormones. Virilised girls may also require surgical intervention to correct the genital abnormalities.

Pituitary disorders

Pituitary insufficiency is rare in the newborn. It may occur in association with other abnormalities, particularly midline developmental defects. Presentation is with signs of glucocorticoid deficiency (hypoglycaemia), prolonged jaundice or signs of hypothyroidism. Growth hormone deficiency generally causes hypoglycaemia but no other signs in the newborn. When it is recognised then treatment is with replacement of the missing hormones.

Parathyroid disorders

The parathyroid glands are responsible for control of calcium metabolism, but abnormalities of the parathyroids are rare causes of hypo- or hypercalcaemia in the newborn. When hypoparathyroidism does occur it may be familial or occur in association with deletions of chromosome 22 (22q11 deletion or DiGeorge syndrome). The symptoms associated with hypocalcaemia are detailed above.

Effects of maternal drug abuse/ use during pregnancy on the newborn

The incidence of drug use within the population has a large geographical variation. As a result the incidence of drug withdrawal symptoms in infants also has a markedly varying incidence. Obviously inner city areas are more likely to be affected but, even within cities, large variation is seen in the incidence of problems.

Opiates and other drugs cross the placenta and so the fetus during pregnancy is likely to be exposed to the same peaks and troughs of drug exposure as the mother. Withdrawal may be manifested before birth. The increased incidence of fetal distress may be related in part to drug withdrawal during labour, but the effects of drugs and their withdrawal on the fetus and newborn are obviously related to the timing of drug doses.

Infants born to mothers who have used illicit drugs during pregnancy are at risk of withdrawal symptoms. However, there are many other problems associated with these pregnancies and infants that must be considered as well as the obvious problem of withdrawal symptoms. Other problems that are more common in these pregnancies are:

- obstetric complications of pregnancy including placental abruption, fetal growth restriction, fetal distress during labour, stillbirth, etc.
- poor attendance for antenatal care
- non-disclosure of information regarding drugs taken during pregnancy
- risk of infectious disease (hepatitis B, hepatitis C and HIV)
- social problems such as poor housing, chaotic lifestyle, care of other infants, etc.
- poor attendance for neonatal follow-up.

Attendance for antenatal care and supervision during pregnancy may be improved by specialty midwifery support and community liaison. It is important to identify these women during pregnancy in order to try to prevent some of the above problems and offer appropriate support. Identification during pregnancy also allows screening for infectious diseases. This is particularly important for hepatitis B and HIV where treatments are available to decrease the chance of the newborn being affected.

Symptoms

Many drugs have been reported to cause problems of withdrawal in the newborn. The most common seen in the UK are opiates in the form of heroin and methadone, but barbiturates, benzodiazepines, cocaine and amphetamines are also frequently seen. Multidrug use is common and usually leads to prolonged difficult withdrawal. Each drug has a different half-life and this leads to different patterns of withdrawal symptoms. In general, methadone produces symptoms for longer periods than heroin (Herzlinger et al 1977), but benzodiazepines may also contribute to this (Sutton & Hinderliter 1990).

The symptoms most frequently seen are jitteriness, irritability and constant high-pitched crying. Infants often fail to settle between feeds and are hyperactive. When feeds are offered they often feed voraciously, although some infants have poor sucking. Vomiting is common. Diarrhoea and an irritant nappy rash are also often seen. Sneezing and yawning are symptoms, and episodes of high temperature in the absence of infection. In rare circumstances infants may have seizures.

Several scoring systems have been developed to guide in giving pharmacological treatment (Finnegan et al 1975). These scoring systems aim to make the assessment more objective. However, most of the symptoms and their severity are difficult to quantify. Infants assessed for signs of drug withdrawal by a scoring system are less likely to be inappropriately treated and may have a shorter hospital stay (Finnegan 1975). It is important not to overtreat infants with drugs as the long term effects of treatment are not clear and treatment may then be difficult to withdraw. Also, treatment in many maternity hospitals means admitting the baby to the neonatal unit and therefore moving him away from the mother. On the other hand, infants who are withdrawing appear to be in discomfort, which we obviously want to relieve; the long term effects of withdrawal symptoms are also unclear. The most useful symptom is whether infants settle and sleep between feeding. If they do then pharmacological treatment may be unnecessary.

Treatment

Treatment can be divided into general care given to the baby and pharmacological treatment. It is important, if at all possible, to keep the baby with his mother. It is vital to encourage bonding with and care of the infant by the mother. The mother is likely to be feeling upset and guilty because of the infant's symptoms and there are frequently already social problems involved with these families. Involving parents in the care of the baby is difficult when he provides little positive behavioural return for their effort. Breastfeeding can be encouraged as long as there is no evidence of HIV or ongoing drug use (cocaine, heroin) that precludes this. This includes methadone as long as the dose is less than 20 mg/day (Committee on Drugs, American Academy of Pediatrics 1989).

A quiet environment with reduced light and noise is helpful keeping stimuli to a minimum. Swaddling is useful and feeds may need to be given frequently. These infants often will take large volumes of milk, which is acceptable so long as vomiting is not a problem. Rocking or cradling is also a useful adjunct.

Pharmacological treatment

Several different treatments have been recommended in the past. Previously the four drugs recommended for use were paregoric (a mixture of alcohol and opiate), phenobarbital, diazepam and chlorpromazine (Committee on Drugs, American Academy of Pediatrics 1983). A number of randomised trials have been performed that attempted to assess the use of various drugs in the treatment of NAS (Theis et al 1997). It seems logical to treat opiate withdrawal with opiates and now the two most commonly used treatments are oral methadone and oral morphine. These appear to control withdrawal seizures much more effectively than previous treatment (Rivers 1999). They can be given in increasing doses if necessary until symptoms are controlled; then the dose is gradually reduced. A possible dosing regimen for oral morphine is:

- initially 0.04 mg/kg morphine sulphate oral every 4 hours
- then 0.03 mg/kg morphine sulphate oral every 4 hours
- then 0.02 mg/kg morphine sulphate oral every 4 hours
- then 0.01 mg/kg morphine sulphate oral every 4 hours.

The dose is reduced every 24 hours if the baby is feeding well and settling better between feeds. If the feeding and settling do not improve, or profuse watery stools and profuse vomiting continue, other treatment needs to be considered. Other medication may sometimes be useful (e.g. clonazepam for benzodiazepine use or chloral hydrate as a general sedative).

Cocaine

Cocaine deserves special mention because its effects on the newborn are different. It is a larger problem in the USA than in the UK but the incidence of its use during pregnancy is unknown. It is present in maternal urine for only 24 hours after exposure, therefore detection is difficult (Zuckerman et al 1989). It can produce significant withdrawal symptoms but these are often less severe and less troublesome than with other drugs. However, it is associated with many other harmful effects on the fetus (Fulroth et al 1989). These include significant fetal growth restriction, brain injury due to haemorrhage or infarction (Hadeed & Siegel 1989), abnormalities of brain development, limb reduction defects and gut atresias. A correlation between cocaine exposure, small head size and developmental scores has been reported (Chasnoff et al 1992).

Discharge and long term effects

Discharge must be planned with the involvement of other support agencies. This may involve a planning meeting involving all agencies involved in the care of the mother and baby.

Although it seems intuitive that exposure to drugs in utero would cause neurodevelopmental impairment, this is not borne out by carefully controlled studies (e.g. Lifschitz et al 1985). These imply that impairment in intellectual outcome in these children relates to other adverse prenatal and postnatal factors. Infants born to these mothers are smaller and have smaller head circumferences (Kandall et al 1976). However, it is difficult to be certain about the exact causes of any long term harmful effects because so many factors are involved, all of which are interlinked. These include:

- the effects of the drugs themselves on the developing fetus
- the use of other harmful substances by mothers who use drugs (e.g. cigarettes and alcohol)
- the effect of pregnancy complications

- the effect of the withdrawal syndrome on the developing neonate
- the effect of treatment to prevent withdrawal symptoms
- the effect of the home environment of the chaotic drug user for the developing child

- genetic effects
- reporting bias, such that negative associations with drug taking are more likely to be reported (Koran et al 1989).

REFERENCES

Chasnoff I J, Griffith D R, Freier C et al 1992 Cocaine/polydrug use in pregnancy: two year follow up. Pediatrics 89:284–289

Collins J W Jr, Hoppe M, Brown K et al 1991 A controlled trial of insulin infusion and parenteral nutrition in extremely low birth weight infants with glucose intolerance. Journal of Pediatrics 118(6):921–927

Committee on Drugs, American Academy of Pediatrics 1983 Neonatal drug withdrawal. Pediatrics 72:895–902

Committee on Drugs, American Academy of Pediatrics 1989 Transfer of drugs and other chemicals into human milk. Pediatrics 84:924–936

Edmondson M B, Stoddard J J, Owens L M 1997 Hospital admission with feeding related-problems after early postpartum discharge of normal newborns. Journal of the American Medical Association 278:299–303

Finnegan L P, Kron R E, Connaughton J F et al 1975 Assessment and treatment of abstinence in the infant of the drug dependent mother. International Journal of Clinical Pharmacology 12:19–32

Fisher D A, Dussault J H, Foley T P et al 1979 Screening for congenital hypothyroidism: results of screening one million North American infants. Journal of Pediatrics 94:700–705

Fulroth R, Phillips B, Durand D 1989 Perinatal outcome of infants exposed to cocaine and/or heroin in utero. American Journal of Diseases in Childhood 143:905–910

Green A, Keffler S 1999 Neonatal biochemical reference ranges. In: Rennie J M, Roberton N R C (eds) Textbook of neonatology, 3rd edn. Churchill Livingstone, Edinburgh, p 1408–1414

Hadeed A J, Siegel S R 1989 Maternal cocaine use during pregnancy: effect on the newborn infant. Pediatrics 84:205–210

Hawdon J M, Ward Platt M P, Aynsley-Green A 1992 Patterns of metabolic adaptation for preterm and term infants in the first neonatal week. Archives of Disease in Childhood 67:357–365

Herzlinger R A, Kandall S R, Vaughan H G 1977 Neonatal seizures associated with narcotic withdrawal. Journal of Pediatrics 91:638–641

Kandall S R, Albin S, Lowinson J 1976 Differential effects of maternal heroin and methadone use on birthweight. Pediatrics 58:681

Koh T H H G, Eyre J A, Aynsley-Green A 1988a Neonatal hypoglycaemia – the controversy regarding definition. Archives of Disease in Childhood 63:1386–1388

Koh T H H G, Aynsley-Green A, Tarbit M et al 1988b Neural dysfunction during hypoglycaemia. Archives of Disease in Childhood 63:1353–1358

Koran G, Graham K, Shear H et al 1989 Bias against the null hypothesis: the reproductive hazards of cocaine. Lancet ii:1440–1442

Lifschitz M H, Wilson G H, Smith E O et al 1985 Factors affecting head growth and intellectual function in children of drug addicts. Pediatrics 75:269–274

Lucas A, Fewtrell M S, Morley R et al 1996 Randomized outcome trial of human milk fortification and developmental outcome in preterm infants. American Journal of Clinical Nutrition 64:142–151

Lucas A, Morley R, Cole T J 1988 Adverse neurodevelopmental outcome of moderate neonatal hypoglycaemia. British Medical Journal 297:1304–1308

Meadow R 1993 Non-accidental salt poisoning. Archives of Disease in Childhood 68:448–452

Oddie S, Richmond S, Coulthard M 2001 Hypernatraemic dehydration and breastfeeding: a population study. Archives of Disease in Childhood 85:318–320

Rivers R 1999 Infants of drug-addicted mothers. In: Rennie J M, Roberton N R C (eds) Textbook of neonatology, 3rd edn. Churchill Livingstone, Edinburgh, p 443–451

Skuza K A, Sills I N, Rapaport R 1996 Prediction of neonatal hyperthyroidism in infants born to mothers with Graves disease. Journal of Pediatrics 128:264–267

Srinivasan G, Pildes R S, Cattamanchi G et al 1986 Plasma glucose values in normal neonates: a new look. Journal of Pediatrics 109:114–117

Sutton L R, Hinderliter S A 1990 Diazepam abuse in pregnant women on methadone maintenance. Implications for the neonate. Clinical Pediatrics (Philadelphia) 29:108–111

Teng C S, Tong T C, Hutchinson J H et al 1980 Thyroid stimulating immunoglobulins in neonatal Graves' disease. Archives of Disease in Childhood 55:894–895

Theis J G W, Selby P, Ikizler Y et al 1997 Current management of the neonatal abstinence syndrome: a critical analysis of the evidence. Biology of the Neonate 71:345–356

Wraith J E, Walker J H 1996 Inherited metabolic disorders diagnosis and initial management. Willink Biochemical Genetics Unit, Royal Manchester Children's Hospital, Manchester

Zuckerman B, Frank D A, Hingson R et al 1989 Effects of maternal marijuana and cocaine use on fetal growth. New England Journal of Medicine 320:762–768

7

Section 7
The Context of Midwifery Practice

SECTION CONTENTS

48 Pharmacology and Childbirth

Jane M. Rutherford

Most women are exposed to drugs of one type or another during pregnancy. These may be prescribed drugs or those bought over the counter. They may be given as part of the management of the pregnancy itself or that of a coincidental medical problem. However, when considering the use of any drugs in a pregnant or breastfeeding woman, it is important to consider the effects of the drug not only on the woman herself, but also on the fetus or neonate. Many drugs have undesirable effects on the fetus and should therefore be avoided during pregnancy. On the other hand, some drugs are given to the woman because of their therapeutic effects on the fetus. For example betamethasone or dexamethasone are given to women at risk of preterm birth because of their effects on fetal lung maturation. It is therefore important to have a working knowledge of the issues surrounding the use of drugs in pregnancy and the puerperium so that women can be correctly informed and advised regarding the potential benefits and risks.

The chapter aims to:

- outline how pregnancy can influence the effects of drugs and their pharmacodynamics

- explain how drugs can affect pregnancy, and the developing embryo and fetus

- detail the use and effects of the commonly used drugs in pregnancy

- discuss the use of drugs in lactation

- outline the legal aspects of midwives' administration and prescription of drugs.

Effects of drugs in pregnancy

Transfer of drugs across the placenta and breast

A drug administered to a pregnant woman or a breast-feeding mother will, in most cases, be present in the blood circulating around her body. Exceptions are certain types of drugs that are not absorbed from the area where they are administered – for example some (but not all) skin creams. The maternal blood will then travel to the placenta or breast, which are organs designed to allow the passage of substances from maternal blood into either fetal blood or milk respectively. Drugs will pass across into the fetus or neonate in greater or lesser quantities depending on the characteristic of the drug molecules themselves. Some drugs will not pass across into the fetus or milk at all, whereas others will pass freely. The factors influencing passage across the placenta and breast are the size of the molecule, the ionisation of the molecule, the lipid or water solubility and the protein binding. In general, large molecules do not cross the placenta and small molecules cross very easily.

Influence of pregnancy on drug dose

There are many physiological changes in pregnancy that influence the way in which the mother's body handles the drugs administered to her. These can result in differences in the circulating concentrations of the drug compared with those in a non-pregnant woman. First, the transit time in the gut is prolonged compared with that in the non-pregnant woman and this may result in changes in absorption of orally administered drugs (Parry et al 1970). Secondly, because the circulating plasma volume is increased, this results in an increased volume in which a defined dose of drug is distributed and therefore a decrease in the plasma concentration of the drug. In addition, because there is an increase in the blood flow to the kidneys (Dunlop 1976), which are responsible for the elimination of many drugs, there may be an increase in the rate of excretion of a drug. The amounts of total body water and fat are increased (McFadyen 1989) and this may alter the distribution of the drug. Some metabolic pathways in the liver increase and therefore may result in quicker metabolism of a drug. There are also major changes in the levels of plasma proteins to which some drugs bind and this may affect the amount of drug that is available to exert its effect on the body.

Adverse effects of drugs in pregnancy

Many drugs have adverse effects during pregnancy. These vary depending on the stage of pregnancy. One of the major problems in giving advice to women is the paucity of information available regarding the effects of drugs in pregnancy and breastfeeding. In most cases it is not ethical to perform randomised trials of drugs in pregnancy where their effects are unknown. Drug companies are also reluctant to promote or to license the use of their drugs because of the potential problems and the cost of subsequent litigation. Therefore, most evidence regarding the safety or otherwise of drugs in pregnancy and breastfeeding is accumulated through inadvertent use, or use in unlicensed circumstances. Indeed, many of the drugs that are now commonly used in pregnancy are still not licensed for use during this time. Because the information is accumulated in this way, there is a bias towards reporting of adverse events. In general, when choosing a drug to use in pregnancy, clinicians should use those agents that have been available for longest and about which most information has been amassed. New agents should be avoided if possible.

Teratogenesis

The word 'teratogen' refers to a substance that leads to the birth of a malformed baby. Organogenesis occurs between approximately 18 and 55 days' postconception (i.e. 4 to 10 weeks of pregnancy). A drug can cause a structural abnormality in a fetus only if it is present in the body during this time. This is an important consideration since it is a stage of pregnancy when a woman may not be aware that she is pregnant or may not have attended her midwife or doctor for advice. It is often the case, therefore, that exposure to a potentially teratogenic drug may have already happened before the woman is seen for the first time.

As discussed above, identifying teratogenic drugs is not an easy process. It is unethical to expose human fetuses to drugs with unknown effects as part of a trial. Drug companies will often try to overcome this by performing animal studies. However, this will neither confirm nor refute that a drug is teratogenic in humans since there is wide interspecies variation. A well-known example of this is the drug 'thalidomide', which was marketed in the 1960s for sickness in pregnancy. Ten thousand cases of limb abnormalities were reported before thalidomide was identified as a teratogen. No toxic effects had been noted in animal experiments because thalidomide is a teratogen only in primates.

Because prospective research on teratogenicity in humans is unethical, we rely on case reports and case studies. These can be misleading, however. If a woman has a baby with an abnormality and she took a certain drug in the first trimester, inevitably an association would be drawn. However, there is a background rate of fetal abnormalities of around 2–3% and an association cannot exclude a chance relationship. Larger cohort studies of several women exposed to the same drug who have offspring with the same abnormality are more reliable indicators.

Some of the commonly used drugs known to be teratogens are detailed in Table 48.1.

Other types of drug effect on pregnancy

Drugs may also exert adverse effects on pregnancy other than as teratogens. Any process that occurs during development of the fetus can be affected. For example beta blockers affect fetal growth (Butters et al 1991), angiotensin-converting enzyme (ACE) inhibitors cause fetal renal failure (Kreft-Jais et al 1988) and iodine affects fetal thyroid function. In addition, some drugs may not cause a problem at one stage of pregnancy but

Table 48.1 Commonly used drugs that are teratogens

Drug	Effect
Lithium	Cardiac defects
Warfarin	Facial anomalies, CNS anomalies
Phenytoin	Craniofacial anomalies
Sodium valproate	Neural tube defects
Carbamazepine	Craniofacial anomalies, neural tube defects
Retinoic acid derivatives	Craniofacial, cardiac and CNS anomalies

may do so at another. There is a risk that the commonly used antibiotic, trimethoprim, is teratogenic when given in the first trimester because it interferes with folate metabolism; however, it is safe in later pregnancy. On the other hand, non-steroidal anti-inflammatory drugs (NSAIDs) such as ibuprofen and voltarol may be relatively safe if used in the first trimester but can cause premature closure of the ductus arteriosus and oligohydramnios if used in the third trimester.

Where possible, drugs should be avoided in the first trimester. Obviously this is not always possible, and in some women it is imperative for the woman's health that a drug that is known to be teratogenic is not stopped abruptly during pregnancy. For example, a woman with epilepsy who is controlled with sodium valproate should not stop abruptly despite the risk of neural tube defects as a prolonged seizure could have devastating effects on both her and her fetus. Where a woman on long term medication is planning a pregnancy it is advisable for her to attend for prepregnancy counselling where plans can be made to minimise the risk.

If a new drug is to be started in pregnancy, one should be chosen that is 'safe'. Women should be informed about the potential risks of any medication they are prescribed. Where a woman is exposed to a teratogen during the first trimester then prenatal diagnosis, usually with ultrasound, should be offered.

Drugs used in pregnancy

Many drugs are prescribed for therapeutic reasons in pregnancy. It is therefore useful for the midwife to have a working knowledge of the drugs, their possible side-effects and contraindications. In the following sections, where specific references are not given, much of the information is gained from Briggs et al (1998).

Folic acid

It is recommended that all women planning a pregnancy should take folic acid in a dose of 400 µg daily and that this should continue throughout the first trimester. Folic acid is a vitamin that is involved in the process of cell growth and division. Demand for folate increases in pregnancy. It has been shown that periconception folic acid supplementation reduces the risk of neural tube defects (Lumley et al 2000). In addition, folic acid deficiency can lead to maternal anaemia so folic acid supplementation in later pregnancy can also be beneficial. The recommended dose in the general population is 400 µg daily, but in women at risk of neural tube defects (e.g. with a previously affected fetus, or on carbamazepine or sodium valproate) should receive 5 mg daily. There are no risks associated with folic acid at this dose.

Iron preparations

Iron deficiency anaemia is common in pregnancy and iron preparations are frequently prescribed. There are many preparations on the market based on either ferrous sulphate or ferrous gluconate. Some are combined with folic acid. Commonly experienced side-effects are constipation (occasionally diarrhoea) and indigestion. Stools are coloured black. When side-effects are a problem, it may be worth trying a different preparation. It should be noted that absorption of iron is reduced by antacids and by some foods (e.g. tea).

Antacid drugs

Antacids are alkalis that act by reducing the acidity of stomach acid. Modern antacid drugs are mostly based on calcium, magnesium and aluminium salts, which are relatively non-absorbable. They are often combined with alginates, which coat the lining of the oesophagus and stomach and therefore reduce contact with stomach acid. Because they are relatively non-absorbable, they are safe for use in pregnancy. Older antacids such as sodium bicarbonate can cause systemic alkalosis and should be avoided.

Antiemetics

Nausea and vomiting may be particularly troublesome in the first trimester but may occur at other times in pregnancy. Where possible, women with mild 'morning sickness' should be encouraged to try non-pharmacological methods of controlling nausea such as eating small amounts frequently. If vomiting is a significant problem then it is preferable to use an antiemetic drug rather than risk dehydration and, in the most severe cases, malnutrition. Most of the commonly used antiemetics are considered safe to use in pregnancy and, as always, the older preparations have a longer established safety profile.

The drugs fall into three main categories:

Antihistamines e.g. cyclizine. The most common side-effect is drowsiness.

Anticholinergic drugs e.g. prochlorperazine. Rarely, in young people these may cause a dramatic side-effect known as a 'dystonic' reaction or 'occulogyric crisis' where there is uncontrolled spasm of the muscles of the face and neck.

Antidopaminergic drugs e.g. metoclopramide. These may also cause dystonic reactions.

Antibiotics

Antibiotics are one of the most commonly prescribed groups of drugs in pregnancy. They are a diverse group of compounds and have different indications and risks. There are definite indications for the use of antibiotics, but care should be taken as some are safe and others are contraindicated. Table 48.2 indicates some of the antibiotics with which caution should be exercised. Table 48.3 indicates those antibiotics considered safe for use in pregnancy.

Analgesia

It is relatively common for a pregnant woman to require analgesia during pregnancy. This may be for something as simple as a headache or a more significant problem such as rheumatoid arthritis, or for a pregnancy-related condition such as symphysis pubis dysfunction. However, many of the available analgesics, including 'over-the-counter' preparations, are not considered safe in pregnancy, so it is often difficult to control chronic pain satisfactorily.

Table 48.2 Antibiotics that may cause adverse effects in pregnancy

Antibiotic group (examples)	Risk
Tetracyclines (tetracycline, oxytetracycline, doxycycline)	Discoloration and dysplasia of fetal bones and teeth, cataracts when used in second and third trimester
Aminoglycosides (gentamicin, netilmicin)	Risk of ototoxicity but often used in serious maternal infection where benefit outweighs risk
Chloramphenicol	'Grey baby syndrome' when used in second and third trimester
Nitrofurantoin	Haemolysis in fetus at term – avoid during labour and delivery but safe at other times
Quinolones (cliprofloxacin, ofloxacin)	Arthropathy in fetus – most of the evidence for this obtained from animal studies

Table 48.3 Antibiotics that are considered safe in pregnancy

Antibiotic	Notes
Penicillins (benzyl penicillin, phenoxymethylpenicillin, ampicillin, amoxicillin, co-amoxyclav (Augmentin), flucloxacillin)	Alternatives if allergic
Cephalosporins (cephradine, cephalexin, cefuroxime, cephotaxime)	
Erythromycin	
Trimethoprim	Avoid in first trimester

Paracetamol. This is one of the drugs which has a long and unblemished safety record when taken in therapeutic doses. It should be the recommended first line analgesic agent in pregnancy However, in overdose it can be potentially lethal to the mother or fetus, or both, as it causes liver failure.

NSAIDs e.g. ibuprofen, indometacin, voltarol. These drugs may be relatively safe in the first trimester but have the potential to cause fetal renal dysfunction, premature closure of the ductus arteriosus, necrotising enterocolitis and intracerebral haemorrhage (Norton et al 1991). Indometacin has been used on a short term basis as a tocolytic agent and to reduce liquor volume in polyhydramnios, but should not be used in the long term because of the above risks. A possible problem with ibuprofen is that it is available widely as an over-the-counter preparation. These drugs are safe in breastfeeding, however.

Opiate analgesics e.g. pethidine, morphine, diamorphine, codeine, dihydrocodeine. When used in analgesic doses there is no clear evidence of teratogenesis with these drugs. For acute episodes there is probably little risk with the use of these drugs. However, with long term use there is a risk of neonatal withdrawal after birth, with a similar pattern to the withdrawal symptoms as seen with opiate abuse. This neonatal withdrawal can be demonstrated even in women using relatively moderate doses of codeine such as those available in over-the-counter preparations. When given in large doses in labour there is a risk of respiratory depression.

Aspirin

In analgesic doses, aspirin has been shown to increase the risk of maternal, fetal and neonatal bleeding because of its effect as an antiplatelet agent. Aspirin at an analgesic dose is therefore contraindicated in pregnancy. A common analgesic dose is 600 mg every 6 hours. Aspirin in these doses is present in many commercially available cold remedies and analgesic preparations.

However, in *low* doses (75 mg daily) aspirin is used in pregnancy for treatment of women with recurrent miscarriage, thrombophilias (inherited risk of thromboembolism), and prevention of pre-eclampsia and intrauterine growth restriction. In low dose there is evidence to suggest that there is no increased risk of maternal or neonatal haemorrhage (CLASP Collaborative Group 1994). Aspirin exerts its antiplatelet effect for around 10 days after administration and may prolong the bleeding time. Some clinicians therefore prefer to discontinue aspirin 3–4 weeks prior to delivery to prevent complications as a result of this.

Antihypertensives

Antihypertensive drugs may be prescribed in pregnancy for pre-existing hypertension, pregnancy-induced hypertension or pre-eclampsia. Several of the drugs which are used in young women outside pregnancy are contraindicated in pregnancy and it is therefore important to recognise this and arrange for alternative medication if necessary.

Antihypertensives that are contraindicated in pregnancy

ACE inhibitors e.g. captopril, enalapril, lisinopril. These are *contraindicated* in the second and third trimester. There is limited information about their use in the first trimester and women should therefore be changed to other agents. They may cause oligohydramnios, fetal anuria and stillbirth.

Diuretics e.g. furosemide (frusemide), bendroflumethiazide (bendrofluazide). These cause a reduction in circulating blood volume. This may potentially compromise uteroplacental circulation and these drugs are therefore not recommended in pregnancy.

Antihypertensives that may be used in pregnancy

Methyldopa. This drug has been available for many years. There is extensive experience with its use in pregnancy and there is no evidence of adverse effects on the fetus. It is one of the first line antihypertensive drugs for use in pregnancy. The disadvantage is the maternal side-effect profile, which includes lethargy, drowsiness and depression. These side-effects may be dose dependent. It is given in two to four divided doses from a starting dose of 250 mg three times daily up to a total of 3 g daily. The onset of action is slow and it is therefore not suitable for acute blood pressure control. Caution should also be taken when stopping methyldopa in women who have been taking it for several weeks as sudden withdrawal may cause insomnia and anxiety symptoms. It should therefore be stopped gradually. It is safe in breastfeeding.

Beta blockers e.g. propranolol, atenolol, labetalol (which also has some alpha-blocking activity). These act by reducing heart rate and stroke volume and therefore reducing cardiac output. Although they cross the placenta and may slightly reduce fetal heart rate, there is no significant change in variability. If commenced before 28 weeks' gestation they have been shown to cause a reduction in fetal growth in up to 25% of cases (Butters et al 1991). They are therefore good antihypertensive drugs for use in the third trimester, but caution should be taken earlier in pregnancy. Beta blockers are contraindicated in women with asthma as they may cause bronchoconstriction. Beta blockers are excreted into breastmilk and some (e.g. atenolol) may actually be concentrated in breastmilk. However, there are no reports of adverse effects on neonates and they are therefore considered safe in breastfeeding.

Calcium channel blockers e.g. nifedipine, nicardipine. These reduce blood pressure mainly by vasodilatation. Nifedipine is increasingly used as an agent in pregnancy. Nifedipine can be given in a rapid release formulation orally to reduce blood pressure quickly in acute situations. However, care should be taken as serious hypotensive reactions have been reported, especially in association with magnesium sulphate (Waisman et al 1988). In general, nifedipine should be given in slow release formulations as these have a more gradual onset and longer period of action. The major side-effect is a headache, which may cause difficulty when determining symptoms of pre-eclampsia. Nifedipine is considered safe in breastfeeding.

Hydralazine. This is a useful drug for management of hypertension in the acute situation. It can only be administered intravenously. It is given either by slow bolus injection or by infusion. It acts as a vasodilator. It is safe in pregnancy and breastfeeding.

Drugs for diabetes mellitus

Sulfonylureas (oral hypoglycaemic agents) e.g. glibenclamide, gliclazide. These drugs should be avoided since they cross the placenta and exert an effect on the fetus.

Metformin. This is occasionally used in infertility treatment in women with polycystic ovarian syndrome (PCOS). It is usually discontinued in pregnancy and is not generally used for diabetic control during pregnancy, although it is said not to cross the placenta.

Insulin. This is the mainstay of diabetic treatment in pregnancy. It is a naturally occurring hormone and most of the available preparations of insulin, which are synthetic human insulins or pork-derived insulins, are safe in pregnancy. Bovine insulin should be avoided, however.

Drugs used in asthma

The drugs commonly used in the treatment of asthma include: inhaled bronchodilators (e.g. salbutamol, salmeterol, ipratropium), inhaled chromoglycate, inhaled and oral corticosteroids and theophyllines. All of these drugs are considered safe. Indeed, in either an acute asthmatic attack or in an exacerbation of asthma, the benefits of the medication outweigh the risks to mother and fetus.

Anticoagulants

A degree of anticoagulation may be required in some women in pregnancy in several situations, such as a history of a previous thromboembolic problem, an acute event, a known thrombophilia or heart valve replacement. There are two main anticoagulant drugs: heparin and warfarin.

Warfarin. This drug crosses the placenta and is a teratogen, the critical time of exposure being 6–9 weeks' gestation. The risk of 'fetal warfarin syndrome' is around 10% of those exposed but there is also an increase in central nervous system abnormalities. The characteristics of fetal warfarin syndrome are: nasal hypoplasia, epiphyseal abnormality, eye defects, shortening of the extremities, deafness, developmental retardation, congenital heart disease and scoliosis. Women on long term warfarin should therefore be aware of the risks and should be asked to inform their doctor immediately they become pregnant. In the second and third trimester there is a risk of fetal intracerebral haemorrhage.

Generally, women on warfarin should be converted to heparin as soon as they become pregnant and will continue on heparin throughout pregnancy. Some women, in particular those with mechanical prosthetic heart valves, may require warfarin in later pregnancy because of the major risk to the mother of inadequate anticoagulation despite the risks to the fetus. Warfarin is safe in breastfeeding and may be safely commenced in postpartum women.

The drug has a very gradual onset of action and requires a loading dose to be given over 2 or 3 days.

The dose required is very variable and it is judged by monitoring the INR (international normalised ratio) in the blood. This gives an index of the prothrombin time in the patient compared with a standard control, which indicates how much longer it takes for certain coagulation pathways to be activated. In other words, it indicates how quickly or slowly the blood is clotting. Also, many other drugs can interact with warfarin so care should be taken when prescribing to women on warfarin.

Heparin. This does not cross the placenta and it is not excreted into breastmilk. It is therefore safe in pregnancy and breastfeeding. In its 'unfractionated' form, which can be given either intravenously or subcutaneously, it is a mixture of large molecules of differing sizes. Because of the variability of the molecular size, the anticoagulant activity can vary. The effectiveness of heparin is monitored by measuring the activated partial thromboplastin time (APTT); this is a measure of the activity of the intrinsic coagulation pathway, which is where heparin exerts its effect. The dose can be altered to keep it within a set level. Heparin is used in pregnancy both for prophylaxis of thromboembolic disease (subcutaneous) and for acute treatment (usually intravenous).

Side-effects of heparin include bleeding, and bruising at the injection site. Some patients have allergic reactions to heparin, which are usually skin rashes. In addition, in some patients there is heparin-induced thrombocytopenia, so all patients who are commenced on heparin need to have a platelet count after a short period of treatment. Long term heparin therapy is associated with osteoporosis, and this in particular is a reason to weigh up the benefits versus the risk of treatment.

Heparin is now also available in low molecular weight (LMW) preparations such as enoxaparin, dalteparin, tinzaparin. LMW heparins have a more predictable anticoagulant response and are usually given by once-daily subcutaneous injection. In general medical practice they are replacing unfractionated heparin for most uses. Certainly in pregnancy they are useful in prophylaxis and in ongoing treatment after an acute event. There is, however, little evidence regarding their use for treatment of an acute event. There are other benefits: there is a lower incidence of thrombocytopenia and osteoporosis (Lin & Hu 2000). Because there is less known regarding the dose requirement in pregnancy, many clinicians would monitor the effectiveness of LMW heparin by measuring the anti-Xa activity about 4 hours after a subcutaneous dose. (LMW heparins exert their greatest effect on the coagulation pathway by affecting factor Xa.) One of the disadvantages in pregnancy is that, because of the long duration of action of the drug, most anaesthetists are not happy to site epidural or spinal blocks within 8–12 hours of an injection because of the risk of haematoma formation.

Tocolytics

At present there are no 'perfect' agents for abolishing uterine activity in women in preterm labour. No agents have been shown to prolong pregnancy significantly. However, tocolytic agents are beneficial for short term use, either for transfer to a centre with neonatal facilities or for allowing 48 hours for corticosteroids to be given. All of the following agents have been shown to be effective for short term use.

Beta sympathomimetics e.g. ritodrine, terbutaline, salbutamol. These are associated with significant maternal side-effects such as palpitations, tremor, nausea, vomiting, headaches, thirst, restlessness, chest pain and breathlessness. Tachycardia is common. The serious complication of pulmonary oedema is a risk but is usually associated with fluid overload. Blood sugar levels may rise and should be monitored; this is a particular risk in women with diabetes where the serious complication of diabetic ketoacidosis may follow. Serum potassium may also fall and urea and electrolytes should also be monitored. Because of these significant side-effects, great care should be taken when administering these drugs and the minimum dose required should be given. For example, ritodrine is given as an intravenous infusion and should be titrated down to the lowest possible rate to abolish uterine activity.

NSAIDS e.g. indometacin. Maternal side-effects include gastrointestinal bleeding, peptic ulceration, thrombocytopenia and allergic reactions. Renal function may also be impaired. Fetal side-effects when used in the long term include oligohydramnios, fetal renal impairment, premature closure of the ductus arteriosus, intraventricular haemorrhage and necrotising enterocolitis.

Calcium channel blockers e.g. nifedipine. These have the advantage of oral administration and fewer side-effects than some of the other agents. Profound maternal hypotension is a risk (Tsatsaris et al 2001).

Magnesium sulphate. This is commonly used in North America. Flushing, nausea, vomiting, palpitations and headaches are common maternal side-effects. Pulmonary oedema and ARDS are rare complications. Magnesium levels need to be monitored because of the risk of hypermagnesaemia, which may cause respiratory depression.

Oxytocin antagonists e.g. atosiban. These are a new class of drugs that appear to have fewer side-effects than other agents, but with similar efficacy.

Corticosteroids

Corticosteroids may be administered in pregnancy for pre-existing maternal disease such as asthma, rheumatoid arthritis and other inflammatory diseases. In these patients the most usual agent is prednisolone, which crosses the placenta in relatively small quantities. It is considered safe for use in pregnancy as there is no evidence of adverse effect on the developing fetus. As the drugs are generally used for significant maternal disease the benefits of administration far outweigh the risks.

If corticosteroids are administered, even in moderate doses, throughout pregnancy then there is a risk of maternal adrenal suppression. This results in a failure of the normal mechanism of increased endogenous corticosteroid production in labour. Women who are on long term steroid treatment should therefore receive extra corticosteroids in labour to compensate for this. This is usually given as intravenous hydrocortisone.

The other use of corticosteroids in pregnancy is for fetal lung maturation in actual or threatened preterm delivery. In this case betamethasone or dexamethasone is used, both of which cross the placenta in higher concentrations than prednisolone. Betamethasone and dexamethasone are generally given as intramuscular injections in divided doses over 24–48 hours. Different units use widely differing regimens. Treatment with antenatal corticosteroids has been shown to be associated with a substantial reduction in the incidence of respiratory distress syndrome (Crowley 1999). The most significant effect is noticed if 48 hours has elapsed between administration of the drug and delivery. There is a significant reduction in perinatal mortality and intraventricular haemorrhage. There is no clear evidence of adverse effects on the fetus or on long term follow-up of children exposed to steroids. There is no clear evidence either to suggest how often courses of steroids should be repeated (if at all) in women at continuing risk of preterm labour.

Magnesium sulphate

Magnesium sulphate has been used in the treatment of eclampsia in North America for many years. More recently, following a study that produced convincing evidence of its effectiveness (Eclampsia Trial Collaborative Group 1995), it has become widely used in the UK for the treatment of eclampsia. It probably exerts its effect by acting as a cerebral vasodilator, thereby reversing cerebral vasospasm and increasing cerebral blood flow. Magnesium sulphate can be given intramuscularly or intravenously. There is no consensus as to the dosing regimen, but care should be taken to avoid magnesium toxicity. Because of this, some units monitor serum magnesium levels and aim to keep then below the threshold for toxicity, which is around 5 mmol/L. The clinical signs of magnesium toxicity are loss of the patellar reflexes, a feeling of flushing, somnolence, slurred speech, respiratory difficulty and, in extreme cases, cardiac arrest. The 'antidote' to magnesium sulphate is calcium gluconate, which is given intravenously when there is evidence of magnesium toxicity.

Some principles for managing drugs during pregnancy are listed in Box 48.1.

Drugs used in labour and the immediate puerperium

Prostaglandins

Prostaglandins are lipid molecules responsible for multiple physiological subcellular reactions. They also play a part in some pathological processes. The prostaglandins important in labour and the puerperium are PGE and PGF. They can be administered by any route but have significant side-effects when given orally.

Prostaglandin E_2. This is generally given by the vaginal route because of the relative lack of side-effects from this route. It is used for induction of labour

> **Box 48.1** Principles of managing drugs in pregnancy
>
> - Avoid drugs where possible in the first trimester
> - Provide prepregnancy counselling where feasible
> - Do not stop long term drugs abruptly without medical advice
> - Choose safe options where possible
> - Inform women of the possible risks (if any) when starting new drugs
> - Establish a prenatal diagnosis of fetal abnormality, where possible, when a woman has been exposed to a teratogen in the first trimester

and acts on both the cervix and the myometrium. The action on the cervix is not completely understood, but there is probably an alteration in the composition of the cervix as occurs in cervical ripening (Arias 2000). It is given in the form of gel or tablets that are modified-release preparations. Repeat doses should not be given within the time interval determined by the preparation because of the risk of uterine hyperstimulation. There is a potentiation of myometrial stimulation with oxytocin; therefore oxytocin should not be given within at least 3–6 hours of prostaglandin because of the risk of uterine hyperstimulation.

Prostaglandin $F_{2\alpha}$. This is used for the treatment of postpartum haemorrhage. It acts on the myometrium as a powerful contractile agent. The available preparation is carboprost, which is an analogue of $PGF_{2\alpha}$. This is given either intramuscularly or intramyometrially in cases of uterine atony.

Oxytocin

Oxytocin is a naturally occurring hormone that exerts a stimulatory effect on myometrial contractility. The effect of oxytocin on the myometrium is mainly dependent on the concentration of oxytocin receptors present. Receptors are not present in non-pregnant myometrium; they appear at around 13 weeks of pregnancy and increase in concentration until term. The highest concentration is in the uterine fundus. Synthetic oxytocin is given antenatally to aid uterine contractility, either in induction of labour or in augmentation of labour, or postpartum for prevention or treatment of uterine atony.

It can be given by any parenteral route. In labour it is generally given by intravenous infusion in order that the amount given can be titrated against its effect. It takes 20–30 minutes for oxytocin to reach a steady state and the rate of infusion of oxytocin should therefore not be increased at time intervals less than 30 minutes. The half-life of oxytocin is 10–12 minutes (Arias 2000). For treatment and prevention of postpartum haemorrhage, larger doses of oxytocin can be given either by intravenous or intramuscular bolus or by intravenous infusion. Care should be taken when administering intravenous bolus doses, which should be given by slow injection.

The major side-effect of oxytocin is water retention and hyponatraemia, which is particularly relevant in women with pre-eclampsia. This effect is compounded when the vehicle for administration of oxytocin is 5% dextrose.

Ergometrine

This is used in the treatment and prevention of postpartum haemorrhage. It is a powerful constrictor of smooth muscle and therefore causes myometrial contraction. It does, however, have the significant side-effects of nausea, vomiting and hypertension. In women with pre-eclampsia it is generally considered to be contraindicated except in exceptional circumstances because of the risk of severe hypertension.

It can be given intramuscularly or intravenously. One of the benefits of ergometrine is that it has a sustained action, up to 2–3 hours. In many areas Syntometrine (oxytocin 5 IU/ml with ergometrine 0.5 mg) is given intramuscularly for the third stage of labour. This has the advantage of the speed of action of oxytocin (within 3 minutes) and the sustained action of ergometrine. The disadvantage is the side-effect profile of the ergometrine.

Drugs and breastfeeding

It is important to remember that the concerns with drugs do not cease after delivery. This applies not only to health care professionals but also to the women themselves who may be more relaxed about what they take after the baby has been born.

Most drugs will pass into breastmilk in greater or lesser concentrations. This is not, however, the most important factor in determining the potential effect on the baby – it is the concentration in the infant's serum that matters. This in turn will depend on the metabolism of the drug within the infant, which will be different to that in the adult.

The amount of a substance passing into breastmilk will also depend on the timing of dosing in relation to feeds. Whether the drug is water or fat soluble will determine whether there are higher concentrations in foremilk or hindmilk, and the feeding pattern of the infant will affect how much of the drug is received. Thus a mother taking a largely fat-soluble drug will pass more to an infant that feeds for prolonged periods than to one who feeds little and often because of the relative amounts of the hindmilk consumed.

A detailed list of drugs and whether or not they are safe in breastfeeding is outside the scope of this chapter. Details can be found in the Further reading list.

Drugs that may affect milk production

Some drugs may adversely affect milk production and are therefore not recommended in breastfeeding. The most commonly encountered drugs that have this effect are:

- oestrogen: the combined contraceptive pill is therefore contraindicated
- bromocriptine and cabergoline
- large doses of thiazide diuretics (e.g. bendroflumethiazide (bendrofluazide)), although the normal pharmacological doses are probably safe
- ergotamine (used in treatment of migraine).

The law, midwives and medicines

Midwives are subject to legislation relating to the prescription, supply and administration of medicines and to the Midwives' rules (UKCC 1998, rule 41). Midwives are also expected to comply with their Code of practice (UKCC 1998, see paragraphs 15–25).

The Medicines Act 1968

In the UK, the legislation relating to the prescribing, supply and administration of medicines is set out in the Medicines Act 1968 and in subsequent secondary legislation. Medicines are divided into three categories:

- prescription-only medicines (POM)
- pharmacy medicines (P)
- general sale list (GSL).

Specific drugs, including those normally available only on a prescription issued by a medical practitioner, may be supplied to midwives for use in their practice. Midwives are therefore recognised as being exempt from certain restrictions on the sale or supply of medicines under this Act. The products that a midwife can supply and administer have to be from an approved list and include:

- antiseptics
- aperients
- sedatives and analgesics
- local anaesthetic
- oxytocic preparation
- approved agents for neonatal and maternal resuscitation.

The Misuse of Drugs Act 1971

This Act covers drugs liable to misuse. Drugs subject to the Act's control are termed 'controlled drugs' and are separated into three classes, A, B or C, depending upon their level of control. Medicinal products containing controlled drugs are still subject to the Medicines Act and are all listed as POMs.

The Misuse of Drugs Regulations

The Misuse of Drugs Regulations 1973, the Misuse of Drugs (Amendment) Regulations 1974, the Misuse of Drugs Regulations 1985 and the Misuse of Drugs (Northern Ireland) Regulations 1986 have permitted registered midwives to possess and administer controlled drugs in their professional practice. Subsequent POM Orders specify the list of drugs that can be supplied to midwives for administration without a doctor's prescription.

Supply order procedure and standing orders

Midwives must use the supply order procedure to obtain drugs for use in their practice. With an increase in the illicit use of controlled drugs and the reduction in home births, midwives may prefer not to store and carry controlled drugs themselves but instead ask individual women planning to birth at home to seek a prescription for pethidine from their GP. In circumstances where a woman is transferred to hospital, drugs obtained under the supply order procedure may not be used. Instead, local policies permit hospital-based midwives to have similar powers to midwives working in the community. These powers are normally covered by 'standing orders'. The medicines permitted under standing orders must be signed by a consultant registered medical practitioner and a senior midwife.

Patient group directions and nurse prescribing

In 1989 the first Crown report (DoH 1989) was published. This extended the power of prescribing a very limited set of medicines to district nurses and health visitors. It also recommended the supply of certain medicines under group protocols.

In 1998 a report (DoH 1998) was published to tighten regulations relating to group protocols. As a consequence the POM Amendment Order 2000 came into force clarifying the meaning of a 'patient group direction' (PGD), which replaced the use of group protocols. In England a Health Service Circular was issued (HSC 2000/02b) to instruct Chief Executives to 'ensure that any current or new patient group directions comply with new legal requirements' (p. 2). This circular also clarified that midwives are already exempt from certain requirements of the Medicines Act and that:

These exemptions which allow them to administer or supply certain specified medicines without the directions of a doctor, will continue and are *not* affected by the new provisions of PGDs (para 15).

This was a particularly important statement to ensure that the status quo in relation to standing orders should remain, as controlled drugs are not permitted under PGDs.

A more recent Crown report (DoH 1999) recommended extending the authorised list of prescribers and establishing two new categories of prescribers:

Independent prescribers. These are responsible for initial assessment and diagnosis.

Dependent prescribers. These are authorised to prescribe certain medicines when the condition has been diagnosed or assessed by an independent practitioner. This activity of 'dependent' prescribing has now been superseded by the term 'supplementary' prescribing (see www.doh.gov.uk/nurseprescribing).

Supplementary prescribing. From 2003 pharmacists (in addition to nurses and midwives) who have trained to prescribe, will be able to prescribe for the first time. The DoH describes supplementary prescribing as 'a voluntary prescribing partnership between an independent prescriber and a supplementary prescriber, to implement an agreed patient-specific clinical management plan with the patient's agreement'.

Unlike the restriction to certain groups of nursing following the first Crown report, midwives are now included in the list of professionals that can apply to be independent prescribers. The formulary to be used by nurse and midwife authorised prescribers is somewhat limited, however, and when seconding staff to an approved course (the first course was approved in 2002) employers will need to consider whether designating midwives as independent prescribers has any advantages for clients over the current arrangements for the administration of medicines. Further details can be found on the following websites: www.npc.ppa.nhs.uk and www.npc.co.uk.

Administration of medicines and record keeping

It is obviously vital that, for the safety and well-being of the woman, all prescriptions for medication are legible and clear in their instruction. It is equally important that prescribed medicines are given at the appropriate time. This may be crucial in achieving the correct concentration of drug in the circulation. When drugs are administered this should be recorded in a legible fashion. Clarity and legibility are essential for safety. Where women are self-medicating, care should be taken to explain to the woman the importance of dosage and timing and ideally she should record her own medications. Occasionally it may be necessary, for example in psychiatric patients, to observe them taking oral medication.

To minimise the risk of human error in the administration of medicines, employers will normally have written policies, protocols and procedures. It is essential that midwives comply with these, and if in doubt about a drug or its dosage prescribed by another practitioner then advice should be sought before it is administered. The consent of the recipient, or parent of a baby, must be obtained before any medicine is given. As well as carefully checking that the drug and dosage are correct, the midwife must also check the expiry date.

The Midwives rules and code of practice (UKCC 1998) and Guidelines for the administration of medicines (UKCC 2000) emphasise the importance of accurate record keeping. Midwives must adhere to the rules, code of practice and local policy in relation to record keeping. Each midwife's supervisor of midwives will periodically audit records to maintain and improve standards of practice.

REFERENCES

Arias F 2000 Pharmacology of oxytocin and prostaglandins. Clinical Obstetrics and Gynecology 43:455–468

Briggs G G, Freeman R K, Yaffe S J 1998 Drugs in pregnancy and lactation, 5th edn. Williams & Wilkins, Baltimore

Butters L, Kennedy S, Rubin P C 1991 Atenolol in essential hypertension during pregnancy. British Medical Journal 301:587–589

CLASP Collaborative Group 1994 CLASP: a randomised trial of low dose aspirin for the prevention and treatment of pre-eclampsia among 9364 pregnant women. Lancet 343:619–629

Crowley P 1999 Prophylactic steroids for preterm birth. *Cochrane Database of Systematic Reviews*, Issue 1. Update Software, Oxford

DoH (Department of Health) 1989 Report on nurse prescribing and supply. Advisory group chaired by Dr June Crown. HMSO, London

DoH (Department of Health) 1998 Review of prescribing, supply and administration of medicines: a report on the supply and administration of medicines under group protocols. Stationery Office, London

DoH (Department of Health) 1999 Final report on the prescribing, supply and administration of medicines. Chaired by Dr June Crown. Stationery Office, London

Dunlop W 1976 Investigations into the influence of posture in renal plasma flow and glomerular filtration rate during late pregnancy. British Journal of Obstetrics and Gynaecology 83:17–23

Eclampsia Trial Collaborative Group 1995 Which anticonvulsant for women with eclampsia? Evidence from the Collaborative Eclampsia Trial. Lancet 345:1455–1463

Kreft-Jais C, Plouin P F, Tchobroutsky C, Boutry J 1988 Angiotensin-converting enzyme inhibitors during pregnancy: a survey of 22 patients given captopril and 9 given enalapril. British Journal of Obstetrics and Gynaecology 95:420–422

Lin R, Hu Z-W 2000 Hematologic disorders. In: Carruthers S G, Hoffman B B, Melmon K L, Nierenberg D W (eds) Melmon and Morelli's clinical pharmacology, 4th edn. McGraw-Hill, New York, p 737–797

Lumley J, Watson L, Watson M, Bower C 2000 Periconceptional supplementation with folate and/or multivitamins for preventing neural tube defects. Cochrane Database of Systematic Reviews, Issue 1. Update Software, Oxford

McFadyen I R 1989 Maternal changes in normal pregnancy. In: Turnbull A, Chamberlain G (eds) Obstetrics. Churchill Livingstone, London, p 151–171

Medicines Act 1968 HMSO, London

Misuse of Drugs Act 1971 HMSO, London

Misuse of Drugs Regulations 1973, 1974, 1985, 1986 HMSO, London

Norton M E, Merrill J, Cooper B A B, Kuller J A, Clyman R I 1991 Neonatal complications after the administration of indomethacin for preterm labour. New England Journal of Medicine 329:1602–1607

Parry E, Shields R, Turnbull A C 1970 Transit time in small intestine in pregnancy. Journal of Obstetrics and Gynaecology of the British Commonwealth 77:900–901

Tsatsaris V, Papatsonis D, Goffinet F, Dekker G, Carbonne B 2001 Tocolysis with nifedipine or beta-adrenergic agonist: a meta-analysis. Obstetrics and Gynecology 97:840–847

UKCC (United Kingdom Central Council for Nursing, Midwifery and Health Visiting) 1998 Midwives rules and code of practice. UKCC, London

UKCC (United Kingdom Central Council for Nursing, Midwifery and Health Visiting) 2000 Guidelines for the administration of medicines. UKCC, London

Waisman G D, Mayorga L M, Camera M I, Vignolo C A, Martinotti A 1988 Magnesium plus nifedipine: potentiation of hypotensive effect in pre-eclampsia? American Journal of Obstetrics and Gynecology 171:417–424

FURTHER READING

Briggs G G, Freeman R K, Yaffe S J 1998 Drugs in pregnancy and lactation, 5th edn. Williams & Wilkins, Baltimore

A detailed discussion of the data available on individual drugs in pregnancy and lactation. Each drug is dealt with in alphabetical order. A good reference text.

British National Formulary Number 41, March 2001.

This is published every 6 months by the British Medical Association and the Royal Pharmaceutical Society of Great Britain. A compilation of prescribing information and pharmaceutical company information regarding individual drugs and preparations of drugs.

Rubin P C 2000. Prescribing in pregnancy, 3rd edn. BMJ Books, London

A short, readable text discussing the use of drugs in pregnancy.

49 Complementary and Alternative Medicine in Maternity Care

Denise Tiran

CHAPTER CONTENTS

This chapter aims to provide student and qualified midwives with an introduction to the subject of complementary and alternative medicine (CAM) and its application to the care of pregnant and childbearing women. Several, but not all, of the most commonly used complementary therapies are discussed in relation to the relief of physiological discomforts of pregnancy, care in labour and the early puerperium. Professional accountability is addressed and cautions, precautions and contraindications are discussed.

After reading this chapter students will have an understanding of the principal complementary therapies in use in Britain today and an appreciation of their application to the care of pregnant and childbearing women, where appropriate. Students will also be able to acknowledge the parameters of their personal professional practice with regard to CAM and be aware of other sources of information.

Introduction

Complementary and alternative medicine is a growing area of health care within Britain and is increasingly popular with consumers and professionals. Use of natural remedies and consultations with CAM practitioners have been sought by at least one in three people in the UK (Stone 1999).

Until the late 1980s these therapies were very much considered to be alternative, even 'fringe', medicine and a report published by the British Medical Association in 1986 derided them as a passing trend not worthy of debate (BMA 1986). However, as a result of consumer demand, a working party was set up in 1993 to examine the situation and the British Medical Association then published a further report entitled Complementary medicine: a guide to good practice (BMA 1993). This second report acknowledged that there was some validity in using alternative therapies and recommendations were made regarding some of the professional issues of concern.

Within maternity care, the use of complementary therapies has been driven by consumers who are looking for strategies to help them cope with the discomforts of pregnancy and labour. It is therefore incumbent on midwives, as the primary caregivers, to be aware of the range of alternatives available and to be able to advise women accordingly – or to know where to turn for more expert assistance if they feel unable to help appropriately.

As CAM became more available and demand for therapies increased, the Foundation for Integrated Medicine (FIM) was set up. Following a series of working parties, the document *Integrated healthcare: the way forward for the next five years?* was produced (FIM 1997). Four main issues were debated: education and training, regulation and registration, research and development, and delivery and availability of CAM services. Despite concerns within the conventional health care fields, CAM has gradually begun to be more accepted and, indeed, to be *integrated* into mainstream care.

Classification of complementary and alternative therapies

There are in excess of two hundred therapies that are complementary or alternative to mainstream health care systems. In December 2000, the House of Lords Select Committee on Science and Technology published its sixth report on CAM and classified the most commonly used therapies into three main categories. At the time of writing there continues to be debate regarding the appropriateness of these categories, for although the report seemed to add credibility to some therapies others were relegated to lower categories than had previously been the case, on somewhat nebulous grounds.

Group 1. This group has been classified as those therapies that are professionally organised, with good standards of basic and ongoing education, national statutory or voluntary self-regulation and disciplinary codes of practice. These are homeopathy, herbal medicine, acupuncture, osteopathy and chiropractic.

Osteopaths and chiropractors are now regulated by statute, since 1993 and 1994 respectively, and their titles are protected in much the same way as the title of midwife or doctor. Both of these aspects of complementary medicine require qualified practitioners to undertake the treatment and, although pregnant women may choose to consult them for problems such as backache, sciatica or symphysis pubis diastasis (separation of the symphysis pubis from the ischial bones), they are unlikely to be therapies provided by midwives. Craniosacral therapy, an extremely gentle 'offshoot' of osteopathy, is especially beneficial for infants and children.

Acupuncturists register with one of three main organisations, according to whether they are already doctors, physiotherapists or lay practitioners (including nurses and midwives), but all 2000 acupuncturists in Britain are registered with the British Acupuncture Accreditation Board. Homeopathy, the only therapy to have been available on the National Health Service since its inception in 1948, is largely classified into medical and non-medical (lay) homeopaths and is regulated by the Faculty of Homeopaths and the Society of Homeopaths respectively. Most medical herbalists are trained and registered with the National Institute of Medical Herbalists (NIMH), with education being at undergraduate level. There are now several midwives in Britain who practise acupuncture, homeopathy or herbal medicine within their normal care of pregnant and childbearing women.

Group 2. This group is classified as those therapies which are considered to be *complementary* to other forms of health care. It includes aromatherapy, reflexology, massage, shiatsu, nutrition, hypnotherapy, Alexander technique, Bach flower remedies, counselling, stress management, yoga, meditation and healing. Education and regulation of therapists is variable, although the aromatherapists and reflexologists have instigated a form of self-regulation via the Aromatherapy/Reflexology Organisations Councils, both of which have as their members the combined schools and registers of relevant practitioners throughout the country. Most of the other therapies have several regulatory organisations, but, significantly, it is not a legal requirement in the UK to be registered in order to practise, or even to be adequately trained. Sixteenth-century English Common Law allows anyone to do anything unless it *contravenes* an existing law, whereas most of Europe uses Napoleonic Law, which prevents people from doing anything unless it is *permitted* by law. An exploration of the use of aromatherapy and reflexology within midwifery practice follows later in this chapter, and readers interested in finding out more about the remaining therapies should consult the list of further reading.

Group 3. This is subdivided into 3a – traditional systems such as Traditional Chinese Medicine (TCM), Ayurvedic medicine, Tibetan medicine, anthroposophical medicine and naturopathy – and 3b – other alternatives including crystal therapy, dowsing, iridology, kinesiology and radionics. It is not the intention of this chapter to discuss these therapies further but interested readers are referred to the list of recommended reading. It is, however, interesting to note that, while TCM, which includes acupuncture, is relegated to group 3, *Western-style* acupuncture is included in group 1. This may be due to medicopolitical distinctions and a continuing desire to treat people in the reductionist manner of orthodox medicine rather than a true representation of the nature of the practices.

Complementary medicine and maternity care

Women may have used complementary therapies prior to pregnancy, either by self-administering natural remedies or by consulting an independent practitioner, or they may wish to do so during pregnancy and for the birth. Expectant mothers are keen to use complementary therapies because they provide a range of additional strategies for pregnancy and labour (Tiran 2001) at a time when pharmaceutical preparations are largely contraindicated and physiological discomforts are dismissed by the medical profession as 'minor disorders'. Also, many women wish to achieve as natural a birth as possible without recourse to drugs for pain relief in labour and may request the presence of a CAM practitioner at the birth. Demand for and interest in natural remedies is high and their use may empower mothers to retain control of their bodies. General dissatisfaction with many aspects of conventional health care and its dependence on technology, not least in maternity care the 'conveyor belt' feeling, a continuing necessary evil of a defensive system of routine obstetrics and its 'just in case' philosophy, has over the years resulted in the publication of policy documents such as the Changing Childbirth report (DoH 1993). Midwives and obstetricians in busy maternity departments often have insufficient time to individualise care. Even where there are schemes in place to address some of the problems, such as case-load or team midwifery, staff shortages often prevent the allocation of quality time to each mother for the provision of holistic care.

Complementary medicine is based on the philosophy of holism and an appreciation of the innate interaction between the body, mind and spirit of the individual. Health care consumers in general are rebelling, perhaps subconsciously, against the reductionist approach to orthodox medicine, which views the body as the sum of its parts but fails to recognise the impact of the total life experience on an individual's health. Within midwifery, Tiran (1999a) has proposed a framework for holistic care and demonstrated the value of incorporating complementary therapies within this framework.

Midwives are keen to implement CAM therapies into their practice and in 1997 it was estimated that approximately 34% of midwives had used some form of complementary therapy (NHS Confederation 1997). It is the view of this author that midwives are the professionals best placed to provide CAM therapies to pregnant, childbearing and newly delivered mothers and their babies. Also the Nursing and Midwifery Order (2001) forbids anyone other than a midwife or doctor, or one in training under supervision, from taking sole responsibility for the care of a childbearing mother, except in an emergency. Thus, any therapies used at this time must be *complementary*, rather than *alternative*, to conventional maternity care. In order to avoid the poor continuity of care so lamented prior to the Changing Childbirth report (DoH 1993), yet to enable women to access CAM therapies, it would seem eminently appropriate that, where possible, women are advised on complementary strategies by the professionals already legally providing maternity care.

Where women choose to consult independent complementary practitioners they should ensure that the therapist has a thorough understanding of pregnancy physiopathology *and* the conventional maternity services. Access to private practitioners should preferably be through personal recommendation, although midwives would be wise to refrain from naming individuals unless they can vouch for their expertise. Mothers wishing to find a practitioner can be advised to ask, at the time of making the first appointment, for the place, date and type of qualifications of their chosen therapist as well as relevant experience of treating pregnant women. Mothers should also enquire whether or not the practitioner has current personal professional indemnity insurance cover, from which it is reasonable to assume that she has adequate qualifications to practise. Any therapist who is unwilling to disclose this information should be rejected.

If the CAM practitioner is to be present during labour, he or she must acknowledge that the midwife or doctor, or both, legally remains the person responsible for the woman's care. Communication and education are vital between conventional providers of maternity care and complementary practitioners specialising in treating pregnant and childbearing women and their babies, and one organisation aimed at achieving this is the Complementary Maternity Forum (Tiran 1999b).

When a midwife wishes to incorporate some aspect of complementary medicine within her own practice, she must nevertheless continue to work within the parameters laid down by the Midwife's code of practice (UKCC 1998). The Nursing and Midwifery Council cannot regulate the practice of complementary therapy except when it is used in conjunction with midwifery, nursing or health-visiting registration. The midwife must be able to demonstrate that she is 'adequately and appropriately' trained to use the therapy, although this does not necessarily mean that she must be a fully qualified practitioner. It is permissible, for example, to learn to use a small selection of aromatherapy essential oils without being a trained aromatherapist, but the midwife remains accountable for her practice and must be able to justify her actions.

Midwives should refer to the UKCC/NMC documents on the Code of professional conduct (NMC 2002), Guidelines for administration of medicines (UKCC 2000) and the Midwives' rules and code of practice (UKCC 1998). The use of any therapy must not be at the expense of normal midwifery responsibilities, but rather should be considered an adjunct to other care. Informed maternal consent is essential, although this does not necessarily have to be written consent. Women have the right to utilise and self-administer natural remedies, and midwives should try to act as the mothers' advocate. If there is any doubt regarding the appropriateness of using a particular therapy then midwives are duty bound to consult relevant practitioners for advice. In units where midwives wish to implement the use of a therapy alongside their existing practice, it is wise to develop policies and protocols to protect both the women and the midwives. Communication and liaison with colleagues are vital to avoid conflict and attempt to dispel scepticism.

Box 49.1 illustrates the point that adequate training is essential for midwives wishing to incorporate CAM into their practice.

Box 49.1 Adequate education and training of midwives using CAM therapies is essential

I recently met with a small group of midwives who were implementing the use of reflexology into their practice. During discussion I heard that the midwives were using a reflexology technique to turn breech presentation fetuses to cephalic. On further questioning, however, it transpired that the midwives had attended a study day organised by a beauty therapy school and that a male therapist, who was not specialising in caring for pregnant women, had shown them how to perform a simple technique on the little toes which he said would cause the fetus to turn.

I asked the midwives to explain further and was concerned to learn that what they were doing was not, in fact, reflexology but was a form of acupressure, based on the Bladder 67 point as used in moxibustion (see p. 924). The midwives were totally unaware of this fact and, indeed, were not even able to identify exactly which *reflexology* points they thought they were stimulating. They had happily returned to their unit and started to use the 'reflexology' (an assumption made presumably because they were working on the feet) on women with breech presentations. There were no guidelines outlining parameters for their practice and, because of her own lack of knowledge, the manager/supervisor was allowing them to pursue a potentially unsafe practice.

Acupuncture

Acupuncture is one of the 'top five' complementary therapies as classified by the Foundation for Integrated Medicine (FIM 1997) and the House of Lords (2000). There are currently about six maternity units in Britain that provide acupuncture as part of their maternity services, although women may choose to visit an independent practitioner if they experience problems during pregnancy.

Acupuncture is a component of TCM, but in Britain is seen as a discrete therapy in its own right, often being practised in a Western 'reductionist' manner rather than as an element of an holistic system of care. It is based on the principle that the body has Qi or 'energy' lines, called meridians, flowing through it from top to hand or toe. Most of these pass through a major organ, after which the meridian is named (e.g. the Kidney meridian). There are 12 major meridians, and 365 points on these in total. When the body, mind and spirit are in equilibrium the energy flows along the meridians unimpeded and, to use the Chinese terminology, the 'Yin' and 'Yang' energies of the individual are balanced. However, when stressors of any sort affect the person, blockages occur at certain points (called acupuncture or 'tsubos') on specific meridians. These points can be stimulated to release and rebalance the energies, either by the insertion of acupuncture needles, or by other means. Sometimes thumb pressure is applied to the points (called acupressure, or the similar practice of *shiatsu*, the Japanese equivalent); on other occasions, heat is applied via moxa sticks (see Moxibustion, p. 924); or suction can be used by covering the points with special cups (cupping). Acupuncture needles may also be stimulated by mild electric pulsations; this is similar to transcutaneous nerve stimulation used for pain relief in labour.

Certain acupuncture points are contraindicated during pregnancy as they may initiate labour (Box 49.2); however, these points are good to stimulate for helping inefficient contractions in labour. These points include the fourth point on the Large Intestine 4 meridian (LI-4) point, in the webbing between thumb and forefinger, the Gall Bladder 21 (GB-21) point, on the edge of the clavicle, which is an easy point to overstimulate when performing shoulder massage, the Spleen 6 (SP-6) point on the inner calf and a range of points around the sacral and abdominal areas.

> **Box 49.2** Case scenario: 'A little knowledge is a dangerous thing'
>
> The complementary therapy (CT) midwife saw Jean in her clinic for the treatment of severe nausea and vomiting persisting to 19 weeks' gestation. Jean knew about certain possible natural remedies for the problem and had tried ginger but this had made the sickness worse. The CT midwife advised her about acupressure to the PC-6 point. However she was horrified when Jean said that her husband had told her about the acupuncture point in the webbing between forefinger and thumb (LI-4 point) and started to stimulate it vigorously.
>
> The issue here was that Jean was unaware of the potential stimulation of uterine contractions from the LI-4 point. Similarly she did not have sufficient knowledge to identify that some women experience an exacerbation of sickness if they use ginger, because, in TCM terms, ginger is 'hot' but they need cooling (for example with peppermint) in order to rebalance their energies.

Uses

Many antenatal conditions respond well to acupuncture or acupressure, including many of the physiological symptoms of pregnancy.

Nausea and vomiting. One condition that has been well researched is nausea and vomiting, which can be treated simply by exerting pressure on the Pericardium 6 (PC-6), also called Neiguan, point on the inner wrist. Some of the research has been carried out on pregnant women (Belluomini et al 1993; Dundee et al 1988, Evans et al 1993), whereas other trials have been done on people with postoperative or chemo- or radiotherapy-induced sickness (Al-Sadi et al 1997, Dundee & McMillan 1991, Dundee & Yang 1990, Dundee et al 1989, McMillan 1994). Commercial wristbands aimed at people with travel or motion sickness can be purchased, and tiny magnetised coils are also available, but it is important that these are positioned correctly for them to be effective.

The PC-6 point is found by measuring with the *mother's own fingers* three fingers' width up from the inner wrist crease where the hand joins the arm, approximately where the buckle of a watch strap might rest. The point is between the tendons and there should be a slight dip and some sensation of tenderness or bruising when the point is pressed, which is worse the more severe the sickness. The bands or magnets should be placed on both wrists prior to rising in the morning and should remain in position for the duration of the problem. However, although this is a simple means of relieving sickness for many women, a fully qualified traditional acupuncturist would take into account all imbalances within the body and may need to work on other points, for example points on the Stomach, Spleen or Conception Vessel meridians.

Moxibustion. The use of moxibustion for breech presentation is gaining popularity in the UK. In this technique, a stick of dried mugwort herb is used as a heat source over the Bladder 67 acupuncture point on the outer edges of the little toes. This is thought to stimulate adrenocortical output, resulting in increases in placental lactogens and changes in prostaglandin levels and leading to both increased myometrial sensitivity and contractility. This in turn leads to a rise in the fetal heart rate and fetal movements, so causing the fetus to turn itself to cephalic. Although the technique originated in China, where a success rate of over 90% was reported between 1979 and 1984 (Cooperative Research Group 1984), trials conducted by an Italian obstetrician and his colleagues have also shown statistically significant results ranging from 66% to 87% (Cardini & Weixin 1998; Cardini et al 1991). The number of cephalic deliveries at term is greatest in the moxibustion group in these trials, despite the number of spontaneous versions and reversions, and appears to be more successful than ECV. Although a few midwives now offer moxa to turn breech presentations, this is worthy of further development within midwifery practice for it provides a cost-effective alternative to caesarean section, is possibly safer than ECV and enables the mother to feel in control of her situation.

Labour. Acupuncture is also useful in labour, especially for pain relief, induction and acceleration (Kubista et al 1975, Ledergerber 1976, Perera 1979, Ying et al 1985, Yip et al 1976) and retained placenta. Most midwives use full-body acupuncture, inserting needles around the body in the most appropriate points, but auricular (ear) acupuncture could readily be learnt without a complete acupuncture training. The first acupuncture labours were conducted by Dr Ehrstroem in Sweden in 1972 and Darras in France in 1974. Labour acupuncture in the UK was available as early as 1987 when Irene Skelton used it in her midwifery practice (Skelton 1988). Martoudis & Christofides (1990) in Cyprus found that, by using one auricular acupoint and one on the hand, analgesia took effect within 40 minutes and lasted for an average of 6 hours. This technique is cheaper, safer, quicker to insert and has fewer side-effects than epidural analgesia, and could readily be applied to midwifery practice.

Homeopathy

Homeopathy is considered by many of its practitioners to be a form of 'energy' medicine; it uses minute, highly diluted doses of substances that, if given in the full dose, would actually cause the symptoms being treated. Most homeopathic medicines are in tablet form but they do not work pharmacologically and will not interact with prescribed drugs, although certain drugs may inactivate the homeopathic tablet. Homeopathy treats the whole person and takes into account the personality of the individual, including the factors that make the symptoms better or worse, and sees as significant factors that may appear to be the most inconsequential of symptoms.

Homeopathy is a gentle form of medicine well suited to the 'acute' nature of pregnancy and childbirth, but it is important that the remedies are used appropriately. When homeopathic remedies are developed the full dose of the substance is tested on groups of healthy volunteers to obtain a symptom picture that relates to the proposed remedy; this remedy can then be used to treat people who present with that symptom picture. An example of this is to consider the effects of an overdose of coffee late at night: insomnia compounded by an overactive mind, irritability, headaches, etc. Homeopathic Coffea may be used to treat someone with insomnia accompanied by the other symptoms of too much coffee. However, incorrect administration of a remedy may cause a 'reverse proving' in which, rather than treating the existing problem, the symptom picture of the remedy used is triggered in the woman. Although homeopathic remedies are available in pharmacies and health food stores, women should ensure they obtain accurate advice to help them make a decision regarding the most appropriate remedy for their condition. Only one tablet should normally be taken at one time. An increase in dosage means an increase in the frequency of administration, for the remedy acts as a stimulus to self-healing rather than as a chemical suppression or reversal of a symptom, as in the case of pharmaceutical drugs. Advice on packaging to take two tablets is nothing more than a commercial ploy, as two tablets have no more effectiveness than one.

Uses

Arnica. A very small number of remedies are classified as universal – that is, they are suitable for almost everyone suffering a particular symptom. The most well known of these is Arnica montana, found in tablet and cream form and effective for the treatment of bruising, shock and trauma, both external and internal. Newly delivered mothers with perineal trauma would benefit from administration of Arnica tablets to reduce trauma, although the cream should not be applied to the open wound, only to bruising surrounding the perineum. Similarly, in combination with homeopathic Hypericum for wound healing, Arnica can be useful for women who have had surgery such as caesarean section. Little research has been undertaken, however, despite numerous anecdotal accounts of its value; indeed, one trial of posthysterectomy patients found no statistically significant difference between women treated with Arnica and those without (Hart et al 1997), and other investigators found similar results in relation to other forms of trauma (Ernst & Pittler 1998, Linde et al 1997, Vickers et al 1998).

Pulsatilla. Pulsatilla is also beneficial in pregnancy and seems to be suited to women with a mild and tearful disposition who are apprehensive. Haemorrhoids, varicosities and heartburn often respond well to a short course of Pulsatilla, and slow progress in labour can be corrected in women with poor uterine contractions causing emotional distress, fainting and palpitations. Its use as a means of turning breech has been reported (Perko 1997), although the mechanism of action is not understood and no research reports have been found.

Homeopathy can be used for physiological discomforts of pregnancy, labour and the puerperium as well as some of the pathological conditions, although in an emergency some conflict could arise about the most appropriate system of medicine to use (Box 49.3).

Box 49.3 Case scenario: 'Professional boundaries must be identified'

A mother books a home birth with her community midwife, and wishes to be accompanied in labour by her homeopath who has been providing care during the pregnancy. Labour progresses so rapidly that a second midwife is unable to reach the house in time before the baby is born. The virtually precipitate delivery causes the baby to have a very low Apgar score and the midwife attempts resuscitation, to no avail. Suddenly the homeopath pushes her out of the way and proceeds to administer to the baby a substance which she calls the 'death remedy'. Almost immediately the baby starts to gasp and the Apgar score rises to 9.

It is not possible to know why the baby suddenly started to breathe – it may have been a delayed effect of the midwife's resuscitation, or a spontaneous resolution, the homeopathy may have been effective or the substance may simply have caused the baby to gasp and inhale air. However, when an independent practitioner is present it is important that discussion takes place with the midwife so that individual boundaries can be identified before an emergency occurs.

Herbal medicine

Phytotherapy, or the medicinal use of herbs and other plants, is similar in mode of action to modern pharmaceuticals; indeed, many drugs are developed from discoveries about the healing properties of plants. Unfortunately, in order for a product patent to be granted, pharmaceutical companies need to identify the active ingredient and then isolate and synthesise it – a process which removes the component from the whole plant and its synergistic action. It is this isolation and synthesis that causes side-effects of drugs to occur, whereas in the original plant there may well be other constituents that act to prevent those side-effects.

Safety

There is a common misconception that just because herbal remedies are natural they are automatically safe. This is untrue. If herbal medicine (or any other form of complementary therapy) has the power to act therapeutically, it also theoretically has the power to harm if used incorrectly. Conversely, pregnant women eschew all drugs, often even those prescribed for specific complaints, in the mistaken belief that all drugs are harmful. The issue here is that *all* substances must be used appropriately – and expectant mothers may need expert help to select the necessary remedy for their particular condition. There are many herbal remedies that should be avoided during pregnancy or breastfeeding, because they may induce uterine bleeding, miscarriage or other systemic effects on the mother or fetus.

St John's wort

One of the herbal remedies that has been much debated in the professional and public press is St John's wort (*Hypericum perforatum*), which has gained a reputation as an antidepressant, especially useful for seasonal affective disorder. Research seems to indicate the effect of one constituent, hyperforin, on serotonin (Singer et al 1999), noradrenaline (norepinephrine) and dopamine (Nathan 1999). However, Ondrizek et al (1999a, b) suggest that St John's wort may damage oocytes (as may also echinacea or *Ginkgo biloba*) and inhibit sperm motility, and so recommend avoiding it during the preconception period and the first trimester of pregnancy. Research from Germany persuaded the Department of Health to publish a report (DoH 2000) advising doctors that St John's wort is contraindicated in women on the contraceptive pill, are pregnant or breastfeeding, or taking certain medications such as anticoagulants and transplant antirejection drugs. On the other hand, Dr Fugh Berman, who advises the US government on the use of herbal medicines (2001, personal communication) believes this is an overreaction in Britain and that there is insufficient evidence to support this action. However, until more research findings are available, midwives in Britain should advise pregnant and breastfeeding women and new mothers who have restarted the contraceptive pill to refrain from administering St John's wort for self-diagnosed depression.

Raspberry leaf

Raspberry leaf is a popular herbal remedy that has long been advocated by pregnant women as helping them to prepare for the birth. It is thought that certain constituents within the leaves of the raspberry have an effect on the uterine muscle making it more efficient, possibly preventing postmaturity, easing discomfort in labour and enhancing uterine action. Very little research has been carried out to test this theory, although recent investigations in Australia appear to suggest that women who take raspberry leaf products are less likely to have pre- and post-term gestation, and may be less likely to require ARM, caesarean section, forceps or ventouse delivery than those in control groups (Parsons et al 1999, Simpson et al 2001). It is, however, recognised that further research is necessary.

Qualified medical herbalists may use raspberry leaf to treat threatened miscarriage but midwives should advise women not to take it as a routine until the third trimester. The tea, made from dried raspberry leaves, is more effective than tablets although some brands of capsules can be opened to release the dried leaf from within, so that a tea can be made. Expectant mothers should start with just one cup of the tea or one tablet daily, giving themselves a few days to become accustomed to the effects before increasing the dose, to a maximum of four cups or tablets daily. When a mother has inadvertently commenced with the full dose, extremely strong Braxton–Hicks contractions have been reported. There is no evidence that these are harmful to the fetus, but the mother may experience considerable discomfort. The tea can be drunk during labour, as long as uterine activity is normal and no hypertonic contractions occur; it is best avoided if medical augmentation (e.g. oxytocin) is administered. Any tea or tablets that the mother may have left over after the birth can be taken postnatally to aid involution.

The uses of herbal medicine in pregnancy and childbirth are summarised in Table 49.1.

Osteopathy and chiropractic

These two therapies are now considered to be professions supplementary to medicine since the passing of the Osteopaths Act in 1993 and the Chiropractors Act in 1994. It is unlikely that midwives will practise osteopathy or chiropractic although some clinics for pregnant women have a midwife in attendance, but it may be appropriate for midwives to advise a mother to seek treatment outside the conventional maternity services.

Table 49.1 Uses of herbal medicine for pregnancy and childbirth*

Condition	Useful herbs
Nausea and vomiting	Peppermint, spearmint or camomile tea, ginger capsules or tea
Threatened miscarriage	Crampbark or chasteberry, raspberry leaf or lady's mantle
Varicose veins/haemorrhoids	Marigold or witch hazel compress
Constipation	Dandelion root or lime blossom
Heartburn and indigestion	Anise, caraway, lemon balm, camomile
Labour progress/exhaustion	Raspberry leaf, ginseng, rosemary
Contraction pain	Motherwort, skullcap
Perineal care	Comfrey, marigold, lavender
Engorgement/mastitis	Cabbage leaves, fennel

* **NB** These are examples of herbal remedies that may be appropriate for certain conditions during the childbearing period; midwives should advise on using these remedies only if they are adequately and appropriately trained to do so.

Both forms of treatment involve rebalancing of the neuromusculoskeletal system so that the whole body can be in alignment. Disorders, trauma or alterations in the body structure can cause imbalances in the whole system, which in turn can lead to a predisposition to other conditions. An example of this would be a pelvic injury causing misalignment in the spine and tension in the upper vertebrae, skull and soft tissues of the brain, thus leading to interference with pituitary hormonal output, resulting in infertility.

The main difference between osteopathy and chiropractic is that osteopaths are concerned with mobility of joints whereas chiropractors deal with relative positions of joints. Different manipulative techniques are used and most chiropractors use more X-rays to aid diagnosis (although not for pregnant women). Osteopaths also use more soft tissue massage prior to manipulation.

Uses

Both osteopathy and chiropractic are useful for treating a range of problems in pregnancy, including sickness, heartburn and constipation, but are notably valuable in the effective treatment of backache, sciatica and symphysis pubis diastasis (Daly et al 1991, Fallon 1993, Harrison et al 1997, Schwartz et al 1985, Stern et al 1993). Other problems related to laxity of the joints caused by relaxin and progesterone, such as groin pain, legs 'giving way' and general pelvic instability, will also respond well to treatment. Chiropractic and osteopathy can also be useful in labour (Diakow et al 1991, Melzack and Belanger 1989, Melzack & Schaffelberg 1987, Sutton & Scott 1997).

Craniosacral therapy

Craniosacral therapy, or cranial osteopathy, is gaining credibility and acceptance as a means of treating babies suffering the effects of excessive moulding following instrumental delivery, including fractiousness, irritability, sleeplessness, poor feeding and, in older children, hyperactivity (Hayden 2000).

Aromatherapy

Aromatherapy is the use of highly concentrated essential oils extracted from plants. Although these oils are aromatic, the term 'aromatherapy' is a misnomer, for the therapy is not simply about the smells of the oils, but utilises the chemical constituents within them for their therapeutic properties. Essential oils enter the body by a variety of means, depending on the method of administration. The most frequently used methods are via the skin, usually as massage, but also in the bath or in compresses or creams, via the mucous membranes in pessaries or suppositories, or via the respiratory tract in inhalations and vaporisers. Simply inhaling the aromas means that some essential oil molecules enter the body and will reach the limbic centre in the brain, the circulation and major organs. All essential oils act in the same way as pharmaceutical drugs, being absorbed, metabolised and excreted via the same pathways, and are therefore likely to interact with prescribed medications.

Safety

Essential oils can be very therapeutic when used appropriately, but also have the potential to be toxic if incorrectly administered or abused. There are many oils that should be avoided during pregnancy, although some may be used in labour. There is no direct human evidence that essential oils cause problems in pregnancy, but animal research suggests the possibility of teratogenicity, mutagenicity, poor ovum implantation and spontaneous abortion (Delgado et al 1993a, b, Nogueira et al 1995, Toaff et al 1979), although other authorities dispute these effects (Pages et al 1990, Tisserand & Balacs 1995). Essential oils have been associated with inducing abortions when these were not medically available, but Balacs (1992) states that those traditionally used for this purpose, such as pennyroyal, are totally contraindicated in clinical aromatherapy. In any case, their toxicity is more likely to be attributed to hepatotoxicity and systemic poisoning than to any complications of attempted abortion.

Currently, essential oils are largely *assumed* to be safe for use by pregnant women simply because there is no real evidence to the contrary, but midwives should continue to be cautious when advising expectant mothers about their uses. Other possible side-effects include phototoxicity, especially with the citrus oils (Meyer 1970, Naganuma et al 1985), skin irritation, notably with camomile (McGeorge & Steele 1991, Van Ketel 1987) and tea tree (De Groot & Weyland 1993, Southwell et al 1997), and carcinogenicity (Anthony 1987, Zangouras et al 1981) – although later work seems to contradict this last issue (Bannerjee et al 1994, Zheng et al 1992). Reports of oral toxicity have appeared in the professional press, usually following accidental ingestion and overdose. Gastrointestinal administration is not advocated widely in Britain as it is not yet fully understood how or at what rate the oils are absorbed and indemnity insurance for practitioners is difficult to obtain. Other systemic effects include alterations in the blood pressure, temperature or fluid balance. For a more in-depth exploration of the safety of essential oils in pregnancy, see Tiran (2000).

Uses

Despite the above concerns the use of aromatherapy in midwifery practice is certainly increasing and one of the largest clinical aromatherapy trials has now been completed in the maternity unit at the John Radcliffe Hospital in Oxford (Burns et al 1999). Here more than 8000 mothers, over a 9 year period, were offered a small selection of essential oils for relief of pain and other discomforts in labour. Maternal satisfaction was significant and aromatherapy is now an established part of labour ward care in this unit. The incidence of side-effects was less than 1%, all of which were minor and none of which affected the fetuses or babies. Dale & Cornwell (1994) demonstrated the value of lavender oil for perineal discomfort after episiotomy and some units now offer this to women in the postnatal wards (Tiran 2001).

Aromatherapy, especially when administered via massage, is also useful for helping women to relax and for balancing their mood swings, but has far more to offer than just psychological effects. Specific complaints of pregnancy can be treated with essential oils – for example adding cypress oil to a sitz bath or bidet for haemorrhoids, citrus oils in abdominal massage for constipation or camomile in the bath water to aid sleep. All essential oils are antibacterial and some are also antifungal, antiviral or antimicrobial. Tea tree has gained credibility as an extremely effective combatant to candidal and other infections and is now also being used for people with HIV and for fighting methicillin resistant *Staphylococcus aureus* (MRSA) (Carson & Riley 1994, 1995, Carson et al 1996, Sweet 1997, Williams et al 1998, Zarno 1994).

Aromatherapy is hugely popular amongst the general public and midwives will frequently come into contact with women who have already used essential oils. It is worrying that the oils are so easily accessible to a general public that believes the oils to be harmless but nice-smelling and that the majority of people use them indiscriminately. Although not wishing to alarm or discourage pregnant women from using what can be a relaxing and refreshing adjunct to normal maternity care, midwives should ensure that their knowledge is accurate, up to date, research based and appropriately applied to pregnancy physiology. If the rules of drug administration are related to essential oil administration it will help midwives to consider how they should use the oils or advise women about aromatherapy (Box 49.4).

> **Box 49.4** 'Rules' for the correct administration of essential oils during pregnancy and childbirth*
>
> The correct essential oil should be prescribed and administered:
>
> - to the correct person
> - at the correct time
> - in the correct dose
> - by the correct route
> - in the correct frequency
> - and recorded accurately and contemporaneously in the notes.
>
> The person administering the essential oil must be aware of:
>
> - the uses and effects
> - precautions and contraindications
> - possible complications and side-effects.
>
> * **NB** Midwives are reminded to comply with the parameters laid down by the UKCC (1998) and should not administer essential oils to pregnant and childbearing women unless they are adequately and appropriately trained to do so.

Reflexology

Reflexology, or reflex zone therapy, involves a precise manipulation of the feet, which are thought to represent a map of the whole body. Every part of the body is reflected on one or both feet and therefore by working on specific parts of the feet, other areas of the body can be treated. Reflexology is *not* a foot massage, although it can be extremely relaxing. It is a powerful therapy that can be very effective when used appropriately, although there are some contraindications, precautions and possible complications of treatment. Reflexology can also be performed on the hands, as well as the tongue, face and back. It is widely thought to work along the meridians used in acupuncture, although there are several other theories regarding its mechanism of action (Crane 1997, Lett 2000, Tiran 2002a)

Uses

During pregnancy, reflexology can be effective in relieving physiological discomforts as well as specific complaints, and in labour is invaluable in easing pain. Antenatal conditions that respond particularly well include constipation (Eriksen 1992), headaches and migraine (Lafuente et al 1990, Launso et al 1999), sinus congestion, carpal tunnel syndrome, heartburn, insomnia, stress and anxiety, backache and sciatica (Tiran 1996). The destressing effects of the treatment can reduce hypertension and regulate cardiac function (Frankel 1997), and a case of hypertension in pregnancy treated with reflexology was reported by Yongsheng & Xiaolian (1995). Both postnatal and antenatal retention of urine may respond to reflexology (Tiran 1996), which has also been shown to have an effect on micturition (Eichelberger 1993) and on renal blood flow (Sudmeier et al 1999).

There would appear to be a strong correlation between first trimester nausea and vomiting and a history of neck problems, especially a previous whiplash injury, or lower back problems. By working on the foot zones for the neck and back, the severity of the nausea and sickness can be reduced and women can be enabled to cope with any milder symptoms which persist (Tiran 2002b).

Research by Motha & McGrath (1993) has shown that expectant women who receive regular reflexology during pregnancy experience an easier, less painful labour than might otherwise have been the case. Danish midwives have also long used reflexology as an analgesic during labour (Feder et al 1993). Anecdotal evidence suggests that reflexology can also be effective for induction of labour and at least one trial is currently in progress to evaluate its use for stimulating contractions in women who are postdates. Stimulation of the foot zones corresponding to the pituitary gland can also assist the separation of a physiologically retained placenta. Similarly, lactation can be encouraged by treating these zones. One theory that has been put forward is that when a mother has had an intravenous cannula sited in the back of the hand this can impair lactation, for the back of the hand just below the fingers corresponds to the reflex zone for the breast (Lett 2000).

Conclusion

It can be seen that there is a wide variety of different complementary and alternative therapies, many of which can be applied to the care of pregnant and childbearing women. Some could be incorporated into midwifery practice relatively easily; this would have the advantage of the therapies being used alongside conventional care and would avoid the fragmentation that might result from the therapies being administered by an independent practitioner. A complementary therapy specialism within midwifery is advocated (Tiran 1995) so that every maternity department in the country has access to a complementary therapy midwife, for it is not feasible for each individual midwife to have sufficient comprehensive and contemporary knowledge of the subject. Midwifery has become such a diverse profession with many different specialisms that complementary medicine should be considered as another area of expertise within it. Many of the issues pertinent to using CAM therapies for pregnant women are different from using them for people who are ill, and midwives must take account of these and the steps necessary to address them. The benefits of complementary medicine for expectant, labouring and newly delivered mothers are such that midwives must also acknowledge that women wish to use natural remedies and it is far preferable that accurate advice or treatment (or both) is offered by the health care professionals already caring for them. Complementary medicine is becoming even more integrated into existing conventional care and is having both direct and indirect effects on general health care provision; it is definitely here to stay.

REFERENCES

Al-Sadi M, Newman B, Julious S A 1997 Acupuncture in the prevention of postoperative nausea and vomiting. Anaesthesia 52:658–661.

Anthony P 1987 Metabolism of estragole in rat and mouse and influence of dose size on excretion of the proximate carcinogen l-hydroxy-estragole. Food and Chemical Toxicology 25:799–806, cited by Tisserand R, Balacs T 1995 Essential oil safety: a guide for health professionals. Churchill Livingstone, London, p 120

Balacs 1992 Safety in pregnancy. International Journal of Aromatherapy 4(1):12–15

Bannerjee S, Sharma R, Kale R K, Rao A R 1994 Influence of certain essential oils on carcinogen-metabolising enzymes and acid-sulphydryls in mouse liver. Nutrition and Cancer 21(3):1679–1691

Belluomini J et al 1993 Acupressure for nausea and vomiting of pregnancy: a randomized blinded study. Obstetrics and Gynecology 84:245

British Medical Association 1986 Alternative therapy: report of the Board of Education. BMA, London

British Medical Association 1993 Complementary medicine: new approaches to good practice. Oxford University Press, Oxford

Burns E, Blamey C, Errser S, Lloyd A J, Barnetson L 1999 The use of aromatherapy in intrapartum midwifery practice: an evaluative study. OCHRAD, Oxford

Cardini F, Weixin H 1998 Moxibustion for correction of breech presentation: a randomized controlled trial. Journal of the American Medical Association 280(18):1580–1584

Cardini F, Basevi V, Valentini A, Martellato A 1991 Moxibustion and breech presentation: preliminary results. American Journal of Chinese Medicine XIX(2):105

Carson C F, Riley T V 1994 Susceptibility of Propionibacterium acnes to the essential oil of Melaleuca alternifolia. Letters in Applied Microbiology 19(1):24–25

Carson C F, Riley T V 1995 Antimicrobial activity of the major components of the essential oil of Melaleuca alternifolia. Journal of Applied Bacteriology 78(3): 264–269

Carson C F, Hammer K A, Riley T V 1996 In vitro activity of the essential oil of Melaleuca alternifolia against Streptococcus spp. Journal of Antimicrobial Chemotherapy 37(6):1177–1181

Chiropractors Act 1994 HMSO, London

Cooperative Research Group of Moxibustion Version of Jangxi Province 1984 Clinical observation on the effects of version by moxibustion. Abstracts from the second national symposium of acupuncture and moxibustion and acupuncture anaesthesia, Beijing, China. All China Society of Acupuncture and Moxibustion, Beijing, p 150

Crane B 1997 Reflexology – the definitive practitioners' manual. Churchill Livingstone, London

Dale A, Cornwell S 1994 The role of lavender oil in relieving perineal discomfort following childbirth; a blind randomized clinical trial. Journal of Advanced Nursing 19(1):89–96

Daly J M, Frame S P, Rapoza P A 1991 Sacroiliac subluxation: a common, treatable cause of low back pain in pregnancy. Journal of Manipulative and Physiological Therapeutics 13(3):60–65

Darras J C 1974 Acupuncture update – symposium held in New York by National Acupuncture Research Society, October

De Groot A C, Weyland J W 1993 Contact allergy to tea tree oil. Contact Dermatitis 28(2):309

Delgado I F, Carvalho S H P, Nogueira A C M et al 1993a Study on the embryo-fetotoxicity of beta-myrcene in the rat. Food and Chemical Toxicology 31(1):31–35

Delgado I F, de Almeida G, Nogueira A C M, Souza C A M, Costa A M N, Figueiredo L H 1993b Peri- and postnatal developmental toxicity of beta-myrcene in the rat. Food and Chemical Toxicology 31(9):623–628

Diakow R P, Gadsby T A, Gadsby J B, Gleddie J G, Leprich D J, Scales A M 1991 Back pain during pregnancy and labour. Journal of Manipulative and Physiological Therapeutics 14(2):116–118

DoH (Department of Health) 1993 Changing childbirth. Report of the Expert Maternity Group. HMSO, London

DoH (Department of Health) 2000 Complementary medicine information pack for primary care clinicians. DoH, London

Dundee J, Yang J 1990 Prolongation of the anti-emetic action of P6 acupuncture by acupressure in patients having cancer chemotherapy. Journal of the Royal Society of Medicine 83:360–362

Dundee J, Sourial F, Ghaly R, Bell P 1988 Acupressure reduces morning sickness. Journal of the Royal Society of Medicine 81:456

Dundee J, Ghaly R, Fitzpatrick K et al 1989 Acupuncture prophylaxis of cancer chemotherapy-induced sickness. Journal of the Royal Society of Medicine 82:268

Dundee J, McMillan C M 1991 Positive evidence of P6 acupuncture anti-emesis. Postgraduate Medical Journal 67:417–422

Eichelberger G 1993 Study on foot reflex zone massage: alternative to tablets. (German) Krankenpflege – Soins Infirmiers 86:61–63

Eriksen L 1992 Zoneterepi mod kronisk forstoppelse (zone therapy in chronic constipation). Sygeplejersken 92(26):7

Ernst E, Pittler M H 1998 Efficacy of homeopathic arnica – a systematic review of placebo-controlled trials. Archives of Surgery 133(11):1187–1190

Evans A T et al 1993 Suppression of pregnancy-induced nausea and vomiting with sensory afferent stimulation. Journal of Reproductive Medicine 38(8):603–606

Fallon J 1993 Orthopaedic and neurological conditions of pregnancy and the chiropractic management of care. International Chiropractors Association International Review of Chiropractic: 25–30

Feder E, Liisberg G B, Lenstrup C et al 1993 Zone therapy in relation to birth. In: Proceedings of the International Confederation of Midwives 23rd International Congress, Vancouver, Canada, vol 2, p 651–656

FIM (Foundation for Integrated Medicine) 1997 Integrated healthcare: a way forward for the next five years? FIM, London

Frankel B S M 1997 The effect of reflexology on baroreceptor reflex sensitivity, blood pressure and sinus arrhythmia. Complementary Therapies in Medicine 5:80–84

Harrison D E, Harrison D D, Troyanovich S J 1997 The sacroiliac joint: a review of anatomy and biomechanics with clinical implications. Journal of Manipulative and Physiological Therapeutics 20(9):607–617

Hart O, Mullee M A, Lewith G, Miller J 1997 Double-blind placebo-controlled randomized clinical trial of homeopathic arnica 30C for pain and infection after total abdominal hysterectomy. Journal of the Royal Society of Medicine 90(2):73–78

Hayden E C 2000 Osteopathy for children, 3rd edn. Self-published, Gloucester

House of Lords Select Committee on Science and Technology 2000 Report of the sixth committee on complementary and alternative medicine. HMSO, London

Kubista E, Kucera H, Muller-Tyl B 1975 Initiating contractions of the gravid uterus through electroacupuncture. American Journal of Chinese Medicine 3(4):343

Lafuente A, Noguera M, Puy C, Molins A, Titus F, Sanz F 1990 Effekt der Reflexonbehandlung am Fuss bezuglich der prophylaktischen Behandlung mit Flunarizin bei an Cephalea Kopfschmerzen leidenen Patienten. Erfahrungsheilkunde 11:713–715

Launso L, Brendstrup E, Arnberg S 1999 An exploratory study of reflexological treatment for headache. Alternative Therapies in Health and Medicine 5(3):57–65

Ledergerber C P 1976 Electroacupuncture in obstetrics. Acupuncture and Electrotherapeutics Research 2:105

Lett A 2000 Reflex zone therapy for health professionals. Harcourt London

Linde K, Clausius N, Ramirez G et al 1997 Are the clinical trials of homeopathy placebo effects? A meta-analysis of placebo controlled trials. Lancet 350(9081):834–843

McGeorge B S, Steele M C 1991 Allergic contact dermatitis of the nipple from Roman chamomile ointment. Contact Dermatitis 24(2):139–140

McMillan C 1994 Transcutaneous electrical nerve stimulation of Neiguan antiemetic acupuncture points in controlling sickness following opioid analgesia in major orthopaedic surgery. Physiotherapy 80(1):5–9

Martoudis S, Christofides K 1990 Electroacupuncture for pain relief in labour. Acupuncture in Medicine 8(2):51

Melzack R, Belanger E 1989 Labour pain: correlation with menstrual pain and acute low back pain before and after pregnancy. Pain 36:225–229

Melzack R, Schaffelberg D 1987 Low back pain during labour. American Journal of Obstetrics and Gynecology 156(4):901–905

Meyer J 1970 Accidents due to tanning cosmetics with a base of bergamot oil. Bulletin de la Societe Francaise de dermatologie et de Syphiligraphie 77(6):881–884

Motha G, McGrath J 1993 The effects of reflexology on labour outcome. Report of the Association of Reflexologists, London

Naganuma M, Hirose S, Nakayama Y et al 1985 A study of the phototoxicity of lemon oil. Archives of Dermatological Research 278(1):31–36

Nathan P J 1999 The experimental and clinical pharmacology of St John's wort (Hypericum perforatum L). Molecular Psychiatry 4(4):333–338

NHS Confederation 1997 Complementary medicine in the NHS: managing the issues. NHS Confederation, Birmingham

Nogueira A C, Carvalho R R, Souza C A M, Chahoud I, Paumgartten F J R I 1995 Study on the embryofetotoxicity of citral in the rat. Toxicology 96(2):105–113

Nursing and Midwifery Council (NMC) 2002 Code of professional conduct. NMC, London

Ondrizek R R, Chan P J, Patton W C, King A 1999a An alternative medicine study of herbal effects on the penetration of zone-free hamster oocytes and the integrity of sperm deoxyribonucleic acid. Fertility and Sterility 71(3):517–522

Ondrizek R R, Chan P J, Patton W C, King A 1999b Inhibition of human sperm motility by specific herbs used in alternative medicine. Journal of Assisted Reproduction and Genetics 16(2):87–91

Osteopaths Act 1993 HMSO, London

Pages N, Fournier G, Le Luyer F, Marques MC 1990 Essential oils and their potential teratogenic properties: the case of *Eucalyptus globulus* essential oil – preliminary study on mice. Plantes Medicinales et Phytotherapie 24(1):21–26

Parsons M, Simpson M, Ponton T 1999 Raspberry leaf and its effect on labour: safety and efficacy. Journal of the Australian College of Midwives 12(3):20–25

Perera W 1979 Acupuncture in childbirth. British Journal of Acupuncture 2(1):12

Perko S J 1997 Homeopathy for the modern pregnant woman and her infant. Benchmark Homeopathic Publications, San Antonio, Texas, USA

Schwartz Z, Katz Z, Lancet M 1985 Management of puerperal separation of the symphysis pubis. International Journal of Gynaecology and Obstetrics 23:125–128

Simpson M, Parsons M, Greenwood J, Wade K 2001 Raspberry leaf in pregnancy: its safety and efficacy in labour. Journal of Midwifery and Women's Health 46(2):51–59

Singer A, Wonnemann M, Muller W E 1999 Hyperforin, a major antidepressant constituent of St John's wort, inhibits serotonin uptake by elevating free intracellular Na^+. Journal of Pharmacology and Experimental Therapeutics 290(3):1363–1368

Skelton I 1988 Acupuncture and labour – summary of results. Midwives' Chronicle and Nursing Notes, May:134

Southwell I A, Markham C, Mann C 1997 Skin irritancy of tea tree oil. Journal of Essential Oil Research 9:47–52

Stern P J, O'Connor S M, Silvano A M 1993 Symphysis pubis diastasis: a complication of pregnancy. Journal of Neuro-musculo-skeletal System 1(2):74–78

Stone J 1999 Using complementary therapies within nursing: some ethical considerations. Complementary Therapies in Nursing and Midwifery 5:46–50

Sudmeier I, Bodner G, Egger I, Mur I, Ulmer H, Herold M 1999 Changes of renal blood flow during organ-associated reflexology measured by colour Doppler sonography. Forschende Komplementarmedizin 6(3):129–134

Sutton J, Scott P 1997 Understanding and teaching optimum fetal positioning seminar. Birth Concepts, Tauranga, New Zealand

Sweet M 1997 Alarm in hospitals over rapid spread of a nasty germ they can't destroy. Sydney Morning Herald 15 March

The Nursing and Midwifery Order 2001. HMSO, London

Tiran D 1995 Complementary therapies education in midwifery. Complementary Therapies in Nursing and Midwifery 1:41–44

Tiran D 1996 The use of complementary therapies in midwifery practice: a focus on reflexology. Complementary Therapies in Nursing and Midwifery 2:32–37

Tiran D 1999a A holistic framework for maternity care. Complementary Therapies in Nursing and Midwifery 5:127–135

Tiran D 1999b Complementing your care: about the special interest groups Part 2 – Complementary therapies in maternity care national forum. Complementary Therapies in Nursing and Midwifery 5(3):85–86

Tiran D 2000 Clinical aromatherapy for pregnancy and childbirth, 2nd edn. Churchill Livingstone, London

Tiran D 2001 Complementary strategies for antenatal care. Complementary Therapies in Nursing and Midwifery 7:19–24

Tiran D 2002a Reviewing theories and origins. In: Mackereth P, Tiran D (eds) 2002 Clinical reflexology: a guide for health professionals. Elsevier, London

Tiran D 2002b Supporting women during pregnancy and childbirth. In: Mackereth P, Tiran D (eds) Clinical reflexology: a guide for health professionals. Elsevier, London

Tisserand R, Balacs T 1995 Essential oil safety: a guide for health professionals. Churchill Livingstone, London

Toaff M E, Abramovici A, Sporn J, Liban E 1979 Selective oocyte degeneration and impaired fertility in rats treated with the aliphatic monoterpene Citral. Journal of Reproduction and Fertility 55:347–352

UKCC (United Kingdom Central Council for Nursing, Midwifery and Health Visiting) 2000 Guidelines for the administration of Medicines. UKCC, London

UKCC (United Kingdom Central Council for Nursing, Midwifery and Health Visiting) 1992 Scope of professional practice. UKCC, London

Van Ketel W G 1987 Allergy to *Matricaria chamomilla*. Contact Dermatitis 8(2):143

Vickers A J, Fisher P, Smith C, Wyllie S E, Rees R 1998 Homeopathic arnica 30X is ineffective for muscle soreness after long distance running: a randomized double blind placebo controlled trial. Clinical Journal of Pain 14(3):227–231

Williams L R, Stockley J K, Yan W, Home V N 1998 Essential oils with high antimicrobial activity for therapeutic use. International Journal of Aromatherapy 8(4):30–40

Ying Y, Lin J, Robins J 1985 Acupuncture for the induction of cervical dilatation in preparation for first trimester abortion and its influence on HCG. Journal of Reproductive Medicine 30(7):530

Yip S, Pang J, Sung M 1976 Induction of labour by acupuncture electrostimulation. American Journal of Chinese Medicine 493:257

Yongsheng Xu, Xiaolian S 1995 Hypertension of pregnancy treated with foot reflexology: a case report. China Reflexology Symposium Report, Ankang City, Shoanxi Province, p 68

Zangouras A et al 1981 Dose-dependent conversion of estragole in the rat and mouse to the carcinogenic metabolite 1'-hydroxyestragole. Biochemical Pharmacology 30:1383–1386

Zarno V 1994 Candidiasis. International Journal of Aromatherapy 6(2):20–23

Zheng G, Kenney P M, Lam L K T 1992 Inhibition of benzo(a)pyrene-induced tumorigenesis by myristicin, a volatile aroma constituent of parsley leaf oil. Carcinogenesis 13(10):1921–1923

FURTHER READING

Geraghty B 1997 Homeopathy for midwives. Churchill Livingstone, Edinburgh

An introduction to homeopathy that can be used as a quick reference for midwives with some understanding of the principles of the therapy.

Mackereth P, Tiran D (eds) 2002 Clinical reflexology: a guide for health professionals. Churchill Livingstone, Edinburgh

Explores some of the issues of current debate relating to the use of reflexology being integrated into mainstream health care; includes chapters on specific clinical specialities including maternity care.

Tiran D 2000 Clinical aromatherapy for pregnancy and childbirth. 2nd edn. Churchill Livingstone, Edinburgh

An updated, comprehensive, research-based review of the principles and practice of using essential oils, specifically related to the care of pregnant and childbearing women.

Tiran D 2001 Natural remedies for morning sickness and other pregnancy problems. Quadrille, London

Easy-to-read exploration of using complementary and alternative remedies, aimed at pregnant and childbearing women

Tiran D 2003 Nausea and vomiting in pregnancy: an integrated approach to care. Churchill Livingstone, Edinburgh

An in-depth exploration of the evidence for the care of women with gestational sickness, from both a conventional and various complementary approaches, culminating in a debate on integrating the two approaches for the benefit of the mother.

Tiran D, Mack S (eds) 2000 Complementary therapies for pregnancy and childbirth, 2nd edn. Baillière Tindall, London

Comprehensive introduction to the subject with chapters on the main therapies in use today, written either by midwives actively using the therapy within midwifery or by practitioners who specialise in treating pregnant and childbearing women.

West Z 2000 Acupuncture in pregnancy and childbirth. Churchill Livingstone, Edinburgh

Application of acupuncture principles aimed at complementary practitioners, but useful for midwives with a knowledge of acupuncture

USEFUL ADDRESS

Complementary Maternity Forum
c/o Denise Tiran (Chair) School of Health
University of Greenwich, Mansion Site, Avery Hill
Campus
Bexley Road, Eltham
London SE9 2UG
Tel 020 8331 8494

50 Community, Public Health and Social Services

Chris McCourt

CHAPTER CONTENTS

A midwife needs knowledge of community health and social services for three main reasons: to appreciate better the social context of health and how this impinges on her or his role; to be able to advise a woman appropriately about other services that may be helpful for her, and to refer appropriately to other services when her input would be beneficial.

The chapter aims to:

- discuss community health and social services in the context of a broad theoretical understanding of health and illness

- provide information that will be useful for midwives in key areas of these services

- discuss the principles, structures, policies and practices that influence the character of each

- discuss the role of the midwife in public health and health promotion

- provide a framework for continuing learning, updating of relevant information and developing local knowledge and networks.

Introduction

The factors influencing the health of mothers and children are broad and complex. Their impact begins long before pregnancy and will continue long after a woman's discharge from the maternity services. Community health and social services, therefore, play an important role in the cycles of family life in many societies. Social services, community- and hospital-based health services have been through several phases of integration and separation in the UK since their establishment in the early part of the twentieth century. Currently, they are provided under quite separate institutional arrangements but much of recent health policy has focused on developing more 'seamless' and community-based models for providing care. To some extent, these policy changes and the structures described in this chapter are products of our tendency to view health within a narrow and mechanistic framework. In consequence, health, social and other personal services, hospital- and community-based services are categorised separately, so that effort is then needed to piece them back together. The boundaries in many of the issues discussed in this chapter are fuzzy and should be so, since that is the way health and illness are influenced and experienced by people, as part of their lives.

The importance of viewing maternal and child health in its social context

It is a common but misplaced assumption that it is provision of health care that is mainly responsible for our health. Evidence from a range of research disciplines, including epidemiology, social science and natural sciences, indicates that health should be viewed much more as an ecological concept; it is a product of many factors, including living environment and conditions, nutrition, occupation and education, and is profoundly influenced by maternal health. The health of mothers receiving maternity care, and of their babies, is most likely to be influenced by such issues as their nutritional status, their housing and working conditions and the level of social support they can call on. This means that the role of maternity services is additional and relatively short term. Midwives cannot change many of these issues but must work with them and may often be involved in assisting the woman in ameliorating or coping with the effects of social and economic circumstances on her health.

The importance of the social context on women's health is reflected particularly clearly in the different social class patterns of health (Acheson 1998, Townsend et al 1988). A key example of this is birthweight; this is a useful indicator, since it is readily measurable, and is an important predictor of future health status (Oakley 1992). Although it may at first sight seem to be an indisputably physiological matter, research shows that low birthweight is strongly associated with poverty, inequality and lack of social support. The physical health of the mother will have been influenced by similar factors, which have a very long term effect. Birthweight is a good example of the multifaceted nature of health as well as the importance of social context on health (Barker 1998, Richards et al 2001, Roberts 1997).

What is meant by community?

'Community' is a very broad term that is currently widely used in policy developments in Euro-American societies. It is attractive partly because of its rather open definition that can encompass a range of ideas. Generally, community is identified along three dimensions: place, relationships and sentiment or sense of belonging (Turton & Orr 1993). All contribute something to the concept, but the degree of importance attached to each is variable. When discussing health and social services, these aspects of community are all relevant, but community tends to be defined by service providers very much in service terms (i.e. the location of a service, the way in which it is delivered and its scale). Popular images of community care often take it to mean care provided at home, rather than in an institution of some type, and provided by family, friends or neighbours rather than professionals or paid workers. To clarify these different concepts of community care – with very different implications for social policy – Bulmer (1987) drew a distinction between care 'in' the community and care 'by' the community, mostly care provided unpaid by friends, kin or neighbours, which is also referred to by service providers as 'informal' care.

The different areas of health services

Historically, the role of medicine has in many respects been peripheral to the concerns of public health, since it is mainly responsive to disease and concerned with the diagnosis and treatment of ill health (McKeown 1979, Stacey 1988). This is reflected in the separation of different health-related activities into the institutional spheres of social services, hospital services and community (or primary) health services. Before the health service reorganisation of 1974 in the UK, domiciliary midwives were employed by local authorities, whereas hospital midwives were employed by health authorities (Robinson 1990). Until this point, domiciliary or community midwives were in closer contact with the Medical Officer of Health, who was responsible for public health in a local area, since community health and social services were combined.

Maternity care, and particularly midwifery, occupies a different role from much of conventional health care, since childbirth is an important life event and transition and pregnant women are generally understood to be healthy people, requiring care and observation for possible problems, rather than curative treatment. Nevertheless, in the latter half of the twentieth century, maternity services in the UK and other industrialised countries were organised increasingly along the lines of acute medical services, based mainly in hospitals, with women routinely referred to them by their GPs (Hunt & Symonds 1995). Women were generally categorised into those deemed high or low risk on an agreed set of medical indicators. Care for women classified as of 'low risk' was then in many cases referred back to community health services – the GP and midwife – for shared care. Midwives have been divided along similar lines into those working in hospitals and those working mainly in the community. The latter have tended in recent years in the UK to provide mainly antenatal and postnatal care, while also caring for the small proportion of home and 'domino' births (meaning *domiciliary in and out* – a community-based midwife accompanies the woman to hospital once in labour and home again about 6 hours following birth).

Following the 'Changing Childbirth' report (DoH 1993), a number of services in the UK have moved towards greater integration of community- and hospital-based midwifery, for example through caseload practice (Flint 1993, Page 1995) or community-based group practice (Sandall et al 2001). Additionally, during the 1990s, UK government attempts to shift appropriate areas of health care back into a community base

led to a renewed emphasis on primary care (DoH 1997a, 1997b, see also Ch. 3).

The structure and role of community health and social services

As indicated in the introduction to this chapter, the structure of these services has been subject to a number of policy changes and varies from one country to another. The structure of the health service is described in more detail in Chapter 53.

The origins of the current system in the UK

Prior to 1946 in the UK, health and social services were largely privately paid for or charitable. The Poor Law had been the main instrument for caring for people who were disabled, chronically ill or destitute, and its operation had become punitive over time in order to discourage people from claiming relief. The nineteenth century, with rapid industrialisation and urbanisation, saw the growth of hospitals as places to provide health care, but it was not until the twentieth century that hospitals came to be seen as a desirable option in care for women giving birth (Donnison 1988). The foundations of the current welfare and health system were set down in the years following the Second World War and were in many ways responding to the enormous social changes taking place at that time. The NHS Act 1946 created the National Health Service, with free health care provided according to need, while the National Assistance Act 1948 replaced the Poor Law with a system of means-tested welfare benefits and a duty for local authorities to provide residential care for those in need. At this point, the emphasis was very much on creating the institutional structures for welfare; relatively little attention was given to community-based services – that is, supports to people living in their own homes (Clements 1996).

Health services

Between 1974 and 1993 in the UK, health authorities were the main providers of health services, incorporating hospitals and some community services such as community midwifery. After the NHS and Community

Care Act 1990, their role became mainly one of planning and contracting for care on behalf of the local population, although they maintained responsibility for direct provision of some services, especially those based in community settings. Hospitals, and some community-based services such as those for people with long term care needs, developed NHS Trust status, working independently within the health service and, in theory at least, competing with other service providers.

Following the 1997 government White Paper, 'The new NHS, modern, dependable' (DoH 1997a), this system was reformed again to remove the concept of an internal health care market and to devolve organisation of care as far as possible to a community level. The new policy introduced Primary Care Groups – involving all GPs and, to a lesser extent, 'community nurses' – to commission services for their local population on behalf of the local health authority (Carnell & Kline 1999, DoH 1997a). These groups were expected to develop into Primary Care Trusts, commissioning and providing services for their local community. The concept of competition, introduced in 1990, was replaced with that of cooperation: between different professions, between local and regional levels, between primary and secondary care and between the health service and other agencies. In the new structure, with an emphasis on the Primary Care Groups and Trusts planning and providing community health services, different professionals were expected to work increasingly as a community health team, although their employment conditions remained the same.

Local authorities

Local authorities have a key role in planning, monitoring and developing services for the needs of the local community in a range of departments, including education, social services, housing and environmental services. As we have seen, all these areas have an influence on health, giving the local authority a potentially powerful role in enhancing the health and welfare of its population. In practice, the different departments have not always worked together effectively in a health-promoting role, partly because the health implications of such public services have been under-recognised. Following the NHS and Community Care Act 1990, these authorities, like health authorities,

were given a more strategic role in planning services for local needs and purchasing these from independent service providers as well as continuing to provide them where appropriate. Knowledge of local authority social services is the most relevant for midwives, since social services departments have legal duties to assess people's needs for support in the community and to provide or arrange for services which are assessed as being needed. The local authority social services are responsible for assessing the overall community health and care needs of its population and producing regular community care plans. They also take a lead role in child protection issues.

New structures for collaboration across community health and social services

During the late 1990s in the UK, government policy showed increasing recognition of research exploring the complex links between social conditions and health and the need for broad social policies to tackle these. Critical research on health education indicated that attempts to change individual knowledge and behaviour were ineffective without attention to the context of people's lives. This was reflected in the publication of a health promotion strategy, 'Our healthier nation' (DoH 1998) and in new policy schemes such as Sure Start (www.surestart.gov.uk) and the New Deal for Communities (www.regeneration.dtlr.gov.uk).

The Sure Start scheme is particularly relevant for midwives, since it focuses on the importance of the early years and maternal and infant health for future health, development and well-being. A number of projects were developed in areas of social and economic deprivation. Their aim is to improve the health and well-being of families and children, from before birth to 4 years of age. Sure Start projects work with all families with young children but focus particularly on supporting socially disadvantaged families, with the intention of 'breaking the cycle of disadvantage' in the important early years of development. Examples of Sure Start schemes include family support, nutritional advice, play facilities and provision of health care assistants in the community to support new parents (see Box 50.1 below, also Carnell & Cline 1999).

Schemes such as the New Deal for Communities are more broadly based regeneration schemes applied to areas with high levels of, often multiple, disadvantages and low levels of 'social capital': informal and other social resources for communities to build on. Following the lessons of earlier attempts to ameliorate the negative effects of poverty with single measures, these projects integrated areas such as health, housing, employment, leisure, child care, education and nutrition or food access schemes – all areas of disadvantage that tend to have a cumulative or 'spiral' effect.

The midwife's role in relation to community health and social services

Since midwives have expertise in the care of normal pregnancy and birth, they are in a good position to provide general care and support to the woman during a period of great personal and social adjustment as well as physical change. In addition to clinical skills, midwives provide information and advice and, in many cases, social support. Such a role has the potential to provide a positive impact on the general health and well-being of women and their families during a period of change and development. Midwifery care is relatively short term, and arrangements for care do not always facilitate continuity of carer, but interventions during certain critical periods may have a long term impact, however small. A good example of this is the midwife's role in health promotion and in supporting women in feeding their babies (Crafter 1997).

When a woman needs more general sources of advice and social support than those provided through the maternity services, midwives may still play a key role in providing relevant information and advice and in referring her to other professionals and organisations for support. This role is underpinned by:

- developing and updating broad health knowledge
- developing local community knowledge and contacts
- reflection and awareness of one's own impact as a practitioner.

Public health role of midwives

Recent UK government policy has recognised the difficulties caused in practice by the institutional split between health and social and community services and advocated returning maternity services towards a more seamless model of care. The Standing Nursing and Midwifery Advisory Committee (for England and Wales, with similar committee reports for Scotland and Northern Ireland) in 1998 advised a stronger public health role for the midwife, through changing the organisation of care and expanding or reviewing the scope of the midwife's roles and responsibilities. Although it did not set out the precise nature of this expanded role, or how it would be achieved, it recommended more integrated models of care, with midwives working across hospital and community service boundaries, for example, with personal or group practice caseloads. The report also advocated a stronger public health role, in collaboration with other primary care practitioners, with an increased focus on working with all women on health promotion and in services to provide additional support to socially disadvantaged women (DoH/SNMAC 1998).

The health promotion role advocated for midwives was particularly through health education for women and through focusing care on women with particular needs for support arising from problems such as domestic violence or substance abuse, which can negatively affect the long term health of mothers and children. This emphasis on health promotion was reflected in the policy document 'Making a difference' (DoH 1999a). This report proposed that maternity services increase integrated care and health promotion work, with midwives working across traditional boundaries, collaborating with other primary care practitioners and taking on expanded roles to support women's health.

Although much of midwives' work is primary, preventive health care, there has been little involvement of midwifery in the new focus on primary health services. Midwives clearly could and should have the important role in public health that is now advocated by government policy. It is unclear how this role will develop in the UK, although there are a number of local projects developing more integrated public-health-focused roles. While health visitors and midwives have tended to work separately in recent years, one following on from the other, such community projects and the proposals for extended public health roles for midwives may involve them in more collaborative ways of working together. One such example is given in Box 50.1.

Box 50.1 Sure Start scheme to support new mothers

Midwives working in West London have teamed up with a local Sure Start programme to develop ways of promoting maternal and infant health. The Coningham Sure Start programme, for example, is pioneering a scheme to increase breastfeeding and reduce smoking in new mothers by providing hands-on support from a health care assistant. The health care assistant works closely with midwives and health visitors, visiting women at home and running groups, on a long term basis, from pregnancy to the months following birth. Developing the project has brought together midwives who work with a personal caseload of women in a socially deprived area and health visitors who work with a strong public health focus as part of the Sure Start team. Previously contact was limited, despite the overlap of roles and interests in promoting the health of mothers and babies, due to the handover of care at about 10–28 days following birth, and by working for different organisations. Community-based schemes like this one, with midwives able to follow women across traditional boundaries such as hospital–community or high–low risk and to plan and provide care around their needs, may be one basis for midwives to develop the more health-promoting focus that has always been seen as an ideal.

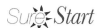

The aim of Sure Start is:

To work with parents-to-be, parents and children to promote the physical, intellectual and social development of babies and young children – particularly those who are disadvantaged – so that they can flourish at home and when they get to school, and thereby break the cycle of disadvantage for the current generation of young children.

The legal framework

Community health and social services operate within a legal framework (Acts of Parliament) set out by government. Local and health authorities are provided with guidance to follow in interpreting and implementing the legislation. Guidance is normally mandatory, for example Executive Letters issued by the Department of Health, whereas guidelines are advisory (e.g. good practice guides), to assist with the complexities of putting policy into practice. UK legislation also operates within the framework of European (EU) legislation and policy directives and is increasingly expected to develop in line with this framework.

Relevant legislation

The main relevant legislation in the UK at the time of writing is shown in Box 50.2. The central pieces of legislation for practitioners in the UK are the NHS and Community Care Act 1990 – which set out a general framework for health and social services – and the NHS (Primary Care) Act 1997, which amended this, replacing competition with collaboration and increasing further the role of primary care. The key aims were to integrate the different services better and to improve organisation of services for people with care needs, particularly since many services are now community based. Many health problems have long term consequences and needs for support are not easily divided into health and social care needs. This was reflected in the 2001 review of the NHS, which proposed a departmental structure that combined health and social care.

Care management

Under the 1990 NHS and Community Care Act, anyone who comes to the attention of the local authority as having possible needs for support is entitled to an assessment followed, where appropriate, by a plan for care, which may include a 'package' of services. This approach is referred to as 'care management'. The principle of care assessment is that the needs of the person should be central and services should be sought to respond to these needs, rather than fitting people into the services. A midwife can request or assist a woman or family with care needs in requesting a care assessment. The needs for support – and the possible solutions – can be quite wide ranging, including 'home help' and additional child care. Assessment should involve the woman, her family where appropriate, and all relevant professionals, who may include the community midwife. If she, or her

> **Box 50.2** The legal framework for community health and social services

- The NHS and Community Care Act 1990 – which set out the framework for community health and social services and duties of local authorities
- The NHS (Primary Care) Act 1997 – which set out the extended role and shape of primary services
- The Housing Act 1977 – which established local authority housing departments with a duty to provide housing for homeless people in certain circumstances (and as amended by subsequent Housing Acts)
- The Disabled Persons Services, Consultation and Representation Act 1986 – which set out the rights of disabled people to receive assessment for community services
- The Race Relations Act 1976 (and Amendment Act 2000), the Sex Discrimination Act 1975 and the Disability Discrimination Act 1995 – which established rights for people of different ethnic groups and people with disabilities and protection against discrimination based on ethnicity, disability or gender, including pregnancy
- The Children Act 1989 – which replaced the previous confusing array of legislation around the welfare and protection of children
- The Mental Health Act 1983 – which provided a framework for services for people with mental health problems, including community services and the terms under which people in distress can be admitted to hospital or treated without their consent and the rules and procedures for discharge from compulsory admissions.

child, is considered to have care needs, a care manager will be appointed to ensure that adequate and suitable support services are arranged. Care managers are often social workers but they may be other professionals (including home care organisers, community nurses or midwives) according to the nature of the individual's needs.

A time frame for undertaking assessments was not specified, but some cases are responded to as emergencies and services can be provided on this basis while awaiting a proper assessment. It is important to try to anticipate needs (such as a woman needing home help after birth or an infant needing support for physical impairments) well in advance and encourage the woman to make an application. Some services may be charged for on a means-tested basis and there is considerable variation in this according to where people live. Needs for care are not tightly defined because they are meant to be broad, but generally the policy is aimed at people (adults and children) who have physical, sensory or intellectual impairments, chronic health problems or mental health problems, or who care for people with such problems. Pregnant women and those who have recently given birth are included. Those who are providing regular and substantial care for friends or relatives, informal carers, are entitled to a linked assessment of how they are affected by their caring responsibilities (Clements 1996, Dimond 1997).

Maternity rights and benefits

In most countries, women are entitled to a series of benefits and have particular rights during pregnancy and childbirth regarding employment. In EU countries these have increased in recent years. Midwives are in an ideal position to advise women of their general rights and entitlements and to respond in a timely fashion to requests for information on rights and benefits and on where to go for further help.

The Benefits Agency (BA)

The Benefits Agency works at national level on behalf of the UK government's Department of Work and Pensions (formerly the Department of Social Security). It assesses needs for financial support, in line with national legislation, and provides payments, exemption certificates and loans where appropriate. It is responsible for the administration of maternity benefits of various types. Local offices and telephone lines are provided for information and enquiries.

Although the overall framework of rights and benefits is relatively stable, details may change from year to year, so that it is important to stay equipped with up-to-date booklets and leaflets. A checklist of sources of information and advice is important, as is regular renewal of the forms and information leaflets provided by the BA. For these reasons, it is crucial not to rely on a textbook; however, the following section summarises the system of rights and benefits in the UK in operation from May 2000, and is valid as of April 2002.

Maternity rights

Women's rights at work are set out in UK law and in EU directives. Where the two differ, UK law is generally expected to comply with EU directives, unless it provides for greater rights. Maternity rights also operate within the broader framework of employment and discrimination law (IDS 2000). They include employment protection, health and safety, paid time off for health care, rights to maternity and parental leave and rights to return to work (Box 50.3). Detailed but clear and accessible information on maternity rights is available in the following booklets and guidelines:

- *DTI URN/1101 Maternity rights*: A guide for employers and employees
- *Maternity Rights PL507 (REV 1)*: A short guide for employers and employees.

These can be mail ordered or downloaded as computer files from the Department for Trade and Industry website: www.dti.gov.uk.

For those with computer access – at home, at work or perhaps through a local library or community centre – the government has set up an interactive website that can be used for general information and more personalised advice: www.tiger.gov.uk. This will be an excellent resource for midwives as well as for pregnant women.

Maternity benefits

These include monetary and non-monetary benefits (benefits in kind or exemptions). The key monetary benefits related to maternity are set out in Box 50.4. The changes in family circumstances due to childbirth may also mean changes in entitlement for families that rely on housing benefit, working families tax credit or income support because of low incomes. Generally, each additional child increases entitlement and may sometimes mean the difference between qualifying for a benefit and not. Since women may

> **Box 50.3** UK maternity and employment rights from 30th April 2000 – key points
>
> **Protection of employment**
>
> A woman with a contract of employment cannot be dismissed from her job for being pregnant or on maternity leave. She maintains general employment rights including protection against discrimination.
>
> **Health and safety**
>
> Employers are responsible for ensuring health and safety at work for women who are pregnant or breastfeeding, or, if not practicable, must provide suitable alternative work or suspension on full pay.
>
> **Leave**
>
> A woman is entitled to paid leave for antenatal health care, including home visits and parent education or preparation classes. An employer may request verification of appointments. All employees are entitled to maternity leave for a minimum of 18 weeks, which can start from the birth or at any time from 29 weeks of pregnancy and a minimum 2 week period is compulsory (4 weeks in factories). Those who have been in continuous employment for a minimum of 1 year (until 29 weeks of pregnancy) are entitled to unpaid extended absence of up to 29 weeks from the week of actual birth. Additionally, either parent may take unpaid parental leave to care for dependants.
>
> **Right to return**
>
> A woman has a right to return to her previous job, on no less favourable terms, provided she complies with limited conditions of notice and returns within the statutory periods of leave. There are some limited exceptions to this rule.

seek advice on any of these benefits, or general advice about coping with new economic demands, it is important to obtain a full set of advice leaflets. Entitlements and benefits are liable to change from one year to another owing to legal and policy changes as well as inflationary increases in benefit levels, so it is important to update all leaflets, and one's own information sources, annually. Detailed information

---

Box 50.4 Monetary maternity benefits in the UK – from 30 April 2000: key points

Statutory Maternity Pay (SMP)

This is payable to women in continuous employment and earning above the statutory limit for National Insurance contributions for 26 weeks before the qualifying week (15 weeks before the expected week of confinement (EWC)). Payment is at a level equivalent to 90% of earnings for 6 weeks followed by 12 weeks at a lower rate, set annually, and can commence at any time from 11 weeks before the EWC, or earlier if the baby has been born. It is administered by employers, who must be given 3 weeks' notice of the intended date for taking leave.

Many employers, especially large organisations, operate more generous schemes than the statutory minimum. The woman should check these terms and whether they apply to her with her employer or personnel department in good time.

Maternity Allowance

This is paid to women not entitled to SMP but who have paid National Insurance contributions during the qualifying period. It is paid weekly for

18 weeks, at a level comparable to the lower rate of SMP. Application must be made on form MA1 accompanied by forms MATB1 and SMP1 (which is issued by the employer) from 26 weeks of pregnancy and before leaving work. Women not entitled to either SMP or MA may be able to claim Incapacity Benefit or Income Support during their leave period.

Surestart Maternity Grants

Women who receive income support, income-based jobseekers allowance, working families or disabled person's tax credit can claim a single payment to assist in the costs of a new baby. The grant is payable from 29 weeks of pregnancy and must be claimed before the baby is 3 months old or within 3 months of adoption.

Child Benefit

All primary carers of children under 16 (or in full-time education until 19) are entitled to Child Benefit. It is payable for each child, with a higher rate for the first child and for lone parents. The Child Benefit claim form must be accompanied by the child's birth certificate.

---

on maternity benefits can be found in the information booklets NI 17A Guide to maternity benefits and BC1 Children and benefits, which are available from local BA offices and most post offices.

Checking entitlements

If in doubt, women should be advised to check their entitlement. Up-to-date details of benefits and entitlements can be obtained by using the local BA office or an independent advice agency. Some local authorities employ welfare rights advisors, who have in-depth knowledge of rights and benefits and who can undertake casework where needed.

Pregnant and childbearing women are also entitled to a range of non-monetary benefits, such as 'welfare foods', some of which are universal (i.e. all are entitled) while others are available only to those who are entitled to income support or family credit. Current provision can be checked with the welfare foods helpline: 0800–056–2665.

Forms and certificates to be supplied by the midwife or GP

Midwives or GPs are responsible for providing the certificates that the woman will need to exercise her employment rights and claim relevant benefits. These include:

- form MATB1: proof of expected date of confinement
- form MATB2: certificate of confinement
- form MA1: for application for statutory maternity pay or maternity allowance
- form FW8: for exemptions from prescription and related charges.

Complete the checklist given in Box 50.5, to help in raising awareness of how to access and update the information a midwife needs for giving advice or referral to specialist advisors, and to function as a ready reminder of where to go for information.

Box 50.5 Advice and information checklist

Benefits Agency helpline

Benefits Agency local office

Citizens' Advice Bureau (local office)

Welfare Rights Officer

Law Centre

Local authority social services/neighbourhood office

Surestart local office

Interpreting or language advice service

Maternity Alliance enquiry line

The community health services

Community health services encompass what is generally known as primary health care, which is based on the GP practice and, increasingly, the Primary Care Group or Trust. They include community-based services for health promotion, such as child health clinics and school health services, and for longer term health needs, such as mental health centres. Since the 1970s, policy has favoured the development of a team approach, with services based in larger GP practices or health centres. Although GP practices may employ professionals such as practice nurses or counsellors, members of primary care teams have tended to practise quite separately, under different employing organisations, and have limited liaison or knowledge of each other's roles (Bowling 1981). The primary care team, therefore, remains an ideal concept in many areas. Despite these difficulties in developing interprofessional care, the philosophy relates closely to the reality of health needs, which do not fit easily into professional or organisational categories. This was acknowledged in the 1997 Government White Paper that introduced Primary Care Groups and Trusts (DoH 1997a).

The GP and the GP practice

In the UK, GPs provide much of the everyday health care for families and act as the key gatekeepers for secondary health care. GPs are independent professionals, who contracted into the health service after its inception in 1946, while maintaining much of their independent status. They receive a fee from their local health authority based on the number of patients on their list, plus some allowances for ancillary work and for particular areas of work such as health screening, maternity care and contraceptive services. Although their fee structure reflects recent health service emphasis on improving preventive health care, the fact that additional fees are received suggests that, historically, this has not been seen as a core part of their work. This structure is likely to change with the advent of Primary Care Trusts and more emphasis on designing services around the needs of the local population (DoH 1997a & b; see also Ch. 53).

GPs and maternity care

In the early part of the twentieth century GPs had little involvement in maternity care, since birth was largely managed by midwives and regular antenatal care was not established. Many women could not afford a doctor's fees and some doctors, in any case, had arrangements with local midwives, delegating care for uncomplicated births (Leap 1993, Robinson 1990). After increasing in importance during the century, the role of GPs in childbirth in particular declined from the 1970s, so that GPs now express concern about losing their skills in maternity care. The Peel report (MoH 1970) and the Short report (House of Commons 1980) advocated a shift of all maternity services to consultant-led hospital units and the closure of small GP-led units or cottage hospitals, despite lack of research evidence that they were less safe (Tew 1990). Much of current maternity care is offered as 'shared care' – shared between the consultant and the GP – but communication between obstetricians and GPs tends to be nominal in this system and much of the hands-on care, in both locations, is given by midwives. Except where GP units remain, or where a GP has a particular interest in birth, GPs are now mainly involved in antenatal care, which they may share with a practice-linked community midwife, group practice or caseload midwife. The advent of Primary Care Trusts offers an opportunity for GPs and midwives to develop community-based services in partnership.

Health visitors and child health services

Health visitors specialise in health promotion and advice for families with children under 5 years and, sometimes, older people. The health visitor's role can, however, be applied to the positive or preventive health needs of the local community in general. It is distinguished from that of the GP in that it focuses on health education and prevention of ill health rather than responding to illness and so is proactive – looking for health needs – rather than reactive. The health visitor tends to work, therefore, with people who do not define themselves as ill, and who are not actively seeking health care. Four key principles of health visiting were outlined in 1977 and confirmed by the Health Visitor's Association and the Standing Conference on Health Visitor Education in 1992:

- the search for health needs
- stimulation of awareness of health needs
- influence on policies affecting health
- facilitation of health-enhancing activities (Turton & Orr 1993).

According to these principles, health visiting means working with communities and taking political action, in addition to working with individuals and families. In practice, the collective aspects of their role have been less well developed, perhaps because of their origins, or the general tendency for health to be viewed in a narrow sense and for health education to focus on individual behaviour. However, the Sure Start initiative provides a route through which health visitors are increasingly becoming involved in such community-oriented, health promotion work (Cowley 2002).

Health visitors are qualified midwives or nurses who may have approved maternity care training and who undertake further, college-based, training for 12 months, plus 9 weeks of supervised health visitor practice. Health visiting in the UK had its origins in the nineteenth century social reform movement that was a response to the problems of rapid industrialisation, urbanisation and poverty (Robertson 1988). Concerns about public health also led to improvements in general sanitation (especially sewerage and water supply) and housing conditions. The most important moves towards improving public health and decreasing the high mortality due to infectious diseases were, therefore, set in place as a result of careful observation of living conditions, before the precise mechanisms of infection were understood (McKeown 1979). Modern health visitors continue this public health role, but since living conditions for many people have

improved and mortality has declined it has focused increasingly on psychosocial care and on the health effects of inequality as well as the more traditional concepts of public health.

Health visitors visit families to give advice or support and run health clinics, which parents can visit for checks on young children's development and progress, general advice with baby and child care and health and immunisations. In some areas, depending on workload, health visitors visit women during pregnancy to offer health advice and preparation for parenthood, or provide parent education classes jointly with community midwives. They may also play a role in providing preventive support or referral for problems such as postnatal depression.

After a baby's birth, the midwife or another professional present at the birth completes a birth notification form, which notifies the Registrar of births and deaths and triggers the production of a set of child health records. The health visitor undertakes a primary visit at around 10–28 days following the birth (i.e. the point at which local midwifery services discharge most women from their care). The parents are given a child health record book to keep, along with general information about community health services, and are invited to visit the child health clinic regularly.

This broad possible remit of health visitors, including screening, health education and prevention roles for the local population, gives them a less clearly defined professional identity than some other health professionals. Despite the importance of the social context of health, their role has been questioned in recent years (Baker et al 1987). They are increasingly encouraged to work with existing or potential social support networks, rather than to attempt to provide all support themselves or adopt the role of experts. This connects to a wider debate about the nature and effectiveness of health education and promotion programmes. This is reflected in their roles within Sure Start projects, or developing links with wider regeneration projects that reflect a broad health promotion role and a renewed emphasis on tackling the problems of poverty and social exclusion (see Box 50.1, also Cowley 2002). However, like other professionals, health visitors also have to balance potentially conflicting roles of providing support and monitoring or surveillance of families. Such dilemmas are faced most acutely when considering child protection issues.

Health education and preventive health care

While community health services such as health visiting and midwifery aim to focus on preventive health care, they differ from much of the health services that are provided in industrialised countries, which tend to react to ill health and favour acute care in terms of expenditure. They also encounter the basic problems confronting health professionals in attempting to provide health education and preventive care by anticipating or looking for health needs. While advice is often welcomed and valued, particularly during pregnancy and the early days of child care, it may also be viewed by some women as an unwarranted interference in their lives.

Preventive health care has been described as operating on three levels:

- *primary:* before a disease process starts (e.g. immunisation or advice on nutrition)
- *secondary:* to alleviate or arrest disease (e.g. screening, diagnosis and treatment)
- *tertiary:* to limit or alleviate the effects of disease or illness (e.g. rehabilitation).

Health education is relevant at all levels of prevention, but is particularly aimed towards preventing the initial development of ill health. Pregnancy and adaptation to parenthood are important life changes and a time when adults are particularly responsive to information and often seek it out actively. None the less, health education, as traditionally conceived, has the important limitation of tending to focus on individual lifestyles and desired behavioural changes, outside the context of the constraints on people's lives and the ways in which such conditions affect health. For example, the 'Health of the nation' document (DoH 1992a) set out clear priority areas and targets for reduction of morbidity and mortality, but was criticised for its emphasis on altering individuals' behaviour in the absence of structural changes to promote healthy lifestyles or increase individual choices. The following government document 'Our healthier nation' (DoH 1998) responded with a far greater emphasis on the conditions that produce ill health.

Noting this constraint, Crafter (1997) distinguishes health education, which largely involves working with individuals or groups to enhance or change knowledge, with the aim of helping people to make informed and positive health choices, from health promotion, a broader concept that recognises the importance of social and environmental influences on health. To promote positive health, it is increasingly acknowledged that health education must work hand in hand with efforts to change the structural and environmental factors influencing health, either directly or through the choices people feel able to make. Principles for health education are set out internationally by the World Health Organization and these have shifted since the 1980s towards involving individuals and communities in planning and implementing health care. The Ottawa charter, for example, states:

> health promotion works through effective community action in setting priorities, making decisions, planning strategies and implementing them to achieve better health. At the heart of this process is the empowerment of communities, and the ownership and control of their own endeavours and destiny
>
> (WHO 1986, p. 1, quoted in Jones & Sidell 1997).

Immunisation

Immunisation is an important aspect of preventive health care globally and will be a topic of concern to many new parents. There are different forms of immunisation, but they all function through stimulation of the immune system in order to enhance resistance to a particular mechanism of infection. Vaccines are available for a range of diseases, some of which have severe symptoms (e.g. polio), whereas others are important for protection against congenital defects. Immunisation against rubella (German measles) is a good example of protecting a vulnerable group, namely pregnant women, by means of protecting the general population. While the disease produces only mild symptoms in children and adults, it has severe implications for early fetal development. Immunisation thus has a dual role in public health:

- *population protection:* decreasing the incidence of an infectious disease
- *individual protection:* decreasing the individual's likelihood of contracting a disease or the severity of symptoms experienced where protection is not complete.

Although population protection is arguably the most important function of immunisation, epidemiologists have pointed out that, historically, its role in improving public health and decreasing mortality has been overestimated in relation to more general measures such as improved nutrition and sanitation (McKeown 1979).

A series of immunisations focusing on the most common and the most potentially damaging childhood illnesses is offered to all children in the UK from about 8 weeks of age. Since women may ask for advice about immunisation during their postnatal care, it is important for midwives to increase their own knowledge of its benefits and limitations, recommended practice and contraindications for certain individuals. Women can be referred to their health visitor for detailed advice but it will be useful for midwives to discuss current immunisation schedules and policies with local health visitors regularly and to update knowledge of the current evidence on the benefits and risks.

Since immunisations can, rarely, have serious side-effects, parents should always be advised about contraindications and precautions when they are encouraged to take up immunisation. Parents are particularly likely to raise questions about vaccinations that have been subject to controversy. The pertussis vaccine, which protects against whooping cough, was a focus of concern regarding severe side-effects during the 1970s, which led to a significant fall in take-up rates. Subsequent studies have failed to confirm the level of risk conclusively and policy documents have emphasised the high level of risk from the disease itself in relation to possible vaccination risks. The combined measles, mumps and rubella vaccine (MMR), introduced during the 1990s as a mass immunisation programme, has also been controversial, with some professionals arguing that the programme was speculative and unnecessary in view of possible side-effects and others arguing that considerable research has shown few ill effects and considerable benefits. Currently, although a number of parents may enquire about separate vaccinations, Department of Health advice is that combined immunisation is safer, and separate vaccines are not provided by the NHS (DoH 2001). In all such cases, the complexity of influences on public health means that definitive evidence on the benefits and risks of immunisation is hard to obtain. Current policy remains that, on the balance of evidence, the benefits to public and individual health greatly outweigh possible risks (Charlish 1996, DoH 1992b).

Social services

The local authority social services departments hold the main responsibility for community care arrangements, liaison with health services and support for specific needs and problems such as child care and protection, although the services arranged to meet such needs may be provided by a range of organisations. Facilities provided or contracted for by social services include home care, respite care, and day and residential child care.

Social workers

Social workers play a key role in community care and also have specific statutory duties with respect to mental health and child protection. As care managers, they effectively act as gatekeepers to other services, such as home help or assistance with child care. They also provide direct support to clients, using a casework approach. Most social workers have a generic role that is concerned with a range of client groups although some work as specialists, particularly those working in hospital-based or multidisciplinary teams. This is more common in mental health social work, where some qualify as Approved Social Workers and are obliged to carry out statutory assessments under sections of the Mental Health Act 1983.

Social work, like health visiting, has its origins in social reform movements. Formal training was introduced relatively recently (training for generic work began only in 1964, although training for psychiatric social workers started at the London School of Economics in 1929) and was university based from the start. The approach of social work in the UK today was laid out when local authority social services departments were created following the Seebohm report in 1970 (Clements 1996). The main areas of social work relevant to midwives' work are their child care and protection and their mental health roles. These roles operate within the frameworks of the Children Act 1989 and the Mental Health Act 1983.

Child protection and families needing support

In general, the aim of social services is to provide support to families that will help them to manage their situation and prevent the need for more extensive services or interventions. A good example of this would be the provision of respite care (care for short breaks), home care, and aids and adaptations in the home for parents whose child has a disability, which may avoid the need for residential care. These aims are not always met in practice owing to funding shortfalls or simply because of problems in coordination of services. Midwives can promote good practice by advising women of their rights to apply for assessment for services and supporting them in the assessment process.

The Children Act 1989 focused on the needs of the child and emphasised that child care services or proceedings should always consider their welfare and interests as paramount. For example, it states that court orders should be made only where it is in the interests of the child to do so. The policy aims to support families so that they can remain together where possible and provides guidance on appropriate social service responses where this may not be in the interest of the child. It introduced the term 'accommodation' (instead of care) where parents voluntarily seek residential care for their children and reformed the procedures for 'involuntary' care. It also replaced the concept of parental rights with that of parental responsibility.

The Children Act 1989 has helped to clarify child care policy generally by giving a clear definition of a child's need:

- if he is unlikely to achieve or maintain, or to have the opportunity of achieving or maintaining a reasonable standard of health or development without the provision for him of services by a local authority.
- if his health or development is likely to be significantly impaired, or further impaired, without the provision for him of such services
- if he is disabled (Children Act Section 17(10)).

This definition can help professionals to form a view of what children need to thrive, whatever their social or cultural background. When a child has needs by virtue of disability or other problems, social services departments have a duty to respond. Since midwives have close contact with women and their families in the perinatal period, they may have an important role in identifying where families need additional support and advising those with special needs (DoH 2000).

Child protection procedures

Midwives need some awareness of child protection procedures (Fig. 50.1) since they are likely to be in contact with families that pose serious concerns about the child's welfare. The distinction between the need for support and the need for child protection is a difficult one and, in many situations, adequate and timely support for a family can prevent the need for child protection measures. The transition to parenthood is an important life event for all parents, and life events, even where they are wanted and viewed positively, can be major sources of stress and emotional distress (Marris 1974, Percival & McCourt 2000). Child care and adjustment to parenthood present a challenge to most parents and there is no clear and simple line between those who are able and those who are unable to cope with the demands of a new baby. However, there are circumstances that have been shown to be strongly associated with parents' capacity to care for a child, in particular families with multiple problems (Cleaver et al 1999). Care or supervision orders are sought only where there is concern about significant harm to the child. In cases of serious and urgent concern (for example, suspicion of serious non-accidental injury) anyone can apply for an Emergency Protection Order. This allows a limited period for the social services department to remove a child from home or to keep him or her in a safe place, to assess the child's situation. In less urgent cases, an Assessment Order can be sought where there is concern and the child is repeatedly not produced for assessment. Where appropriate, such assessments will be followed by a strategy meeting or a case conference, or both, to consider the concerns and plan responses, as set out in the Children Act 1989 (DoH 1991a). Case conferences are generally convened by social services child protection teams, who should inform and involve all relevant health professionals including the GP and, where appropriate, midwives (DoH 1999b).

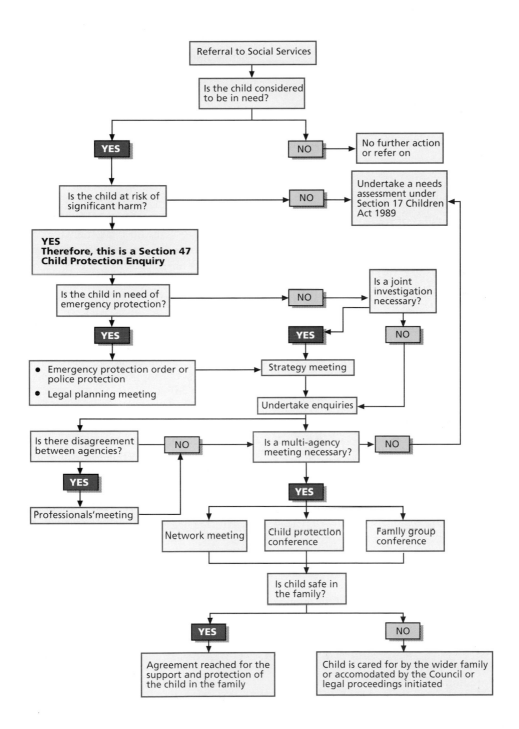

Fig. 50.1 The child protection process. (From Hammersmith and Fulham Area Child Protection Committee, with permission.)

Basic principles for the effective conduct of child protection procedures have been drawn from inquiries into child protection problems. They include (DoH 1991b):

- good and clear record keeping
- communication between professionals
- listening to the child
- taking an open approach
- working with families where possible.

Midwives may become concerned about potential child abuse antenatally, influenced by factors in the woman's history, her current mental state or her living situation. This may include concerns about domestic violence towards the woman herself, and research has shown that there are strong associations between situations of domestic violence and child abuse (Cleaver et al 1999). Antenatal care is a good point at which to work with a woman and to provide support, or assist the woman in obtaining the support she needs, in order to prevent possible problems arising after the baby is born. Indeed many of the family problems that are often associated with higher levels of abuse are those where parents, mothers in particular, would benefit from high levels of ante- and postnatal support. Interventions to support women with mental health problems, substance abuse problems and those who suffer from social isolation, poor support or domestic violence (including emotional or psychological as well as physical abuse) are important preventive and health promoting measures. Their importance for midwives is reflected in the recent 'Making a difference' report (DoH 1999a).

When midwives are seriously concerned antenatally, or detect signs of possible abuse after a baby is born, procedures laid down by the local Area Child Protection Committee should be followed. In the first instance, concerns can be raised with the supervisor of midwives or with the named senior midwife with responsibility for child protection, who should ensure that the appropriate social services officers are contacted. Cases are normally referred to the Area Child Protection Committee. In emergencies out of hours, police Child Protection Teams may be involved (DoH 1992c). The midwives' code of practice also provides basic guidelines to appropriate conduct.

Identifying possible child abuse

Abuse is difficult to define and even more difficult to judge. It is equally challenging for professionals to define responses that are appropriate and in the best interests of the child, yet health and social services professionals have responsibilities to take action where there is concern (DoH 1991a, b). The incidence of abuse is difficult to measure since it depends on reporting or detection; that is likely to be related to social awareness and policy as much as anything else.

Recent UK research has shown that, although abuse is very widespread, it is by no means confined to particular social groups; when child protection cases reach court proceedings, high rates of identifiable parental problems such as mental illness, domestic violence or substance misuse are found. Domestic violence is an important issue in its own right and is also associated with increased risk of child abuse. For both reasons, it is important for health professionals to respond to signs of possible domestic violence. Women may often present problems but in an indirect rather than overt manner, such as repeated visits to health providers complaining of vague illness symptoms, or through self-harm or symptoms of mental distress (National Children's Bureau 1995, Turton & Orr 1993). Rates of child abuse are particularly high where families are experiencing multiple problems. None the less, the majority of mothers with such problems are able to care for their children well, particularly if they have support from their partner or family, and supportive services to turn to (Cleaver et al 1999).

This evidence lends further weight to the current emphasis in child protection on prevention and efforts to work with families. It is helpful if problems are not seen as resulting from a dichotomy in parenting styles but as occurring on a continuum from calm and confident parenting through the normal range of most parents to those who have great difficulties and potential for abuse. It also highlights the potential value of appropriate midwifery support in pregnancy. It is important for midwives to respond to early signs of stress or distress in pregnant and postnatal mothers and their families, by being ready to listen and to provide advice and information or referrals to other sources of support, including self-help groups. Health visitors in some areas use systems for risk scoring as a method of screening, including risk for depression. These may be useful if they are used to trigger a positive and constructive response and when support services can be offered. However, great care is needed in using such systems to avoid unwarranted labelling of families as potential abusers and this risk must be balanced against the possible benefits of positive intervention (Robertson 1988).

Robertson (1988) argued that health visitors dealing with child protection should work within a framework of cross-cultural and societal violence and should maintain a focus on prevention. By this she meant understanding that child abuse is not just an individual issue but takes place within the framework of social and cultural conditions and values. Professionals should focus on the basic needs of the child and on the child per se and avoid relying on subjective judgements about what constitutes good or appropriate parenting, which are strongly influenced by cultural norms (Cloke & Naish 1992, DoH 1991a, Narducci 1992). It is tempting to believe, particularly as a service provider,

that one's own knowledge and values are naturally right or superior.

Child abuse can be identified in various forms and, although problems tend not to fall into neat categories in practice, these may be of use in assessing possible abuse. The categories used in government policy are listed in Box 50.6.

Signs and symptoms of abuse are not always clear. Bruising, for example, may be the result of a range of causes and suspicion of abuse is more likely if the bruising forms a particular pattern. The signs are more likely to be taken seriously if a number of symptoms are found together or where inconsistent accounts of accidents are given and where there are delays in seeking care (Robertson 1988). Although midwives are not expected to have the expertise of social workers, further reading on signs of abuse and appropriate responses is strongly recommended. In situations of concern it is always important to discuss this with health service colleagues such as the GP, health visitors and the local social work team.

Box 50.6 Categories of child abuse (DOH 1999b)

Physical abuse

May involve hitting, shaking, throwing, poisoning, burning or scalding, drowning, suffocating, or otherwise causing physical harm to a child. Physical harm may also be caused when a parent or carer feigns the symptoms of, or deliberately causes ill health to a child whom they are looking after.

Sexual abuse

Involves forcing or enticing a child or young person to take part in sexual activities, whether or not the child is aware of what is happening. The activities may involve physical contact, including penetrative (rape or buggery) or non-penetrative acts. They may include non-contact activities, such as involving children in looking at, or in the production of, pornographic material or watching sexual activities, or encouraging children to behave in sexually inappropriate ways.

Emotional abuse

Is the persistent emotional ill treatment of a child as to cause severe and persistent effects on the

child's emotional development. It may involve conveying to children that they are worthless or unloved, inadequate, or valued only in so far as they meet the needs of another person. It may feature age or developmentally inappropriate expectations being imposed on children. It may involve causing children frequently to feel frightened or in danger, or the exploitation or corruption of children. Some level of emotional abuse is involved in all types of ill treatment of a child though it may occur alone.

Neglect

The persistent failure to meet a child's basic physical or psychological needs, or both, which is likely to result in the serious impairment of the child's health or development. It may involve a parent or carer failing to provide adequate food, shelter and clothing, failing to protect a child from physical harm or danger, or failing to ensure access to appropriate medical care or treatment. It may also include neglect of, or unresponsiveness to, a child's basic emotional needs.

Fostering and adoption

Midwives often provide care for women whose pregnancy was not planned. This is more common than many professionals may realise and it is important not to make assumptions about the woman's feelings about her pregnancy. For example, in a study of women's experiences of maternity services, between 22 and 40% of women in the groups studied had mixed or negative initial feelings about the pregnancy (McCourt & Page 1996). In many cases women will be happy about an unplanned pregnancy, whereas others may be ambivalent and need support and possibly non-directive counselling to assist them in making decisions and plans for the future. For some women, this may involve relinquishment of the child for adoption. It is important to remember that such women share ordinary needs for information and support in pregnancy and childbirth, as well as having additional needs for support around relinquishing their child. Midwives can make a difference to how women feel in quite simple ways, such as avoiding judgmental or insensitive comments or approaches to care, by offering women a chance to discuss their situation privately but openly, and by providing advice on where they might find more specialised support.

Adoption procedures were reformed by the Children Act 1989 so that there is now a greater emphasis on open adoption where possible, so that relinquishing mothers may remain in agreed forms of contact with their children. Practice in child care agencies has also developed in recent years so that children who are adopted, fostered or placed in residential care are given more opportunity to understand and talk about their personal history. Fostering (on a short or long term basis) may be a consideration for mothers who are unable to care for their babies after birth but who do not wish to relinquish their children for adoption. The Children Act also increases flexibility for family members to care for children or remain in contact with them where mothers are unable to do so.

Other community services

Child care services

Child care services may be valuable for a range of needs, not just when parents are working or studying.

They may be important in providing support to families experiencing stress, for example due to poor or temporary housing, caring responsibilities or postnatal depression. Child care services for children under 5 years old are mainly the responsibility of social services, although education departments may manage local authority provision for children aged between 3 and 5. They generally provide a limited number of places but are responsible for the registration and inspection of all other facilities for the under 5s in their local area, including privately owned nurseries and individual childminders. Some services, often run by voluntary agencies, are also geared to the needs of families under stress. These include family centres, where parents and children can attend together and receive parenting support, and schemes such as Homestart or Newpin as well as an increasing range of Sure Start programmes that are available to all families but mainly operating in areas of social deprivation.

Social services departments often provide under-5s advisors, and health visitors also generally have good knowledge of local facilities. Local authorities often publish guides to local child care facilities, not only day care but resources for parents and small children to use together, such as playgroups or toy libraries and crèche facilities linked to adult education or sports activities. These can be of great value for parents who might otherwise feel isolated. The government website www.childcarelink.gov.uk gives some useful information on finding child care.

Interpreting, advocacy and link workers

Women and families from minority ethnic communities have two closely related sets of needs from maternity and other community health and social services (see Ch. 2). First are the ordinary needs, which they share with women of all backgrounds but which are often attended to more poorly owing to language or cultural barriers or to discrimination. Second are the particular needs resulting from their minority status, which may include language access and more specialised services. In practice, both are likely to be related. For example, women in a small scale study of a refugee community in West London voiced concerns about lack of information, advice, choices and sensitive personal care. These concerns were widely shared amongst local women but they were experienced as far more severe problems by women from ethnic minorities (Harper-Bulman & McCourt 1997, 2002).

Women who are refugees may also be socially isolated and need practical support in adjusting to life in a new country. Many will have come from situations of fear and conflict, only to meet with the difficulties of the asylum process on arrival. There is debate around the psychological health status of refugees, between those who emphasise the likelihood of post-traumatic stress and the need for psychological interventions such as counselling, and those who argue that medical approaches to the needs of refugees are not necessarily or always appropriate. None the less, midwives are in a good position to work with women in a health-promoting way. Sensitive care that provides good levels of support, tuned in to the woman and family's self-perceived needs, may make a difference. In addition to consulting with the women and families as much as possible about their needs, it might be argued that minority groups (particularly refugees) will benefit particularly from continuity of care and carer (McCourt & Pearce 2000).

Housing

Many women experience housing problems during pregnancy as they are faced with the need for stable and adequate accommodation for a new or growing family. Housing is important for both the physical and psychological health of parents and children. Local authorities in the UK have a statutory duty to provide housing for families who are homeless, including pregnant women, but this may involve temporary accommodation that is not well suited to caring for a child. The duty to provide accommodation for those in unsuitable housing is less clear cut and many families join long waiting lists, with priority given to those with the highest 'points' for several categories of need. Local authorities may also nominate families to the waiting lists of housing associations, trusts and cooperatives, some of which also operate their own application systems. Midwives may be asked to support applications for housing or improved housing, usually by writing letters.

Accommodation with support may be available or offered for mothers and babies in certain circumstances, including refuges for women experiencing domestic violence and supported accommodation for

mothers of school age, or those experiencing depression or other mental health problems. Shortage of specialist mother and baby facilities, however, may limit what can be offered to women who need such support. The emphasis is, where possible, on providing care for mothers and babies together or, when children need accommodation without their mothers, on gaining support from the wider family if possible or providing foster care.

Voluntary and independent services

Voluntary organisations have always played an important part in providing community health and social services and have in many cases been a major influence on their development, by showing what can be done and by campaigning for particular interest groups or services. They are linked to a long tradition of charitable work undertaken before the advent of the modern welfare state and were traditionally often linked with religious groups, as were the early hospital services in many countries. Voluntary organisations have shifted over time from being primarily charitable to a mutual or self-help focus, with many organisations founded by relatives of people in need of long term services and, more recently, service user organisations. Government policy in the 1980s in the UK strongly encouraged broadening the range of organisations providing services, including private companies. Voluntary and private providers of care are often referred to in policy terms as 'the independent sector'.

Voluntary organisations have generally combined two rather different roles effectively: that of campaigning or providing information and advice and that of providing community health or social services, or both. Services provided were often innovative, or responded to a gap in provision, which would, if effective, gradually be adopted by the statutory service providers. Following the NHS and Community Care Act 1990, they were encouraged to take on a far greater role in service provision and in some areas are now key providers of essential services such as residential and day child care (Box 50.7).

Services for mothers with disabilities

A range of services are provided by local authorities and voluntary or mutual support groups for women

Box 50.7 Voluntary organisations relevant for pregnant women and families with young children

- Informal and mutual support groups – often locally based or focused on a particular issue, e.g. local postnatal support groups facilitated by health visitors or community workers, or developing from formal parent education classes
- Parent and baby or toddler groups and clubs – these are generally locally, informally run and play an important part in preventing social isolation
- Childbirth groups which combine campaigning with practical and social support, e.g. National Childbirth Trust, Maternity Alliance
- breastfeeding support groups, which provide practical and moral support to women establishing breastfeeding, e.g. La Leche League
- Postnatal depression and women and mental health groups
- Minority ethnic community groups, refugee organisations and women's groups, which play a valuable role for women and families who may need practical and social support, including language services

- Groups for people who have suffered pregnancy loss or bereavement including mutual support, advice and counselling organisations, e.g. the Stillbirth and Neonatal Death Society (SANDS) or the Foundation for the Study of Infant Deaths (FSID)
- Groups for families under stress or needing support, e.g. Newpin, Homestart
- Groups for parents of children with disabilities or chronic health problems
- Support and counselling for relinquishing mothers and those whose children are in residential or foster care – such support is often now provided by voluntary adoption and fostering agencies, e.g. British Association for Adoption and Fostering (BAAF)
- Groups for parents with baby crying problems, e.g. Cry-Sis
- Groups for single parents, e.g. Parentpack, Gingerbread

A number of directories of local and national organisations are published and will be valuable to keep to hand for reference. See also links on the website: www.tiger.gov.uk

with disabilities, including those who are mothers. Although many are informal, and benefit from being so, it is important to remember the framework of rights and procedures provided by the NHS and Community Care Act 1990 and subsequent Disability legislation. In addition to service information, it is important for midwives to enhance their own awareness of disability issues, in order to provide a good service to all women whatever their needs. Issues for mothers with physical disabilities are considered in Chapter 2. Here, we provide some introductory information on issues for women with learning disabilities and those with mental health problems.

Learning disability

Midwives need awareness of learning disability issues both to support parents who may have some form of learning disability but also, increasingly, to provide

information and support to all pregnant women offered screening for different disabilities. The issues surrounding parents with learning disabilities are particularly sensitive since social policy in the UK and other industrialised societies has historically been strongly influenced by eugenic ideas and focused on preventing people with disabilities from reproduction or parenthood. Many individuals are still sterilised, if not through force then by persuasion, or are encouraged to terminate pregnancies. In this context, disabled activists and academics have argued that the availability of screening and termination for impairments reflects and contributes to assumptions that physical or intellectual impairment is always and only a negative thing. Such a cultural environment is likely to impact on the feelings of people with such impairments, particularly when approaching the issue of parenthood. A number of theorists have, therefore, identified three different models of disability: the medical (or individual deficit model), the religious (or moral) model and the social oppression model. The last of these models recognises that disability occurs as a result of social forces rather than simply because of the person's impairment. What may be disabling for particular individuals with impairments are features of that environment, for example emphasis on literacy, design of buildings, or stigmatising attitudes (Barnes et al 1999, Oliver 1996).

The category 'learning disability' (formerly called 'mental handicap' and in the US referred to as 'mental retardation') covers a wide span and includes people who will need very high levels of support in becoming parents. Professional knowledge of learning disability, like 'lay' knowledge, is often very limited, partly because of the history, before recent philosophical and policy changes, of keeping people with disabilities socially segregated. Mental handicap hospitals were built in the UK in the early part of the twentieth century (rather like the psychiatric asylums built before them) as geographically isolated institutions that functioned rather like self-sufficient communities (Alasewski 1986). It will be valuable to learn more about learning and other disabilities, not only to counter discriminatory practice and provide education and support for mothers with learning disabilities, but also to be in a better position to advise and counsel parents about antenatal screening and diagnostic tests (Dixon 1997).

Mental health and illness

The prevalence of mental health problems amongst women is acknowledged to be high, and mental health problems are far more widespread within the population than many people imagine, since mental illness is often associated with distorted media-based images of psychosis or violence. The majority of mental health problems are responded to by the community health and social services, by GPs, community psychiatric nurses, counsellors, health visitors or social workers.

Amongst women, the experience of depression is very widespread and, like other health problems, is strongly associated with stress factors such as poverty, lack of supportive partners, housing problems and caring for young children without employment outside the home (Brown & Harris 1978, Oakley 1992). Researchers differ in how far they view postnatal depression as one manifestation of depression in women or as a distinct form, and this is partly linked to the continuing lack of clear understanding of causes of depression or other forms of mental illness (see Ch. 35). Recent research suggests that much postnatal depression begins antenatally (or earlier) and is associated with a range of possible predisposing or precipitating factors, which include personal history and previous experience of pregnancy and birth (Ball 1994, Cox & Holden 1994). Ball argues that, because such depression is likely to be multicausal, midwives should focus their attention on the areas where they might make a difference to women. She identified a range of issues related to social support and the manner in which birth and postnatal care are managed that may help to prevent depression developing in women who are vulnerable.

The use of screening schedules, such as the Edinburgh Postnatal Depression Scale (Cox & Holden 1994), may have some value if they can lead to targeting of additional support and advice to the woman. Effective sources of support are not necessarily formal ones provided by health professionals, but good midwifery care may be particularly important to women who lack ordinary sources of support. Oakley and colleagues also found, in a study of social support and pregnancy, that women offered such support by midwives appeared to be better prepared to seek and obtain support from other people, including their partners (Oakley 1992).

Conclusion

This chapter has highlighted key areas of community health and social services with which midwives need to be familiar. Some are important for general awareness and some for more specific roles such as providing advice, support or referral. A textbook can only provide an introduction and these areas have seen radical and rapid change in recent years. The references and further reading suggestions will provide some pointers for developing further knowledge.

REFERENCES

Acheson D 1998 Independent enquiry into inequalities in health. Stationery Office, London.

Alasewski A 1986 Institutional care and the mentally handicapped. Croom Helm, London

Baker G, Bevan J M, McDonnell L, Wall B 1987 Community nursing. Research and some recent developments. Croom Helm, London

Ball J 1994 Reactions to motherhood: the role of postnatal care. Cambridge University Press, Cambridge

Barker D J P 1998 Mothers, babies and health in later life. Churchill Livingstone, Edinburgh

Barnes C, Mercer G, Shakespeare T 1999 Exploring disability, a sociological introduction. Polity Press, Cambridge

Bowling A 1981 Delegation in general practice. A study of doctors and nurses. Tavistock, London

Brown G W, Harris T 1978 Social origins of depression. A study of psychiatric disorder in women. Tavistock, London

Bulmer M 1987 The social basis of community care. Allen & Unwin, London

Carnell J, Kline R (eds) 1999 Community practitioners and health visitors' handbook. Radcliffe Medical, Abingdon

Charlish A 1996 Vaccination and immunisation. What does your child need? Thorsons, London

Children Act 1989, HMSO, London

Cleaver H, Unell I, Aldgate J 1999 Children's needs – parenting capacity. The impact of parental mental illness, problem alcohol and drug use, and domestic violence on children's development. Stationery Office, London

Clements L 1996 Community care and the law. Legal Action Group, London

Cloke C, Naish J (eds) 1992 Key issues in child protection for health visitors and nurses. Longman, UK

Cowley S 2002 Public health in policy and practice. A sourcebook for health visitors and community nurses. Baillière Tindall, Edinburgh

Cox J, Holden J (eds) 1994 Perinatal psychiatry. Use and misuse of the Edinburgh Postnatal Depression Scale. Gaskell, London

Crafter H 1997 Health promotion in midwifery. Principles and practice. Arnold, London

DoH (Department of Health) 1991a Working together under the Children Act 1989 (guidelines). HMSO, London

DoH (Department of Health) 1991b An introduction to the Children Act 1989, a new framework for the care and upbringing of children. HMSO, London

DoH (Department of Health) 1992a The health of the nation. HMSO, London

DoH (Department of Health) 1992b Immunisation against infectious disease. HMSO, London

DoH (Department of Health) 1992c Child protection. Guidance for senior nurses, health visitors and midwives. HMSO, London

DoH (Department of Health) 1993 Changing childbirth: report of the expert maternity group. HMSO, London

DoH (Department of Health) 1997a The new NHS: modern, dependable. Cm 3807. Stationery Office, London

DoH (Department of Health) 1997b NHS (Primary Care) Act. DoH, London

DoH (Department of Health) 1998 Our healthier nation. A contract for health. Cmd 3852. Stationery Office, London

DoH (Department of Health) 1999a Making a difference: strengthening the nursing, midwifery and health visiting contribution to health and healthcare. DoH, London

DoH (Department of Health) 1999b Working together to safeguard children. Stationery Office, London

DoH (Department of Health) 2000 Framework for the assessment of children in need and their families. Stationery Office, London

DoH (Department of Health) 2001 Measles, mumps and rubella vaccine: www.doh.gov.uk/mmr.htm

DoH (Department of Health)/SNMAC 1998 Midwifery: delivering our future. Report by the standing nursing and midwifery advisory committee. DoH, London

Dimond B 1997 Legal aspects of care in the community. Macmillan, London

Dixon K 1997 Practical tips for supporting pregnant women with learning disabilities. MIDIRS Midwifery Digest 7(1):40–42

Donnison J 1988 Midwives and medical men. A history of the struggle for the control of childbirth. Historical Publications, Barnet, Herts

Flint C 1993 Midwifery teams and caseloads. Butterworth Heinemann, London

Harper-Bulman K, McCourt C 1997 Report on Somali women's experiences of maternity care. Thames Valley University, London. Online. Available: www.health.tvu.ac.uk/cmp

Harper-Bulman K, McCourt C 2002 Somalia refugee women's experiences of maternity care in west London: a case study. Public Health 12:365–380

House of Commons Social Services Committee 1980 Perinatal and neonatal mortality (the Short report). HMSO, London

Hunt S, Symonds S 1995 The social meaning of midwifery. Macmillan, London

IDS (Incomes Data Services) 2000 Maternity and parental rights, employment law handbook. IDS, London

Jones L, Sidell M 1997 The challenge of promoting health. Exploration and action. Macmillan/Open University, Basingstoke

Leap N, Hunter B 1993 The midwife's tale: an oral history from handy women to professional midwife. Scarlett Press, London

McCourt C, Page L 1996 Report on the evaluation of one-to-one midwifery. Centre for Midwifery Practice, Thames Valley University, London. Online (summary). Available: www.health.tvu.ac.uk/cmp

McCourt C, Pearce A 2000 Does continuity of carer matter to women from minority ethnic groups? Midwifery 16:145–154

McKeown T 1979 The role of medicine: dream, mirage or nemesis? Blackwell, Oxford

Marris P 1974 Loss and change. Routledge & Kegan Paul, London

MoH (Ministry of Health) 1970 Domiciliary midwifery and maternity bed needs: the report of the standing maternity and midwifery advisory committee (the Peel report). HMSO, London

Narducci T 1992 Race, culture and child protection. In: Cloke C, Naish J (eds) Key issues in child protection for health visitors and nurses. Longman, London, ch 2, p 12–22

NCB (National Children's Bureau) 1995 Children and domestic violence. NCB, London NHS and Community Care Act 1990 HMSO, London

Oakley A 1992 Social support and motherhood. The natural history of a research project. Blackwell, Oxford

Oliver M 1996 Understanding disability: from theory to practice. Cassell, London

Page L 1995 Effective group practice in midwifery: working with women. Blackwell Science, Oxford

Percival P, McCourt C 2000 Becoming a parent. In: Page L (ed) The new midwifery. Science and sensitivity in practice. Churchill Livingstone, Edinburgh, p 185–222

Richards M, Hardy R, Kuh D, Wadsworth M E J 2001 Birth weight and cognitive function in the British 1946 birth cohort: longitudinal population based study. British Medical Journal 322(7280):199–200

Roberts H 1997 Socioeconomic determinants of health: children, inequalities and health. British Medical Journal 314(7087):1122–1125

Robertson C 1988 Health visiting in practice. Longman, Edinburgh

Robinson S 1990 Maintaining the role of the midwife. In: Garcia J, Kilpatrick R, Richards M (eds) The politics of maternity care. Clarendon, Oxford

Sandall J, Davies J, Warwick C 2000 Evaluation of the Albany Midwifery Practice. Kings College, London

Stacey M 1988 The sociology of health and healing. Unwin & Hyman, London

Tew M 1990 Safer childbirth? A critical history of maternity care. Chapman & Hall, London

Townsend P, Davidson N, Whitehead M 1988 Inequalities in health. Penguin, London

Turton P, Orr J 1993 Learning to care in the community, 2nd edn. Edward Arnold, London

FURTHER READING

Bowling A 1981 Delegation in general practice. A study of doctors and nurses, Tavistock, London

Not up to date but useful for the background to general practice and the working relationships between GPs and nurses.

Charlish A 1996 Vaccination and immunisation. What does your child need? Thorsons, London

A consumer- rather than academically oriented book that sets out all the views expressed in debates about immunisation and focuses on parental concerns.

Texts on health visiting are useful for midwives since they focus on relevant areas of work such as health advice, preventive care and monitoring, and child health and development. Read some introductory texts to increase your understanding of health visitors' aims and ways of working and explore how these relate to the approach of midwives.

Social science textbooks will also be useful, as will those more directly related to analysis of maternity care, the health of mothers and babies and accounts of research into health beliefs, practices and social conditions. For example:

Cornwell J 1984 Hard earned lives. Tavistock, London

Oakley A 1993 Essays on women, medicine and health. Edinburgh University Press, Edinburgh

Stacey M 1988 The sociology of health and healing. Unwin & Hyman, London

It is also important to obtain a good and up-to-date range of local and national directories of organisations and services. For example:

MIDIRS Directory of Maternity Organisations. MIDIRS, Bristol, UK (Updated regularly by means of the addition of inserts when new information is received.)

Whitfield C (ed) People who help. A guide to voluntary and other support organisations, Profile Productions, London (Updated regularly.)

A number of guides to the legislation, aimed at health professionals, are published. For example:

DoH (Department of Health) 1999 Working together to safeguard children. Stationery Office, London

It is important to check that they reflect the most up-to-date guidance and legislation that is still in force.

Copies of all the relevant legislation and associated guidelines should be found in a good college library but they are increasingly easy to obtain from government websites, either by mail order or by downloading file copies. Key websites are given in Useful addresses (below).

USEFUL ADDRESSES

The Department of Health:
www.doh.gov.uk

The Department of Trade and Industry – employee rights:
www.dti.gov.uk

The Department of Work and Pensions (formerly Department of Social Security) – rights and benefits:
www.dwp.gov.uk

51 Supervision of Midwives and Clinical Governance

Jean Duerden

CHAPTER CONTENTS

Supervision of midwives empowers midwives to work within the full scope of their role, offering a framework for scrutiny of professional standard practice, through a non-confrontational, confidential, midwife-led review of a midwife's level of knowledge, understanding and competence (ENB 1999a). The philosophy of midwifery supervision and the standards it develops reflect the key themes of clinical governance described in NHS First Class Service (DoH 1998). These themes are:

- professional self-regulation
- clinical governance
- lifelong learning.

The chapter aims to:

- describe the supervision of midwives and how it supports the clinical governance framework
- review the various aspect of clinical governance
- promote the supervision of midwives as a mechanism for quality assurance, sensitive to the needs of mothers and babies
- assist midwives in using supervision effectively.

Supervision of midwives

A short history of the supervision of midwives

Supervision of midwives was introduced early last century with the passing of the Midwives Act in 1902. Under the Act, the Central Midwives Board (CMB) was established and, through that board, the inspection of midwives. The inspectors of midwives so created were not practising midwives, as are the supervisors of midwives today, but middle class women, 'ladies', used to supervising subordinates (Kirkham 1995) and who had domestic standards much higher than those of the working class midwives. As a result, they were extremely critical of the poor environments in which many of the midwives then lived. These lady inspectors attempted to impose their middle class standards on the midwives, and had little understanding of the needs of midwives who had to undertake the domestic work in their own homes themselves. They expected the midwives to 'use plenty of clean linen' (Kirkham 1995, quoting Nursing Notes July 1907:106) despite the fact that the women they attended could not afford such linen. Similarly, the midwives struggled to comply with the Midwives rules that instructed them to summon medical aid even though there was no possibility of the family paying the doctor's fee. It was not until 1918 that this matter was resolved when a further Midwives Act required midwives to notify the Local Supervising Authority (LSA), via the supervisor of midwives, that they had summoned medical aid. If summoned by a midwife the GP could be paid.

The LSA officers were the Medical Officers of Health. They passed on the bulk of their LSA work to non-medical inspectors who were at liberty to inspect the midwives in any way they felt appropriate. They could follow them on their rounds, visit their homes, question the patients they had cared for and even investigate their personal lives (Kirkham 1995), in addition to inspecting their equipment. Records could not be checked; these were rarely made as many midwives were illiterate, notwithstanding their immense practical knowledge and independence. Midwives who disobeyed or ignored the rules would be disciplined. The Midwives Act also called for the LSA to investigate midwives who were guilty of negligence, malpractice or misconduct, personal or professional, and to report these midwives to the CMB for disciplinary action. The LSA also had to report any midwife convicted of an offence, suspend a midwife from practice if likely to be a source of infection, report the death of any midwife and submit a roll of midwives annually to the board.

The roll of midwives was introduced with the 1902 Act, which demanded the registration of midwives. Midwives must have their names on the roll of midwives, in order to continue practising. Training for midwives was established at the same time, but it was not until the 1910 Act that registration was permitted only on successful completion of an approved training course for midwives. Despite the training, it was not until 1936 that another revision of the Midwives Act led to the LSA being required to provide a salaried midwifery service. The amended Act empowered the CMB to set rules requiring midwives to attend refresher courses. It also determined the qualifications required to be a supervisor. Medical supervisors had to be medical officers, and non-medical supervisors were midwives, the latter under the control of the former. By 1937, the Ministry of Health had recognised the difficulties that midwives were experiencing by not having been supervised by midwives, and these changes were detailed in a Ministry of Health letter (MoH 1937), changing the title from 'inspector of midwives' to 'supervisor of midwives', and requiring the supervisors to be experienced midwives. For some reason, it was thought appropriate that they should not be engaged in midwifery practice. A real change of heart had taken place since the 1902 Act, as the letter referred to the supervisor of midwives as 'counsellor and friend' rather than 'relentless critic' and expected the supervisor to display 'sympathy and tact'.

Further revisions of the Midwives Act took place and in 1951 the most significant change wrought was for supervisors of midwives to ensure that midwives attended statutory refresher courses and to supply the names of those midwives who should attend. This statutory requirement continued until 2001 when rule 37 of the Midwives rules (UKCC 1998a) was superseded by Post-Registration Education and Practice (PREP) requirements (UKCC 1997).

Supervision of midwives did not move away from the auspices of the medical officers of health until 1974 when the National Health Service (Reorganisation) Act (1973) nominated Regional Health Authorities as LSA, and District Health Authorities nominated supervisors of midwives for appointment by the LSA. In 1977 the medical supervisor role was finally abolished and all supervisors were required to be *practising* midwives. Shortly afterwards, supervision was introduced into the hospital environment as well as in the community, and in 1979 the framework for the United Kingdom Central Council for Nursing, Midwifery and Health Visiting (UKCC) and the National Boards of England, Scotland, Wales and Northern Ireland was established. The National Boards were required to provide advice and guidance to the LSA, leading to the abolition of the Central Midwives Board in 1983.

Rather surprisingly, courses for supervisors of midwives were not introduced until 1978 when induction courses became a requirement for any supervisor of midwives appointed after 1974. Today, these courses are much more rigorous and undertaken at first degree or master's level. Midwives must complete the course successfully before being eligible for appointment as a supervisor of midwives. The requirement for training as a supervisor of midwives *prior* to appointment did not exist until as recently as 1992 when the English National Board for Nursing, Midwifery and Health Visiting (ENB) developed an open learning programme (ENB 1992). In 1993 the revised Midwives rules (Rule 44(2) UKCC 1993) stipulated that this preparation take place prior to appointment, meaning that all four UK countries had to introduce training for supervisors, but only England and Wales used the ENB open learning programme with associated study days. Scotland and Ireland had a less structured training, which has become more rigorous over recent years.

In 1994, the Midwives code of practice (UKCC 1994) was revised to include a section that emphasised the relationship between midwife and supervisor of midwives as a partnership, rather than as one of controlling. The last amendment of the Midwives rules (UKCC 1998a) involved a change in rule 44 to address both preparation and updating for supervisors of midwives.

The introduction of supervision of midwives in 1902 resulted in improvement in standards in midwifery and created a situation in which women were exposed to safe practitioners. Midwives were obliged to notify their intention to practise each year so that the roll of midwives was regularly updated and monitored. The midwifery inspectors could report to the LSA Officer any midwives whose standards were considered unsatisfactory and who were a danger to the public. In such cases the LSA officer could suspend the midwife from practice.

Many of these functions continue today, although in a much more supportive fashion. The principal function of supervisors of midwives continues to be the protection of the public, but the main ethos is support for midwives. Midwives still have to notify their intention to practise midwifery each year to the LSA, and each LSA office maintains a database of all midwives practising within the LSA area. Information from the notifications of intention to practise is added to the details of registration on the UKCC register. From April 2002 this body became the Nursing and Midwifery Council (NMC) (DoH 2001a).

Supervision of midwives in the twenty-first century

Midwives today enjoy the benefits of having a named supervisor of midwives to whom they can relate and look for support, and with whom they can share their concerns. The Midwives code of practice (UKCC 1998a, paragraph 34) details how midwives and supervisors of midwives should work towards a common aim of providing the best possible care for mothers and babies. It also mentions the mutual responsibility they have for effective communication between themselves.

There is always a supervisor of midwives on call at any time who can be contacted if there are any practice concerns, or if there has been a critical incident. There are certain times when a supervisor of midwives must be called, according to the Midwives' code of practice (UKCC 1998a, paragraph 39) – such as in the event of an unexpected stillbirth.

Record keeping in midwifery must be accurate, contemporaneous and provide a good account of events (UKCC 1998b). Supervisors of midwives are responsible for ensuring good record-keeping standards. They regularly check the midwifery records at their NHS Trust, and feed back to midwives on their standards of record keeping. This assists midwives in perfecting their notes and helps them to avoid problems that could lead to litigation.

Although the Midwives rules (UKCC 1998a) talk about the inspection of equipment and premises, much less heed is paid to inspecting the bags of community midwives than was the case in earlier years. Much more emphasis is placed on discussion, support and professional development needs and being there for the midwives when they are in need, providing a confidential framework for a supportive relationship (Box 51.1).

Supervisory reviews

The annual supervisory review provides dedicated time for the midwives to sit down with their supervisors of midwives and reflect on their practice over the

---

Box 51.1 Activities of a supervisor of midwives

- Supporting best practice and ensuring evidence-based midwifery care
- Being a confident advocate for midwives and mothers
- Acting as an effective change agent
- Providing leadership and guidance
- Acting as a role model
- Undertaking the role of mentor
- Empowering women and midwives
- Facilitating a supportive partnership with midwives
- Supporting midwives through dilemmas
- Helping midwives' personal and professional development
- Facilitating midwives' reflection on critical incidents
- Supporting midwives through supervised practice
- Maintaining an awareness of local, regional and national NHS issues
- Giving advice on ethical issues
- Liaising with clinicians, management and education
- Maintaining records of all supervisory activities

(From ENB 1999b, with permission of the English National Board for Nursing, Midwifery and Health Visiting)

---

preceding year. If midwives are concerned about any aspects of their practice they can discuss them frankly with their supervisors within the confidential arena of the supervisory review knowing that they will be offered support and guidance, rather than criticism.

Although it is customary for only one supervisory review a year, this is not fixed in tablets of stone and midwives are able to access their supervisor of midwives as, and when, they need or want to. As many supervisors of midwives hold clinical posts, they often work alongside the midwives they supervise and have more regular contact on an informal basis.

Critical incidents

If midwives have been involved in critical incidents, they will be encouraged to meet with their supervisors and reflect on the incidents, the events leading up to the incidents and the outcomes. The named supervisor of midwives is there to support the midwife, and acts on behalf of the LSA, not the NHS Trust. If the incident is sufficiently serious, another supervisor of midwives may be asked to carry out a supervisory enquiry, again on behalf of the LSA, but a midwifery manager might undertake a management enquiry on behalf of the NHS Trust. The named supervisor will support the midwife throughout the enquiry, and will help to identify any weaknesses in practice and ascertain whether there were any knowledge gaps. Such gaps can then be addressed through appropriate learning, and a learning contract can be prepared to address these deficiencies, supported by the supervisor of midwives. The contract will have a specific time frame, and regular meetings with the named supervisor to monitor progress will be accommodated. An appropriate mentor of the midwife's choice will be allocated to support the midwife in the work area and there will be liaison with the head of midwifery education at the local university if academic input is required. These are the only individuals who need to be aware of the difficulties that the midwife has experienced, and every effort will be made by them to maintain confidentiality at all times to protect the integrity of the midwife concerned.

Local Supervising Authorities

A practising midwife, with experience as a supervisor of midwives, performs the LSA 'Responsible Midwifery Officer' role in every LSA in England. Currently, each health authority is an LSA. Following the Health Authorities Act of 1995, 100 health authorities were formed in April 1996 and the statutory LSA function was handed down to them from the eight regional health authorities. Rather than appoint 100 LSA Responsible Midwifery Officers to carry out the LSA function, the health authorities formed consortia and each consortium appointed a practising midwife to carry out the LSA function within the consortium. There are 11 LSA Responsible Midwifery Officers in England acting on behalf of all the LSAs. Each of the 99 health authorities was an LSA until April 2002, when they merged to form 28 Strategic Health Authorities

(DoH 2001b) with the same number of LSAs. In the other UK countries the LSA Responsible Officer is not necessarily a midwife. In Scotland, 16 link supervisors of midwives perform much of the LSA function for the Health Board LSA Officers, as well as carrying out their substantive posts, which are usually head of midwifery. In Wales, the Health Authorities have appointed practising midwives, similar to the Scottish system, but the midwives are referred to as 'lead supervisors of midwives'. In Northern Ireland, the four Health Boards have 'link supervisors of midwives' to carry out the LSA function on behalf of the LSA Officers at the Health Boards. There are also heads of midwifery from a NHS Trust in each Health Board area (Duerden 2000a, p. 146).

The LSA role has no management responsibility to NHS Trusts, but it acts as a focus for issues relating to midwifery practice (ENB 1999a) and its strength lies in its influence on quality in local midwifery services. All LSA Officers have to be aware of the wider NHS picture and contemporary issues. The National Forum of LSA Responsible Midwifery Officers meets every 2 months in England to ensure a national framework in which the responsible officers can contribute informed advice on issues impacting on midwifery, such as structures for local maternity services and post-registration education for midwives.

Each LSA is responsible for ensuring that statutory supervision of all midwives is exercised to a satisfactory standard within its geographical boundary (ENB 1999a). This is a requirement of the Nursing and Midwifery Order 2001 and the Midwives rules and code of practice (UKCC 1998a).

The duties of the Responsible Midwifery Officer are detailed in Box 51.2.

Risk management and the supervision of midwives

The next chapter relates to risk management and should be read in context with this section. All of the functions of a supervisor of midwives could be considered to have a risk management element, as the framework for supervision is based on safety and good outcomes. The supervisor of midwives acts as an advocate for the consumer by monitoring the professional performance of midwives, thereby ensuring a safe standard of midwifery practice and enhancing the quality of care for a mother and her family. Supervision is a

separate function from the management of the midwifery service and, although some supervisors may have responsibility for both, their responsibility for supervision is to the LSA.

Supervisors of midwives, in fulfilling their role of protecting the public, must be aware of the current safety culture in their units and be prepared to inform NHS Trust Executives of the risks being taken by staffing their maternity unit both inadequately and inappropriately.

The safety culture of the midwifery profession is bound by the Midwives rules and code of practice (UKCC 1998a) and the Code of professional conduct (NMC 2002), by which all midwives must abide. The Code of professional conduct states that, in the exercise of professional accountability, staff should acknowledge any limitations in their knowledge and competence, and decline any duties or responsibilities unless able to perform them in a safe and skilled manner. It is not always easy to refuse when there is no one else to carry out the tasks, especially if this means that clients' needs will not be met, but the onus is placed on the individual by the Code. The supervisor of midwives has to ensure that the rules and the codes are honoured, and take action in the event of breach of any of them. Supervision should, through its development and use, enable practitioners to make a real contribution to any organisation's ability to manage risk effectively.

It is impossible to be a supervisor of midwives without practising risk management. Supervisors can ensure the best outcome for mother and baby by influencing how midwives practise. When supervision is carried out effectively, with a particular regard to the monitoring of midwives' practice and competence, the perceptions of risk can be related to midwifery practice, as can the principles of risk management.

Supervision and management

These two entities are often confused and yet they are distinctly separate. This confusion is probably a legacy from the introduction of supervision of midwives into hospitals in 1973 when the midwifery managers became supervisors of midwives. To many midwives the positions appeared synonymous – indeed many of the supervisors themselves failed to distinguish between the two roles (RCM 1994). Today there are

Box 51.2 Duties of the responsible midwifery officer

- Provides advice and guidance to supervisors of midwives
- Provides a framework of support for supervisory and midwifery practice
- Ensures each midwife meets the statutory requirements for practice
- Selects and appoints supervisors of midwives and deselects if ever necessary
- Provides education and training for prospective supervisors of midwives
- Provides continuing education and training for supervisors of midwives
- Ensures appropriate ratios of midwives to supervisors of midwives in each trust
- Provides advice on midwifery matters to health authorities
- Manages communications within supervisory systems
- Investigates cases of alleged misconduct
- Receives reports of maternal deaths
- Assesses the retraining requirements of non-practising midwives wishing to return to midwifery practice
- Leads the development of standards and audit of supervision
- Determines whether to suspend a midwife from practice, in accordance with Rule 38 of the Midwives rules and code of practice (UKCC 1998)

- Prepares an annual report of supervisory activities within the report year, including audit outcomes and emerging trends affecting maternity services for Health Authorities and Trusts.
- Maintains a list of current supervisors
- Provides a framework for supporting supervision and midwifery practice
- Publishes details of how to contact supervisors
- Publishes details of how the practice of midwives will be supervised
- Receives notifications of intention to practise
- Operates a system that ensures midwives meet statutory requirements for practice
- Ensures supervisors have access to education and training
- Leads the development of standards and audit of supervision
- Manages communications with supervisors
- Conducts regular meetings for supervisors to develop key areas of practice
- Facilitates inter-Trust activities, such as provision of cover by supervisors of midwives from other NHS Trusts
- May suspend a midwife, if appropriate
- Conducts investigations and initiates legal action in cases of practice by persons not qualified to do so under the Nursing and Midwifery Order 2001.

more supervisors of midwives in clinical posts than in management, so the differences are much clearer to midwives. Much work has been done in recent years to educate midwives, and supervisors of midwives, about the different roles, and to increase awareness of the benefits of statutory supervision. There is now a trend for any midwifery managers who are also supervisors of midwives not to supervise the midwives they manage.

There is no hierarchy within supervision; from the moment of appointment, supervisors of midwives have full supervisory responsibilities. They will be helped into their role by more experienced supervisors, but there is no seniority or ranking of supervisors.

There should not be any conflict between supervision and management as, when acting in either capacity, the objectives are clear and separately defined. The aims of supervision are to ensure the safety of mothers and babies and support midwives in order to achieve high standards of practice, whilst the aim of management is to achieve a high quality service to meet contract specifications and make the best use of resources (ENB 1992). If there is a critical incident to be investigated, the same person cannot act as both manager and supervisor, as the former is acting on behalf of the NHS Trust and the latter as advocate for the midwife, with responsibility to the LSA (Duerden 2000b, p. 37).

Box 51.3 Responsibilities of a supervisor of midwives

Each supervisor of midwives is expected to carry out a number of responsibilities:

Administrative

- Receive and process notification of intention to practise forms
- Ensure that midwives have access to the statutory rules and guidance, and local policies to inform their practice
- Report to the LSA serious cases involving professional conduct where the UKCC rules and codes have been contravened and when it is considered that local action has failed
- To achieve safe practice
- Contribute to activities such as confidential enquiries, risk management strategies, clinical audit and clinical governance

Interactive

- Provide guidance on maintenance of registration, identify and accredit opportunities for updating in relation to statutory requirements
- Create an environment that supports the midwife's role and empowers practice through evidence-based decision making
- Monitor standards of midwifery practice through audit of records and assessment of clinical outcomes

- Monitor local maternity services to ensure that appropriate care is available to all women and babies
- Investigate critical incidents and identify any action required, whilst seeking to achieve a positive learning midwife and agree appropriate experience for the midwives involved, liaising with the LSA as appropriate

Developmental

- Be available for midwives to discuss issues relating to their practice and provide appropriate support
- Arrange regular meetings with individual midwives, at least once a year, to help them to evaluate their practice and identify areas of development
- Participate in the identification and preparation of new supervisors of midwives
- Identify when peer supervisors are not undertaking the role to a satisfactory standard and take appropriate action
- Ensure that every practising midwife has a named supervisor and that systems are in place for this to be changed by either party when appropriate.

(From ENB 1999b, with permission of the English National Board for Nursing, Midwifery and Health Visiting)

Despite this, confusion continues to exist, particularly on the issue of suspension (Shennan 1996) and the difference between suspension from duty, a management procedure, and suspension from practice, a recommendation to the LSA by a supervisor of midwives.

The responsibilities of a supervisor of midwives are detailed in Box 51.3.

Clinical governance

Clinical governance is defined in First Class Service (DoH 1998, p. 33) as 'a framework through which NHS organisations are accountable for continuously improving the quality of their services and safeguarding high standards of care by creating an environment in which excellence in clinical care will flourish'.

Professional self-regulation and lifelong learning are the other key themes within this document. None of these is new to midwives as they have all been integral to the supervision of midwives for some time past. The philosophy for the supervision of midwives and the standards it develops reflect these key themes.

Supervision of midwives promotes and develops safe practice and ensures the dissemination of good, evidence-based practice and innovation (ENB 1999b). Since 1955, supervision of midwives has ensured a statutory framework for continued professional development, and compulsory refreshment of midwifery knowledge has led to a lifelong learning programme for midwives throughout their careers. Supervision has provided a formal focus of support and reflection with a confidential review of professional development needs.

It is evident, therefore, that the supervision of midwives contributes to an effective framework of clinical governance, minimising risk, reducing patient complaints, and contributing to a multidisciplinary collaboration in producing practice guidelines (ENB 1999a).

The government has set clear national standards backed by consistent monitoring arrangements. The 11 LSA responsible midwifery officers, through their supervisory audit visits to each maternity unit, regularly monitor standards of practice against documented evidence such as that produced by the Confidential Enquiry into Stillbirths and Deaths in Infancy (CESDI) and the Confidential Enquiry into Maternal Deaths (CEMD). National standards are also developed through National Service Frameworks (NSF) and the National Institute for Clinical Excellence (NICE). Any pertaining to maternity services can also be monitored in this way. Where there are unacceptable variations in clinical midwifery practice, or care is inappropriate for women's needs, the LSA Responsible Midwifery Officer, as an outside assessor, is in a position to recommend remedial action (Duerden 2000a, p. 143). Similarly, the LSA can contribute to the dissemination of information from NICE to ensure the implementation of the most effective care.

The clinical governance framework

The DoH report First Class Service (DoH 1998) described a clinical governance framework (3.11) to:

- modernise and strengthen professional self-regulation and build on the principles of performance
- strengthen existing systems for quality control, based on clinical standards, evidence-based practice and learning the lessons of poor performance
- identify and build on good practice
- assess and minimise the risk of untoward events
- investigate problems as these arise and ensure lessons are learnt
- support health professionals in delivering quality care.

All of these aspects of clinical governance are covered within the ambit of supervision of midwives. Supervisors of midwives monitor midwifery practice and they are able to discuss with midwives the regulation of midwifery practice and ensure full understanding of accountability to themselves, to the Nursing and Midwifery Council and to the NHS Trust that employs them.

The principles of lifelong learning are deep rooted in supervision with its history of regular refresher courses.

Systems for quality control, based on clinical standards, evidence-based practice and learning the lessons of poor performance, are met through supervisory audit. Evidence-based practice is a term that might be considered to be over- and inappropriately used, but it is crucial to the government's programme of quality improvement activities within clinical governance: 'Evidence-based practice is supported and applied routinely in everyday practice' (DoH 1998, p. 36). Supervisors of midwives have a responsibility to monitor midwifery practice. Not only must they ensure that the practice within their own clinical area is evidence-based, but they must also challenge areas of practice that are carried out, out of a sense of tradition, without any evidence for maintaining them. They must furthermore ensure that the midwives concerned not only understand the meaning of evidence-based practice, but that they also know where and how to find evidence and evaluate it adequately, being able to differentiate between poor and high quality studies.

Supervisors of midwives are in an excellent position to identify good practice and also to learn of examples of good practice in other maternity units that can be adopted within their own NHS Trust, as such examples are shared through the supervisory network. Where midwives have ideas for changing and improving practice, supervisors of midwives should be able to empower the midwives to introduce such change and support them in their initiatives acting as their advocate with senior staff. A supervisor of midwives should be amongst the membership of every labour ward forum (RCOG/RCM 1999) providing a useful opportunity for the sharing of new ideas and encouraging midwives to attend in order to promulgate their suggestions for changing practice.

Through regular monitoring of midwifery practice, especially by supervisors of midwives who work in the clinical environment, areas of risk can be identified and addressed. Critical incident analysis is a crucial part of the supervisor's role. Following any untoward event or 'near miss', some sort of incident form will be completed. All untoward events involving midwives are recorded, investigated and monitored by supervisors.

The link between clinical governance and statutory supervision of midwives is illustrated in Figure 51.1.

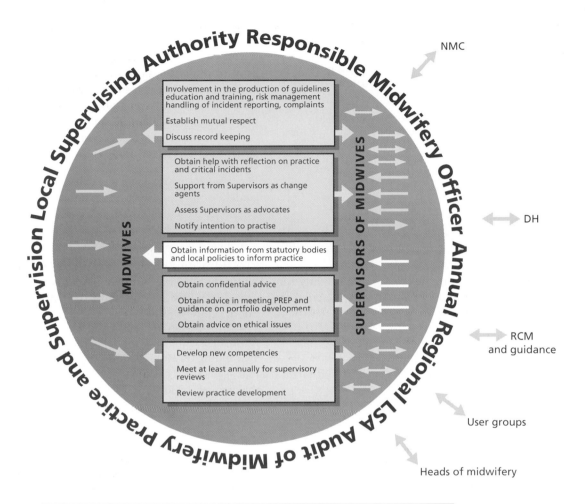

Involvement in the production of guidelines education and training, risk management handling of incident reporting, complaints

Establish mutual respect

Discuss record keeping

Obtain help with reflection on practice and critical incidents

Support from Supervisors as change agents

Assess Supervisors as advocates

Notify intention to practise

Obtain information from statutory bodies and local policies to inform practice

Obtain confidential advice

Obtain advice in meeting PREP and guidance on portfolio development

Obtain advice on ethical issues

Develop new competencies

Meet at least annually for supervisory reviews

Review practice development

MIDWIVES

SUPERVISORS OF MIDWIVES

Supervising Authority Responsible Midwifery Officer Annual Regional LSA Audit of Midwifery Practice and Supervision Local

NMC

DH

RCM and guidance

User groups

Heads of midwifery

"We believe that it (Supervision of Midwives) is a valued and valuable system and one which we see as being an integral part of clinical governance in the future".

Lord Hunt January 2000

Annual Regional LSA Audit of Midwifery Practice and Supervision audits recommendations of:

- CEMD (Confidential Enquiries into Maternal Deaths in the UK)
- CESDI (Confidential Enquiries into Stillbirths and Deaths in Infancy)
- Towards Safer Childbirth
- Saving Lives
- Making a Difference
- Fitness for Practice
- Clinical Concerns of Midwives

Fig. 51.1 The link between clinical governance and statutory supervision of midwives. (Model devised by Carol Paeglis, supervisor of midwives, and practice development nurse/midwife, Airedale Hospitals NHS Trust, with permission of Carol Paeglis and Rachel Wilson, medical illustrator, Airedale Hospitals NHS Trust.)

Quality

The NMC examines and certifies the knowledge base of those admitted to professional registers, but knowledge does not remain constant: the knowledge and skills of the experienced midwife differ from those of the midwife recently admitted to the register.

Most hospitals have regular perinatal audit meetings, designed to review the outcomes of clinical care and identify possible areas for improvement. These are excellent arenas for supervisors of midwives to monitor midwifery practice and take appropriate action where suboptimal care has been demonstrated.

The results of research should inform our decisions about health care. It is, however, evident from the conclusions of Chalmers et al (1989) that research findings appear often to be only slowly and incompletely reflected in practice. Many journals available to midwives provide a great deal of up-to-date information on research findings relevant to practice, but access to information alone does not always influence putting research findings into clinical practice. Support and advocacy from a supervisor will often be necessary.

Another body that, through the modernisation programme, monitors quality and performance in NHS Trusts, is the Commission for Health Improvement (CHI). With the regular monitoring visit of the LSA Responsible Midwifery Officer, plus a visit by CHI, it is understandable that midwifery staff can sometimes feel overwhelmed and over-inspected. In addition to these visits, there will be visits from the Royal Colleges to assess the practice area for medical staff training. The ENB assessed the practice area for the education and training of student midwives, a role that is now to be undertaken by the LSA Responsible Midwifery Officers. This rigorous monitoring means that, from a clinical governance perspective, there can be confidence in the standard of care provided in each maternity unit.

NICE is a government-appointed body that sets standards and guidelines for clinical practice in all specialties. At the time of writing, two sets of guidelines have been published that dictate practice for midwives and obstetricians. The first covers electronic fetal monitoring and the second the induction of labour. Supervisors of midwives have a role here in ensuring that midwives implement these guidelines.

The former has created problems for some midwives who feel insecure if they do not undertake CTG monitoring on every woman admitted in labour for at least 20 minutes, and supervisors of midwives have had to support midwives through a change of practice that will enhance woman-centred care, rather than medicalising a problem-free labour.

Policies, protocols and guidelines

Many maternity units will have protocols, policies and guidelines in place to govern the way in which care should be provided. These terms sometimes lead to confusion, and may be used interchangeably.

A *protocol* is a written system for managing care that should include a plan for audit of that care. Ballière's midwives' dictionary (Tiran 1997) describes a protocol as 'a multidisciplinary planned course of suggested action in relation to specific situations'; protocols determine individual aspects of practice and should be researched using the latest evidence. Most protocols are binding on employees as they usually relate to the management of consumers with urgent, possibly life-threatening, conditions (Beresford 1999). A protocol may exist for the care of women with antepartum haemorrhage, but not for the care of women in labour without complication. If midwives work outside a protocol they could be considered to be in breach of their employment contract.

Guidelines, or *procedures*, are usually less specific than protocols and may be described as suggestions for criteria or levels of performance that are provided to implement agreed standards (see Ch. 52).

Policies are general principles or directions; they are usually without the mandatory approach for addressing an issue, but might be considered mandatory in some NHS Trusts. They are often set at national level, such as the indicators of success in the report Changing Childbirth (DoH 1993).

It is essential that supervisors of midwives ensure that midwives clearly understand the different definitions.

Midwives' contribution to clinical governance

The Midwifery Action Plan (DoH 2001c), written in response to Making a Difference, a strategy for nursing, midwifery and health visiting (DoH 1999), gives the following suggestions (p. 13) about how midwives can contribute to clinical governance:

- auditing and reflecting on own practice
- identifying issues and participating in critical incident reporting
- reviewing and applying the outcomes of risk management reviews to own practice
- making best use of available support from supervisors of midwives.

Using supervision effectively

Partnership

To benefit from supervision, mutual respect between supervisors of midwives and midwives is essential. Midwives should work in partnership with their supervisors of midwives and make the most of supervision (Fig. 51.2) (ENB 1999b), so that it can be effective for not only themselves but also for the mothers and

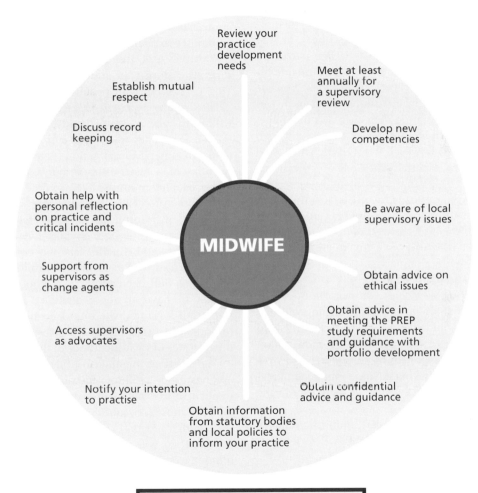

Review your practice development needs

Meet at least annually for a supervisory review

Establish mutual respect

Discuss record keeping

Develop new competencies

Obtain help with personal reflection on practice and critical incidents

MIDWIFE

Be aware of local supervisory issues

Support from supervisors as change agents

Obtain advice on ethical issues

Access supervisors as advocates

Obtain advice in meeting the PREP study requirements and guidance with portfolio development

Notify your intention to practise

Obtain confidential advice and guidance

Obtain information from statutory bodies and local policies to inform your practice

Ask yourself these questions:

How can I contact my supervisor?

How often do I seek out my supervisor?

Do I make the most of supervision?

Would I consider becoming a supervisor?

Fig. 51.2 Making the most of supervision. (From ENB 1999b, with permission of the English National Board for Nursing, Midwifery and Health Visiting.)

babies for whom they care. When supported by a supervisor of midwives, a midwife can practise safely with confidence.

The primary responsibilities of a midwife are to ensure the safe and efficient care of mothers and babies, maintain personal fitness for practice and maintain registration with the professional body (ENB 1999b). The supervisory relationship enables, supports and empowers midwives to fulfil these responsibilities.

Accountability and advocacy

A midwife's accountability is described in the Midwives code of practice (UKCC 1998a, paragraph 1): 'As a practising midwife, you are accountable for your own practice in whatever environment you are practising.' There will be occasions when midwives have difficulty appreciating their own accountability, especially when carrying out the instructions of medical staff. It is clear, however, from all the UKCC and NMC publications, especially the Code of professional conduct (NMC 2002) that accountability cannot be either delegated to or borne by others; it simply rests with the practitioner. A registered midwife is accountable to the NMC as well as to the employing NHS Trust. The dilemmas that this might create can be discussed with a supervisor of midwives for greater clarity and understanding.

When acting as advocates for women exercising their choice, which might not be in keeping with the NHS Trust policy, midwives may wish to seek the help of their supervisor or the supervisor of midwives on call. The supervisor can help by supporting midwives in caring for women, giving advice about documentation and even initiating a review of the policy in the light of new evidence.

Just as NHS Trust policies can inhibit a woman's choice, so too can the availability of services. Examples of this are home births and water births. Women may demand either of these services when the NHS Trust either cannot or does not provide them. Home birth services are occasionally temporarily withdrawn during staffing crises, and some NHS Trusts will not support women giving birth in water. Women will sometimes opt for a home birth when their obstetric history would place them outside the criteria for this. Situations such as these will challenge a midwife's responsibilities, both as a midwife and as an employee. This is another useful time to seek out

the support of a supervisor of midwives to talk through the issues.

Choice

Midwives are able to choose their supervisor of midwives, usually from a list provided by the contact supervisor. A midwife should consider carefully with which supervisors they can form an open and honest relationship, and whether or not there would be mutual respect. The supervisor should also be able to appreciate the environment in which the midwife is currently practising (ENB 1999b).

Midwives prioritised the qualities required in a supervisor during an audit of supervision (Duerden 1995). The results in priority order were: approachable; clinically experienced; in touch and up to date; willing to take action; a good listener; a good role model; a good advocate; wise; empathetic and sympathetic. In Supervision in Action (ENB 1999b, p. 7) the qualities of a supervisor of midwives are listed as approachable; committed to woman-centred care; a source of professional knowledge and expertise; visionary and inspiring; able to resolve conflict; motivated and thorough; articulate; sympathetic and encouraging; and, finally, fair and equitable. These lists make a supervisor of midwives sound like the perfect being, and, realistically, it is impossible for one person to have all these qualities. It is, however, important for a midwife to judge which qualities are important in a supervisor of midwives and to consider the qualities of each supervisor in the proffered list.

The ability to maintain confidentiality is not listed amongst the qualities described above, but it is implicit in the role of the supervisor of midwives. A midwife must feel confident at all times that discussions with a supervisor of midwives will remain confidential. There will always be times when the supervisor of midwives may need to take action in the interest of safety, in which case discussion would take place about the need to share the information. Similarly, the midwife might be encouraged to take the initiative to raise the issue with the midwifery manager.

Support

In the modern NHS, change occurs at an alarming rate. This can be very stressful for midwives, especially if it means a change in practice or the work area. The supervisor of midwives is well placed to advise and guide midwives who are challenged by change, and any concerns that a midwife might have should be shared with the named supervisor. Similarly, the supervisor can act as advocate for the midwife in debate amongst professional groups, especially if the practice being suggested is not evidence-based. At all times, the supervisor of midwives' responsibility is to protect the public and ensure the highest standards of care and professional practice by midwives.

Supervisory reviews

The annual supervisory review should be used by midwives to reflect on their midwifery practice in a confidential arena where aspirations and goals for the future can be shared. Both midwife and supervisor should value the meeting, as this is the opportunity to take time out and consider personal learning needs and professional development requirements in order to achieve goals. Midwives are responsible for meeting their own PREP requirements before reregistering with the NMC (UKCC 1999) and these requirements can be discussed with the supervisor of midwives during the review. The supervisor will probably have information about the NHS Trust professional development budget and will be able to guide the midwife if further academic study is being considered.

This secure environment should provide an opportunity to evaluate practice, and share any practice issues causing concern. If it is felt to be necessary, the supervisor will investigate the matter in confidence and take appropriate action. If a midwife feels that, because of allocation to one practice environment for a protracted time, midwifery skills are being lost, the supervisory review can be used to consider mechanisms for gaining relevant experience in other areas and receiving the necessary professional update.

A midwife may have a particular interest in research or audit. Using the supervisor of midwives as a sounding board can assist the midwife greatly in making decisions, and guidance can be obtained.

There cannot always be a perfect supervisory relationship, but to get the most out of supervision the relationship must have the essential elements of mutual respect and confidentiality. Research by Stapleton et al (1998) clearly demonstrated that midwives who feel empowered by their supervisor of midwives feel in turn able to empower their clients. Being valued and supported by supervisors and having achievements recognised will enhance professional confidence and practice. The supervisory decisions perceived as empowering are those made by consensus between the supervisor and the midwife (Stapleton et al 1998). If this relationship is not recognised by either midwife or supervisor, then the opportunity to change supervisor should be taken by the midwife – possibly with the encouragement of the supervisor of midwives, who will know that there can be no success without the necessary rapport and confidence in the supervisory relationship. It benefits some midwives to change their supervisor every few years, whereas others feel the need for a longer term relationship.

An over-secure relationship should also be avoided, however, as the supervisor is not there to attend to the midwife's every need. At all costs, dependency should be avoided. Midwives are accountable for their own practice and continuous professional development. They should not be seeking out their supervisors all the time, but should recognise that all supervisors of midwives have substantive posts to which supervision is an addendum. For many, this means that much of supervision is carried out in personal time, so demands made on the supervisor should be considered, and arrangements made to meet at mutually convenient times. When the named supervisor of midwives is not available, there is always an on-call supervisor to deal with emergencies.

Box 51.4 is a summary of how to get the best from supervision.

Conclusion

With the support of supervisors of midwives, midwives can expect to practise confidently and competently, but they must value supervision in order to gain its maximum benefit and to receive the empowerment it can provide. The changing role of the midwife, described in this book, highlights the need for support through the change programme. We are privileged in this country to have supervision of midwives, and in that the government has recognised its value and guaranteed its continuance through the changing legislation and development of the new Nursing and Midwifery Council.

Box 51.4 Getting the best from supervision

- Make yourself known to your supervisor of midwives if the supervisor does not contact you first.
- Make sure you know the local arrangements to contact your supervisor.
- Make sure you know the supervisor's specific areas of expertise. Who, for example, can provide advice on issues such as educational opportunities, research evidence, or ethical considerations?
- Discuss with your supervisor your ideas for new approaches or developments.
- Explore the feasibility and opportunities for implementation.
- Alert your supervisor to potential problems at an early stage, so the supervisor is aware of the action you intend to take and can support you.

- Enlist the help of your supervisor to open doors that may be closed to you – for example, when the care you are giving requires cooperation or authorisation by personnel or departments with which you do not normally have contact, such as the Chief Executive of the NHS Trust or the Primary Care Trust.
- Discuss with your supervisor your preferences for your professional development, after you have identified what you feel would best enhance your practice.
- Be aware of the value of discussing complicated issues in clarifying your thoughts and drawing upon your pooled knowledge and experience.
- If you feel unhappy with the advice or action taken by your supervisor, ask to discuss the issue again, or approach another supervisor.

(From ENB 1997, with permission of the English National Board for Nursing, Midwifery and Health Visiting.)

REFERENCES

Chalmers I, Enkin M, Keirse M J N C 1989 Effective care in pregnancy and childbirth. Oxford University Press, Oxford

DoH (Department of Health) 1993 Changing childbirth: report of the expert maternity group. HMSO, London

DoH (Department of Health) 1998 First class service. HMSO, London

DoH (Department of Health) 1999 Making a difference: strengthening the nursing, midwifery and health visiting contribution to health and healthcare. HMSO, London

DoH (Department of Health) 2001a Establishing the new Nursing and Midwifery Council, April 2001. Stationery Office, London

DoH (Department of Health) 2001b Shifting the balance of power Launch of the NHS Modernisation Agency Speech by Secretary of State 24th April 2001. Stationery Office, London

DoH (Department of Health) 2001c Making a difference – the nursing, midwifery and health visiting contribution. The midwifery action plan. Stationery Office, London

Duerden J M 1995 Audit of the supervision of midwives in the North West Regional Health Authority. Salford Royal Hospitals NHS Trust DMI, Salford

Duerden J M 2000a The new LSA arrangements in practice. In: Kirkham M (ed) Developments in the supervision of midwives. Books for Midwives Press, Manchester, p 143, 146

Duerden J M 2000b Audit of supervision of midwives. In: Kirkham M (ed) Developments in the supervision of midwives. Books for Midwives Press, Manchester, p 37

ENB (English National Board for Nursing, Midwifery and Health Visiting) 1992 The supervisor's role in professional development. Module 4, Preparation of supervisors of midwives: an open learning programme. ENB, London

ENB (English National Board for Nursing, Midwifery and Health Visiting) 1997 Module 1, Preparation of supervisors of midwives: an open learning programme. ENB, London

ENB (English National Board for Nursing, Midwifery and Health Visiting) 1999a Advice and guidance to local supervising authorities and supervisors of midwives. ENB, London

ENB (English National Board for Nursing, Midwifery and Health Visiting) 1999b Supervision in action – a practical guide for midwives. ENB, London

Health Authorities Act 1995 HMSO, London

Kirkham M 1995 The history of midwifery supervision. In: Supervision Consensus Conference proceedings. Books for Midwives Press, Hale, Cheshire, p 3

Midwives Act 1902, 1910, 1918, 1936, 1951 HMSO, London

MOH (Ministry of Health) 1937 Circular 1620 Supervision of midwives. HMSO, London

National Health Reorganisation Act 1973 HMSO, London

Nurses, Midwives and Health Visitors Act 1979, 1992, 1997 HMSO, London

NMC (Nursing and Midwifery Council) 2002 Code of professional conduct. NMC, London

RCM (Royal College of Midwives) 1994 Supervision of midwives and midwifery practice. Paper 6. Future practices of midwifery. RCM, London

RCOG/RCM (Royal College of Obstetricians and Gynaecologists & Royal College of Midwives) 1999 Towards safer childbirth – minimum standards for the organisation of labour wards. RCOG, London

Shennan C 1996 Midwives perception of the role of a supervisor of midwives. In: Kirkham M (ed) Supervision of midwives. Books for Midwives Press, Hale, Cheshire, p 169–174

Stapleton H, Duerden J, Kirkham M 2000 Implications of current supervision. In: Kirkham M (ed) Developments in the supervision of midwives. Books for Midwives Press, Manchester

Tiran D 1997 Midwives' dictionary, 9th edn. Baillière Tindall, London

UKCC (United Kingdom Central Council for Nursing Midwifery and Health Visiting) 1993 Midwives rules. UKCC, London

UKCC (United Kingdom Central Council for Nursing Midwifery and Health Visiting) 1994 Midwives code of practice. UKCC, London

UKCC (United Kingdom Central Council for Nursing Midwifery and Health Visiting) 1997 Midwives refresher courses and PREP. UKCC, London

UKCC (United Kingdom Central Council for Nursing Midwifery and Health Visiting) 1998a Midwives rules and code of practice. UKCC, London

UKCC (United Kingdom Central Council for Nursing Midwifery and Health Visiting) 1998b Guidelines for records and record keeping. UKCC, London (reprinted NMC 2002)

UKCC (United Kingdom Central Council for Nursing Midwifery and Health Visiting) 1999 The continuing professional development standard. UKCC, London

FURTHER READING

ENB (English National Board for Nursing, Midwifery and Health Visiting) 1999 Supervision in action – a practical guide for midwives. ENB, London

This useful little book helps midwives to get the most out of supervision. It is very user friendly and explains the supervision of midwives very succinctly from the perspective of the midwife rather than the supervisor of midwives.

Kirkham M (ed) 1996 Supervision of midwives. Books for Midwives Press, Hale, Cheshire

This book contains a comprehensive examination of the supervision of midwives beginning with a fascinating history of supervision and also giving some examples of good practice within supervision.

Kirkham M (ed) 2000 Developments in the supervision of midwives. Books for Midwives Press, Manchester

Following on from the previous book, this edition explores how the supervision of midwives has developed in recent years, describing research and audit of supervision, changes in practice and education and training for supervisors of midwives.

Stapleton H, Duerden J, Kirkham M 1998 Evaluation of the impact of the supervision of midwives on professional practice and the quality of midwifery care. ENB, London

This is the report of a large study of differing models of supervision practised in five very varied geographical areas in England. It describes how midwives evaluated their personal supervision and gives some challenging descriptions from punitive to supportive supervision.

52 Risk Management

Robina Aslam   Sue Brydon

Midwives work in an environment that entails risks to mothers, to babies, to their employer and to themselves. They must understand the basic principles of risk management and how it applies specifically to their practice.

Although its original application in health care lay in an attempt to reduce litigation, risk management is now seen by most practitioners and NHS Trusts as a vehicle for enhancing the quality of client care as part of modern clinical governance.

This chapter aims to:

- discuss the origins and approaches to risk management
- describe the role played by risk management in clinical governance
- outline the practice of risk management in a clinical setting
- give an overview of reporting procedures associated with risk management and, most particularly, untoward incident and near miss reporting
- briefly review the role of the Clinical Negligence Scheme for Trusts.

Although the text is written with reference to UK standards (e.g. the Code of professional conduct issued by the Nursing and Midwifery Council (NMC 2002)) and British professional bodies (e.g. the Royal College of Midwives), the principles are universally applicable.

Introduction

The various meanings of 'risk management'

In the context of midwifery, the term 'risk management' can be used in a number of senses. In its broadest sense, it means a formal process for identifying, assessing and responding to risk so that the decisions taken about childbirth and its associated care lead to the elimination (insofar as is possible) of undesired outcomes and the promotion of desired outcomes. In its narrowest sense, it means 'what an NHS risk manager does'.

Risk management has been used by industry for several decades. In an industrial context, risk management is typically used as part of a company's overall strategy to enhance the quality of the service offered. An airline, for example, needs to ensure that the service it offers is as safe as is humanly possible – in other words, that the risks of harm to passengers are minimal. But it also has to offer a service that is attractive, convenient, comfortable and affordable. Because of the need to strike the right balance between safety, quality and price, risk management is necessarily integrated with other facets of the management process such as quality management. This is an example of the broader sense in which risk management is used. This broader approach – using risk management as part of a broader strategy to enhance the service to the client – is now gaining ground in the NHS. Risk management is coming to be seen as part of a wider suite of processes, collectively known as *clinical governance*.

It is necessary, however, also to be aware that the term 'risk management' is frequently used in the NHS in a much narrower sense. Risk management was originally introduced into the NHS in the mid 1990s with the central aim of reducing litigation risk. As a result, the job descriptions of 'risk managers' were originally drawn up to meet this particular perceived threat and the use of the term 'risk management' is often used to mean what a risk manager does in practice, particularly in regard to reducing litigation risk.

In this chapter, risk management will be examined both as a broad philosophy and in the more restrictive sense in which it is sometimes used in the NHS. As will be seen, these two approaches are rapidly converging – or, more correctly, the narrower approach is giving way to the broader approach. The practice of care in the NHS is becoming much more client/patient orientated and many traditional views about clinical negligence compensation are being reconsidered. Furthermore, it is becoming clearer to clinicians and litigation-funders alike that the best way to achieve the goals of the Health Service as a whole and, at the same time, to reduce litigation risk is to use the available resources to provide the best possible service to the client – risk management should be used positively to deliver that service rather than seeking primarily to counter the threat of litigation.

Risk and the midwife

The Code of professional conduct of the Nursing and Midwifery Council (NMC 2002) provides in Section 8: 'As a registered nurse or midwife, you must act to identify and minimise the risk to patients and clients.' It is essential that midwives take their responsibilities in respect of risk seriously, but midwives must interpret these responsibilities within their own professional context. This context includes the fact that childbirth is, by and large, a reasonably safe and natural process. Midwives are rightly keen to be seen as facilitators of that natural process. Indeed, the government supports this model of midwifery; Changing Childbirth (DoH 1993) placed women at the centre of care and gave them control of the process through informed choice.

Although childbirth is reasonably safe, a number of factors have, in recent years, amplified the perceived risks:

- *Screening tests* – pregnant women were once simply congratulated on the happy circumstances in which they found themselves. Now they are assessed for various risks and offered various screening options. The results of these tests are often expressed in the language of risk (e.g. a 1 in 500 chance of such-and-such an outcome).
- *Litigation statistics* – it is undeniable that midwives work in the department with the highest litigation risk. But again, this statistic needs to be put in perspective. It does not mean, of course, that there are any more incidents here than in other departments. What it does mean is that the compensation payable (which can include round-the-clock care for the claimant over a lifetime) is likely to be much greater than, say, for an accident in a health care of the elderly department.

- *The increasing medicalisation of childbirth* – midwives who promote a natural approach to childbirth work in hospitals staffed by medical practitioners, who tend to apply a medical model of care whereby pregnancy is defined as a potentially dangerous condition requiring close monitoring.

Midwives must use risk management responsibly. In particular, midwives must be aware that the terminology of risk can be disempowering. Clients may see themselves no longer as independent actors but as reliant on 'medical' professionals to steer them safely through a dangerous condition. As Thomas (1998) writes:

> Most women begin their pregnancies full of anticipation and excitement and they value midwives who help them to feel special and unique. This positive feeling, however, can quickly change when, at the booking appointment, the woman is introduced to the concept of risk. As part of her introduction to antenatal care, she will be offered screening tests which help her determine whether her baby is normal. It may never have crossed her mind that the baby would be anything but normal and she has to try and make sense of the meaning of being 'at risk'. Instead of feeling like a unique individual, she may feel more like a statistic; a member of an at-risk population simply because she is pregnant.

Ultimately, the real challenge for the midwife is this: to use risk management as a tool in the planning and provision of safe systems of care, whilst at the same time supporting the view that pregnancy and birth is a safe process for the majority. To do this the midwife will need to understand the risks, using the evidence as it becomes available, and to put those risks into proper perspective. This will enable the midwife to explain risks to the mother in a way that allows constructive debate and decision making without creating anxiety, which in itself can lead to unnecessary intervention.

A brief historical review of risk management in midwifery

The original view of risk management: a response to litigation risk

Approximately 400 people die or are seriously injured every year as a result of medical errors (DoH 2000). The financial costs are also high. The NHS pays out about £400 million annually in litigation costs. Some 30% of this vast cost to the NHS arises from midwifery/obstetric work. Analysis also shows (DoH 2000) that the vast majority of mistakes – probably more than 75% – are caused by 'systems failures'. This means that no one individual can be said to have caused the incident. The real cause of the mistake was a failure of one or more of the following: communication, supervision, checking, staffing levels, equipment, etc.

As a result of such statistics, it was clearly seen that the most significant improvement in health care outcomes could be produced not by new medicines or treatments, but by tightening up on the management of the system, particularly in midwifery and obstetric departments.

Risk management was seen as the key to reducing litigation risk. Since the litigation risk was the mainspring for the introduction of risk management into the midwifery/obstetric context, it was natural that those who developed the early ideas were clinical negligence lawyers and medical practitioners with experience of reviewing legal claims. A consequence of this was that 'risk management' was seen in these early days almost entirely in terms of minimising litigation risk. For example, Clements (1995) suggested: 'Risk management is the reduction of harm to the organisation, by the identification and as far as possible elimination of risk'. Dineen (1997) explicitly links 'risk management' with clinical negligence litigation.

The development of a broader view of risk management: enhancement of client care

Many people – both policy makers and employees of the NHS – were uneasy about risk management, which was designed to protect the 'organisation' (i.e. the Trust) against the 'patient'. As a consequence, an alternative approach to risk management developed – the 'enhancement of client care' model. Aslam (1999), for example, says: 'enhancement of client care, rather than litigation avoidance, should be the principal driving force in implementing risk management procedures'. This alternative approach places little direct emphasis on saving the hospital from litigation; rather, it takes as its starting point the provision of a quality service in the interests of all parties, but especially mothers and babies. It involves balancing risks against opportunities in clinical decisions so that – like an airline company – it provides a safe, satisfying and convenient service.

This latter approach is now broadly supported by the professional institutions as well as the Government. For example, in its Clinical governance advice no. 2 (RCOG 2001), the RCOG says of risk management:

> Others have summarised the aims of clinical risk management as: to reduce the frequency of adverse events and harm to patients, to reduce the chance of a claim being made and to control the cost of claims that are made. This focus on litigation and cost-containment reflects the original, somewhat defensive view of risk management – that its purpose is to protect a hospital from claims, rather than to improve the wellbeing of patients. A more positive and broader view of clinical risk management, reflected in the RCOG's chosen definition, is that it represents one approach to improving the quality of care, which places special emphasis on care episodes with unexpected outcomes and where patients may have been harmed or disturbed. The approach to risk management outlined here reflects this philosophy of using detailed study of adverse events to promote reflective practice and to improve subsequent care, rather than a 'litigation management' approach.

Although the use of the term 'risk management' to describe processes that are exclusively aimed at reducing litigation risk has not disappeared – and, indeed, will not disappear because Trusts must, of course, take reasonable precautions to safeguard themselves from spurious litigation – it is far less common than before. Significantly, even the scheme designed specifically to reduce litigation risk – the Clinical Negligence Scheme for Trusts (described in the following section) – now promotes 'standards' aimed primarily at enhancing client care; it is tacitly and implicitly assumed that reduced litigation risk will naturally and inevitably be a by-product of enhancing client care.

The Clinical Negligence Scheme for Trusts

One of the most significant changes in the structure of the NHS took place in the early 1990s with the establishment of NHS Trusts. The legislation that established the Trusts also required them to meet the considerable litigation costs. In order to manage this most effectively, a system of pooled insurance – known as the Clinical Negligence Scheme for Trusts (CNST) – was established in 1994 and came into effect in 1995–6. It is administered by a special health authority, the NHS Litigation Authority (NHSLA).

The establishment of the CNST was a defining moment for NHS risk management. Although membership of CNST is optional, the vast majority of Trusts did in fact join and so the CNST requirements were, in essence, requirements placed on all Trusts. These requirements were published as standards that participating Trusts are required to meet. The standards were expressed in terms of processes, most of which clearly fell within the general realm of 'risk management'. Thus, risk management was no longer an optional extra for Trusts striving for excellence, but was now a core activity. Indeed, because discounts on the insurance premiums are available for improved compliance with the standards (level 1 is the basic requirement for cover, 2 is good and 3 is the top level of attainment), risk management has become an activity with significant funding implications.

The CNST publishes two sets of standards – a general set for Trusts as a whole and a special set of standards for maternity services. In the introduction to the latest Standards for maternity services (NHSLA 2002), the rationale for this is explained as follows: 'In response to the fact that maternity services in England account for a significant proportion of the number and cost of claims reported to the NHSLA each year, it has been decided to develop risk management standards exclusively aimed at this area … All Trusts providing maternity services will in future be assessed specifically against these standards…'.

Throughout this chapter, reference will be made to the CNST standards.

The modern context of risk management: a strand within clinical governance

The Government has most recently promoted a view of risk management that begins to resemble that used in many other industries: risk management as part of the overall provision of a quality, customer-focused service.

This integrated system for managing health care is called 'clinical governance' (DoH 1999). It originated in A First Class Service (DoH 1998), which sought to put quality at the heart of health care and has been defined as 'a system through which NHS Organisations are accountable for continuously improving the quality of their services and safeguarding high standards of care, by creating an environment in which clinical excellence will flourish' (Scally & Donaldson 1998).

As a result of the Health Act 1999, Trust chief executives are now personally obliged to implement, maintain and improve clinical governance within their Trusts. They are under a duty to identify a clinical governance lead, often a senior clinician. The essential feature of clinical governance is the integration of all those processes that improve client care including:

- improving clinical quality by building on good practice
- development of clinical risk reduction programmes
- the promotion of evidence-based practice
- detection and open investigation of adverse incidence and near misses
- collection of performance data to monitor care and support the delivery of care
- dealing appropriately with poor clinical performance so as to minimise harm to clients, babies and staff
- continuing professional development of staff
- appropriate complaints management
- effective communication between staff, consumers of the service and individual departments.
- consumer involvement in service planning
- health and safety management.

The formal system of clinical governance simply places a responsibility on all to have the appropriate systems in place and to ensure that such systems are effective. It should be pointed out of course that, even prior to the introduction of the current system of clinical governance, midwifery already had systems that operated in that spirit. These include:

- statutory supervision
- the setting of standards
- evidence-based policies and protocols
- research and audit
- consumer participation (the Maternity Liaison Group)
- statutory refresher courses
- mandatory study days and updating sessions.

The professional institutions have all welcomed clinical governance. The Royal College of Midwives' paper Assessing and managing risk in midwifery practice (RCM 2000) says, for example: 'Clinical governance is to be integrated with risk management to raise standards of care. The fundamental aims of this process are to raise standards of care and define best practice, thereby improving quality outcomes. It also has the potential to reduce medical negligence claims.'

The risk management process

Generic model

Many of the principles of risk management are generic; the basic principles apply equally to operating a passenger airline as they do to midwifery. Risk management is often described using a 'process model' such as that shown in Figure 52.1. This model can be described as follows.

Identifying risks. Risks are those factors that may affect our prospects of achieving an optimal result. The types of question that need to be asked are: 'what could go wrong?', 'how could it happen?' and 'what outcomes could result?' (Williams 2002). Information on risk in midwifery can be gleaned from a variety of sources. Personal experience is a relatively uncertain form of data acquisition, despite reflective practice models (e.g. Clements 2000). More reliable will be incident reporting and published surveys such as Confidential Enquiries into Stillbirths and Deaths in Infancy (Maternal and Child Health Research Consortium 2000).

Assess risks. Those factors that generate the greatest risk need to be assessed in order to gain some indication

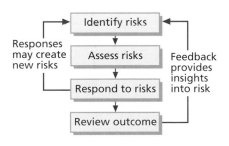

Fig. 52.1 Simple generic risk management model.

of how high those risks are. The risk of an outcome is generally considered to be the product of the probability of that outcome multiplied by the severity of that outcome if it were to occur. Thus, life-threatening outcomes must be kept at very low levels of probability to be acceptable, whereas outcomes such as vaginal/perineal lacerations and short term discomforts may be tolerated at much higher levels of probability.

Respond to risks. In the most dangerous situations, such as a fetus in distress, risk response may be dramatic – for instance by opting for an emergency caesarean section. In less risky situations, monitoring may be required. Responses must be guided by the need to minimise the risks without sacrificing the aspirations of the client; for example, if a client expresses a sincere desire to have a natural childbirth, the midwife should refer to the possibility of medical intervention only when this is becoming increasingly advisable.

Review outcome. As part of an ongoing commitment to improving service, performance is reviewed in order to improve the service provided.

There are two 'feedback loops' in the model. The first (emanating from 'respond to risks') requires the midwife to identify whether the response to existing risk itself has created any new risks. For example, if a drug is administered to control one problem, it may have side-effects, which also need to be risk managed. The second feedback loop involves an input from experience into the way that the individual and team as a whole identify, assess and respond to risks for future clients.

Learning, the organisation and the wider world

There is very considerable scope for learning from practice. Every birth – including each successful birth – has its own unique features and midwives in the team can learn from their own experiences and those of others in the team. The scope for this is practically unlimited; there are more than 100 million childbirths annually worldwide. Tapping into the experiences in all these births requires a significant reporting infrastructure. This is dealt with below in relation to incident reporting and the new National Patient Safety Agency.

Reactive and proactive risk management

Reactive risk management involves learning from one's mistakes. There are, of course, great benefits to be had from learning from mistakes – and the incident reporting programme (described below) seeks to exploit these benefits. However, the generic model presented in Figure 52.1 encourages a more proactive approach. The aim is to identify and manage risks before they occur so as to avoid harm rather than to learn from it. It is sometimes said that proactive risk management helps us to learn from our mistakes without having to make them.

Of course, all midwives should aspire to proactive risk management by continually striving to develop new and better forms of care, subjecting each to a rigorous risk assessment before implementation. But it is necessary also to be realistic and to recognise that many risk factors are well understood only after having caused adverse outcomes. In practice historical data are relied upon to identify, assess and respond to risk. But it is essential always to be alert to identify new risks and to manage them before they become unfortunate statistics.

Guidelines

Although the generic model applies to every situation, and although proactive risk management is desirable, it is nevertheless unrealistic and indeed inappropriate for each midwife (or doctor or other health professional) to consider the application of the generic model in each and every clinical situation. Not only is there not usually enough time to carry out detailed individual assessments in most routine cases, but the individual carer is unlikely to have a sufficient in-depth knowledge of the relevant data to enable them to make full assessments. Therefore, in order to assist carers in their choice of care, guidelines are developed for day-to-day use. These provide a much more efficient and effective way of ensuring that staff act in line with acceptable evidence-based practice.

Guidelines are now drawn up in most maternity units for most critical or common conditions. For those Trusts subscribing to CNST, guidelines are mandatory. The CNST standards for maternity services (NHSLA 2002) require that:

4.1.1 There are referenced, evidence-based multidisciplinary guidelines for the management of all key conditions or situations on the labour ward...

4.1.2 The Trust has a policy on the use of antenatal and intrapartum fetal monitoring which includes guidelines on performing fetal blood sampling

4.1.3 There are clear guidelines for when high dependency care for the mother is necessary...

Some aspects of practical risk management

Identifying risks in a clinical setting

Risks occur in many forms. The following classification is just one way of classifying these risks:

- *Clinical presentation risks* – these include medical, obstetric or social complications such as diabetes, obesity, hypertension, smoking, drug abuse, maternal age and breech presentation.
- *Choice risks* – these include choices made by women such as home birth, caesarean section, and the refusal or acceptance of interventions such as induction of labour.
- *Systems failures* – these include ineffective communication, poor training of staff, ineffective referral or supervision procedures, provision of faulty or ineffective equipment, and poor or inappropriate staffing.
- *Professional misinterpretation risks* – this is failure by a clinician to recognise a problem; although professionals (as in every discipline) sometimes make inappropriate decisions, many situations within this category are equally well classified as system failures (e.g. lack of training or supervision).

Doing risk management: who, when and what?

Risk management is not just for 'risk managers'; it is for everyone. Midwives have informally been involved in risk management since the profession began. The following are examples of situations where risk management principles apply.

Involving clients in decision making. This includes ensuring that:

- clients are fully consulted and involved in decision making
- client preferences are respected.

Identifying risks at an early stage. This is done by:

- a booking history
- screening tests.

Dealing with risks when they arise. This includes:

- properly educating, training and updating midwives
- basing practice upon evidence rather than tradition
- guidelines being made available for all critical and common situations
- ensuring there is a system in place for referring developing situations to senior staff (e.g. a consultant midwife).

A system of feedback. This includes:

- proper reporting of practice whether or not there is any untoward event, together with proper investigation of serious incidents
- audit and review of records
- a fair and responsive system for dealing with possibly unsafe practitioners
- staff reflecting upon and sharing experiences in a no-blame environment so as to create a self-reflective organisation with memory.

A means of managing clients who have experienced an untoward incident. This includes:

- full, timely and open response to any enquiries by the client.

Evidence-based practice and communication

It is important that decisions concerning the management of an individual client's care are made with their full and informed consent (except, of course, in unavoidable emergencies). This frequently means that the risks must be fully and clearly explained to the client. For example, if the woman's inclination is to have a totally natural childbirth, but the fetus is in a breech presentation, the risks and contingency plans need to be explained in a way that:

- addresses all the key issues (i.e. does not simply deal with the carer's preferred plan)
- provides clear advice on the benefits and risks of each option
- supports the decision of the woman, whatever that decision might be.

Clearly this not only involves good communications skills, but also requires that the midwife must fully understand the risks before attempting to communicate them to the client. Understanding of risks requires the midwife continually to update herself and to take a critical interest in research as published to ensure that the information being given is up to date, balanced and appropriate to the context.

The midwife needs also to be able to put risk data into perspective for the client. For example if, following screening, the risk of the baby having a particular condition is '1 in 200', some clients may consider this a remote risk, whereas others may consider it a high risk. Some clients may wish to have a second, more invasive test, which carries a new risk of damaging the fetus and that new risk may also be expressed as a probability, say '1 in 50'. It is difficult for many people to comprehend these probabilities, and to decide what to do. The problem becomes even more acute when the client is in a state of emotional shock; significant communication skills are required by the midwife to ensure not only that the risk data are presented but that their significance is fully understood.

Untoward incidents: reporting and staff issues

Reporting of untoward incidents

Reporting of untoward incidents is a key part of the risk management process. The Royal College of Obstetricians and Gynaecologists' definition of risk management specifically refers to the study of adverse incidents in understanding risk (RCOG 2001): 'It is an approach to improving the quality of care which places special emphasis on care episodes with unexpected outcomes.'

In broad terms, incident reporting is designed to:

- identify the frequency of and the correlated factors associated with adverse incident
- identify systems failures with a view to rectifying them so as to reduce risk
- ensure that teams of clinicians reflect critically on their own performance and that of their team
- develop 'an organisation with a memory' (i.e. one in which common mistakes are learned by all and past mistakes inform future action).

The reporting framework

Effective management requires feedback on performance and, over recent decades, most maternity units have operated reporting systems – with a greater or lesser degree of formality. As a result of the following two factors, adverse incident reporting is now essentially imperative:

1. CNST 'Standard 2: Learning from experience' (NHSLA 2002) insists on a sophisticated reporting system. The key requirements in relation to the forms are:

2.1.1 A system is in place for reporting adverse incidents and near misses in all areas of the maternity service

2.1.2 The incident form gathers significant data about the event … [it then lists out a variety of factual circumstances to be reported]

2.1.3 The incident form contains clear guidance on its completion and subsequent action required. Fact only and no opinion must be recorded … Near misses are to be reported.

2.1.4 Summarised adverse incident forms are provided regularly to the Maternity Services Risk Management Group for review and action.

2. The government (Building a safer NHS for patients – DoH 2001) is now promoting adverse incidents reporting as a key element in its drive to improve patient safety. Building a safer NHS for patients provides what is called a 'blueprint for the new national system for learning from adverse events and near misses'. This is based on the proposals set out in An Organisation with a Memory (DoH 2000). By 'organisation' is meant not just the individual Trust, but the NHS as a whole through reporting back to the National Patient Safety Agency (established in 2001–2), which liaises and interfaces with international bodies and similar agencies in other countries.

According to Building a safer NHS for patients the key drivers for the development of a coordinated national reporting system are:

to address the question of patient safety comprehensively and decisively by:

- Establishing a clear and strong focus on patient safety within the overall NHS quality programme

- Creating an effective system for identifying, recording, reporting and analysing adverse events and near misses in all NHS clinical services...

- Enabling lessons learnt to be available at a local, national and international level so that risk can be reduced and recurrence prevented through changes in practice and in service organisation and delivery...

Incident report forms

Incident reporting forms have developed considerably over recent years. Added impetus comes from the requirements of CNST and Building a safer NHS for patients. Most Trusts have come to the view that a single Trust-wide form is appropriate, not least because it creates a sense of a common interest in reducing risk.

A typical example is the form issued by United Lincolnshire Hospitals NHS Trust. This is shown in Figure 52.2. The following features can be seen:

- The form is in a common style for use across the Trust and is not specifically used for midwifery.
- The incident types are classified.
- Some of the incident types are 'non-clinical' (e.g. thefts and assaults).
- The risk management department assesses whether non-clinical departments need to be informed (e.g. the health and safety advisor, fire safety officer, etc.) and whether 'further action is required', or whether an 'IR2 to follow', or both.

The IR2 is a second standard form – an incident investigation form. This sets out a procedure whereby an 'investigating officer', who may be a midwife in the risk management department, restates the incident facts and the action taken. This action may include:

- recommending new procedures or the enhancement of existing procedures
- general training for staff or specific retraining for the individual involved.

There is a growing body of literature on the analysis of incident report forms to which reference may be made (e.g. Vincent et al 2002).

Incident reporting: concerns of midwives

Risk management procedures such as adverse event and near miss reporting may cause concern to staff,

including midwives. Some may see it as a means for fostering rivalry and distrust amongst staff. However, the Government guidance has been at pains to promote a blame-free approach to reporting.

Adverse incident reporting is, first and foremost, a device for learning about the *system* and seeking to prevent systems failures. For example, Building a safer NHS (DoH 2001) quotes Saul Weingart who says: 'Improvement strategies that punish individual clinicians are misguided and do not work. Fixing the dysfunctional system, on the other hand, is the work that needs to be done.' The report continues: 'To help promote effective use of the system, it needs to be embedded in an open no-blame reporting culture, designed and built in a way that addresses potential barriers to reporting.' Many Trusts are now seeking actively to allay the concerns of staff members about the effect of reporting an adverse incident in which they have been involved. In 2001, for example, the United Lincolnshire Hospitals NHS Trust issued its new incident-reporting policy. The Assistant Director of Nursing for Risk Management and Clinical Improvement wrote (United Lincolnshire Hospitals Trust 2001):

> There has been a change in policy and staff who fill in the adverse incident form (IR1) have to send the form directly to the Risk Management Department for their hospital site and not to their manager first ... We have also just amended the policy to reinforce the message that the Trust wants staff to feel confident that they can inform management when they have been involved in an adverse event and the aim of the adverse incident reporting system is not to apportion blame, but to learn from the experience and improve practice throughout the organisation as a result.

Nevertheless, no Trust can say categorically that no action will be taken. That is simply unrealistic – indeed, a Trust Chief Executive's legal obligation (as part of his or her general clinical governance obligations) is to have appropriate procedures in place for dealing with staff whose performance needs correction. The same article (United Lincolnshire Hospitals Trust 2001) sets out the position in Lincolnshire – a position that is repeated to a great extent in hospitals around the country:

> It is recognised that the fear of disciplinary action may stop staff from reporting an incident. Disciplinary action should not result from a report of an adverse incident, except in one or more of the following cases:

Serial No.		United Lincolnshire Hospitals **NHS**	Confidential
		NHS Trust	

Incident Report Form (IR 1)

➤ Use this form to record **ALL** incidents, accidents and dangerous occurrences

➤ Unexpected death or serious injury involving patients, staff and others must be reported immediately by telephone to the Senior Nurse with site responsibility.

➤ Any equipment involved in an incident must be retained in safe keeping pending further investigation

DETAILS OF INCIDENT

Date: Time: .   (24 hr clock)   HOSPITAL:

Directorate/Division: Ward/Dept/Location:

A) Actual Outcome
- ☐(1) Death or multiple deaths
- ☐(3) Moderate injury/ill health
- ☐(5) Loss/damage of property worth £ ....
- ☐(2) Severe injury/ill health
- ☐(4) Minor injury/ill health
- ☐(6) No injury/ill health/damage or other loss

B) Potential Outcome
- ☐(1) Death or multiple deaths
- ☐(3) Moderate injury/ill health
- ☐(5) Loss/damage of property worth £ ....
- ☐(2) Severe injury/ill health
- ☐(4) Minor injury/ill health
- ☐(6) No injury/ill health/damage or other loss

C) Incident Type (Tick one box)

☐(1) Medical record error	☐(14) Self harm	☐(27) Contact with a hazardous substance
☐(2) Diagnosis error/deficiency	☐(15) Patient absconded	☐(28) Trapped/crushed by something
☐(3) Incorrect treatment administered	☐(16) Tissue damage on admission	☐(29) Electric Shock
☐(4) Error/omission in clinical procedure	☐(17) Tissue damage post admission	☐(30) Struck by a moving vehicle
☐(5) Drug prescribing error	☐(18) Needlestick/sharps injury	☐(31) Asphyxiation
☐(6) Drug dispensing error	☐(19) Cut by sharp (non medical)	☐(32) Fire/explosion
☐(7) Drug administration error	☐(20) Slip, trip or fall on floor	☐(33) Assault by person(s)
☐(8) Consent error or omission	☐(21) Fall from height of ....metres	☐(34) Abuse/threatening behaviour
☐(9) Intentional injury/malicious activity	☐(22) Struck by a moving/falling object	☐(35) Theft/fraud
☐(10) Breach of confidentiality	☐(23) Struck against something	☐(36) Other criminal activity
☐(11) Hospital acquired infection	☐(24) Moving and handling of patient	☐(37) Security incident
☐(12) Equipment/operational problem	☐(25) Moving and handling of a load	☐(38) Hot/cold contact
☐(13) Contact with machinery	☐(26) Blood transfusion incident/error	☐(39) Near miss (specify in D)

D) Incident Description (Give brief details – information must be factual and free from personal opinion)

E) Remedial Action Undertaken or Required (Describe what has or will be done to prevent recurrence) - **IR 2 TO FOLLOW**   YES / NO

ANONYMOUS REPORTS MAY BE SENT DIRECTLY TO THE RISK MANAGEMENT DEPARTMENT
(Please continue overleaf)

Fig. 52.2 Example incident-reporting form. (From United Lincolnshire Hospitals NHS Trust, with permission.)

DETAILS OF PERSON AFFECTED (if applicable)

F) Person is: ☐(1) Patient ☐(2) Staff ☐(3) Trainee/Volunteer ☐(4) Visitor/Member of the Public ☐(5) Contractor ☐(6) Other employee

NAME: Mr/Mrs/Miss

Date of Birth if not a patient

ADDRESS:

Patient Addressograph Label

Postcode .... Tel No.

DETAILS OF ANY INJURY AND/OR TREATMENT (if applicable)

G) Site of Injury: (e.g. lower back, right eye, abdomen, left ankle etc.)

H) Nature of injury:
☐(1) Abrasion ☐(2) Bruise/swelling ☐(3) Burn/scald ☐(4) Laceration ☐(5) Puncture wound
☐(6) Sprain/strain ☐(7) Dislocation ☐(8) Concussion ☐(9) Fracture ☐(10) Amputation
☐(11) Infection ☐(12) Other (specify) ....

I) Treatment: ☐(1) None ☐(2) First aid ☐(3) Resident Doctor ☐(4) GP ☐(5) A&E ☐(6) Occ. Health ☐(7) Other

Is staff absence expected? **YES / NO / DON'T KNOW** **If YES**, give estimate in days .... Days

NAME AND CONTACT DETAILS OF ANY WITNESSES

Person completing form: (Capitals):

Signature: .... Date: ....

THIS FORM MUST BE SENT TO THE RISK MANAGEMENT DEPARTMENT IMMEDIATELY

RISK MANAGEMENT DEPARTMENT

DATE RECEIVED: ....

Is this a R.I.D.D.O.R INCIDENT	YES / NO	H&S Advisor Informed	Date informed:
Is this a MEDICAL DEVICE/EQUIPMENT/PLANT INCIDENT	YES / NO	Medical Devices Agency /NHS Estates Informed	Date informed:
Is this a FIRE INCIDENT	YES / NO	Fire Safety Officer Informed	Date informed:

Further Action Required: YES / NO   DETAILS: ....

IR 2 to follow: YES / NO   Review Date: ....

- Where there have been repeated incidents involving the same individual despite training or other intervention
- Where there is evidence of breaking the law
- Where in the view of the professional registration body the action causing the incident is far removed from acceptable practice
- Where there is a failure to report an incident in which a member of staff was either involved or about which they were aware.

Possible reform

In mid 2001 the Secretary of State for Health announced plans for a White Paper in 2002 (not available at the time of writing) setting out reforms to the system for dealing with clinical negligence.

These plans were prompted by the following:

- the National Audit Office report published in May 2001 (NAO 2001) showing that the NHS paid out 1% of its entire turnover (1% of £40 billion) to lawyers
- the report in July 2001 by Professor Ian Kennedy and others on the Bristol Royal Infirmary Enquiry (Kennedy 2001) recommending an urgent review of compensation systems for those who suffer harm arising out of medical care and – most importantly – a review of the entire system, which is perceived to be defensive and does not allow the open reporting of 'sentinel events'.

These proposed reforms will have an impact on risk management in practice. Risk managers – whose role is already moving away from its original defensive remit – will be further involved in the provision of improved services although the emphasis may turn sharply away from litigation risk (especially if a no-fault compensation scheme is introduced).

Conclusion

Midwives have traditionally seen childbirth as a reasonably safe and natural process. The advent of risk terminology, widespread screening and the increased medicalisation of midwifery has changed matters. Risk is now a key factor to be considered in midwifery practice.

Risk management was first introduced into the NHS as a device for reducing litigation risk. The focus has changed over the past decade and the term 'risk management' is now largely used to mean risk reduction processes for the enhancement of client care.

The CNST was formed in the mid 1990s as a funding body for clinical negligence. Most Trusts have joined the CNST. They must therefore abide by the CNST standards, which contain detailed rules about the risk management processes that the Trust must operate. Maternity services are unique in having their own set of standards.

One of the most visible areas of risk management is that of 'incident reporting'. In this chapter, we have examined some of the requirements laid down by the CNST and the involvement of central government through the National Patient Safety Authority. 'Reporting' is to be done within a culture that focuses on improving the system rather than blaming the individual.

The precise direction risk management will take in the future is somewhat uncertain. The government is currently considering a range of proposals for reforming clinical negligence compensation. One thing that is certain, however, is that risk management will continue to play an important role in delivering a quality health service and that midwives will continue to play a key role in managing risk to provide enhanced client care.

REFERENCES

Aslam R 1999 Risk management in midwifery practice. British Journal of Midwifery 7(1):41–44

Clements C 2000 Critical incident analysis of the third stage of labour. British Journal of Midwifery 8(8):500–504

Clements R V 1995 Implementing risk management: essentials of clinical risk management. Quality in Health Care 4:129–134

Dineen M 1997 Clinical risk management and midwives. Modern Midwife 7(11):9–13

DoH (Department of Health) 1993 Changing childbirth. Report of the Expert Maternity Group. HMSO, London

DoH (Department of Health) 1998 A First class service – quality in the new NHS (consultation document). HMSO, London

DoH (Department of Health) 2000 An organisation with a memory. HMSO, London

DoH (Department of Health) 2001 Building a safer NHS for patients. HMSO, London

Health Act 1999 HMSO, London

Kennedy I (chairman) 2001 Learning from Bristol: the report of the public inquiry into children's heart surgery at the Bristol Royal Infirmary 1984–1995. Command paper CM 5207. Stationery Office, London

MCHRC (Maternal and Child Health Research Consortium) 2000 Confidential Enquiry into Stillbirth and Death in Infancy, seventh report. MCHRC, London

NAO (National Audit Office) 2001 Handling clinical negligence claims. Report HC 403. Stationary Office, London

NHSLA (NHS Litigation Authority) 2002 Clinical Negligence Scheme for Trusts clinical risk management standards for maternity services (June 2002 version). NHS Litigation Authority, London

NMC (Nursing and Midwifery Council) 2002 Code of professional conduct. NMC, London

RCM (Royal College of Midwives) 2000 Assessing and managing risk in midwifery practice (RCM clinical risk management paper). RCM Midwives Journal 7:224–225

RCOG (Royal College of Obstetrics and Gynaecology) 2001 Clinical risk management for obstetrics and gynaecology – clinical governance advice no. 2. Online. Available: www.rcog.org.uk/mainpages.asp?PageID=317

Scally G, Donaldson L 1998 Clinical governance and the drive for quality improvement in the new NHS in England. British Medical Journal 317:61–65

Thomas B G 1998 The disempowering concept of risk. Practising Midwife 1(12):18–21

United Lincolnshire Hospitals Trust 2001 United hospitals news, no. 8. ULHT, Lincoln

Vincent C, Taylor-Adams S, Chapman J et al 2002 How to investigate and analyse clinical incidents. British Medical Journal 320:771–781

Williams J 2002 The tools of risk management and their application to midwifery practice. In: Wilson J, Symon A (eds) Clinical risk management in midwifery. Books for Midwives, Oxford, ch 8, p 109–123

53 Organisation of the Health Services in the United Kingdom

Margaret A. Crichton

The main source of health services in the UK comes from the NHS. The independent sector provides health care for fee-paying patients and companies and is sometimes used by the NHS to reduce waiting times for operations. Midwives need to understand how the NHS was conceived and developed so that they can play their part in shaping its future. This chapter will outline the changes in the NHS from its inception to the beginning of the new millennium.

The NHS was set up over 50 years ago by an Act of Parliament in 1946 leading to its inception in 1948. It is now the largest organisation in Europe. Until recently it was recognised as being one of the best health care systems in the world (Caines 1999, WHO 2001). Health services need constant modification and improvement to meet population needs and expectations in the twenty-first century. Of increasing importance is the interrelationship between health, education and socioeconomic factors such as deprivation. Many of the recent changes in the health service are an attempt to address the wider health environment.

The chapter aims to:

- give a brief account of how the NHS was conceived, delivered and financed and how it became the organisation of health care in the United Kingdom

- describe the new acts and reports affecting the NHS and how these will impinge on midwifery practice

- consider the future to try and envisage how the NHS may grow and develop.

Central Government

The system of government for the UK is one of democracy. Central government is divided into two chambers: the House of Commons and the House of Lords. The UK is divided into 659 constituencies, each of which elects one Member of Parliament (MP) to the House of Commons. Candidates from different parties stand for election in each constituency and the one with the most votes from the public eligible to vote is elected. The House of Commons therefore consists of elected MPs. The incumbent Prime Minister determines which MPs should serve as cabinet ministers and those who will be appointed to more junior posts. These two sets of MPs form the 'front bench' of the governing party, the remainder being called 'back bench' MPs.

A cabinet minister heads a particular ministry or department. For example the Secretary of State for Health heads the Department of Health (DoH). Health matters in Wales are dealt with by the Welsh Office, in Scotland by the Scottish Executive Health Department and in Northern Ireland by the Department of Health, Social Services and Public Safety. (Further details can be found on each country's website in Useful addresses, p. 999.) The House of Lords is made up of peers of the realm, bishops and judges. Peers may be appointed (life peers) or they may have inherited their peerage. A government White Paper on reform of the House of Lords closed to consultation on 31 January 2002 (House of Commons 2002). The reform states that in future the second chamber (i.e. The House of Lords) is to remain as the upper chamber to the House of Commons although its membership will, in the main, be by nomination from the political parties.

It is Parliament that passes legislation on how the country will be run through primary legislation (Acts of Parliament), or secondary legislation (Statutory Instruments) (see Ch. 6 for legislation affecting midwifery). It is these two systems of legislation that govern the organisation of health care in the United Kingdom, though the government of each of the four countries of the UK will decide how best to implement policies for its people.

The civil service

The civil service provides the administrative and executive support to the Government. It is staffed by permanent civil servants and is divided into departments and ministries. Each UK country has a number of chief professional officers including a chief medical officer and a chief nursing officer. Nursing and midwifery officers, all of whom are civil servants, support the chief nursing officer and ministers.

The National Health Service – the first 50 years

Birth of the NHS to 1973

The NHS was the dream child of Aneurin Bevan. He was a politician who had not previously been involved in central government, nor had he any experience of health matters. However, he passionately wanted to provide a free health service for all so that the poor did not have to go without treatment because they could not afford to pay. A system of health care, free at the point of delivery, was set up as a tripartite structure. The three parts were: hospital services, provided by hospital management committees, community services (including district nursing, midwives and ambulances), run by local authorities, and GPs, who were contracted to medical executive committees.

The National Health Service Act was passed in 1946 and became operational on 5 July 1948. It remained unchanged until a new Act in 1973. There were several difficulties with the system, not least of all cost. An increase in National Insurance contributions was insufficient to pay for all health services and general taxation was used to provide for the bulk of the cost. It must have been quite difficult to foresee exactly how much such a system would cost on a day-to-day basis, especially as the Second World War had only just ended. There was still food rationing and the country had sustained much structural damage, there were few building materials and no new hospitals.

The health service grew rapidly from its inception and one of the major changes occurred in 1952 when a 1 shilling (5 pence) charge for prescriptions was introduced by the Conservative Government and there was a £1 charge for dental care.

Major NHS reforms 1974–1990

Since the advent of the NHS in 1948, successive governments have reorganised the way the NHS has been directed and managed. A flow chart of the main reports or acts, their influence and the change they produced can be seen in Figure 53.1. There have been numerous White and Green Papers produced for discussion prior to the actual implementation of the reports, and detailed explanations of these can be found in Ham (1993), Levitt et al (1995) and West (1997).

1974 three-tier management

The NHS continued from 1948 to 1973 largely unchanged, in spite of a number of changes of government, until the Conservative Government of 1974 reorganised the service. This was because of the *National Health Service Reorganisation Act of 1973*. This Act abolished the tripartite system and integrated all health services under a single management structure, though GPs, dentists, optometrists and pharmacists were still contracted to the health service not employed by it. Sir Keith Joseph became Secretary of State and it was he who headed the Department of Health and Social Security.

The reorganisation of 1974 culminated from (a) a review of the medical services (MSRC 1962) chaired by Porritt, (b) a first Green Paper on a unified health service (MoH 1968) chaired by Robinson, (c) a second Green Paper on a unified health service (DHSS 1970) chaired by Crossman and (d) a White Paper on reorganisation of the health service (NHS 1972) chaired by Joseph.

Under Sir Keith Joseph a three-tier system of the management of the NHS was established through regional, area and district health authorities. Community services, which included district nurses, community midwives, health visitors and the ambulance services, were transferred from local authority to health service management. Family practitioner services were organised separately in England and Wales, but not in Scotland or Northern Ireland, a nuance that persisted until the 1990s.

Community health councils, representing the voice of the public, were also made accountable to the area health authorities (AHAs) rather than regional health authorities (RHAs) in order that the users of the service could influence decision making about public services at a local level. Although the three-tier system was retained the boundaries had been expanded in an effort to unify the system and to encourage better communication between the different tiers of the health

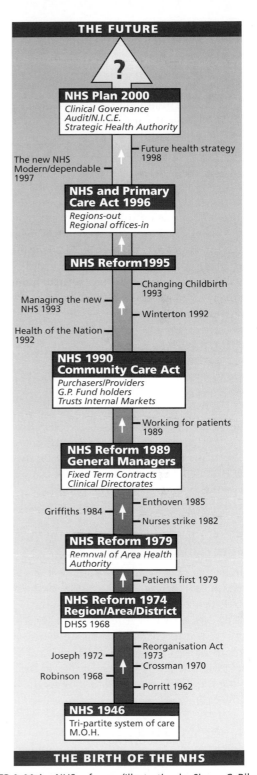

Fig. 53.1 Major NHS reforms. (Illustration by Simon C. Riley.)

care service. The new system was based on population figures, to provide services for communities.

The 14 regional health authorities covering populations of 3.5 million were responsible for the planning of services with two tiers of management below, the area and district health authorities (DHAs). However area health authorities were to move towards a fusion with the local authorities by the setting up of liaison committees, the idea being to coordinate both health and welfare systems.

There were also many critics who felt that the government was trying to play 'nanny' in overseeing the system. As a consequence, community health councils were set up at district level in the hope of making the service more democratic; however, they were not given management responsibility, which limited their powers. The district health authorities were to manage the health services at grass roots level serving populations of 500 000 with a remit to provide an integrated health service for the population they served.

The 1974 reforms were planned by Conservative Government but implemented by the incoming Labour Government. One aim of the plan was to provide district general hospitals with supporting community services. As a consequence many smaller units were closed, as the professions within the NHS demanded that the fullest range of services were required to support the accident and emergency services of the district general hospital. It should be noted that many doctors, nurses and midwives opposed the closure of small units, which provided a local easily accessible service for the community.

Two-tier management, 1979–1983

The incoming Conservative Government of 1979 was swift to set its first reform of the NHS with the publication of Patients First (DHSS and Welsh Office 1979). It was, however, reluctant to disrupt the service totally again as it was estimated that the 1974 reforms had cost more than 9 million pounds (Levitt et al 1995).

The government was concerned that in the 5 years since the introduction of the last reforms the delivery of patient care had not noticeably improved. Patients First (DHSS 1979) was a consultative document, which suggested that the area health authority tier should be removed to allow discussions and decisions about care to be made nearer the patient. An interesting aspect of Patients First (DHSS and Welsh Office 1979)

was that it recognised that the area was the best place to make decisions about health care, but was not the place to manage it, and so AHAs were removed.

During this time there was a great deal happening in the maternity services. The Short report (House of Commons 1980) agreed with the Peel report (MoH 1970) that there should be 100% bed availability for births in hospital. The report recommended that home births should be phased out but the skills of the midwife maintained. In the restructuring, RHAs were to remain in the background to allow the new DHAs to be established in natural communities, which already had good transport facilities. Links with local authorities and coterminus boundaries were desirable but not essential – a complete move away from the philosophy of 1974 when such associations were considered to be of paramount importance.

The intention of a new reorganisation was to reduce the massive cost of running the service, and so the privatisation of some services such as laundry, catering and domestic services was implemented. Although early on both politicians and professionals found the three-tier system unwieldy, it was not until 1979 that the Royal Commission on the NHS presented its report, again to a changing government (West 1997). The DHAs did not actually come into being until April 1982. They were given a great deal of power but service management remained problematic as no named member of the district management team was given responsibility for taking action. The theory of management by mutual consent led to many doctors feeling that they had the right to rule. As a result the Secretary of State commissioned a management enquiry in 1983.

Griffiths report and general management, 1983–1990

The then Secretary of State Norman Fowler asked the Sainsbury's managing director Roy Griffiths to look at the managerial issues of the health service. The published report (DHSS 1983) stated that NHS management was poor, as it appeared that there was no operational head of the organisation at local level. Griffiths advocated that there should be a general manager for each health authority in an effort to create accountable management. This person would have responsibility for making and evaluating decisions taken and be responsible for the smooth running of the whole service. Fixed-term contracts were introduced so that a manager could be removed if there was a failure to meet targets (DHSS 1983).

It became the norm for non-nursing/non-medical personnel to take on the general manager role and this was unpopular with the professions because they were used to being managed by nursing or medical staff. Many such managers were appointed from the private sector or were ex-military. Some critics thought that the then Prime Minister, Margaret Thatcher, was pushed into reform because of the nurses' strike in 1982 (BNHS 1998). Alternatively it may have been because the Royal Colleges were publicly demanding more money for the NHS. Walton & Hamilton (1995) felt that it was during these years that the Royal College of Midwives (RCM) and the Association of Radical Midwives (ARM) set out basic principles of care, which were later encompassed within the Winterton report (House of Commons 1992) and Changing Childbirth (DoH 1993a).

The NHS and Community Care Act 1990

The report 'Working for Patients' (Secretaries of State 1989) suggested further wide-ranging changes. The reforms were embodied in the NHS and Community Care Act (1990), introduced in April 1991, which established an internal competitive market within the NHS. Hospitals were enabled to be self-governing by becoming NHS Trusts and GPs could also apply to be independent. Hospital Trusts could then sell contracts, and were described as 'providers', while DHAs and GP fundholders could buy services, thereby becoming the 'purchasers'. West (1997, p. 22) describes this system of buying and selling care as 'competition without privatisation'.

Levitt et al (1995) and West (1997) have stated that this was the most radical change to the NHS from its inception. Both felt that it was the beginning of the end of the welfare state. The Conservative Government, and particularly Margaret Thatcher, made a concentrated effort to reassure the public that the NHS was *not* going to be 'ripped asunder' but managed more effectively so that funding improved patient care.

Purchasers and providers

By introducing this 'internal market' purchasers could then decide from which providers they would buy services. This altered the status of care, as patients whose GPs were fundholders could have any of their health care outside the NHS as well as from NHS hospitals. It took 5 years for all health care nationwide to come under the auspices of a Trust. In those years there were accusations of double standards of care as not all hospitals were successful in gaining Trust status in the first wave of implementation.

The idea of separating the purchasers and providers of health care was never really understood by users, or many health care workers, despite the money it had cost to introduce the changes. The reason for introducing the change was to try and reduce the rising, some would say spiralling, costs of health care by purchasers being able to buy good quality care from within or outside the NHS for a better price.

Family health service authorities (FHSAs). The 1990 Act disbanded the family practitioner committees of the DHAs, and set up a network of new authorities, the family health service authorities (FHSAs). The main task of the FHSA was to administer the family practitioner services, issue contracts and investigate complaints.

Clinical directorships. Although it was not specifically mentioned in the Act, it was at this time that the concept of clinical directorships became widespread as part of the ways that Trusts organized themselves.

The Health of the Nation 1992

During this time there was an increasing acknowledgement of the importance of public health and the need for greater public involvement in shaping the health services. The Health of the Nation report (DoH 1992) was introduced in an effort to target the main causes of early deaths that were preventable (e.g. coronary heart disease, cancer, mental illness, HIV/AIDS and accidents). This paper was influential in that it introduced the concept of good health for everyone, not just the provision of free health care. Mortality and morbidity rates would be monitored and the causes of early deaths reduced by preventative medicine and education. This was a milestone in the history of promoting the concept of health for all.

During 1993 the DoH produced several papers in an effort to improve services and offer ideas for future change. Changing Childbirth (DoH 1993a) was dynamic in providing opportunities for midwives to implement the kind of care women really wanted from the maternity services.

Vision for the future (DoH 1993b) brought in more of the changes of the NHS and Community Care Act of 1990 and Managing the New NHS (DoH 1993c) highlighted specific changes that would be required in organisation and management to remove the 14 RHAs and bring about the merger of DHAs and FHSAs into health authorities.

The Patient's Charter (DoH 1993d) was brought in by the government, plus a separate one for maternity services (DoH 1994). Both set standards that had to be monitored, for example respecting patient dignity, privacy and cultural beliefs.

The Health Authorities Act 1995 and NHS Primary Care Act 1996

Reorganised tiers of management

On 1 April 1996 the regional health authorities were finally disbanded following the Health Authorities Act 1995. RHAs were replaced by eight regional offices of the NHS Executive. A key difference was that staff in these departments were now civil servants, not NHS employees. Their roles were to monitor the performance of health authorities. They were also to retain the public health function and be responsible for research and development.

The NHS Primary Care Act 1996

This was passed to encourage innovation through more flexibility in primary care. Health authorities were to contract with practices rather than individual GPs.

The New NHS and Making a Difference

In 1997 a new Labour Government came to power with a commitment to abolish the internal market, and in December of that year published a White Paper containing its proposals.

The new NHS: modern, dependable

This White Paper spelled out the promises of the government's manifesto (DoH 1997). The mission was to retain what was good in health care but to eliminate the bad. The separation between planning and

purchasing care was retained; primary care was to be strengthened and management decentralised. GP fundholding was to cease and be replaced by primary care groups (PCGs), which would be teams of GPs and community nurses who would work together to shape services for patients. This was to be achieved by an ethos of partnership to do away with competition. There was to be the setting of national standards through national service frameworks (NSFs) and health improvement plans (HIPs). In time Primary Care Groups were to become Primary Care Trusts and there were plans for health authorities to merge.

Making a difference (DoH 1999a)

This document highlights the importance of good leadership within the NHS. It is rightly assumed that, when change takes place, improvement can only be enhanced with strong leaders at the helm.

People's health needs and expectations of the NHS had altered, technology had advanced and the NHS had to change in order to meet the different needs of the clientele it served. Return to practise courses were given high priority and the government invested a large amount of money in order to help nurses, midwives and health visitors return. New education programmes for all learners were designed and initiated. Some authors had observed that there were students who did not feel prepared to deal with complicated pregnancies and needed more time to assimilate their skills (Fraser et al 1997, Maggs & Rapport 1996). More modern career pathways were instigated with new positions such as consultant midwife posts.

The quality of care was to be enhanced. The introduction of clinical governance and audit were the forerunners to setting standards of care, which could then be used to audit performance.

Midwives' role in public health

The expansion of roles, particularly into public health, was clearly seen in midwifery. The escalation of teenage pregnancies in the UK was alarming, as highlighted in 1999 by the Prime Minister when he launched the Social Exclusion Unit's report, 'Tackling Teenage Pregnancy' (DoH 1999b). It became clear that midwives needed to expand their public health role. The change required better use of midwifery skills, better partnerships in schools with school nurses and health visitors to support good lifestyles, safe sexual practices and the responsibility of parenting. Midwives were also expected to work more with disadvantaged groups (e.g. non-English-speaking women, drug users, those with mental illness and women in deprived or violent home situations). Midwives need to be enabled to meet women's needs, as was evident in the Kath Locke Centre project (Ferguson & Thomson 1999). Midwives are also actively participating in Sure Start schemes (DFEE 1999; see also Ch. 50).

The NHS Plan (England)

July 2000 saw reform of the NHS on a massive scale, with publication of the 'NHS Plan' (DoH 2000). All four countries of the United Kingdom were required to produce their own plans developed from the same central principles. The plan is thought to be the most radical reform of the NHS since its inception. Over the next 10 years the government intends to have measures in place to put patients and people at the centre of the health service by increasing funding by over 6.3% in the years to 2004.

Aims of the plan

The plan is about investment and the reform is built around the needs of patients, who must have more say in their own treatment and be able to influence the way the NHS works. For the first time, patients will not only have a say but they will have power. The intention is to have more medical consultants to increase productivity with increased payments and more doctors, nurses, midwives and health visitors. There will be targets for much shorter waiting times for hospital and GP appointments.

It is anticipated that there will be more hospital beds, cleaner wards, better food and facilities in hospitals, with national equality targets. Improved care for the elderly will be a priority and, most importantly, the NHS will still be free at the point of delivery. The main tasks of the plan are that power will devolve from government to local health services and there will be new relationships between the NHS and the DoH.

Modern contracts for all doctors, both in general practice and in hospitals, will be implemented and NHS staff will have greater opportunities to extend roles, with increased funding for training and improving skills.

For the first time there will be proactive contracts with private investors to supply services and set targets for those conditions that cause the highest morbidity and mortality amongst people.

The DoH will set national standards matched by regular reviews by the Commission for Health Improvement (CHI). The National Institute of Clinical Excellence (NICE) is charged with ensuring that effective clinical interventions are available throughout the NHS, and the Modernisation Agency will spread best practice through regional and local boards. New Care Trusts have been formed between the NHS and social services and there will be leadership centres to train managerial and clinical leaders for the tasks ahead.

The government's intention is to bring about improvements in the NHS workforce, in the quality of health care, reducing inequalities, promoting public health, investment in facilities and information technology.

Shifting the balance of power

From 1 April 2002 half a century of centralised health care drew to a close. The day-to-day management of the NHS moved from the 95 health authorities to 28 strategic health authorities (SHAs). These are the local headquarters of the NHS and their main functions are to coordinate and monitor local health services, build capacity and support performance improvement. The real power and resources will move to the frontline of health care as Primary Care Trusts (PCTs) will hold the majority of the NHS budget and be free to commission care with providers increasingly informed by patient choice (DoH 2001a).

PCTs are free-standing, legally established statutory bodies accountable to their SHA and are key NHS organisations in partnership with NHS acute hospitals Trusts, workforce development confederations and others. The four regions of the country – North, South, Midlands/Eastern and London – each have a Directorate of Health and Social Care. Lobbying by regional and Trust nurses has ensured a nurse appointment at directorate level. The staff will however be less involved locally than were the former regional office staff as they will be engaged in the overall management of services and project management. They will only intervene if the SHAs are failing in their responsibilities.

Implementation of the plan

The vision of the plan is to provide a service designed and built around patients and will provide a framework for reviewing HIPs, primary care, investment plans, service and financial agreements and joint investment plans.

Modernisation agency

All targets and milestones will be monitored by the Modernisation Agency. The first Director, David Fillingham, believes that the Agency belongs to the NHS and the staff working within it. The proposal is that in the first 10 years an entire modernisation movement will occur, which will engage everyone working in the service. Guidance has been issued on local modernisation reviews and the power to be released to frontline staff who, in conjunction with service users, will develop local services.

The Agency will identify problems, and help those Trusts that are struggling, share good practice and train staff. The greatest aim is to see the service through the eyes of patients. The remaining health authorities will take over the responsibilities of NHS regional offices and be accountable for the management of local health care systems. There will be partnership between the Agency, regional offices and the Commission for Health Improvement.

NHS and social services care trusts

Further support to the NHS plan will be provided through the Health and Social Care Act 2001, which will deal mainly with long term care issues. Crucial changes will be made to NHS funding, creating new opportunities for investment in the health service. Local health authorities will have new powers to manage local health economies. Demarcations between health and social care will be removed.

The Plan for Scotland, Wales and Northern Ireland

Each member country will make its own interpretation of the plan and produce a document based on the concepts of the original plan. Scotland's plan for modernisation is called 'Our national health: a plan for action, a plan for change' (NHS Scotland 2000). The document is very similar to the English plan but addresses some of the issues peculiar to the geography and people of the country. One of their targets for action is to increase the number of breastfeeding mothers at 6 weeks' postnatal to 50% by 2005. Parenting skills schemes known as 'Starting Well, Sure Start Scotland' are aimed at reducing incidents of postnatal depression and domestic violence – areas in which it is thought midwives can help. Further information can be accessed on the website www.scotland.gov.uk.

The Welsh response to the plan is again very similar. One of the midwifery targets is that midwives will be able to update their skills continuously to bring about change. There will be new career structures and new strategies for recruiting and retaining staff. The Welsh website can be accessed at www.wales.gov.uk.

In Northern Ireland the plan has not yet been implemented but consultation is under way with all interested parties. So far one major theme is that midwives should be using evidence-based practice in their work. The website for further information is www.niassembly.gov.uk.

The next few years will be interesting, not only in reviewing each of the plans, but also to see what the audits reveal of the changes within the service and whether they can demonstrate if the objectives have been met.

Delivering quality standards

The Commission for Health Improvement is a non-departmental public body covering England and Wales. It was established under the Health Act 1999 and its associated regulations and started operating in April 2000. The commission is independent of the government but has statutory powers. Its aims have been to improve the quality of patient care by assisting the NHS to address unacceptable variations and ensure consistently high standards of care.

- CHI works with Trusts to ensure that patients receive the highest standards of care.
- CHI gathers information over a 24 week period from a wide variety of sources, staff, patients, GPs and any other related sources.
- In every Trust and health authority, clinical governance reviews will be undertaken every 4 years.

Investigation by CHI should be a positive experience looking into major systems failures within the NHS.

The overall service is assessed and the subsequent report identifies where services can be improved. CHI's intention is to lead, review and assist health care systems and in time become a collection point for good practice, which it will share with the rest of the NHS. It is not about apportioning blame – it is there to help by publishing summaries of all reviews and investigative reports, which are available on the CHI website www.chi.nhs.uk/eng. After only 2 years since CHI was established the government announced that it will legislate to create a new health inspectorate called the Commission for Healthcare Audit and Inspection (CHAI) to replace CHI. Its remit will be to inspect not only the NHS, by taking over the functions of CHI, but also private health care.

There is also a very important point to remember, that improvements do not always cost money: they can be achieved by treating each other with respect and dignity. A first class service (DoH 1998) was a consultation paper dealing with the delivery of quality standards within the NHS. In the new plan this is again highlighted and it is the intention of the government to ensure that clear national standards for service care are supported by evidence-based guidance to raise quality standards. NICE will provide clear, consistent guidance for clinicians based on the expertise of professionals, NHS managers and service users. NICE will assess both existing and new interventions for clinical and cost effectiveness and produce and disseminate techniques to support frontline staff. Patients will be able to make use of that guidance through new technology available to the NHS.

National service frameworks have been set up so that patients will know what to expect in areas of major concern or disease groups. These can be viewed as 'blueprints' for how care should be provided and are a key component of plans to tackle inequality of service across the country.

To ensure that quality standards are consistent in local practice there will be a new system of clinical governance. In order to help NHS staff deal with change, there will be increased opportunities for lifelong learning to maintain and develop skills, overseen by modern self-regulatory systems. Education and training should be multidisciplinary to aid clinical team working (DoH 2001b).

Professional self-regulation must instil confidence in the public over the standards and conduct of health professionals. It must act swiftly and openly when things go wrong. The NHS is a public service accountable to both users and taxpayers for providing value for money. To assess what matters to patients a new national framework for assessing performance will judge how each part of the NHS is performing in delivering services.

The focus will be on key areas: health improvement, effective delivery of care, fair access to services, patient and care experiences and health outcomes of care. This is reinforced with a White Paper addressing inequalities in health 'Saving lives: our healthier nation' (DoH 1999c) aimed at not only improving health but also to reduce any inequalities. Community health councils are facing a period of transition as new arrangements are made subject to legislation. A document entitled 'Involving patients and the public in healthcare: a discussion document' (DoH 2001a) outlines proposals to abolish the community health councils (CHCs). It is proposed that these will be replaced by a variety of methods such as patients' forums, patients' councils and scrutiny committees who will provide a voice for local people to express their views on the NHS as well as monitor local health services. From 1 April 2002 all Trusts were required to have patients' advice and liaison services (PALS) whose staff will act as patient advocates (www.doh.gov.uk/involvingpatients/listening.htm).

Fitness for practice (UKCC 1999) was a report that highlighted the question of balance between theory and practice in training. Since the early 1980s, when nursing and midwifery education moved into higher education, this important point had been raised. The placement areas are affected by staffing levels and motivation of the staff to teach students. Partnership between education and practice is as important today as it ever was (Collington 2001). The recommendations of the report make it clear that a flexible innovative programme must be available in all four countries within the United Kingdom in order to achieve balance between education and practice and help the newly qualified nurses and midwives become competent to practice.

Implications for maternity services

The NHS plan is a radical reform of a service that is preparing for the twenty-first century, trying to maintain what is good and workable and changing the things that have not worked in the past.

The government have promised increased NHS spending and that may well indicate more doctors, midwives and nurses to help reduce some of the stress in certain areas. It has introduced an element of competition between Trusts, an audit system that will measure standards and publish findings. It has committed itself to improving facilities for patients and staff and allowing more money for training of staff and extra facilities for an improved environment. The better Trusts will be rewarded and have a greater say in the assessing and supporting of the poor Trust performers. There will be clearer lines of promotion for midwives, occupational health facilities and child care provision will be more available and accessible to working midwives.

In the main, it will mean that the emphasis is on partnership. Throughout the plan the theme is on renewed partnerships within the various services. Midwives will be expected to increase their role in clinical tasks, to lead care, make referrals to consultants and discharge or transfer women to community care. Since the closure of isolated GP maternity units following the Peel report (MoH 1970), there has been public pressure and government support for local midwife-led birthing centres (see Ch. 3). A greater involvement in public health is also highlighted with emphasis on child health services and Sure Start projects (DFEE 1999).

From the patients' perspective, women are better informed. Much information is now available online; NHS Direct Online gives 24 hour cover including information on midwifery matters. The complaints procedure is continually being reviewed. All patients using the services will be asked to assess their treatment/management as an audit tool and all difficulties encountered addressed by the providers of care.

Midwives in action plan (ENB 2001)

A resource has been produced to enable midwives to develop their skills further in both leadership and public health roles, which are key to Making a Difference (DoH 1999a) and the success of the Midwifery Action Plan. It has been developed by a group of expert midwives along with former English National Board officers. Midwives will be encouraged to step outside their traditional boundaries, to think and work for the interests of women in a holistic way (ENB 2001).

Conclusion

The NHS plan is a massive undertaking and it will be some time before all the ideas bear fruit, and still more time for them to be adequately audited. This radical reform is an effort to improve the service and to make it cost effective not only for the people who use it, but for those who work in it. It will be constantly assessed and audited and it will be very interesting to see whether it does achieve its objectives. In midwifery the report entitled Vision 2000 (RCM 2000) echoes many of the concepts in the NHS plan, such as partnership, leadership and continuity of care.

Roch urged in 1996 that midwives *must* be politically aware, understand legislation and be proactive in encouraging good practice. Midwives must have knowledge and understanding of what women want and what we as midwives give them in order to be instrumental in gaining the most well-researched, evidence-based practice available to enhance care. Midwives need to be assertive in obtaining that information and be political in their endeavours to take advantage of the offer to contribute to the programme of NHS reform (the NHS Plan, DoH 2000). To echo the sentiments of Karlene Davis (RCM 2000), midwifery care stands at a crossroads. Midwives can take this golden opportunity and make a difference to the care we give because we *have* contributed to a better, safer, cost effective service.

REFERENCES

BNHS (British National Health Service) 1998 Can it survive? Online. Available: www.trauma-illness.com

Caines K 1999 In: Holdaway K, Kogan H (eds) Healthcare management handbook. Institute of Health Service Management, London

Collington V C 2001 The 3rd Zepherina Veitch lecture: prepared for practice. Midwives Journal 4(8):250–253

DFEE (Department for Education and Employment) 1999 Sure Start. DFEE, London

DHSS (Department of Health and Social Security) 1970 The future structure of the NHS. White Paper (chairman Crossman) (separate Welsh report). HMSO, London

DHSS (Department of Health and Social Security) 1983 NHS management enquiry (chairman Griffiths). DHSS, London

DHSS (Department of Health and Social Security) and Welsh Office 1979 Patients first. HMSO, London

DoH (Department of Health) 1989 Working for patients. HMSO, London

DoH (Department of Health) 1992 The health of the nation. A strategy for health in England. HMSO, London

DoH (Department of Health) 1993a Changing childbirth: report of the Expert Maternity Group parts 1 and 2. HMSO, London

DoH (Department of Health) 1993b Vision for the future. HMSO, London

DoH (Department of Health) 1993c Managing the new NHS. Management Executive letter EL(93)72. DoH, London

DoH (Department of Health) 1993d The patient's charter. HMSO, London

DoH (Department of Health) 1994 The patient's charter: The maternity services. HMSO, London

DoH (Department of Health) 1997 The new NHS: modern, dependable. Stationery Office, London

DoH (Department of Health) 1998 A first class service. Quality in the new NHS. HMSO, London

DoH (Department of Health) 1999a Making a difference: Strengthening the midwifery and health visiting contribution to health and healthcare. DoH, London

DoH (Department of Health) 1999b Tackling teenage pregnancy. Social Exclusion Unit report. DoH, London

DoH (Department of Health) 1999c Saving lives: our healthier nation. DoH, London

DoH (Department of Health) 2000 NHS plan: a plan for investment, a plan for reform. DoH, London

DoH (Department of Health) 2001a Involving patients and the public in healthcare: a discussion document. DoH, London. Online Available: www.doh.gov.uk/involvingpatients/listening.htm

DoH (Department of Health) 2001b Shifting the balance of power in the NHS: securing delivery. DoH, London

ENB (English National Board) 2001 ENB News, October. ENB, London

Ferguson, K Thomson A M 1999 An evaluation of the Kath Locke maternity project. School of Nursing, Midwifery and Health Visiting, University of Manchester

Fraser D, Murphy R, Worth-Butler M 1997 An outcome evaluation of the effectiveness of pre-registration midwifery programmes of education. ENB, London

Ham C 1993 The new national health service. Radcliffe Medical Press, Oxford

Health Act 1999 Stationery Office, London

Health and Social Care Act 2001 Stationery Office, London

Health Authorities Act 1995 HMSO, London

House of Commons Social Services Committee 1980 Perinatal and neonatal mortality: second report from the Social Service Committee (chairwoman R Short). HMSO, London

House of Commons 1992 Health Committee, second report. Maternity services (chairwoman N Winterton). HMSO, London

House of Commons 2002 House of Lords reform. The government White Paper on House of Lords reform – completing the reform. HMSO, London

Levitt R, Wall A, Appleby J 1995 The reorganised NHS. Chapman & Hall, London

Maggs C, Rapport F 1996 Getting a job and growing confidence in the dual experience of newly qualified midwives prepared by the pre-registration route. Nursing Times Research 1(1):68–78

MSRC (Medical Services Review Committee) 1962 A review of the medical services in Great Britain (chairman Sir A Porritt). Social Assay, London

MoH (Ministry of Health) 1968 The administrative structure of medical and related services in England and Wales. Green Paper (chairman Robinson). HMSO, London.

MoH (Ministry of Health) 1970 Domiciliary midwifery and maternity bed needs: the report of the Standing Maternity Advisory Committee (chairman Peel). HMSO, London

National Health Service Act 1946 HMSO, London

National Health Service Reorganisation: England 1972 White Paper (chairman K Joseph). HMSO, London (separate Welsh report)

National Health Service Reorganisation Act 1973 HMSO. London

NHS (National Health Service) Scotland 2000 Our national health: a plan for action, a plan for change. Scottish Executive Health Department, Edinburgh, Scotland. Online. Available: www.scotland.gov.uk/library3/health/onh.pdf

NHS and Community Care Act 1990 HMSO, London

NHS Primary Care Act 1996 HMSO, London

RCM (Royal College of Midwives) 2000 Vision 2000. RCM, London

Roch S 1996 Equal opportunities for midwives – too much to ask? Modern Midwife 6(3):4–5

UKCC (United Kingdom Central Council for Nursing, Midwifery and Health Visiting) 1999 Fitness for practice: the UKCC Commission for Nursing and Midwifery Education (chairman Sir L Peach). UKCC, London

Walton I, Hamilton H 1995 Midwives and Changing childbirth. Books for Midwives, Hale, Cheshire

West P A 1997 Understanding the National Health Service reforms. The creation of incentives? Oxford University Press, Buckingham

WHO (World Health Organization) 2001 Online. Available: www.who.int/health-services-delivery

USEFUL ADDRESSES

CHI www.chi.nhs./uk/eng
DoH www.doh.gov.uk
NHS www.nhs.uk
NORTHERN IRELAND www.niassembly.gov.uk

RCM www.rcm.org.uk
SCOTLAND www.scotland.gov.uk
WALES www.wales.gov.uk
WHO www.who.int/health-service-delivery

54 International Midwifery

Della Sherratt

CHAPTER CONTENTS

The chapter outlines the issues and agendas facing midwifery from an international perspective. Its focus is on the major events and global issues that have helped raise the profile of midwives and their profession.

The chapter aims to:

- consider the issues facing midwifery in different cultural settings and the practicalities of midwives working outside their own country

- describe the major international events and organisations relevant to midwifery, in particular the International Confederation of Midwives (ICM), the global Safe Motherhood Initiative (SMI) and the Baby Friendly Hospital Initiative (BFHI)

- outline some of the issues facing midwives in other countries, their education and working conditions and highlight some of the main barriers to providing quality midwifery care.

In such a short chapter it is not possible to give an in-depth analysis of the global situation, nor describe in detail midwifery in every country. When reference is made to the situation in a named country, it is as an example to assist understanding and not to criticise the midwives working there. The aim is to increase understanding and foster a sense of unity and respect for a shared philosophy that underpins the profession, despite the different models, health or education systems in use throughout the world.

Introduction

Today, the effects of globalisation mean that, more than at any other time in history, the issues and problems of the world increasingly find their way into both the workplace and the home. As in other professions, an increasing number of midwives today choose to spend part of their professional career in another country. Others find themselves in other countries for a variety of reasons, such as accompanying their partners, etc. In addition, demographic shifts and ageing populations have led to workforce shortages, especially in the public sector and acutely the health sector. One of the strategies to fill such a shortage has been to recruit health workers from other countries. Additionally, the increased global focus on safe motherhood has resulted in increased opportunities for midwives to be active in international projects and initiatives. Finally, the last decade has uniquely seen unprecedented massive population shifts and displacements due to natural disasters or conflict. Sudden and often unexpected population shifts frequently result in calls for assistance from health care staff from other countries, as the receiving countries often do not have spare capacity to meet this increased demand. The rise in migration of staff across nations is one of the major issues currently facing health service planners in a number of countries. For whatever the reason, more midwives than in previous years will at some time in their working career find themselves working in another country with different cultures, traditions and resources. On moving to this new environment some midwives may find themselves initially ill at ease and overwhelmed by their experience, despite having developed a high level of professional expertise in their own country. Sadly, preparation for this area of practice often remains poor. This chapter will first try to explore some of the issues as well as practicalities of working in another country, as well as working in an international setting, then will try to outline some of the current international agendas. It aims to be of benefit to those who wish to explore this field of practice, as well as those who would just like to know what is happening to midwifery globally.

The practicalities of working in another country

Before departure

One of the first practical issues to address is obtaining permission to work and ensuring that the correct visa is obtained. This can be difficult as many countries have stringent regulations for issuing work visas and it may be necessary to produce an official letter of invitation from the employing agency or company. Without the correct documents and letter of invitation, it can be complicated to gain entry into the country and obtain permission to stay and work there; therefore it is always advisable to check the requirements carefully. Most embassies or consulates will provide the necessary information and advice on documentation needed to apply for the correct visa.

Attention to health and personal safety is another essential practicality that must be taken care of before departure. It is essential to have adequate medical insurance cover. Where possible, always ensure insurance cover will allow an unscheduled return home to deal with personal difficulties, as trying to arrange this very quickly from another country can be traumatic. Many agencies or employers will be sympathetic and may include this as a benefit in the terms and conditions of the contract, if one exists.

When responding to advertisements for a specific post, these details should be clarified before accepting the position. Information on necessary immunisations, health precautions and so on is readily available from the WHO. Many countries also have a national travellers' help-line or institution that will also be able to offer advice.

The issues that are frequently least easy to deal with are the actual feeling and psychological practicalities of working in another culture. However, adaptation to working in a different country with different customs, beliefs and traditions can be difficult. Midwives may find such feelings difficult to accept, as they conflict with their internal view of themselves as a capable, flexible practitioner. A great deal of illness, however, can result from the stress of working in such conditions. The potential for such illness needs to be acknowledged by those going to other countries to work, as well as those recruiting staff from other countries. Therefore speaking to and if possible spending some time with someone who has worked in the same area can be very helpful and rewarding. One of the difficulties of preparing for such stress is that it is not easy to predict how well one will cope in a given situation at any specific time. The factors that help adaptation are different in every situation. Experience of working in different cultures and countries can help, but each situation is new and must be seen as such. Increasingly, organisations are providing courses or workshops for health workers who would like to consider this work, to help explore some of these issues before making a definite decision. The International Health Exchange in the UK and the International Red Cross are two such organisations and they provide excellent courses for those intending to work internationally and those wishing to consider it. Information on such courses is often available in quality primary or international health care journals. Also there is an increase in the number of university programmes that include elective periods where a short time can be spent in another country undertaking a small project or work experience.

One factor that can influence adaptation to working in another country is the careful consideration of the motives for undertaking this type of work. More research is required on how and why midwives choose to work in another country, in order to help identify the factors that will assist with their adequate preparation. On the whole, as with all career choices, there are varied and complex reasons why someone would choose this particular path. Some find themselves in a certain place at a certain time, able and willing to respond to opportunities as they are presented. Others have a burning desire to travel and experience the wider world – that is to say, they have moral, humanitarian, personal or family reasons for choosing this particular professional path. Whatever the reasons, it is the responsibility of each midwife to explore carefully her personal motives for choosing this type of work.

There is no one valid reason, only an issue of individual choice. However, midwives must apply a certain level of objectivity to ensure the right choice is being made about the suitability, type, as well as place of work that is appropriate for them. It is all too easy to become quickly disillusioned with the new environment if the main motive for seeking this type of work was travel, but the project or place chosen makes travel difficult or impossible.

Clarification of motives is also helpful when faced with unfamiliar, frustrating or difficult situations. Working in another country, in a culture that is unfamiliar, is very different from visiting on holiday or for pleasure or interest. However, such work does have its rewards. It can help to develop a wider view of midwifery, motherhood and health. It often assists with reflection by allowing the opportunity to view one's own practice through different eyes. Most midwives who have done such work feel that it allows them to develop greater flexibility, innovation and self-confidence. Of course, much will depend upon the type of work undertaken, but the advantages and the friendships that develop whilst undertaking such work often outweigh the difficulties.

Working in a different culture

Recent changes in midwifery practice that foster an individual- or woman-centred approach to care can assist midwives to function in different cultures. The requirement to provide culturally sensitive care is embodied in the International code of ethics for midwives (ICM 1993). *Culturally sensitive care* is care that makes a positive acknowledgement that each woman belongs to a specific family located within a particular society and culture at a particular time, and is discussed in greater depth elsewhere.

The issue facing midwives from another country developing culturally sensitive care may be the difficulty around language and being unable to listen to women, as frequently cultural traditions and beliefs are vocalised in particular practices, taboos, stories and even folk songs. Also in some countries, particularly in Asia, the cultural beliefs and taboos surrounding pregnancy and birth can make listening to women's stories particularly difficult. Frequently myths and beliefs, especially around birth, are not spoken about directly, for fear of evoking bad spirits or bringing bad luck. Just to acknowledge the pregnancy might be viewed as dangerous. This too raises obstacles to the receipt of any midwifery care. For example, encouragement of antenatal care, promotion of health in pregnancy, or even advice on planned pregnancies is problematic in a culture where to do so is unacceptable.

In the circumstances outlined above, the only way forward is to work with the local community, especially women's groups and community or religious leaders. Where such leaders are usually men, this can raise other gender-laden issues. For the midwife there may be tensions in how to work with or through male leaders in a way that will empower women. Here some additional gender training or gender sensitivity courses may help and it is always essential first to identify, together with the women, what existing strategies women have for dealing with such issues. Assisting the male leaders and the community to consider practices and beliefs, and the effects that these may have on childbearing women, is possible, and where this approach has been used it has had positive results.

When working on empowerment issues it is important to remember that notions of empowerment are also culturally bound. Women from different cultures have different ideas about what they see as empowerment (Chitnis 1988, Collins 1994, Dawit & Busia 1995). Given the opportunity however, women from all cultures have clear ideas about what they think would assist them to give birth in a way that is safe and yet culturally sensitive, and therefore acceptable to them.

Use of appropriate technology

In addition to adopting the right approach, midwives also need to concern themselves with the appropriate use of technology. Careful consideration is necessary when taking new technology from one country to another. For example, in many industrialised settings it is no longer considered essential to give iron supplementation routinely to well-nourished pregnant women. In resource-poor countries, however, haemorrhage before, during and after birth remains the major cause of death in countries owing to poor nutrition and social deprivation (Royston & Armstrong 1989). In these situations, faced with high maternal mortality and high levels of undernutrition, it is clearly appropriate to have a protocol that promotes routine iron supplementation to all pregnant women.

Equally, there are problems in training doctors to undertake surgical procedures such as caesarean sections without simultaneously providing good anaesthetics and analgesia, hygiene and sanitation for hospitals that offer these facilities. This is not to say such training should not take place. Clearly the facts show that too many women still die because of lack of appropriate emergency obstetric care, lack of equipment or lack of appropriately skilled staff to use the equipment (WHO 1991a). However, importing systems, technologies and tools that do not get appropriately adapted can adversely affect the quality of care. Although in themselves the tools may be good, if they are not adapted to meet the cultural complexity of the receiving country they may be ineffective, or used in

an inappropriate way. For example, there is almost universal acceptance that the partograph is a useful and effective tool, yet it is not without its difficulties. For midwives working in a country or a culture where the counting of time is not in units of minutes or hours, the idea of charting events on a graph can be very difficult.

There has been some work in simplifying the partograph and a modified partograph is being recommended in the most recent WHO material, Management of complications in pregnancy and childbirth (WHO 2000). However, work is still needed to simplify the tool further for use by those who have conceptual difficulty with time or graphic displays of information. Midwives working in an international arena, therefore, need to ensure that the technology they take with them to other countries is appropriate and that correct training and systems are provided for its effective implementation and use.

The role of the consultant midwife

Beware the 'expert'

Although the above is an issue of concern for all midwives, it is particularly problematic for those working as international midwifery consultants or expatriate project workers, trainers or managers. The temptation to allow oneself to be seen as the 'expert', the one who knows all, is sometimes difficult to resist. In the eyes of the new community, women and local midwives, there is a serious risk of being perceived as or being identified along with the project managers, donors and politicians, rather than being with the local midwives and women. The international midwife will then be able to work as one of the former groups, but may not be allowed entry into local knowledge and systems. The above issues apply to all who work in the field, regardless of cultural or educational background, or even of the position and status or experience of the midwife.

This issue of being viewed as an outside expert is particularly problematic when working in countries that do not have recent experience of personal autonomy or personal responsibility. Midwives in countries that have a particular political tradition of being controlled from the centre are more familiar at looking towards those in power or to those who they see as 'experts' to dictate the actual activities of care provided. They are not familiar with democracy or participation in decision making and may feel slightly afraid or unsure when introduced to such approaches. Therefore locals may initially resist or misinterpret requests, or not respond to opportunities to share their ideas with the newcomer.

Encouraging participation

It is important for the consultant to avoid falling into the trap of being seen as the person who knows all and who will tell the local women what or how something needs to be done. For the consultant faced with enthusiastic individuals eager for change, tight work schedules, needs that often far outweigh resources or expectations that they will be the one to sort out the problems, or all of these, it is not always easy to hold firm to principles of facilitation and participatory approaches to decision making. In these situations, advocacy can easily stray into paternalism (or maternalism) and then only the voice of the 'expert' midwife is heard. The midwife's role is always to encourage women to find their own voice and always to ensure that it is the local women's voice that is being heard; for the international consultant this includes the voices of the local midwives. The key skills for the consultant midwife are listening, supporting and participating in the daily lives and tasks of those they work with, be they receivers of care, or working colleagues.

The midwife working as a consultant in whatever field or country needs patience, humility, a good sense of humour and a great deal of self-determination and self-esteem to carry out the role effectively. The role of the consultant midwife can be lonely; therefore any one taking on this role should ensure that they have a good personal support system from family, friends or long-standing colleagues (preferably ones with similar experiences).

International issues

International Confederation of Midwives (ICM)

The International Confederation of Midwives is now one of the foremost actors in the global arena working to improve maternity services by empowering of midwives through strengthening professional associations

and promoting good practice. The ICM, a non-governmental organisation (NGO), started in 1919 as the International Midwives' Union. The purpose of the union was to 'improve the services available to childbearing women through campaigning for a stronger, better educated and properly regulated midwifery profession' (ICM 1994, p. 1). In the early 1960s the ICM gained accreditation by the United Nations (UN) and works closely with UN organizations especially WHO. It has more than 85 member associations that cover approximately 66 countries; Council admits new members on demonstration they meet the criteria for membership and payment of a membership fee, calculated against the number of midwives in the association and taking into account the economic situation of the country.

The ICM has a small but friendly office that relocated from the UK to The Hague, The Netherlands in 1999. The office welcomes both visitors and enquiries from midwives and midwifery organisations from anywhere in the world. Information on the history of the ICM, along with other information and leaflets, is obtainable from ICM HQ (see Useful addresses, p. 1018). The ICM also produces a regular newsletter free to its member associations, but is available to individuals on payment of a modest subscription.

ICM accomplishments

In recent years, the ICM has been proactive in a variety of global initiatives. By working collaboratively with other agencies, it has contributed to the increasing acceptance of the midwife as the key provider of quality maternity care. Working with WHO and the International Federation of Gynaecologists and Obstetricians (FIGO) the ICM developed the International definition of the midwife, first devised in 1966, the latest revision being in 1992 (WHO/FIGO/ICM 1966, 1992).

Other achievements of the ICM include the development of the International code of ethics (ICM 1993 and revised in 1999) and the instituting and coordination of the International Day of The Midwife (annually on 5 May). Although each country and midwifery organisation may choose to devise their own celebrations, the ICM Board draws up the major themes. The intention is to assist midwives and midwifery associations to unite under a central banner to promote the role and responsibilities of the midwife under a specific theme. Recent themes have included 'safe motherhood', 'equity for women' and 'the midwife as the key health promoter'. Currently ICM are finalising an internationally agreed set of core competencies for a midwife that will supplement the International definition of the midwife.

Perhaps one of the most rewarding accomplishments of ICM is the bringing together of groups of midwives from different countries for workshops, seminars and the triennial congress. The meetings, particularly the triennial congresses, are valuable not only for allowing midwives internationally to meet, debate and network, but also have been a useful vehicle for promoting midwives and midwifery in the host country. The opening ceremony of the triennial international congress with midwives dressed in their national costumes remains a favourite and moving spectacle for all who attend.

Immediately prior to the congress, ICM hosts a collaborative precongress workshop, usually for 3 days leading to the opening ceremony; these too have been extremely beneficial for those attending and for raising certain issues in the international arena. A report of these collaborative precongress workshops, which usually include useful background papers or information and material for the midwives attending the workshops, is always published. Initially these workshops were exclusively on an invitation basis, and were mainly for midwives from least developed countries and in a practical way contributed to capacity-building midwifery. The action orientation of these workshops has allowed midwives from a variety of countries to develop plans and activities for improving the midwifery services to women nationally and globally. The 1990 congress in Kobe, Japan took as its theme 'midwifery education for safe motherhood' and it was at the precongress workshop that the now popular Midwifery modules for safe motherhood (published by WHO in 1996) were first formulated. In 1993, in Vancouver, Canada, the precongress workshop theme was 'midwifery practice: measuring, developing and mobilising quality care', and in 1996 in Oslo, Norway, preparing 'national safe motherhood' plans was the focus of attention. The Oslo precongress workshops also offered, for the first time, a parallel workshop for the preparation of midwife consultants, where midwives could request attendance but on a self-funding basis. This precongress activity ran parallel

to and interacted with the regular precongress workshop working on national safe motherhood planning. The Oslo congress was also significant for the launching of the Midwifery modules for safe motherhood (WHO 1996a). In 1999, the congress was held for the first time in a low resource country, The Philippines. Their colleagues in the Australian Midwives Association assisted the hosting association of midwives. The precongress collaborative workshop focused on HIV, reproductive tract infections (RTIs) and STIs. The theme for the 2002 congress was 'midwives and women together for the family of the world' and the precongress collaborative workshop focused on the role of the midwife in reducing gender-based violence to adolescent girls and women. The congress in 2005 will take place in Brisbane, Australia.

The ICM has been an active participant and influence on the global Safe Motherhood Initiative (SMI) from its outset in Nairobi in 1987. The Confederation endeavours to continue with this important activity by working with WHO, UNICEF, UNFPA, FIGO and other agencies to promote safe motherhood through assisting the development and strengthening of midwifery and midwifery organisations.

Safe Motherhood Initiative

The global SMI was officially launched in Nairobi in February 1987. The global programme is supported by ICM, WHO, UNICEF and the World Bank as well as many NGOs, associations and multi- and bilateral aid agencies.

The aim of SMI was to achieve a reduction of 50% in the global number of maternal deaths by 2000. One of the specific ways in which it was envisaged that the goals of SMI would be achieved was through the development of strategies that enable women to have more control over their lives. This point was further strengthened following the International Conference on Population and Development in Beijing and the UN Conference on Women Platform of Action, Cairo 1995; both of these called for the rights of women to be further strengthened and respected. Various strategies have been employed to achieve the goal of safe motherhood. These include ensuring access to safe water, culturally appropriate family planning services, including advice and methods, and promotion of free prenatal, intranatal and postnatal care and services.

> **Box 54.1** Definition of a skilled attendant
>
> A skilled attendant refers exclusively to people with midwifery skills (for example midwives, nurses and doctors) who have been trained to proficiency in the skills necessary to manage normal deliveries and diagnose, manage* and refer obstetric complications.
>
> ---
>
> * Manage was added following the Tunis conference on skilled attendance at birth, November 2000.
> (From Reduction of maternal mortality: a joint WHO/UNPF/UNICEF/World Bank statement 1999 WHO Geneva.)

Other strategies have focused on improving the sociopolitical and legal status of women, increasing their access to wealth and ending gender decimation, especially in education and access to health care.

More recently, strategies have focused on the calls for ensuring all women have access to a 'skilled attendant' at birth. A skilled attendant is seen as someone with midwifery skills (Box 54.1); to most people this is a professional midwife, someone who has the competency for provision of normal care, is able to manage or initiate first line care for emergencies and is linked to a facility where specialist obstetric and neonatal care is available. The call for skilled attendant for all came about as result of the failure of the 'risk approach' to antenatal care to demonstrate the ability to reduce maternal mortality. Criticism of the risk approach strategy for reducing maternal mortality, whereby pregnant women identified as having risk factors were provided with specialist obstetric care, focused around the lack of specificity, sensitivity and predictability of the risk factors used. As Maine (1990) and others have demonstrated the risk approach has limitations: that even though we know that some women with certain histories and medical conditions, etc., have a potentially higher risk than others of developing a complication, research shows that a significant proportion of life-threatening problems occur in women identified as being at low risk using most of the risk-scoring systems. Consequently, reductions in maternal mortality can be achieved only if all pregnant woman have access to a skilled attendant and emergency obstetric care. The same is true when considering reductions in

perinatal mortality and morbidity. A historical review of the literature supports what Loudon (2000) and others found: that only countries that have strengthened access to skilled care in pregnancy and during childbirth have managed to reduce their maternal mortality significantly. This evidence was presented and discussed during an intentional consensus meeting held in Tunis in 2000. The result of this consultation has been to sharpen the focus and call for skilled attendance for childbirth. Skilled attendance is seen as the presence of a health practitioner with midwifery skills and an enabling environment where systems are in place to allow the practitioner to provide skilled care; these systems include a regular safe supply of drugs and equipment, as well as supportive supervision, and close links for easy referral to a facility able to offer higher level medical obstetric and neonatal services, amongst others (Graham et al 2001).

Although the initial focus of SMI was only maternal mortality, in recent years this focus has shifted slightly and is now on women's health and reproductive health for all, especially adolescents. Today, through the human rights approach, there is also concern for morbidity. Studies in India and Bangladesh give morbidity rates as high as 15 to 16 times that of mortality rates (Goodburn 1995). A great deal of the morbidity was found to be due to unsafe and unhygienic practices based on superstitions and taboos, such as putting mustard oil into the vagina to try to hasten cervical dilatation and ensure a speedy exit through the birth canal, or use of excessive fundal pressure to deliver the placenta, in the belief that it is the placenta that harbours or attracts the evil spirits.

Many of the global activities around safe motherhood can be found in the Safe Motherhood Newsletter, available free of charge from the Department of Reproductive Health and Research at WHO Headquarters in Geneva (see Useful addresses, p. 1018).

Major global actions under the safe motherhood banner

- *1987* – The Safe Motherhood Initiative was launched in Nairobi.
- *1989* – The first global study on maternal mortality was published (Royston & Armstrong 1989) and WHO's global factbook on maternal mortality (WHO 1991b). The factbook is a compendium of

data collected from all over the world. Both are available from WHO, Geneva.

- *1987* – The partograph, a tool for effective monitoring of labour, was launched. In 1990 to 1991 a large multicentre trial was undertaken to review the effectiveness of this tool, with reasonably positive results. The report concluded that the tool had potential benefits for the timely management of prolonged labour (WHO 1994a).

- *1990* – The ICM triennial congress was preceded by a workshop to discuss 'midwifery education for safe motherhood'. The results of the precongress workshop were recommendations for action to strengthen the curriculum of midwives (WHO/UNICEF/ICM 1991). This report recommended making the curriculum more community based and including management of selected obstetric emergencies.

- *1994* – WHO produced the Mother–baby package: a practical guide to implementing safe motherhood in countries (WHO 1994b). In this package it is recognised that the key to successful safe motherhood is 'appropriately trained midwifery personnel living and working in the community'. The package makes strong recommendations for countries to give priority to developing the midwifery skills of their health personnel, especially those providing community-based care. The recommendations included strengthening of midwifery skills in all aspects of maternity care provision. Importantly these skills must include the immediate management of selected obstetric emergencies such as haemorrhage, prolonged and obstructed labour, puerperal sepsis and hypertension in pregnancy. They also detail the minimum package for basic maternity care, in terms of both what services should be available and the requisite equipment.

- *1996* – WHO launched the Midwifery education modules for safe motherhood (WHO 1996a). There are five modules and these include teachers' and students' notes. Each module deals with a specific aspect of maternal mortality. There is one on the community, which discusses how to understand the community, how to measure maternal mortality and how to work with the community to devise culturally and locally applicable solutions to preventing maternal mortality. The other four modules deal with the four major causes of maternal

mortality: obstructed labour, pre-eclampsia and eclampsia, postpartum haemorrhage and puerperal sepsis (incomplete abortion added in 2002). They are complete training packs and include games, puzzles and quizzes to help both the teacher and the student. They have been thoroughly field tested in more than one country and are available free from WHO, Geneva.

- *1996* – WHO held a technical working group on normal delivery (WHO 1996b). A working group of internationally credible obstetricians and midwives together reviewed the evidence for all the current practices and interventions used throughout the world in caring for women having a normal delivery. Their conclusions supported the ones found by the Oxford Perinatal Epidemiological Group. Following the same format as in Effective care in pregnancy and childbirth (Chalmers et al 1987), they listed the practices according to the scientific evidence (WHO 1996b). This document along with other safe motherhood documents is also available from WHO, Geneva.

- *2000* – WHO launched its new initiative for safe motherhood, 'Making Pregnancy Safer'. This followed after the statement by the WHO, UNFPA, UNICEF and the World Bank entitled reducing maternal mortality (1999), in which, as stated elsewhere, attention was drawn to the emerging consensus that in order to achieve the reduction in maternal mortality there must be an increased proportion of all deliveries attended by a skilled attendant. Also, skilled attendants must be able to provide quality prenatal care that must include: assisting all families to format appropriate plans for birth, including plans for immediate referral to a hospital offering comprehensive emergency obstetric and neonatal care in case this becomes needed; norms for the management of normal childbirth; avoidance of iatrogenic complications; and immediate management of life threatening complications. The WHO's strategy for Making Pregnancy Safer is built around assisting countries strengthen their health systems and apply the lessons learnt to date from the global action on safe motherhood according to each country's needs and resources. More information on WHO's new initiative can be found on the WHO website, accessed via the Reproductive Health and Research pages (see Useful addresses, p. 1018).

Other global events significant to Safe Motherhood

- *1990* – there was global action towards improving the health and well-being of children and the international congress, World Summit on the Health of the Child. This summit put the child on the world's agenda (UNICEF 1990). At the UN General Assembly in 1990, the Convention on the Rights of the Child (UN 1990) entered into international law. Both at the World Summit and by signing The Convention on the Rights of the Child, governments agreed that they would take steps to increase the health of children throughout the world. Article 6, which deals with survival and development, lays down the need for effective prenatal care and the right to have the delivery conducted by appropriately trained health personnel. Other articles deal with non-discrimination (effectively outlawing practices such as gender selection, female fetocide and discriminatory feeding practices based on gender), the best interests of the child, separation from the family and family reunification. By 1997, The Convention on the Rights of the Child had been ratified by all members of the UN, except for the Cook Islands, Oman, Somalia, Switzerland, the United Arab Emirates and the United States (UNICEF 1997a).
- *1993* – The UNICEF annual report on The progress of nations (UNICEF 1993), charting the progress to date of achieving 'health for all by the year 2000,' reported explicit concern that the targets set in Alma Ata (now Almaty) in 1976 would not be met by the year 2000. Although there had been concern from many quarters, this publication did act to prompt some countries like Bangladesh into making different plans.
- *1994 and 1995* – Many interesting conferences were held including the International Conference on Population and Developments in Cairo 1994, the World Summit for Social Democracy, Copenhagen 1995 and the Fourth World Conference on Women in Beijing 1995. They all had safe motherhood as an integral issue. At all these conferences, governments from all over the world declared an intent to improve the health of women. This included provision for strengthening the health services to women, particularly in and around childbirth.

One important initiative, which has helped focus global attention on the continuing need to develop safe motherhood programmes, has been the WHO and UNICEF survey on the 1990 maternal mortality figures (WHO 1996c). The revised estimates for 1990 show the figures for maternal mortality to have been drastically underestimated in some countries. Globally, estimates suggest that there were some 8000 more deaths than was initially thought. Furthermore, it demonstrated that the anticipated decline in maternal mortality was not occurring at the rate required to reach the year 2000 target. In some countries there had been either a levelling off, or even a rise. This is of concern to all involved in safe motherhood. It underlines the fact that there is no room for complacency in the attempts to make motherhood safer, if not completely safe. Therefore, the training of health personnel in effective midwifery skills is an urgent, continuing and priority need.

To summarise, safe motherhood is not just about ensuring that women do not die in childbirth. It is also about empowering women to take control over their own bodies to enable them to achieve optimum health. This must include being empowered to make effective and informed choices about if and when they will embark upon pregnancy. If they choose to become pregnant, then they should have access to all services, education and support (including community support) needed to achieve a healthy outcome; this may include access to safe abortion in countries where abortion is not against the law. It also includes the need for women, families and society to be assured that the newborn child can reach healthy adult maturity, for without this the pressures on women to conceive many babies will not reduce and family planning strategies will be impeded.

The strategies required to achieve all of these will vary from country to country. The strategies are as much, or more, concerned with the sociological perspectives of women's health as they are with the provision of effective health services. As Thompson & Bennett (1996) outline in their precongress paper, the provision and access to health care has only a small effect on the overall determinants for the health of women. It would appear that by far the most important factors for improving women's health are changes in the cultural practices, eliminating gender inequalities and improving the environment in which the woman lives, which includes elimination of poverty and improved nutrition. This inevitably means that, in addition to developing appropriate technical midwifery skills, midwives must also involve themselves in political action to address these issues, which have a direct effect on improving women's health.

The role of the midwife in Safe Motherhood

There have been many reports, symposia, conferences, events, books and articles on the subject of the Safe Motherhood Initiative and safe motherhood programmes. However, what all midwives must remember is that safe(r) motherhood, in its broadest and narrowest sense, is still not an option for many thousands of women in the world. Although women in highly industrialised countries are subject to a different lack of control over their own bodies from women in developing or transitional market economy countries, both are denied their rights. They are denied the right to choose and denied their right to exercise control over their own birth processes. Some Western countries are making progress in this field. New Zealand along with Holland are perhaps two countries in the forefront of ensuring that women have the right to choose what type of assistance they want during pregnancy and childbirth and where and when they want it. The UK is another, following the Changing Childbirth initiative (DoH 1993). Other countries are also developing similar initiatives and are trying to give choice to women for care in pregnancy and birth. However, in too many countries the health systems, structures and medicalisation of this care militate against effective implementation of safe motherhood programmes. For this reason, midwives must become more politically active and learn to relate to, work with and seek to influence the leaders and major decision makers, both at the local and at the national level.

It is with humility that midwives can boast that, throughout the Safe Motherhood Initiative, in many countries they have played and continue to play a pivotal role in helping achieve the goals of SMI; yet more is still required.

Breastfeeding and Baby Friendly Hospital Initiative (BFHI) and Saving Newborns Lives (SNBL)

The Baby Friendly Hospital Initiative is driven by UNICEF and WHO and is now considered to be one of the most effective mechanisms for creating strong political commitment to breastfeeding. Unfortunately, and despite scientific evidence showing the importance of breastfeeding for maternal, infant and child health, global indicators demonstrate that the decline of breastfeeding in the 1950s and the trend towards bottle feeding has continued in the 1990s (Saadeh 1993). This is despite the research supporting the promotion of exclusive breastfeeding in the first 4–6 months, particularly for the control of diarrhoeal disease and upper respiratory tract infections. Following a review of the then available scientific evidence, Saadeh (1993) concluded that: 'the results showed that breastfeeding can save more infant lives and prevent more morbidity than any other intervention strategy' (p. 2).

The BFHI was launched in 1991 following the joint WHO/UNICEF statement on breastfeeding in 1989, which outlined the 'ten steps to successful breastfeeding' (WHO/UNICEF 1989). The 'ten steps' (see Ch. 40) have become the management tool and criteria for awarding BFHI status. UNICEF now provides a training package for hospitals who wish to work towards the award of the status 'baby friendly hospital'. WHO also provides a similar course for breastfeeding counselling. Both courses have been implemented into a growing number of countries, with some countries incorporating them into their own national breastfeeding programmes.

Difficulties to be overcome to achieve exclusive breastfeeding

Despite these global initiatives, the lack of exclusive breastfeeding for 4–6 months and the practice of discarding the colostrum remain the two major difficulties to be overcome in many countries. Very often such practices, influenced by strong cultural superstitions and belief systems, cannot be overcome by simply presenting mothers with scientific evidence. A recent report suggests that the promotion of exclusive breastfeeding is still being hampered by inappropriate advertising and violations of the International Code of Marketing Breastmilk Substitutes (UNICEF 1997b). The aim of the code is to eliminate inappropriate marketing of breastmilk substitutes (WHO 1981). Despite almost universal agreement that it is unacceptable and immoral to import and promote formula feed to countries where the water supply is not safe, violations of the code continue. The International

Baby Food Action Network (IBFAN) and others seek to promote and protect as well as to identify violations of the International Code of Marketing of Breastmilk Substitutes.

The newborn

More recently, attention has been given for the need to ensure that safe motherhood includes care for the newborn. Save the Children are taking a particular lead on this with the launch of the global Saving Newborns Lives (SNBL) initiative. More information on this initiative can be found on their website (see Useful addresses, p. 1018).

International agenda

Midwifery identities

Listening to midwives at many and varied conferences and meetings worldwide, it would appear that the global concerns of midwives and the constraints they face have changed little since Kwast & Bentley published their paper in 1991. The paper presented at the ICM precongress workshop in 1990 detailed the constraints and problems facing midwives worldwide, which include both the shortage and maldistribution of midwives and the economic and training problems facing midwifery in many countries.

Midwives need specific policies and legislation to practise

One of the most common and urgent needs facing midwives in many countries is the need for specific (if not separate) policies and legislation to enable them to practise. Where separate policies and practices for midwifery are not identified, midwives can be hampered if they have to practise under nursing protocols and legislation. For example, many of the procedures the midwife requires in order to practise essential life-saving skills, as identified in the WHO Mother–baby package (WHO 1994b) and reinforced in the review of evidence for skilled attendant at childbirth by BFHT, are not always allowed under nursing policies or legislation.

By far the most common and continuing issue that faces midwives internationally is their right to practise, and to practise as autonomous practitioners. The manifestations of this issue will vary depending on the country concerned. For many, the domination of the medical profession will be the most difficult barrier to overcome. It is heartening to read, for example, that, as far back as 1985, WHO and some obstetricians recognised the pivotal role of the midwife in providing quality maternity care (Wagner 1994). However, too often the relationship between the two professions remains contentious and leads to the fragmentation of care and services for women and babies. The principle of providing holistic care to mothers and babies as a unit is still more observed in rhetoric than in practice in many countries. For many countries, especially in Russia and the whole Eastern bloc, maternity services for pregnancy and childbirth are still dominated by medical practice, with almost 100% of all deliveries taking place in a hospital environment under medical supervision. Indeed, in some of these countries midwives are faced with falsifying records to indicate that the birth was conducted by a medical officer when in fact it was a midwife who conducted the delivery.

In addition, the unique nature of midwifery practice, as separate and distinct from nursing, is still not universally accepted. In countries such as many in Africa there are logical and rational reasons for having nurse–midwives, and midwifery can appropriately be a qualification obtained after training as a nurse, especially where the nurse–midwife may be the only health care person available in a rural setting (Box 54.2). Yet even in these situations there are still issues that must be addressed. The two professions have a distinctive, if overlapping, body of knowledge and practice. They both need valuing for their individual contribution to a nation's health, and legislation and structures must reflect this. The legislation must be sensitive to the particular situation in a country, yet still allow the midwife to undertake all the skills necessary for saving life.

Licence to practise is an issue of safeguarding the public and therefore a matter for government concern and good stewardship; so government must ensure that the professional standards are set and remain under central control. Governance, however, must not be confused with political interference or dominance in the determination of professional standards. It is the responsibility of governments to ensure that frameworks exist that will ensure that individual health practitioners have appropriate education. Therefore governments may set the criteria for educational institutions or even the curriculum itself.

Box 54.2 Tanzania; midwives not sufficient staff and not always providing adequate or acceptable care

Many women in our country still live in rural areas, whereas most skilled attendants (midwives) work in urban areas. Therefore many births are still attended by TBAs or family members. The reasons why midwives prefer working in urban areas include: lack of infrastructure, lack of incentives, high workload in rural areas where the midwife must do more than midwifery, poor safety and professional isolation. Not only is there a need to address these issues, there is also a need to strengthen the skills, knowledge and attitude among the skilled providers. Women are reported to have preference for TBAs' services rather than skilled midwifery services because of the bad attitudes of those skilled attendants (midwives) and that, although trained, many woman feel the midwives still have insufficient and inadequate skills. There is also lack of updating of skills specifically for those few in the rural areas.

(Report of Tanzanian midwifery representative at WHO technical meeting on strengthening midwifery services to support Making Pregnancy Safer, November 2001.)

Education and training, however, are only one element; there must also be adequate and appropriate supportive supervision to ensure that service providers are enabled to carry out their function. For example, where trained traditional birth attendants (TBAs) are considered essential to fulfil a need in the country, their role should be regarded as integral to the rest of the maternity service provision and not seen as something outside the formal services or replacing the need for sufficient numbers of appropriately qualified (skilled) midwives. It is also important to ensure that where TBAs are used they are adequately prepared for their role, are properly supervised and encouraged to work closely with qualified midwives. Without this, the TBA will always remain outside the formal health structures and will be vulnerable and may not be valued for her expertise. More importantly she or he may feel unable or unwilling to seek appropriate help if and when it is required. Questions such

as whether there is a place in modern midwifery for such workers, or whether the TBA should be a support worker for the trained midwife, have not yet been resolved in many countries. What has been made clear, though, is that they cannot and should not, be seen as a replacement for a skilled health worker (WHO/UNPF/UNICEF/World Bank 1999).

Education of midwives

The education of midwives is yet another matter of debate and concern in many countries, for a variety of reasons. As previously stated, in some countries the preparation of midwives may follow on from nursing. Although there are good reasons for this in some situations there are also a number of disadvantages, particularly where nursing does not have a sufficiently strong public health basis. The arguments for and against midwifery following nursing will depend on the individual country. Although there are a number of advantages for having health practitioners dually qualified or multiskilled, it may be useful to also consider one or two of the more common reasons against this. The midwifery-following-nursing model can result in midwifery being seen as an adjunct to nursing. The consequence in some countries is that midwifery is afforded very little time within the curriculum, as happens in Japan where the midwifery component lasts only 6 months. It may also lead to fragmentation of care between an institutionalised intrapartum service and separate community-based prenatal care. Role confusion can occur in some countries where the prenatal services are provided by community health workers or public health workers, completely separately from midwives who offer intranatal care. Often these workers have minimal midwifery input into their curriculum.

Training must be skills based. Midwifery is essentially a practical profession where practice is underpinned by evidence, scientific principles and knowledge and sound practical application. The skills required by the midwife may vary from country to country, depending on the specific needs of the country. The results of field testing of the ICM core competencies (presented at the 2002 triennial ICM congress) should elicit a list of common skills required. In addition to the usual midwifery skills, the list may include other additional skills that may not be seen as usual for midwives – for example, being able to undertake a manual removal of the placenta competently. However, midwives should be aware that, in some resource-poor settings, midwives may find themselves in a situation where knowledge and skills alone are all that are available to save the woman's life. For example, faced with a woman having a severe haemorrhage after delivery, the competent midwife, if trained correctly, should be able to apply aortic compression. This is where the midwife, using her clasped hand, exerts downward pressure on the abdominal aorta to reduce the flow of blood to the uterus (Fig. 54.1). The correct application of aortic pressure may be the only option available for a midwife to stem the flow of the haemorrhage until medical assistance is available. Training for these and other life-saving skills must focus on achieving competence. Very often in some countries, although the theoretical knowledge may be taught well in the initial programmes, there is little or no opportunity to practise the skills in the clinical situation. All too frequently, newly trained midwives find themselves lacking in confidence and competence in these skills.

Direct entry programmes. With the above in mind, many countries such as the USA and Canada are exploring direct entry into midwifery. Direct entry programmes are well established in some countries such as France, the UK and Holland. Some feel that such programmes offer a greater opportunity for midwives to be acknowledged as autonomous practitioners and true partners in the team required for safe pregnancy and childbirth (Box 54.3). Direct entry programmes would allow more appropriate programmes to be developed based on a fitness-for-purpose model (Fig. 54.2). The fitness-for-purpose approach to curriculum planning looks at the required competencies of a midwife for that particular situation or country. From this, a programme is devised that demonstrates how the specific outcomes and the necessary skills, knowledge and attitudes to practise competently will be met. These should be pertinent to the country in which the training takes place and conform to the International definition of the midwife (WHO/FIGO/ICM 1992). Such outcomes can then be used for assessment and evaluation of the curriculum. Attempts are being made to strengthen the skills of midwives in many countries. However, this is complicated by the fact that identification of who is a midwife is not always easy. In a survey across the 10 countries that make up the WHO South-East Asia Region, there are approximately 18 different categories of worker providing maternity services, of which only seven have the word 'midwife' in their job title (WHO/SEARO 1996). Some, such as the border

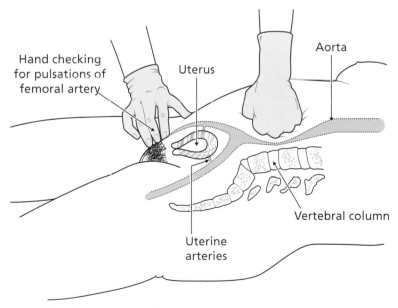

Fig. 54.1 Aortic compression (based on WHO 1996a).

Hand checking for pulsations of femoral artery

Uterus

Aorta

Vertebral column

Uterine arteries

Box 54.3 Midwifery in Canada: an autonomous direct entry profession by Bridget Lynch from the Canadian Midwives Association

In Canada midwifery is legislated and regulated at a provincial rather than federal level. Since the early 1990s six of ten provinces have legislated midwifery as a direct entry health profession, with legislation pending in two more provinces. Midwives in Canada are independent practitioners who provide primary care to low risk women and their newborns from conception to 6 weeks' postpartum. Midwives are required by provincial regulation to attend women, as appropriate, in a woman's choice of birthplace; whether in the home, in a birth centre, or in hospital. The midwives' scope of practice includes admitting and discharge privileges in the hospital setting. Continuity of care, with a small group of midwives known to a woman providing care throughout her pregnancy, birth and the postpartum, is fundamental to the Canadian model of midwifery.

The route of entry to the profession is through a Bachelor of Science in Midwifery, offered in both francophone and anglophone university settings. There is also a process offered by provincial colleges, the regulators of the profession, to assess and register midwives who have been educated in jurisdictions outside of Canada. In several provinces, aboriginal midwives and the practice of aboriginal midwifery are recognized and protected through legislation. Midwifery services are funded through the public health care system.

(For more information on midwifery in Canada, visit the website of the Canadian Association of Midwives at: www.canadianmidwives.org.)

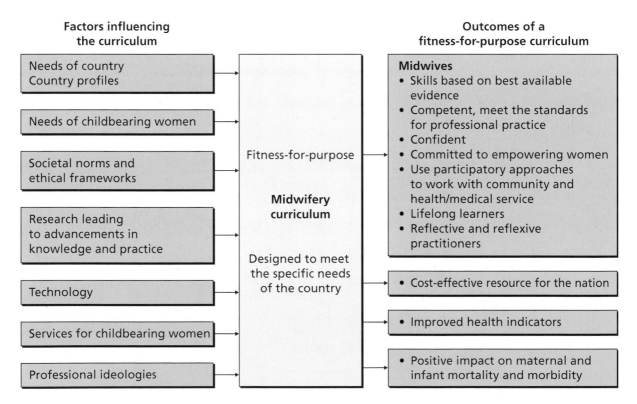

Fig. 54.2 Fitness-for-purpose curriculum model.

midwives in Bhutan, have only 3 months' training in midwifery and provide delivery-only care.

One of the main difficulties facing the preparation of midwives is the lack of sufficient numbers of appropriately trained midwife teachers. Many countries, including some European countries such as Germany, are without a standardised approved preparation for their midwife teachers. It was partly the debate about strengthening midwifery education and in recognising the needs of midwives teachers in some countries for additional teaching material that led WHO to fund the development of the Midwifery modules for safe motherhood (WHO 1996a). Currently, issues around the omission of research from the midwifery curriculum are also hotly debated, and its lack is recognised as being detrimental to the preparation of critically thinking midwives. Midwives must be able to be both proactive and responsive to the needs of individual mothers and babies. Many countries are now addressing these deficiencies, but are being hampered by medical, particularly obstetric and paediatric, domination. Such medical dominance makes undertaking appropriate midwifery research problematic. Without midwives who are active researchers, not simply research assistants or data gatherers for medical research but midwives engaged upon midwifery research, it is difficult to build up sufficient evidence-based practice. Therefore it is essential that some midwives become researchers as well as research users. It is imperative that each country has a mechanism by which some midwives are able to receive adequate preparation as researchers to ensure that country-specific midwifery research is carried out. Such research is not only essential for evidence-based practice but also needed by governments and other decision makers to allow them to improve their maternity services. WHO is preparing a toolkit 'Strengthening midwifery' in resource-poor countries to support Making Pregnancy Safer. This toolkit, which is being developed with the assistance and support from ICM as well as other UN agencies, will deal with many of these issues.

Employment and the working environment

Another major problem facing many midwives worldwide includes issues surrounding employment and the environments in which midwives work. Changes such as the rise in HIV and increasing migration to city dwellings (bringing with it the demise of family support networks for childbearing women) will require different approaches to the provision of maternity services. Mass urbanisation, with its overcrowding, increased poverty and deprivation often leading to higher crime and violence, has resulted in an increased concern for the safety of midwives at work. Even in some Western countries, midwives fear for their personal safety and are reluctant to go out to labouring women at night without some form of security cover.

These demographic changes also bring with them an explosion of demands on the health services. The resulting economic burden laid on communities and countries in these circumstances means that adequate remuneration is increasingly an issue for many midwives. This is not only in terms of monetary rewards, because hospital budgets cannot match the huge demands on the services and sometimes are unable to pay their workers' salaries, but also in terms of reduced opportunities and restrictions on practice. South Africa is one country faced with such issues. Since the move to free health care following the political changes that marked the end of apartheid, and coupled with the effects of mass urbanisation, South Africa is facing huge problems in all of its public services. These include struggling with an overstretched health service where demand exceeds hospital and district budgets. Midwives working in similar situations are being faced with many problems (Box 54.4).

Finally, in many countries, health service funding often fails to take into account remuneration for community practice, budgets being based on formal structured care from hospitals or health centres. In all of these situations, community services and the setting up of independent community practice become difficult and often devalued. Even some Western countries, including the UK, some states in the USA and Canada and Norway, are facing similar problems with independent midwifery. The problem for independent midwifery practice in the more industrialised countries, however, is frequently one of payment for such care, as insurance companies can be reluctant for a variety of reasons to pay for this type of service. Often the reason relates to their close association with the medical profession, who are not always supportive of

---

Box 54.4 Midwives in Zimbabwe

Midwives in Zimbabwe have a long tradition and have done a great deal to strengthen midwifery care to ensure they meet the changes in society. One of the greatest challenges Zimbabwe has had to face in recent years has been the incredible rise in HIV/AIDS. The midwifery curricula have been revised to take on board HIV/AIDS and counselling. Currently the country is busy strengthening midwifery education and services through offering a master's degree with specialisation in MCH and Midwifery. However, these gains are being wiped out due to the current crisis, namely increased migration of midwives to other countries who are offering better salaries and packages including improving safety. Due to the HRH shortage, the need for capacity building is greater than ever in the country. Sometimes even in the large hospitals there are not sufficient midwives and nurses and others are left to assist the woman during birth. The midwife then becomes a supervisor of staff rather than carrying out the skills she has been trained to do.

(Report of Zimbabwe midwifery representative at WHO technical meeting on strengthening midwifery services to support Making Pregnancy Safer, November 2001.)

---

midwifery-led care. As funding of health care becomes increasingly reliant on insurance schemes this is likely to become an increasing problem.

The success of the midwives in The Netherlands and the New Zealand midwives' initiatives to have their services recognised as a legitimate option for pregnant women does offer hope. However, these successes were as a result of hard-fought battles. In The Netherlands, two out of three babies are now born with midwifery-only care (Smulders & Limburg 1995), but the medical profession continues to try to gain control by establishing criteria for women who in their opinion require hospital care for birth. In New Zealand, the midwives' fight in 1999 to have the Nurses' Amendment Act passed was not without fierce opposition (Donley 1995). In each case, although circumstances may be different, the force of medical opposition was enormous

and the midwifery profession had to unite and work in partnership with women to achieve success. In both accounts the force of the women's support was paramount. This can be achieved only if women are free and able to offer this support – free in that they are not excessively burdened with malnutrition, ill health and poverty. Unfortunately in some countries many women are still being denied such freedom.

Scope of midwifery practice increased in some countries

Increasingly, turbulence, war and political upheaval are posing new problems for midwifery. The recent stories that have emerged, from Rwanda and former Yugoslavia, of the attempts to carry out what has become termed ethnic cleansing give graphic testimony to the impact such upheaval causes to women. Violence against women is more than ever on the international agenda, despite the UN Convention on the elimination of all forms of discrimination against women (UN 1979) and the Declaration on violence against women (UN 1993).

Female genital mutilation is still a concern in many countries, as is the damage inflicted on women as a result of lack of appropriate health care in pregnancy and childbirth. Morbidity, especially pelvic floor problems, incontinence and vesicovaginal fistulae, and the provision of appropriate and safe reproductive health care for refugees and displaced persons, are perhaps the most pressing concerns for research and innovations by midwives in the new millennium.

Conclusion

Midwives must be more politically aware and active. It is not possible to reflect all the issues or the different approaches being made by midwives in different countries in one short chapter. What is possible though, is to heighten all midwives' awareness that today, more than ever, globalisation does have an impact on midwifery. As such, midwives from both a theoretical and a practical point of view should be aware and keep abreast of what is happening in other countries. Globalisation and the impact of technology require midwives in all countries to be aware of just what is going on in the world. In addition, midwives must become more politically active if they are to bring about safe(r) motherhood in their own and other countries. It is clear that what is required to bring about safe motherhood in most countries is sufficient well-trained midwives and the resources to provide holistic quality care, including emergency obstetric care. Such care must be available close enough for the women to gain access, as well as influence, the provision of care to ensure it is culturally acceptable. This requires action by community leaders, policy makers and politicians. Therefore midwives must become active in political debates concerning structures of society, especially the rights of women and women's empowerment. In addition, if they are to be true advocates for mothers and newborn, they must also be able to identify and influence local leaders and key decision makers in the community. This is more likely to succeed if done through rational considered discussion and community grass roots action.

Awareness of one's own culture, both personal and professional, will help in adopting appropriate and culturally sensitive models for action, including models of care. Midwives must accept that their own cultural baggage will alter their perspective on best practice and fitness for purpose. Therefore, adopting an advocacy role and participatory approaches is not only good practice, but is the only way forward. This will require all midwives to ensure that, at all times, it is the women they serve who are in the front and making the decisions. If midwives are to provide appropriate effective care anywhere in the world, they must always listen to and respect the women they seek to serve.

REFERENCES

Chalmers I, Keirse M J N C, Enkin M W 1991 Effective care in pregnancy and childbirth. Oxford University Press, Oxford

Chitnis S 1988 Feminism: Indian ethos and Indian convictions. In: Ghandially S (ed) Women in Indian society: a reader. Sage, London

Collins P 1994 Shifting the centre: race, class, and feminist theorizing about motherhood. In: Glenn E, Chang G, Forcey L (eds) Mothering ideology, experience, and agency. Routledge, New York.

Dawit S, Busia A 1995 Thinking about culture: some programme pointers. In: Gender development, Oxfam Journal 5(1):7–11

DoH (Department of Health) 1993 Changing childbirth: report of the expert maternity group. HMSO, London

Donley J 1995 Independent midwifery in New Zealand. In: Murphy-Black T (ed) Issues in midwifery. Churchill Livingstone, Edinburgh

Goodburn E 1995 Maternal morbidity in rural Bangladesh: an investigation into the nature and determinants of maternal morbidity related to delivery and the puerperium. Bangladesh Rural Advancement Committee, Dhaka

Graham W, Bell J, Bullough C H W 2001 Can skilled attendance at delivery reduce maternal mortality in developing countries? In: De Brouwere V, Lerberghe W V (eds) Safe motherhood strategies: a review of the evidence. Studies in Health Services Organization & Policy 17:97–130

ICM (International Confederation of Midwives) 1993 International code of ethics for midwives. ICM, London

ICM (International Confederation of Midwives) 1994 A birthday for midwives: seventy five years of international collaboration. The International Confederation of Midwives 1919–1994. ICM, London

Kwast B, Bentley J 1991 Introducing confident midwives: midwifery education – action for safe motherhood. Midwifery 7:8–19

Loudon I 2000 Maternal mortality in the past and its relevance to the developing world today. American Journal of Clinical Nutrition (1S):241S–246S

Maine D 1990 Safe motherhood programmes: options and issues. Centre For Population and Family Health, Columbia University, New York

Royston E, Armstrong S 1989 Preventing maternal deaths. WHO, Geneva

Saadeh R 1993 breastfeeding: the technical basis and recommendations for action. WHO, Geneva, p 2

Smulders B, Limburg A 1995 Obstetrics and midwifery in the Netherlands. In: Kitzinger S (ed) The midwifery challenge, new edn. Pandora, London

Thompson J, Bennett R 1996 Women are dying: midwives in action. ICM/WHO/UNICEF Pre-Congress Workshop, May 1996, Oslo, Norway

UN (United Nations) 1979 Convention on the elimination of all forms of discrimination against women. UN, New York

UN (United Nations) 1990 The convention on the rights of the child. UN, New York

UN (United Nations) 1993 Declaration on violence against women. UN, New York

UNICEF (United Nations Children's Fund) 1990 World summit rights of the child. UNICEF, New York

UNICEF (United Nations Children's Fund) 1993 The progress of nations. UNICEF, New York

UNICEF (United Nations Children's Fund) 1997a The state of the world's children: 1997 summary. UNICEF, New York

UNICEF (United Nations Children's Fund) 1997b Cracking the code (code no. 16027). UNICEF, Essex

Wagner M 1994 Pursing the birth machine: the search for appropriate birth technology. Ace Graphics, Australia

WHO (World Health Organization) 1981 International code of marketing of breastmilk substitutes. WHO, Geneva

WHO (World Health Organization) 1991a Essential elements of obstetric care at first referral level. WHO, Geneva

WHO (World Health Organization) 1991b Maternal mortality: a global factbook. WHO, Geneva

WHO (World Health Organization) 1994a The application of the WHO partograph in the management of labour. Maternal Health and Safe Motherhood Programme, Division of Family Health, WHO, Geneva

WHO (World Health Organization) 1994b Mother–baby package: a practical guide to implementing safe motherhood in countries. Health and Safe Motherhood Programme, Division of Family Health, WHO, Geneva

WHO (World Health Organization) 1996a Midwifery modules for safe motherhood. Maternal Health and Safe Motherhood Programme, Division of Family Health, WHO, Geneva

WHO (World Health Organization) 1996b Normal birth. Maternal Health and Safe Motherhood Programme, Division of Family Health, WHO, Geneva

WHO (World Health Organization) 1996c Revised 1990 estimates of maternal mortality: a new approach by WHO and UNICEF. WHO, Geneva

WHO (World Health Organization) 2000a Management of complications in pregnancy and childbirth, WHO, Geneva

WHO (World Health Organization) 2000b Making pregnancy safer: a paper for discussion. World Health Organization, Department of Reproductive Health and Research, Geneva.

WHO/FIGO/ICM (World Health Organization/International Federation of Gynaecologists and Obstetricians/ International Confederation of Midwives) 1996, 1992 International definition of a midwife. WHO, Geneva

WHO/SEARO (World Health Organization/South-East Asia Regional Office 1996 Standards for midwifery practice for safe motherhood. Working paper 1 An inter-country consultation, November 1996. WHO/SEARO, New Delhi, India

WHO/UNICEF (World Health Organization/United Nations Children's Fund) 1989 Protecting, promoting and supporting breastfeeding: the special role of maternity services. WHO, Geneva

WHO/UNICEF/ICM (World Health Organization/United Nations Children's Fund/International Confederation of Midwives) 1991 Midwifery education action for safe motherhood: report of a collaborative pre-congress workshop, Kobe, Japan 5–6 October 1990. WHO, Geneva

WHO/UNPF/UNICEF/World Bank (World Health Organization/United Nations Population Fund/United Nations Children's Fund/World Bank) 1999 Reducing maternal mortality. WHO, Geneva

FURTHER READING

Jeffrey P, Jeffrey R, Lyon A 1988 Labour pains and labour power: woman and childbearing in India. Zed Books, London

Koblinsky M, Timyan J, Gay J (eds) 1992 The health of women: global perspective. Westview, Boulder, CO

Murphy-Black T 1995 Issues in midwifery. Churchill Livingstone, Edinburgh

Murray S (ed) 1996 Midwives and safer motherhood. Mosby, London

Murray S (ed) 1996 Baby friendly/mother friendly: international perspectives on midwifery. Mosby, London

Taylor D 1991 The children who sleep by the river. WHO, Geneva

USEFUL ADDRESSES

Department of Reproductive Health and Research
World Health Organization
1211 Geneva 27
Switzerland
www.who.int/reproductive_health/making pregnancy safer

International Confederation of Midwives HQ
Eisenhowerlaan 138
2517 KN
The Hague The Netherlands

Save the Children SNBL initiative
http://www.savethechildren.org/health/healthsaving newbornlives1

55 Vital Statistics

Linda K. Brown   V. Ruth Bennett   Mary McGowan

Registration of births and deaths is so much taken for granted in the developed world that it may come as a surprise that it became a requirement in England only in the nineteenth century. Even today a few births and deaths escape registration in the UK; in countries where communication is less easy, many more may be uncounted. The collection of these vital statistics allows for analysis of the rates of birth and death in different population groups. The information is essential for planners at national and local level who must forecast the needs of the community for health facilities, schooling, housing and so on.

The chapter aims to:

- describe the collection of data on births and deaths and the legal requirements for registration

- emphasise the role of the midwife, who, being a person present at virtually every birth, is a key witness who can supply details of births and deaths occurring within her practice and encourage families to discharge their responsibilities

- explain how the various mortality statistics that are of interest to midwives are calculated

- review the causes and trends within each death rate category.

Notification of birth

Legislation

Provision for the early notification of birth was first made in 1907 but it did not become a statutory requirement until 1915. When the early Acts were repealed the legislation was included in the Public Health Act 1936 and slightly amended by the National Health Service Act 1946.

Notification

It is the duty of the father or any other person in attendance, or present within 6 hours after the birth, to give notice in writing to the appointed medical officer in the district in which the child is born. This must be done within 36 hours of birth for any child born after 24 completed weeks of pregnancy, whether alive or dead. The health authority supplies prepaid addressed envelopes and forms (unless electronic) for the notification of birth. It is usual for the midwife to undertake completion of the form. In addition to biographical information about the mother and her baby, the midwife will record the period of gestation, any congenital malformation and factors that may put the baby at risk.

The purpose of notification is to enable the health visitor to call at the home as soon as the midwife ceases to visit. An 'at-risk' register is compiled from the details on the cards and is used for providing appropriate care for the children concerned. The birth information is also made available to the Registrar of Births and Deaths of the district in which the birth took place.

Registration of birth

The original Births and Deaths Registration Act was passed in 1837 but updated by the Act of 1953. This Act now governs the registration of births.

Births must be registered within 6 weeks (3 weeks in Scotland), although under certain circumstances that time might be extended by the Registrar of Births and Deaths. There is a statutory fine for those who fail to register.

Place of registration

Every birth must be registered in the district in which it took place. This usually means a visit to the Register Office but some hospitals arrange for Registrars to visit the maternity wards regularly so that the new mothers may register there.

It is possible to make a Declaration of the birth to a Registrar in another Registration District in England or Wales. This will then be sent to the Registrar of the district where the birth occurred, who will do the registration and send the certificates to the parent through the post.

Responsibility to register

The primary duty to register a birth rests with the mother of the child, although in the case of a married couple the father may attend to register. If a mother is unmarried and wishes the father's name and details to be included, the couple should attend together to give details to the Registrar. If this is not possible, the mother could register the baby with her details only, and then the couple could re-register the birth later, adding the father's particulars. An unmarried father may also attend alone to register if he takes with him a Statutory Declaration made by the mother that he is the father of the child, or certain other court orders. (It is also a requirement of law for parents who marry after the birth to re-register the child as a married couple.)

A number of other people, including a senior administrator at the hospital where the child was born, or someone present at the birth, which could be the midwife, are qualified to register a birth and, in the absence of a better informant, may be required to do so. However, it is always preferable for the parents to attend as they will give the most accurate information.

Naming a child

Whether or not a couple is married, the same general rules apply to the choosing of their child's names. They may in fact opt for any surname. It could be the same as or different from their own or a double-barrelled combination of their names.

With an unmarried mother, however, the midwife may be in a unique position to give advice, being in touch with the couple so early. If the child of an unmarried couple is given the father's surname and they subsequently part, it is not possible to change that name on the Birth Certificate. If, however, the child has the mother's surname and she later marries the father, it is possible on re-registration to change the child's name to his at that stage. It might be thought prudent therefore to choose the mother's surname. It sometimes happens, however, that the father will put undue pressure on the mother to use his surname but the midwife could make the mother aware that she can sidestep the issue by registering the baby on her own.

It would have to be without the father's details, but these could be added later on re-registration without legitimisation (that is, without the marriage of the parents), and the surname could then be changed to that of the father. The extra time for reflection could help to resolve the dispute.

Forenames are of course a free choice as well (although a Registrar may refuse to register an offensive name). There is a facility to add or change the forenames in the registration if a new name is chosen and used within 1 year. This can either be done by a Certificate of Naming or, if the child has been baptised, with a Certificate of Baptism signed by the minister of religion. Both these certificates may be obtained from the Register Office.

Statistics

At the time of registration, the Registrar also collects further information that is not entered in the Register but is used for statistical purposes and passed to the Office of National Statistics. This relates to dates of birth and marriage of the parents and previous children born, live or still, and is kept confidential. In addition, brief and simple questions on the employment of the parents may be asked. This further information is not confidential and may be used in an identifiable form.

Birth Certificates

Short (now A4) Birth Certificate. This is issued free of charge at the time of registration. It gives the baby's name, sex, date of birth and the Registration District.

Full Birth Certificate. This may also be obtained for a prescribed fee. This is a copy of the complete entry in the Register.

NHS numbers no longer appear on certificates, but on registration the parent or other informant will be given a form for them to register the child on a doctor's list under the NHS. This form is called FORM FP58. Procedures for the issue of NHS numbers were changed in the autumn of 2002. Numbers are now issued shortly after birth in the maternity unit and passed on to the Registrars (electronically) by Child Health offices with the regular notifications of births. This new system, called NN4B, yields significant benefits on various fronts and in particular in the case of sick babies who are transferred from hospital to hospital (see the www.nhsia.nhs.uk/nn4b website).

Stillbirths

Definition of stillbirth

The definition of a stillbirth is given in section 41 of the Births and Deaths Registration Act 1953 and the Still-Birth (Definition) Act 1992 in the following terms:

> 'still-born child' means a child which has issued forth from its mother after the twenty-fourth week of pregnancy and which did not at any time after being completely expelled from its mother breathe or show any other signs of life.

Registration of stillbirths

In order to register a stillborn baby, the mother or other informant must have a Medical Certificate of Stillbirth. A medical practitioner or midwife who is present at the stillbirth or who examines the body of a stillborn child may write and sign this certificate. A midwife would be unwise to offer to complete the stillbirth certificate unless she had personally witnessed the birth.

Informants who have responsibility to register a stillbirth are the same as those in the case of a live birth (see above) and it has been possible since 1997 to make a declaration of the stillbirth to a Registrar in another district.

The Registrar will record the details in the Stillbirth Register and issue an authority for burial or cremation. She will also give a short free Certificate of Stillbirth similar to that for a live birth. The informant can also buy a full certificate, which is a copy of the entry in the Register. The chosen names for the child now appear on both these certificates.

In the case of stillbirths the event cannot be re-registered to add the father's name, nor to add or change a name for the baby.

Burial of a stillborn baby

Parents may make private arrangements for the baby to be buried or cremated but it is also possible for the hospital to undertake this on their behalf. Midwives who counsel the mother and father should encourage them to think about this carefully and to choose the arrangement that suits their need. Chapter 37 discusses support of the grieving parents.

Duties of a midwife concerning stillbirth

Notification of stillbirth. This is the same as is required for live birth.

Certificate of Stillbirth. The midwife will ensure that this has been completed, usually by the doctor (see above).

Registration of stillbirth. The midwife explains to the parents that the birth must be registered and the procedure for burial or cremation.

The supervisor of midwives. The midwife responsible for the care of the woman and her baby must notify the supervisor of midwives of the stillbirth (UKCC 1998, p. 35).

Registration of deaths

This is the responsibility of the family. They should notify the Registrar of any child who has died after having been born alive. (In the rare event of a woman dying in childbirth, they will of course notify her death.)

Funeral arrangements

In the case of a neonatal death (see below) the funeral arrangements are the responsibility of the parents. There is a small death grant payable on the death of a child under 3 years but this will in no way offset the costs incurred. If there is hardship the midwife may refer the family to the social worker. Midwives should be familiar with local policy as in a few cases the hospital administrator may agree to meet some of the cost.

Both a Birth Certificate and a Death Certificate are required. The midwife will need to make sure that the parents are aware of this in order to spare them unnecessary distress.

In the case of a stillbirth where the parents wish to make private arrangements for the funeral, the midwife may need to explain that no death grant is payable.

In the case of a baby born dead before the completion of 24 weeks of pregnancy there is no procedure of notification or registration, but if the parents wish the child to have a funeral then they will need a letter from the doctor or midwife stating that the baby was born before the legal age of viability and showed no signs of life (see also Ch. 37).

Birth and death rates

Vital statistics relate to life and death events, and specifically to the systematic collection of numerical data in order that they may be summarised and studied. In measuring health there are difficulties in finding objective data to quantify; therefore it is pertinent to study the numbers of deaths occurring at different ages and their causes. This helps to explain why there are so many different types of death rate. The statistics of special interest to midwives are:

- birth rate
- miscarriage rate
- stillbirth rate
- perinatal death rate
- neonatal death rate
- postneonatal death rate
- infant death rate
- maternal death rate.

Figure 55.1 shows graphically the periods relating to these different types of death.

Definition of 'rate'

Crude figures give little idea of the real frequency of events. If they are related to a specific number within the population, it becomes possible to compare 1 year's figures with another. If a particular group is studied, for example women in their fertile years, it is possible to identify the degree of risk in relation to certain events.

To calculate the rate of, for instance, stillbirth, the number of actual stillbirths in a year is compared with the number of total births (both live and still). This ratio is then related to a group of 1000 of those total births. The mathematical formula is as follows:

$$\frac{\text{no. of stillbirths}}{\text{no. of total births}} \times 1000 = \frac{\text{stillbirth rate per}}{1000 \text{ total births}}$$

Perinatal death

Definitions

Perinatal death. This is either a stillbirth or a death occurring in the 1st week of life (early neonatal death).

Perinatal death (or mortality) rate. This is the number of stillbirths and early neonatal deaths per 1000 total births.

Causes and predisposing factors

The perinatal death rate is often taken as the primary indicator of success or failure in obstetric care. These

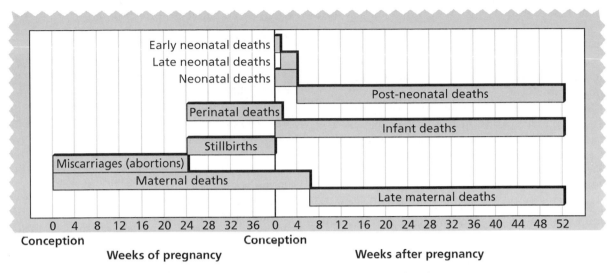

Fig. 55.1 Subdivision of deaths occurring during pregnancy and within 1 year of birth.

deaths are those that are closest to the event of birth. Some of them are caused by such factors as hypoxia in labour and intracranial trauma during delivery. Others may be the result of genetic factors or of events in pregnancy. The main identifiable causes are:

- low birthweight (preterm and small for gestational age babies)
- intrauterine hypoxia
- respiratory depression at birth
- intracranial injury
- congenital abnormality.

It may be impossible to attribute a perinatal death to any one of the listed causes, but a combination of predisposing factors increases the risk of death. These include:

- socioeconomic disadvantage
- poor maternal health (including effects of smoking, alcohol consumption, drug abuse and poor diet)
- multiple pregnancy
- antepartum haemorrhage
- pre-eclampsia
- breech presentation.

Trends

When new figures are published each year, small improvements are welcome but real encouragement is found in viewing the decline in rates over a number of years. These are often plotted in graphical form (Fig. 55.2). In looking for reasons for these trends it is important to take account of a wide range of factors such as the establishment of the NHS in 1948. The passing of the Abortion Act 1967 has resulted in the termination of many pregnancies for congenital abnormalities and thus the removal of deaths from

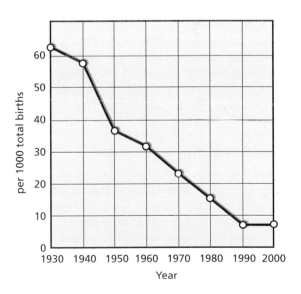

Fig. 55.2 Graph showing the perinatal death rates for England and Wales, 1930–2000.

these causes from the perinatal mortality statistics. Conversely, the redefinition in 1992 of the age of legal viability as being 24 weeks' instead of 28 weeks' gestation has brought more babies within the definition of stillbirth and a consequent increase in perinatal mortality figures.

Rates are consistently higher than average in social classes IV and V as defined by the occupation of a parent, usually the father (5 and 6 in the new socioeconomic classification (ONS 2001)).

Reasons for improvement

Improved care in pregnancy. Improved identification of the unborn baby at risk allows it to be monitored and born at the optimum time. Mothers also receive more information about healthy diet, cutting down on smoking and alcohol and care of their own health.

Improved care in labour. This aims at maintaining the mother and baby in good condition. Skilled midwifery care aims to minimise intervention and to promote the normal process of labour as far as possible. If assistance becomes needed, medical help may be required and technological aids may become useful.

Improved neonatal care. This results in more survivors and in a better quality of life for those who do survive. Intensive neonatal care helps babies born after less than 28 weeks of pregnancy to survive, whereas in earlier years little attempt would have been made to prolong life.

Better socioeconomic conditions. These result in improvement in both survival and health of babies. Health professionals must be wary of assuming, however, that improvement is continuous. The level of unemployment, for example, may rise and have unhappy effects for families.

Perinatal mortality in the world

Statistics published by WHO (1996) reveal a sharp contrast in rates of perinatal death. Babies in developing countries are five times as likely to die before or just after birth as those in the industrialised world. The rate in western Africa is almost 10 times that in North America. Thirty per cent of the world's births occur in south-central Asia and this region accounts for almost 40% of perinatal deaths. Undoubtedly the poorer socioeconomic conditions of these countries contribute to the loss of 7.5 million babies.

Neonatal death

Definitions

A neonatal death is one occurring in the first 28 days of life. Neonatal deaths are divided into early neonatal deaths, which occur during the first 7 days of life, and later neonatal deaths, which occur during the next 21 days. The reason for this is that the causes of early deaths are more similar to those of stillbirth, whereas the causes of later deaths are different.

The rates of neonatal deaths are calculated per 1000 live births.

Causes of late neonatal death

Some of the causes are similar to those of earlier deaths because babies whose deaths are attributable to birth trauma or perinatal events may survive beyond the 1st week. After this time there is a greater likelihood of death occurring because of infection, intraventricular haemorrhage, necrotising enterocolitis or iatrogenic disorders.

Infant death

An infant death is one occurring in the 1st year of life. By definition this includes all neonatal deaths; the remainder are termed postneonatal deaths. The infant mortality rate is calculated per 1000 live births. This rate is taken as one of the best measures of a nation's health.

Causes of postneonatal death

Some of the important causes that a midwife should be aware of are non-accidental injury, infection and, in older babies, accidents in the home. Sudden infant death also accounts for a significant number; these are unexpected deaths in which no cause is identified (see CESDI below).

Trends and reasons for improvement

There has been a dramatic reduction since the beginning of the 20th century in the number of infants who die under the age of 1 year. In 1900 in England and Wales the infant mortality rate was between 140 and 160 per 1000, whereas in 1985 the rate was 9.4 per 1000. By 1995 this had fallen further to 6.0 per 1000 live births. Improvement has been due to a number of factors including:

- better housing and standard of living
- immunisation
- antibiotics and chemotherapeutic agents
- prevention of cross-infection
- health education
- intravenous therapy
- appointment of paediatricians, neonatal specialists, health visitors and others.

CESDI

A Confidential Enquiry into Stillbirths and Deaths in Infancy (CESDI) was established in England, Wales and Northern Ireland in 1992. In the first few years attention was focused on intrapartum deaths with a separate analysis of sudden, unexplained infant deaths (SIDS).

More recently (MCHRC 1998) a study was made of antepartum term stillbirths (SATS), which account for around one-third of perinatal deaths (Persad et al 1995). Two features occurred more frequently in the cases than in the case controls: having any antenatal problem noted and being a mother of non-white origin. Concern was expressed about discrepancies between mothers' reports and the medical record, for instance some mothers who admitted smoking were recorded at the booking interview as non-smokers.

A particular study was initiated to examine sudden unexpected deaths in infancy (SUDI) between the ages of 1 and 52 weeks (Fleming et al 2000). Of 418 deaths, 93 were explained and nearly half of these showed signs of illness severe enough to need medical attention in the 24 hours before they died, using the criteria of the Cambridge Baby Check (Morley et al 1991). Overall, many factors were examined and a number of recommendations emerged:

- the risk is lower for infants sleeping in the supine position
- infants should be protected from tobacco smoke
- infants should not be heavily wrapped and be kept warm but not sweaty
- parents are encouraged to share a bedroom with the baby for the first 6 months
- parents should be taught to recognise significant features of illness in babies
- parents should never share a settee or armchair to sleep with the baby

- bed sharing can be dangerous after drinking alcohol or using drugs
- immunisation decreases rather than increases the risk of SIDS.

Fleming et al (2000, p. ix) comment that, although sudden infant death has fallen substantially since the 'back to sleep' campaign in 1991, SUDI remain the largest single group of deaths in the postneonatal period. Robinson (1996a) points out the international success of the campaign but also stresses the continuing adverse influence of poverty.

Statistics for CESDI are collected through a rapid reporting system in which midwives may participate. The form should be filled out as soon after the death as possible and sent to the district coordinator (Wallace 1994).

Maternal death

The ninth International Classification of Diseases, Injuries and Causes of Death (ICD9) defines maternal death as 'the death of a woman while pregnant or within 42 days of delivery, miscarriage or termination of pregnancy, from any cause related to or aggravated by the pregnancy or its management, but not from accidental or incidental causes' (Lewis & Drife 2001). WHO estimates that at least 600 000 women die every year from pregnancy-related causes, though the rate is difficult to calculate with accuracy (Clark 2002). Whereas the lifetime risk of maternal death for a woman in a developed country is 1 in 1800, in Africa it is 1 in 16, in Asia 1 in 65 and in Latin America 1 in 130 (WHO 1998). The global causes of maternal death are haemorrhage, infection, obstructed labour, eclampsia and the consequences of unsafe abortion. The 'Safe Motherhood Initiative' was originated to address the scandalous loss of maternal life but has sadly had little impact on outcomes, although awareness has been heightened. More recently WHO (2002) has launched the initiative 'Making Pregnancy Safer' (MPS), which addresses three targets:

- prevention and management of unwanted pregnancy and unsafe abortion
- skilled care during pregnancy and childbirth
- access to referral care when complications arise.

All these are of direct concern to midwives and their practice.

The reports on Confidential Enquiries into Maternal Deaths (CEMD)

These triennial reports on maternal deaths in the UK (from 1952 to 1985 they covered only England and Wales) analyse virtually every maternal death. They constitute the longest uninterrupted series of such enquiry in the world. The information is entirely confidential so that contributory factors can be examined without fear of recrimination. Practice in respect of each complication can be assessed and the report makes recommendations that have been most valuable. Any individual obstetrician, midwife or general practitioner is unlikely to see many mothers die in his or her care (Mander 2001) and cannot therefore rely on personal experience; the availability of a national report shares the knowledge that has been gained.

The UK maternal mortality rate is calculated as the number of deaths occurring per 100 000 or per million maternities – that is, pregnancies that resulted in a birth, live or still. The rate includes deaths due to abortion, although abortions are not included in 'maternities' since it is impossible to calculate an accurate number. In October 1992 the definition of stillbirth was altered from one occurring after 28 weeks of pregnancy to one at 24 weeks or later and this affected the calculation of the total number of maternities (as well as the number of stillbirths).

Four groups of deaths are defined:

1. 'True' maternal death may be regarded as the *direct maternal death*, which is one 'resulting from obstetric complications of the pregnant state (pregnancy, labour and puerperium), from interventions, omissions, incorrect treatment or from a chain of events resulting from any of the above'.

2. *Indirect obstetric deaths* are those 'resulting from previous existing disease or disease that developed during pregnancy and which was not due to direct obstetric causes, but which was aggravated by the physiologic effects of pregnancy'.

3. Deaths from other causes that happen to occur in pregnancy or the puerperium are defined as *coincidental (fortuitous) deaths*. The term 'coincidental' is now preferred to 'fortuitous' as being more appropriate and sensitive.

4. *Late deaths* are those due to direct or indirect causes that occur between 42 days and one year after abortion, miscarriage or delivery. This last category was added for the 1991–1993 triennial report (DoH et al 1996) and for part of the previous one.

The report identifies the causes of maternal deaths and reveals the trends in incidence. It reveals substandard care and names the disciplines responsible. Where shortage of resources has contributed to the death, this is mentioned. The authors of the report are careful to stress that avoiding the elements of substandard care that are discussed would not necessarily have averted the death concerned.

Causes

In the report relating to the years 1997–1999 (Lewis & Drife 2001), the six main causes of direct maternal death were as follows:

- thrombosis and thromboembolism
- early pregnancy death (ectopic pregnancy, miscarriage, termination)
- pregnancy-induced hypertension
- sepsis
- amniotic fluid embolism
- haemorrhage.

Figure 55.3 shows the causes of direct maternal death in the UK for the triennium from 1997 to 1999.

Trends

Broadly speaking the maternal mortality rate has fallen in each triennium but has levelled off somewhat since 1987. In the 1997–1999 triennium the rate was 11.4 direct and indirect deaths per 100 000 maternities. For the first time, indirect deaths outnumbered direct deaths and the highest cause of maternal death overall was identified as suicide. Cardiac deaths equalled deaths from thrombotic conditions.

Deaths from *thrombosis and pulmonary embolism* continue to be the largest group of direct deaths. There was a dramatic fall in deaths from thromboembolism following caesarean section, but a *rise* in this type of death in other women. Body mass index (BMI) should be calculated at booking (see Ch. 12) to identify women with a BMI over 30 kg/m^2. Midwives should alert medical staff to any chest or leg symptoms in the puerperium in order to exclude deep vein thrombosis.

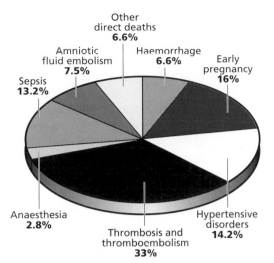

Fig. 55.3 Causes of direct maternal deaths: UK 1997–1999. Data from Lewis & Drife 2001.)

Pre-eclampsia and eclampsia were responsible for 15 deaths in the recent triennium. The use of magnesium sulphate has been accepted as the anticonvulsant of choice. The report cautions that automated blood pressure recording systems may underestimate blood pressure in pre-eclampsia and readings should be compared with those obtained by conventional mercury sphygmomanometers.

Deaths from *haemorrhage* have fallen, but, because of the speed with which collapse can occur with obstetric haemorrhage, the report recommends that a woman at high risk of haemorrhage is cared for in a hospital with a blood bank on site. A clear protocol is needed, including arrangements for women who refuse blood transfusion because of religious beliefs (DoH et al 1996).

Causes of *substandard care* in the 1997–1999 triennium include:

- lack of communication and teamwork
- failure to appreciate the severity of the illness
- wrong diagnosis, incorrect or suboptimal treatment
- failure to refer to a senior person or hospital.

A number of factors were identified as bearing a higher risk. Young mothers who died were almost always severely socially excluded; many of them were homeless or victims of domestic violence and abuse.

Women of higher maternal age and parity were at greater risk of death. Those in certain ethnic groups were more at risk: women from the Indian subcontinent are three times as likely to die as white women, and black women one-and-a-half times as likely. Six travellers were included in the report. It was clear that women in the lower social classes are also at higher risk.

A chapter in the report concerns midwifery practice and should be studied carefully by midwives. The midwife should be at the forefront of helping to plan models of care provision. Each woman should have a flexible, individual care plan from the moment of booking and this should be reviewed constantly with ongoing risk assessment. Women who miss an antenatal appointment should be followed up actively, especially if they fail to appear twice. Those who do not speak English should be provided with an interpreter; it is not acceptable to use family members, particularly children.

The midwife is in an ideal position to give advice on a healthy lifestyle, including helping obese women to lose weight. The report recommends that all women are informed of how to wear a seatbelt while pregnant, namely using a three-point seatbelt 'above and below the bump'. All women should be asked in privacy about domestic violence. The midwife is enjoined to develop an understanding of each woman's social and cultural background and to act as her advocate. This should include being prepared to refer across professional boundaries, for instance telephoning the GP or calling in a community psychiatric nurse for a woman suffering from mental illness.

This latter highlights the need to be alert for psychiatric illness and not use 'postnatal depression' as a blanket term for all mental health problems (see Ch. 35). There is a high risk of recurrence of psychiatric illness and midwives need to know of the possible rapid deterioration that may occur. They should summon appropriate help.

Midwives involved in some of the cases in the report are criticised for failing to challenge decisions made by junior medical staff. This happened in a case of death due to hypertension in which there was also a failure to alert senior staff (p. 262). This problem is not new. Robinson (1996b), commenting on a case of uterine rupture in a GP unit following the use of prostaglandins in a highly parous woman, considered that the midwives should have raised their voices in protest and exhorted them to be more assertive. This includes demanding training in any procedures that are not understood and owning up to limitations.

The Confidential Enquiries have had a significant effect in reducing the number of maternal deaths since the middle of the twentieth century. The latest report identifies the fall in deaths from thromboembolism following caesarean section as a case in point. By fully cooperating with the detailed enquiries following the death of a mother, midwives can make an active contribution to the prevention of future deaths and the continuing improvement of outcomes.

Conclusion

Midwives everywhere are concerned at the loss of a woman's life at or near the time of giving birth. The WHO 'Safe Motherhood Initiative' (see Ch. 54) has brought this into high profile. Just as tragic is the loss of infant life at the time when the new baby should be welcomed into the family. Although the problem is greater in the developing world, there is no room for complacency in industrialised countries. Each midwife needs to be aware of local circumstances and seek to apply best practice to the utmost of her ability. This may include initiating research and applying available evidence to ensure that appropriate care is given (see Ch. 5).

REFERENCES

Abortion Act 1967 HMSO, London

Births and Deaths Registration Act 1953 HMSO, London

Clark PA 2002 Maternal and neonatal morbidity and mortality: progress to date. MIDIRS Midwifery Digest 12(1):32–35

DoH et al (Department of Health, Welsh Office, Scottish Home and Health Department, Department of Health and Social Security, Northern Ireland) 1996 Report on confidential enquiries into maternal deaths in the United Kingdom 1991–1993. HMSO, London

Fleming P, Blair P, Bacon C, Berry J (eds) 2000 Sudden unexpected deaths in infancy: the CESDI SUDI studies. 1993–1996. Stationery Office, London

Lewis G, Drife J (eds) 2001 Why mothers die 1997–1999. The fifth report of the Confidential Enquiries into Maternal Deaths in the United Kingdom. RCOG Press, London

Mander R 2001 Death of a mother: taboo and the midwife. Practising Midwife 4(8):23–25, reprinted in MIDIRS Midwifery Digest 12(1):132–135

MCHRC (Maternal and Child Health Research Consortium) 1998 Confidential enquiry into stillbirths and deaths in infancy: 5th annual report. MCHRC, London

Morley C J, Thornton A J, Cole T J, Hewson P H, Fowler M A 1991 Baby Check: a scoring system to grade the severity of acute illness in babies under six months old. Archives of Disease in Childhood 66:100–106

National Health Services Act 1946 HMSO, London

ONS (Office for National Statistics) 2001 The national statistics socio-economic classification. Online. Available: www.statistics.gov.uk (accessed 2 April 2002)

Persad P, Hiscock C, Mitchell T 1995 The study of antepartum term stillbirths (SATS). MIDIRS Midwifery Digest 5(4):479–480

Public Health Act 1936 HMSO, London

Robinson J 1996a The emperor's new clothes. British Journal of Midwifery 4(11):609–610

Robinson J 1996b Death of a mother. British Journal of Midwifery 4(7):381–382

Still-Birth (Definition) Act 1992 HMSO, London

UKCC (United Kingdom Central Council for Nursing, Midwifery and Health Visiting) 1998 Midwives' rules and code of practice. UKCC, London

Wallace V 1994 New reporting system for perinatal deaths. MIDIRS Midwifery Digest 4(2):231

WHO (World Health Organization) 1996 Perinatal mortality: a listing of available information. Maternal health and safe motherhood programme (WHO/FRH/MSM 96.7). WHO, Geneva

WHO (World Health Organization) 1998 World Health Day 1998 information kit. WHO, Geneva

WHO (World Health Organization) 2002 Making pregnancy safer. Discussion paper. Online. Available: www.who.int/reproductivehealth/mps/discussion_paper.pdf (accessed 2 April 2002)

FURTHER READING

Clark P A 2002 Maternal and neonatal morbidity and mortality: progress to date. MIDIRS Midwifery Digest 12(1):32–35

Clark discusses in detail the global causes of death in mothers and young babies with a realistic appraisal of the reasons that progress has been so slow and disappointing and with positive proposals for the future. Midwives will find their overall appreciation of the challenges helped by this overview.

Fleming P, Blair P, Bacon C, Berry J (eds) 2000 Sudden unexpected deaths in infancy: the CESDI SUDI studies 1993–1996. Stationery Office, London

This detailed report of the study into deaths between 1 and 52 weeks of age reveals a number of facts that midwives would do well to note. Important conclusions are drawn about various theories associated with sudden infant death, including some that have not been substantiated, such as the 'toxic mattress' theory. Useful suggestions are made that can be used by midwives in teaching and guiding parents about the care of their baby, including the use of the Cambridge Baby Check for signs of illness.

Lewis G, Drife J 2001 Why mothers die 1997–1999. The fifth report of the Confidential Enquiries into Maternal Deaths in the United Kingdom. RCOG Press, London

This report should be studied in detail by midwives as well as all others involved in the care of women in pregnancy, labour and the puerperium. In particular the chapter on midwifery practice (Ch. 17) is of enormous value. It will help midwives appreciate their crucial role as well as point to ways in which they can contribute significantly to ensuring a safe outcome. The previous reports (published by the Departments of Health) are also worth looking at and midwives should be alert for the publication of each succeeding report.

Mander R 2001 Death of a mother: taboo and the midwife. Practising Midwife 4(8):23–25, reprinted in MIDIRS Midwifery Digest 12(1):132–135

This report of a research study confronts the problem of the lack of personal experience on the part of any one midwife in addressing the possibility of maternal death and the recognition that even discussing it is taboo. The author recommends a new openness in order to increase confidence and appropriate care.

MCHRC (Maternal and Child Health Research Consortium) 1998 Confidential Enquiry into Stillbirths and Deaths in Infancy (CESDI): 5th annual report. MCHRC, London

This report covers the years 1996 and 1997. A one-in-ten random sample of all deaths notified to the consortium was examined. Other specific studies were considered, including analysis of non-SIDS sudden unexplained deaths in infancy and a case-controlled study of antepartum term stillbirths. Focus groups were used to study three particular aspects; the one of greatest interest to midwives reviewed 22 cases of planned home birth associated with the death of the baby. Recommendations for practice are made that will be useful for assessing local protocols. Midwives will find this report and its predecessors and successors invaluable sources of information.

www.safemotherhood.org

This website is an invaluable resource for keeping up to date with the latest developments in trends of maternal and infant deaths and the measures being taken to improve matters for the world-wide community.

Glossary of Selected Terms

Abortion Termination of pregnancy before the fetus is viable, i.e. before 24 weeks' gestation in the UK.

Abruptio placenta Premature separation of a normally situated placenta. Term normally used from viability (24 weeks).

Acardiac twin One twin presents without a well-defined cardiac structure and is kept alive through the placental circulation of the viable twin.

Acridine orange A stain used in fluorescence microscopy that causes bacteria to fluoresce green to red.

Aetiology The science of the cause of disease.

Amenorrhoea Absence of menstrual periods.

Amniotic fluid embolism The escape of amniotic fluid through the wall of the uterus or placental site into the maternal circulation, triggering life-threatening anaphylactic shock in the mother. (The word 'embolism', denoting a clot, is a misnomer.)

Amniotomy Artificial rupture of the amniotic sac.

Anterior obliquity of the uterus Altered uterine axis. The uterus leans forward due to poor maternal abdominal muscles and a pendulous abdomen.

Antigen A substance which stimulates the production of an antibody.

Anuria Producing no urine.

Atresia Closure or absence of a usual opening or canal.

Augmentation of labour Intervention to correct slow progress in labour.

Bandl's ring An exaggerated retraction ring seen as an oblique ridge above the symphysis pubis between the upper and lower uterine segments which is a sign of obstructed labour.

Basal body temperature The temperature of the body when at rest. In natural family planning, it is taken as soon as the woman wakes from sleep and before any activity occurs or after a period of at least one hour's rest.

Beneficence To do good.

Bicornuate uterus A structural abnormality of the uterus.

Birth centres These may be freestanding (away from hospital) or in hospital grounds or in the hospital. The emphasis is on providing a less medical environment and supporting normal birth.

Bishops Score Rating system to assess suitability of cervix for induction of labour.

Burns Marshall Manoeuvre A method of breech delivery involving traction to prevent neck from bending backwards.

Calendar calculation The fertile phase of the menstrual cycle is calculated in accordance with the length of the woman's 6–12 previous cycles.

Cardiotocograph Measurement of the fetal heart rate and contractions on a machine that is able to provide a paper print of the information it records.

Caseload practice Generally this refers to a personal caseload where named midwives care for individual women.

Central venous pressure line An intravenous tube which measures the pressure in the right atrium or superior vena cava, indicating the volume of blood returning to the heart and by implication, hypovolaemia.

Cephalopelvic disproportion Disparity between the size of the woman's pelvis and the fetal head.

Cerclage Non-absorbable suture inserted to keep cervix closed.

Cervical eversion Physiological response by cervical cells to hormonal changes in pregnancy. Cells proliferate and cause cervix to appear eroded.

Cervical intraepithelial neoplasm (CIN) Progressive and abnormal growth of cervical cells.

Cervical ripening Process by which the cervix changes and becomes more susceptible to the effect of uterine contractions. Can be physiological or artificially produced.

Cervicitis Inflammation of the cervix.

Choanal atresia (Bilateral) membranous or bony obstruction of the nares; baby is blue when sleeping and pink when crying.

Choroid plexus cyst Collection of cerebrospinal fluid within the choroids plexi, from where cerebrospinal fluid is derived.

Coloboma A malformation characterised by the absence of or a defect in the tissue of the eye; the pupil can appear keyhole-shaped. It may be associated with other anomalies.

Colposcopy Visualisation of the cervix using colposcope.

Commensal Micro-organisms adapted to grow on the skin or mucous surfaces of the host, forming part of the normal flora.

Conjoined twins Identical twins where separation is incomplete so their bodies are partly joined together and vital organs may be shared.

Couvelaire uterus (uterine apoplexy) Bruising and oedema of uterine tissue seen in placental abruption when leaking blood is forced between muscle fibres because the margins of the placenta are still attached to the uterus.

Cryotherapy Use of cold or freezing to destroy or remove tissue.

Deontology Duty-based theory.

Deoxyribonucleic acid (DNA) The substance containing genes. DNA can store and transmit information, can copy itself accurately and can occasionally mutate.

Diastasis symphysis pubis A painful condition in which there is an abnormal relaxation of the ligaments supporting the pubic joint.

Dichorionic twins Twins who have developed in their own separate chorionic sacs.

Diploid Containing two sets of chromosomes.

Disseminated intravascular coagulation/ coagulopathy A condition secondary to a primary complication where there is inappropriate blood clotting in the blood vessels, followed by an inability of the blood to clot appropriately when all the clotting factors have been used up.

Dizygotic (dizygous) Formed from two separate zygotes.

Doering rule The first fertile day of the cycle is determined by a calculation based upon the earliest previous temperature shift. This is an effective double check method to identify the onset of the fertile phase.

Dyspareunia Painful or difficult intercourse experienced by the woman.

Echogenic bowel Bright appearances of bowel, equivalent to the brightness of bone. Also associated with intra-amniotic bleeding and fetal swallowing of blood-stained liquor.

Echogenic foci in the heart Bright echoes from calcium deposits in the fetal heart, often the left ventricle. These do not affect cardiac function.

Ectopic pregnancy An abnormally situated pregnancy, most commonly in an uterine tube.

Embryo reduction (see Fetal reduction).

Endocervical Relating to the internal canal of the cervix.

Epicanthic folds A vertical fold of skin on either side of the nose which covers the lacrimal caruncle. They may be common in Asian babies, but may indicate Down syndrome in other ethnic groups.

Erbs palsy Paralysis of the arm due to the damage to cervical nerve roots 5 & 6 of the brachial plexus.

Erythematous Reddening of the skin.

Erythropoiesis The process by which erythrocytes (red blood cells) are formed. After the tenth week of gestation, erythropoiesis production rises and seems to be involved in red cell production in the bone marrow during the third trimester.

External cephalic version (ECV) The use of external manipulation on the pregnant woman's abdomen to convert a breech to a cephalic presentation.

False-negative rate The proportion of affected pregnancies that would not be identified as high-risk. Tests with a high false-negative rate have low sensitivity.

False-positive rate The proportion of unaffected pregnancies with a high-risk classification. Tests with a high false-positive rate have low specificity.

Ferguson reflex Surge of oxytocin, resulting in increased contractions, due to stimulation of the cervix, and upper portion of the vagina.

Fetal reduction The reduction in the number of viable fetuses/embryos in a multiple (usually higher multiple) pregnancy by medical intervention.

Fetofetal transfusion syndrome (Twin to twin transfusion syndrome (TTTS)) Condition in which blood from one monozygotic twin fetus transfuses into the other via blood vessels in the placenta.

Fetus-in-fetu Parts of a fetus may be lodged within another fetus. This can only happen in monozygotic twins.

Fetus papyraceous A fetus that dies in the second trimester of the pregnancy and becomes compressed and parchment-like.

Fibroid Firm, benign tumour of muscular and fibrous tissue.

Fraternal twins Dizygotic (non-identical).

Fundal height The distance between the top part of the uterus (the fundus) and the top of the symphysis pubis (the junction between the pubic bones). This assessment is undertaken to assess the increasing size of the uterus antenatally and decreasing size postnatally.

Group practice Generally refers to a small group of midwives who provide care for a group of women.

Haematuria Blood in the urine.

Haemostasis The arrest of bleeding.

Haploid Containing only one set of chromosomes.

HELLP syndrome A condition of pregnancy characterised by haemolysis, elevated liver enzymes and low platelets.

Herpes gestationis An autoimmune disease precipitated by pregnancy and characterised by an erythematous rash and blisters.

Homan's sign Pain is felt in the calf when the foot is pulled upwards (dorsiflexion). This is indicative of a venous thrombosis and further investigations should be undertaken to exclude or confirm this.

Homeostasis The condition in which the body's internal environment remains relatively constant within physiological limits.

Hydatidiform mole A gross malformation of the trophoblast in which the chorionic villi proliferate and become avascular.

Hydropic vesicles Fluid filled sacs, or blisters.

Hypercapnia An abnormal increase in the amount of carbon dioxide in the blood.

Hyperemesis gravidarum Protracted or excessive vomiting in pregnancy.

Hypertrophy Overgrowth of tissue.

Hypovolaemia Reduced circulating blood volume due to external loss of body fluids or to loss of fluid into the tissues.

Hypoxia Lack of oxygen.

Hysteroscope An instrument used to access the uterus via the vagina.

Induction of labour Intervention to stimulate uterine contractions before the onset of spontaneous labour.

Intraepithelial Within the epithelium, or among epithelial cells.

Intrahepatic cholestasis of pregnancy (ICP) An idiopathic condition of abnormal liver function.

LAM A method of contraception based upon an algorithm of lactation, amenorrhoea and 6 months' time period.

Lanugo Soft downy hair which covers the fetus in utero and occasionally the neonate. It appears at around 20 weeks' gestation and covers the face and most of the body. It disappears by 40 weeks' gestation.

Løvset manoeuvre A manoeuvre for the delivery of shoulders and extended arms in a breech presentation.

Macrosomia Large baby.

Malposition A cephalic presentation other than normal well-flexed anterior position of the fetal head, e.g. occipito posterior.

Malpresentation A presentation other than the vertex, i.e. face, brow, compound or shoulder. (Breech may be included in this category.)

Mauriceau-Smellie-Veit manoeuvre A manoeuvre to deliver a breech which involves jaw flexion and shoulder traction.

McRoberts manoeuvre A manoeuvre to rotate the angle of the symphysis pubis superiorly and release the impaction of the anterior shoulder in shoulder dystocia. The woman brings her knees up to her chest.

Midwife-led care Midwives or a midwife take the lead role in care of a woman or group of women.

Miscarriage Spontaneous loss of pregnancy before viability (see Abortion).

Monoamniotic twins Twins who have developed in the same amniotic sac.

Monochorionic twins Identical twins who have developed in the same chorionic sac.

Monozygotic (monozygous) Formed from one zygote (identical twins).

Multifetal reduction (see Fetal reduction).

Naegele's rule Method of calculating the expected date of delivery.

Natural Family Planning (NFP) Methods of contraception based on observations of naturally occurring signs and symptoms of the fertile and infertile phases of the menstrual cycle.

Neoplasia Growth of new tissue.

Neutral thermal environment (NTE) The range of environmental temperature over which heat production, oxygen consumption and nutritional requirements for growth are minimal, provided the body temperature is normal.

Non-maleficence Do no harm.

Oedema The effusion of body fluid into the tissues.

Oligohydramnios Abnormally low amount of amniotic fluid in pregnancy.

Oliguria Producing an abnormally small amount of urine.

One-to-one midwifery One midwife takes responsibility for individual women. A partner backs up the named midwife. It integrates a high level of continuity of caregiver and midwifery-led care. It is geographically based and includes women who are both 'high risk' and 'low risk'.

$PaCO_2$ Measures the partial pressure of dissolved carbon dioxide (CO_2). This dissolved CO_2 has moved out of the cell and into the bloodstream. The measure of $PaCO_2$ accurately reflects the alveolar ventilation.

PaO_2 Measures the partial pressure of oxygen in the arterial blood. It reflects how the lung is functioning but does not measure tissue oxygenation.

Paronychia An inflamed swelling of the nail folds; acute paronychia is usually caused by infection with staphylococcus aureus.

Peak mucus day A retrospective assessment of the last day of highly fertile mucus which is seen or felt around ovulation.

Pedunculated Stem or stalk.

Pemphigoid gestationis (see Herpes gestationis).

Perinatal Events surrounding labour and the first seven days of life.

pH A solution's acidity or alkalinity is expressed on the pH scale, which runs from 0–14. This scale is based on the concentration of H^+ ions in a solution expressed in chemical units called moles per litre. When the fetus is hypoxic the increased acid produced raises the acidity of the blood and the pH falls.

Pill free interval The 7 days when no pills are taken during Combined Oral Contraceptive regimen.

Placenta accreta Abnormally adherent placenta into the muscle layer of the uterus.

Placenta increta Abnormally adherent placenta into the perimetrium of the uterus.

Placenta percreta Abnormally adherent placenta through the muscle layer of the uterus.

Placenta praevia A condition in which some or all of the placenta is attached in the lower segment of the uterus.

Placental abruption (see Abruptio placenta).

Polyhydramnios An excessive amount of amniotic fluid in pregnancy.

Polyp Small growth.

Porphyria An inherited condition of abnormal red blood cell formation.

Postnatal period A period of not less than 10 and not more than 28 days after the end of labour, during which the continued attendance of a midwife on the mother and baby is a statutory obligation.

Postpartum After labour.

Pre-eclampsia A condition peculiar to pregnancy which is characterised by hypertension, proteinuria and systemic dysfunction.

Primary postpartum haemorrhage A blood loss in excess of 500 ml or any amount which adversely affects the condition of the mother within the first 24 hours of delivery.

Progestogen Synthetic progesterone used in hormonal contraception.

Prostaglandins Locally acting chemical compounds derived from fatty acids within cells. They ripen the cervix and cause the uterus to contract.

Proteinuria Protein in the urine.

Pruritus Itching.

Ptyalism Excessive salivation.

Puerperal fever/pyrexia A rise in temperature in the puerperium. This is poorly defined in the textbooks but is assumed to be based on the definition of pyrexia which is a rise above the normal body temperature of 37.2°C. Where pyrexia is used as a clinical sign of importance, the elevation in temperature is generally taken as being 38°C and above.

Puerperal sepsis Infection of the genital tract following childbirth; still a major cause of maternal death where it is undetected and/or untreated.

Puerperium A period after childbirth where the uterus and other organs and structures which have been affected by the pregnancy are returning to their non-gravid state. Usually described as a period of up to 6–8 weeks.

Quickening First point at which the woman recognises fetal movements in early pregnancy.

Retraction Process by which the uterine muscle fibres shorten after a contraction. Unique to uterine muscle.

Rubin's manoeuvre A rotational manoeuvre to relieve shoulder dystocia. Pressure is exerted over the fetal back to adduct and rotate the shoulders.

Sandal gap Exaggerated gap between the first and second toes.

Secondary postpartum haemorrhage An 'excessive' or 'prolonged' vaginal blood loss which is usually defined as occurring from 24 hours to 6 weeks after the birth.

Selective fetocide The medical destruction of an abnormal twin fetus in a continuing pregnancy.

Sheehan's syndrome A condition where sudden or prolonged shock leads to irreversible pituitary necrosis characterised by amenorrhoea, genital atrophy and premature senility.

Short femur Shorter than the average thigh bone, when compared with other fetal measurements.

Shoulder dystocia Incidence around 0.3% of deliveries. Failure of the shoulders to spontaneously traverse the pelvis after delivery of the head.

Siamese twins Conjoined twins.

Speculum (vaginal) An instrument used to open the vagina.

Subinvolution The uterine size appears larger than anticipated for days postpartum, and may feel poorly contracted. Uterine tenderness may be present.

Superfecundation Conception of twins as a result of sexual intercourse with two different partners in the same menstrual cycle.

Superfetation Conception of twins as a result of two acts of sexual intercourse in different menstrual cycles.

Surfactant Complex mixture of phospholipids and lipoproteins produced by type 2 alveolar cells in the lungs that decreases surface tension and prevents alveolar collapse at end expiration.

Symphysiotomy A surgical incision to separate the symphysis pubis and enlarge the pelvis to aid delivery.

Symphysis pubis dysfunction (see Diastasis symphysis pubis).

Talipes A complex foot deformity, affecting 1 per 1000 live births and is more common in males. The affected foot is held in a fixed flexion (equinus) and in-turned (varus) position. It can be differentiated from positional talipes because the deformity in true talipes cannot be passively corrected.

Team midwifery Midwives are team-based rather than ward- or community-based. The team takes responsibility for a number of women. Teams may be restricted to hospital or community, or cover both.

Teratogen An agent believed to cause congenital abnormalities, e.g. Thalidomide.

Torsion Twisting.

Trizygotic Formed from three separate zygotes.

Twin to twin transfusion syndrome (see Fetofetal transfusion syndrome).

Uniovular Monozygotic.

Unstable lie After 36 weeks' gestation a lie that varies between longitudinal and oblique or transverse is said to be unstable.

Uterine involution The physiological process that starts from the end of labour that results in a gradual reduction in the size of the uterus until it returns to its non-pregnant size and location in the pelvis.

Utilitarianism Greatest good for greatest number.

Vanishing twin syndrome The reabsorption of one twin fetus early in pregnancy (usually before 12 weeks).

Vasa praevia A rare occurrence in which umbilical cord vessels pass through the placental membranes and lie across the cervical os.

Withdrawal bleed Bleeding due to withdrawal of hormones.

Wood's manoeuvre A rotational or screw manoeuvre to relieve shoulder dystocia. Pressure is exerted on the fetal chest to rotate and abduct the shoulders.

Zavanelli manoeuvre Last choice of manoeuvre for shoulder dystocia. The head is returned to its pre-restitution position then the head is flexed back into the vagina. Delivery is by caesarean section.

Zygosity Describing the genetic make-up of children in a multiple birth.

Index

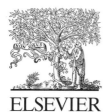

ELSEVIER

  Books *for* **Midwives**

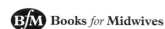

CHURCHILL
LIVINGSTONE

Mosby

THE PRACTISING
MIDWIFE

Baillière Tindall

MIDWIFERY PUBLISHERS OF CHOICE FOR GENERATIONS

For many years and through several identities we have catered for professional needs in midwifery education and practice. Leading publishers of major textbooks such as *Myles Textbook for Midwives* and *Mayes' Midwifery: a Textbook for Midwives*, our expertise spreads across both books and journals to offer a comprehensive resource for midwives at all stages of their careers.

Find out how we can provide you with the right book at the right time by exploring our website, www.elsevierhealth.com/midwifery or requesting a midwifery catalogue from Lorna Peden, Midwifery Market Specialist, Elsevier, 32 Jamestown Road, Camden, London, NW1 7BY, UK.

We are always keen to expand our midwifery list so if you have an idea for a new book please contact Mary Seager, Senior Commissioning Editor at Elsevier, The Boulevard, Langford Lane, Kidlington, Oxford, OX5 1GB, UK (m.seager@elsevier.com).

 Have you joined yet?
Sign up for e-Alert to get the latest news and information.

Register for eAlert at www.elsevierhealth.com/eAlert Information direct to your Inbox

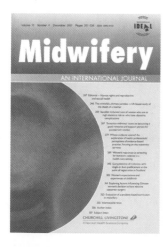

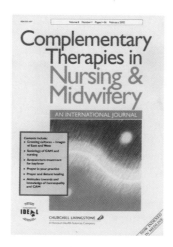